Renal and Adrenal Tumors

Renal and adrenal tumors
biology and management

Edited by

Arie Belldegrun, MD, FACS
*Roy and Carol Doumani Chair in Urologic Oncology,
Professor of Urology, Chief, Division of Urologic Oncology,
Department of Urology, UCLA School of Medicine,
Los Angeles, California 90095-1738, USA*

Alastair W.S. Ritchie, MD, FRCSEd
*Consultant Urological Surgeon, Gloucestershire Royal Hospital,
Great Western Road, Gloucester GL1 3NN, UK*

Robert A. Figlin, MD, FACP
*Professor of Medicine and Urology, Henry Alvin and Carrie L. Meinhardt
Chair in Kidney Cancer Research, Departments of Medicine and Urology,
Divisions of Hematology/Oncology and Urologic Oncology,
University of California, Los Angeles, School of Medicine, USA*

R.T.D. Oliver, MD, FRCP
*Sir Maxwell Joseph Professor in Medical Oncology,
St Barts and The Royal London Hospital School of Medicine,
Queen Mary and Westfield College Smithfield,
London EC1A 7BE, UK*

Edwin Darracott Vaughan, Jr., MD
*James J. Colt Professor and Chairman Emeritus of the Urology Department
at The Weill Medical College of Cornell University, Cornell University Medical Center,
New York, New York 10021, USA*

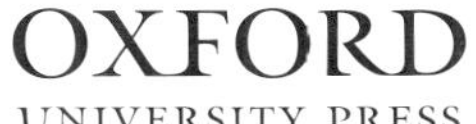

OXFORD
UNIVERSITY PRESS

OXFORD

UNIVERSITY PRESS

Great Clarendon Street, Oxford OX2 6DP

Oxford University Press is a department of the University of Oxford.
It furthers the University's objective of excellence in research, scholarship,
and education by publishing worldwide in

Oxford   New York

Auckland   Bangkok   Buenos Aires   Cape Town   Chennai
Dar es Salaam   Delhi   Hong Kong   Istanbul   Karachi   Kolkata
Kuala Lumpur   Madrid   Melbourne   Mexico City   Mumbai   Nairobi
São Paulo   Shanghai   Singapore   Taipei   Tokyo   Toronto

Oxford is a registered trade mark of Oxford University Press

in the UK and in certain other countries

Published in the United States
by Oxford University Press Inc., New York

© Oxford University Press, 2003

The moral rights of the authors have been asserted

Database right Oxford University Press (maker)

First published 2003

A catalogue record for this title is available from the British Library

Library of Congress Cataloging in Publication Data

Renal and adrenal tumors: biology and management/ edited by Arie Belldegrun.

ISBN 0 19 850822 0 (Hbk : alk : paper)
1. Kidneys–Tumors. 2. Adrenal gland–Tumors. I. Belldegrun, Arie.
RC280.K5 R43 2002   616.99′461–dc21   2002025829

10   9   8   7   6   5   4   3   2

Printed in Italy
on acid-free paper by Legoprint S.p.A.

This book is dedicated to the memory of the late Professor G.D. Chisholm.

Preface

In the past decade there has been an explosion of far-reaching developments in the biological and physical sciences relevant to cancer. This rapid growth of information in the field of oncology can be overwhelming. The burden of this logarithmic growth in our knowledge in both the clinical and basic science realms has led to an expanding number of cancer journals, reviews, and books each with its own limited focus. As a result, the place of a comprehensive textbook that paints a complete picture of a disease becomes all the more important and practical in this age of increased specialization. Nowhere is this more true than for the field of urologic oncology and for renal and adrenal tumors.

The incidence and mortality from renal cell carcinoma (RCC) have continuously risen through the past 50 years. Despite this, survival for patients has notably improved and great strides have been made in the management of patients with renal cell carcinoma. Improvements in radiological imaging leading to earlier diagnosis and improved staging, refinements in existing and introduction of new surgical techniques, better perioperative care, greater knowledge of the underlying molecular genetics and recognition of inherited forms of RCC, and enhanced understanding of the immunobiology of solid tumors have all led to an improved outlook for patients with RCC. Our understanding of the natural history of RCC, the role of nephrectomy, the benefits of immunotherapy and the possibilities of new technologies are evolving and are being integrated with advances in classification and staging. Currently, patients with both localized and metastatic RCC have experienced improvements in outlook and have expanded therapeutic options available to them. For patients with adrenal disease, many of these same trends hold true. Advances in endocrinology, imaging, and diagnosis have improved our ability to tailor treatment for the individual patient. Furthermore, the treatments themselves have evolved with the introduction of newer surgical approaches including partial, laparoscopic, and ablative techniques.

The objective of the present volume is to provide a single, comprehensive source of information on renal and adrenal tumors in a single volume that will be of practical interest for students, residents, physicians, and researchers alike. We have chosen a panel of authors that are internationally recognized for having made major contributions in the areas that they have been asked to discuss. The text is designed both to provide historical perspectives and an overview of basic facts, but also to assess and explore newer developments in our understanding of the clinical, genetic, and molecular aspects of these diseases. We attempt to cover the full totality, ranging from epidemiology through gene therapy. Finally, in both kidney and adrenal tumors there are still many controversial issues. We attempt to clearly distinguish what is generally agreed upon from what is still controversial, giving both sides equal treatment.

Editors:
Arie Belldegrun
Alastair Ritchie
Robert A. Figlin
Tim Oliver
E. Darracott Vaughan

Contents

Part 1, Section 2   Renal cell carcinoma: molecular genetics and immunobiology

Part I, Section 3 Renal cell carcinoma: imaging and management

Part I, Section 4 Renal cell carcinoma: metastatic disease

Part 2, Adrenal tumors

List of Contributors

Nejd F. Alsikafi, MD, Section of Urology, Department of Surgery, University of Chicago, Chicago, Illinois 60637, USA

Jesse Aronowitz, MD, Associate Professor, Departments of Radiation Oncology and Urology, Upstate Medical University, State University of New York, Syracuse, New York, USA

Joseph Baar, MD, PhD, Assistant Professor of Medicine and Surgery, University of Pittsburgh Cancer Institute, Division of Hematology/Oncology, Pittsburgh, Pennsylvania 15213–2582, USA

Shiro Baba, MD, Department of Urology, Kitasato University, School of Medicine 1–15–1, Kitasato, Sagamiharashi, Kanagawa, Japan

N. Bander, MD, Department of Urology, New York Presbyterian Hospital–Weill Medical College of Cornell University; Ludwig Institutes for Cancer Research, New York Branch, New York, New York 10021, USA

Zoran L. Barbaric, MD, Professor of Radiology, Department of Radiology, UCLA School of Medicine, Los Angeles, California 90095-1721, USA.

Ricardo Beduschi, MD, Lecturer, Section of Urology, Department of Surgery, University of Michigan, Ann Arbor, Michigan 48109–0330, USA

Arie S. Belldegrun, MD, FACS, Professor of Urology, Chief of the Division of Urologic Oncology, Director of Urologic Research, Department of Urology, University of California School of Medicine, Los Angeles, California 90095-1738, USA

Léon Berard, 69373 Lyon Cedex 08, France, Groupe Français d'Immunothérapie, Fédération des Centres de Lutte contre le Cancer, 101 rue Tolbiac 75013 Paris, France

Jon D. Blumenfeld, MD, Director of Hypertension, The Rogosin Institute, New York Presbyterian Hospital, Associate Professor of Medicine, Weill Medical College of Cornell University, New York 10021, USA

Murray F. Brennan, MD, Professor and Chairman Department of Surgery, Memorial Sloan-Kettering Cancer Center, New York, New York, USA

Dieter Bruno, MD, Division of Urology, Department of Surgery, Duke University Medical Center, Durham, North Carolina 27710, USA

Ronald M. Bukowski, MD, Director, Experimental Therapeutics, The Cleveland Clinic Taussig Cancer Center, Cleveland, Ohio 44195, USA

Robert M. Carey, MD, MACP, James Carroll Flippin Professor of Medical Science and Dean, University of Virginia School of Medicine, Charlottesville, Virginia 22908, USA

David Y. Chan, MD, Assistant Professor of Urology, James Buchanan Brady Urological Institute, Johns Hopkins Medical Institutions, Baltimore, Maryland 21287, USA

Alfred E. Chang, MD, Professor of Surgery, Chief, Division of Surgical Oncology, Associate Director of Clinical Affairs, University of Michigan, Ann Arbor, Michigan 48109, USA

Sachiko T. Cochran, MD, FACR, Department of Radiological Sciences, UCLA School of Medicine, Los Angeles, California 90095-1721, USA

John M. Corman, MD, Section of Urology, Virginia Mason Medical Center, Assistant Clinical Professor of Urology, University of Washington, Seattle, Washington, USA

Jean B. deKernion, MD, Fran and Ray Stark Professor of Urology, Chair, Department of Urology, UCLA School of Medicine, Los Angeles, California 90095-1738, USA

C. Divgi, MD, Nuclear Medicine Service, Memorial Sloan–Kettering Cancer Center, New York, New York, USA

Graeme Eisenhofer, MD, Pediatric and Reproductive Endocrinology Branch and Clinical Neurocardiology Section, National Institutes of Health, Bethesda, Maryland 20892, USA

Paul J. Elson, ScD, The Cleveland Clinic Foundation, 9500 Euclid Ave., Cleveland, OH 44195, USA

Robert A. Figlin, MD, FACP, Department of Medicine, Division of Hematology–Oncology, UCLA School of Medicine, Jonsson Comprehensive Cancer Center, Los Angeles, California, USA

Jean Emmanuel Filmont, MD, Division of Nuclear Medicine, Department of Medical and Molecular Pharmacology, UCLA School of Medicine, Los Angeles, California, USA

Robert C Flanigan, MD, Albert J Jr and Claire R Speh Professor and Chair, Department of Urology, Loyola University Medical Center and Hines VA Hospital, Maywood, Illinois 60153, USA

Sophie D. Fosså MD, Department of Clinical Research, The Norwegian Radium Hospital, Montebello, 0310 Oslo, Norway

Stephen J. Freedland, MD, Resident in Urology, Division of Urologic Oncology, Department of Urology, University of California School of Medicine, Los Angeles, California 90095-1738, USA

Reza Ghavamian, MD, Director Division of Urologic Oncology, Albert Einstein College of Medicine/Montefiore Medical Center, Bronx, New York 10467, USA

Inderbir S. Gill, MD, MCh, Section of Laparoscopic and Minimally Invasive Surgery, Department of Urology, Cleveland Clinic Foundation, Cleveland, Ohio, USA

Barbara J. Gitlitz, MD, Department of Medicine, Division of Hematology–Oncology, UCLA School of Medicine, Jonsson Comprehensive Cancer Center, Los Angeles, California, USA

Lucy A. Godley, MD, PhD, Section of Hematology/Oncology, Department of Medicine, University of Chicago, Chicago, Illinois 60637, USA

Philip J. Gold, MD, Swedish Medical Center, Swedish Cancer Institute, Seattle, Washington 98104, USA

Graham F. Greene, MD, Associate Professor of Urology, Department of Urology, University of Arkansas College of Medicine, Little Rock, Arkansas 72205-7199, USA

H. Albin Gritsch, MD, Surgical Director, Renal Transplantation, UCLA Medical Center, PO Box 951738, Los Angeles, California 90095-1738, USA

Groupe Français d'Immunothérapie, Medical Oncology Department, Centre Léon Bérard, 69373 Lyon Cedex 08, France

Gabriel Haas, MD, Professor and Chairman, Department of Urology, Upstate Medical University, State University of New York, Syracuse, New York, USA

Peter Hahn, PhD, Associate Professor, Department of Radiation Oncology, Upstate Medical University, State University of New York, Syracuse, New York, USA

Andreas Hinkel, MD, Department of Urology, Ruhr-Universität Bochum, Marienhospital, Widurner Strasse 8, Herne 44627, Germany

David M.J. Hoffman, MD, Department of Medicine, Division of Hematology–Oncology, UCLA School of Medicine, Jonsson Comprehensive Cancer Center, Los Angeles, California, USA

Masatsugu Iwamura, MD, Department of Urology, Kitasato University, School of Medicine 1–15–1, Kitasato, Sagamiharashi, Kanagawa, Japan

Guihua Jiang, MD, Division of Surgical Oncology, University of Michigan, Ann Arbor, Michigan 48109, USA

Louis R. Kavoussi, Vice-Chairman, Patrick C. Walsh Distinguished Professor of Urology, James Buchanan Brady Urological Institute, Johns Hopkins Medical Institutions, Baltimore, Maryland, 21287 USA

Gyula Kovacs, MD, PhD, DSc, Laboratory of Molecular Oncology, Department of Urology, Universitätsklinikum Heidelberg, Im Neuenheimer Feld 365, D-691290 Heidelberg, Germany

Sherelle Laifer-Narin, MD, Department of Radiological Sciences,UCLA School of Medicine, Los Angeles, California 90095-1721, USA

Qiao Li, PhD, Division of Surgical Oncology, University of Michigan, Ann Arbor, Michigan 48109, USA

John A. Libertino, MD, Chairman, Department of Urology, Lahey Clinic Medical Center, Burlington, Massachusetts 01805, USA

W. Marston Linehan, MD, Urologic Oncology Branch, Division of Clinical Sciences, National Cancer Institute, National Institutes of Health, Bethesda, Maryland 20892, USA

Zhenqi Liu, MD, Assistant Professor of Research, Division of Endocrinology and Metabolism, Department of Medicine, University of Virginia School of Medicine, Charlottesville, Virginia 22908, USA

Jodie K. Maranchie, MD, Urologic Oncology Branch, National Cancer Institute, National Institutes of Health, Bethesda, Maryland 20892, USA

Ken Marumo, MD, Department of Urology, Keio University, School of Medicine, 35 Sinanomachi, Shinjukuku, Tokyo 160-8582, Japan

Nehal Masood, MD, University of Washington Medical Center, Division of Medical Oncology, Seattle, Washington 98109-1023, USA

Anoop M. Meraney, MD, Section of Laparoscopic and Minimally Invasive Surgery, Department of Urology, Cleveland Clinic Foundation, Cleveland, Ohio, USA

James E. Montie, MD, Head, Section of Urology, Professor of Surgery, Department of Surgery, University of Michigan, Ann Arbor, Michigan 48109–0330, USA

Robert J. Motzer, MD, Genitourinary Oncology Service, Division of Solid Tumor Oncology, Department of Medicine, Memorial Sloan–Kettering Cancer Center, New York, New York, USA

MRC Renal Cell Cancer Group, MRC Clinical Trials Unit, Cancer Division, London, NW1 2DA, UK

Peter Mulders, MD, PhD, Department of Urology, University Hospital, Nijmegen, PO Box 9101, 6500 Hb The Netherlands

Masaru Murai, MD, Department of Urology, Keio University, School of Medicine, 35 Sinanomachi, Shinjukuku, Tokyo 160-8582, Japan

Sylvie Négrier, MD, PhD Medical Oncology Department, Centre Léon Berard, 69373 Lyon Cedex 08, France

Maria I. New, MD, Professor and Chairman, Department of Pediatrics, Chief, Division of Pediatric Endocrinology, Harold and Percy Uris Professor of Pediatric Endocrinology and Metabolism, New York Presbyterian Hospital–Weill Medical College of Cornell University, New York, New York 10021, USA

Andrew C. Novick, MD, Urological Institute, The Cleveland Clinic Foundation, Cleveland, Ohio 44195, USA

R.T.D. Oliver, MD, FRCP, Sir Maxwell Joseph Professor in Medical Oncology, St Barts and The Royal London Hospital School of Medicine, Queen Mary, University of London, Smithfield, London EC1A 7BE, UK

E. Oosterwijk, MD, Department of Urology, University Hospital, Nijmegen, PO Box 9101, 6500 Hb The Netherlands

Karel Pacak, MD, Pediatric and Reproductive Endocrinology Branch and Clinical Neurocardiology Section, National Institutes of Health, Bethesda, Maryland 20892, USA

Allan J. Pantuck, MD, Fellow in Urologic Oncology, Division of Urologic Oncology, Department of Urology, University of California School of Medicine, Los Angeles, California 90095-1738, USA

Nicholas Papanicolaou, MD, Department of Radiology, New York Presbyterian Hospital, Cornell University Medical Center, New York, New York 10021, USA

David F. Paulson, MD, Division of Urology, Department of Surgery, Duke University Medical Center, Durham, North Carolina 27710, USA

Christian P. Pavlovich, MD, Brady Urological Institute, Johns Hopkins Bayview Medical Center, Baltimore, Maryland 21224, USA

Aaron P. Perlmutter, MD, James Buchanan Brady Foundation, Department of Urology, New York Presbyterian Hospital, Joan and Sanford I. Weill Medical College of Cornell University, New York, New York 10021, USA

Dix P. Poppas, MD, FACS, FAAP, Chief, Pediatric Urology, The Richmond Rodgers Family Associate Professor of Pediatric Urology, Children's Hospital of New York Presbyterian

Michael Probst-Kepper, MD, PhD German Research Centre for Biotechnology, Molecular Immunology, Braunschweig, Germany

Steven S. Raman, MD, Department of Radiological Sciences,UCLA School of Medicine, Los Angeles, California 90095-1721, USA

Mitchell K. Rauch, MD, Fellow in Urologic Oncology, Division of Urologic Oncology, Department of Urology, University of California School of Medicine, Los Angeles, California 90095-1738, USA

Bruce G. Redman, DO, Division of Hematology–Oncology, University of Michigan, Ann Arbor, Michigan 48109, USA

John F. Redman, MD, Professor of Urology, Department of Urology, University of Arkansas College of Medicine, Little Rock, Arkansas 72205-7199, USA

Alastair W.S. Ritchie, MD, FRCSED, Consultant Urological Surgeon, Gloucestershire Royal Hospital, Great Western Road, Gloucester GL1 3NN, UK

Gregory J. Rubino, MD, Assistant Professor, Division of Neurosurgery, UCLA Medical Center, Los Angeles, California 90095-1738, USA

G. Bino Rucker, MD, The Center for Pediatric Urology, Department of Urology, Children's Hospital of New York Presbyterian Weill Medical College of Cornell University, New York, New York 10021, USA

Donna M. Sayre, MSN, Division of Surgical Oncology, University of Michigan, Ann Arbor, Michigan 48109, USA

Richard D. Schulick, MD, Assistant Professor of Surgery and Oncology, Johns Hopkins Hospital, Baltimore, Maryland 10021, USA

David A. Schulsinger, MD, James Buchanan Brady Foundation, Department of Urology, New York Presbyterian Hospital, Joan and Sanford I. Weill Medical College of Cornell University, New York, New York 10021, USA

Marc Seltzer, MD, Assistant Professor of Nuclear Medicine, Department of Medical and Molecular Pharmacology, UCLA School of Medicine, Los Angeles, California, USA

Ojas Shah, MD, Senior Resident, Department of Urology, New York University School of Medicine, New York, New York 10016, USA

Steven Shichman, MD, Connecticut Surgical Group PC, Hartford Hospital, Hartford, Connecticut, USA

Helmy M. Siragy, MD, Professor of Medicine, Division of Endocrinology and Metabolism, Department of Medicine, University of Virginia School of Medicine, Charlottesville, Virginia 22908, USA

Joel W. Slaton, MD, Department of Urologic Surgery, The University of Minnesota, Minneapolis, Minnesota 55455, USA

Eric J. Small, MD, Departments of Medicine and Urology, UCSF Comprehensive Cancer Center, San Francisco, California.

Mitchell H. Sokoloff, MD, Assistant Professor and Director of Urologic Oncology, Section of Urology, Department of Surgery, University of Chicago, Chicago, Illinois 60637, USA

Andrea Sorcini, MD, Department of Urology, Lahey Clinic Medical Center, Burlington, Massachusetts 01805, USA

R. Ernest Sosa, MD, James Buchanan Brady Foundation, Department of Urology, New York Presbyterian Hospital, Joan and Sanford I. Weill Medical College of Cornell University, New York, New York 10021, USA

M. Steffens, MD, Department of Urology, University Hospital, Nijmegen, PO Box 9101, 6500 Hb The Netherlands

Stephen Stoerkel, MD, Department of Urology, Ruhr-Universität Bochum, Marienhospital, Widurner Strasse 8, Herne 44627, Germany

David A. Swanson, MD, Professor and Chairman, Department of Urology, The University of Texas M.D. Anderson Cancer Center, Houston, Texas 77030, USA

Samir S. Taneja, MD, Assistant Professor, Director of the Advanced Genitourinary Oncology Program, Department of Urology, New York University School of Medicine, New York, New York 10016, USA

Neyssan Tebyani, MD, Resident, Department of Urology, Kaiser Permanente Medical Center, 4900 Sunset Blvd., Los Angeles, CA 90027

Susan Teeger, MD, Department of Radiology, New York Presbyterian Hospital, Cornell University Medical Center, New York, New York 10021, USA

John A. Thompson, MD, University of Washington Medical Center, Division of Medical Oncology, Seattle, Washington 98109-1023, USA

Donald L. Trump, MD, Professor of Medicine, University of Pittsburgh Cancer Institute, Division of Hematology/Oncology, Pittsburgh, Pennsylvania 15213–2582, USA

Robert G. Uzzo, MD, Department of Surgical Oncology, Fox Chase Cancer Center, 7701, Burholme Avenue, Philadelphia, PA 19111, USA

Benoît J. Van den Eynde, MD, PhD, Ludwig Institute for Cancer Research, Brussels Branch, and Université Catholique de Louvain, Unité de Génétique Cellulaire, Brussels, Belgium

E. Darracott Vaughan Jr, MD, James J. Colt Professor of Urology, Department of Urology, New York Presbyterian Hospital, Cornell University Medical Center, James Buchanan Brady Foundation, New York, New York 10021, USA

Nicholas J. Vogelzang, MD, Director of the Cancer Research Center and the Fred C. Buffett Professor of Medicine, Section of Hematology/Oncology, Department of Medicine, University of Chicago, Chicago, Illinois 60637, USA

McClellan M. Walther, MD, Urologic Oncology Branch, Division of Clinical Sciences, National Cancer Institute, National Institutes of Health, Bethesda, Maryland 20892, USA

Jeff A. Wieder, MD, Department of Urology, University of California School of Medicine, Los Angeles, California 90095-1738, USA

Jon M. Wigginton, MD, Investigational Biologics Section, Pediatric Oncology Branch, Center for Cancer Research, National Cancer Institute, Bethesda, Maryland, USA

Robert H. Wiltrout, PhD, Laboratory of Experimental Immunology, Division of Basic Sciences, National Cancer Institute Frederick Cancer Research and Development Center, Frederick, Maryland 21702-1201, USA

J. Stuart Wolf, Jr, MD, FACS, Associate Professor, Department of Urology, University of Michigan, Ann Arbor, Michigan 48109-0330, USA

Mark P.J. Wright, MD, FRCS, Consultant Urological Surgeon, Bristol Royal Infirmary Bristol B52 8HW, UK

Paul Matthew Yonover, MD, Resident, Department of Urology, Loyola University Medical Center and Hines VA Hospital, Maywood, Illinois 60153, USA

Horst Zincke, MD, PhD, Professor of Urology, Mayo Graduate School of Medicine, Mayo Clinic, Rochester, Minnesota 55905, USA

Amnon Zisman, MD, Stephen and Mary Meadow Fellow in Urologic Oncology, Division of Urologic Oncology, Department of Urology, University of California School of Medicine, Los Angeles, California 90095-1738, USA

Part 1, Section 1
Anatomy, epidemiology, and pathology

1. Historical perspective: past, present, and future

Amnon Zisman and Jean B. deKernion

Anonymous

In the last 25 years the knowledge about renal and adrenal tumors has expanded dramatically. What was in the beginning of the century a pioneering surgical craft progressing as a reflection of general surgery has become a multidisciplinary component of the field of urological oncology. Patient care has been influenced by surgical innovations that have continued to evolve, and also by other accomplishments in biochemistry, imaging, immunology, endocrinology, genetics, and molecular biology. These influences set the course for the therapy of renal and adrenal tumors at the start of the third millennium.

In this chapter we will identify trends, key events, and breakthroughs in the care of renal and adrenal tumors. Although the medical history of renal tumors is a continuity, for didactic purposes we will be discussing specific periods and entities so that the interested reader will find it easy to follow the evolutionary trends. It is our belief that reviewing the history of renal and adrenal tumors will intensify the yield and pleasure to be obtained from the following chapters in this book and will give a balanced image of future prospects.

The importance of renal cancer is evidenced not only by the steady rise in its annual incidence (2 per cent) but also by the number of publications dealing with this topic. The number of publications per year in the evaluated ™MEDLINE for the years 1966–99 using the key words hypernephroma, renal cell carcinoma (RCC), and kidney cancer increased by more than one decimal order. The percentage of publications dealing with renal tumors in the *Journal of Urology* also rose significantly from 1 per cent of the published material during 1966 to approximately 10 per cent currently, whereas the overall number of publications in the evaluated ™MEDLINE has risen only by 2.4-fold (Fig. 1.1).

Not only has the number of scientific publications risen but, as in other medical fields, the ways in which patients educate themselves and seek remedy have changed dramatically. The availability and the quality of information open to the public are outstanding as is demonstrated in the following example. During the first day of the year 2000 the authors performed an internet search using the lay terminology 'kidney cancer'. Sixty-three highly relevant sites for patients, caregivers, and researchers were found through two randomly chosen search engines. Retrieval time for the primary site list was 9 seconds, using cable hook-ups, and, for first site entry, an additional 4 seconds. The mean number of relevant 'one step further' links leading to relevant new information was 3.7 ± 1.3 links per site. During a limited time of 30 minutes, 212 different and relevant sites were entered.

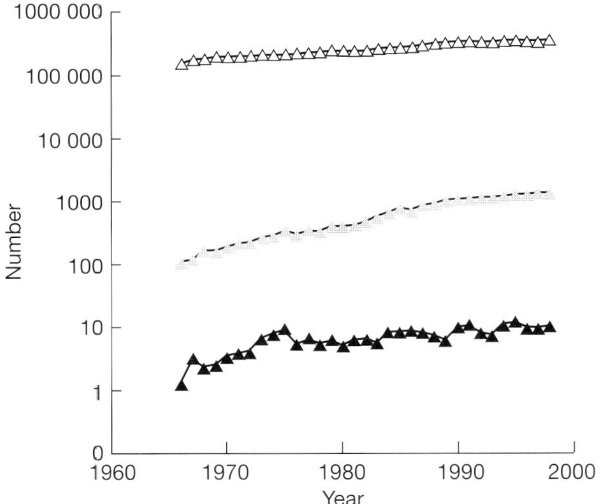

Fig. 1.1 Number of publications in ™MEDLINE: △ overall number of publications △ number of publications using key words 'hypernephroma', 'renal cell carcinoma', 'RCC', and 'kidney cancer'. ▲ number of publications using the same key words in *The Journal of Urology*

Beginnings

The progress in the treatment of renal cancer at the dawn of modern medicine was tightly bound to the establishment of nephrectomy as a standard of care procedure for treating patients with renal tumors. The first nephrectomies were performed in dogs during the seventeenth century. In 1678 Giuseppe Zambeccarrius (1650–1702) performed a nephrectomy in a dog, which survived the surgery. The result of his surgery and Giuseppe's prior observation that some of the healthy appearing dogs had only one kidney on autopsy proved that life may be maintained with only one kidney. Moreover, Roonhuysen in 1672 described the phenomenon of compensatory enlargement of the remaining kidney in an animal model (Moll and Rathert 1999). Experimental nephrectomies in animals led Stephan Blankkard (1650–1702) of Amsterdam to declare, in 1690, that nephrectomy might be performed in humans (Gifford 1973). Scholars of the nineteenth century contributed to the understanding of the macroscopic and microscopic properties of renal tumors. The most important reports were those of Konig, who described the gross appearance of kidney tumors in 1826, the description by Robin (1885) of tubular epithelial proliferation invading and destroying the lamina proprea and extending uninterruptedly to become a cancerous nodulation, and the legendary description of embryoma by Wilms in 1882 (published in Wilms 1899).

The courage, skills, and technology necessary for the performance of nephrectomy in humans, as well as the proper atmosphere for carrying out and reporting such an effort in a publication, evolved during the second half of the nineteenth century, both in Europe and in the United States.

History credits Gustav Simon (1824–76) of Heidelburg with performing the first intentional nephrectomy on August 2, 1869, in a woman anguished with a nonremitting uretero-cutaneous and uretero-vaginal fistula following hysterectomy. The operation took 40 minutes and 50 ml of blood were lost. The patient left her bed on postoperative day 28 and left the hospital 2 months later (Moll and Rathert 1999). Less well known is the fact that the case almost ended in court rather than in the operating theater. In spite of the patient's consent to the revolutionizing surgery, there was great public criticism expressed over the intent to remove a functioning vital organ. At approximately the same period, across the Atlantic, an American surgeon by the name of Erastus B. Wolcott excelled in a range of surgery unusual for his time, such as mastectomy, thoracotomy, oophorectomy, cesarean section, and plastic surgery for burn victims. Dr Wolcott was born in Benton, New York, in 1804 and practiced medicine in the city of Milwaukee, Wisconsin. On June 4, 1861 he performed a right nephrectomy on a 58-year-old male who preoperatively was thought to have a cystic liver tumor. He found a large tumor arising from the lower pole of the kidney, causing organ displacement. The kidney was removed but, unfortunately, the patient passed away on postoperative day 15 because of sepsis. Dr Wolcott was assisted by Dr Chester L. Stoddard who summarized the data in a case report published in the *Philadelphia Medical and Surgical Reporter* of 1861–62. This was the first nephrectomy reported for an oncological indication. In his report Dr Stoddard (1862) referred to the patient's preoperative diagnosis: '…but what the deposit was we were unable to learn, as no reliable chemical or microscopical evidence was presented.' This set a point of historical and scientific reference for the knowledge and the environment in which oncological surgery was performed in that era.

Slowly, nephrectomy was popularized by the surgeons of the late nineteenth century for a wide range of indications, but mostly for the treatment of infectious and benign lesions. Only a minority of procedures were performed for kidney cancer.

By the end of the nineteenth century, the first reports on nephrectomy series were available (Weir 1884; Gross 1885; Kuster 1902). The overall mortality rate for nephrectomy in those days reached 50 per cent. Mortalities resulted mainly from postoperative sepsis and massive bleeding from infectious erosion into the great vessels and delayed bleeding from the pedicle stump due to slipped silk ties.

Just before the First World War the founder of the American Urological Association, Dr Ramon Guiteras, in his two-volume textbook of urology, dedicated only 12 pages to tumors of the kidney (Guiteras 1913). In his time he could already refer to over 600 documented cases of renal tumors. In his chapter he summarized the knowledge that existed in his era, in which one may readily recognize the seeds of future knowledge and development. Included in his chapter is one of the first attempts to classify and pathologically subdivide malignant renal tumors into distinct categories. Although pioneering themes, and naïve and simplistic ideas, are expressed in this monograph, this is one of the earliest manuscripts encompassing a thorough discussion of the topic of kidney cancer in a format that would be basically preserved in textbooks of urology during the entire twentieth century. We choose to regard Guiteras's textbook as a historical document having a great importance as a baseline reference for the future.

Early innovations

Medical and surgical accomplishments during the last three decades of the nineteenth century and during the first half of the twentieth century were influenced by the great discoveries and inventions that promoted surgery and urology in general in steps crucial to the establishment of the straightforward competent approach to renal tumors utilized today. During the early days of nephrectomy, at the end of the nineteenth century, the intraoperative and immediate postoperative mortality was around 50 per cent, primarily due to wound infection and sepsis. This was an era in which operations were carried out without gloves, with very mild sanitation, and with only chemical antiseptics. Anesthesia was light and monitorless. Imaging was not available and preoperative staging was done by physical examination. Antibiotics and blood transfusions were in the realm of science fiction. At the beginning of the twentieth century great technological and scientific breakthroughs happened outside the medical field, which, within a short period of time, influenced and promoted the development of urology in a dramatic fashion. It is beyond the scope of this chapter to detail the evolution of each one of these important modifiers. However, those advances had an impressive impact on intraoperative and perioperative mortality and on patients' long-term survival. The effect of these discoveries on the standard of care for urological patients as well as on those with renal tumors is reflected in periodicals published during the first half of the twentieth century. The advances in microbiology, availability of rubber industry products, and the establishment of the connection between bacteria and infection led finally to the use of gloves, antiseptics, and sterile preparation of surgical equipment, towards the end of the eighteenth century. The great discoveries in physics harnessed radiation as a diagnostic and therapeutic tool for medicine: plain abdominal films were used to delineate the contour of the kidneys and thus it was possible to image large masses and calcifications before the First World War. In 1932 intravenous pyelography was already a commonly used diagnostic procedure for hematuria and renal masses but its risks were not fully appreciated at that time (Cunningham

1932). Radiation therapy, which was not a therapeutic option for renal tumors in 1913 (Guiteras 1913), was used extensively after the First World War and was held to be an effective treatment for the majority of renal malignancies (Gottesman *et al.* 1932). During the Second World War the first series describing the experience with sulfonamide and later penicillin in urology were published. The *Year book of urology* annotated their increased utilization since 1941 (Lowsley 1941*b*) and 1944 (Lowsley, 1944*b*), respectively. The 1950s are definitely reflected in the literature as the decade of antibiotics (Scott 1950) and, since then, antibiotic therapy has continued to develop and has backed up almost all urological procedures up to the present.

The establishment of urology as a safe surgical practice after the Second World War, aided, supported, and backed up by the other medical disciplines, made it possible to address issues specific to renal tumors leading to a more refined and detailed approach to the different entities collectively addressed as renal tumors. For example, during the 1950s, Kolff produced and used the first modern 'artificial kidney', in which extracorporeal dialysis of circulating blood from uremic patients was employed. Seligman and Fine first reported the use of peritoneal dialysis. These were the first steps towards avoiding inevitable death due to uremia, making bilateral nephrectomy feasible. More than 3 decades later organ transplantation came to the stage and further improved the outcome for these rare and desperately ill patients.

Indeed during 4 decades, until the late 1980s, knowledge concerning renal tumors was accumulated and refined mainly by clinicians, surgeons, and pathologists. During these 4 decades great progress was achieved in understanding and classifying renal tumors, with the conclusion that there are in fact three major histological groups of malignant renal tumors (renal cell carcinomas, Wilms' tumor, and upper tract transitional cellcarcinomas) and a group of other rare malignancies, mainly sarcoma. In each group implementation of grading and staging systems correlating with tumor behavior has improved patient selection for surgery and refined the indications for different surgical procedures. Then, during the 1980s and early 1990s, a second round of technological and scientific discoveries again modified the standard of care for renal tumors. We will try to isolate and analyze these trends and their major contributions.

Macro, micro, nano, and pico: the story of the classification of renal tumors

Before the First World War, the assumed origin and classification of renal tumors differed extensively from present knowledge. Nonmalignant tumors were lipomas, fibromas, myxomas, and angiomas but also adenomas, which were believed to arise from the renal tubules and to have two varieties, the small and the large, of which the latter is usually malignant especially if hypervascular. Malignant lesion were *hypernephromas*, originally described by Grawitz (1883) as *struma lipomatodes aberrantae renis*, and were believed to arise from the adrenal gland or from adrenal tissue ectopically situated within the kidney. Hypernephromas were believed to be distinct from *carcinomas*, whereas sarcomas were

reported to be the most frequent type of renal tumor diagnosed and most commonly found in children. In addition, the term *rhabdomyoma* was given by Rokitansky in 1848 to a distinct group of tumors, arising mainly in children aged 1–3 years and manifesting an extremely malignant behavior and characterized by long slender cells. Untreated patients succumbed within 4 years of detection. Relapse after nephrectomy ended uniformly in death and was very common during the first year after surgery. The only treatment according to Guiteras (1913) was nephrectomy: '…as soon as the other kidney has been shown by cystoscopic and ureteral catheterization, with chemical and microscopical examination of the urine, to be sufficiently healthy to carry on the renal function.'

In 1932 50 per cent of cases were metastatic on diagnosis and in 37 per cent of cases the pathological diagnosis was different from the preoperative diagnosis, but the main histological terms for what is known today as renal cell carcinoma (RCC) were cortical adenoma and various variants of hypernephroma: typical, atypical, papillary, adenoumatous, highly malignant, and sarcoma-like (Gottesman *et al.* 1932). A distinction was made between hypernephroma and embryoma (Simpson 1934) based on Wilms' observation (Wilms 1899). This fundamental distinction between early childhood tumors and other renal tumors constitutes the special multimodal niche of Wilms' tumor, to be shared between urologists, pediatric surgeons, and radiation oncologists in the years to come and also medical oncologists after the discovery of cytotoxic drugs 3 decades later. The first documentation for this multimodal approach was a report in the *Annals of Surgery* by Randall of the University of Pennsylvania in 1934 who suggested that better care for children with renal embryonic tumors would be attained by combining radiation therapy and surgery. Twenty years after Guiteras's textbook, it was obvious that childhood tumors were very rare (McCurdy 1934) and highly malignant with 80–90 per cent recurrence after surgery as opposed to the main bulk of renal tumors (85 per cent), which were 'hypernephromas' arising in adults with a 60 per cent recurrence rate (Cunningham 1935*b*). These notes were in agreement with the Minnesota classification (Bell 1938) based on 160 cases of renal tumors found in 30 000 necroscopies as well as with the Columbia University classification published 6 years later, based on 199 nephrectomy cases.

The Minnesota classification is an important document since it also comprises one of the earliest documented reports on the correlation between tumor size and biological behavior: For tumors sized 0–3 cm, 3–5 cm, and >5 cm, the occurrence of metastases was 1/37 (3 per cent), 4/22 (18 per cent), and 66/84 (76 per cent), respectively. Those were also the years in which the adrenal origin of RCC and the term 'hypernephroma' began to be challenged by E.R. Whitmore of Georgetown University (Whitmore 1937), 64 years after wrongly being proposed by Grawitz (1883). Although challenged as early as 1937, this semantic and conceptual mistake established the term 'hypernephroma' in kidney cancer literature for many decades until some convincing histochemical evidence showed that hypernephromas also arise from renal tubular cells (Grayhack 1966).

In 1951 a report from Cornell University based on 295 RCC patients included a classification system similar to the Columbia

University classification mentioned above but including the key words 'renal celled carcinoma' and 'Wilms' tumor' and omitting the term 'hypernephroma' (Foot *et al.* 1951). More classification systems have been proposed since then and most of them are summarized in the different editions of *Campbell's urology*. However, the most recent and perhaps the most challenging classification, which also sheds light on future prospects for renal tumor classification, is the Heidelberg classification of renal tumors (Kovacs *et al.* 1997), which summarizes the conclusions of a workshop entitled 'Impact of molecular genetics on the classification of renal cell tumours' held in Heidelberg in October 1996. The proposed classification subdivided renal cell tumors into benign and malignant parenchymal neoplasms and limited further subcategorization to the most commonly documented genetic alterations known at that time. Benign tumors were subclassified into metanephric adenoma and adenofibroma, papillary renal cell adenoma, and renal oncocytoma. Malignant tumors were subclassified into common renal cell carcinoma; chromophil papillary renal cell carcinoma; chromophobe renal cell carcinoma; collecting duct carcinoma, medullary carcinoma of the kidney, and renal cell carcinoma—unclassified. The power of this classification lies in its association with genetic knowledge and in its correlation with recognizable histological findings but, in our opinion, its main historical importance is that it set the direction for future classification systems in which molecular properties reflecting biological behavior rather than descriptive appearance will be used to classify renal tumors.

Staging and grading: from clinical gut feeling to accurate prediction of outcome

Sporadic reports on different aspects of what would become criteria for *staging* appeared in the literature years before the first published staging system and reflected good clinical judgement and meticulous patient follow-up by surgeons at that time: J.B. Beare and J.R. McDonald reported in the *Journal of Urology* on a poorer prognosis for patients with capsular penetration of tumor with perinephric fat infiltration (Lowsley 1949). The same idea was the basis for a practical guideline in the same years (Scott 1951): 'All the methods are alike so far as survival rates are concerned. With any method the general principle of early ligation of the renal pedicle, gentleness in handling the kidney, and as complete removal of surrounding fat and fascia of the kidney as is possible must be followed.'

The first documented staging system for RCC was developed by R.H. Flocks and M.C. Kadesky at the University of Iowa and published in 1958. This system was based on their experience with 353 patients followed for 5 years or more. The authors detected a difference in the 5-year survival between treated patients in whom the tumor was limited to the capsule (55 per cent), patients with invasion into the pedicle or perinephric fat (41 per cent), patients with lymph node involvement (14 per cent), and patients with distant metastasis (4 per cent) (Flock and Kadesky 1957). In 1963 Robson *et al.* modified the University of Iowa staging system and

used their modified staging system to report on results with radical nephrectomy (Robson *et al.* 1969), which was a surgical modification that ingeniously combined what was learned from previous observations and what was logical according to data obtained from correlating staging and survival. The Robson staging system and the technique for radical nephrectomy were popularized all over the world. His staging system remained for many decades the preferred one for RCC because of its simplicity and clinical applicability whereas radical nephrectomy still remains the gold standard for treatment of RCC nowadays. Dr J.T. Grayhack (1964) who took the office of the editor of the *Year Book of Urology* in 1964 wrote on Robson's findings: 'These results are very good. Whether this is due to the surgical procedure or to some other factor is not certain.'

Since 1978 the TNM (tumor, node, metastasis) classification for malignant tumor has been available (Harmen 1978). In 1983, the new TNM classification proposed by the American Joint Committee for Cancer Staging and End Results Reporting (Beahrs and Myers 1983) recognized tumor size as important. It offered a systematic partition of Robson stage III into subgroups, thereby overcoming a drawback in the Robson system that caused in some of the series reported to use it an equal survival between Robson stage II and III tumors, indicative of an inappropriate assignment of prognostic factors. However the complexity of the 1983 TNM staging system initially restricted its utilization. The TNM staging system was again refined in a joint workshop held by the Union International Contre Le Cancer (UICC) and the American Joint Committee on Cancer (AJCC) in Rochester, Minnesota during Spring, 1997 (Guinan *et al.* 1997). The results of this workshop are believed to be a key milestone in the field of renal tumors. The modified staging system seems already to be having an impact on publications in the field (Belldegrun *et al.* 1999).

The first report on the correlation between *grading* and patient outcome was published in the US in 1932 (Hand and Broders 1932). Since the publication of this key manuscript, reports on at least 10 different grading systems have been published, mainly during the 1970s and 1980s. Each system had its own advantages and disadvantages but all combined nuclear and nucleolar appearances as their major criteria. There was a global consensus that grading systems should be used since correlation with prognosis was evident. However, there is less unanimity concerning which grading system to use. The majority of the pathologists in the US currently use the Fuhrman grading system described in 1982 (Fuhrman *et al.* 1982). The Fuhrman grading system was shown to be deficient in the distinction between grades I and II (Medeiros *et al.* 1988) but there is as yet no better prognostic system than simple grading. Basic cancer research and genetics are constantly examining for grading purposes a large number of more refined and sophisticated prognostic indices. Nuclear morphometry and DNA content in the mid-1980s (Ljungberg *et al.* 1986; Tosi *et al.* 1986; deKernion *et al.* 1989) and an array of molecular markers in the 1990s, of which the more prominent are the von Hippel–Lindau (VHL) and the *P53* genes (Haitel *et al.* 1999), but also many other markers and technologies, such as the proposed RCC marker G250 (Mulders *et al.* 1997), tissue microarrays, and fluorescence *in situ* hybridization (FISH) analysis for mass detection of genetic alterations, are evolving while this chapter is being finalized. As with prostate-specific antigen (PSA) in prostate cancer, it is not unlikely that one of these novelties will pass the test of time and prove clinically significant.

From physical examination as a staging procedure to incidental tumor detection

After the First World War intravenous pyelography (IVP) was available for the work-up of patients with signs and symptoms suggesting the possibility of kidney cancer (Cunningham 1932). In those days the state of the art imaging methods included IVP and retrograde pyelography. IVP was first performed in 1923 (Osborne *et al.* 1923), refined in 1929, and supplemented with nephrotomography after 1954 (Evans *et al.* 1954). Retrograde pyelography was first reported by Voelcker and von Lichtenberg (1906) for the presumably affected side (Cunningham 1935*b*) and also in the evaluation of the contralateral kidney for its ability to support life (Guiteras 1913). In spite of a high index of clinical suspicion and excellent skills in physical examination, the presenting symptoms in the patients subjected to this work-ups were those of obvious stigmata for advanced disease: palpable mass in 83 per cent; mass detected by the patient, 15 per cent; loin pain, 85 per cent; hematuria, 62 per cent; weight loss, 23 per cent; and acute varicocele, 8 per (Cunningham 1935*b*). Twenty per cent of the patients had the classical triad of hematuria, flank pain, and abdominal mass and all of them had metastasis (Cunningham 1938*b*). Thus in that era 50 per cent of patients were metastatic at diagnosis and 24 per cent were thought to be inoperable or too ill to be operated upon. The only active therapy modalities that could be offered to these patients were surgery or radiation. Cunningham (1935*b*) wrote in the *Yearbook of Urology*: '…the size of the mass should be neglected in deciding on operability. Metastasis does not always preclude operation, one should operate first on kidney, then on metastases.' This led surgeons to rely more on their intraoperative findings during exploration rather than on preoperative staging. This practice led quite often to heroic operations on very large tumors, closure without performing the operation, great difficulty in differentiating preoperatively and intraoperatively between benign and malignant lesions (Cunningham 1939), and stumbling into dangerous situations such as an unforeseen need to remove a tumor thrombus from the inferior vena cava (Priestley and Walters 1933).

The first reports of a *chromogenic test for hematuria* by H. Zwarenstein (1943) of the University of Cape Town (Zwarenstein, 1943) has historical importance since the test, and its fast development and assimilation into practice, led by the end of that decade to a rise in the number of hematuria work-ups. In his concluding editorial remarks for the 1940–50 decade W.W. Scott (1950) wrote concerning renal tumors: 'Little has been added in this category except through the increased recognition of the importance of hematuria… Hopefully we look forward to 1950–60.'

We believe that recognizing the importance of hematuria during the 1940s was one of the precursors leading to earlier diagnosis of RCC. The eagerness of urologists at that time for a more precise and early diagnosis was expressed in an essay by D.K. Rose in 1949 in the *Surgical Clinics of North America*. His article reviewed the potential for early diagnosis using three available tools for achieving that goal. These were routine search for hematuria in urological work-ups; *aortography* (first performed intraoperatively by a mistake in 1929 by a Portuguese urologist, Dos Santos (Dos Santos *et al.* 1929), and defined for the purpose of clinical use by Nelson (1942) in Seattle); and *pneumoradiology of the kidney* (*perirenal and presacral gas insufflation*) (Rose 1949). At about the same time, the technique of *percutaneous puncture of cysts* was developed (Lindblom 1946) since it was readily recognized that renal angiography was not accurate in differentiating between renal masses and cysts.

Rose's article heralded the golden era of angiography for kidney tumors. It was refined and evolved for almost 3 decades. The first important publication delineating the angiographic findings in RCC was that of Evans (1957) who claimed 95 per cent correlation between the radiographic findings and the intraoperative and pathological findings.

Also in the early 1950s some authors reported a decline in the number of patients with metastasis at diagnosis (Burford *et al.* 1951) and a reduction in the proportion of patients presenting with the full blown classical triad (Scott 1951). In 1952 a dispute concerning the controversial use of *renal biopsy* became evident. Since then, the urological discussion on the yield and dangers of renal mass biopsy has never ceased. It is, however, worth mentioning that Weyrauch and co-workers (1952) of the Veterans' Administration hospital in San Francisco recommended an open exploration and biopsy with the goal of renal preservation. Weyrauch was primarily interested in differentiating between malignant and benign conditions and not in the preservation of renal units harboring cancer. The guideline for the decades to follow was forming: *any renal mass is malignant unless proven otherwise*. However, the motif suggested by Weyrauch served and evolved in parallel to this guideline for special indications in the form of partial nephrectomy and was to come back to centerstage at the end of the century in the discussion concerning partial nephrectomy with a normal contralateral kidney.

As early as 1963, a search for *markers and prognostic factors for RCC* was launched. Amador and colleagues (1963) proposed elevated urinary lactate dehydrogenase (LDH) and alkaline phosphatase activities as markers for the diagnosis of renal adenocarcinoma. This publication led to discussions concerning tissue specificity and correlation with stage but the 'marker race' was on, always reflecting the cutting edge of basic science achievements in discovering novel molecules with biological significance. In fact, since 1963 the marker race has never stopped and has grown faster and more competitive by the year. Although many molecules have been suggested over the years to have diagnostic or prognostic qualities, currently there is no molecule that offers tissue specificity and proven clinical value. Currently, the expression of at least 13 specific genes and proteins is thought to have the properties of the sought-after marker/prognosticator, nine are possible candidates, and an additional eight are under preliminary investigation (Edited 1999). We estimate that it may be possible that one of these compounds will prove valuable and will also pass the test of time and clinical practice.

A second round of technological advances took place in radiology with the ability to make slice images. The first announcement on renal *ultrasonography* took place in 1969 (Grayhack 1969). By 1973 it became apparent that ultrasonography may differentiate renal masses from cysts and ultrasonography-guided punctures of renal mass were also reported (Grayhack 1973). In 1974, 5 years after the proof of the concept by Hounsfield (Hounsfield 1980), Pickering reported his results with *computerized tomography* (CT) on 10 excised kidneys (Pickering *et al.* 1974). In an editorial comment on this report J.T. Grayhack (1976) wrote: '…this exciting noninvasive technique seems likely to revolutionize our diagnostic efforts.'

And, indeed, in 1980 the yield of cyst aspiration and contrast injection started to be questioned (Gillenwater and Howards 1980) and abandoned as a routine procedure (Amis *et al.* 1987). In 1981 ultrasonography and CT were recognized as precise tools for imaging renal masses and cysts, competing with and even surpassing the yield of angiography in staging RCC (Gillenwater and Howards 1981). During the 1980s, although intravenous digital subtraction angiography was available from 1986 onwards (Gillenwater and Howards 1986), the indications for angiography shrank rapidly because of the use of slice imaging, which has proved to be by far the more accurate, less invasive, and more cost-effective method. The last member to join the slice-imaging family was *nuclear magnetic resonance* introduced in the late 1980s and popularized during the 1990s as a staging technique for RCC (Choyke 1988; Hricak *et al.* 1988). It has the advantage of multiplanar imaging capability. The effects of slice imaging on RCC prognosis were striking since more asymptomatic patients were diagnosed incidentally with a lower stage disease. *Incidental RCC* are found in 0.3 per cent of CT scans performed and 2 per cent of autopsies (Hellsten *et al.* 1990). In current series, 30–61 per cent of RCC are discovered incidentally (Jayson and Sanders 1998). Between 1973 and 1975, only 13–15 per cent of tumors were discovered incidentally (Konnak and Grossman 1985; Ritchie and de Kernion 1988). This had an immediate impact on the size of tumor diagnosed: In the 1980s the number of tumors with a diameter less than 3 cm resected was fivefold larger than in the 1970s (Smith *et al.* 1989) so that the average tumor size decreased from 6.9 cm. before 1985 to 3.5 cm. after 1985 with a local recurrence rate of 2 per cent and a 95 per cent overall survival rate. Obviously, the resulting improved prognosis (Fig. 1.2) seen over time was partly attributed to early detection (Thompson and Peek 1988). However it is wrong to believe that incidental finding of RCC is a phenomenon unique to the last decade of the twentieth century. Bottiger *et al.* in a study on 4563 autopsies defined and set the theoretical grounds for incidental findings of RCC. They found 89 cases of RCC, of which 53 per cent were not expected and in which RCC was not the main clinical diagnosis (Grayhack 1965). Reports of RCC series diagnosed using IVP as a result of work-ups for stone disease and benign prostate hyperplasia (BPH) started to accumulate in the early 1960s (Plaine and Hinman 1965), whereas case reports were present even earlier. As opposed to the slice-imaging era, these reports were anecdotal and did not influence epidemiology or survival.

Future prospects in imaging are exciting. The increased reliance on non-contrast *helical CT* in the diagnosis of acute flank pain (Smith *et al.* 1996; Bove *et al.* 1999) may further increase the number of diagnosed renal tumors. Currently, it seems that slice images have not reached their maximum potential in the field of renal tumors. It has become evident that the images obtained contain a tremendous amount of anatomical information that has only recently been processed and that may be attained by sophisticated image analysis using powerful processors and software capable of three-dimensional reconstructions. These technologies create precise images of parenchymal and hollow organs as seen from their exterior as well as from the interior and also include images of the internal blood supply of normal as well as malignant tissues (Takebayashi *et al.* 2000). Another modality expected to benefit the diagnosis of patients with renal tumors in the future is metabolic imaging. Examples of this are *positron emission tomography* (PET), combining anatomical localization with biochemical radiotracers such as F-18 fluorodeoxyglucose (FTG) designed to detect altered metabolic tissues (Hoh *et al.* 1998), and *immunoscintography* permitting visualization of RCC by using a monoclonal antibody to G250 linked to technetium (^{99m}Tc) (Oosterwijk and Debruyne 1995). PET scanning holds a particularly exciting future as it may be possible with more advanced tracers to detect more informative molecules, for example, DNA sequences inserted into tumor cells by gene therapy and other novel markers of genetic damage, and to integrate the PET images obtained with anatomical images. Given the rapid progress in the past, it is clear that a future technology will be able to further improve the accuracy of detection non-invasively though it remains to be seen whether screening will become a reality.

Nephron-sparing surgery, the golden decade of endourology and minimally invasive medicine

As a result of the developments leading to earlier diagnosis and the feasibility of minimally invasive surgery, fundamental questions are being asked concerning the surgical management of

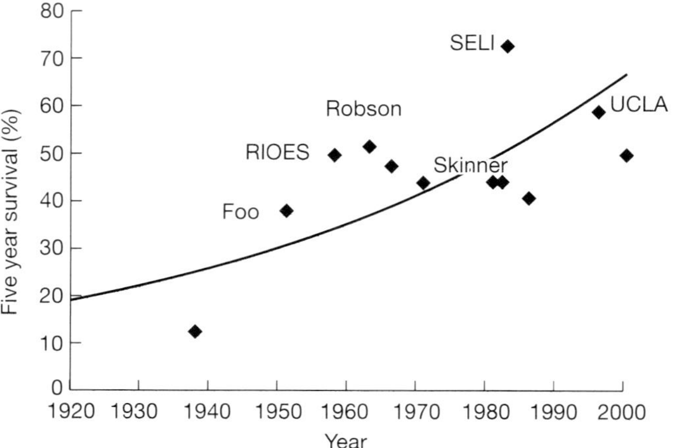

Fig. 1.2 Report of 5 year survival rates of patients with RCC.

RCC: What is the role of partial nephrectomy in the presence of contralateral normal kidney? Is it the best cancer operation? Is there scientific proof that it provides a biological advantage for the patient, apart from the intuitive notion that two is better than one? If all the answers are 'yes', then is ablative surgery equivalent to partial nephrectomy? What are the indications and limitation for minimally invasive surgery, namely, laparoscopic nephrectomy? The chapters dealing with nephron-sparing procedures, laparoscopy, and investigational therapies such as cryosurgery and high-intensity focused ultrasound therapy will provide some specific answers to these unsettled issues, but historical perspective may also contribute to the clarification of the pros and cons of these advances.

The role of partial nephrectomy and partial-nephrectomy-like treatments in patients with contralateral normal kidney is currently being examined after almost 4 decades of performing mainly radical nephrectomy. For historical integrity it should be mentioned that nephron-sparing surgery for renal tumors dates from the late 1800s. Czerny in 1887 was the first to perform a partial nephrectomy for a renal tumor (Herczel 1980). Significant rates of renal bleeding, fistulas, leaks, and postoperative death were the major causes for it being abandoned as a therapy for renal cancer in the presence of normal contralateral kidney (Novick, 1987). Moreover, the alternative was more appealing and logical. The radical approach described by Robson seemed to provide patients with a better cure. Furthermore, alarming data concerning the multicentric nature of RCC (Mukamel *et al.* 1988) further emphasized the advantage of the radical approach. In 1950 partial nephrectomy was revived by Vermooten (1950) for special indications. Ballanger (1962) from France reported on partial nephrectomy (PNx) for cancer in solitary renal units with fairly good survival when compared to radiation therapy. At that time the author claimed to find only 12 similar cases in the literature. It seems that at least some of the cases that had an absolute indication for PNx as we recognize it today were given radiation therapy during the first 50 years of the twentieth century. Since its revival in the 1950s the utilization of PNx has been conservative and it has been carried out with extreme caution when compelling factors prevented the performance of radical nephrectomy. Seen from a historical perspective it is obvious that the limited experience gained with partial nephrectomies for RCC in solitary kidneys and bilateral tumors (Novick *et al.* 1977) provided a justification for the wider application of PNx in the face of normal contralateral kidney 3–4 decades later. At this stage progress in early diagnosis meant that sufficiently early disease stage cases could be diagnosed. Early detection had a substantial impact on the disease biology since the percentage of patients having satellite tumors was reduced dramatically in comparison to studies in the early-1990s. As a consequence, in practice the percentage of partial nephrectomies in the US rose from 8 per cent between 1979 and 1984 to 20 per cent between 1984 and 1988, and 30 per cent between 1989 and1991 (Herr 1994). Drs deKernion and Howards (1995) summarized the situation in an editorial comment: 'We now know clearly and without doubt that renal tumors are multi-focal…however, it seems that these small tumors take many years to develop and thus far have not proven to have an impact on survival of patients with nephron-sparing surgery…at the present

time very small unifocal tumors that are easy to excise by wedge resection or partial nephrectomy can be so managed even when the opposite kidney is normal.'

These trends were followed by urologists and today performing nephron-sparing surgery in the presence of a normal contralateral kidney has become common practice for lesions smaller than 3–4 cm. Performing a radical nephrectomy for solitary small lesions has begun to be regarded as overtreatment as there are now phase II studies that suggest equal survival rates for radical nephrectomy and nephron-sparing surgery in patients with masses less than 3 cm in diameter. UCLA experience also shows that nephron-sparing surgery provides patients with the same prognosis as radical nephrectomy, provided that patients with small and low-grade tumors are chosen (Belldegrun *et al.* 1999). Nevertheless, the reported complication rate for partial nephrectomy is 30 per cent. Its performance mandates a generous flank incision and it is claimed that it is associated with a substantial morbidity during convalescence. Moreover, the lack of objective criteria for defining normal tissue margin during partial nephrectomy results in some cases in surgical margins being positive, forcing a subsequent nephrectomy. The incidence of such cases seems to be operator-dependent.

The same logic as that used to justify partial nephrectomy has led to the first reports of attempts to ablate renal tumors by *in situ* freezing using cryosurgical probes in humans (Onik *et al.* 1993; Uchida *et al.* 1995) and high-intensity focused ultrasound in an animal model (Watkin *et al.* 1997). Substituting partial nephrectomy with real-time monitored ablative procedures is appealing. As these can be done laparoscopically or percutaneously, one may not only reduce the associated morbidity but also make the procedure more accurate oncologically. Today there is a window of opportunity for technology-driven minimally invasive surgery in the increasing proportion of patients who are diagnosed with low-stage tumors. There remains, however, a need for meticulous patient selection to ensure the success of these procedures. It may be that urologists practising today will in the future see further developments so that outpatient ablative surgery can be applied extracorporeally to a microscopic tumor deposit depicted by a non-invasive form of molecular trace imaging.

Nephrectomy, the urological cholecystectomy?

In 1980 Riabinski of Moscow used preoperative transperitoneal laparoscopy in 63 RCC patients in order to evaluate local extension of the tumor (Riabinski *et al.* 1980). It took 10 more years until the first laparoscopic nephrectomy (LapNx) was performed by Dr Ralph Clayman in a pig. One year later he performed the first LapNx in an 85-year-old woman and reported it in the *New England Journal of Medicine* and in *The Journal of Urology* (Clayman *et al.* 1991). A year later Dr Clayman reported on 16 more cases (Clayman *et al.* 1992). At the 1996 World Congress on Endourology and shock wave lithotripsy (SWL) in Melbourne, Australia, 53 cases of LapNx were reported and at the 1998 meeting over 350 cases. The technique has been rapidly mastered by urologists all over the world and its use is expanding rapidly. There is an increased interest in the technique and medium- and long-term follow-up data are starting to accumulate (McDougall *et al.* 1996). The 5-year disease-free rate has reached 91 per cent (Cadeddu *et al.* 1998). By combining laparoscopy and effective surface coagulation, argon beam lasers, harmonic scalpels, and advanced tissue glues may allow the combination of nephron-sparing surgery and minimally invasive urology. Nevertheless, questions concerning the dangers of trocar site implantation have not been answered and there are still concerns about the safety and applicability of renal biopsy before an ablative procedure.

From the legend of Saint Peregrine to combating metastasis with designer cells and molecules

The changing character of the disease has resulted in a striking dichotomy. While many patients are diagnosed and treated earlier for smaller tumors with improved survival, a small proportion of patients continue to present with advanced disease or disease that has progressed after a curative attempt. Chemotherapy has been available for urological use since the early 1960s (Scott 1962) but, despite significant progress in medical oncology, no substantial benefit has been shown to result from using chemotherapy in metastatic RCC patients (deKernion *et al.* 1979; Yagoda *et al.* 1993).

Reports on the spontaneous regression of RCC metastases after nephrectomy are well-known and have convinced clinicians and researchers that the cure of metastatic disease might be induced by pulling the right biological switch. This is a modern equivalent to the legend of Saint Peregrine. At the end of the thirteenth century Peregrine, a young priest, had developed a large bone tumor requiring amputation. On the night before surgery he prayed and he awoke the next morning with no evidence of disease. He died at the age of 80 in 1345 of an unrelated cause (Boyd 1966). William Boyd (1966) described 'The spontaneous regression of cancer, 22 cases of "hypernephroma" regressing, representing 17 per cent of the global experience with the phenomenon in cancer in general.' This was explained by theories associated with hormonal influence and immune modulation. Reports at a rate of 1–2 cases per year continued to be published (deKernion *et al.* 1979; Chalis and Stam 1990) and the incidence of spontaneous RCC regression was estimated to range between 0.3 and 7 per cent of cases (Papac 1996). The validity of the data and the correct definition of the phenomenon were continuously questioned (Kavoussi *et al.* 1986; Merz *et al.* 1993), but the most stimulating aspect of the debate was whether it is possible to induce spontaneous regression in a large number of patients. In 1974 the US National Cancer Institute sponsored a conference on spontaneous regression of cancer in which possible mechanisms were presented. It is possible that the first modern attempt to 'pull the switch' was that of Nairn *et al.* (1963) who tried to prepare a tumor vaccine by using microsomal fractions of renal carcinomas. Others, considering the regression phenomenon in terms of the immunological knowledge of those days and applying it to the

practices of surgical and interventional radiology, attempted the use of angioinfarction and delayed nephrectomy. This represented one of the earliest attempts to apply the concepts of immunotherapy to RCC by exposing the immune system to degraded epitopes of RCC.

Renal angioinfarction was first described in the early 1970s (Grayhack 1974). Many reports on results with renal embolization were available between 1970 and 1980. Angiography and embolization were used at that time to reduce operative blood loss but also to evoke an immune response in metastatic patients. Thus, it was believed that a delayed nephrectomy after the embolization might hinder some systemic advantage for those patients. However, the majority of authors found the procedure morbid with complete response in only 14 per cent of the patients and partial response in 10 per cent (Gillenwater and Howards 1982) leading Gillenwater and Howards (1986) to write in an editorial that, 'Renal infarction and delayed nephrectomy for metastatic renal cell cancer with activation of the immune system appeared attractive and seemed to meet with some success in early reports. Unfortunately, it does not work…'.

However immunotherapy as a concept was not abandoned. Morales and Eidinger (1976) reported objective improvement with intracutaneous injection of bacille Calmette–Guérin (BCG). Then, immunotherapy was given by mixing tumor lysate with BCG or *Candida albicans* preparations and injected intradermally within 1 month after surgery. Initially, results from Europe were striking: disappearance of lung metastases during immunotherapy was observed in five patients. In a larger series published a few years later and using the same approach, Tykka (1981) reported a 24 per cent 5-year survival rate as opposed to 4.3 per cent in untreated patients and a survival advantage of 15 months for the study group (Tykka *et al.* 1974).

In September 1976 Robert Gallo, Doris Morgan, and Frank Ruscetti reported in *Science* the discovery of T-cell growth factor, interleukin 2 (IL-2) (Morgan *et al.* 1976). Using IL-2 to mass-produce cells, Dr Steve Rosenberg was able to show that infusing the treated lymphocytes can destroy tumors in mice. In 1980 he found that incubating lymphocytes for 4 days with IL-2 would transform them into lymphokine-activated killer cells (LAK cells). The first clinical data with IL-2 was acquired. In 1982 Tada Taniguchi of Osaka, Japan, cloned the IL-2 gene (Taniguchi *et al.* 1983) and enabled mass production of IL-2. Large-scale clinical studies were launched, first with IL-2 alone and later with LAK cells (Belldegrun *et al.* 1988*b*). In 1986 Rosenberg *et al.* reported for the first time that tumor-infiltrating lymphocytes (TIL) are 50–100 times more potent than LAK cells in the mouse and are specific for the tumor from which they are extracted. These findings made the route for adoptive immune therapy possible (Belldegrun *et al.* 1988*a*, 1989*a*). In June 1989 the global oncological experience with adoptive immune therapy in general consisted of 650 patients of whom 20 per cent had responded to the therapy (Culliton 1989). In 1995 Dr Rosenberg's group summarized the results. Of 255 metastatic RCC patients receiving high-dose IL-2, 14 per cent had a partial response, 5 per cent a complete response, and 4 per cent died as a result of the therapy (Fyfe *et al.* 1995). The majority of the patients suffered major systemic side-effects (Belldegrun *et al.* 1987, 1989*b*). This produced strong criticism of IL-2-based immunotherapy (Moertel 1986) which resulted in clinical trials using lower-dose IL-2 given subcutaneously (Sleijfer *et al.* 1992).

Clinical trials using alpha-interferon (IFNα) alone and in combination with cytostatic drugs were carried on during the early 1980s (deKernion *et al.* 1983) in parallel with the IL-2-based approach. During the following decade, at least 43 clinical trials using different forms and preparations of IFN alone and 11 in combination with vinblastin were performed and reported (Figlin *et al.* 1985). IFN plus IL-2 regimens were introduced in 1989 at the National Cancer Institute (Rosenberg *et al.* 1989) and in the next 4 years at least 16 additional clinical trials were launched, using the combined regimens (Figlin *et al.* 1991, 1992, 1993; Belldegrun *et al.* 1993*b*; Wirth 1993).

While clinical experience in using IL-2-based therapies was expanding during the late 1980s and the 1990s, different fields of immunology and molecular biology continued to generate discoveries that were translated to clinical trials and expanded the number of therapeutic options for metastatic RCC patients. Therapies beyond immunotherapy in the narrow sense have started to immerge including tumor lysate pulsed dendritic cells plus IL-2 (UCLA clinical trial), antiangiogenic factors (anti-EGFr mAb; UCLA clinical trial), cancer vaccines containing IL-2 genes (Belldegrun *et al.* 1993*a*), and other cytokine genes and corrective gene therapies using the VHL gene and p53 gene in clinical trails. Molecule-based therapy is growing and diversifying.

The emergence of those therapies also contributes to clinical and ethical dilemmas.

● Does immune therapy as a paradigm for molecular based therapy really work?

It is not unusual to encounter criticism of immunotherapy based on low response rates, high toxicity, and, as yet, inability to cure a substantial proportion of metastatic patients. Reports on the 5-year survival rates of advanced RCC patients over the last decades (reviewed by Motzer *et al.* 1999) indicate that overall survival improved, mainly in the immunotherapy area: Motzer *et al.* showed a progressive rise in overall median survival rates for metastatic RCC treated with interferon-based immunotherapy from 4.2 months in 1975–80 to 13.2 months in 1991–96. According to UCLA experience there is also a significant survival advantage for patients receiving immune therapy and the percentage of patients alive 5 years after therapy exceeds by far previously reported survival rates of patients with advanced disease (manuscript in preparation).

● Is surgery for metastatic renal cell carcinoma justified?

Different authorities would give different answers during different periods. However, it is astounding to find out that the answer to this question has come full circle during the last century. In 1913 Guiteras believed that surgery is contraindicated in the face of metastasis. Later, some authors believed that, since surgery was the only solution for RCC and since there were some reports on spontaneous regression of metastasis after the resection of the primary tumor, it was justified to perform nephrectomy and then to extir-

pate or to irradiate the metastatic deposits. However, at the same time it was recognized by many physicians that there were patients too ill to be operated upon. With time it became apparent that this strategy is much more beneficial in patients with solitary metastases appearing 2 years or more after the resection of the primary tumor (deKernion *et al.* 1979). Then immunotherapy stepped on to the stage and asked the same question in a different context. First, the various adoptive therapies using tumor-infiltrating lymphocytes or tumor lysate required the resection of the primary tumor for the preparation of the remedies. Second, the high concentration of transforming growth factor beta (TGFβ) in the primary tumors is believed to pose a powerful inhibitory effect on the effector cells that do not allow the therapy to be effective in the primary tumor. In the mid-1980s some author could not demonstrate an advantage for nephrectomy plus IL-2 therapy over IL-2 therapy alone (Swanson *et al.* 1990). Others criticized nephrectomy in advanced RCC patients since, in some series, as many as 40 per cent of the patients did not meet the entry criteria for IL-2 treatment 6 weeks after debulking nephrectomy (Walther *et al.* 1983). Nephrectomy before IL-2 is currently supported by the UCLA experience showing that the prognosis for metastatic patients receiving nephrectomy and high-dose IL-2 is by far better than for those with high-dose IL-2 alone. Moreover, there is good reason to believe that their quality of life is well preserved for an extended period of time during the course of the disease (Litwin *et al.* 1997).

Adrenal tumors

Adrenal and renal tumors arise in close anatomical proximity and, therefore, for a long period of time were erroneously considered to originate from the same embryonic stem cells. Important and large chapters in physiology, pharmacology, internal medicine and

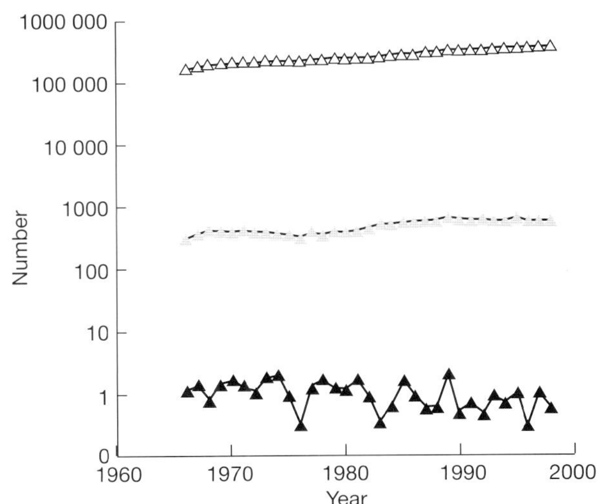

Fig. 1.3 Number of publications in ™MEDLINE: △ overall number of publications △ number of publications using key words 'Adrenal tumor', 'Andrenocortical carcinoma/tumor', and 'pheochromacytoma'. ▲ number of publications using the same key words in *The Journal of Urology*.

primary care, endocrinology, and nephrology are devoted to the art of suspecting and the science of detecting the various adrenal pathological states. Because of their familiarity with the retroperitoneum for more than 150 years, urologists were privileged to have the additional role of managing surgically malignant adrenal growths. These are malignant in the sense of having a metastatic potential as well as in the sense of life-threatening clinical manifestations. The evolution of adrenal surgery shares some similarities and influences with that of renal surgery. However, some aspects are unique.

Although adrenal tumors are relatively rare, the rise in the number of publications dealing with the subject has closely kept up with the global trend of increase in publication number (Fig. 1.3). One of the earliest anatomical considerations of the adrenal was published in the *Opuscula Anatomica* in 1563 (Eustachius 1563) and the partition to medulla and cortex was known at the beginning of the nineteenth century (Cuvier 1800–05). Addison (1855) observed that adrenal destruction in tuberculosis patients was associated with their death. One year later Brown-Sequard (1856) performed bilateral adrenalectomies in animals and concluded that the adrenals were essential for life.

Hyperfunction of the adrenal cortex was suspected by Cushing (1912) but the definite description of Cushing's syndrome was not reported until 1932 (Cushing 1932). Hartman *et al.* (1927) identified the adrenal cortex as the site of essential steroid production. Progressive and sequential advances in the understanding of adrenal steroid production have led to the development of precise diagnostic tests to identify patients with Cushing's syndrome (Orth 1995), adrenocortical forms of hypertension (Biglieri *et al.* 1990), congenital adrenal hyperplasia (New and Speiser 1989), and adrenal carcinoma (Vaughan and Carey 1989).

Medullary adrenal tumor was described by Frankel (1886). The London physiologists Oliver and Sharpey-Schafer (1895) demonstrated a pressor substance from the adrenal medulla, which they named adrenaline, later renamed 'epinephrine' by Abel and Crawford (1897). Kohn was the first to recognize the chromaffin system (Kohn 1902) and Pick (1912) formulated the term 'pheochromocytoma' to describe adrenal medullary tumors with their chromaffin reaction. From the Greek *phaios* means dark or dusty and *chroma* means color. An indication of the status of surgery for pheochromocytoma is given by an editorial comment by Dr JH Cunningham in the *1935 Year Book of Urology*:

The editor has had the opportunity to see Dr. Crile do several of these operations and observe some of the end-results. Aside from the technical surgical skill required and which may be mastered only by a small group of genito-urinary sergeons, the facilities and knowledge intelligently to study these patients prior to and after the operative procedure will limit its employment to a relatively few who have the advantage of expert biologists' and physiologists' assistance in this work. That this new field offers great benefit in the type of cases that it has already been applied to seems without question. It is a great step forward.

(Cunningham 1935*a*)

During the 1930s adrenal surgery became more feasible since replacement therapy from tissue extracts was available in some centers and postadrenalectomy death due to adrenal insufficiency became less frequent. From the description of Waltman Walters

and Edwin J Kepler from the Mayo clinic (Cunningham 1938*a*) it is obvious that the clinical picture of the various virilizing functional adrenal cortex tumors was well recognized and established. However diagnostic studies were cumbersome and sparse: 'Routine laboratory studies have been of little aid in differential diagnosis although a high content of estrogenic substance in the urine is suggestive of adrenal cortical carcinoma provided pregnancy is excluded. Injection of air about the gland has been of aid in localizing some of the adrenal tumors.'

MacKenzie and McEachern (1938) reported on a case of pheochromocytoma and could count no more than 20 cases of operations for pheochromocytoma. Of those, 15 had recovered and were free of attacks. By 1941, 103 reports on pheochromocytoma were available in the literature (Lowsley 1941*a*) and by 1944 enough surgical data was available to draw and publish the first notions on the limitations on anesthetics during anesthesia for pheochromocytoma patients (Lowsley 1944*a*). Four years later Dibenamine (phenoxybenzamine) was introduced for diagnostic and therapeutic purposes (Spear and Griswold 1948) and by 1950 the diagnostic value of increased urinary output of noradrenaline and adrenaline was recognized (Engel and von Euler 1950). These advances, combined with imaging, which allowed some anatomical localization of suprarenal masses by using air insufflation into the retroperitoneum (Scott 1957), gradually diminished the use of histamine and metacholyl tests, used to provoke acute attack in patients suspected to have pheochromocytoma (Scott 1954). During the 1970s and 1980s slice imaging revolutionized the clinical behavior of adrenal tumors (Stewart *et al.* 1978). Imaging techniques became highly accurate and essential (Markisz and Kazam 1989). Quite rapidly, most of the diagnosed masses were those that were incidentally depicted. Radionuclide tracing using cholesterol metabolic tracer analogs ([131]I-19-iodocholesterol) and catecholamine tracers (^{131}I-metaiodobenzylguanidine (MIBG)) (Sisson *et al.* 1981) were already available during the early 1980s and used for metastatic work-up and recurrence detection and follow-up. Belldegrun *et al.* (1986) presented one of the largest series of incidentally diagnosed adrenal tumors and, by correlating pathology and imaging properties, Belldegrun and colleagues laid the foundations for modern management of adrenal tumors. Magnetic resonance imaging (MRI) was tested for use with adrenal pathology in 1988, and contributed to the refinement of incidental adrenal tumor work-up guidelines. The development of precise urinary and plasma tests led to the accurate identification of patients with adrenal medullary disorders (Stein and Black 1991). The diagnosis of the major adrenal disorders is now actually simpler than in the past because of precise diagnostic assays and imaging. The evaluation of a patient for a potential adrenal disorder can be performed efficiently, usually without hospitalization, and the surgical approaches are well within the expertise of the urologist and are now precisely described (Libertino and Novick 1989; Scott *et al.* 1990d. As for renal tumors, the influence and advantages of laparoscopy led to increasing use of laparoscopic adrenalectomy instead of open procedures. Since 1991 laparoscopy has become the procedure of choice for the majority of adrenalectomies with open adrenalectomy reserved for the occasional patient with a large or locally invasive adrenal mass (Gill and Novick 1999).

References

Abel, J. and Crawford, A. (1897). On the blood-pressure raising constituent of the suprarenal capsule. *Johns Hopkins Hosp. Bull.* **8**, 151.

Addison, T. (1855). *On the constitutional and local effects of disease of the suprarenal capsule.* Samuel Highley, London.

Amador, E., Zimmerman, T., and Waker, W. (1963). Urinary alkaline phosphatase activity: I. Elevated urinary LDH and alkaline phosphatase activities for diagnosis of renal adenocarcinoma. *J. Am. Med. Assoc.* **185**, 769–75.

Amis, E., Cronan, J., and Pfister, R. (1987). Needle puncture of cystic renal masses: A survey of the Society of Uroradiology. *Am. J. Roentgenol.* **148**, 297–9.

Ballanger, R. (1962). Partial nephrectomy for cancer of the kidney. *J. Urol. Nephrol.* (*Paris*) **68**, 785–6.

Beahrs, O. and Myers, M. (1983). *American Joint Committee on Cancer: Manual for staging of cancer.* J.B. Lippincot, Philadelphia.

Bell, E. (1938). Classification of renal tumors with observations on frequency of various types. *J. Urol.* **39**, 238–43.

Belldegrun, A., Hussain, S., Seltzer, S., Loughlin, K., Gittes, R., and Richie, J. (1986). Incidentally discovered mass of the adrenal gland. *Surg. Gynecol. Obstet.* **163**, 203–8.

Belldegrun, A., Webb, D.E., Austin, H.A.D., Steinberg, S.M., White, D.E., Linehan, W.M., and Rosenberg, S.A. (1987). Effects of interleukin-2 on renal function in patients receiving immunotherapy for advanced cancer. *Ann. Intern. Med.* **106**, 817–22.

Belldegrun, A., Muul, L.M., and Rosenberg, S. (1988*a*). Interleukin 2 expanded tumor-infiltrating lymphocytes in human renal cell cancer: isolation, characterization, and antitumor activity. *Cancer Res.* **48**, 206–14.

Belldegrun, A., Uppenkamp, I., and Rosenberg, S.A. (1988*b*). Anti-tumor reactivity of human lymphokine activated killer (LAK). cells against fresh and cultured preparations of renal cell cancer. *J. Urol.* **139**, 150–5.

Belldegrun, A., Kasid, A., Uppenkamp, M., Topalian, S.L., and Rosenberg, S.A. (1989*a*). Human tumor infiltrating lymphocytes. Analysis of lymphokine mRNA expression and relevance to cancer immunotherapy. *J. Immunol.* **142**, 4520–6.

Belldegrun, A., Webb, D.E., Austin, H.A.D., Steinberg, S.M., Linehan, W.M., and Rosenberg, S.A. (1989*b*). Renal toxicity of interleukin-2 administration in patients with metastatic renal cell cancer: effect of pre-therapy nephrectomy. *J. Urol.* **141**, 499–503.

Belldegrun, A., Pierce, W., Kaboo, R., Tso, C.L., Shau, H., Turcillo, P., Moldawer, N., Golub, S., deKernion, J., and Figlin, R. (1993*a*). Interferon-alpha primed tumor-infiltrating lymphocytes combined with interleukin-2 and interferon-alpha as therapy for metastatic renal cell carcinoma. *J. Urol.* **150**, 1384–90.

Belldegrun, A., Tso, C.L., Sakata, T., Duckett, T., Brunda, M.J., Barsky, S.H., Chai, J., Kaboo, R., Lavey, R.S., McBride, W.H. *et al.* (1993*b*). Human renal carcinoma line transfected with interleukin-2 and/or interferon alpha gene(s): implications for live cancer vaccines. *J. Natl Cancer Inst.* **85**, 207–16.

Belldegrun, A., Tsui, K., deKernion, J.B., and Smith, R. (1999). Efficacy of nephron sparing surgery for renal cell carcinoma: analsyis based on the new 1997 tumor–node–metastasis system. *J. Clin. Oncol.* **17**, 2868–75.

Biglierie, E.G., Irony, I., Kater, C.E. Adrenocortical forms of human hypertension. In Laragh, J.H., Brenner, B.M., eds. (1990) *Hypertension: Pathology, Diagnosis and Management.* New York, Raven Press.

Bove, P., Kaplan, D., Dalrymple, N., Rosenfield, A., Verga, M., Anderson, K., and Smith, R. (1999). Reexamining the value of hematuria testing in patients with acute flank pain. *J. Urol.* **162**, 685–7.

Boyd, W. (1966). *The spontaneous regression of cancer.* Charles C. Thomas, Springfield, Illinois.

Brown-Sequard, C. (1856). Recherches experimentales sur la physiologie et la patholgie des capsules surrenales. *Arch. Gen. Med.* **2**, 385.

Burford, C., Glenn, J., and Burford, E. (1951). Evaluation of kidney cancer. *Missouri Med. Assoc.* **48**, 17–19.

Cadeddu, J., Ono, Y., Clayman, R., Barrett, P., Janetschek, G., Fentie, D., Mcdougall, E., Moore, R., Kinukawa, T., Elbahnasy, A., Nelson, J., and Kavoussi, L. (1998). Laparoscopic nephrectomy for renal cell cancer: evaluation of efficacy and safety: A multicenter experience. *Urology* **52**, 773–7.

Chalis, G. and Stam, H. (1990). The spontaneous regression of cancer. A review of cases from 1900 to 1987. *Acta Oncol.* **29**, 545–9.

Choyke, P. (1988). MR imaging in renal cell carcinoma. *Radiology* **169**, 572–3.

Clayman, R.V., Kavoussi, L.R., Soper, N.J., Dierks, S.M., Meretyk, S., Darcy, M.D., Roemer, F. D., Pingleton, E.D., Thomson, P.G., and Long, S.R. (1991). Laparoscopic nephrectomy: initial case report. *J. Urol.* **146**, 27–82.

Clayman, R., Kavoussi, L., McDougall, E., Soper, N., Figenshau, R., Chandhoke, P., and Albala, D. (1992). Laparoscopic nephrectomy: a review of 16 cases. *Surg. Laparosc. Endoscopy* **2**, 29–34.

Culliton, B.J. (1989). Fighting cancer with designer cells [news]. *Science* **244**, 1430–3.

Cunningham, J. (1932). The kidney and adrenal: tumors and cysts. *The practical medicine series of year books—Urology* 186–99.

Cunningham, J. (1935*a*). The adrenal. *1935 Year book of Urology* 196–206.

Cunningham, J. (1935*b*). The kidney: malignant tumors. *1935 Year book of Urology* 153–73.

Cunningham, J. (1938*a*). The adrenal. *1938 Year book of Urology* 202–7.

Cunningham, J. (1938*b*). The kidney: tumors. *1938 Year book of Urology* 167–92.

Cunningham, J. (1939). The kidney and adrenal: tumors and cysts. *1939 Year book of Urology* 148–65.

Cushing, H. (1912). *The pituitary body and its disorder: clinical states produced by disorders of the hypophysis cerebri.* J.B. Lippincott, Philadelphia.

Cushing, H. (1932). The basophil adenomas of the pituitary body and their clinical manifestation (pituitary basophilism). *Bull. John Hopkins Hosp.* **50**, 137–95.

Cuvier, G., Baron (1800–05). *Lec[,]ons d'anatomie comparée.* Paris.

deKernion, J. and Howards, S. (1995). *Renal neoplasms.* Mosby, St. Louis.

deKernion, J., Ramming, K., and Smith, R. (1979). Natural history of metastatic renal cell carcinoma: Computer analysis. *J. Urol.* **120**, 148–52.

deKernion, J.B., Sarna, G., Figlin, R., Lindner, A., and Smith, R.B. (1983). The treatment of renal cell carcinoma with human leukocyte alpha-interferon. *J. Urol.* **130**, 1063–6.

deKernion, J.B., Mukamel, E., Ritchie, A.W., Blyth, B., Hannah, J., and Bohman, R. (1989). Prognostic significance of the DNA content of renal carcinoma. *Cancer* **64**, 1669–73.

Dos Santos, R., Lamas, A., and Caldas, J. (1929). Aortography of the aorta and the abdominal blood vessels. *Bull. Mem. Soc. Nat. Chir.* **55**, 587–601.

Edited (1999). Kidney cancer—part II: Molecular markers, diagnosis, staging, prognosis and current treatment modalities. *Future Oncol.* **4**, 974–7.

Engel, A. and von Euler, U. (1950). Diagnostic value of increased urinary output of noradrenaline and adrenaline in pheochromocytoma. *Lancet* **2**, 387.

Eustachius, B. (1563). *Opuscula anatomica Venice vicentius luchinus.*

Evans, A. (1957). Renal cancer: translumbar arteriography for its recognition. *Radiology* **69**, 657–62.

Evans, J., Dubilier, W.J., and Monteith, J. (1954). Nephrotomography: a preliminary report. *Am. J. Roentgenol.* **71**, 213–23.

Figlin, R. A., deKernion, J. B., Maldazys, J. and Sarna, G. (1985). Treatment of renal cell carcinoma with alpha (human leukocyte) interferon and vinblastine in combination: a phase I–II trial. *Cancer Treat. Rep.* **69**, 263–7.

Figlin, R.A., Abi-Aad, A.S., Belldegrun, A., and deKernion, J.B. (1991). The role of interferon and interleukin-2 in the immunotherapeutic approach to renal cell carcinoma. *Sem. Oncol.* **18**, 102–7.

Figlin, R.A., Belldegrun, A., Moldawer, N., Zeffren, J., and deKernion, J. (1992). Concomitant administration of recombinant human interleukin-2 and recombinant interferon alfa-2A: an active outpatient regimen in metastatic renal cell carcinoma [see comments]. *J. Clin. Oncol.* **10**, 414–21.

Figlin, R.A., Pierce, W.C., and Belldegrun, A. (1993). Combination biologic therapy with interleukin-2 and interferon-alfa in the outpatient treatment of metastatic renal cell carcinoma. *Sem. Oncol.* **20**, 11–15.

Flocks, R.H., Kadesky, M.C. (1958). Malignant neoplasms of the kidney: an analysis of 353 patients followed five years or more. *J. Urol.* **79**, 196–201.

Foot, N., Humphreys, G., and Whitmore, W. (1951). Renal tumors: pathology and prognosis in 295 cases. *J. Urol.* **66**, 190–200.

Frankel, F. (1886). Ein Fall von doppelseitigen vollig latent verlaufenen Nebennierentumor und gleichseitigen Nephritis mit Veranderungen am Circulations—Apparat und Retinitis. *Arch. Patholog. Anat. Physiol. Klin. Med.* **8**, 103–25.

Fuhrman, S., Lasky, C., and Limas, C. (1982). Prognostic significance of morphologic parameters in renal cell carcinoma. *Am. J. Surg. Pathol.* **6**, 655–63.

Fyfe, G., Fisher, R., Rosenberg, S., Sznol, M., Parkinson, D., and Louie, A. (1995). Results of treatment of 225 patients with metastatic renal cell carcinoma who recieved high dose recombinant interleukin-2 therapy. *J. Clin. Oncol.* **13**, 688–96.

Gifford, R.R. (1973). Erastus B. Wolcott, M.D. *Invest. Urol.* **10**, 409–10.

Gill, I. and Novick, A. (1999). In *American Urological Association update series* (ed. T.J. Ball), Vol. XVIII, lesson 33, pp. 258–63. American Urological Association, Inc., Houston.

Gillenwater, J. and Howards, S. (1980). The kidney: tumors. *1980 Year Book Urol.* 133–6.

Gillenwater, J. and Howards, S. (1981). The kidney, hypertension and vascular disease: tumor. *1981 Year Book Urol.* 116–33.

Gillenwater, J. and Howards, S. (1982). The kidney: tumors. *1982 Year Book Urol.* 220–44.

Gillenwater, J. and Howards, S. (1986). Adult: renal neoplasms. *1986 Year Book Urol.* 87–92.

Gottesman, J., Perla, D., and Elson, J. (1932). Pathogenesis of hypernephroma. *Arch. Surg.* **24**, 722–51.

Grawitz, P. (1883). Die sogenannten Lipome der Niere. *Virch. Arch. Pathol. Anat.* **93**, 39.

Grayhack, J. (1964). The kidney: tumors. *Year Book Urol.* (*1963–64 Ser.*) 91–104.

Grayhack, J. (1965). The kidney: tumors. *Year Book Urol.* (*1964–65 Ser.*) 101–11.

Grayhack, J. (1966). The kidney: tumors. *Year Book Urol.* (*1965–66 Ser.*) 88–96.

Grayhack, J. (1969). The kidney: tumors. *1969 Year Book Urol.* 73–85.

Grayhack, J. (1973). The kidney: tumors. *1973 Year Book Urol.* 74–90.

Grayhack, J. (1974). The kidney: tumors. *1974 Year Book Urol.* 123–43.

Grayhack, J. (1976). *1976 Year Book Urol.* 167–82.

Gross, S. (1885). Nephrectomy: its indication and contraindications. *Am. J. Med. Sci.* **90**, 79–90.

Guinan, P., Sobin, L., Algaba, F., Badellino, F., Kameyama, S., MacLennan, G., and Novick, A. (1997). TNM staging of renal cell carcinoma. Union Internationale Contre le Cancer (UICC). and the American Joint Committee on Cancer (AJCC). *Cancer* **80**, 992–3.

Guiteras, R. (1913). In *Urology, the diseases of the urinary tract in men and women. A book for practitioners and students*, Vol. I, pp. 480–91. D. Appleton, New York.

Haitel, A., Wiener, H., Blaschitz, U., Marberger, M., and Susani, M. (1999). Biologic behavior of and p53 overexpression in multifocal renal cell carcinoma of clear cell type: an immunohistochemical study correlating grading, staging, and proliferation markers. *Cancer* **85**, 1593–8.

Hand, J. and Broders, A. (1932). Carcinoma of the kidney: the degree of malignancy in relation to factors bearing on prognosis. *J. Urol.* **28**, 199–216.

Harmen, P.E. (1978). *TNM classification of malignant tumours*. Union Internationale Contre le Cancer, Geneva.

Hartman, F., MacArthur, C., and Hartman, W. (1927). A substance which prolongs the life of adrenalectomized cats. *Proc. Soc. Exp. Biol. Med.* **25**, 69.

Hellsten, S., Johnsen, J., Berge, T., and Linell, F. (1990). Clinically unrecognized renal cell carcinoma. Diagnostic and pathological aspects. *Eur. Urol.* **18** (suppl. 2), 2–3.

Herczel, H. (1980). Uber Nierenextirpation beitr 2. *Klin. Chir.* **6**, 485.

Herr, H. (1994). Partial nephrectomy for incidental renal cell carcinoma. *Br. J. Urol.* **74**, 431–43.

Hoh, C., Seltzer, M., Franklin, J., de, K. J., Phelps, M., and Belldegrun, A. (1998). Positron emission tomography in urological oncology. *J. Urol.* **159**, 347–56.

Hounsfield, G. (1980). Computed medical imaging [Nobel Lecture Dec. 8, 1979]. *J. Comput. Assist. Tomogr.* **4**, 656–74.

Hricak, H., Thoeni, R., Carroll, P., Demas, B., Marotti, M., and Tanagho, E. (1988). Detection and staging of renal neoplasm: a reasessment of MR imaging. *Radiology* **166**, 643–9.

Jayson, M. and Sanders, H. (1998). Increased incidence of serendipitously discovered renal cell carcinoma. *Urology* **51**, 203–5.

Kavoussi, L., Levine, S., Kadmon, D., and Fair, W. (1986). Regression of metastatic renal cell carcinoma: a case report and literature review. *J. Urol.* **135**, 1005–7.

Kohn, A. (1902) Das chromaffin Gewebe. *Anat. entwicklungsgeschicte.* **12**, 253.

Konnak, J. and Grossman, H. (1985). Renal cell carcinoma as an incidental finding. *J. Urol.* **134**, 1094–6.

Kovacs, G., Akhtar, M., Beckwith, B.J., Bugert, P., Cooper, C.S., Delahunt, B., Eble, J.N., Fleming, S., Ljungberg, B., Medeiros, L.J., Moch, H., Reuter, V.E., Ritz, E., Roos, G., Schmidt, D., Srigley, J.R., Storkel, S., van den Berg, E., and Zbar, B. (1997). The Heidelberg classification of renal cell tumours [editorial]. *J. Pathol.* **183**, 131–3.

Kuster (1902). *Chirurgie der Niere*. Enke, Erlangen.

Libertino, J. and Novick, J. (1989). Adrenal surgery. *Urol. Clin. N. Am.* **16**, 417–606.

Lindblom, K. (1946). Percutaneous puncture of renal cysts and tumors. *Acta Radiol.* **27**, 68–72.

Litwin, M., Fine, J., Dorey, F., Figlin, R., and Belldegrun, A. (1997). Health related quality of life outcomes in patients treated for metastatic kidney cancer: a pilot study. *J. Urol.* **157**, 1608–12.

Ljungberg, B., Stenling, R., and Roos, G. (1986). DNA content and prognosis in renal cell carcinoma. A comparison between primary tumors and metastases. *Cancer*, **57**, 2346–50.

Lowsley, O. (1941*a*). The kidney and adrenal: the adrenal. *1941 Year Book Urol.* 177–9.

Lowsley, O. (1941*b*). The kidney and adrenal: tumors. *1941 Year Book Urol.* 154–68.

Lowsley, O. (1944*a*). The kidney and adrenal: adrenal. *1944 Year Book Urol.* 160–6.

Lowsley, O. (1944*b*). The kidney and adrenal: tumors. *1944 Year Book Urol.* 113–42.

Lowsley, O. (1949). The kidney and adrenal: tumors. *1949 Year Book Urol.* 151–64.

MacKenzie, D. and McEachern, D. (1938). Tumor of medulla of adrenal (adrenal pheochromocytoma) with removal and relief of paroxysmal hypertension. *J. Urol.* **40**, 467–76.

Markisz, J.A., Kazam, E. (1989). Magnetic resonance imaging of the adrenal glands. In Vaughan, E.D., Jr, Carey, R.M., eds. (1989). *Adrenal disorders*. New York, Thieme Medical publishers.

McCurdy, G. (1934). Renal neoplasms in childhood. *J. Pathol. Bact.* **39**, 623–33.

McDougall, E., Clayman, R., and Elashry, O. (1996). Laparoscopic radical nephrectomy for renal tumor: the Washington University experience. *J. Urol.* **155**, 1180–5.

Medeiros, L., Gelb, A., and LM., W. (1988). Renal cell carcinoma: prognostic significance of morphologic parameters in 121 cases. *Cancer* **61**, 1639–51.

Melicow, M.M. (1944). Classification of renal neoplasms. Clinical and pathological study based on 199 cases. *J. Urol.* **51**, 333–85.

Merz, V., Looser, C., Kraft, R., and Studer, U. (1993). Pseudoregression of pulmonary metastasis after nephrectomy for renal cell carcinoma. *Br. J. Urol.* **71**, 751–3.

Moertel, C. (1986). On lymphokines, cytokines, and breakthroughs [editorial]. *J. Am. Med. Assoc.* **256**, 3141.

Moll, F. and Rathert, P. (1999). The surgeon and his intention: Gustav Simon (1824–1876), his first planned nephrectomy and further contributions to urology. *World J. Urol.* **17**, 162–7.

Morales, A. and Eidinger, D. (1976). Bacille Calmette–Guérin in the treatment of adenocarcinoma of the kidney. *J. Urol.* **115**, 377–80.

Morgan, D., Ruscetti, F., and Gallo, R. (1976). Selective *in vitro* growth of T lymphocytes from normal human bone marrows. *Science* **193**, 1007–8.

Motzer, R., Mazumbar, M., Bacik, J., Berg, W., Amsterdam, A., and Ferrara, J. (1999). Survival and prognostic stratification of 670 patients with advanced renal cell carcinoma. *J. Clin. Oncol.* **17**, 2530–40.

Mukamel, E., Konichevsky, M., Engelstein, D., and Servadio, C. (1988). Incidental small renal tumors accompanying clinically overt renal carcinoma. *J. Urol.* **140**, 22–4.

Mulders, P., Figlin, R., deKernion, J. B., Wiltrout, R., Linehan, M., Parkinson, D., deWolf, W., and Belldegrun, A. (1997). Renal cell carcinoma: recent progress and future directions. *Cancer Res.* **57**.

Nairn, R., Phillip, J., Ghose, T., Proteous, I., and Fothergill, J. (1963). Production of a precipitin against renal cancer. *Br. Med. J.* **1**, 1702–4.

Nelson, O. (1942). Arteriography of abdominal organs by aortic injection: a preliminary report. *Surg. Gynecol. Obstet.* **74**, 655–62.

New, M. and Speiser, P. (1989). In *Adrenal disorders* (ed. E.J. Vaughan and R. Carey). Thieme Medical Publishers, New York.

Novick, A. (1987). Partial nephrectomy for renal cell carcinoma. *Urol. Clin. N. Am.* **14**, 419–33.

Novick, A., Stewart, B., Straffon, R., and Banowsky, L. (1977). Partial nephrectomy in treatment of renal adenocarcinoma. *J. Urol.* **118**, 932–6.

Oliver, G. and Sharpey-Schafer, E. (1895). The physiological effects of extracts on the suprarenal capsules. *J. Physiol.* (*London*) **18**, 230.

Onik, G., Reyes, G., Cohen, J., and Porterfield, B. (1993). Ultrasound characteristics of renal cryosurgery. *Urology* **42**, 212–15.

Oosterwijk, E. and Debruyne, F. (1995). Radiolabeled monoclonal antibody G250 in renal-cell carcinoma. *World J. Urol.* **13**, 186–90.

Orth, D. (1995). Cushing's syndrome. *New Engl. J. Med.* **332**, 791–803.

Osborne, E., Sutherland, C., Scholl, A., and Rowntree, L. (1923). Roentgenography of urinary tract during excretion of sodium iodide. *J. Am. Med. Assoc.* **95**, 1403–9.

Papac, R. (1996). Spontaneous regression of cancer. *Cancer Treat. Rev.* **22**, 395–423.

Pick, L. (1912). Das Ganglioma embryonale sympaticum. *Klin. Wochenschr.* **19**, 16.

Pickering, R., Hatery, R., Hartman, G., and Holly, K. (1974). Computed tomography of excised kidney. *Radiology* **113**, 643–7.

Plaine, L. and Hinman, F. J. (1965). Malignancy in asymptomatic renal masses. *J. Urol.* **94**, 342–7.

Priestley, J. and Walters, W. (1933). Opening of vena cava associated with nephrectomy: report of 4 successful cases. *Proc. Staff Meet., Mayo Clin.* **8**, 302–4.

Riabinski, V., Sotnikov, V., Iadgarov, I., and Erokhin, P. (1980). Laparoscopy in carcinoma of the kidney. *Urol. Nefrol.* (*Mosk.*) **5**, 29–34.

Ritchie, A. W. and deKernion, J. B. (1988). Incidental renal neoplasms: incidence in Los Angeles County, treatment and prognosis. *Prog Clin. Biol. Res.* **269**, 347–57.

Robin, C. (1885). Memoire sur l'épithélioma du rein et sur les minces filaments granuleux de tubes urinipares expulses avec les urines. *Gaz. d'Hôp.* **28**, 186–94.

Robson, C., Churchill, B., and Anderson, W. (1969). The results of radical nephrectomy for renal carcinoma. *J. Urol.* **101**, 297–301.

Rose, D. (1949) Early diagnosis of cancer of the kidney. *Surg. Clin. N. Am.* **29**, 1483–503.

Rosenberg, S., Lotze, M., Yang, J., Linehan, W., Seipp, C., Calabro, S., Karp, S., Sherry, R., Steinberg, S., and White, D. (1989). Combination therapy with interleukin-2 and alpha-interferon for the treatment of patients with advanced cancer. *J. Clin. Oncol.* **7**, 1863–74.

Scott, H.J., Van Way, C.I., Gray, G. and Sussman, C. (1990). In *Surgery of the adrenal gland* (ed. H. Scott). J.B. Lippincott, Philadelphia.

Scott, W. (1950). The kidney and adrenal: tumors. *1950 Year Book Urol.* 89–99.

Scott, W. (1951). The kidney and adrenal: tumors. *1951 Year Book Urol.* 81–94.

Scott, W. (1954). The adrenals. *Year Book Urol.* (*1953–54 Ser.*) 127–42.

Scott, W. (1957). The adrenals. *Year Book Urol.* (*1956–57 Ser.*) 145–63.

Scott, W. (1962). The kidney: tumors. *Year Book Urol.* (*1961–62 Ser.*) 90–102.

Simpson, G. (1934). Carcinoma of kidney. *Br. J. Surg.* **21**, 388–97.

Sisson, J., Frager, M., Valk, T., Gross, M., Swanson, D., Wieland, D., Tobes, M., Beierwaltes, W., and Thompson, N. (1981). Scintigraphy localization of pheochromocytoma. *New Engl. J. Med.* **305**, 12–17.

Sleijfer, D., Janssen, R., de Vries, E., Wilemse, P., and Mulder, N. (1992). Phase II study of subcutaneous interleukin-2 in unselected patients with advanced renal cell cancer on an outpatient basis. *J. Clin. Oncol.* **10**, 1119–23.

Smith, R., Verga, M., McCarthy, S., and Rosenfield, A. (1996). Diagnosis of acute flank pain: value of unenhanced helical CT. *Am. J. Roentgenol.* **166**, 97–101.

Smith, S., Bosniak, M., Megibow, A., Hulnick, D., Horii, S., and Raghavendra, B. (1989). Renal cell carcinoma: earlier discovery and increased detection. *Radiology* **170**, 699–703.

Spear, H. and Griswold, D. (1948). Use of dibenamine in pheochromocytoma, report of a case. *New Engl. J. Med.* **239**, 736–9.

Stein, P. and Black, H. (1991). A simplified diagnostic approach to pheochromocytoma. A review of the literature and report of one institution's experience. *Medicine* (*Baltimore*) **70**, 46–66.

Stewart, B., Bravo, E., Haaga, J., Meaney, T., and Tarazi, R. (1978). Localization of pheochromocytoma by computed tomography. *New Engl. J. Med.* **299**, 460–1.

Stoddard, C. (1862). Case of encephaloid disease of the kidney, removal, etc. *Philadelphia Med. Surg. Rep.* **7**, 126.

Swanson, D., Markowitz, A., and Wishnow, K.E.A. (1990). Primary biological therapy with delayed radical nephrectomy for patients with metastatic renal cell carcinoma [abstract]. *J. Urol.* **143**, 293A.

Takebayashi, S., Hosaka, M., Kubota, Y., Noguchi, K., Fukuda, M., Ishibashi, Y., Tomoda, T., and Matsubara, S. (2000). Computerized tomographic ureteroscopy for diagnosing ureteral tumor. *J. Urol.* **163**, 42–6.

Taniguchi, T., Matsui, H., Fujita, T., Takaoka, C., Kashima, N., Yoshimoto, R., and Hamuro, J. (1983). Structure and expression of a cloned cDNA for human interleukin-2. *Nature* **302**, 305–10.

Thompson, I. and Peek, M. (1988). Improvement in survival of patients with renal cell carcinoma—the role of the serendipitously detected tumor. *J. Urol.*, **140**, 487–90.

Tosi, P., Luzi, P., Baak, J., Miracco, C., Santopietro, R., Vindigni, C., Mattei, F., Acconcia, A., and Massai, M. (1986). Nuclear morphometry as an important prognostic factor in stage I renal cell carcinoma. *Cancer* **58**, 2512–18.

Tykka, H. (1981). Active specific immunotherapy with supportive measures in the treatment of advanced palliatively nephrectomised renal adenocarcinoma. A controlled clinical study. *Scand. J. Urol. Nephrol.* **63** (suppl.), 1–107.

Tykka, H., Hjelt, L., Oravisto, K., Turunen, M., and Tallberg, T. (1974). Disapprearance of lung metastases during immunotherapy in five patients suffering from renal carcinoma. *Scand. J. Respir. Dis.* **89** (suppl.), 123–34.

Uchida, M., Imaide, Y., Sugimoto, K., Uehara, H., and Watanabe, H. (1995). Percutaneous cryosurgery for renal tumours. *Br. J. Urol.* **75**, 132–6.

Vaughan, E. J. and Carey, R. (ed.) (1989). *Adrenal disorders*. Thieme Medical Publishers, New York.

Vermooten, V. (1950). Indications for conservative surgery in certain renal tumors: study based on the growth pattern of clear cell carcinoma. *J. Urol.* **64**, 200–8.

Voelcker, F. and von Lichtenberg, A. (1906). Pyelographie rontgenographie des Nierenbeckens nach Kollargolfullung. *Münch. Med. Wochenschr.* **53**, 105–6.

Walther, M., Alexander, R., Weiss, G., *et al.* (1983). Cytoreductive surgery prior to interleukin-2 based therapy in patients with metastatic renal cell carcinoma. *Urology* **42**, 250–8.

Watkin, N., Morris, S., Rivens, H., and ter Haar, G. (1997). High-intensity focused ultrasound ablation of the kidney in a large animal model. *J. Endourol.* **11**, 191–6.

Weir, R. (1884). Remarks on extirpation of the kidney with cases of nephrectomy for pyonephrosis and nephrectomy for rupture of the kidney. *NY Med. J.* **40**, 721–6.

Weyrauch, H., Wanless, H., Gobel, J., and Scott, K. (1952). Biopsy of kidney for suspected neoplasm. *J. Urol.* **67,** 60–85.

Whitmore, E. (1937). Nature of certain kidney tumors. *South. Med. J.* **30,** 1149–57.

Wilms, M. (1899). *Die Mischgeschwulste der Niere.* Arthur George, Leipzig.

Wirth, P. (1993). Immunotherapy for metastatic renal cell carcinoma. *Urol. Clin. N. Am.* **20,** 283–95.

Yagoda, A., Petrylak, D., and Thompson, S. (1993). Cytotoxic chemotherapy for advanced renal cell carcinoma. *Urol. Clin. N. Am.* **20,** 303–21.

Zisman, A., Pantuck, A.J., Dorey, F., *et al.* (2001). Improved prognostication of renal cell carcinoma using an integrated staging system. *J. Clin. Oncol.* **19,** 1649–57.

Zwarenstein, H. (1943). Simple specific test for occult blood in urine. *Clin. Proc. Cape Town Postgrad. Med. Assoc.* **2,** 125–9.

2. Renal and adrenal anatomy

John F. Redman and Graham F. Greene

The mental picture that emerges when the word anatomy appears in regard to the human anatomy is often that of pungent cadaveric body parts and monochromatic tones of brown. The anatomy as presented in this chapter should be thought of in the context of a living person in whom the vasculature is actually conveying blood and the nerves transmitting impulses and the organs moving with respiration or palpation. Structures easily visualized and understood when widely exposed in the laboratory can be maddeningly elusive when visualized through a limited incision. Further, the expected morphology becomes distorted and obscured by tumor growth, edema, hemorrhage, or inflammation. The knowledge of normal structures and especially relationships are therefore vital in interpreting images and performing surgery.

This chapter will describe the anatomy of the kidney and adrenal glands with coverage of organology, histology, and relationships.

Kidney

Gross anatomy

The kidney in the adult is a relatively large organ that resembles an elongated bean with a lateral convex surface and a medial concave surface (Fig. 2.1). The cranial and caudal aspects of the kidneys are referred to as the upper and lower poles, respectively. The surface of the kidney is smooth but may be normally slightly bosselated due to persistent fetal lobulations. The convex surface of the kidney particularly on the left side may be noted to have a curious gradual bulging in its midsection, which has been termed a dromedary hump. When viewed coronally the ventral surface of the kidney will be noted to have a convex curvature whereas the dorsal surface will be flat. Just ventral to the lateral or convex border of the kidney is a longitudinal depression termed the white line of Brodel (Fig. 2.2). Any other alterations of the surface should be ascribed to other causations such as scarring or tumor. The medial surface of the kidney is depressed in its midsection by an elongated oval opening, the renal hilum, which gives the renal arteries and the renal veins and collecting structures entry and egress to and from the hollow of the interior of the kidney, which is termed the renal sinus (Fig. 2.3). The renal lymphatics and innervation also pass through the renal hilum. The kidney's color is distinctive varying from maroon to purple. Its smooth glistening covering, the capsule, may appear gray when viewed obliquely.

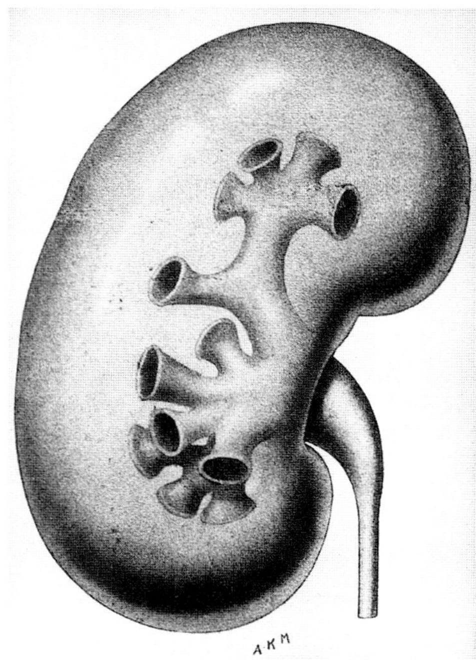

Fig. 2.1 Schematic drawing of right kidney showing contour of kidney and the relationship of the parenchyma to the renal collecting structures. Reproduced with permission from Glenister (1976, Fig. 537(A), p. 415).

Kidneys vary in weight from 90 to 220 g (mean, 150 g). Renal length is 9–15 cm, width 5–7 cm, and depth 3–4 cm.

When the kidney is sectioned longitudinally through the convex border it is quickly appreciated that the renal parenchyma is comprised of two distinct tissues (Fig. 2.3). The outer portion of the parenchyma is tan in coloration with granular appearing red stippling (the glomeruli) and is covered by a thin gray capsule that can be easily stripped from the parenchyma. The outer-parenchyma is referred to as the cortex. Regularly separated in the interior of the renal substance are maroon-colored pyramid-shaped regions of parenchyma collectedly termed the medulla. Each separate portion of the medulla is termed a renal pyramid. From the base of the pyramid to the medial tip the tissue appears to be linearly striped. The intervening tissue that separates each pyramid is a tongue-like extension of renal cortex termed a renal column (of Bertin). The rounded tip of each renal pyramid is referred to as a renal papilla. Although not distinctly separable as

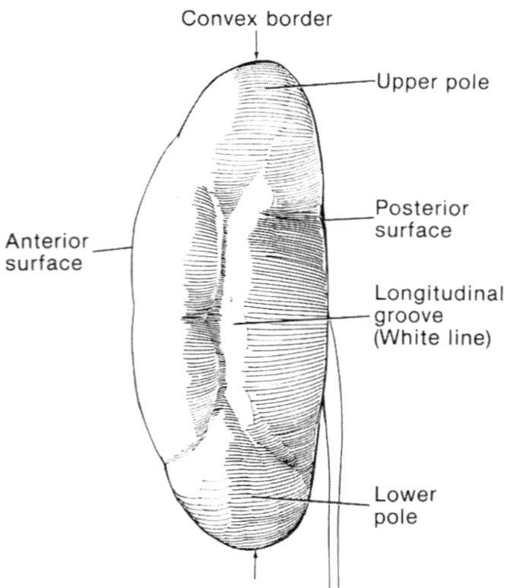

Fig. 2.2 Schematic drawing of kidney as viewed from its convex border or lateral aspect showing relative position of Brodel's white line. Reproduced with permission from Hinman (1993, Fig. 12.27A, Ch. 12, p. 265).

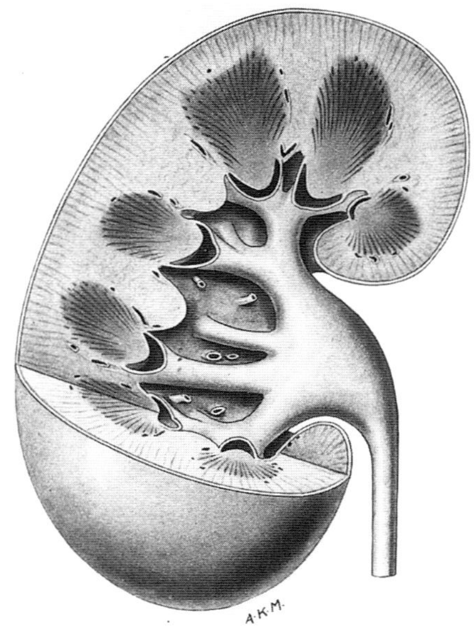

Fig. 2.3 Schematic drawing of kidney that has been cut away to show the hollow of the renal sinus and its relationship to the renal collecting structures. Note the two distinct tissues of the renal parenchyma. The light-colored peripheral cortex and the darker medulla (pyramids). The light-colored intervening tissue between the pyramids are the renal columns (of Bertin). Reproduced with permission from Glenister (1976, Fig. 537(B), p. 415).

such, the parenchyma (cortex and medulla) of the kidney drained by a single papilla is termed a renal lobe. The renal papillae and consequently their renal lobes number 5–18 per kidney.

On longitudinal section it is clearly seen that the kidney does appear to be hollowed out and that the renal capsule as a contiguous layer covers the renal sinus with the exception of the papillae. The renal sinus is filled with fat, vasculature, nerves, lymphatics, and the renal collecting structures.

Renal vasculature

It is an understatement to say that a kidney is a vascular organ. Indeed the kidneys receive one-fourth of the systemic cardiac output with each heartbeat. Without an understanding of the

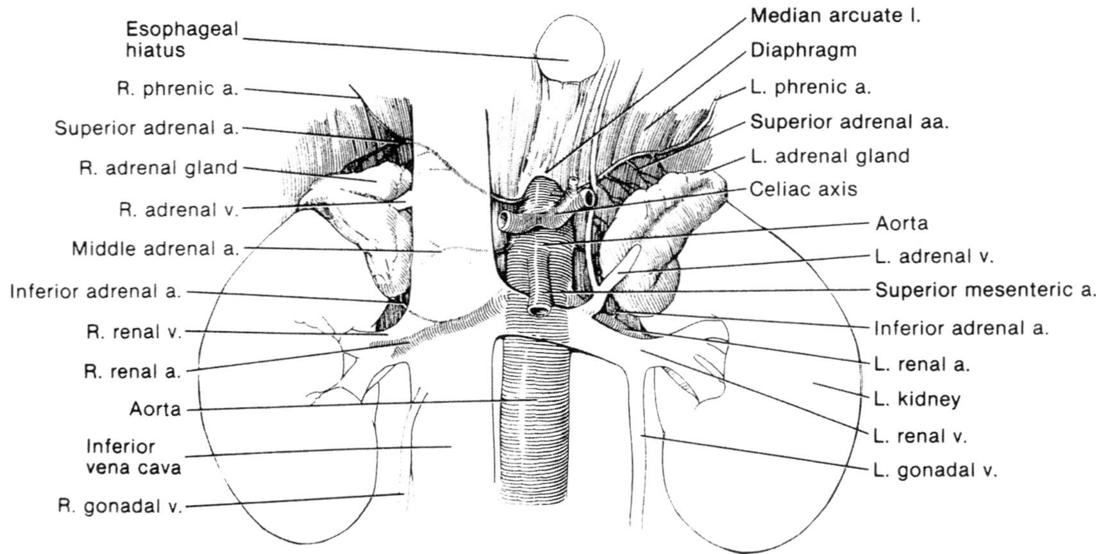

Fig. 2.4 Schematic drawing showing major vascular trunks of the upper abdomen. The renal and adrenal arteries pass dorsal to the large venous structures. Reproduced with permission from Hinman (1993, Fig. 12.49, Ch. 12, p. 290).

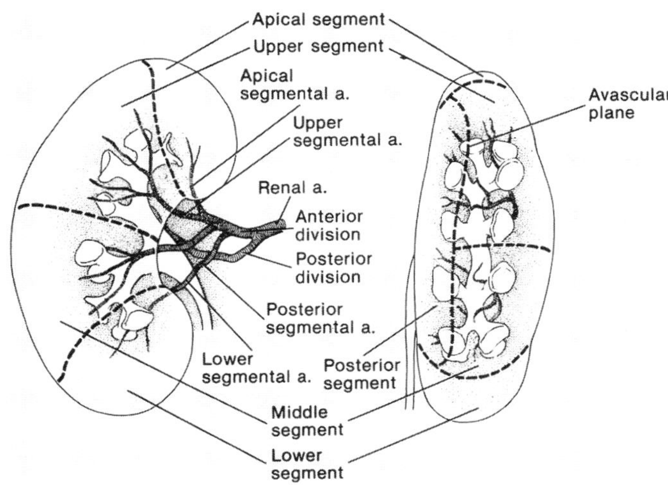

Fig. 2.5 Schematic drawing showing relative position of the anterior and posterior divisions of the renal artery, the segmental arteries, and the resultant renal segments. Reproduced with permission from Hinman (1993, Fig. 12.34A, B, Ch. 12, p. 273).

vasculature of the kidney there can be no understanding of the kidney. Generally, each kidney receives blood through a single artery and is drained by a single vein; however, many variations and anomalies occur.

Arteries

The renal arteries arise from the lateral aspects of the aorta usually opposite each other and just caudal to the origin of the superior mesenteric artery (Fig. 2.4). The right renal artery is longer than the left. *En route* to the kidney an inferior suprarenal artery is given off to course cranially to the adrenal gland. At almost any point between the renal artery's origin and the renal hilum, the main renal artery divides into two trunks termed anterior and posterior divisions (Fig. 2.5). Both divisions usually enter the hilum in its cranialmost aspect. Most commonly, the anterior division enters ventral to the renal pelvis and the posterior division over its dorsal aspect. The anterior division, almost without exception, divides into four segmental arteries: an apical, upper, middle, and lower. In addition to the renal artery *per se*, the kidney may be supplied with arteries, particularly to the poles of the kidney, termed accessory arteries or, as described by Graves, normal segmental arteries of precocious origin.

A general statement can be made about the renal arterial supply to the kidney: within the kidney the arteries are end-arteries with no collateral branches to adjacent segments. The portions of the kidney vascularized by the segmental arteries are termed the renal segments. The posterior division gives origin to the posterior segmental artery, which thus supplies the posterior renal segment. The posterior renal segment is the largest segment and occupies the dorsal portion of the kidney between the dorsal aspects of the apical and the lower segments. The posterior segmental artery courses over the dorsal aspect of the renal pelvis near the origin of the superior major calyx. It then turns and courses caudally giving off generally three groups of branches: upper, middle, and terminal.

The apical segmental artery may arise from the renal artery itself or from either the posterior or anterior division. The apical segment is the smallest segment, only a relatively small cap of tissue, which forms the superior apex of the kidney. In similar fashion the lower segment forms the apex of the lower pole of the kidney, but is considerably more substantial than the apical segment. The lower segmental artery arises from the anterior division and courses ventral to the renal pelvis dividing into an anterior and posterior branch. The posterior branch is a rather constant vessel and is found in close association with the origin of the inferior major calyx.

Although the segmental arterial distribution may result in well-defined renal segments as has been described, it should be stated that many variants exist such that, for instance, the posterior segment may be quite small with the posterior aspect of the kidney being vascularized by segmental branches deriving from the anterior division.

It will be noted on a transverse section of the kidney in its midsection, that is, between the apical and lower segments, that an essentially avascular plane exists between the distribution of the branches of the arteries of the anterior and posterior renal artery divisions. This plane is generally located 1–2 cm dorsal to the lateral or convex border of the kidney. The white line of Brodel, which can be identified running longitudinally just ventral to the convex border, does not represent the site of the avascular plane. Usually, the course of the segmental vessels within the substance

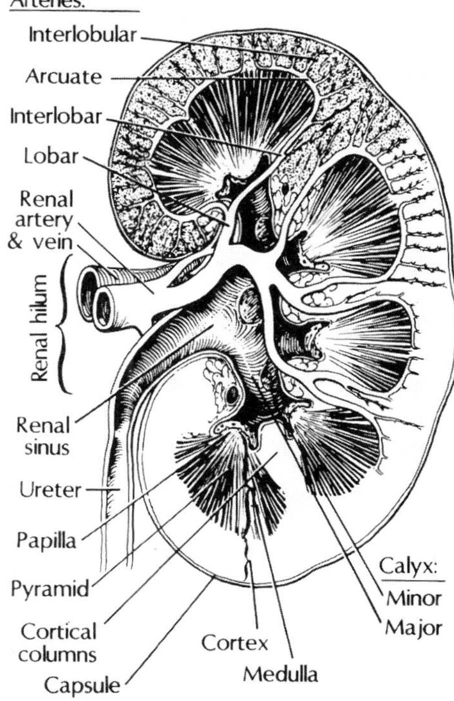

Fig. 2.6 Drawing of longitudinal section of kidney showing the relative spatial arrangements of segmental, interlobar and interlobular arteries in relation to the renal pyramids. Reproduced with permission from Redman (1996, Fig. 1.36, p. 25).

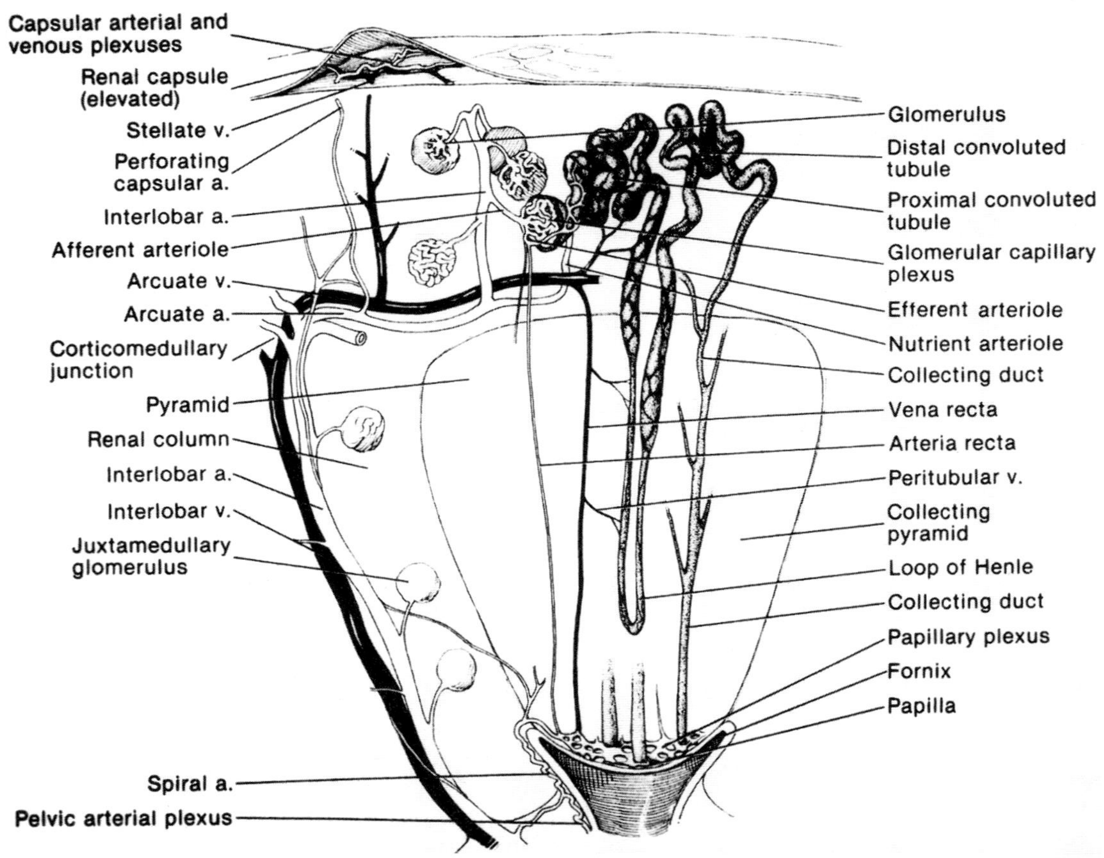

Fig. 2.7 Drawing showing relationships of interlobar and interlobular arteries, afferent anterioles, glomeruli, and vasa rectae to the renal pyramid and uriniferous tubule. Reproduced with permission from Hinman (1993, Fig. 12.35, Ch. 12, p. 275).

of the kidney is in a transverse direction and, accordingly, longitudinal incisions in the renal parenchyma would more likely result in cutting across major vasculature than those made in a transverse manner.

Intrarenal arterial distribution

Shortly before they approach the wall of the renal sinus the segmental arteries give origin to interlobar arteries, which enter the renal parenchyma alongside the minor calyces, that is, the apex of the papilla (Fig. 2.6). The interlobar arteries course alongside the medulla (renal pyramid) within the columns of Bertin and then around the base of the pyramids as arcuate arteries. Both the interlobar and arcuate arteries give origin to the fine vasculature of the renal cortex termed interlobular arteries. The interlobular arteries can terminate in several fashions (Fig. 2.7). Within the so-called inner zone of the renal cortex, that is, the juxtaglomerular cortex, the interlobular arteries can give rise to afferent arterioles to the glomeruli or give origin to vasculature to the papillae itself, the vasa rectae vera. Further, the efferent arterioles from juxtaglomerular glomeruli vascularize the papillae as vasa rectae spuriae. Efferent arterioles from the glomeruli located in the

periphery of the cortex terminate in capillaries in the outer portion or zone of the cortex.

Veins

The renal veins are large veins that drain into the lateral aspect of the inferior vena cava. Like the renal arteries the renal veins enter the renal hilum at its cranial aspect, usually ventral to the arteries. On the right side the renal vein is short, whereas it is long on the left side coursing ventral to the aorta to reach the left side of the vena cava. On the left side the renal vein is unique in that it is usually the site of drainage of three significant (nonrenal) veins. On its caudal and dorsal aspect, just lateral to the aorta, it receives a large lumbar vein, which, because of its location, may not be easily appreciated and can be easily cut across or lacerated. Just proximal to the left kidney, usually opposite each other, entering on the cranial and caudal aspects of the left renal vein, respectively, are the left adrenal and gonadal veins. The renal veins differ from the arteries in that multiple anastomotic channels ultimately form several large lobar veins, usually three, that join to form the renal vein within the renal sinus.

The kidney also has an extensive renal capsular drainage which communicates with peripheral stellate veins just under the capsule

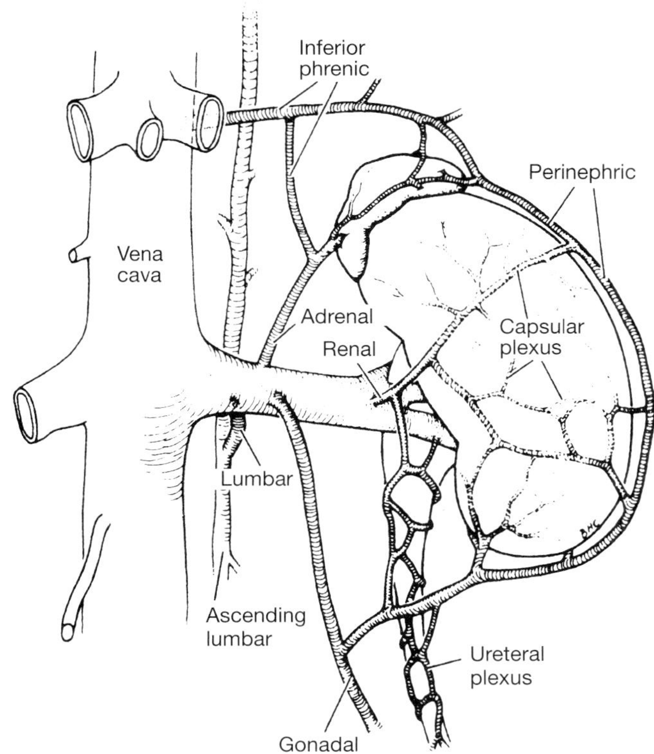

Fig. 2.8 Venous drainage of the kidney showing potentials for extensive collaterals. Note the inferior phrenic vein draining into the left adrenal vein and lumbar vein draining into the renal vein medial to the gonadal vein. Reproduced with permission from Kabalin (1998, Fig. 2.34, p. 78).

of the kidney (Fig. 2.8). The capsular veins communicate with veins in the perirenal fat and subsequently to the surrounding musculature as well as the adrenal, renal, and gonadal veins. With proximal obstruction of the renal vein, the capsular veins and their tributaries can be greatly and significantly enlarged.

Intrarenal vein distribution

The intrarenal venous distribution is not segmental but is characterized by small arcades of veins that course longitudinally through the substance of the kidney and that anastomose, at varying levels, with horizontally oriented venous arcades that parallel each other throughout the renal parenchyma. The longitudinal venous arcades join to form the venous trunks within the hilum which then conjoin to form one or more renal veins which join the vena cava. The key point of the arrangement is that there is free circulation throughout the renal venous system and therefore ligation of a vein does not hinder venous drainage of that portion of the kidney. Further, all but one of the larger renal veins draining each kidney may be ligated if necessary with impunity without impairing the overall renal venous drainage.

Lymphatics

Lymphatic drainage of the kidney begins in the lymphatic channels that course along the intrarenal vasculature beginning at the interlobular arteries, progressing centrally to ultimately form

4–5 relatively large lymphatic channels, which course over the main renal veins and arteries to chains of lymph nodes: on the left side, the left para-aortic nodes, and on the right side the right para-aortic or interaortocaval nodes. Lymphatic drainage is also to nodes located pre- and retrocavally and pre- and retroaortically (Fig. 2.9). Lymphatic drainage is ultimately to the cisterna chyli, which is located on the right side of the L1–L2 vertebral bodies, and then through the thoracic duct, which drains into the left subclavian vein. Lymphatic channels are also to be found perirenally and in the renal capsule. These lymphatics course over the surface of the kidney to drain to the renal hilar lymphatic chains.

Innervation

The innervation of the kidney is autonomic, which is mediated through the greater, lesser, and least thoracic splanchnic nerves through the celiac and aortorenal ganglia. Innervation is also through the second lumbar ganglia. The renal innervation itself is through renal nerves that course along the renal arteries to form the renal plexuses located on the ventral aspects of the renal arteries.

Histology

As stated the renal parenchyma consists of the renal cortex and the renal medulla. The renal cortex may be divided for histologic description into an outer and an inner zone. The inner zone is also termed the juxtamedullary cortex. Likewise, the renal medulla or pyramid may be divided into an outer and inner zone. The inner zone is the papilla. Further, the outer zone of the medulla may be described as having an outer and inner stripe. The renal parenchyma contains the uriniferous tubules (nephrons and collecting ducts), renal vasculature, lymphatics, and nerves with a supporting connective tissue.

The basic functional unit of the kidney is the nephron, which consists of the renal or Malpighian corpuscle and the renal tubules, which number approximately 2 million per kidney (Fig. 2.10). The renal corpuscle is comprised of a tuft of anastomosing capillaries termed the glomerulus, which is surrounded by the invaginated and enlarged blind end of the renal tubule termed Bowman's or the glomerular capsule. The capillary tuft is fed by an afferent arteriole and drained by an efferent arteriole. The capillaries themselves are formed of fenestrated endothelial cells overlain by a basement membrane that in turn is overlain by a complex pedicled epithelial cell termed a podocyte. Between the interdigitations of the podocytes are interstices called filtration slits. At the bases of the capillary tufts within the basement membrane are located mesangial cells, which support the endothelium. The glomerular capsule is lined by squamous epithelial cells with nuclei that bulge into the lumen of the space, termed the urinary space, between the podocytes and the capsule. The glomerular (Bowman's) capsule is contiguous with the proximal convoluted tubule.

The renal tubule is that portion of the nephron extending from the glomerular capsule to the collecting ducts. The intervening component parts of the nephron from proximal to distal are: the proximal tubule, which has a convoluted and straight part; the

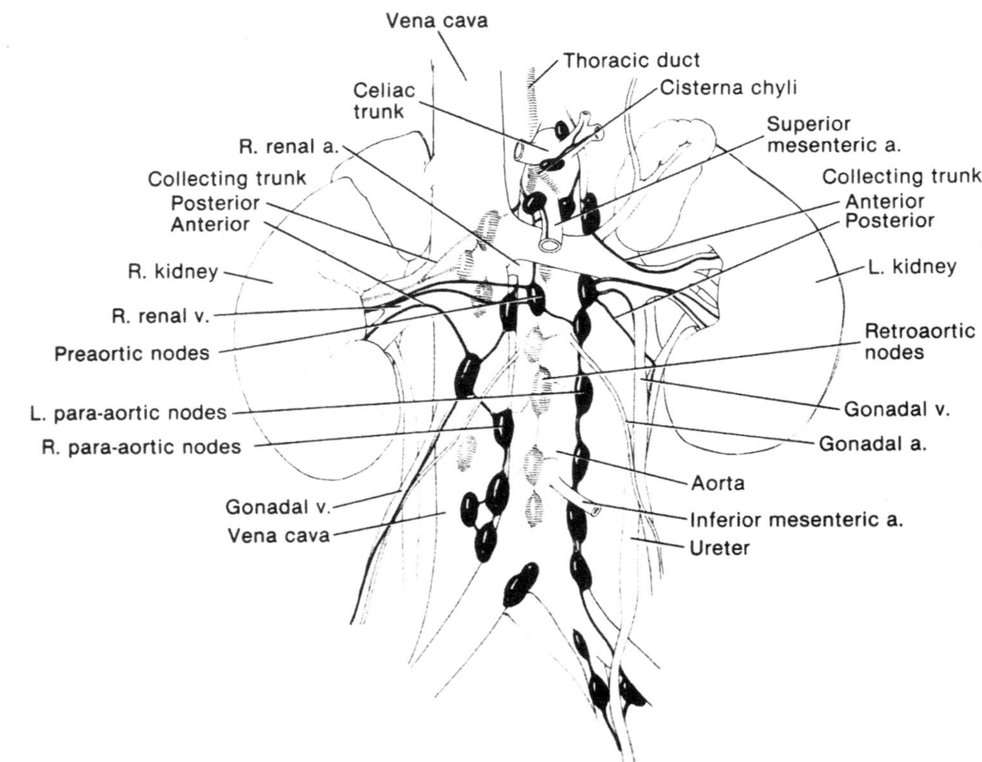

Fig. 2.9 Schematic drawing of renal lymphatic trunks and potential nodal drainage of renal lymphatics. Reproduced with permission from Hinman (1993, Fig. 12.41, Ch. 12, p. 282).

loop of Henle, which has a descending and an ascending limb; and the distal tubule, which has a straight and convoluted portion. Although the glomerular capsule is lined with squamous epithelial cells, the proximal tubule is lined with cuboidal epithelial cells with a brush border of microvilli. The lumen of the loop of Henle in its thick part is formed of cuboidal to squamous epithelium, while the thin segment is primarily lined with squamous epithelium. The distal tubule is lined with cuboidal epithelium largely devoid of microvilli. The collecting ducts, which ultimately drain to the ducts of Bellini at the tip of the papilla, are lined with cuboidal to columnar epithelium.

A unique grouping of cells is found at the junction of the afferent and efferent arterioles of the glomerular tuft and the distal convoluted tubules. This grouping of cells is known as a juxtaglomerular apparatus (Fig. 2.11). The cells are unique in the way they change as the afferent arteriole approaches the glomerular capsule. The smooth muscle cells of the arteriolar walls adjacent to the glomerular capsule assume a cuboidal epithelial appearance and contain granules; these are termed juxtaglomerular cells. In the portion of the distal convoluted tubule that lies adjacent to the glomerular hilum, the lining epithelial cells become greatly thickened and columnar on the side of the tubule adjacent to the glomerulus. This area of thickened epithelium is termed the macula densa. A cushion of cells, called lacis cells, fills the area between the juxtaglomerular cells and macula densa and are contiguous with the mesangial cells of the tuft.

To review the zones of the kidney and the structures that predominate in those areas: within the outer zone of the cortex will be found nephrons whose loops of Henle will be short, extending only into the outer zone of the medulla; within the inner zone of the cortex are juxtamedullary glomeruli whose Henle's loop will extend deep into the inner zone of the medulla (papilla); within the outer zone of the medulla will also be found dense capillary plexuses of vasa recta; and within the inner zone of the medulla will be found a less dense capillary plexus, but larger collecting ducts ultimately draining into the ducts of Bellini in the cribiform area of the papilla.

Renal collecting structures

Gross anatomy

The renal collecting structures from the tips of the papilla to the ureter consist of the calyces, infundibula, and renal pelvis (Fig. 2.12).

The tip of each papilla is covered by the proximal portion of the renal collecting structure termed a calyx, which by definition means cap (Fig. 2.12(a)). The calyx conforms to the papilla and thus assumes the configuration of a depressed ring. The periphery of the ring when viewed on coronal section forms an arch between the papilla and the renal columns of Bertin and is termed the

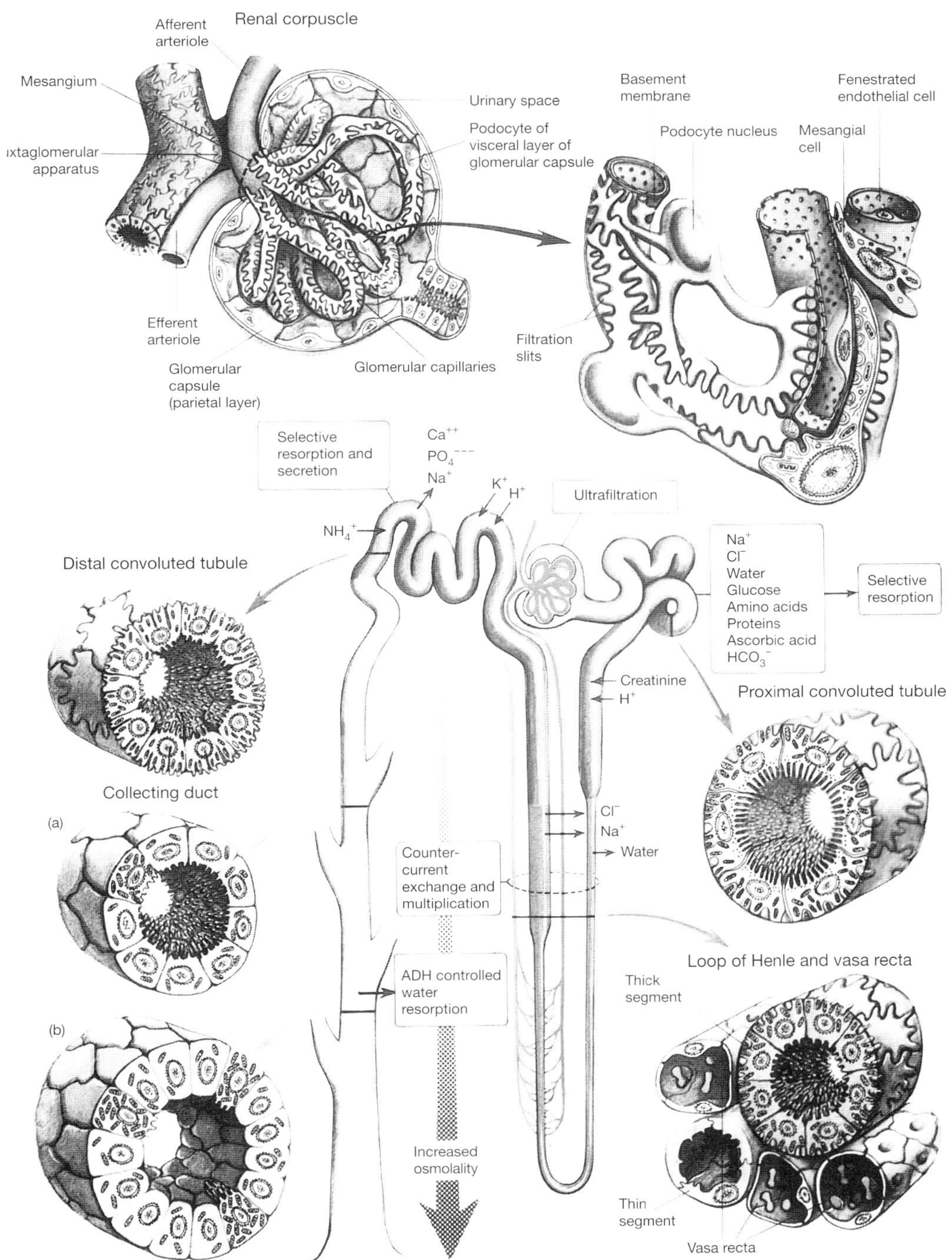

Fig. 2.10 Schematic drawing showing uriniferous tubule with detail of histology of its component parts. Reproduced with permission from Gray (1980, Fig. 8.152D, p. 1393).

fornix. The midmost part of the calyx covering the papilla is fenestrated with the entrances of the collecting ducts of Bellini and is termed the cribiform plate. If two papillae fuse, a compound papilla, and then drain into one large calyx, that calyx is termed a compound calyx (Fig. 2.12(a), (b)). However, if two papillae are closely aligned but separate, a so-called conjoined papilla, the receiving calyx would be termed a conjoined calyx and would be characterized by two distinct sets of circumferential fornices.

Calyces are connected to the rest of the renal collecting structures by short necks. The cup and the neck together are referred to as a minor calyx (Fig. 2.12(c)). Although the caliceal neck may join the renal pelvis directly, there generally is an intervening long

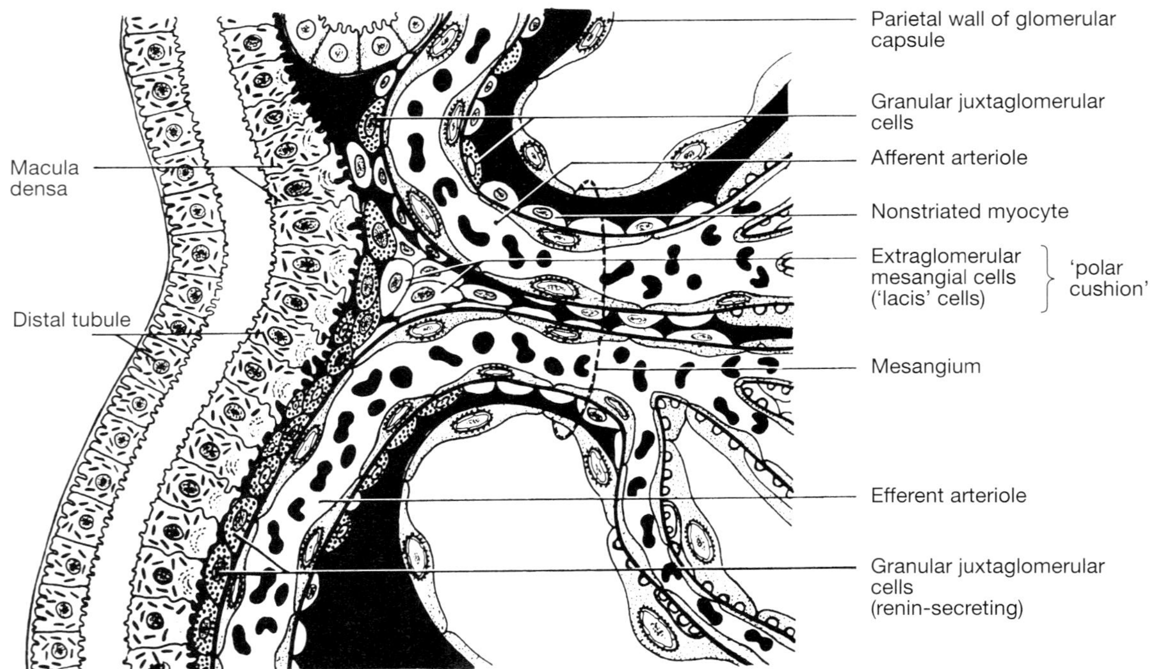

Fig. 2.11 Drawing showing detail of juxtaglomerular apparatus. Reproduced with permission from Gray (1980, Fig. 8.154, p. 1395).

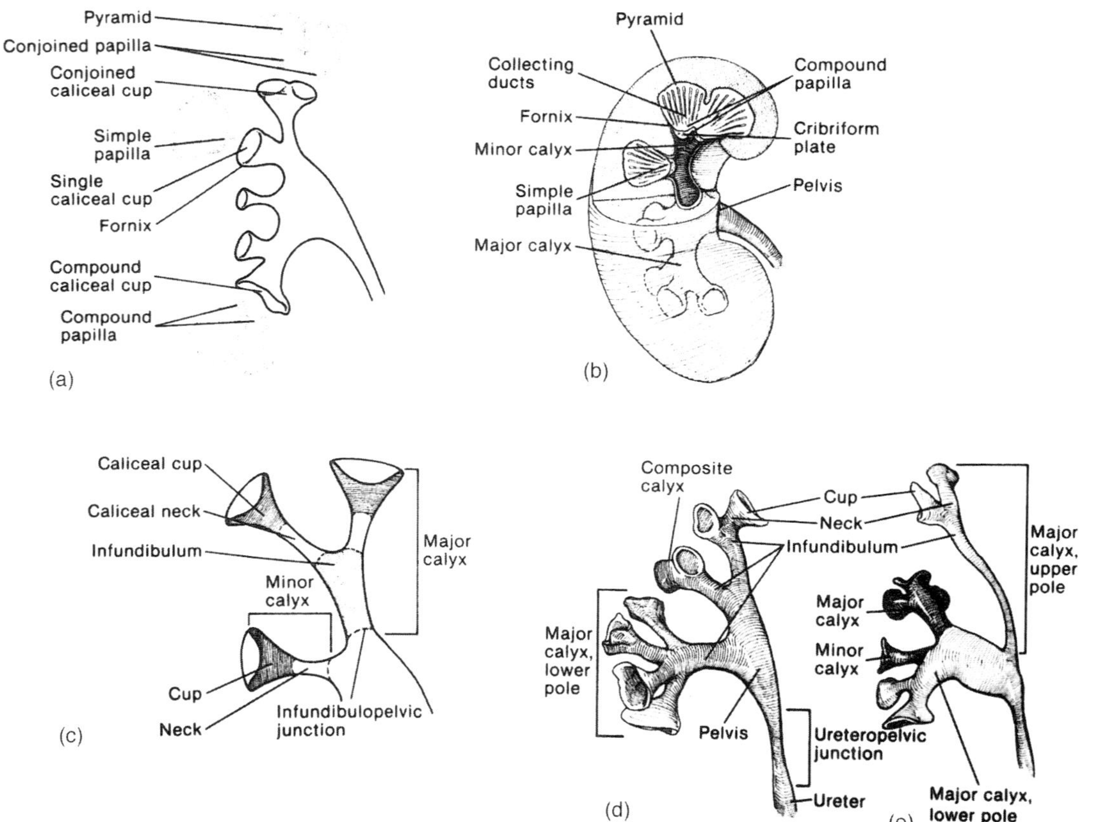

Fig. 2.12 (a) Drawing showing simple, conjoined, and compound papilla. (b) Drawing showing collecting structures in relation to the parenchyma. (c) Drawing showing characteristics of minor and major calyces. (d) and (e). Drawing showing various configurations of major calyces. Reproduced with permission from Hinman (1993, Fig. 12.28, Ch. 12, p. 266).

neck draining two or more calyces. This elongated neck is termed an infundibulum. The infundibulum and its connecting calyces is referred to as a major calyx. Generally, each kidney has 2–3 major calyces (Fig. 2.12(d) and (e)).

The calyces are usually found in two longitudinal rows and are described as anterior or posterior calyces, respectively, the calyces being separated in their orientation to each other by about 70° (75° on the right side and 60° on the left) in the midsection of the kidney.

There is considerable variation in renal pelves both in size and in their relation to the renal sinus. That is, the pelvis may be small and entirely situated within the sinus, therefore an intrarenal pelvis, or capacious, and located for the most part outside the renal sinus, and therefore an extrarenal pelvis. The juncture of the renal pelvis with the ureter is termed the ureteropelvic junction, which is normally funneled and dependent.

Vasculature

The renal pelvis *per se* is vascularized via a renal pelvic artery deriving from the renal artery or from its divisional arteries. The calyces and infundibula are supplied by interlobar arteries.

Lymphatics

The lymphatics draining from the renal calyces, infundibula, and renal pelvis generally join the lymphatics of the kidney (Fig. 2.9).

Innervation

Renal pelvic innervation is by autonomic nerves via the renal and aortic plexuses.

Histology

The renal pelvis and calyces are characterized histologically by three layers: an adventitia; a muscular coat; and mucosa. The muscular coat is comprised of two layers, an outer circular and an inner longitudinal layer, although these layers are not always clearly discernible as such. The mucosa or urothelium is composed of transitional epithelium, which overlies a fibroelastic subepithelial layer.

Adrenal

Gross anatomy

The adrenal or suprarenal glands are paired organs that, though quite similar in many ways, differ from left to right (Fig. 2.4). The color is distinctive and is often described as cadmium yellow, which contrasts sharply with the surrounding fat. The right adrenal gland is triangular in shape while the left adrenal is elongated and crescentic or palm-leaf shaped and slightly larger than the right. The weight varies between 4 and 8 g. Each gland has been described as having a medial head, a body, and a lateral tail. On sectioning the adrenal it will be noted that it is comprised of a cadmium yellow cortex overlying a maroon- or brown-colored medulla. The ventral surface of the gland is flat. In the midsec-

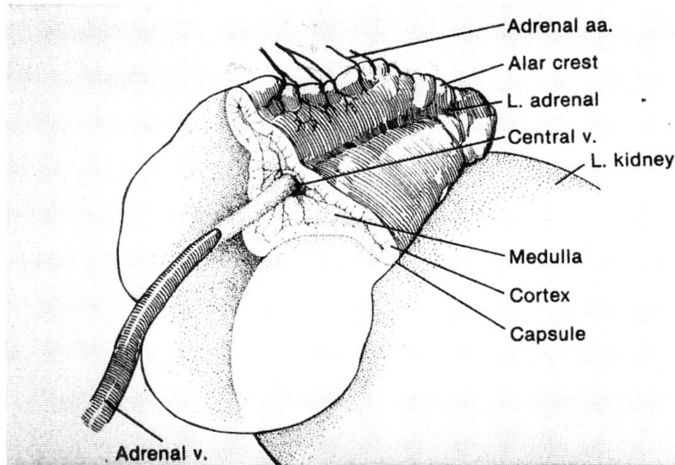

Fig. 2.13 Schematic drawing of left adrenal gland. Note triangular appearance of gland on cross-section with the ventral flattened base and thinned flattened edge, the ala. Reproduced with permission from Hinman (1993, Fig. 12.48, Ch. 12, p. 290).

tion, running the length of the gland ventrally, is a shallow depression, the anterior groove. It is from this groove that the central vein of the adrenal will be seen to emerge. On cross-section it is also apparent that the gland has a triangular appearance with flared flattened edges at its base, the base of the triangle being the ventral surface (Fig. 2.13). At the apex of the triangle is a ridge that runs the length of the gland dorsally, which is termed the alar crest. On the lateral sides of the gland the flared edges appear compressed the length of the gland, the edges being termed the ala.

Adrenal vasculature

Arteries

The adrenal gland has three primary sources of vasculature termed suprarenal arteries: the superior, middle, and inferior (Fig. 2.14). The superior suprarenal artery arises as a branch from the inferior phrenic artery, which arises from the ventrum of the aorta just caudal to the median arcuate ligament of the diaphragm. As the inferior phrenic arteries course over the cranial medial extent of the gland, multiple short arteries are given off to enter the adrenal cortex. The middle suprarenal artery is a relatively short artery on the left, but long on the right, which arises from the lateral aspect of the aorta at about the level of the origin of the celiac axis artery. Almost immediately it divides into multiple small branches that enter the gland on its caudomedial aspect. The inferior suprarenal artery arises from the renal artery and, running the extent of the caudal aspect of the gland, gives off multiple short arteries that enter the cortex. As the arteries approach the cortex, ultimately as many as 50–60 small branches may enter each gland.

Within the adrenal gland the artery forms a subcapsular plexus of arteries that within the zona glomerulosa gives rise to straight vessels that pass with few branches through the zona fasiculata to again form a rich plexus of vessels within the zona reticularis. Short vessels then enter from the plexus to the medulla to again

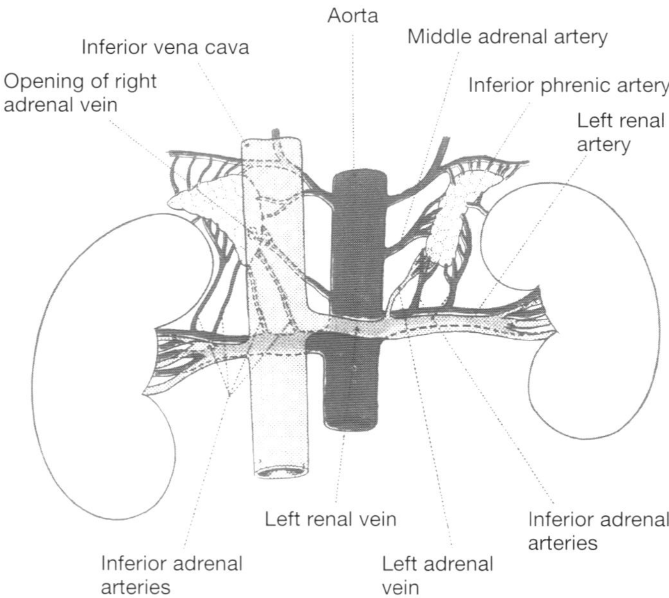

Fig. 2.14 Schematic drawing showing suprarenal vessels. Note position of medial aspect of the right adrenal gland dorsal to the inferior vena cava. Reproduced with permission from Coupland (1976, Fig. 628, p. 497).

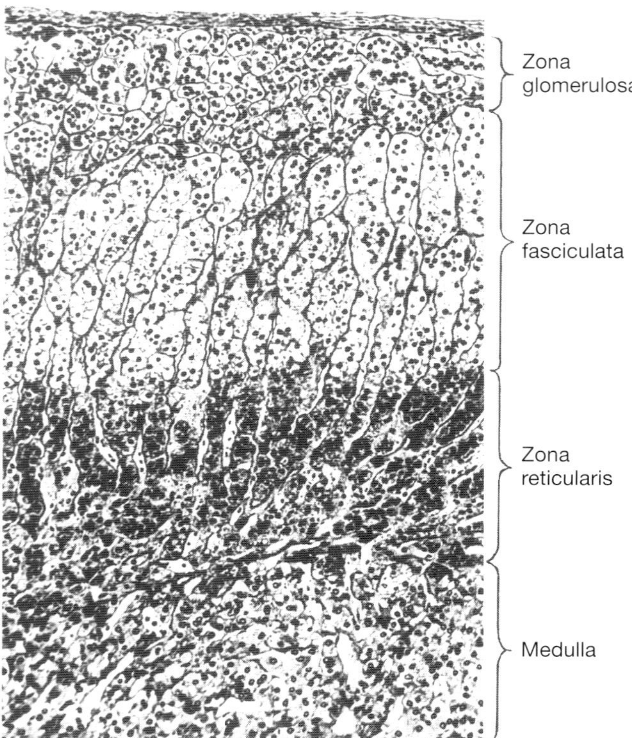

Fig. 2.15 High-power photomicrograph of adrenal gland showing the zonal configuration of the cortex. Reproduced with permission from Coupland (1976, Fig. 626, p. 496).

form a medullary plexus that drains to the central or medullary vein. From the capsular artery are also given off medullary arterioles that pass through the adrenal cortex directly to the medulla to form medullary capillary plexuses that drain then by venous sinuses to the central vein.

Veins
Medullary capillary plexuses drain into venous sinuses in the medulla, which then drain to a muscular central adrenal or suprarenal vein. A unique feature of the adrenal vein is a cuff that the adrenal cortical tissue forms by invaginating around the vein as it traverses the medulla. The cuff also surrounds the main tributaries of the vein.

On the right side the vein is short and drains directly into the vena cava on its dorsal lateral aspect. On the left side the vein is long and is joined by the inferior phrenic vein before joining the renal vein just opposite the left gonadal vein and just proximal to the hilum of the left kidney. It should be noted that the left phrenic vein also drains into the inferior vena cava just caudal to the diaphragm.

Lymphatics

The adrenal cortex is drained by lymphatics, which accompany the suprarenal arteries to drain to para-aortic nodes. The lymphatics of the adrenal cortex and medulla accompany the suprarenal veins as one or two trunks to the renal hilum to follow the renal lymphatics to the para-aortic lymph nodes (Fig. 2.9).

Innervation

The adrenal gland is richly innervated; however, innervation is only to the medulla and is autonomic. Sympathetic preganglionic fibers from the T10–L1 spinal cord via the greater splanchnic nerve and the celiac ganglia pass through the cortex to innervate the chromaffin cells of the adrenal medulla.

Histology

The adrenal cortex is divided histologically into three zones (Fig. 2.15). Just beneath the adrenal capsule there is a relatively thin zona glomerulosa, which is comprised of small polyhedral cells that form glomerular-like groupings or curved columns of cells. The intermediate layer of the cortex is the thick zona fasciculata in which large polyhedral cells form two-cell-layer thick columns that parallel the venous sinusoids. The innermost layer of cortex is the zona reticularis, which is comprised of round cells that form branching or anastomosing columns.

The adrenal medulla is comprised of chromaffin cells (pheochromocytes) that form groups of cells or columns arranged around the venous sinuses.

Renal and adrenal relationships

Equally as important as understanding the organs and their vasculature and innervation is appreciating their relationships within the body. For ease of understanding, the relationships of the adrenal gland, kidney, and renal collecting structures will be considered together beginning with the relationships of the adrenal gland to the kidney.

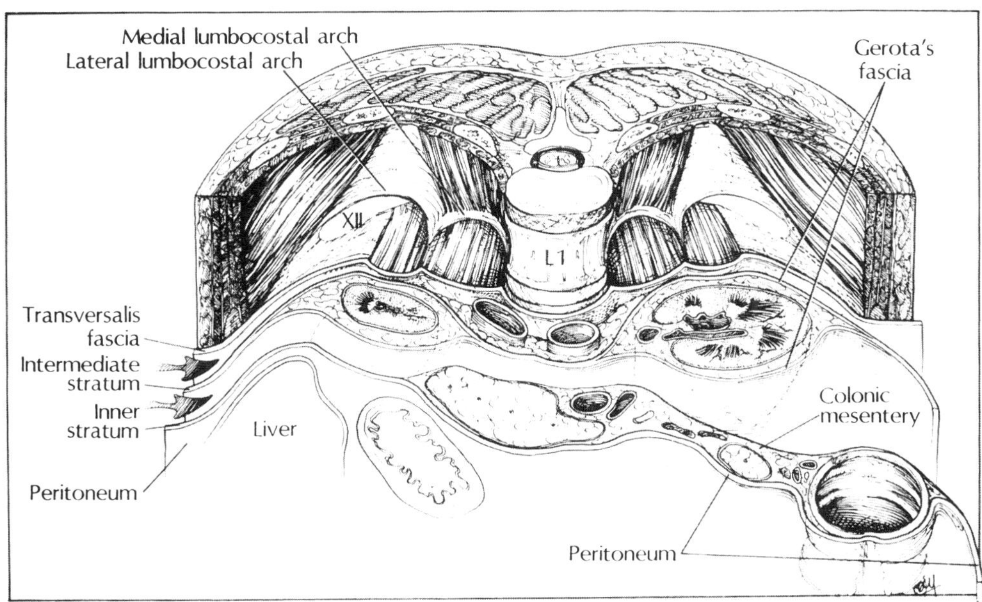

Fig. 2.16 Drawing of retroperitoneal connective tissue in relation to the dorsal body wall, kidneys, and abdominal viscera. Reproduced with permission from Redman (1996, Fig. 1.16, p. 13)

Relationships of the adrenal gland to the kidney

On the right side the adrenal gland is located decidedly cranial to the kidney and at times may be separate from the kidney itself, though there is usually contact with the medial and ventral aspects of the apical segments. In addition, a portion of the medial aspect of the gland may lie dorsal to the inferior vena cava. On the left side the adrenal gland is situated over the medial aspect of the kidney to such an extent that at times the adrenal may be intimately related to the capsule of the left kidney. Further, the head of the left adrenal may extend almost to the renal vein itself as it accompanies the course of the adrenal vein.

Retroperitoneal connective tissue relationships to the kidney and adrenal gland

Although in proximity to the body wall musculature dorsally and the abdominal viscera ventrally, it is generally accepted that the kidneys and adrenal glands are well encased and cushioned by an abundant quantity of fatty tissue supported by connective tissue. To clearly understand the fibrofatty retroperitoneal connective tissue of the upper abdomen it is helpful to consider the retroperitoneal connective tissue in terms of three strata: outer, inner, and intermediate (Fig. 2.16). The outer stratum is the transversalis fascia, which is contiguous over the musculature of the upper abdomen, that is, the transversus abdominis, quadratus lumborum, psoas major, and diaphragm. The inner stratum is the supporting connective tissue of the peritoneum and is a persistent layer in areas once covered developmentally by peritoneum, that is, the dorsal surface of the ascending and descending colon, duodenum, and pancreas. All the intervening fibrofatty tissue is the intermediate stratum. The intermediate stratum is characterized by specializations or condensations. In the upper retroperitoneum, the most evident specialization is the perirenal fascia

most commonly referred to as Gerota's fascia. As viewed sagittally, Gerota's fascia appears fusiform, tapering sharply cranial to the adrenal gland and caudally tapering sharply at the level of the iliac crest. Medially, the dorsal and ventral layers of the fascia fuse and cross ventrally over the great vessels to meld with the Gerota's fascia of the contralateral kidney. When no kidney has been present in the retroperitoneum, Gerota's fascia does not develop.

Between the renal capsule and Gerota's fascia is found fat, which is termed perirenal fat. The fatty layer surrounding the Gerota's fascia, particularly dorsally between the transversalis fascia and Gerota's fascia, is termed pararenal fat. Even in obese subjects the fat is scant ventral to the kidney.

Dorsal relationships of the kidney and adrenal glands

The kidneys and adrenal glands dorsally are in relation to the dorsal musculature of the upper abdomen (Fig. 2.17(a)). It should be remembered that the lower pole of the right kidney generally lies 1–2 cm caudal to the lower pole of the left kidney. Although there can be extreme variations, the longitudinal axes of the kidney usually extend from the T12 to L1 vertebral bodies. The cranial aspects of both kidneys and adrenal glands are overlain dorsally by the diaphragm. On the left side the upper one-third to one-half of the kidney may be overlain by the diaphragm, while on the right side the upper one-fourth to one-third of the kidney overlies the diaphragm. The portion of the kidney not overlain by the diaphragm is covered dorsally from lateral to medial by the dorsal aponeurosis of the transversus abdominis muscle and the quadratus lumborum and psoas major muscles, respectively.

Ventral relationships of the kidneys and adrenal glands

The ventral relationships of the kidneys and adrenal glands are to the abdominal viscera and peritoneum and as expected differ from right to left (Fig. 2.17(b)). The ventral surface of the right

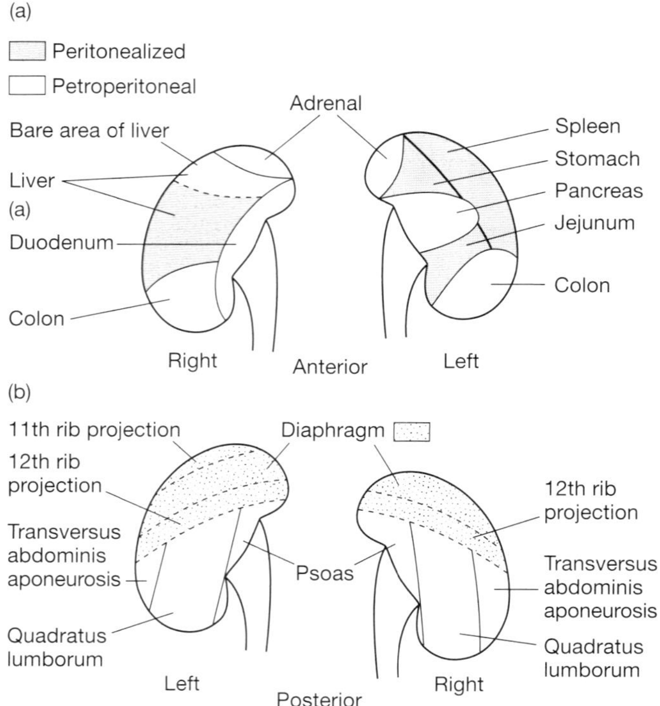

Fig. 2.17 (a) Drawing showing dorsal relationships of kidneys to dorsal abdominal wall musculature and diaphragm. (b) Drawing showing ventral relationships of kidneys to viscera. Reproduced with permission from Kabalin (1998, Fig. 2.25, p. 72).

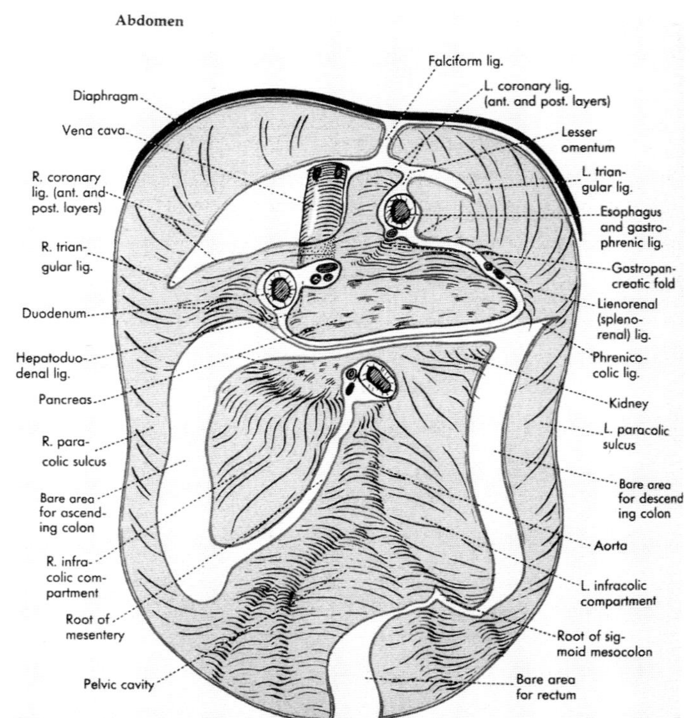

Fig. 2.18 Drawing showing sites of peritoneal reflection following excision of intraperitoneal viscera. Reproduced with permission from Rosse and Gaddum-Rosse (1997, Fig. 23.20, p. 536).

kidney is overlain by three visceral structures. The craniolateral two-thirds is covered by the liver. The cranial one-fourth of the kidney is overlain by the bare area of the liver, whereas the remaining cranial portion is covered by the liver, which is separated from the kidney by the peritoneum. The caudal one-third of the kidney is overlain by the hepatic flexure of the transverse and descending colon. The medial aspect of the kidney ventrally is covered by the second or descending part of the duodenum.

The left kidney is covered on its ventral surface by five visceral structures. The craniolateral two-thirds of the kidney is covered by the spleen contained within the peritoneal cavity. The craniomedial two-thirds is overlain from cranial to caudal by the stomach, pancreas, and jejunum, the stomach and the jejunum being contained within the peritoneal cavity. The caudal one-third of the kidney is covered by the splenic flexure of the colon.

Relationships of the peritoneum and its reflections to the kidney and adrenal glands

Within the retroperitoneum the colon and duodenum on the right side and the colon and pancreas on the left side may be reflected from the kidney by pursuing the plane of fusion fascia formed between the two leaves of primitive peritoneum. Developmentally, peritoneum enveloped both the ventral surface of the kidney and the dorsal aspects of the visceral structures. The disappearance of the peritoneum as the ascending and descending colon, duodenum, and pancreas assumed their final position over the dorsal wall of the abdomen left only the supporting connective tissue of the peritoneum, the inner stratum of retroperitoneal connective tissue.

Intraperitoneally, just as from a retroperitoneal approach, the peritoneum may be similarly reflected from the ventral surface of the kidney along with the colon, duodenum, and pancreas by incising the peritoneum along the lateral aspect of the colon at the white line of Toldt, which represents a site of peritoneal fusion (Fig. 2.18). On the right side a peritoneal incision can be carried medially around the cecum and cranially along the root of the mesentery to the ligament of Treitz. The incision may be carried around the hepatic flexure cranially and then medially along the cranial peritoneal reflection of the transverse colon. The colon and its mesentery along with the duodenum can be freed from the surface of the kidney by pursuing the fusion fascial plane between the inner and intermediate stratum of retroperitoneal connective tissues. The cranial aspect of the right kidney as well as the right adrenal gland and infrahepatic vena cava may be exposed by reflecting the liver medially by first incising the peritoneal reflections on to the lateral aspect of the liver, which are termed the triangular ligament and, more medially, the coronary ligaments. The triangular ligament extends medially and obliquely, cranially and caudally, as the coronary ligaments.

On the left side an incision may be made along Toldt's white line on the lateral aspect of the descending colon followed by an incision of the phrenicocolic ligament. Then, either turning the dissection medially to incise the root of the transverse mesocolon or cranially to incise respectively the splenorenal and

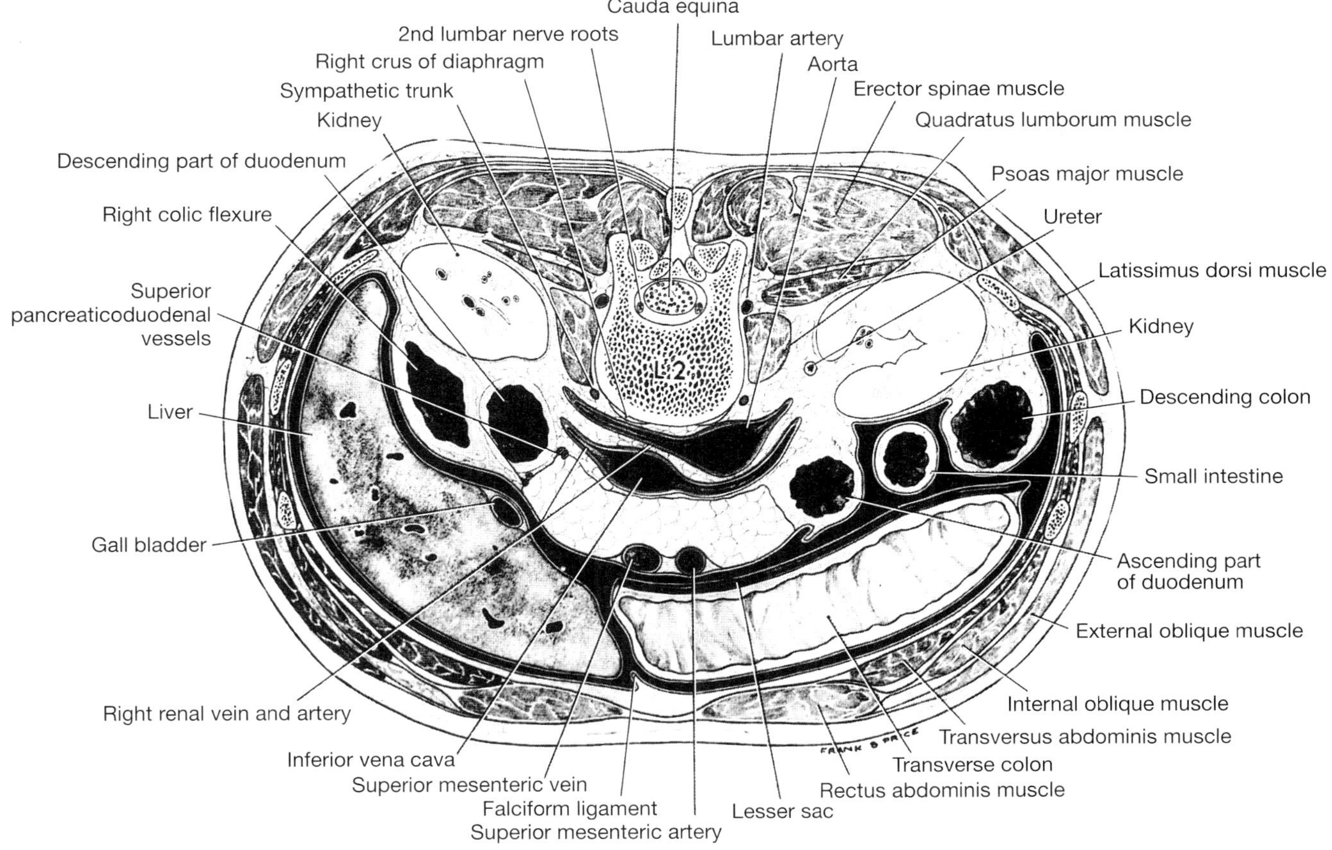

Fig. 2.19 Cross-section of abdomen at second lumbar vertebrae. Note the position of the kidney in relation to the vertebral body, the great vessels, and the psoas major and quadratus lumborum muscles. Reproduced with permission from Glenister (1979, Fig. 538, p. 415)

gastrophrenic ligaments allows the retraction medially of the descending colon, pancreas, and spleen to expose the ventral surface of the left kidney and adrenal gland.

Spatial relationships of the kidney to the body and rotational axes of the kidney

It is quite easy when viewing the kidneys in the context of textbook illustrations to assume that the kidney and adrenal glands lie in the same plane as the great vessels with the kidneys lying flat on a flat bed of muscle. A most useful exercise to understand the correct relationships is to examine anatomic illustrations or radiographic tomography showing transverse cross-sections of the body from the level of the T12–L3 vertebrae. It will be noted at the T12 level that the kidneys lie well dorsal of the great vessels on either side of the vertebral body which is covered by diaphragm. At the L2 vertebral cross-sectional level it will be noted that the kidneys still lie dorsal to the great vessels (Fig. 2.19). The muscles, as opposed to laying flat, actually are at virtual right angles to each other with the psoas major muscles separating the kidney from the vertebral bodies. The psoas will be noted to be oriented per-

pendicular to the quadratus lumborum muscle. On cross-section these rotational axes may be quantified in that a line drawn through the frontal plane of the kidney, that is, from the convex border through the renal hilum, will intersect the coronal plane at approximately 30° (Fig. 2.20(a)). Although there is considerable variation in the orientation and morphology of the renal collecting structures, it has been determined, particularly as an aid to percutaneous access to the calyces, that the axes of the calyces can be determined in relationship to the frontal plane of the kidney. Although not exact, on the right side the anterior calyces lie at angles of 45° from the frontal plane of the kidney, whereas the posterior calyces lie at an angle of 30° (Fig. 2.20(a)). On the left side the anterior and posterior calyces lie at an angle approximately 30° dorsal or ventral to the frontal plane, respectively.

When viewed from the coronal or anterior projection the kidneys will be noted not to lie with their long axes oriented in a vertical axes as commonly illustrated but to be tilted at their upper poles to form a 15° angle with the midsagittal plane (Fig. 2.20(b)). When viewed from the sagittal or lateral projection, it will be noted that the kidneys are tilted dorsally at their upper poles approximately 10° from the vertical plane (Fig. 2.20(c)).

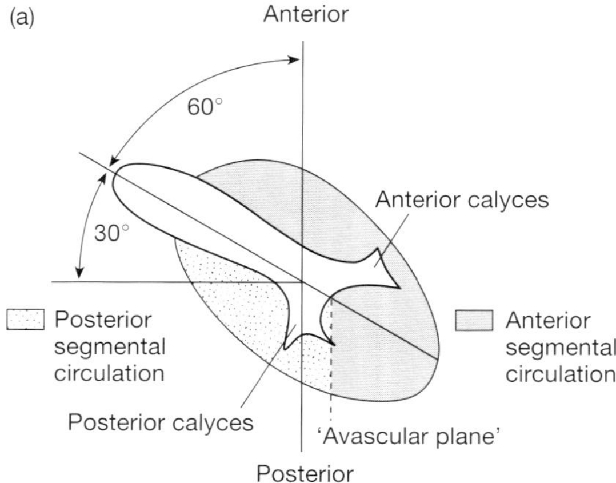

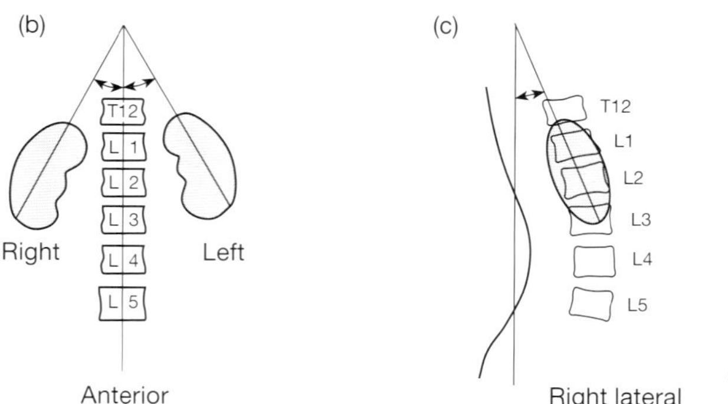

Fig. 2.20 (a) Drawing showing rotational axes of kidney and calyces in relation to the coronal plane. (b) Drawing showing medial tilt of upper poles of the kidneys as viewed from the anterior projection. (c) Drawing showing dorsal tilt of upper pole of kidney when viewed from a lateral projection. Reproduced with permission from Kabalin (1998, Fig. 2.26, p. 72)

References

Coupland, R.E. (ed.) (1979). Endocrine system. In *Textbook of human anatomy*, 2nd edn. Mosby, St Louis.

Dobbie, J.W. and Symington, T. (1966). The human adrenal gland with special reference to the vasculature. *J. Endocrinol.* **34**, 479.

Glenister, T.W. (1976). Urogenital system. In *Textbook of human anatomy*, 2nd edn. (ed. W.I. Hamilton) Mosby, St Louis.

Graves, F.T. (1955). The anatomy of the intrarenal arteries and its application to segmental resection of the kidney. *Br. J. Surg.* **2**, 132.

Gray, H. (1980). Splanchnology. In *Gray's Anatomy*, 36th British edn (ed. P.L. Williams and R. Warwick), Chapter 8. W.B. Saunders, Philadelphia.

Hayes, M.A. (1950). Abdominopelvic fascia. *J. Anat.* **87**, 119.

Hinman, F. (1993). Kidney, ureter, and adrenal glands. In *Atlas of urosurgical anatomy*, Chapter 12, pages 235–307. W.B. Saunders, Philadelphia.

Kabalin, J.N. (1998) Surgical anatomy of the retroperitoneum, kidneys, and ureters. In *Campbell's urology*, 7th edn (ed. P.C. Walsh, A.B. Retik, E.D. Vaughan, Jr, and A.J. Wein), Vol. 1, Chapter 2. W.B. Saunders, Philadelphia.

Redman, J.F. (1996). Anatomy of the genitourinary system. In *Adult and pediatric urology*, 3rd edn (ed. J.Y. Gillenwater, J.T. Grayhack, S.S. Howards, and J.W. Duckett), Chapter 1, Vol. 1. Mosby-Year Book, St. Louis.

Rosse, C. and Gaddum-Rosse, P. (1997). The abdomen in general. In *Hollinshead's textbook of anatomy*, 5th edn (ed. C. Rosse, P. Gaddum-Rosse), Chapter 23. Lippincott–Raven, Philadelphia.

Tighe, J.R. (1982). Histology and ultrastructure. In *Scientific foundation of urology* (ed. G.D. Chisholm and D.I. Williams). Year Book Medical, Williams, Inc, Chicago.

Tobin, C.E. (1944). The renal fascia and its relation to the transversalis fascia. *Anat. Rec.* **89**, 295.

3. Diagnosis and management of the incidental renal mass

Allan J. Pantuck, Mitchell K. Rauch, Amnon Zisman, and Arie Belldegrum

Introduction and epidemiology

Malignant tumors of the kidney comprise 2 per cent of cancer incidence and mortality in the US (Landis *et al.* 1998) with 31 200 new cases estimated to occur in the year 2000 causing approximately 11 900 deaths (Greenlee *et al.* 2000). In general, no distinction has been made in the past between parenchymal and pyelocalyceal tumors from an epidemiological standpoint, and little information is available to separate the two incidence rates. By conservative estimate, however, more than 80 per cent of these tumors will arise in the renal parenchyma (Devasa *et al.* 1990) and the vast majority will be adenocarcinomas (renal cell carcinomas). The incidence of renal cell carcinoma (RCC) at autopsy has been reported to be approximately 2 per cent (Hellsten *et al.* 1990).

The incidence rate of RCC has increased steadily throughout the world (Chow *et al.* 1999; Liu *et al.* 1997; Nakata *et al.* 1998). According to incidence, mortality, and survival data from the US National Cancer Institute's Surveillance, Epidemiology, and End Results (SEER) program, there has been an increase in the incidence of RCC in the US in all age groups with the greatest increase occurring in patients with localized tumors (Chow *et al.* 1999). This suggests a migration towards earlier stages as a result of earlier detection. This phenomenon may be explained in part by the increased number of asymptomatic, incidental tumors being detected as a result of the widespread use of non-invasive abdominal imaging modalities including ultrasound (US), computerized tomography (CT), and magnetic resonance imaging (MRI) (Jaysen and Sanders 1998). In 1973, only 13 per cent of tumors were discovered incidentally (Konnak and Grossman 1985), compared to 61 per cent of renal tumors in 1998 (Jaysen and Sanders 1998). Although mortality rates for RCC actually rose between 1975 and 1995 (Chow *et al.* 1999), reflecting rising rates of patients presenting with regional extension and distant metastasis, 5-year survival for patients of all races with RCC increased from 52 per cent in 1974–76 to 60 per cent in 1989–95 (Greenlee *et al.* 2000).

The increase in the incidental detection of pre-symptomatic tumors brings to the foreground several important issues, as their clinical significance, tumor characteristics, and optimal treatment remain controversial. With an increase in incidentally discovered masses, one would expect that earlier detection should have a significant impact on patient prognosis. At UCLA, we analyzed the presenting symptoms of 663 patients with RCC and divided them into three groups—true incidental (22 per cent), classic triad (hematuria, flank pain, and abdominal mass), and constitutional symptoms (weight loss, fever, night sweats, anorexia, cough, malaise)—in order to determine the effect of presenting symptoms on patient survival. The median survival rates for patients with incidental tumors, triad-associated tumors, and constitutional symptoms were 117, 56, and 29 months, respectively ($p < 0.05$). Furthermore, the incidental tumors at UCLA were smaller in size, significantly lower grade, and tended to present at earlier stages than symptomatic tumors (Tsui *et al.* 2000).

Although several recent studies have suggested that incidental and symptomatic RCC have equal proportions of early-stage lesions and therefore share similar prognoses (Jaysen and Sanders 1998), the literature for the most part supports the notion that incidental renal carcinomas are of lower stage and are associated with improved survival (Konnak and Grossman 1985; Thompson and Peek 1988). In a recent retrospective review, 161 patients with the diagnosis of RCC were analyzed (Sweeney *et al.* 1996). In this study, the groups were divided into incidental and symptomatic masses. The incidentally detected tumors had lower pathological stage, lower histological grade, and overall 5-year survival was 53 per cent for symptomatic and 85 per cent for incidentally detected masses. Another study has noted a slightly higher 5-year survival for masses diagnosed by ultrasound compared to other radiographic modalities (Aso and Homma 1992).

Retrospective analysis of the histopathology of incidental RCC has shown no difference in the nuclear grade, DNA ploidy, or survival when compared to symptomatic tumors stage for stage, and it is quite possible that the improved prognosis of incidental renal masses is merely a consequence of early detection. At UCLA, lower-stage lesions have similar grade distributions for both incidental and symptomatic lesions (Tsui *et al.* 2000). Interestingly, however, symptomatic stage IV tumors demonstrated more high-grade histology than the incidental tumors of the same stage, suggesting an alternative hypothesis, that the underlying histology and natural history of incidental lesions may be inherently less aggressive than lesions that produce symptoms. Another interesting trend worth noting is that, as the number of incidentally detected renal masses increases, so apparently does the incidence of benign renal tumors discovered at the time of nephrectomy. Two recent studies of solid renal masses treated by nephrectomy have demonstrated a 14 per cent incidence of benign renal tumors (Silver *et al.* 1997; Dechet *et al.* 1999). The majority of these tumors were oncocytomas, and the overall incidence of benignity increased to 22 per cent when only tumors 4 cm or less were considered (Dechet *et al.* 1999). At present, it is impossible to identify these cases preoperatively.

Considering the improved prognosis of incidental RCC, the increase in the number of benign masses and the difficulty in their preoperative diagnosis, the excellent results associated with partial nephrectomy (Morgan and Zincke 1990), and the possibility that these lesions themselves may have a less aggressive natural history, it becomes apparent that not all solid renal masses are optimally treated by radical nephrectomy. Given these results, changes in the approach to the management of these masses have occurred. Traditionally, renal parenchymal-sparing procedures were reserved for patients with a functional or anatomical impairment of the contralateral kidney. Currently, appropriately located lesions 4 cm or less are treated effectively and with excellent long-term survival by partial nephrectomy, even in patients with a normal contralateral kidney, and novel methods of minimally invasive, nephron-sparing surgery are being tried with very encouraging results. In this chapter, we will consider the differential diagnosis, radiographic evaluation, treatment options, and future trends in the management of the patient with an incidentally detected renal mass.

Differential diagnosis

The differential diagnosis of an incidentally detected renal mass includes both benign and malignant processes. Malignant renal masses include RCC, sarcoma, lymphoblastoma, metastatic disease (especially lung, breast, prostate, colon, testes) and urothelial-based tumors of the pelvis and collecting system. Of these, RCC account for the majority of such masses.

Conventionally, there have been four main histologic subtypes of RCC: clear cell; granular cell; tubulopapillary; and sarcomatoid. In 1997, a combined European and American work group developed a new histopathological classification system (Table 3.1) which takes into account advances in the understanding of the underlying genetic abnormalities in the subtypes of RCC (Storkel *et al.* 1997). The sarcomatoid pattern is no longer considered a distinct subtype, as sarcomatoid changes have been noted to occur in all types of RCC. Instead, the sarcomatoid pattern is considered to be a manifestation of high-grade carcinoma involving the individual type from which it arose. Renal carcinoma is typically

Table 3.1 UICC histological classification for renal tumors

Malignant neoplasms
    Clear cell carcinoma
    Papillary renal carcinoma
    Chromophobe renal carcinoma
    Collecting duct carcinoma
    Renal cell carcinoma unclassified

Benign neoplasms
    Oncocytoma
    Papillary adenoma
    Metanephric adenoma

unilateral, but bilaterality, either synchronous or asynchronous, occurs in approximately 2 per cent of cases (Moertel *et al.* 1961).

Sarcoma of the kidney accounts for only 2–3 per cent of all renal malignancies. Unless the tumor contains fat or bone (liposarcoma or osteosarcoma), differentiation from RCC by radiodensity is nearly impossible. Renal lymphoblastic processes are typically a manifestation of a systemic lymphoma, lymphosarcoma, or leukemic disease. Managing the underlying disease process best treats these tumors. CT may have findings that are suggestive of the diagnosis; however, a tissue diagnosis is usually required. Urothelial tumors, of which 90 per cent are transitional cell carcinomas (TCC), are rarely found incidentally. More commonly, these tumors present with symptoms such as gross hematuria.

Lesions classified as benign include simple cysts, oncocytoma, adenoma, angiomyolipoma, fibroma, and lipoma. Simple cysts (thin-walled and filled with clear fluid) are found commonly, comprising nearly 70 per cent of asymptomatic renal mass lesions and are of no clinical significance. Complex cysts can be classified according to Bosniak's (1995) classification. Complex cysts are usually explored in order to ascertain their true malignant potential. Renal oncocytoma has become a recognized clinical and pathologic entity with almost invariably benign clinical behavior. Oncocytomas are found in 3–7 per cent (Lieber 1993) of all renocortical tumors, although their incidence appears to be rising in more recent series (Silver *et al.* 1997; Dechet *et al.* 1999). These tumors may have a typical gross appearance—usually tan or light brown (mahogany) in color, well circumscribed, round, and encapsulated—and contain a central dense fibrous band with fibrous trabeculae extending out in a stellate pattern. The central scar can sometimes be imaged preoperatively by CT or MRI suggesting the diagnosis of oncocytoma. The typical angiographic picture is seen on the arterial phase of the angiogram revealing a spoke-wheel or stellate pattern.

Differentiation between a typical renal oncocytoma and oncocytic RCC can be a difficult pathologic task based on nuclear morphology. The management of renal oncocytomas, therefore, must be influenced by two characteristic features: (1) the unreliability and nonspecificity of current radiographic studies; (2) the presence of malignant elements and oncocytoma cells in the same tumor. Therefore a needle core biopsy suggestive of oncocytoma cannot reliably justify a non-operative approach (see discussion below and Case study 1).

Case study 1 During a routine executive physical examination, a 55-year-old male underwent abdominal ultrasonography, which revealed a left renal mass. A CT scan revealed a solid, enhancing mass as seen in Fig. 3.1. Due to a history of hypertension, atherosclerotic cardiovascular disease, and mild azotemia (creatinine 1.7), a nephron-sparing approach was used. Intraoperative ultrasonography was used to remove this mass. Pathology revealed oncocytoma.

The existence of benign renal tubular epithelial lesions (cortical adenoma) less than 3 cm in diameter remains controversial. Bell (1950) found a direct correlation between size and malignant potential, noting that tumors less than 3 cm in size had little propensity for metastasis. Murphy and Mostofi (1970) concluded that renal adenomas are benign tumors, distinguishable from true

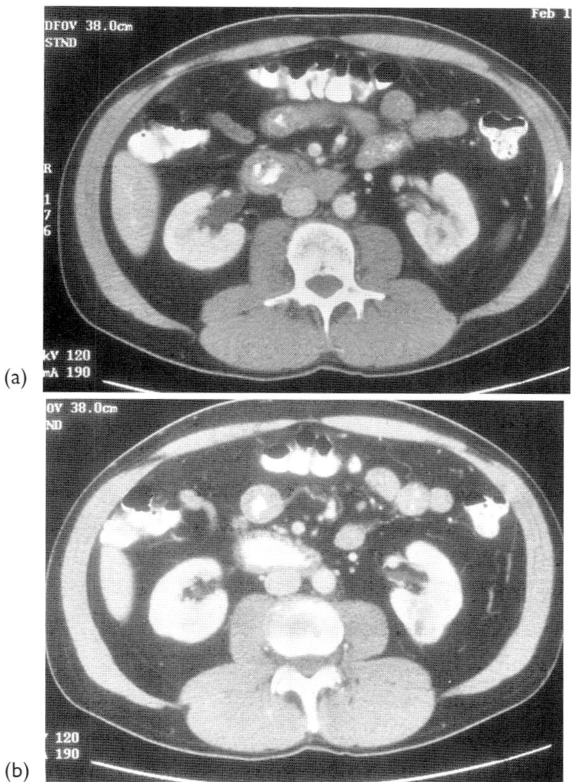

Fig. 3.1 CT scan of the patient in Case study I showing a solid, enhancing mass on the (right or left) kidney.

adenocarcinomas. Bennington and Beckwith (1975) presented an alternative view, arguing that all tubular cell adenomas are malignant, simply representing an early stage of RCC. The majority of cortical adenomas are of the papillary type and they histologically resemble low-grade papillary RCC. Furthermore, the cytogenetics of papillary adenoma suggest that they represent an early form of papillary RCC (Brown *et al.* 1997). For this reason, most renal parenchymal tumors are treated as true RCC.

Renal angiomyolipoma, is a benign solid renal tumor composed of elements of fat, muscle, and abnormal blood vessels. They are often yellow and gray and have a propensity for profuse hemorrhage, large size, and multiplicity. The diagnosis can often be made on CT scan by virtue of the characteristic fat density (−20 to −80 Hounsfield units). On sonography, the tumor is highly echogenic due to the numerous fatty interfaces, and on angiography the tumor is highly vascular. Since incidentally discovered angiomyolipomas are asymptomatic by definition, management is determined by the size of the mass. Oesterling *et al.* (1986) reviewed the world literature of angiomyolipomas and concluded that asymptomatic lesions smaller than 4 cm in diameter do not require therapy but should be observed for evidence of tumor growth or for the development of symptoms or bleeding.

Fibromas may arise from fibrous tissue found in the renal parenchyma, the perinephric tissue, or the renal capsule. These are rare benign tumors, often found on the periphery of the kidney. A radical nephrectomy is usually performed because of the uncertainty of the diagnosis on preoperative evaluation.

Renal lipomas are among the rarest of renal tumors. Their origin is unclear, but they probably originate from fat cells within the renal capsule or parenchyma. The gross characteristics are the same as those of any lipoma. The treatment is surgical excision, usually requiring total nephrectomy because of their large size.

Management

Role of biopsy in the evaluation of the renal mass

Since the majority of incidental masses found today are accurately diagnosed by non-invasive cross-sectional imaging tests, the role of percutaneous renal biopsy is limited. Seeding of the puncture sight with tumor has been described with large core biopsies, but small (18-gauge) core biopsies probably carry a negligible risk (Kiser *et al.* 1986). This small risk should be weighed against the potential value of a biopsy's ability to provide an unequivocal diagnosis of cancer. Unfortunately, in a large series of 301 fine needle aspirations of solid renal masses (Juul *et al.* 1985), 8 per cent were false-negative biopsies. In a review of the literature, the sensitivity and specificity for cytology fine needle biopsies of renal masses were 80–92 per cent and 83–100 per cent, respectively. Reported positive and negative predictive values range between 90 and 95 per cent (Niceforo and Coughlin 1993). Importantly, the rate of obtaining adequate cytological and histological specimens for analysis was 70–98 per cent, leaving many biopsies as 'indeterminate'.

Dechet and associates (1999) published a best case scenario of intraoperative biopsy with direct access to the kidney. In this series, accuracy was only 75 per cent with the largest degree of uncertainty involving benign lesions for which there was a 20 per cent false-positive rate. Given these limitations, open exploration is the best approach except in rare circumstances. If clinical or radiographic evidence exists to suggest a diagnosis other than primary RCC, such as metastatic disease, primary lymphoblastic process, or renal abscess, then biopsy may be considered. In general, renal biopsy is therefore not recommended for the incidental renal mass and, in most cases, a biopsy would not obviate the need for a surgical procedure.

Observation

As more small incidentally detected RCC are being discovered in elderly patients or in patients with extensive co-morbidities, a 'watchful waiting' approach has become a viable option in selected patients. This approach is based on experience accumulated in studying the growth rate and behavior of small incidentally found renal tumors. In a series of 40 patients with 43 small renal tumors all of which were less than 3.0 cm, none developed metastases with an average follow-up of 3.5 years. Tumor kinetics for the masses in the series showed variable growth rates of 0 to 1.3 cm/year. The majority of the patients eventually underwent surgery, but 14 patients were still being followed at the time of publication because of advanced age or poor physical condition (Bosniak 1995). In another series of over 100 proven small renal parenchymal neoplasms (< 3.0 cm) that have been followed expectantly over the past 10 years, only two cases (< 2.0 per cent) have been associated with metastatic disease (Bosniak *et al.* 1995). In both of those cases, patients presented with widespread meta-stases, and the renal lesion was found on subsequent evaluation. Although the natural biology of RCC is inherently unpredictable, these results suggest that many well-marginated, small tumors grow slowly and do not metastasize until they are larger.

When contemplating expectant management of an incidentally discovered solid renal mass, several factors must first be consid-ered. These include the age of the patient, the patient's clinical condition and associated co-morbidities, and the size and CT appearance of the tumor when first discovered. In general, watch-ful waiting should never be the standard recommended therapy for any renal lesion. However, if small (< 2 cm), homogeneous (nonnecrotic) lesions are discovered in elderly or frail patients who are considered to be poor surgical candidates, then these patients can be followed with periodic radiographic studies. Minimally invasive, alternative therapeutic options for these patients are evolving as will be discussed below.

Radical nephrectomy versus a nephron-sparing approach

Surgery remains the only effective method of treatment of primary renal carcinoma, and the objective of the procedure must be to excise all tumors with an adequate surgical margin. Although the definition varies, radical nephrectomy generally implies the excision of Gerota's fascia and its contents, including the kidney and adrenal gland. This historical standard surgical approach accomplishes several objectives: (1) the ipsilateral adrenal gland, which historically was involved in 10 per cent of cases , is excised; (2) lymphatic metastases, which may diffuse through the perirenal fat, are removed; (3) a more adequate margin away from the tumor is achieved, especially when the tumor invades the perirenal fat.

This approach was developed in the era when the diagnosis of a renal mass was based primarily on intravenous pyelography, and the difficulty in accurately defining the status of the primary tumor and the ipsilateral adrenal gland justified wide excision of normal tissue along with the tumor. However, consideration of the increase in the detection of localized tumors combined with the development of high-resolution CT scanning, which allows for accurate preoperative clinical staging of tumors, brings the necess-ity of radical nephrectomy for all renal masses under scrutiny. For example, a contemporary series from the Mayo Clinic evaluated the incidence of ipsilateral adrenal metastasis in a prospective manner and found only a 2 per cent rate (Kletscher *et al.* 1996). Of greater significance, all of these lesions could to be identified preoperatively by CT or MRI.

Although radical nephrectomy is still considered the standard treatment for localized RCC with a normal contralateral kidney, it is now well established that open partial nephrectomy is an effective form of therapy in selected patients. Nephron-sparing surgery was originally described in the late 1880s and quickly abandoned secondary to significant complications, including bleeding, urinary fistulae, and death. In the past decade, enthusi-asm for renal-sparing surgery has been stimulated by advances in renal imaging, the growing incidence of incidentally detected tumors, and improved surgical techniques that limit warm ischemia time. Renal parenchyma-sparing surgery had been rec-ommended only for patients with a solitary kidney, a poorly func-tioning contralateral kidney, bilateral RCC (see Case study 2), or where the remaining kidney is at risk for future functional impair-ment (that is, renal artery disease, stone disease, chronic pyelo-nephritis, nephrosclerosis, diabetes mellitus). Extended experience has now established that nephron-sparing surgery can be per-formed safely with low morbidity, good preservation of renal function, and long-term cure in many patients. The principal dis-advantage of nephron-sparing surgery for RCC is the risk of post-operative local tumor recurrence, the rate of which has ranged from 2 to 9 per cent (Licht and Novick 1993). The etiology of local recurrence can be due to incomplete resection of the initial lesion, unrecognized satellite lesions, and *de novo* tumor formation.

Case study 2 A 46-year-old woman underwent CT scan of the abdomen and pelvis after an automobile accident, which revealed a solid 2.5 cm left renal mass as well as a 6.5 cm right renal mass (see Figs 3.2 and 3.3). Left exploration was undertaken with intraoperative ultrasonography reveal-ing three masses, two not seen on preoperative imaging. These were excised. Final pathology revealed low-grade RCC. Given the bilaterality and multiplicity of the tumors, a right partial nephrectomy was then successfully performed revealing low-grade RCC with negative margins.

In properly selected patients, one can reduce the risk of local recurrence. Licht et al. (1994) found no local or systemic recur-rences after nephron-sparing surgery in patients with small (< 4.0 cm), unilateral, stage T1–2 tumors. The mean follow-up for these 50 patients was 4 years. If the mass was discovered inci-dentally, there was an improved prognosis. Hafez et al. (1997) reported on 327 patients with an average follow-up of nearly 5 years who underwent nephron-sparing surgery for sporadic localized RCC. Local tumor recurrence occurred in 4 per cent of patients. The higher the pathologic (p) stage, the more likely it was that local tumor recurrence occurred. No patients with

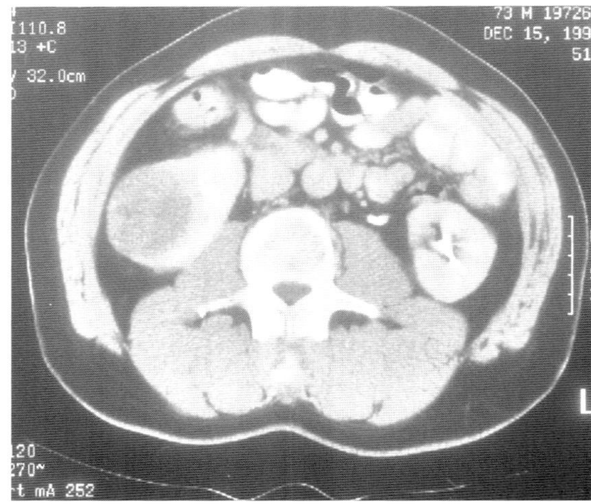

Fig. 3.2 CT scan of the patient in Case study 2 showing a solid 6.5 cm right renal mass.

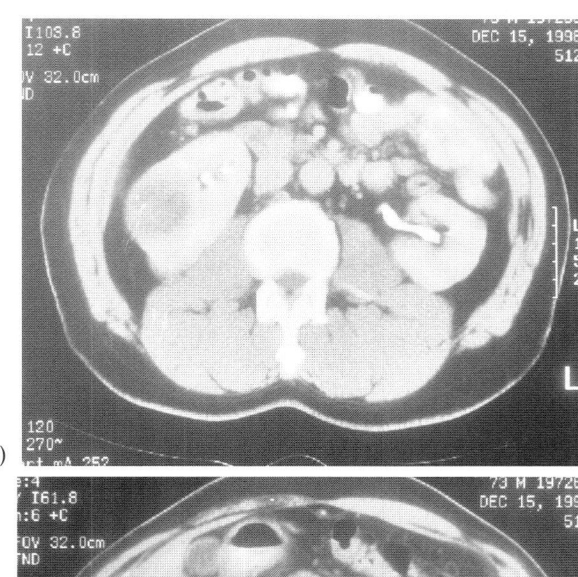

(a)

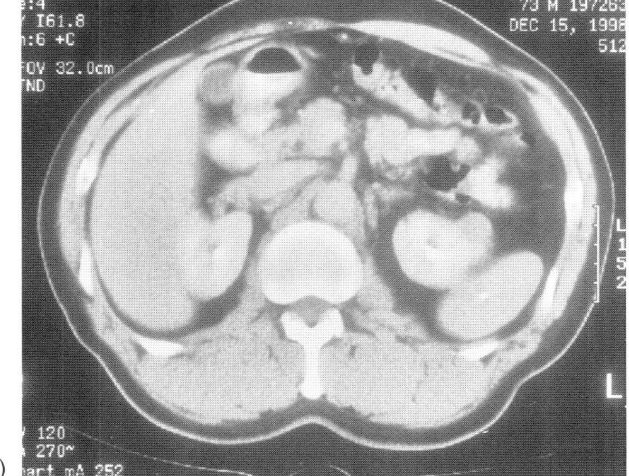

(b)

Fig. 3.3 CT scan of the patient in Case study 2 showing a 6.5 cm right renal mass (A) and a 2.5 cm left renal mass (B).

Table 3.2 1997 AJCC TNM classification of renal cell carcinoma

T1	Tumor < 7 cm in greatest dimension limited to the kidney
T2	Tumor > 7 cm in greatest dimension limited to the kidney
T3	Tumor extends into major veins, adrenal, or perinephric tissues but not beyond Gerota's fascia
T3a	Tumor invades adrenal gland or perinephric tissue but not beyond Gerota's fascia
T3b	Tumor grossly extends into renal vein(s) or vena cava below the diaphragm
T3c	Tumor grossly extends into vena cava above the diaphragm
T4	Tumor invades beyond Gerota's fascia
N0	No regional lymph node metastasis
N1	Metastasis to a single lymph node
N2	Metastasis in more than one regional lymph node
M0	No distant metastasis
M1	Distant metastasis

34–86 years). Patients were followed for an average of 57 months during which tumor recurrence, metastasis, and patient deaths were recorded. For the purposes of comparison, a matched group of 125 patients undergoing radical nephrectomy between 1987 and 1997 were selected to match the partial nephrectomy group.

The partial and radical groups were similar in terms of the revised TNM (tumor–node–metastasis; 1997) staging system (Table 3.2), with the majority of tumors being T1 (less than 7 cm). The cancer-specific survival rates of patients undergoing partial nephrectomy increased from 72 per cent in group 1 to 98 per cent in group 2. When comparing cancer-specific survival rates for patients with T1 lesions under both the 1987 and 1997 TNM staging criteria, no statistically significant difference in survival was noted based on the different staging classifications ($p = 0.53$). Lesions greater than T1 under the 1997 TNM and greater than T2 under the 1987 criteria yielded a survival rate of 66 per cent. Patients with T2 lesions (1997 TNM) demonstrated a significant decrease in survival when compared to patients with T1 lesions ($p < 0.001$). In comparing the outcomes of partial versus radical nephrectomies, no statistically significant differences in survival were seen for patients with T1 RCC treated with either type of surgery. In contrast, for patients with lesions greater than T1, survival rates were significantly higher in patients treated with radical as opposed to nephron-sparing surgery. These data support the excellent cancer control obtained with nephron-sparing surgery in appropriately selected patients. In addition, our data indicate that radical and partial nephrectomy provide equally effective curative treatment for such patients with T1 (1997 TNM) lesions less than 7 cm and a normal contralateral kidney.

Partial nephrectomy

Preoperative evaluation should include a careful review of all imaging studies. If one suspects renal vein involvement, MRI with gadolinium-enhanced vascular sequences should be obtained to evaluate the renal vein and inferior vena cava (IVC). Renal arteriography should be utilized selectively in patients undergoing nephron-sparing surgery. It is usually unnecessary in patients with peripheral tumors, but patients with centrally located masses may benefit.

pT1 tumors had recurrences; 2 per cent of pT2, 8.2 per cent of pT3, and 10.6 per cent of pT3b tumors recurred. The peak postoperative intervals until local tumor recurrence were 6 to 24 months and longer than 48 months. Velagapudi et al. (1993) have also reported excellent results with nephron-sparing surgery for patients with small (mean diameter = 3.2 cm), unilateral, stage T1–2 tumors. All 60 patients, with a mean follow-up of 4.8 years, were cancer-free at last follow-up.

When directly comparing radical versus nephron-sparing surgery, Butler *et al.* (1995) showed similar efficacy in patients with favorable prognostic features. In this study, 42 patients were treated with nephron-sparing surgery and 46 with radical nephrectomy; there was only one tumor recurrence in each group. The cancer-specific 5-year survival rates were 100 per cent after nephron-sparing and 97 per cent after radical nephrectomy.

Recently we reviewed the UCLA experience with nephron-sparing surgery in the era of altered staging criteria and expanded indication (Belldegrun *et al.* 1999). Between 1980 and 1997, 146 patients underwent partial nephrectomy for unilateral, solitary, or bilateral tumors. For the purpose of the study, these patients were divided into two subgroups: 38 patients undergoing surgery between 1980 and 1986 (group 1) and 108 patients between 1987 and 1997 (group 2). The mean patient age was 62.4 years (range

The choice of approach and incision for nephron-sparing surgery is largely a matter of surgeon preference. An extra-peritoneal flank approach offers excellent exposure and allows for complete mobilization of the kidney. The entire kidney should then be inspected for multiple nodules not seen on preoperative imaging studies (see Case study 2).

Several recent reports (Marshall *et al.* 1992; Walther *et al.* 1994) have established the role of intraoperative ultrasonography as a useful adjunct when performing partial nephrectomies. This is particularly useful for a centrally located mass that is not palpable or able to be seen at the time of surgery. In addition, satellite lesions have been seen with intraoperative ultrasound that were not appreciated preoperatively. Occasionally, intraoperative ultrasound has changed a planned partial nephrectomy to a radical nephrectomy by showing more tumors than evident on pre-operative imaging. At our institution a 12 megahertz ultrasound probe is used with color flow Doppler, which provides even greater anatomic resolution especially when major vessels are involved.

A variety of surgical techniques are available for performing nephron-sparing surgery, including simple enucleation, polar seg-mental nephrectomy, wedge resection, hemi-nephrectomy, and extracorporeal partial nephrectomy with autotransplantation. The technical aspects of each of these procedures are covered in detail elsewhere in this text. Many renal carcinomas are completely encapsulated by a distinct pseudocapsule of fibrous tissue that can allow complete tumor removal by enucleation with maximal con-servation of nephrons. Some reports have shown excellent short-term clinical results, with low local recurrence rates. (Novick *et al.* 1986) However, histological studies have shown frequent microscopic penetration of the pseudocapsule, increasing the risk of local recurrence. Tumor excision with a surrounding rim of normal parenchyma may be the safest approach to ensure com-plete tumor resection, leaving simple enucleation for selected highly individualized cases. In general, the specimen should include the tumor circumscribed by a rim of normal appearing parenchyma and abundant perinephric soft tissue overlying the mass. Multiple deep margins of the mass should be sent for frozen section analysis to verify adequate pathological margins.

Follow-up after partial nephrectomy

Table 3.3 summarizes the local recurrence rates and survival of patients with stage T1 unilateral renal carcinoma and a normal opposite kidney, stratified by tumor size, after partial or radical nephrectomy at UCLA. Knowledge of rates of local tumor recurrence and patterns of metastasis is useful in developing guidelines for patient follow-up after surgery. Hafez *et al.* (1997) developed guidelines for follow-up of patients who have under-gone nephron-sparing surgery. The follow-up should be tailored according to the initial pathological stage (Table 3.4). All patients should be evaluated yearly with a medical history, physical exam-ination, and selected laboratory studies. Many patients with stage T1 RCC require no additional monitoring; however, more careful follow-up is justified for patients with tumors between 4 and 7 cm, which carry a higher risk of recurrence. Patients with stage T2 disease should undergo a yearly chest X-ray and abdominal CT every 2 years. The same recommendations are offered for patients with stage T3 RCC with the additional recommendation that abdominal CT be done every 6 months for the first 2 years postoperatively.

Minimally invasive surgery for the incidental renal mass—the future is now

The field of minimally invasive surgery for RCC is one of rapid advancement involving exciting new technologies. Laparoscopic nephrectomy was introduced in 1991 by Clayman *et al.* (1991)

Table 3.3 Local recurrence rates and survival of patients with stage T1 unilateral renal carcinoma and normal opposite kidney, stratified by tumor size, after partial or radical nephrectomy

Tumor size (cm)	Partial nephrectomy				Radical nephrectomy			
	N	Tumor recurrence	Death	Months	N	Tumor recurrence	Death	Months
< 2.5	15	0	0	44	12	0	0	31
2.5–4	38	1	0	51	40	1	1	45
4–7	10	1	0	64	27	1	1	35

N, number of patients; Death, number of deaths from cancer; Months, months of follow-up.

Table 3.4 Postoperative surveillance after partial nephrectomy for localized RCC

Pathological tumor stage	History, examination, blood tests	Chest X-ray	Abdominal CT
T1N0M0	Yearly	—	—
T2N0M0	Yearly	Yearly	Every 2 years
T3abN0M0	Every 6 mos. for 3 years, then yearly	Every 6 mos. for 3 years, then yearly	Every 6 mos. for 3 years, then every 2 years

and there has been much experience gained with this procedure since then. Although laparoscopic nephrectomy has become an accepted surgical modality for benign disease with well established perioperative benefits of reduced morbidity (Kerbl *et al.* 1994), laparoscopic radical nephrectomy for RCC has yet to become a well-accepted oncologic alternative. Specific concerns in regard to the principles of cancer surgery include the threat of tumor spillage leading to potential local and port site tumor recurrence, as well as the inability to pathologically stage patients since most kidneys are removed by a process of *in situ* renal morcellation that does not permit adequate evaluation of the tumor or its surgical margins.

In initial reports, small patient numbers and short-term follow-up limited efficacy and survival comparisons to standard surgical approaches (McDougall *et al.* 1996). However, better data with intermediate follow-up is beginning to emerge. Cadeddu *et al.* (1998) presented the results on 157 patients undergoing laparoscopic nephrectomy at five institutions. During the mean follow-up of 19 months, no patients developed a laparoscopic port site or renal fossa tumor recurrence, and there was a 91 per cent actuarial estimate for 5-year disease-free rate and no cancer deaths occurred. Other authors have had similar results (Barrett *et al.* 1998). Still limited by scant long-term follow-up, the inability to pathologically stage patients may become problematic when comparing the efficacy and long-term cancer-specific survival rate of laparoscopic nephrectomy to those of open radical nephrectomy. However, early data regarding the feasibility, safety, and efficacy are encouraging.

Laparoscopic nephrectomy may find that, although it does not become the overall standard approach, certain selected populations may derive additional benefit from this less invasive alternative to open nephrectomy. Hsu *et al.* (1999) retrospectively compared the outcome of laparoscopic and open nephrectomy in the octagenerian and nonagenarian populations. Eleven patients 80 years or older undergoing retroperitoneal laparoscopic nephrectomy were compared to six similarly aged patients undergoing open nephrectomy. The laparoscopic group compared favorably to the open group in regard to median surgical time and blood loss. However, they also had a quicker resumption of oral intake, decreased narcotic requirement, shorter hospital stay, and faster convalescence. A pilot study of laparoscopic cytoreductive nephrectomy prior to systemic immunotherapy for patients with metastatic RCC was recently published (Walther *et al.* 1999a). The timing of surgery and biologic therapy has been controversial, and opponents of performing cytoreductive surgery first cite concerns regarding delay in systemic therapy or the inability to administer immunotherapy because of surgical morbidity and/or disease progression. In this study, patients with metastatic RCC underwent open nephrectomy or laparoscopic nephrectomy with tumors removed using either morcellation or via a small incision. Patients whose tumors were morcellated had reduced postoperative parenteral narcotic requirements and shorter hospitalizations. Furthermore, time to treatment with interleukin-2 (IL-2) was shortest in the morcellation group with median time to treatment of 37 days. Although selected patients may benefit from this minimally invasive approach, prospective, randomized trials are necessary to fully define these benefits.

Similarly to the situation with total nephrectomy, in an effort to reduce the morbidity of open nephron-sparing surgery, laparoscopic partial nephrectomy has now been well described in several institutions. Clayman and colleagues recently described their experience with this procedure (McDougall *et al.* 1998). Their conclusions were that laparoscopic wedge resection and polar partial nephrectomy are feasible, albeit currently tedious techniques. Wedge resection of superficial, small (< 2 cm) tumors is technically easier and efficient. In a separate study, seven patients underwent laparoscopic wedge resection of the kidney for renal tumors up to 2 cm in diameter (Janetschek *et al.* 1998). The authors describe their experience using bipolar coagulation, argon beam laser, fibrin glue, and an ultrasonic dissector. Tissue retrieval was performed using an entrapment sack through a 10 mm port and showed negative surgical margins in all patients with RCC. Two of seven patients had benign multilocular cysts and were spared the morbidity of open surgery. No patients experienced postoperative hemorrhage or urinary fistula. Interestingly, blood loss was greatest using the ultrasonic dissector, emphasizing the fact that currently available surgical tools cannot always achieve adequate hemostasis. With further development of instrumentation to provide for a reliable and hemostatic procedure, more will be done in the future. Although there is increased risk of bleeding currently, we believe that laparoscopic partial nephrectomy should be discussed with patients as a possible surgical option.

The increasing popularity of these minimally invasive approaches has stimulated investigation into the use of cryotherapy to target and ablate selected, small renal tumors. Cryoablative technology has recently improved, with better ultrasound monitoring and advanced delivery systems. The availability of reliable intraoperative lapraoscopic ultrasound that can provide precise positioning of the cryoprobe and allow for the necessary visualization of the tumor margin and the advancing edge of the evolving iceball as it freezes the tumor has made cryotherapy a viable alternative (Novick *et al.* 1999; Zegel *et al.* 1998).

Currently, investigators are exploring several approaches, including the use of cryotherapy during open surgery, laparoscopic surgery, and as a percutanous technique. Delworth *et al.* (1996) investigated the feasibility of renal cryotherapy on two patients with tumors involving solitary kidneys. Both patients tolerated renal cryotherapy well with no change in renal function and no postoperative complications. Follow-up MRI revealed a decrease in the size of one patient's 3 cm RCC, whereas there was a 10 per cent enlargement in the size of the second patient's 10 cm angiomyolipoma. Gill and Novick (1999) reviewed the worldwide experience of laparoscopic renal cyrotherapy, comprising approximately 50 cases of which 32 were performed at the Cleveland Clinic. Initial review of their first 10 cases, which were performed on patients with an average tumor size of 2.3 cm, showed minimal blood loss, and mean cyroablative time of less that 13 minutes (Gill *et al.* 1998). Mean operative time was 2.4 hours and most patients were discharged within 24 hours. Currently, 6-month follow up is available for 12 patients, all of whom have had negative CT-directed biopsies of the cryoablated site and have demonstrated no significant complications related to the cryotherapy involving the kidney or surrounding organs. They offer cryotherapy to selected patients with less than 4 cm, peripheral, exophytic, localized tumors away from the collecting system. Percutaneous renal cyrotherapy was performed in two patients with symptomatic metastatic RCC (Uchida *et al.* 1995). Both patients showed tumor shrinkage during limited follow-up.

Another area of active research is radiofrequency (RF) ablation of renal tumors. Radio-frequency interstitial tissue ablation (RITA) is a US Fedral Drugs Administration (FDA)-approved device for the treatment of liver lesions. Walther *et al.* (1999*b*) are currently performing a phase II study evaluating RITA of small renal lesions. Currently, prior to partial nephrectomy, tumors are being treated with RF, then excised. Early data show excellent tumor control. McGovern and collegues (1999) described a single case of percutaneous RF ablation of a 3.5 cm renal mass under ultrasound guidance in an 84-year-old man who refused open surgery. This outpatient procedure was performed under conscious sedation. Follow-up imaging at 1 and 3 months revealed nonenhancement of the treated region and no evidence of bleeding or urinoma. As with cryotherapy, additional study with extended follow-up will be necessary to determine the long-term efficacy and future role of radiofrequency ablation.

Conclusion

The problem of the incidental renal mass and its management will continue to confront clinicians with increasing frequency well into the new century. Newer, minimally invasive approaches will be used more in the future, especially for the treatment of small (< 4 cm) peripheral lesions and in selected groups of patients who are poor surgical risks or who require maximal renal preservation. With increasing follow-up of patients, we will realize the true value and potential expanded applications of these newer technologies. This is certainly an exciting area of urology and one that will continue to interest us for some time to come.

References

Aso, Y. and Homma, Y. (1992). A survey on incidental renal cell carcinoma in Japan. *J. Urol.* **147**, 340–3.

Barrett, P., Fentie, D., and Taranger, L. (1998). Laparoscopic radical nephrectomy with morcellation for renal cell carcinoma: the Saskatoon experience. *Urology* **52**, 23–38.

Bell, E. (1950). *Renal disease.* Lea and Febiger, Philadelphia.

Belldegrun, A., Tsui, K., deKernion, J., *et al.* (1999). Efficacy of nephron sparing surgery for renal cell carcinoma: analsyis based on the new 1997 tumor–node–metastasis system. *J. Clin. Oncol.* **17**, 2868–75.

Bennington, J. and Beckwith, J. (1975) Tumors of the kidney, renal pelvis, and ureter. *Atlas of tumor pathology.* Armed Forces Institute of Pathology, Washington, DC.

Bosniak, M.A. (1995). Observation of small incidentally detected renal masses. *Sem. Urol. Oncol.* **13**. 267–72.

Bosniak, M.A., Birnbaum, B.A., Krinsky, G.A., *et al.* (1995). Small renal parenchymal neoplasms: further observations on growth [see comments]. *Radiology* **197**, 589–97.

Brown, J., Anderl, K., Borell, T., *et al.* (1997). Simultaneous chromosome 7 and 17 gain and sex chromosome loss provide evidence that renal metanephric adenoma is related to papillary renal cell carcinoma. *J. Urol.* **158**, 370–4.

Butler, B.P., Novick, A.C., Miller, D.P., *et al.* (1995). Management of small unilateral renal cell carcinomas: radical versus nephron-sparing surgery. *Urology* **45**, 34–40; discussion 40–1.

Cadeddu, J.A., Ono, Y., Clayman, R.V., *et al.* (1998). Laparoscopic nephrectomy for renal cell cancer: evaluation of efficacy and safety: a multicenter experience. *Urology* **52**, 773–7.

Chow, W.H., Devesa, S.S., Warren, J.L., *et al.* (1999). Rising incidence of renal cell cancer in the United States. *J. Am. Med. Assoc.* **281**, 1628–31.

Clayman, R.V., Kavoussi, L.R., Soper, N.J., *et al.* (1991). Laparoscopic nephrectomy: initial case report. *J. Urol.* **146**, 278–82.

Dechet, C., Sebo, T., Farrow, G., *et al.* (1999). Prospective analysis of intraoperative frozen needle biopsy of solid renal masses in adults. *J. Urol.* **162**, 1282–4.

Delworth, M., Pisters, L., Fornage, B., *et al.* (1996). Cryotherapy for renal cell carcinoma and angiomyolipoma. *J. Urol.* **155**, 252–4.

Devasa, S., Silverman, D., McLaughlin, J., *et al.* (1990). Comparison of the descriptive epidemiology of urinary tract cancers. *Cancer Causes Control* **1**, 1133–41.

Gill, I.S. and Novick, A.C. (1999). Renal cryosurgery. *Urology* **54**, 215–19.

Gill, I.S., Novick, A.C., Soble, J.J., *et al.* (1998). Laparoscopic renal cryoablation: initial clinical series. *Urology* **52**, 543–51.

Greenlee, R.T., Murray, T., Bolden, S., and Wingo, P.A. (2000). Cancer statistics, 2000. *CA Cancer J. Clin.* **50**, 7–33.

Hafez, K.S., Novick, A.C., and Campbell, S.C. (1997). Patterns of tumor recurrence and guidelines for followup after nephron sparing surgery for sporadic renal cell carcinoma. *J. Urol.* **157**, 2067–70.

Hellsten, S., Johnsen, J., Berge, T., *et al.* (1990). Clinically unrecognized renal cell carcinoma. Diagnostic and pathological aspects. *Eur. Urol.* **18** (suppl. 2), 2–3.

Hsu, T.H., Gill, I.S., Fazeli-Matin, S., *et al.* (1999). Radical nephrectomy and nephroureterectomy in the octogenarian and nonagenarian: comparison of laparoscopic and open approaches. *Urology* **53**, 1121–5.

Janetschek, G., Daffner, P., Peschel, R., *et al.* (1998). Laparoscopic nephron sparing surgery for small renal cell carcinoma [see comments]. *J. Urol.* **159**, 1152–5.

Jayson, M. and Sanders, H. (1998). Increased incidence of serendipitously discovered renal cell carcinoma. *Urology* **51**, 203–5.

Juul, N., Torp-Pedersen, S., Grønvall, S., *et al.* (1985). Ultrasonically guided fine needle aspiration biopsy of renal masses. *J. Urol.* **133**, 579–81.

Kerbl, K., Clayman, R.V., McDougall, E.M., *et al.* (1994). Transperitoneal nephrectomy for benign disease of the kidney: a comparison of laparoscopic and open surgical techniques. *Urology* **43**, 607–13.

Kiser, G.C., Totonchy, M., and Barry, J.M. (1986). Needle tract seeding after percutaneous renal adenocarcinoma aspiration. *J. Urol.* **136**, 1292–3.

Kletscher, B.A., Qian, J., Bostwick, D.G., *et al.* (1996). Prospective analysis of the incidence of ipsilateral adrenal metastasis in localized renal cell carcinoma. *J. Urol.* **155**, 1844–6.

Konnak, J.W. and Grossman, H.B. (1985). Renal cell carcinoma as an incidental finding. *J. Urol.* **134**, 1094–6.

Landis, S.H., Murray, T., Bolden, S., *et al.* (1998) Cancer statistics, 1998. *CA Cancer J. Clin.* **48**, 6–29.

Licht, M. and Novick, A. (1993). Nephron-sparing surgery for renal cell carcinoma. *J. Urol.* **149**, 1–7.

Licht, M.R., Novick, A.C., and Goormastic, M. (1994).Nephron sparing surgery in incidental versus suspected renal cell carcinoma [see comments]. *J. Urol.* **152**, 39–42.

Lieber, M.M. (1993). Renal oncocytoma. *Urol. Clin. N. Am.* **20**, 355–9.

Liu, S., Semenciw, R., Morrison, H., Schanzer, D., and Mao, Y. (1997). Kidney cancer in Canada: the rapidly increasing incidence of adenocarcinoma in adults and seniors. *Can. J. Public Health* **88** (2), 99–104.

Marshall, F.F., Holdford, S.S., and Hamper, U.M. (1992). Intraoperative sonography of renal tumors. *J. Urol.* **148**, 1393–6.

McDougall, E., Clayman, R.V., and Elashry, O.M. (1996). Laparoscopic radical nephrectomy for renal tumor: the Washington University experience. *J. Urol.* **155**, 1180–5.

McDougall, E.M., Elbahnasy, A.M., and Clayman, R.V. (1998). Laparoscopic wedge resection and partial nephrectomy—the Washington University experience and review of the literature. *J. Soc. Laparoendosc. Surg.* **2**, 15–23.

McGovern, F.J., Wood, B.J., Goldberg, S.N., *et al.* (1999). Radiofrequency ablation of renal cell carcinoma via image guided needle electrodes. *J. Urol.* **161**, 599–600.

Moertel, C., Dockerty, M., and Baggenstoss, A. (1961). Multiple primary malignant neoplasms: III. Tumors of multicentric origin. *Cancer* **14**, 238–48.

Morgan, W. and Zincke, H. (1990). Progression and survival after renal conserving surgery for renal cell carcinoma, experience in 104 patients and extended followup. *J. Urol.* **144**, 852–7.

Murphy, G. and Mostofi, F. (1970). Histologic assessment and clinical progress of renal adenoma. *J. Urol.* **103**, 31–6.

Nakata, S., Ohtake, N., Kubota, Y., Imai, K., Yamanaka, K., Ito, Y., Hirayama, N., and Hasegawa, K. (1998). Incidence of urogenital cancers in Gunma Prefecture, Japan: a 10-year summary. *Int. J. Urol.* **5** (4), 364–9.

Niceforo, J. and Coughlin, B.F. (1993). Diagnosis of renal cell carcinoma: value of fine-needle aspiration cytology in patients with metastases or contraindications to nephrectomy. *Am. J. Roentgenol.* **161**, 1303–5.

Novick, A.C., Zincke, H., and Neves, .RJ. (1986). Surgical enucleation for renal cell carcinoma. *J. Urol.* **135**, 235–8.

Novick, A., Gill, I., and Hobart, M. (1999). Laparoscopic renal cryoablation in 32 patients. *J. Urol.* **161** (suppl.), 191A.

Oesterling, J.E., Fishman, E.K., Goldman, S.M., *et al.* (1986). The management of renal angiomyolipoma. *J. Urol.* **135**, 1121–4.

Silver, D.A., Morash, C., Brenner, P., *et al.* (1997). Pathologic findings at the time of nephrectomy for renal mass. *Ann. Surg. Oncol.* **4**, 570–4.

Storkel, S., Eble, J.N., Adlakha, K., *et al.* (1997). Classification of renal cell carcinoma: Workgroup No. 1. Union Internationale Contre le Cancer (UICC) and the American Joint Committee on Cancer (AJCC). *Cancer* **80**, 987–9.

Sweeney, J.P., Thornhill, J.A., Graiger, R., *et al.* (1996). Incidentally detected renal cell carcinoma: pathological features, survival trends and implications for treatment [see comments]. *Br. J. Urol.* **78**, 351–3.

Thompson, I. and Peek, M. (1988). Improvement in survival of patients with renal cell carcinoma: the role of serendipitiously detected tumor. *J. Urol.* **140**, 487–90.

Tsui, K.H., Shvarts, O., Smith, R.B., Figlin, R., deKernion, J.B., and Belldegrun, A. (2000). Renal cell carcinoma: prognostic significance of incidentally detected tumors. *J. Urol.* **163**, 426–30.

Uchida, M., Imaide, Y., and Sugimoto, K. (1995). Percutaneous cryosurgery for renal tumors. *Br. J. Urol.* **75**, 132–6.

Velagapudi, S., Rackle, H., and Zincke, H. (1993). Conservative surgery in patients with unilateral renal cell cancer and a normal contralateral unit: experience with 60 patients. *J. Urol.* **149**, 44A.

Walther, M.M., Choyke, P.L., and Hayes, W. (1994). Evaluation of color doppler intraoperative ultrasound in parenchymal sparing surgery. *J. Urol.* **152**, 1984–7.

Walther, M.M., Lyne, J.C., Libutti, S.K., *et al.* (1999a). Laparoscopic cytoreductive nephrectomy as preparation for administration of systemic interleukin-2 in the treatment of metastatic renal cell carcinoma: a pilot study. *Urology* **53**, 496–501.

Walther, M.M., Shawker, T., Choyke, P.L., Libutti, S., and Lineham, W.M. (1999b). *A phase II trial to evaluate radiofrequency interstitial tissue ablation (RITA) for the treatment of renal cancer.* American Urological Association, Dallas.

Zegel, H.G., Holland, G.A., Jennings, S.B., *et al.* (1998). Intraoperative ultrasonographically guided cryoablation of renal masses: initial experience. *J. Ultrasound Med.* **17**, 571–6.

4.   Epithelial tumors of the kidney

Stephen Stoerkel and Andreas Hinkel

Introduction

The purpose of tumor pathology is to understand etiology and pathogenesis and to classify tumor diseases, to determine patients' prognosis, and thus to guide clinicians to plan and justify their therapeutic regimens.

A multitude of tumors has been described in the kidney, such as benign renal tumors (for example, cystic lesions, adenomas, angiomyolipomas, and oncocytomas), tumors of the renal pelvis (for example, papillomas, and transitional cell carcinomas), para-enal tumors (mostly sarcomas), embryonal tumors (for example, nephroblastomas and related tumors), renal cell carcinomas (RCC), and other primary or secondary tumorous lesions of the kidney (Glenn 1980). The focus of this chapter is on epithelial renal tumors only.

Morphological classification of epithelial renal tumors has been a debatable field since the first description by Grawitz in 1883. In the past, the World Health Organization (WHO) had avoided sub-dividing renal tumors other than into adenoma and carcinoma. Recent progress in understanding the pathology of kidney tumors has led to a new morphological classification, which has been adopted in part by the WHO (Storkel *et al.* 1997).

Today, the most frequent epithelial kidney tumors can be subdi-vided into adenomas, of the oncocytic, papillary, and meta-nephrogenic types, and carcinomas, of the clear cell, papillary, chromophobe, collecting duct associated, transitional cell, and neuroendocrine types. Some additional rare and extraordinary types also exist. The classification no longer includes granular RCC, as this phenotype is part of several tumor types mentioned above. Even spindle cell RCC has been deleted as an entity, as spindle cells result from the dedifferentiation process that can develop in all types of renal carcinomas.

All kidney tumor types have a distinct histogenesis and thus express a specific immunohistological marker profile. While clear cell carcinomas and papillary carcinomas derive from the proximal tubule, oncocytomas and chromophobe carcinomas are related to the collecting duct along with collecting duct carcinomas.

Recent data have shown that each pathomorphological kidney tumor entity expresses specific chromosomal aberrations that fit completely the above-mentioned pathomorphological pheno-types. Besides structural and numerical chromosomal aberrations, some oncogenes and suppressor genes (von Hippel–Lindau (VHL)-gene, met-oncogene) are involved in the carcinogenesis of parenchymal renal tumors. Here for the first time a kidney tumor model combining both morphological and genetic features is presented, starting with the precursor cells in the renal tubule system via an adenoma stage to a fully developed RCC stage. Although some steps in this model are still hypothetical, it offers a better understanding of the puzzling kidney cancer complex. This novel view makes possible future research that may lead to more specific kidney cancer therapies.

Epidemiology

Renal cell carcinoma is the most common malignant tumor of the kidney and comprises 3 per cent of all human malignancies (Wingo *et al.* 1995). In Western industrial countries every 10th male and every 14th female will suffer from an RCC. In 1994 2.4 per cent of all deaths from cancer could be traced to RCC. RCC affects men and women in a 2–3:1 ratio to the disadvantage of the male population (Ernstoff *et al.* 1997).

The age-related incidence increases continuously from 35 years of age and peaks in the sixth decade (80 per cent of all RCC are discovered between ages 40 and 69 years). RCC (predominantly of the clear cell type) can appear in childhood and young adult-hood, possibly indicating a hereditary history (Petersen 1994).

RCC are discovered all over the world within any ethnic group, with an overall rising incidence. The highest incidence is found in Scandinavia measuring up to 7.5 per 100 000 inhabitants (La Vecchia *et al.* 1992; Tavani and La Vecchia 1997).

Despite the predominance of sporadic cases, hereditary RCC do exist and are discovered increasingly. The most well known disease is the von Hippel–Lindau syndrome (autosomal dominant), which is characterized by multiple and often bilateral develop-ment of clear cell RCC mainly in young male patients. Moreover, there are a few families suffering from RCC of the clear cell type without von Hippel–Lindau syndrome. Hereditary forms of papil-lary RCC have been described. More recently, hereditary renal oncocytomas have been detected. In addition, there is an asso-ciation between sickle cell anemia and collecting duct carcinoma, the adult form of polycystic kidney disease, and RCC of the clear cell type and the so-called end stage kidney and RCC of both clear cell and papillary type. The risk of developing kidney cancer is nine times higher in patients with chronic renal failure than in the normal population (Takahashi *et al.* 1993).

Etiology

Several epidemiologic studies have found a weak correlation between tobacco smoking and RCC, although the carcinogen has not yet been identified (Weir and Dunn 1970; Kantor 1977). Other substances that may have cancer-promoting properties are cadmium (Kolonel 1976) and thorium dioxide, which has been used as a radiographic agent (Thorotrast®) (Wenz 1967). The use of diuretics (for example, furosemide) as well as beta-blockers has also been incriminated as promoting the development of renal tumors. However, it remains unclear whether the antihypertensive drugs or hypertension itself is the actual risk factor (Mellemgaard *et al.* 1992; McLaughlin *et al.* 1995). Furthermore, obesity seems to be associated with a higher incidence of RCC (Mellemgaard *et al.* 1995; Boeing *et al.* 1997). Both effects, that of antihypertensive medication/hypertension and that of obesity, are more pronounced in the female than in the male population. In animal models the role of specific carcinogens such as nitroso compounds and arylamide compounds in inducing epithelial renal cell tumors has been clarified. There is only one substance that has unequivocally been shown to be nephrocarcinogenic: The metabolism of trichloroethene allows the formation of carcinogenic agents that cause renal adenomas and carcinomas in animal models (Henschler and Bonse 1977). Moreover, those genotoxic metabolites (*N*-acetyl-*S*-dichlorovinyl-L-cysteine) have also been detected in the urine of workers with occupational exposure to trichloroethene (Birner *et al.* 1993; Bernauer *et al.* 1996), some of whom developed RCC after a long period of intense exposure (Henschler *et al.* 1995; Vamvakas *et al.* 1998). However, the formation of toxic metabolites and the subsequent increased cancer risk are dependent on the polymorphism of certain glutathione transferases (GSTM1 and GSTT1) (Bruning *et al.* 1997*b*) and associated with somatic gene mutation, for example, of the VHL gene (Bruning *et al.* 1997*a*).

Histological classification

The classification of kidney tumors, initially described by Grawitz (1883), has changed during the last decade (Mostofi 1981; Thoenes *et al.* 1986) due to progress in pathology and genetics (Bostwick and Eble 1997; Storkel 1993). Parts of this tremendous increase in knowledge were published in monographs such as the *Atlas of tumor pathology*, Series 2, Fascicle no. 11 (Murphy *et al.* 1994) and 'Histological typing of kidney tumors' (Mostofi and Davie 1998) in *WHO, International histological classification of tumors.*

Nevertheless, in 1997 a consensus conference organized by the Union Internationale Contre le Cancer (UICC) and the American Joint Committee on Cancer (AJCC) defined a new kidney cancer classification that forms the basis of the following discussion (Storkel *et al.* 1997; Fig. 4.1). This new classification has its main roots in the cytologically and histologically oriented but, more recently, cytogenetically proven classification of Thoenes and co-workers (1986), which has been modified and extended (Storkel *et al.* 1989*a*; Thoenes *et al.* 1990; van den Berg *et al.* 1993). This

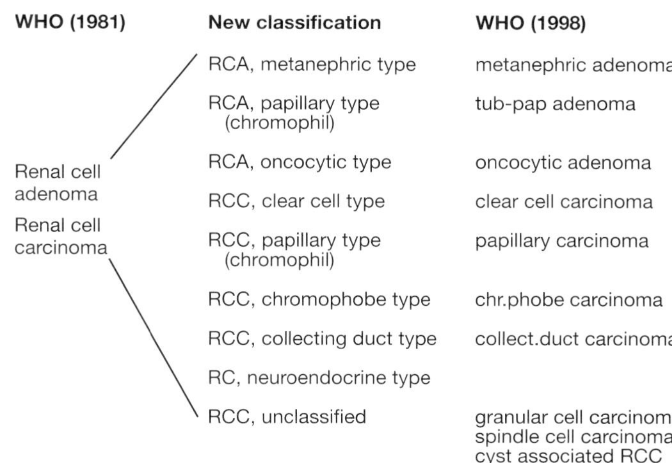

Fig. 4.1 Classification of kidney cancers

classification does not identify a separate granular cell subgroup as identified in the WHO classification as these cells are only seen as a component of other subtypes (Hartwick *et al.* 1992; Storkel *et al.* 1997). Table 4.1 presents an overview of the incidence of 2350 tumors in large surgical series according to the new classification. Morphological definition of adenoma and carcinoma of the kidney is still an unsolved problem. There is consensus on the grouping of oncocytic, metanephric, and some papillary types as an adenoma. All other types (clear cell, papillary (chromophil), chromophobe, duct Bellini, neuroendocrine, spindle cell/ pleomorphic, and unclassified) are malignant or potentially malignant and therefore termed carcinoma. There are extremely rare cases of multiple, synchronous, papillary (chromophil) or oncocytic tumors measuring only a few millimeters in diameter, termed renal adenomatosis. Apart from the misinterpretation of Bell's 3 cm rule (1938) in the literature Thoenes and co- workers (1986) have created a pragmatic proposal for routine diagnostics that includes grading and size of the tumor: Tumors with a

Table 4.1 Incidence of epithelial neoplasms of the kidney in a series of 2350 tumors of adults

Tumor type	ICDO no.	Incidence (per cent)
1. RCC, clear cell type	8312/3	73
2. RCC, papillary (chromophil) type	8320/3	12
3. RCA, oncocytic type	8290/0	5
4. RCC, chromophobe type	8310/3	5
5. RCC, duct Bellini type	8319/3	< 1
6. Transitional cell carcinoma (primarily intrarenal)	8120/3	< 1
7. Neuroendocrine tumors (carcinoid, small cell RCC, PNET)	8240/3, 8041/3, 9473/3	< 1
8. RCA, metanephric (embryonal)	—	< 1
9. RCC, spindle cell/pleom. type	8033/3	< 1
10. RCC, unclassified	8312/3	< 1

diameter below 1 cm and malignancy grade 1 are termed adenomas, tumors with a diameter between 1 and 3 cm and malignancy grade 1 are termed tumors of low metastatic potential or of unknown dignity, and tumors more than 3 cm in diameter with malignancy grade 1 as well as tumors of any size presenting with malignancy grade 2 or higher are termed carcinoma.

Pathologic staging

The TNM (tumor–node–metastasis) classification of the Union International Contre le Cancer (UICC) is internationally binding. It has recently been changed. The major difference between the 1992 and the 1997 TM classifications is the increased size of T1 tumors, which may now measure up to 7 cm in diameter provided they don't extend outside the kidney. The 1992 and the 1997 TNM classifications are displayed in Table 4.2.

Patients suffering from RCC stages I and II according to the TNM stage groupings have an excellent prognosis after radical nephrectomy, with a 5-year-survival rate of 90–100 per cent, a very low rate of local recurrences, and a probability of lymph node or distant metastasis of below 15 per cent. Patients with locally advanced non-metastasized RCC (T3) are at high risk for recurrences. Their 5-year-survival rate after radical surgery is about 60 per cent. Stage IV RCC has a very poor prognosis. Distant metastasis especially is almost predictive of a life expectancy of less than 3 years, even after radical tumor nephrectomy (Giuliani *et al.* 1990; Goepel and Rubben 1991). Although 5-year-survival rates are very favorable for T1 and T2 tumors, a significant number of late recurrences is observed when 10- and 15-year-survial rates are taken into account. After such long follow-up periods survival rates do not differ significantly between tumors classified as T1–T3b N0 M0 at the time of initial diagnosis (Dinney *et al.* 1992).

While many urologists support the 1997 TNM classification because of a better stratification of patients with a very favorable prognosis (Javidan *et al.* 1999), others feel uneasy calling a tumor T1 that measures 7 cm in diameter (Kinouchi *et al.* 1999*a*). As

Table 4.2 Comparison of 1992 and 1997 UICC TNM classifications of renal cell carcinoma (bold face indicates changes in classification)

TNM (1992)	TNM (1997)
Primary tumor (T)	
TX Primary tumor cannot be assessed	TX Primary tumor cannot be assessed
T0 No evidence of primary tumor	T0 No evidence of primary tumor
T1 Tumor ≤ 2.5 cm in greatest dimension limited to the kidney	**T1 Tumor ≤ 7 cm in greatest dimension limited to the kidney**
T2 Tumor > 2.5 cm in greatest dimension limited to the kidney	**T2 Tumor > 7 cm in greatest dimension limited to the kidney**
T3 Tumor extends into major veins or invades adrenal gland or perinephric tissues but not beyond Gerota's fascia	T3 Tumor extends into major veins or invades adrenal gland or perinephric tissues but not beyond Gerota's fascia
T3a Tumor invades adrenal gland or perinephric tissues but not beyond Gerota's fascia	T3a Tumor invades adrenal gland or perinephric tissues but not beyond Gerota's fascia
T3b Tumor grossly extends into renal vein(s) or vena cava below diaphragm	T3b Tumor grossly extends into renal vein(s) or vena cava below diaphragm
T3c Tumor grossly extends into vena cava above diaphragm	T3c Tumor grossly extends into vena cava above diaphragm
T4 Tumor invades beyond Gerota's fascia	T4 Tumor invades beyond Gerota's fascia
Regional lymph nodes (N)	
NX Regional lymph nodes cannot be assessed	NX Regional lymph nodes cannot be assessed
N0 No regional lymph node metastasis	N0 No regional lymph node metastasis
N1 Metastasis in a single lymph node, ≤ 2 cm in greatest dimension	**N1 Metastasis in a single regional lymph node**
N2 Metastasis in a single lymph node, > 2 cm but not > 5 cm in greatest dimension; or multiple lymph nodes, none > 5 cm in greatest dimension	**N2 Metastasis in more than a single regional lymph node**
N3 Metastasis in a lymph node > 5 cm in greatest dimension	
Distant metastasis (M)	
MX Distant metastasis cannot be assessed	MX Distant metastasis cannot be assessed
M0 No distant metastasis	M0 No distant metastasis
M1 Distant metastasis	M1 Distant metastasis

TNM (1992)				TNM (1997)			
Stage grouping							
	T	N	M		T	N	M
Stage I	1	0	0	Stage I	1	0	0
Stage II	2	0	0	Stage II	2	0	0
Stage III	1	1	0	Stage III	1	1	0
	2	1	0		2	1	0
	3	0, 1	0		3	0, 1	0
Stage IV	4	any	0	Stage IV	4	**0, 1**	0
	any	2, 3	0		any	**2**	0
	any	any	1		any	any	1

regards nephron-sparing surgery, tumors should not exceed 4 cm in diameter in order to be resectable (Belldegrun *et al.* 1999; Hafez *et al.* 1999).

However, tumor size alone is not a definite predictor of prognosis. Prognosis is mainly determined by tumor biology. Therefore, staging according to the TNM system has to be combined with histopathologic and biologic features in order to be conclusive for clinical decision-making. Patients suffering from poorly differentiated RCC as compared to well differentiated tumors have a markedly worse prognosis, even if the primary tumor is small (Storkel *et al.* 1990; Ditonno *et al.* 1992). Sarcomatoid variants are seen in all histological subtypes of RCC, and are associated with poor prognosis (Storkel *et al.* 1997). Moreover, classical RCC originating from the collecting duct (duct Bellini carcinomas) are very aggressive regardless of their size, and develop into systemic disease rapidly (Weiss *et al.* 1995). However, in chromophobic RCC grade 1 and 2 (G1–2) the probability of metastatic spread is extremely low. Papillary RCC are frequently (up to 40 per cent) associated with multifocality and tend to present at a lower stage than clear cell RCC, thus having a better overall prognosis (Amin *et al.* 1997).

Morphology of epithelial renal tumors

RCC, clear cell type (synonym: RCC, conventional type)

Gross features

Clear cell RCC are characterized by a multinodular and multicolored tumor mass with a predominantly yellow cut surface and additional gray and white foci. The yellow nodes correspond to well differentiated and the white nodes to moderately or poorly differentiated tumor areas. In most of the cases a solid growth pattern is detected in clear cell RCC. However, some patients present with cystic conventional type RCC composed of multiple cysts, varying in size up to 2–3 cm in diameter. Tumor regression results in white sclerotic septa, focal calcifications, circumscript potentially liquefied necroses, and irregular hemorrhages (Helpap 1993).

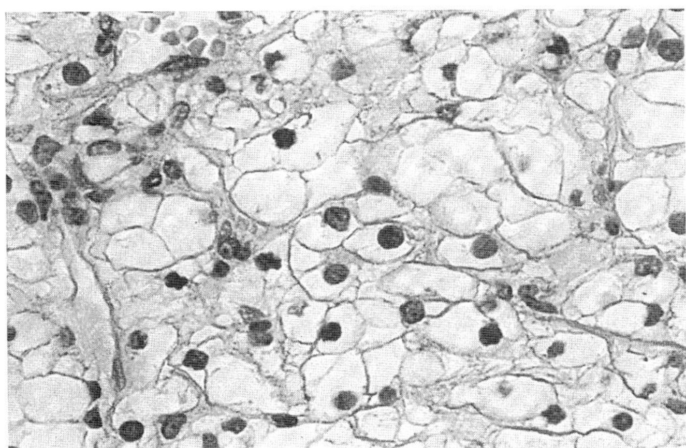

Fig. 4.2 RCC, clear cell type

Microscopic features

Light microscopy reveals a clear cytoplasm in the basic clear cell type, more or less empty after staining with hematoxylin and eosin (H & E) (Fig. 4.2). This is the result of an intense intracytoplasmic accumulation of glycogen, phospholipids, and neutral lipids due increased glucose-6-phosphate levels, activated glycolysis, and reduced gluconeogenesis. Simultaneously, the clear cells present a stepwise decrease of cholesterol deposits with an increasing malignancy grade (Saito *et al.* 1991; Steinberg *et al.* 1992). The nuclei of well differentiated tumor cells are condensed and hyperchromatic. However, in less differentiated tumor cells nuclei appear polymorphic accompanied by prominent nucleoli (Farrow *et al.* 1968). Nuclear features correlate with DNA content (Storkel 1989). Ultrastructurally, brush border equivalents and pinocytotic vesicles can be found occasionally as well as basal infoldings, analogous to those observed in the epithelial cells of the proximal tubule. In addition, there are two eosinophilic variants associated with higher grades of malignancy. Those variants are characterized by cytoplasmic eosinophilia or cytoplasmic granularity, respectively, either in the vicinity of the nucleus or more or less diffusely distributed within the cytoplasm due to the augmentation of mitochondria. Sarcomatoid or pleomorphic phenotypes are often found in clear cell RCC. Usually they are associated with more differentiated tumor tissue, but exclusive sarcomatoid differentiation can also be detected (Ro *et al.* 1987; Remmele 1997). There is a positive correlation between the extent of intratumoral and peritumoral lymphocytic infiltration and increasing grade of malignancy (Storkel *et al.* 1992a).

RCA/RCC, papillary (synonym: RCC, chromophilic cell type)

Gross features

Papillary renal cell tumors are characterized by a ball-shaped outline and a dotted pattern. Tumors with a diameter up to some millimeters, usually adenomas, tend to be beige- or white-colored, while larger tumors, usually carcinomas, exhibit extended greasy brown-colored central necrosis resulting from poor vascular supply and consecutive hemorrhages. Sometimes there are yellow glittering spots consisting of foamy cell accumulations mainly in the tumor periphery just beneath the fibrous pseudocapsule.

Microscopic features

Using light microscopy, the basic cell type in papillary tumors exhibits a less basophilic stained cytoplasm and overlapping centrally located small nuclei (cell type 1) (Matsumoto *et al.* 1992; Fig. 4.3). Electron microscopy reveals a cytoplasm covered with few organelles only, predominantly endoplasmic reticulum. Rudimentary microvilli develop from the apical cell pole as well as extensive basal infoldings covered with basal membrane material, resembling cellular features of the proximal tubule. Increasing dedifferentiation results in enlarged nuclei with prominent nucleoli and an eosinophilic or granular cytoplasm due to an accumulation of mitochondria (cell type 2). In general, the tumors express a papillary or tubulopapillary growth pattern, but become solid in undifferentiated tumor areas. The papillary stalks are often crowded with characteristic lipid-loaded macrophages and focal psammoma bodies. Developing tumors are often associated

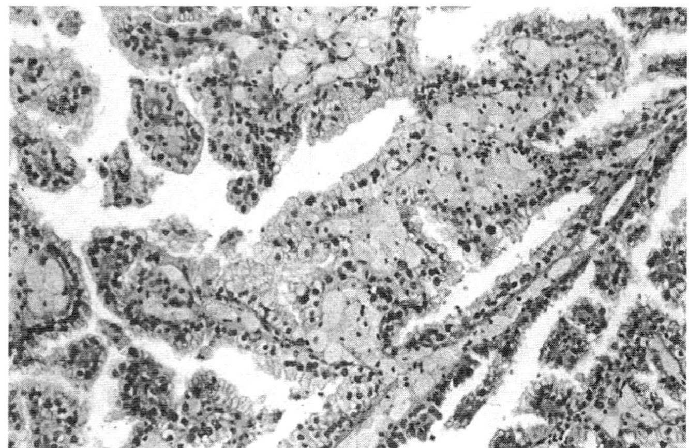

Fig. 4.3 RCC, papillary type

with cortical scars and absence of peritumoral capsule formation (Spiegel *et al.* 1991).

Renal cell adenoma (RCA)/RCC, chromophobic cell type

Gross features
Depending on size, chromophobic renal cell tumors consist of one or more solid tumor nodules with a slightly lobulated surface. In unfixed conditions the cut surface appears homogeneously orange, turning beige or sandy after formalin fixation. The uniform pale cut surface interspersed with a few hemorrhages is a very characteristic gross feature of this predominantly well differentiated tumor type, while a slight brown-colored cut surface is usually associated with moderately or poorly differentiated tumors (Thoenes *et al.* 1985).

Microscopic features
The basic chromophobic cell type is characterized by large polygonal cells with a transparent slightly reticulated cytoplasm and prominent cell membranes resembling the appearance of a plant cell (Thoenes *et al.* 1985; Fig. 4.4). Another diagnostic hallmark is the lack of cytoplasmatic coloring with routine dyes but a diffuse

cytoplasmatic staining reaction with Hale's iron colloid, which is a characteristic feature of this special tumor type only (Bonsib *et al.* 1993). Electron microscopically, the cytoplasm is crowded by loose glycogen deposits and numerous invaginated or studded vesicles, 150–300 nm in diameter, resembling those of the intercalated type b cells of the cortical collecting duct (Eble 1990; Storkel *et al.* 1989*b*). Immunohistochemical results point in the same direction (Ortmann and Vierbuchen 1989; Ortmann *et al.* 1991). Increased malignancy of chromophobic tumors is also associated with an increased cytoplasmic eosinophilia or granularity due to augmentation of mitochondria as mentioned above. Well differentiated tumors show condensed hyperchromatic, and sometimes binucleated nuclei becoming more atypical with increasing grade of malignancy or dedifferentiation, respectively. In general, the growth pattern is compact. Sometimes cribriform patterns are detected, associated with focal psammoma-like calcifications.

RCC, ductus Bellini type (synonym: collecting duct carcinoma; special types: medullary carcinoma in children; collecting duct carcinoma associated with sickle cell trait)

Gross features
Ductus Bellini carcinomas are usually large tumors located in the medulla or central parts of the kidney with extension into the perinephric fat and invasion of the renal pelvis (Dimopoulos *et al.* 1993). The white-colored and firm cut surface is interspersed with necroses and presents an irregular border with peritumoral cortical satellite nodules and parenchyma infarctions as a result of severe angioinvasiveness (Rumpelt *et al.* 1991). Regional spread with infiltration of the adrenal glands and lymph node metastases are common.

Microscopic features
Light microscopically, the basic cell type of duct Bellini carcinoma exhibits medium-sized tumor cells with a basophilic, sometimes light cytoplasm due to a pronounced formation of endoplasmic reticulum and varying degrees of glycogen deposits (Kennedy *et al.* 1990). Anaplastic nuclei are usually found. Electron microscopically, the lateral and basal cell membranes are oriented linearly without interdigitations and invaginations resembling features of principal cells of the medullary collecting duct. An eosinophilic (granular) cell variant as well as spindle cell/ polymorphic/sarcomatoid cell type is often found (Baer *et al.* 1993). In general, the growth pattern is tubular, combined with a microcystic, pseudopapillary, and solid pattern associated with intense desmoplastic stromal reaction as well as granulocytic infiltration (Fig. 4.5).

RCC, transitional cell type

Gross features
RCC of the transitional cell type express the same morphologic spectrum as those observed in other parts of the urinary tract. The solid or planar tumors occupy intensively medullary and central parts of the kidney and present a few papillary formations at the site of renal pelvis infiltration only. They consist of variably sized, single to multiple, tan–gray, nodular or papillary structures

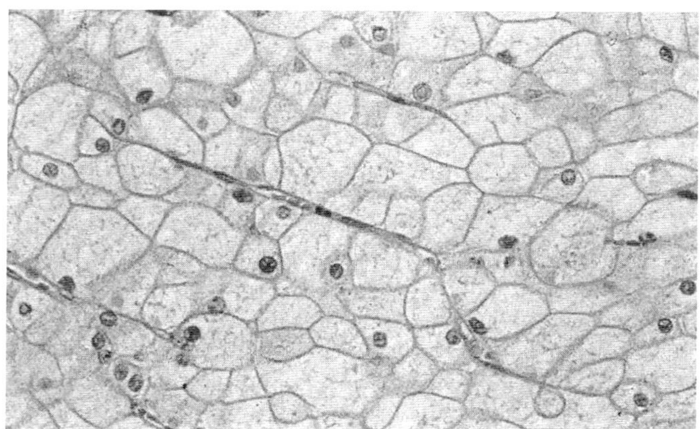

Fig. 4.4 RCC, chromophobic cell type

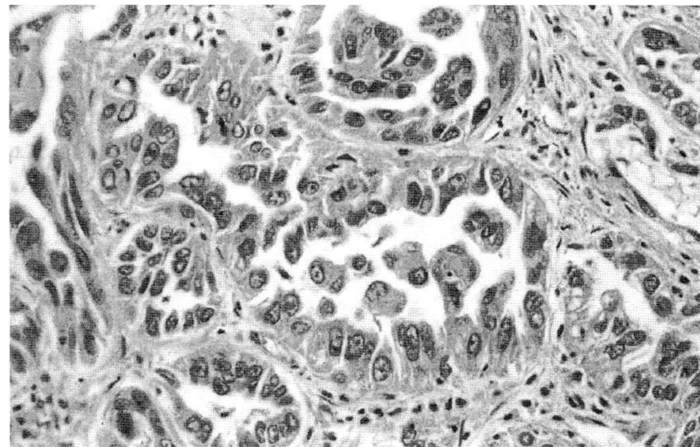

Fig. 4.5 collecting duct cell type

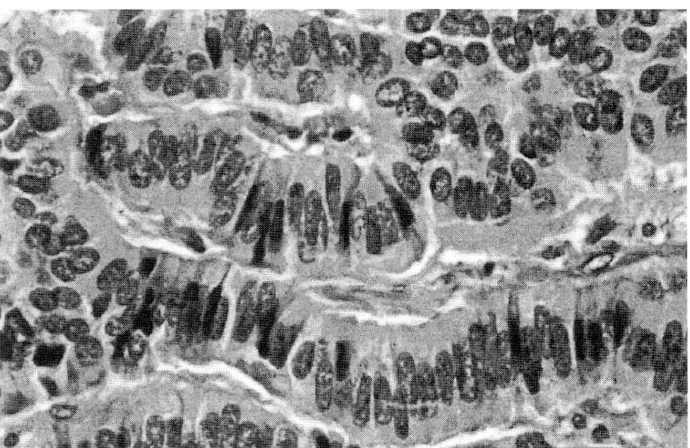

Fig. 4.7 RCC, neuroendocrine cell type

intermingled with focal necrosis and hemorrhages. Hilar infiltration and transrenal extension through the capsule into the perinephric fat are often found, similar to the findings in RCC, duct Bellini type.

Microscopic features
The light microscopical spectrum of transitional cell carcinoma of the kidney ranges from cells closely resembling normal urothelium (grade 1) to pleomorphic or undifferentiated transitional cell carcinoma cells (grade 3/4; Fig. 4.6). Nuclear atypia, number of mitoses, altered polarity, and cytoplasmic pleomorphism in general increase with dedifferentiation (Remmele 1997). Electron microscopically, straightened cell membranes, some pleomorphic microvilli, and a loss of desmosomes can be demonstrated on the cell surface. Invasion takes place in narrow irregular trabeculae, sometimes accompanied by an inflammatory reaction of the connective tissue stroma.

RCC, neuroendocrine cell type

Gross features
These aggressive tumors are usually large in size at the time of operation, and present with a widespread and diffuse destruction

of the kidney parenchyma, invasion of the renal pelvis and perirenal fatty tissue, and pronounced hemangio- and lymphangioinvasion. Neuroendocrine RCC are not sharply demarcated and are of solid consistency. The gray-colored tumor masses are often interspersed with dark and mollificated necroses (Gouillou *et al.* 1993).

Microscopic features
The RCC of neuroendocrine type show a broad spectrum of differentiation ranging from less differentiated small cell variants (oat cell type) to the well differentiated classical eosinophilic columnar cell type (carcinoid) (Huettner *et al.* 1991; Fig. 4.7). Ultrastructurally, these tumors contain various amounts of intracytoplasmic membrane-bound granules with dense cores ranging from 150 to 400 nm in diameter. Silver stains (that is, Bodian or Grimelius stain) can be utilized successfully for staining these hormone precursors. The small cell variant nuclei are hyperchromatic and oval with abundant mitoses. However, the nuclei of more differentiated forms are round in shape with less anaplasia. A mixture of broad trabeculae and anastomosing cords embedded in a well vascularized stroma form the characteristic growth pattern of neuroendocrine RCC (Ishikawa and Kovacs 1993).

RCA, oncocytic cell type

Gross features
True RCA of the oncocytic type (oncocytomas) are solitary, in rare instances multiple, round and slightly lobulated solid tumors with a tan to brown cut surface and a stellate central scar in the case of bigger tumors only. After removing the peritumoral fibrous capsule, a gyrus-like pattern appears with twisted venous vessels within the invaginations. Necroses have never been found, but focal bleeding and invasion of adjacent structures are present.

Microscopic features
Light microscopically, this basic cell type is characterized by isomorphic tumor cells with a coarsely granulated eosinophilic cytoplasm due to accumulations of enlarged mitochondria (Fig. 4.8), which express pathologic cristae structures, and a disturbed intramembranous arrangement of molecules, typical

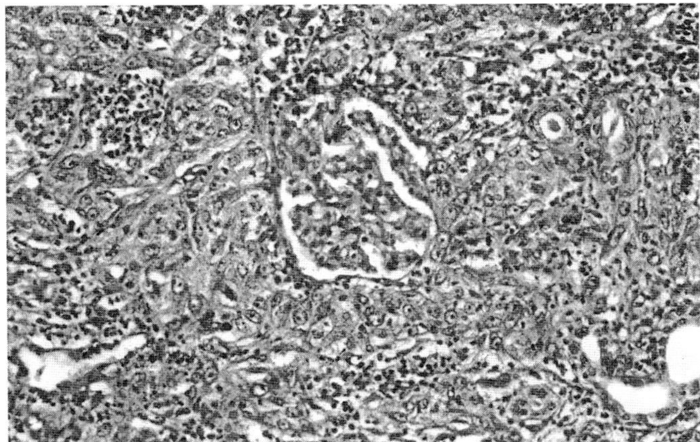

Fig. 4.6 RCC, urothelial cell type

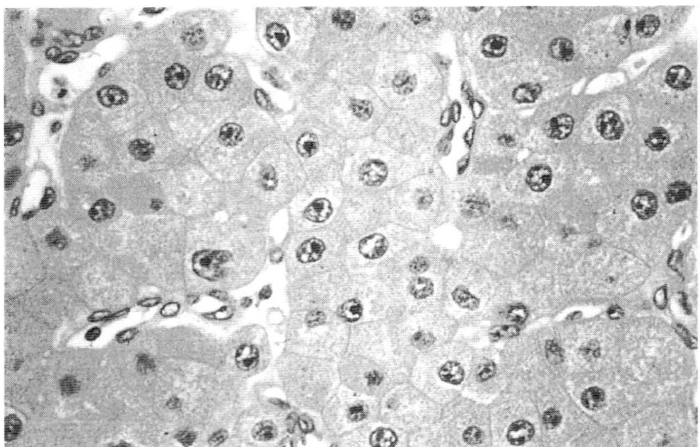

Fig. 4.8 RCC, oncocytic cell type

for oncocytomas only. Usually round, vesicular, centrally located nuclei can be found. They focally become polymorphic as a result of polyploidization. An increase of binucleated cells with overlapping nuclei is of differential diagnostic importance. The growth pattern is solid and trabecular with typical acinar or nest-like formations close to the regressive zones in the central tumor areas (Barnes and Beckman 1983). Tubulocystic areas and hemorrhages, but no necroses, can be found. Peritumoral and centrally radiating large-sized blood vessels as well as entrapped kidney tubules in the tumor periphery are also of diagnostic importance. Ultrastructurally and immunohistochemically, oncocytomas show similarity to intercalated cells of the collecting duct system (Storkel *et al.* 1988).

RCA, *metanephric type (special type: metanephric adenofibroma)*

Gross features
These rare tumors present as single, solid, well demarcated tumors with a light brown to sandy cut surface of glassy quality. They are sharply demarcated and composed of several nodules arising in

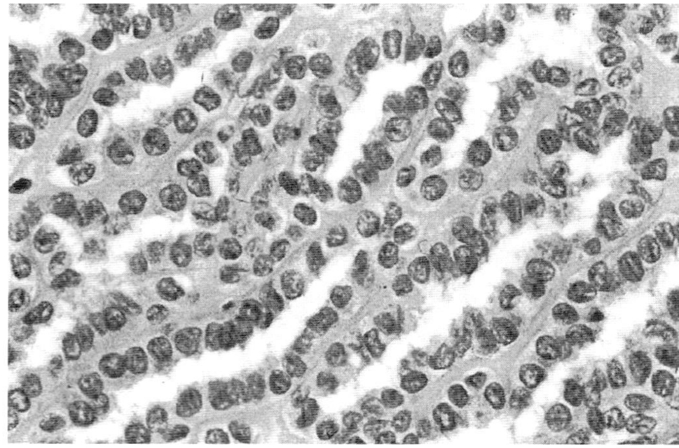

Fig. 4.9 RCC, metanephric cell type

the cortex and streakened with small fibrous septa. Necroses and mollifications are absent (Storkel *et al.* 1992*b*).

Microscopic features
Metanephric adenomas are composed of densely packed small tumor cells with overlapping nuclei and invisible cell borders in solid appearing areas, turning to a polar orientation in case of more differentiated tubular or tubulopapillary structures (Nagashima *et al.* 1991; Fig. 4.9). Electron micorscopically, the cytoplasmic equipment is scanty with only a few organelles, rudimentary apical microvilli, and some basal membrane formations. The nuclei are innocent in appearance. Only a few typical mitoses are found. The tumor stroma is not, or scarcely, developed, and psammoma-like calcified bodies are typical, especially for sclerotic zones in the tumor periphery.

Immunohistochemistry of kidney tumors

Immunohistochemistry can be very helpful in the differential diagnosis of renal neoplasms, as each tumor entity is characterized by a special antigen pattern (Banner *et al.* 1990). In general, most of the kidney cancers present antigens that are associated with specific segments or cell types in the tubular and collecting duct system, offering histogenetic relationships. Table 4.3 includes commercially available antibodies for diagnostics that allow characterization of tissue and cellular antigens involved in differentiation and histogenesis.

Pathomorphologic classification and cytogenetic correlation

New cytogenetic and molecular genetic data confirm the morphologic classification of epithelial kidney tumors outlined above and present the first evidence for tumor initiation and tumor progression, according to an adenoma–carcinoma sequence (Anglard *et al.* 1991; Kovacs 1993; Presti *et al.* 1993; van den Berg 1993; van der Hout *et al.* 1993) (Fig. 4.10). They are also associated with chromosomal abnormalities in non-neoplastic renal tissue (Casalone *et al.* 1992; Dal Cin *et al.* 1992).

Renal cell carcinomas of the clear cell type can be divided into sporadic and hereditary forms (Gnarra *et al.* 1993; LaForgia *et al.* 1993). They have in common either the partial (p-segment) or complete loss of chromosome 3 or a gene mutation in that area, resulting in the loss of one or more tumor suppressor genes (Tory *et al.* 1989; Zbar *et al.* 1987). Whilst the VHL gene is located at 3p25–26 (the gene is almost completely cloned; Latif *et al.* 1993), there are some regions of interest for suppressor genes in sporadic cases, located at 3p21–22 and 3p13–14 (Shuin *et al.* 1994). Recent studies have shown that multiple somatic gene mutations in sporadic renal cell cancers and surrounding normal kidney tissue can be induced by long-lasting and high-dosage exposure to trichloroethylene, an industrial solvent used in the metal industry (Bruning *et al.* 1997*a*). Whether the VHL-

Table 4.3 Immunohistochemical differential diagnosis of kidney tumors

Tumor type	CK 8–18	CK 13	CK 19	VIM	UEA 1	CD 34	Des Min	Actin	HMB 45	NSE + S 100	Chro mogr	N-CAM	CLA	MIB 1
RCC, clear cell type (incl. multiloc. cyst. RCC)	+	–	(+)	+	–	–	–	–	–	–	–	–	–	+/+++
RCC, papillary type (chromophil)	+	–	(+)	+	–	–	–	–	–	–	–	–	–	+/+++
RCA, oncocytic type	+	–	(+)	–	–	–	–	–	–	–	–	–	–	(+)
RCC, chromophobe type	+	–	(+)	–	+	–	–	–	–	–	–	–	–	+/
RCC, ductus Bellini type	+	–	+	(+)	+	–	–	–	–	–	–	–	–	+
RCC, neuroendocrine type	+	–	–	–	–	–	–	–	–	+	+	–	–	+/+
RCA, metanephric type	(+)	–	(+)	+	–	–	–	–	–	–	–	–	–	(+)
Nephroblastoma (incl. cystic variants)	(+)	–	–	+	–	–	(+)	(+)	–	(+)	–	+	–	+
Cystic nephroma	+	–	+	+	(+)	–	+	–	–	–	–	–	–	(+)
Leiomyoma/leiomyo-SA	(+)	–	–	+	–	–	+	+	–	–	–	–	–	(+)/+
Rhabdomyo-SA	(+)	–	–	+	–	–	+	–	–	(+)	–	–	–	+
Hemangioma/Hemangio-SA	(+)	–	–	+	+	+	–	–	–	–	–	–	–	(+)/+
Hemangiopericytoma	–	–	–	+	–	–	–	–	–	–	–	–	–	
Angiomyolipoma (incl. Epitheloid variant)	(+)	–	–	+	–	(+)	(+)	+	+	(+)	–	–	–	+
Lipoma/Lipo-SA	–	–	–	+	–	–	–	–	–	+	–	–	–	(+)/+
Chondro-SA	–	–	–	+	–	–	–	–	–	+	–	–	–	+/+
MFH	(+)	–	–	+	–	(+)	+	+	–	–	–	–	–	+
Malignant lymphoma	–	–	–	+	–	(+)	–	–	–	–	–	–	+	+/+

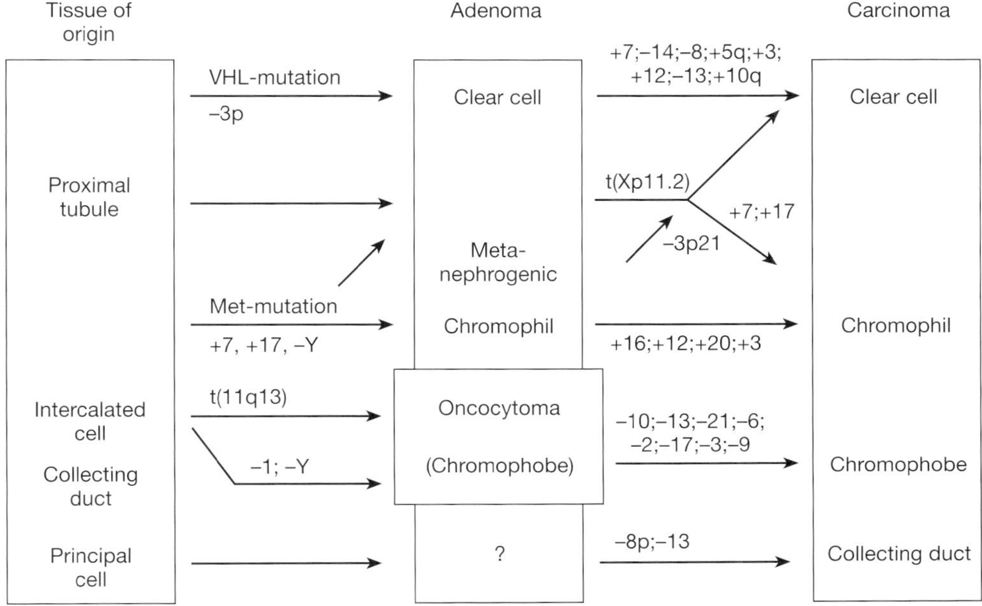

Fig. 4.10 Genetic model of renal carcinoma development

mutation alone or in combination with different mutated, lost, or amplified genes can initiate the whole spectrum of clear cell carcinoma is not known. That is why in our model a hypothetical clear cell adenoma is proposed. In case of dedifferentiation of clear cell carcinomas (from G1 to G3) there is an overexpression of chromosome 7, 5q, and 10 (Morita *et al.* 1991). Metastases are associated with an amplification of the 1q segment. It is remarkable with respect to genotype/phenotype correlation that, in rare cases of oncocytic phenotype developing in clear cell carcinomas, a translocation t(6;11)(p21;q13) has been found, the breakpoint of which is identical in oncocytic adenoma.

Renal cell adenomas of the papillary (chromophil) type present with trisomy 7 and tri- or tetrasomy 17 (Kovacs 1989; Presti *et al.* 1991). In addition, during progression towards papillary RCC there is an overexpression on chromosomes 16, 12, and 3q, which is complicated by trisomy 10 in case of further dedifferentiation (G3). Recent data have shown that mutation of the met-oncogene seems to be the primary genomic lesion. Bilateral synchronous and asynchronous tumors are described (Henn *et al.* 1993). Also translocation cases (X;1) exist (Meloni *et al.* 1993).

Renal cell carcinomas of the chromophobe type are characterized by a massive loss of chromosomes, that is −1, −2, −6, −10, −13, −17, and −21 (Kovacs and Kovacs 1992; Kovacs *et al.* 1992). These data were confirmed by fluorescence *in situ* hybridization (FISH) and comparative genomic hybridization (CGH) analysis (Speicher *et al.* 1994).

The rare cases of *renal cell carcinoma of the ductus Bellini type* present aberrations on chromosomes 8p- and 13; contradictory results were first published and revealed monosomy 1, 6, 14, 15, and 22 (Fuzesi *et al.* 1992).

There are no proven data on *carcinomas of the neuroendocrine type* in the kidney. Numerical and structural aberrations of chromosome 13 seem to be involved.

Renal cell adenomas of oncocytic type form a cytogenetically heterogeneous group. There is one group characterized by loss of chromosome −Y and −1 and telomeric associations, and another group characterized by reciprocal translocation t(5;11)(q35;q13) (Kovacs *et al.* 1987; Crotty *et al.* 1992; Dobin *et al.* 1992; van den Berg *et al.* 1994). This raises the question whether there exists a genetic relationship between oncocytic adenoma and chromophobe carcinoma (adenoma–carcinoma sequence) as a result of increasing genetic alterations. The morphologic spectrum of phenotypically oncocytoid/oncocytic tumors of the kidney is large (Fig. 4.10). It includes mesenchymal tumors such as angioleiomyolipoma and epithelial tumors, starting with the classical oncocytoma ranging to the eosinophilic and oncyocytic variant of chromophobe RCC.

There are only a few data on *renal cell adenomas of the metanephric type*. Numerical or structural aberrations were not found but recent investigations indicate that mutation of the met-oncogene is involved at the beginning.

Summarizing the pathomorphologic and cytogenetic data there is a fascinating picture of the subtypes of epithelial renal tumors, which opens the door to a better understanding of the complex initial mechanisms of tumor differentiation and progression. For the first time it allows the creation of a model that also describes the morphologically based entities cytogenetically (Fig. 4.11). This

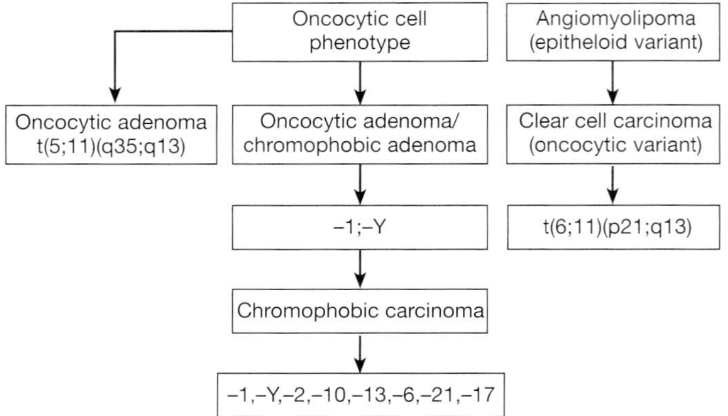

Fig. 4.11 Genotypes of oncocytic kidney tumors

offers new starting points for basic science for possibilities research into differential therapy. Novel immunologic and gene therapeutic studies based on the above-mentioned results are underway.

Other prognostic indicators

Nuclear morphometry assesses nuclear parameters, such as increased nuclear area and variations in nuclear shape, and provides independent information about an unfavorable prognosis (Delahunt *et al.* 1994). The proliferation index of RCC, as determined by immunohistochemical staining with either Ki-67 or MIB-1, seems to correlate with both local tumor stage and long-term survival (de Riese *et al.* 1993; Hofmockel *et al.* 1995). However, DNA content, as determined by flow cytometry or image analysis, is inconclusive for predicting prognosis in RCC (Flint *et al.* 1995). Moreover, apoptosis markers such as BCL-2, p21, or P53 have not been proven to be of prognostic value in RCC.

Decreasing expression of alpha-catenin, which is an intracellular ligand of cadherins, seems to independently correlate with an adverse prognosis (Shimazui *et al.* 1997). An imbalance between matrix metalloproteinases (MMP-2 and -9) and their endogenous inhibitors (TIMP-1 and -2) seems to promote metastasis (Kugler *et al.* 1998). Urokinase plasminogen activator inhibitor (uPAI-1) overexpression, which is regulated by the VHL gene, also correlates with increased metastatic potential and poor survival (Hofmann *et al.* 1996, Los *et al.* 1999).

In several recently published articles, new markers have been described that may hold potential as prognostic indicators: The expression of cyclin A has been found to correlate with venous invasion, high nuclear grade, and high proliferation index. Statistical analysis has revealed that cyclin A is an independent prognostic marker in all clinical stages of RCC (Aaltomaa *et al.* 1999). Elevated soluble CD95 (Fas) detected in the serum of RCC patients might also be an independent prognostic factor indicating lower probability of survival (Kimura *et al.* 1999). The expression of CD44H, which is involved in interaction between the cells and the extracellular matrix, has been associated with aggressive behavior of RCC. It might serve as an independent prognosticator for both overall and disease-free survival (Paradis *et al.* 1999). Transforming growth factor beta(TGFβ, which may be down-regulated by the VHL gene, seems to promote the growth of RCC *in vitro* and *in vivo* (Ananth *et al.* 1999). Platelet endothelial cell adhesion molecule (PECAM-1) expression by endothelial cells facilitates the migration of leukocytes into tumor deposits and thus promotes an immune response (Anastassiou *et al.* 1996). An isoform of the glycolytic enzyme pyruvate kinase, named Tu M2-PK, is strongly expressed in RCC as compared to normal kidney tissue. It is correlated with tumor stage and, moreover, seems to fall to normal levels within 11 weeks of complete surgical removal of RCC. In metastatic or recurrent disease Tu M2-PK remains high or rises, respectively (Oremek *et al.* 1999; Wechsel *et al.* 1999). However, the intriguing findings about those potential new markers remain to be confirmed by other investigators.

Clinical aspects

Radical versus nephron-sparing surgery

The results of nephron-sparing surgery are excellent in selected patients. Kidney-preserving surgery for small tumor lesions is equally as effective as radical nephrectomy in terms of local cancer control and long-term survival (Novick 1998; Belldegrun *et al.* 1999). There are elective and non-elective indications (for example, solitary kidney, bilateral tumors) to perform organ-preserving surgery. Bilateral tumors represent fewer than 5 per cent of all RCC cases. Most of these tumors are sporadic non-hereditary RCC (87.5 per cent) and present synchronously in both kidneys (Grimaldi *et al.* 1998). Therapy-related complications are more frequent in patients with a solitary kidney undergoing nephron-sparing surgery than in those with a normal contralateral kidney (Duque *et al.* 1998). Surgery of small central lesions by nephron-sparing surgery is technically more demanding than in peripheral lesions but can be performed equally effectively as by the radical surgical approach (Hafez *et al.* 1998). Intraoperative frozen sections may not only be useful in demonstrating complete tumor resection but also in determining tumor stage in patients undergoing elective nephron-sparing surgery (Campbell *et al.* 1996). The follow-up after organ-preserving RCC surgery should be more rigorous in patients with pathological (p) stage T2 or T3 including chest X-rays every year and abdominal CT scans (pT2: every 2 years; pT3: every 6 months for the first 2 years, every 2 years thereafter). PT1 tumors only require yearly medical history, physical examination, and laboratory work-up (Hafez *et al.* 1997).

However, there is some objection to such a therapeutic approach due to the existence of satellite tumors that may represent both intrarenal spreading of a primary tumor and synchronous multifocal tumor lesions. The overall incidence of satellite tumors in unifocal RCC is about 6.5 per cent and still amounts to almost 4 per cent in T1 and T2 lesions (Oya *et al.* 1995; Kinouchi *et al.* 1999*b*). It increases significantly when comparing tumors below 2 cm to tumors between 2 and 4 cm in diameter (Wunderlich *et al.* 1999*a*).

There is also controversy about the maximum size of RCC suitable for nephron-sparing surgery. Tumors measuring below 2.5 cm in diameter show significantly lower frequencies of capsular invasion, lymph node, and distant metastasis as well as lower grading than tumors larger than 2.5 cm or even 4 cm in diameter (Miller *et al.* 1999). Cancer-free survival in resected tumors measuring below 4 cm is significantly better than in those between 4 and 7 cm (Lerner *et al.* 1996; Hafez *et al.* 1999).

Organ-preserving surgery has also been performed for RCC in von Hippel–Lindau disease and metastatic RCC showing small intrarenal tumor lesions. Initial results are satisfactory. However, recurrence and progression rates are high (Steinbach *et al.* 1995; Krishnamurthi *et al.* 1996).

Adrenalectomy

In large nephrectomy series the overall incidence of adrenal involvement in histologically confirmed RCC is about 3–4 per cent. Adrenal metastasis is associated with advanced tumor stage, high progression rate, and poor survival (Sagalowsky *et al.* 1994; Shalev *et al.* 1995; Li *et al.* 1996; Sandock *et al.* 1997; von Knobloch *et al.* 1999). Therefore, the overall advantages of routine adrenalectomy are minimal, as most of the patients will be overtreated, and those patients in whom adrenal metastasis is histologically detected will probably not benefit from the removal of the gland.

It is widely accepted in clinical decision-making that the risk of adrenal metastasis is correlated with left-sided RCC, upper pole RCC, advanced T stage, poor differentiation, multifocality, and large tumor diameter (Sagalowsky *et al.* 1994; Shalev *et al.* 1995; Li *et al.* 1996; Wunderlich *et al.* 1999*b*). Thus, In many institutions adrenalectomy is performed in upper pole, multifocal, and large tumors only, or if adrenal involvement is suspected after preoperative ultrasound or CT scan.

However, some investigators found no preferential localization of the primary tumor within the kidney in case of adrenal involvement (Kozak *et al.* 1996; von Knobloch *et al.* 1999). The role of preoperative CT scan for the detection of adrenal metastasis remains unclear. Some studies claim a high sensitivity of abdominal CT scan in detecting adrenal involvement (Wunderlich *et al.* 1999*b*) or non-involvement (Gill *et al.* 1994), respectively, while others found preoperative imaging diagnosis to be unreliable with respect to small adrenal metastases (von Knobloch *et al.* 1999). However, due to the scarcity of adrenal metastases, the distinct populations in those series are small, not allowing statistically significant analysis.

Lymph node dissection

Due to the extension use of modern imaging techniques, especially ultrasound, RCC are detected earlier today. Thus, the prognosis of RCC patients has improved. The controversy over the extent of lymph node dissection is based on different findings about the frequency of lymph node metastases in RCC patients. In publications from the early 1990s, reporting on large numbers of patients diagnosed with RCC in the late 1970s and the 1980s, the frequency of lymph node metastasis ranged between 10 and

17.5 per cent (Giuliani *et al.* 1990; Herrlinger *et al.* 1991). Since then, there have been repeated discussions as to whether extensive lymph node dissection contributes to a favorable outcome after surgery. Radical lymph node excision can best be performed from a median laparotomy. However, most urologists prefer the lumbar approach for radical nephrectomy.

In an autopsy study, lymph node metastasis was found to be connected with distant metastasis in nearly all the cases (94 per cent). Independent lymph node involvement was detected in fewer than 1 per cent of the patients, suggesting a rather limited value for extensive lymph node dissection (Johnsen and Hellsten 1997). The preliminary results of a randomized European Organization for Research and Treatment of Cancer (EORTC) trial on the therapeutic value of lymph node dissection confirm these data. In patients suffering from localized RCC without enlarged lymph nodes or distant metastasis, as confirmed by CT scans, the incidence of histopathologically detected lymph node invasion was 3.3 per cent (Blom *et al.* 1999). Although the morbidity appears to be acceptable and pathological staging is improved after radical lymph node dissection, the therapeutic value remains unproven (Mickisch 1999). Other investigators confirm the findings of the EORTC, but emphasize that to date there is no curative treatment for metastatic RCC and that at least 4 per cent of the RCC patients without distant metastasis benefit from radical lymph node dissection (Schafhauser *et al.* 1999).

Hilar invasion

The localization of some tumors in the center of the kidney rather than the periphery may facilitate invasion into the hilar structures. Besides the venous involvement, invasion into the lymphatic vessels may be detected histologically.

Arising from the medulla, duct Bellini carcinoma aggressively infiltrates into the central kidney structures, invading vessels and lymph nodes as well as the adrenal gland (Storkel 1999). In those cases a more aggressive surgical approach combining wide excision and extensive lymph node resection may be justified, given a clinical M0 stage after preoperative chest X-ray, ultrasound, and CT scans.

Immunogenicity of RCC

Although RCC are supposed to be immunogenic and immunotherapeutic regimens are widely applied, little is known about the reactions involved in immune recognition and response to the tumor cells *in vivo.*

Mononuclear infiltrates of RCC contain T lymphocytes predominantly. The amount of tumor-infiltrating lymphocytes (TIL) increases with stage and grade (Banner *et al.* 1990; Kolbeck *et al.* 1992; Eskelinen *et al.* 1993). However, the antitumor activity of those lymphocytes is silenced. Only 3 per cent of the TIL are activated, expressing IL-2 receptor (CD25) (Storkel *et al.* 1992*a*). A decrease of CD4+ cells and an increase in CD8+ cells within the TIL are correlated with rising histological grade and pathognomonic for impaired local immune status and poor prognosis (Igarashi *et al.* 1992). However, changes in the ratio between CD4 and CD8 cells may also reflect sensitization and activation of TIL

(Kowalczyk *et al.* 1997). Specific interaction of T lymphocytes with tumor cells via the T-cell receptor (TCR) complex induces interferon-gamma production and lymphocyte proliferation (Finke *et al.* 1994). Analysis of the TCR repertoire of TIL reveals the recurrence of single T-cell clones in different tumor localization within a patient, suggesting specific TCR-mediated tumor cell recognition and subsequent intratumoral lymphocyte selection and proliferation (Choudhary *et al.* 1995; Olive *et al.* 1997; Angevin *et al.* 1997). TCR and signaling defects, for example, , decrease of the TCR zeta chain or p561ck tyrosine kinase, are induced by exposure of lymphocytes to tumor cells and might be one of the major mechanisms of immune escape (Finke *et al.* 1993). However, they can be reversed by cytokine-based immunotherapy (Gratama *et al.* 1999). Other immunosuppressive mechanisms associated with unfavorable outcome in RCC are the suppression of both TIL and dendritic cells (DC) via IL-10 secretion by tumor cells (Nakagomi *et al.* 1995; Wittke *et al.* 1999). IL-6 and macrophage colony-stimulating factor (M-CSF) inhibit the acquisition of an antigen-presenting phenotype by DC precursors (Menetrier-Caux *et al.* 1998). Moreover, TIL may be inhibited by TGFβ secreting tumor cells, which themselves have become resistant to negative growth control by TGFβ (Ramp *et al.* 1997).

Essentials of routine treatment

Radical tumor nephrectomy is still the treatment of choice in RCC (Ljungberg *et al.* 1998). The complication rates after radical surgery are low, and it allows for local tumor control and long-term survival in patients with localized tumors. *Nephron-sparing surgery* has evolved into an alternative surgical approach for very small tumor lesions. However, the significant probability of local recurrence and metastatic spread, even in tumors as small as 2–4 cm in diameter, has to be taken into account. Intraoperative frozen sections are mandatory, not only to reconfirm complete tumor resection but also tumor stage during nephron-sparing surgery. Nevertheless, by preventing end stage renal failure and dialysis, organ-preserving surgery makes it possible to maintain good quality of life in patients presenting with bilateral RCC.

Adrenalectomy should routinely be performed in upper pole RCC as well as in all other large tumors. Although many patients may be overtreated by removing the adrenal gland, the procedure allows for a correct staging and prognostic determination, while long-term following indicated it is not harmful (Hellstrom *et al.* 1997).

To date, there are no data supporting the general application of *extensive lymph node dissection.* Although it may improve pathological staging and survival in those patients in whom extrarenal tumor is completely removed by resection of the lymph nodes, the benefits do not outweigh the more intense clinical efforts.

Dedifferentiated (for example spindle cell) RCC are not a contraindication against *adjuvant immunotherapy.* Complete remissions are achievable by a combined approach of surgery and cytokine-based immunotherapy in selected patients presenting with a good performance status (Cangiano *et al.* 1999).

RCC of ductus Bellini or neuroendocrine type are very aggressive tumors. The life expectancy of patients suffering from such tumors is limited. In the case of complete surgical removal, however, long-term survival is possible. Therefore, these patients require a closer follow-up than other RCC patients.

Metanephrogenic adenomas and oncocytomas are benign renal tumors. After resection they do not require any additional treatment or follow-up. However, differential diagnosis in those cases may be difficult (oncocytoma versus eosinophilic type of chromophobic RCC, metanephrogenic adenoma versus Wilms' tumor in adults).

References

Aaltomaa, S. Lipponen, P., Ala-Opas, M., Eskelinen, M., Syrjanen, K., and Kosma, V.M. (1999). Expression of cyclins A and D and p21 (waf1/cip 1) proteins in renal cell cancer and their relation to clinicopathological variables and patient survival. *Br. J. Cancer* **80**, 2001–7.

Amin, M.B., Corless, C.L., Renshaw, A.A., Tickoo, S.K., Kubus, J., and Schultz, D.S. (1997) Papillary (chromophil) renal cell carcinoma: histomorphologic characteristics and evaluation of conventional pathologic prognostic parameters in 62 cases. *Am. J. Surg. Pathol.* **21**, 621–35.

Ananth, S., Knebelmann, B., Gruning, W., Dhanabal, M., Walz, G., Stillman, I.E., and Sukhatme, V.P. (1999). Transforming growth factor beta1 is a target for the von Hippel–Lindau tumor suppressor and a critical growth factor for clear cell renal carcinoma. *Cancer Res.* **59**, 2210–16.

Anastassiou, G., Duensing, S., Steinhoff, G., Zorn, U., Grosse, J., Dallmann, I., Kirchner, H., Ganser, A., and Atzpodien, J. (1996). Platelet endothelial cell adhesion molecule-1 (PECAM-1): a potential prognostic marker involved in leukocyte infiltration of renal cell carcinoma. *Oncology* **53**, 127–32.

Angevin, E., Kremer, F., Gaudin, C., Hercend, T., and Triebel, F. (1997). Analysis of T-cell immune response in renal cell carcinoma: polarization to type 1-like differentiation pattern, clonal T-cell expansion and tumor-specific cytotoxicity. *Int. J. Cancer* **72**, 431–40.

Anglard, P., Tory, K., Brauch, H., Weiss, G.H., Latif, F., Merino, M.J., Lerman, M.I., Zbar, B., and Linehan, W.M. (1991). Molecular analysis of genetic changes in the origin and development of renal cell carcinoma. *Cancer Res.* **51**, 1071–7.

Baer, S.C., Ro, J.Y., Ordonez, N.G., Maiese, R.L., Loose, J.H., Grignon, D.G., and Ayala, A.G. (1993). Sarcomatoid collecting duct carcinoma: a clinicopathologic and immunohistochemical study of five cases. *Hum. Pathol.* **24**, 1017–22.

Banner, B.F., Burnham, J.A., Bahnson, R.R., Ernstoff, M.S., and Auerbach, H.E. (1990). Immunophenotypic markers in renal cell carcinoma. *Mod. Pathol.* **3**, 129–34.

Barnes, C.A. and Beckman, E.N. (1983). Renal oncocytoma and ist congeners. *Am. J. Clin. Pathol.* **79**, 312–18.

Bell, E.T. (1938). Classification of renal tumors with observations on the frequency of the various types. *J. Urol.* **39**, 238–46.

Belldegrun, A., Tsui, K.H., deKernion, J.B., and Smith, R.B. (1999). Efficacy of nephron-sparing surgery for renal cell carcinoma: analysis based on the new 1997 tumor–node–metastasis staging system. *J. Clin. Oncol.* **17**, 2868–75.

Bernauer, U., Birner, G., Dekant, W., and Henschler, D. (1996). Biotransformation of trichloroethene: dose-dependent excretion of 2,2,2-trichloro-metabolites and mercapturic acids in rats and humans after inhalation. *Arch. Toxicol.* **70**, 338–46.

Birner, G., Vamvakas, S., Dekant, W., and Henschler, D. (1993). Nephrotoxic and genotoxic N-acetyl-S-dichlorovinyl-L-cysteine is a urinary metabolite after occupational 1,1,2-trichloroethene exposure in humans: implications for the risk of trichloroethene exposure. *Environ. Health Perspect.* **99**, 281–4

Blom, J.H., van Poppel, H., Marechal, J.M., Jacqmin, D., Sylvester, R., Schroder, F.H., and de Prijck, L. (1999). Radical nephrectomy with and without lymph node dissection: preliminary results of the EORTC randomized phase III protocol 30881. *Eur. Urol.* **36**, 570–5.

Boeing, H., Schlehofer, B., and Wahrendorf, J. (1997). Diet, obesity and risk for renal cell carcinoma: results from a case control-study in Germany. *Z. Ernahrungswiss.* **36**, 3–11.

Bonsib, S.M., Bray, C., and Timmerman, T.G. (1993). Renal chromophobe cell carcinoma: limitations of paraffin-embedded tissue. *Ultrastruct. Pathol.* **17**, 529–36.

Bostwick, D.G., and Eble, J.N. (1997). *Urologic surgical pathology*. Mosby, St Louis.

Bruning, T., Weirich, G., Hornauer, M.A., Hofler, H., and Brauch, H. (1997a). Renal cell carcinomas in trichloroethene (TRI) exposed persons are associated with somatic mutations in the von Hippel-Lindau (VHL) tumor suppressor gene. *Arch. Toxicol.* **71**, 332–5.

Bruning, T., Lammert, M., Kempkes, M., Thier, R., Golka, K., and Bolt, H.M. (1997b). Influence of polymorphisms of GSTM1 for risk of renal cell cancer in workers with long-term high occupational exposure to trichloroethene. *Arch. Toxicol.* **71**, 596–9.

Campbell, S.C., Fichtner, J., Novick, A.C., Steinbach, F., Stockle, M., Klein, E.A., Filipas, D., Levin, H.S., Storkel, S., Schweden, F., Obuchowski, N.A., and Hale, J. (1996). Intraoperative evaluation of renal cell carcinoma: a prospective study of the role of ultrasonography and histopathological frozen sections. *J. Urol.* **155**, 1191–5.

Cangiano, T., Liao, J., Naitoh, J., Dorey, F., Figlin, R., and Belldegrun, A. (1999). Sarcomatoid renal cell carcinoma: biologic behavior, prognosis, and response to combined surgical resection and immunotherapy. *J. Clin. Oncol.* **17**, 523–8.

Casalone, R., Casalone, P.G., and Minelli, E. (1992). Significance of the clonal and sporadic chromosome abnormalities in non-neoplastic renal tissue. *Hum. Genet.* **90**, 71–8.

Choudhary, A., Davodeau, F., Moreau, A., Peyrat, M.A., Bonneville, M., and Jotereau, F. (1995). Selective lysis of autologous tumor cells by recurrent gamma delta tumor-infiltrating lymphocytes from renal carcinoma. *J. Immunol.* **154**, 3932–40.

Crotty, T.B., Lawrence, K.M., Moertel, C.A., Bartelt, D.H., Hatts, K.P., Dewald, G.W., Farow, G.M., and Jenkins, R.B. (1992). Cytogenetic analysis of six renal oncocytomas and a chromophobe cell renal carcinoma. *Cancer Genet. Cytogenet.* **61**, 61–6.

Dal Cin, P., Aly, M.S., Delabie, J., Ceuppens, J.L., van Gool, S., van Damme, B., Baert, L., van Poppel, H., and van den Berghe, H. (1992). Trisomy 7 and trisomy 10 characterize subpopulations of tumor infiltrating lymphocytes in kidney tumors and in surrounding kidney tissue. *Proc. Natl. Acad. Sci., USA* **89**, 9744–8.

Delahunt, B., Becker, R.L., Bethwaite, P.B., and Ribas, J.L. (1994). Computerized nuclear morphometry and survival in renal cell carcinoma: comparison with other prognostic indicators. *Pathology* **26**, 353–8.

de Riese, W.T., Crabtree, W.N., Allhoff, E.P., Werner, M., Liedke, S., Lenis, G., Atzpodien, J., and Kirchner, H. (1993). Prognostic significance of Ki-67 immunostaining in nonmetastatic renal cell carcinoma. *J. Clin. Oncol.* **11**, 1804–8.

Dimopoulos, M.A., Logothetis, C.J., Markowitz, A., Sella, A., Amato, R., and Ro, J. (1993). Collecting duct carcinoma of the kidney. *Br. J. Urol.* **71**, 388–9.

Dinney, C.P., Awad, S.A., Gajewski, J.B., Belitsky, P., Lannon, S.G., Mack, F.G., and Millard, O.H. (1992). Analysis of imaging modalities, staging systems, and prognostic indicators for renal cell carcinoma. *Urology* **39**, 122–9.

Ditonno, P., Traficante, A., Battaglia, M., Grossi, F.S., and Selvaggi, F.P. (1992). Role of lymphadenectomy in renal cell carcinoma. *Prog. Clin. Biol. Res.* **378**, 169–74.

Dobin, S.M., Harris, C.P., Reynolds, J.A., Coffield, K.S., Klugo, R.C., Peterson, R.F., and Speights, V.O. (1992). Cytogenetic abnormalities in renal oncocytic neoplasms. *Genes Chromosom. Cancer* **4**, 25–31.

Duque, J.L., Loughlin, K.R., O'Leary, M.P., Kumar, S., and Richie, J.P. (1998). Partial nephrectomy: alternative treatment for selected patients with renal cell carcinoma. *Urology* **52**, 584–90.

Eble, J.N. (ed.) (1990). *Tumors and tumor-like conditions of the kidneys and ureters*. Churchill Livingstone, New York.

Ernstoff, M.S., Heaney, J.A., and Peschel, R.E. (1997). *Urologic cancer*. Blackwell Science, Cambridge.

Eskelinen, M., Lipponen, P., Aitto-Oja, L., Hall, O., and Syrjanen, K. (1993). The value of histoquantitative measurements in prognostic assessment of renal adenocarcinoma. *Int. J. Cancer* **55**, 547–54.

Farrow, G.M., Harrison, E., and Utz, D.C. (1992). Sarcomas and sarcomatoid and mixed malignat tumors of the kidney in adults—part III. *Cancer* **22**, 556–63.

Finke, J.H., Zea, A.H., Stanley, J., Longo, D.L., Mizoguchi, H., Tubbs, R.R., Wiltrout, R.H., O'Shea, J.J., Kudoh, S., Klein, E., *et al.* (1993). Loss of T-cell receptor zeta chain and p561ck in T-cells infiltrating human renal cell carcinoma. *Cancer Res.* **53**, 5613–16.

Finke, J.H., Rayman, P., Hart, L., Alexander, J.P., Edinger, M.G., Tubbs, R.R., Klein, E., Tuason, L., and Bukowski, R.M. (1994). Characterization of tumor-infiltrating lymphocyte subsets from human renal cell carcinoma: specific reactivity defined by cytotoxicity, interferon-gamma secretion, and proliferation. *J. Immunother. Emphasis Tumor Immunol.* **15**, 91–104.

Flint, A., Grossman, H.B., Liebert, M., Lloyd, R.V., and Bromberg, J. (1995). DNA and PCNA content of renal cell carcinoma and prognosis. *Am. J. Clin. Pathol.* **103**, 14–19.

Fuzesi, L., Cober, M., and Mittermayer, C. (1992). Collecting duct carcinoma: cytogenetic characterization. *Histopathology* **21**, 155–60.

Gill, I.S., McClennan, B.L., Kerbl, K., Carbone, J.M., Wick, M., and Clayman, R.V. (1994). Adrenal involvement from renal cell carcinoma: predictive value of computerized tomography. *J. Urol.* **152**, 1082–5.

Giuliani, L., Giberti, C., Martorana, G., and Rovida, S. (1990). Radical extensive surgery for renal cell carcinoma: long-term results and prognostic factors. *J. Urol.* **143**, 468–73.

Glenn, J.F. (1980). Renal tumors. In *Campbell's urology* (ed. J.H. Harrison, R.F. Gittes, A.D. Perlmutter, *et al.*). W.B. Saunders, Philadelphia.

Gnarra, J.R., Glenn, G.M., Latif, F., Anglard, P., Lerman, M.I., Zbar, B., and Linehan, W.M. (1993). Molecular genetic studies of sporadic and familial renal cell carcinoma. *Urol. Clin. N. Am.* **20**, 207–16.

Goepel, M. and Rubben, H. (1991). Adjuvant therapy in renal cancer. *World J. Urol.* **9**, 232–6.

Gratama, J.W., Zea, A.H., Bolhuis, R.L., and Ochoa, A.C. (1999). Restoration of expression of signal-transduction molecules in lymphocytes from patients with metastatic renal cell cancer after combination immunotherapy. *Cancer Immunol. Immunother.* **48**, 263–9.

Grawitz, P. (1883). Die sogenannten Lipome der Niere. *Virch. Arch. Pathol. Anat. Physiol. Klin. Med.* **93**, 39–63.

Grimaldi, G., Reuter, V., and Russo, P. (1998). Bilateral non-familial renal cell carcinoma. *Ann. Surg. Oncol.* **5**, 548–52.

Guillou, L., Duvoisin, B., Chobaz, C., Chapuis, G., and Costa, J. (1993). Combined small cell and transitional cell carcinoma of the renal pelvis. *Arch. Pathol. Lab. Med.* **117**, 239–43.

Hafez, K.S., Novick, A.C., and Campbell, S.C. (1997). Patterns of tumor recurrence and guidelines for followup after nephron sparing surgery for sporadic renal cell carcinoma. *J. Urol.* **157**, 2067–70.

Hafez, K.S., Novick, A.C., and Butler, B.P. (1989). Management of small solitary unilateral renal cell carcinomas: impact of central versus peripheral tumor location. *J. Urol.* **159**, 1156–60.

Hafez, K.S., Fergany, A.F., and Novick, A.C. (1999). Nephron sparing surgery for localized renal cell carcinoma: impact of tumor size on patient survival, tumor recurrence and TNM staging. *J. Urol.* **162**, 1930–3.

Hartwick, R.W., el Naggar, A.K., Ro, J.Y., Srigley, J.R., McLemore, D.D., Jones, E.C., Grignon, D.J., Thomas, M.J., and Ayala, A.G. (1992). Renal oncocytoma and granular cell carcinoma. A comparative clinicopathologic and DNA flow cytometric study. *Am. J. Clin. Pathol.* **98**, 587–93.

Hellstrom, P.A., Bloigu, R., Ruokonen, A.O., Vainionpaa, V.A., Nuutinen, L.S., and Kontturi, M.J. (1997). Is routine ipsilateral adrenalectomy during radical nephrectomy harmful for the patient? *Scand. J. Urol. Nephrol.* **31**, 19–25.

Helpap, B. (1993). *Atlas der Pathologie urologischer Tumoren*. Springer Verlag, Berlin.

Henn, W., Zwergel, T., Wullich, B., Thonnes, M., Zang, K.D., and Seitz, G. (1993). Bilateral multicentric papillary renal tumors with heteroclonal origin based on tissue-specific karyotype instability. *Cancer* **72**, 1315–18.

Henschler, D. and Bonse, G. (1977). Metabolic activation of chlorinated ethylenes: dependence of mutagenic effect on electrophilic reactivity of the metabolically formed epoxides. *Arch. Toxicol.* **39**, 7–12.

Henschler, D., Vamvakas, S., Lammert, M., Dekant, W., Kraus, B., Thomas, B., and Ulm, K. (1995). Increased incidence of renal cell tumors in a cohort of cardboard workers exposed to trichloroethene. *Arch. Toxicol.* **69**, 291–9,

Herrlinger, A., Schrott, K.M., Schott, G., and Sigel, A. (1991). What are the benefits of extended dissection of the regional renal lymph nodes in the therapy of renal cell carcinoma? *J. Urol.* **146**, 1224–7.

Hofmann, R., Lehmer, A., Buresch, M., Hartung, R., and Ulm, K. (1996). Clinical relevance of urokinase plasminogen activator, its receptor, and its inhibitor in patients with renal cell carcinoma. *Cancer* **78**, 487–92.

Hofmockel, G., Tsatalpas, P., Muller, H., Dammrich, J., Poot, M., Maurer-Schultze, B., Muller-Hermelink, H.K., Frohmuller, H.G., and Bassukas, I.D. (1995). Significance of conventional and new prognostic factors for locally confined renal cell carcinoma. *Cancer* **76**, 296–306.

Huettner, P.C., Bird, D.J., Chang, Y.C., and Seiler, W.M. (1991). Carcinoid tumor of the kidney with morphologic and immunohistochemical profile of a hindgut endocrine tumor: report of a case. *Ultrastruct. Pathol.* **415**, 655–61.

Igarashi, T., Murakami, S., Takahashi, H., Matsuzaki, O., and Shimazaki, J. (1992). Changes on distribution of CD4+/CD45RA- and CD8+/CD11-cells in tumor-infiltrating lymphoctyes of renal cell carcinoma associated with tumor progression. *Eur. Urol.* **22**, 323–8.

Ishikawa, I. and Kovacs, G. (1993). High incidence of papillary renal cell tumors in patients on chronic haemodialysis. *Histopathology* **22**, 135–9.

Javidan, J., Stricker, H.J., Tamboli, P., Amin, M.B., Peabody, J.O., Deshpande, A., Menon, M., and Amin, M.B. (1999). Prognostic significance of the 1997 TNM classification of renal cell carcinoma. *J. Urol.* **162**, 1277–81.

Johnsen, J.A. and Hellsten, S. (1997). Lymphatogenous spread of renal cell carcinoma: an autopsy study. *J. Urol.* **157**, 450–3.

Kantor, A.F. (1977). Current concepts in the epidemiology and etiology of primary renal cell carcinoma. *J. Urol.* **117**, 415.

Kennedy, S.M., Merino, M.J., Linehan, W.M., Roberts, J.R., Robertson, C.N., and Neumann, R.D. (1990). Collecting duct carcinoma of the kidney. *Hum. Pathol.* **21**, 449–56.

Kimura, M., Tomita, Y., Imai, T., Saito, T., Katagiri, A., Tanikawa, T., Takeda, M., and Takahashi, K. (1999). Significance of serum-soluble CD95 (Fas/APO-1) on prognosis in renal cell cancer patients. *Br. J. Cancer* **80**, 1648–51.

Kinouchi, T., Saiki, S., Meguro, N., Maeda, O., Kuroda, M., Usami, M., and Kotake, T. (1999*a*). Impact of tumor size on the clinical outcomes of patients with Robson stage 1 renal cell carcinoma. *Cancer* **85**, 689–95.

Kinouchi, T., Mano, M., Saiki, S., Meguro, N., Maeda, O., Kuroda, M., Usami, M., and Kotake, T. (1999*b*). Incidence rate of satellite tumors in renal cell carcinoma. *Cancer* **86**, 2331–6.

Kolbeck, P.C., Kaveggia, F.F., Johansson, S.L., Grune, M.T., and Taylor, R.J. (1992). The relationships among tumor-infiltrating lymphocytes, histopathologic findings, and long-term clinical follow-up in renal cell carcinoma. *Mod. Pathol.* **5**, 420–5.

Kolonel, L.N. (1976). Association of cadmium with renal cancer. *Cancer* **37**, 1782.

Kovacs, A. and Kovacs, G. (1992). Low chromosome number in chromophobe renal cell carcinomas. *Genes Chromosom. Cancer* **4**, 267–8.

Kovacs, A., Storkel, S., Thoenes, W., and Kovacs, G. (1992). Mitochondrial and chromosomal DNA alterations in human chromophobe renal cell carcinomas. *J. Pathol.* **167**, 273–7.

Kovacs, G. (1989). Papillary renal cell carcinoma: a morphologic and cytogenetic study of 11 cases. *Am. J. Pathol.* **134**, 27–34.

Kovacs, G. (1993). Molecular differential pathology of renal cell tumors. *Histopathology* **22**, 1–8.

Kovacs, G., Szucs, S., Eichner, W., Maschek, H. J., Wahnschaffe, U., and deRiese, W. (1987). Renal oncocytoma. A cytogenetic and morphologic study. *Cancer* 59, 2071–7.

Kowalczyk, D., Skorupski, W., Kwias, Z., and Nowak, J. (1997). Flow cytometric analysis of tumour-infiltrating lymphocytes in patients with renal cell carcinoma. *Br. J. Urol.* 80, 543–7.

Kozak, W., Holtl, W., Pummer, K., Maier, U., Jeschke, K., and Bucher, A. (1996). Adrenalectomy—still a must in radical renal surgery? *Br. J. Urol.* 77, 27–31.

Krishnamurthi, V., Novick, A.C., and Bukowski, R. (1996). Nephron sparing surgery in patients with metastatic renal cell carcinoma. *J. Urol.* 156, 36–9.

Kugler, A., Hemmerlein, B., Thelen, P., Kallerhoff, M., Radzun, H.J., and Ringert, R.H. (1998). Expression of metalloproteinase 2 and 9 and their inhibitors in renal cell carcinoma. *J. Urol.* 160, 1914–18.

LaForgia, S., Lasota, J., Latif, F., Boghosian-Sell, L., Kastury, K., Ohta, M., Druck, T., Atchison, L., Canizzaro, L.A., Barnea, G., Schlessinger, J., Modi, W., Kuzmin, I., Tory, K., Zbar, B., Croce, C.M., and Huebner, K. (1993). Detailed genetic and physical map of the chromosome region surrounding the familial renal cell carcinoma chromosome translocation, t(3;8)(p14.2;q24.1). *Cancer Res.* 53, 3118–24.

Latif, F., Tory, K., Gnarra, J., Yao, M., Duh, F.M., Orcutt, M.L., Stackhouse, T., Kuzmin, I., Modi, W., Geil, L., Schmidt, L., Zhou, F., Li, H., Wie, M.H., Chen, F., Glenn, G., Choyke, P., Walther, M.M., Wenig, Y., Duan, D.R., Dean, M., Glavac, D., Richards, F.M., Crossey, P.A., Ferguson-Smith, M.A., Paslier, D.L., Chumakov, I., Cohen, D., Chinault, C., Maher, E.R., Linehan, W.M., Zbar, B., and Lerman, M.I. (1993). Identification of the von Hippel–Lindau disease tumor suppressor gene. *Science* 260, 1317–20.

La Vecchia, C., Levi, F., Lucchini, F., and Negri, E. (1992). Descriptive epidemiology of kidney cancer in Europe. *J. Nephrol.* 5, 37–43.

Lerner, S.E., Hawkins, C.A., Blute, M.L., Grabner, A., Wollan, P.C., Eickholt, J.T., and Zincke H. (1996). Disease outcome in patients with low stage renal cell carcinoma treated with nephron sparing or radical surgery. *J. Urol.* 155, 1868–73.

Li, G.R., Soulie, M., Escourrou, G., Plante, P., and Pontonnier, F. (1996). Micrometastatic adrenal invasion by renal carcinoma in patients undergoing nephrectomy. *Br. J. Urol.* 78, 826–8.

Ljungberg, B., Alamdari, F.I., Holmberg, G., Granfors, T., and Duchek, M. (1998). Radical nephrectomy is still preferable in the treatment of localized renal cell carcinoma. A long-term follow-up study. *Eur. Urol.* 33, 79–85.

Los, M., Zeamari, S., Foekens, J.A., Gebbink, M.F., and Voest, E.E. (1999). Regulation of the urokinase-type plasminogen activator system by the von Hippel–Lindau tumor suppressor gene. *Cancer Res.* 59, 4440–5.

Matsumoto, T., Iijima, T., Kuwabara, N., Wakumoto, Y., Fukushima, T., Sakamoto, Y., Kitagawa, R., Takeda, K., Oonuma, Y., and Suzuki, S. (1992). Papillary renal cell carcinoma. Report of two cases. *Acta Pathol. Jpn* 42, 298–303.

McLaughlin, J.K., Chow, W.H., Mandel, J.S., Mellemgaard, A., McCredie, M., Lindblad, P., Schlehofer, B., Pommer, W., Niwa, S., and Adami, H.O. (1995). International renal-cell cancer study. VIII. Role of diuretics, other anti-hypertensive medications and hypertension. *Int. J. Cancer* 63, 216–21.

Mellemgaard, A., Moller, H., and Olsen, J.H. (1992). Diuretics may increase risk of renal cell carcinoma. *Cancer Causes Control* 3, 309–12.

Mellemgaard, A., Lindblad, P., Schlehofer, B., Bergstrom, R., Mandel, J.S., McCredie, M., McLaughlin, J.K., Niwa, S., Odaka, N., Pommer, W., *et al.* (1995). International renal-cell cancer study. III. Role of weight, height, physical activity, and use of amphetamines. *Int. J. Cancer* 60, 350–4.

Meloni, A.M., Dobbs, R.M., Pontes, J.E., and Sandberg, A.A. (1993). Translocation (X;1) in papillary renal cell carcinoma—a new cytogenetic subtype. *Cancer Genet. Cytogenet.* 65, 1–6.

Menetrier-Caux, C., Montmain, G., Dieu, M.C., Bain, C., Favrot, M.C., Caux, C., and Blay, J.Y. (1998). Inhibition of the differentiation of dendritic cells from CD34(+) progenitors by tumor cells: role of interleukin-6 and macrophage colony-stimulating factor. *Blood* 92, 4778–91.

Mickisch, G.H. (1999). Lymphatic metastases in renal cell carcinoma. What is the value of operation and adjuvant therapy? *Urology* 38A, 326–31.

Miller, J., Fischer, C., Freese, R., Altmannsberger, M., and Weidner, W. (1999). Nephron-sparing surgery for renal cell carcinoma—is tumor size a suitable parameter for indication? *Urology* 54, 988–93.

Morita, G., Saito, S., Ishijawa, J., Ogawa, O., Yoshida, O., Yamakawa, K., and Nakamura, Y. (1991). Common regions of deletions on chromosomes 5q, 6q and 10q in renal cell carcinoma. *Cancer Res.* 51, 5817–20.

Mostofi, F.K. (ed.) (1981). Histological typing of kidney tumors. In *International histological classification of tumours*, no. 25. WHO, Geneva.

Mostofi, F.K. and Davie, C.J. (ed.) (1998). Histological typing of kidney tumors. In *WHO, international histological classification of tumours*, 2nd edn. Springer, Berlin.

Murphy, W.M., Beckwith, J.B., and Farrow, G.M. (1994). Tumors of the kidney, bladder, and related urinary structures. In *Atlas of tumor pathology*, 3rd Series, Fascicle 11. Armed Forces Institute of Pathology, Washington, DC.

Nagashima, Y., Arai, N., Tanaka, Y., Yoshida, S., Sumino, K., Ohaki, Y., Matsushita, K., Morita, T., and Misugi, K. (1991). Two cases of renal epithelial tumour resembling immature nephron. *Virch. Arch. A* 418, 77–81.

Nakagomi, H., Pisa, P., Pisa, E.K., Yamamoto, Y., Halapi, E., Backlin, K., Juhlin, C., and Kiessling, R. (1995). Lack of interleukin-2 (IL-2) expression and selective expression of IL-10 mRNA in human renal cell carcinoma. *Int. J. Cancer* 63, 366–71.

Novick A.C. (1998). Nephron-sparing surgery for renal cell carcinoma. *Br. J. Urol.* 82, 321–4.

Olive, C., Nicol, D., and Falk, M.C. (1997). Characterisation of gamma delta T cells in renal cell carcinoma patients by polymerase chain reaction analysis of T cell receptor transcripts. *Cancer Immunol. Immunother.* 44, 27–34.

Oremek, G.M., Teigelkamp, S., Kramer, W., Eigenbrodt, E., and Usadel, K.H. (1999). The pyruvate kinase isoenzyme tumor M2 (Tu M2-PK) as a tumor marker for renal carcinoma. *Anticancer Res.* 19, 2599–601.

Ortmann, M. and Vierbuchen, M. (1989). Lektinhistochemie an Nieren und Nierentumoren. *Verh. Dtsch. Ges. Pathol.* 73, 339–49.

Ortmann, M., Vierbuchen, M., and Fischer, R. (1991). Sialylated glycoconjugates in chromophobe cell renal carcinoma compared with other renal tumors. Indication of its development from collecting duct epithelium. *Virch. Arch. B* 61, 123–32.

Oya, M., Nakamura, K., Baba, S., Hata, J., and Tazaki, H. (1995). Intrarenal satellites of renal cell carcinoma: histopathologic manifestation and clinical implication. *Urology* 46, 161–4.

Paradis, V., Ferlicot, S., Ghannam, E., Zeimoura, L., Blanchet, P., Eschwege, P., Jardin, A., Benoit, G., and Bedossa, P. (1999). CD44 is an independent prognostic factor in conventional renal cell carcinomas. *J. Urol.* 161, 1984–7.

Petersen, R.O. (1994). *Urologic pathology*, 2nd edn. J.B. Lippincott, Philadelphia.

Presti, J.C., Rao, P.H., Chen, Q., Reuter, V.E., Li, F.P., Fair, W.R., and Jhanwar, S.C. (1991). Histopathological, cytogenetic, and molecular characterization of renal cortical tumors. *Cancer Res.* 51, 1544–52.

Presti, J.C., Reuter, V.E., Cordon-Cardo, C., Mazumdar, M., Fair, W.R., and Jhanwar, S.C. (1993). Allelic deletions in renal tumors: histopathological correlations. *Cancer Res.* 53, 5780–3.

Ramp, U., Jaquet, K., Reinecke, P., Nitsch, T., Gabbert, H.E., and Gerharz, C.D. (1997). Acquisition of TGF-beta 1 resistance: an important progression factor in human renal cell carcinoma. *Lab. Invest.* 76, 739–49.

Remmele, W. (ed.) (1997). *Pathologie*, Vol. 5, 2nd edn. Springer, Berlin.

Ro, J.Y., Ayala, A.G., Sella, A., Samuels, M.L., and Swanson, D.A. (1987). Sarcomatoid renal cell carcinoma: a clinicopathologic study of 42 cases. *Cancer* 59, 516–26.

Rumpelt, H.J., Storkel, S., Moll, R., Scharfe, T., and Thoenes, W. (1991). Bellini duct carcinoma—further evidence for this rare variant of renal cell carcinoma. *Histopathology* 18, 115–22.

Sagalowsky, A.I., Kadesky, K.T., Ewalt, D.M., and Kennedy, T.J. (1994). Factors influencing adrenal metastasis in renal cell carcinoma. *J. Urol.* 151, 1181–4.

Saito, S., Orikasa, S., Ohyama, C., Satoh, M., and Fukushi, Y. (1991). Changes in glycolipids in human renal cell carcinoma and their clinical significance. *Int. J. Cancer* **49**, 329–34.

Sandock, D.S., Seftel, A.D., and Resnick, M.I. (1997). Adrenal metastases from renal cell carcinoma: role of ipsilateral adrenalectomy and definition of stage. *Urology* **49**, 28–31.

Schafhauser, W., Ebert, A., Brod, J., Petsch, S., and Schrott, K.M. (1999). Lymph node involvement in renal cell carcinoma and survival chance by systematic lymphadenectomy. *Anticancer Res.* **19**, 1573–8.

Shalev, M., Cipolla, B., Guille, F., Staerman, F., and Lobel, B. (1995). Is ipsilateral adrenalectomy a necessary component of radical nephrectomy? *J. Urol.* **153**, 1415–17.

Shimazui, T., Bringuier, P.P., van Berkel, H., Ruijter, E., Akaza, H., Debruyne, F.M., Oosterwijk, E., and Schalken, J.A. (1997). Decreased expression of alpha-catenin is associated with poor prognosis of patients with localized renal cell carcinoma. *Int. J. Cancer* **74**, 523–8.

Shuin, T., Kondo, K., Torigoe, S., Kishida, T., Kubota, Y., Hosaka, M., Nagashima, Y., Kitamura, H., Latif, F., Zbar, B., Lerman, M.I., and Yao, M. (1994). Frequent somatic mutations and loss of heterozygosity of the von Hippel–Lindau tumor suppressor gene in primary human renal cell carcinomas. *Cancer Res.* **54**, 2852–5.

Speicher, M.R., du Manoir, S., Schoell, B., Schrock, E., Ried, T., Storkel, S., Kovacs, A., Cremer, T., and Kovacs, G. (1994). Specific loss of chromosomes 1,2,6,10,13,17 and 21 in chromophobe renal cell carcinomas revealed by comparative genomic hybridization. *Am. J. Pathol.* **145**, 356–64.

Spiegel, D.M., Yuen Ko, J.L., Hou, S.H., Brandt, T.D., Grant, T.H. (1991). Incidence of renal cell carcinoma and natural history of acquired renal cystic disease in end stage renal disease. *Am. J. Nephrol.* **11**, 166–7.

Steinbach, F., Novick, A.C., Zincke, H., Miller, D.P., Williams, R.D., Lund, G., Skinner, D.G., Esrig, D., Richie, J.P., deKernion, J.B., *et al.* (1995). Treatment of renal cell carcinoma in von Hippel–Lindau disease: a multicenter study. *J. Urol.* **153**, 1812–16.

Steinberg, P., Storkel, S., Oesch, F., and Thoenes, W. (1992). Carbohydrate metabolism in human renal clear cell carcinomas. *Lab. Invest.* **67**, 506–11.

Storkel, S. (1989). DNA Image Cytometrie humaner Nierenzelltumore mit dem Leitz Miamed-DNA. *Mitt. Wiss. Tech.* **9**, 214–19.

Storkel, S. (1993). *Karzinome und Onkozytome der Niere.* Gustav Fischer Verlag, Stuttgart.

Storkel, S. (1999). Epithelial tumors of the kidney. Pathological subtyping and cytogenetic correlation. *Urology [A]* **38**, 425–32.

Storkel, S., Pannen, B., Thoenes, W., Steart, P.V., Wagner, S., and Drenckhahn, D. (1988). Intercalated cells as a probable source for the development or renal oncocytoma. *Virch. Arch. B* **56**, 185–9.

Storkel, S., Thoenes, W., Jacobi, G.H., and Lippold, R. (1989*a*). Prognostic parameters in renal cell carcinoma—a new approach. *Eur J. Urol.* **416**, 416–22.

Storkel, S., Steart, P.V., Drenckhahn, D., and Thoenes, W. (1989*b*). The human chromophobe cell renal carcinoma: probable relation to intercalated cells of the collecting duct. *Virch. Arch. B* **56**, 237–45.

Storkel, S., Thoenes, W., Jacobi, G.H., Engelmann, U., and Lippold, R. (1990) suppl. Prognostic parameters of renal cell carcinoma. *Eur. Urol.* **18** (suppl. 2), 36–7.

Storkel, S., Keymer, R., Steinbach, F., and Thoenes, W. (1992*a*). Reaction patterns of tumor infiltrating lymphocytes in different renal cell carcinomas and oncocytomas. *Prog. Clin. Biol. Res.* **378**, 217–23.

Storkel, S., Husmann, G., and Thoenes, W. (1992*b*). Zur Diagnose und Differentialdiagnose des metanephroiden Nierentumors des Erwachsenen—ein unbekannter Nierentumor. *Verh. Dtsch. Ges. Pathol.* **76**, 306.

Storkel, S., Eble, J.N., Adlakha, K., Amin, M., Blute, M.L., Bostwick, D.G., Darson, M., Delahunt, B., and Iczkowski, K. (1997). Classification of renal cell carcinoma. *Cancer* **80**, 985–7.

Takahashi, S., Shirai, T., Ogawa, K., Imaida, K., Yamazaki, C., Ito, A., Masuko, K., and Ito, N. (1993). Renal cell adenomas and carcinomas in hemo-

dialysis patients: relationship between hemodialysis period and development of lesions. *Acta Pathol. Jpn* **43**, 674–82.

Tavani, A. and La Vecchia, C. (1997). Epidemiology of renal-cell carcinoma. *J. Nephrol.* **10**, 93–106.

Thoenes, W., Storkel, S., and Rumpelt, H.J. (1985). Human chromophobe cell renal carcinoma. *Virch. Arch. B* **48**, 207–17.

Thoenes, W., Storkel, S., and Rumpelt H.J. (1986). Histopathology and classification of renal cell tumors (adenomas, oncocytomas and carcinomas). The basic cytological and histomorphological elements and their use for diagnostics. *Pathol. Res. Pract.* **181**, 125–43.

Thoenes, W., Rumpelt, H.J., and Storkel, S. (1990). Klassifikation der Nierenzelltumoren und ihre Beziehung zum Nephron-Samelrohrsystem. *Klin. Wochenschr.* **68**, 1102–11.

Tory, K., Brauch, H., Linehan, M., Barba, D., Oldfield, E., Filling-Katz, M., Seizinger, B., Nakamura, Y., White, R., Marshall, F.F., Lerman, M.I., and Zbar, B. (1989). Specific genetic change in tumors associated with von Hippel–Lindau disease. *J. Natl. Cancer Inst.* **81**, 1097–101.

Vamvakas, S., Bruning, T., Thomasson, B., Lammert, M., Baumuller, A., Bolt, H.M., Dekant, W., Birner, G., Henschler, D., and Ulm, K. (1998). Renal cell cancer correlated with occupational exposure to trichloroethene. *J. Cancer Res. Clin. Oncol.* **124**, 374–82.

van den Berg, E. (1993). Order and complexity in renal cell tumors. Proefschrift. University of Groningen, pp. 91–6.

van den Berg, E., van der Hout, A.H., Oosterhuis, J.W., Storkel, S., Dijkhuizen, T., Dam, A., Zweers, H.M.M., Mensink, H.J.A., Buys, C.H.C.M., and de Jong, B. (1993). Cytogeetic analysis of epithelial renal cell tumors; relationship with a new histopathological classification. *Int. J. Cancer* **55**, 223–7.

van den Berg, E., Dijkhuizen, T., Storkel, S., Brutel de la Reviere, G., Dam, A., Mensink, H.J.A., Oosterhuis, J.W., and de Jong, B. (1994). Chromosomal changes in renal oncocytomas—evidence that t(5;11)(q35;q13) may characterize a second subgroup of oncocytomas. *Cancer Genet. Cytogenet.* **79**, 164–8.

van der Hout, A.H., van den Berg, E., van der Vlies, P., Dijkhuizen, T., Storkel, S., Oosterhuis, J.W., de Jong B., and Buys, C.H.C.M. (1993). Loss of heterozygosity at the short arm of chromosome 3 in renal cell cancer correlates with the cytological tumour type. *Int. J. Cancer* **53**, 353–7.

von Knobloch, R., Seseke, F., Riedmiller, H., Grone, H.J., Walthers, E.M., and Kalble, T. (1999). Radical nephrectomy for renal cell carcinoma: is adrenalectomy necessary? *Eur. Urol.* **36**, 303–8.

Wechsel, H.W., Petri, E., Bichler, K.H., and Feil, G. (1999) Marker for renal cell carcinoma (RCC): the dimeric form of pyruvate kinase type M2 (Tu M2-PK). *Anticancer Res.* **19**, 2583–90.

Weir, J.M. and Dunn, J.E. Jr (1970). Smoking and mortality: a prospective study. *Cancer* **25**, 105.

Weiss, L.M., Gelb, A.B., and Medeiros, L.J. (1995). Adult renal epithelial neoplasms. *Am. J. clin. Pathol.* **103**, 624–35.

Wenz, W. (1967). Tumors of the kidney following retrograde pyelography with colloidal thorium dioxide. *Ann. NY Acad. Sci.* **145**, 806.

Wittke, F., Hoffmann, R., Buer, J., Dallmann, I., Oevermann, K., Sel, S., Wandert, T., Ganser, A., and Atzpodien, J. (1999). Interleukin 10 (IL-10): an immunosuppressive factor and independent predictor in patients with metastatic renal cell carcinoma. *Br. J. Cancer* **79**, 1182–4.

Wingo, P.A., Tong, T., and Bolden, S. (1995). Cancer statistics. *CA J. Cancer Clin.* **45**, 8.

Wunderlich, H., Schlichter, A., Kosmehl, H., and Schubert, J. (1999*a*). The histopathological heterogeneity of small renal cell carcinoma. *Anticancer Res.* **19**, 1497–500.

Wunderlich, H., Schlichter, A., Reichelt, O., Zermann, D.H., Janitzky, V., Kosmehl, H., and Schubert, J. (1999*b*). Real indications for adrenalectomy in renal cell carcinoma. *Eur. Urol.* **35**, 272–6.

Zbar, B., Brach, H., Talmage, C., and Linehan, M. (1987). Loss of alleles of loci on the short arm of chromosome 3 in renal cell carcinoma. *Nature* **327**, 721–4.

5. Paraneoplastic manifestations of renal cell carcinoma

Nehal Masood, Philip J. Gold, and John A. Thompson

The triad of hematuria, pain, and a palpable mass is the classic initial presentation for renal cell carcinoma (RCC), but is present in only 10 per cent of patients (de Kernion *et al.* 1995). More often, nonspecific signs and symptoms, such as fever, malaise, anorexia, and weight loss, may precede other evidence of RCC by weeks to years, or may be found incidentally during routine evaluation (Table 5.1). Many symptoms of RCC are caused by the elaboration by the tumor of specific polypeptide hormones. These substances are responsible for the 'paraneoplastic' effects of the cancer, rather than the direct invasion of vital structures by the tumor or its metastases. Other etiologies for paraneoplasia include peptide production by normal cells in response to tumor, antibody made in response to tumor, and other mechanisms. These paraneoplastic effects of the tumor may occur in potentially curable RCC, and they may not necessarily represent metastatic disease. Effective therapy of the underlying carcinoma typically causes the paraneoplastic syndrome to remit. In contrast, few paraneoplastic syndromes respond to medical therapies, with the notable exception of hypercalcemia. Recurrence of a paraneoplastic syndrome may herald relapse, either local or metastatic.

Recognition of paraneoplastic syndromes is an important component of the diagnosis and management of RCC, as roughly 10–40 per cent of RCC patients will develop a paraneoplastic syndrome during the course of their illness (Mc Dougal and Garnick 1995). The incidence of the most common paraneoplastic syndromes is listed in Table 5.2. Paraneoplastic syndromes may be categorized according to whether or not endocrinopathy is present.

Table 5.1 Presenting characteristics of patients with renal cell carcinoma

Characteristic	Incidence (%)
Hematuria	40–60
Flank or abdominal pain	40
Palpable mass	30
Weight loss	20–30
Anemia	20
Triad of hematuria + palpable mass + pain	10
Fever	2–12

Table 5.2 Incidence of the most common paraneoplastic syndromes associated with renal cell carcinoma

Paraneoplastic syndrome	Incidence (%)
Cachexia	33
Nephropathy	27
Hypertension	25
Anemia	20–40
Hyperglycemia	10–20
Nonmetastatic hepatic dysfunction (Stauffer's syndrome)	3–20
Erythrocytosis	1–8
Amyloidosis	3–5
Synovitis	1
Neurological dysfunction	1
Dermatitis	1

Endocrine paraneoplastic syndromes

Hypercalcemia

Albright (1941) reported the first case of RCC associated with hypercalcemia. Transient reversal of the hypercalcemia followed irradiation of a solitary pelvic metastasis. Hypercalcemia is the most common of all paraneoplastic syndromes, affecting 10–20 per cent of patients with cancer, and has been reported in up to 20 per cent of patients with RCC (Muggia 1990). In most patients with malignancy, the development of symptomatic hypercalcemia carries a grim prognosis. The median survival of all cancer patients with symptomatic hypercalcemia is 4–5 weeks. Two categories of hypercalcemia have been identified in patients with RCC.

Non-metastatic hypercalcemia (humoral hypercalcemia of malignancy)
Hypercalcemia in patients with solid tumors and no bony metastases is a phenomenon that has undergone considerable research over the last 20 years. Several humoral mediators of bone resorption have been identified, and many investigators have identified the presence of a substance that mimics the effects of parathyroid hormone (PTH). Goldberg *et al.* (1964) described a 64-year-old woman with metastatic RCC and hypercalcemia without bony metastases. At autopsy, a tumor extract was made, which reacted as PTH on immunoassay. More recently, investigators have molecularly cloned a PTH-like peptide purified from a variety of cancer cell lines, which has near homology with PTH (Strewler *et al.*

1987; Suva *et al.* 1987). Gotoh *et al.* (1993) used a parathyroid hormone-related peptide (PTHrP) specific monoclonal antibody to identify PTHrP in the tumors of 40 of 42 cases of RCC, although this did not correlate significantly with the serum calcium level. Other humoral factors apart from PTHrP have also been described as contributing to the humoral hypercalcemia of malignancy, including osteoclast activating factor (OAF), transforming growth factor alpha (TGFα), interleukin-1, and tumor necrosis factor (Muggia 1990).

PTHrP mimics many of the effects of PTH on renal tubular function by binding to and activating the PTH receptor. This leads to alterations in normal calcium homeostasis, including increased bone resorption, decreased renal calcium clearance, increased nephrogenous cyclic adenosine monophosphate levels, and increased phosphorous excretion. Ectopic PTHrP mimics primary hyperparathyroidism, except that patients with the RCC-related syndrome have decreases in renal calcium reabsorption, intestinal calcium absorption, and 1,25(OH)$_2$-vitamin D synthesis (Fahn *et al.* 1991).

Transforming growth factor alpha (TGFα) has also been shown to mediate the humoral hypercalcemia of malignancy. TGFα is produced by several solid tumors, and has biologic properties in common with epidermal growth factor, a substance known to stimulate osteoclastic bone resorption (Mundy *et al.* 1985). Some investigators believe that PTHrP and TGFα work in concert to produce the humoral hypercalcemia of malignancy. TGFα is thought to act by increasing osteoclast activity and by inhibiting bone formation. PTHrP acts predominantly by activating osteoclasts, and by inhibiting renal phosphate reabsorption (Mundy 1990). Additionally, the stimulation of normal host immune cells by the tumor may result in the elaboration of other cytokines, such as tumor necrosis factor and interleukin-1, which may work in concert with PTHrP and TGFα to cause hypercalcemia.

The clinical manifestations of hypercalcemia are influenced by many factors, including the duration of hypercalcemia, performance status, age, prior chemotherapy, hepatic or renal dysfunction, as well as sites of metastatic disease (Warrell and Bockman 1989). Many of the signs and symptoms, such as nausea, anorexia, fatigue, lethargy, and confusion, are nonspecific, and the physician must have a high index of suspicion for the presence of hypercalcemia. This is of importance, as the symptoms are generally reversible with therapy.

Neurologic manifestations of hypercalcemia include weakness, diminished deep tendon reflexes, altered mental status, and impaired neuromuscular function. Initial lethargy, mild confusion, and personality changes can progress to stupor and coma. Treatment of the hypercalcemia will generally improve the mental status, but there may be a delay of several days (Barjorunas 1990).

Hypercalcemia is associated with changes in cardiac electrophysiology that may result in prolonged PR and QRS intervals, as well as shortening of the QT interval. As calcium concentration climbs, the T wave widens, which prolongs the QT interval. This may ultimately cause bradyarrhythmias, complete heart block, and possibly asystole (Muggia and Heinemann 1970).

Hypercalcemia may depress the autonomic nervous system, thereby causing gastrointestinal toxicity, including anorexia, nausea, and vomiting. Constipation, obstipation, and abdominal pain may also develop. Unlike primary hyperparathyroidism, peptic ulcer disease and pancreatitis are uncommon manifestations in patients with the hypercalcemia of malignancy, as these syndromes may be related to the duration of hypercalcemia (Habener 1989).

Renal manifestations include tubular defects resulting in loss of urinary concentrating ability, which causes polyuria. The polyuria then contributes to volume depletion, which decreases the glomerular filtration rate and promotes calcium reabsorption in the proximal tubule, thereby worsening the hypercalcemia. Additional renal complications include metabolic alkalosis, azotemia, and nephrocalcinosis (Barjorunas 1990).

Other manifestations of hypercalcemia include bone pain, either from osteolytic metastases or humorally mediated bone resorption as outlined above (Myers 1977). Metastatic calcification is more common in long-standing hypercalcemia than in the hypercalcemia of malignancy (Habener 1989).

Initial therapy for patients with symptomatic hypercalcemia is aggressibe intravascular volume replacement with normal saline, as most patients are severely dehydrated. Once intravascular volume has been replaced, loop diuretics such as furosemide can be added to promote urinary calcium excretion. Following initial fluid replacement, therapy is directed at normalizing calcium homeostasis by inhibiting osteoclastic bone resorption. Many agents are available, including calcitonin, plicamycin, glucocorticoids, and indomethacin (Ritch 1990). However, the bisphosphonates, including etidronate and pamidronate, are the most effective agents. These drugs are thought to work by several mechanisms, including inhibition of hydroxyapatite crystal growth and direct osteoclast cytotoxic effects (Singer 1990). Pamidronate may be administered in doses of 60–90 mg intravenously every 3 weeks. Toxicity is acceptable, with rare instances of allergic reactions and hypocalcemia (Berenson *et al.* 1996). Newer bisphosphonates such as Zoledronate are more potent inhibitors of calcium resorption and are associated with less inhibition of mineralization than other bisphosphonates (Green *et al.* 1994).

Resection of the underlying RCC is the most effective way of treating asymptomatic hypercalcemia (Ritch 1990). This is of special significance for patients with no evidence of metastasis who have the humoral hypercalcemia of malignancy, as resection may remove the source of PTHrP production.

Metastatic hypercalcemia

The hypercalcemia seen in RCC is usually associated with bony metastases. Fifty-two per cent of patients with RCC and hypercalcemia had bony metastases in one series (Chasan *et al.* 1989). Metastatic hypercalcemia does not represent a true paraneoplastic syndrome, as the hypercalcemia is the direct result of osteolytic bone disease by the metastatic process. The etiology of metastatic hypercalcemia has not been completely defined, but prostaglandin secretion by tumor cells has been linked to bone resorption. Local and systemic factors mediating bone resorption have also been described (Mundy 1990). The presentation, clinical course, and therapy of metastatic hypercalcemia are similar to those of the humoral hypercalcemia of malignancy (non-metastatic hypercalcemia). However patients with metastatic hypercalcemia may not respond to nephrectomy, in contrast to patients with non-metastatic hypercalcemia. Additionally, hypercalcemia associated with bony disease may be ameliorated by radiotherapy.

Hypertension

Hypertension is present in up to 25 per cent of patients with RCC, and renin production by the hypernephroma has been documented in 37 per cent (Mc Dougal and Garnick 1995; Lindop and Fleming 1984). The excess renin and hypertension associated with RCC is generally refractory to antihypertensive therapy, but may respond to nephrectomy. Hollifield *et al.* (1975) reported the first case of hypertension and RCC that improved following nephrectomy. A patient with poorly controlled hypertension was found to have a renal mass on intravenous pyelography (IVP). No renal artery stenosis was present angiographically, and renal vein levels of renin were elevated on the side with the hypernephroma. The patient's renin levels and blood pressure normalized following nephrectomy. The RCC in this case was found to have renin levels markedly higher than the surrounding tissues. Other potential mechanisms for hypertension in RCC include polycythemia, compression of the renal artery, or arteriovenous shunting secondary to tumor vascularity, as renin levels may rise when tumor growth exceeds blood supply.

Erythrocytosis

RCC is the most common cause of ectopic erythropoietin (Epo) production, with elevated levels measured in up to two-thirds of patient (Sufrin *et al.* 1977). However, this manifests as erythrocytosis in only a small percentage of patients with RCC, as anemia is more common than erythrocytosis (Kazal and Erslev 1975). The hemoglobin must be taken into account when evaluating elevated erythropoietin levels, as tissue hypoxia is the main stimulus for Epo production. The etiology for erythrocytosis is felt to be increased Epo production or production of a biologically analogous substance by the hypernephroma. This erythropoiesis-stimulating factor may be identical to Epo, although mutant proteins may prevent quantification by enzyme-linked immunosorbent assay (ELISA) (Laski and Vugrin 1987).

More recently, Gross *et al.* (1994) found elevated Epo levels in only one of 49 patients with RCC. Additionally, none of the 14 tumor lines studied demonstrated *in vitro* production of Epo. These results, while not confirmed in other studies, cast doubt on the potential use of serum erythropoietin levels as a marker for recurrent RCC.

Occasionally, there may be diagnostic uncertainty between ectopic erythropoietin production secondary to RCC and polycythemia vera. Patients with RCC typically have a normal or slightly enlarged spleen, as opposed to the marked splenomegaly characteristic of polycythemia vera. Hyperviscosity syndromes are rare, and may be treated with phlebotomy prior to nephrectomy. Bone marrow evaluation may show erythroid hyperplasia; reticulocyte counts and the erythrocyte sedimentation rate may also be elevated. The erythrocytosis typically resolves following nephrectomy or resection of metastases, but it may return with disease recurrence (Rosenblum 1987).

Human chorionic gonadotrophin

Renal cell carcinoma has been associated with elevations of gonadotrophic hormones. Several cases have been reported, though there is no direct evidence of tumor production of these hormones. Golde *et al.* (1974) reported the case of a 45-year-old woman with evidence of masculinization. She had elevated serum levels of human chorionic gonadotrophin (HCG), follicle-stimulating hormone (FSH), and testosterone. Following nephrectomy for RCC, the levels returned to normal Male gynecomastia and increased urinary gonadotrophins associated with RCC have been reported, with resolution of the endocrine abnormality postnephrectomy (Laski and Vugrin 1987).

Prolactin

Elevated levels of prolactin have been reported in at least two cases of RCC. In one case, a 49-year-old woman with galactorrhea was diagnosed with RCC. Postoperative prolactin levels normalized, and tumor cells were found to produce a material that reacted with anti-prolactin antibodies (Turkington 1971).

Adrenocorticotrophin (ACTH)

Cushing's syndrome secondary to ectopic ACTH production by RCC has been described, although it is quite rare, especially in comparison to small cell lung carcinoma. The mechanism is the enzymatic conversion of inactive proopiomelanocortin (POMC) to ACTH by the tumor. This causes symptoms of cortisol excess, including weakness, muscle atrophy, fatigue, hypertension, glucose intolerance, etc. The diagnosis is made by documenting increased basal cortisol levels with the loss of normal diurnal variation, increased urinary free cortisol and ketogenic steriod levels, failure to suppress cortisol secretion by high-dose dexamethasone suppression test, and the documentation of elevated ACTH levels (ectopic ACTH is identical to the native protein). Resection of the tumor causes symptoms to remit, but occasionally medicines that interfere with adrenal steroid synthesis are required, such as bromocripine, aminoglutethimide, ketoconozole, and mitotane (Wallach *et al.* 1992).

Riggs and Sprague (1961) of the Mayo Clinic first reported this possible association, where three patient out of 232 with Cushing's syndrome were also found to have hypernephroma. In one case, the syndrome resolved following nephrectomy (Riggs and Sprague 1961). There remains no conclusive evidence that Cushing's syndrome is a paraneoplastic process in RCC.

Hyperglycemia

Two cases of hyperglycemia have been associated with RCC, raising the possibility that hyperglycemia may represent another paraneoplastic manifestation of RCC (Palgon *et al.* 1986; Jobe *et al.* 1993). In both cases, a patient with controlled diabetes mellitus was found to have RCC. After radical nephrectomy, all laboratory values returned to normal. No specific etiology was found, but the possibility of ectopic glucagon production was considered. Other potential mechanisms include ectopic ACTH production, hyperprolactinemia causing insulin resistance, and the potential for the production of an insulin receptor antagonist (Jobe *et al.* 1993).

Non-endocrine paraneoplastic syndromes

Constitutional symptoms

Nonspecific symptoms such as cachexia and malaise are common presenting features in up to a third of patients with RCC (McDougal and Garnick 1995). The etiology is not well understood, but the cancer cachexia associated with RCC is probably cytokine-mediated. Tumor necrosis factor alpha (TNFα) is the cytokine most commonly associated with cachexia. TNFα has been shown to alter fat metabolism in cultured adipocytes, and may play a role in the regulation of appetite (Laski and Vugrin 1987). Other cytokines including IL-1, IL-6, and gamma interferon have also been implicated in cancer cachexia. The cachexia may improve after resection of the tumor, but it typically represents widespread disease.

Fever has been reported in 20–30 per cent of patients with RCC and is the presenting sign of malignancy in approximately 2–12 per cent (Laski and Vugrin 1987). Until recently, no specific pyrogen had been isolated as a potential cause of fever in these patients. Interleukin-6 has been identified as a cytokine that may stimulate acute phase reactants in patients with RCC. This may in turn cause paraneoplastic syndromes such as fever and hepatic dysfunction. Several human RCC cell lines have been reported to secrete IL-6 (Jobe *et al.* 1993). Additionally, 18/71 (25 per cent of patients with RCC studied were found to have elevated serum concentrations of IL-6 (Tsukamoto *et al.* 1992). The level of cytokine did not correlate with tumor stage, but patients with metastatic disease had higher serum levels. Fever was documented in 78 per cent of patients with elevated IL-6 levels. Interestingly, two patients with localized RCC had a resolution of elevated IL-6 levels post-nephrectomy (Tsukamoto *et al.* 1992) Other studies of the fever associated with RCC have implicated IL-1, TNFα and the interferons, which may modulate hypothalamic function (Tsukamoto *et al.* 1992). While there is firm evidence associating IL-6 with the fever of RCC, the role of other cytokines has not been defined.

Hematologic syndromes

Anemia is present in 20–40 per cent of patients with RCC, though it is more prevalent in advanced disease (McDougal and Garnick 1995). The anemia is typically normochromic and normocytic, similar to the anemia of chronic disease. It is probably the result of marrow suppression secondary to inflammatory cytokines secreted by the RCC (Laski and Vugrin 1987). Ferritin has been proposed as a possible marker for RCC. Kirkali *et al.* (1995) found elevated levels of ferritin in both the tumor and renal vein in patients with RCC. They hypothesize that production of ferritin by RCC may serve as a marker for disease, but their results are inconclusive.

Autoimmune hemolytic anemia (AIHA) has been associated with RCC, but the mechanism is unknown. Stimulation of cross-reacting red cell antibodies by the tumor has been proposed as a possible mechanism, as has immune complex disease. Resection of the hypernephroma may improve the anemia. In contrast to idiopathic AIHA, the hemolytic anemia associated with malignancy is often poorly responsive to steroids, and splenectomy may be necessary for refractory cases (Rosenblum 1987).

Acquired dysfibrinogenemia has been reported in at least one case of RCC. A patient with localized RCC presented with prolonged thrombin and Reptilase times. Polymerization of fibrinogen was found to be abnormal secondary to increased sialic acid residues. Following nephrectomy, there was normalization of the coagulopathy, but it recurred when the patient developed metastases (Dawson *et al.* 1985). It is unclear whether acquired dysfibrinogenemia represents a true paraneoplastic syndrome, as only one case has been reported.

Hepatic paraneoplastic syndrome

The non-metastatic hepatic dysfunction syndrome associated with RCC was first reported by Stauffer (1961) of the Mayo Clinic. This syndrome is characterized by abnormal hepatic dysfunction in the absence of hepatic metastases. The abnormalities resolve with resection of the primary RCC, but have been shown to recur with the presence of non-hepatic metastases (Stauffer 1961). The incidence of Stauffer's syndrome varies from 3 to 20 per cent (Rosenblum 1987). Patients classically present with hepatosplenomegaly, fever, fatigue, and weight loss. Several biochemical abnormalities are present, including elevated transaminases, elevated alkaline phosphatase, hypoprothrombinemia, prolonged partial thromboplastin time, and elevated alpha-2 globulin levels (Laski and Vugrin 1987; Rosenblum 1987; Hanash 1982).

The etiology of Stauffer's syndrome remains undefined. Hepatic biopsies reveal a nonspecific hepatitis, and there is no evidence of biliary obstruction to explain the elevated alkaline phosphatase (Hanash 1982). A specific isoenzyme of alkaline phosphatase, the Regan isoenzyme, has been proposed as an abnormal enzyme of tumor origin that may account for the elevated alkaline phosphatase serum levels. However, the Regan isoenzyme was found to be elevated in only 1 of 14 patients evaluated (Laski and Vugrin 1987). The isoenzyme does not explain the other manifestations of this syndrome. IL-6 has been shown to stimulate hepatocyte production of several proteins, including C-reactive protein, haptoglobin, and fibrinogen (Tsukamoto *et al.* 1992). IL-6 is frequently secreted by RCC cell lines and may be detected in the serum of approximately half of patients with metastatic RCC (McClellan *et al.* 1998). In a series of 119 patients with metastatic RCC, IL-6 levels were found to be significantly higher in patients with paraneoplastic fever and weight loss (Blay *et al.* 1997). Patients with detectable serum IL-6 had significantly higher serum C-reactive protein, haptoglobin, alkaline phosphatase, and gamma-glutamyl transferase levels. It is possible that the production of these acute phase reactants may contribute to hepatic dysfunction. Nevertheless, the exact nature of the hepatotoxin thought to cause Stauffer's syndrome has yet to be characterized.

Renal syndromes

The glomerulonephropathies associated with RCC are attributed to the formation of immune complexes. An antigen common to RCC and normal renal tubular epithelium was demonstrated in a patient with glomerulonephritis in a setting of RCC (Cronin *et al.* 1976). The changes in renal histopathology associated with RCC are described as minimal-change glomerulonephritis, membranous glomerulonephritis, and IgA nephropathy (Magyarlaki *et al.* 1999). An immunohistochemical analysis of resected kidneys of 60 patients with RCC showed that 27 per cent had immune complex nephropathy (11 IgA nephropathy and 5 focal segmental glomerulosclerosis), Preoperative proteinuria and/or hematuria observed in 11 of 16 cases disappeared in 6 patients with IgA nephropathy within a 2–3 month follow-up after nephrectomy. Light-chain nephropathy has been reported in at least one patient with RCC; 2 years following nephrectomy the light-chain excretion resolved (Enia *et al.* 1981). Ninet *et al.* (1994) describe one case of extramembranous glomerulonephritis that resolved following nephrectomy for RCC.

Neurological syndromes

Polyneuromyopathy and polymyositis have been reported with RCC and are thought to be caused by an autoimmune mechanism (Darnell 1996). Other neurological conditions associated with RCC include subacute necrotic myelopathy and myopathy (Handforth *et al.* 1994; Solan *et al.* 1994). A case of myasthenia gravis occurred in a 38-year-old man who presented with bladder dysfunction and RCC, although anti-acetylcholine receptor antibodies were not detected. There was full recovery after nephrectomy (Torgerson *et al.* 1999). Other rare neurologic paraneoplastic syndromes associated with RCC include limbic encephalitis (Bell *et al.* 1998) amyotrophic lateral sclerosis (Evans *et al.* 1990) and lower motor neuronopathy (Evans *et al.* 1990). Each condition has been reported to resolve after nephrectomy.

Amyloidosis

RCC is the most common nonlymphoid malignancy associated with systemic amyloidosis, with an incidence of 3–5 per cent (Mc Dougal and Garnick 1995). Berger and Sinkoff (1957) found evidence of amyloid in eight patients out of a consecutive series of 273 patients with RCC. The mechanism of amyloid formation remains undetermined. The typical presentation is that of secondary or reactive amyloidosis, as is seen in chronic inflammatory disease, with elevation of serum AA protein. One hypothesis is that the relatively slow growth and frequent necroses of RCC result in prolonged immune stimulation, resulting in increased serum AA production (Rosenblum 1987). Alternatively, RCC has been shown to be associated with marrow plasmacytosis, as in other malignancies. The plasma cells are reactive and not malignant, but may in some way contribute to amyloid formation (Laski and Vugrin 1987).

Synovitis

A case report of a 60-year-old was described who presented with oligoarthritis and Baker's cyst and subsequently was diagnosed with RCC (Schultz *et al.* 1999). The arthritic symptoms were resolved after surgical resection of the renal mass. By analyzing the pattern of T-cell antigen receptor gamma gene from T-lymphocytes infiltrating the carcinoma and the synovial tissue from the Baker's cyst, it was suggested that the T lymphocytes induced chronic synovitis by cross-reacting with synovial tissue components.

Miscellaneous paraneoplastic syndromes

Several other clinical syndromes have been reported as paraneoplastic manifestations of RCC, but there is no apparent specificity for hypernephroma. Leukocytoclastic vasculitis has been reported, but no specific hormone or marker has been identified (Hoag 1987; Mautner *et al.* 1993). Other cutaneous markers of malignancy associated with RCC include bullous pemphigoid (Blum *et al.* 1997), pemphigus foliaceus (Bowman and Hogan 1999), and paraneoplastic pityriasis lichenoides chronica (Lazarov *et al.* 1999). Hypertrophic pulmonary osteoarthropathy has also been associated with RCC, but not with the frequency of other malignancies such as adenocarcinoma of the lung and mesothelioma (Wallach *et al.* 1992).

Summary

RCC is associated with a wide variety of paraneoplastic syndromes. At this time, however, we have an understanding only of those paraneoplastic manifestations that result in the production of an identifiable hormone that causes an endocrinopathy. With the notable exception of hypercalcemia, conventional medical therapies do little to improve symptoms or survival in patients with paraneoplasia. The primary approach remains surgical, and resection removes the source of the paraneoplastic syndrome. The recurrence of the syndrome is a harbinger of relapsed disease. While many different syndromes have been reported, conclusive, non-anecdotal evidence of tumor production of biologically active proteins is present in only a few syndromes. This hinders the potential for finding markers of paraneoplasia and therefore markers of disease progression. The pathophysiology of paraneoplastic syndromes will need to be studied in more detail in order to improve our understanding of this phenomenon and to improve therapeutic options for patients.

References

Albright, F. (1941). Case records of the Massachusetts General Hospital case 39061. *New Engl. J. Med.* **225**, 789–96.

Barjorunas, D. (1990). Clinical manifestations of cancer-related hypercalcemia. *Sem. Oncol.* **17**, 16–25.

Bell, B., Tognoni, P., and Bihrie, R. (1998). Limbic encephalitis as a paraneoplastic manifestation of renal cell carcinoma. *J. Urol.* **160**, 828.

Berenson, J., Lichtenstein, A., Porter, L. *et al.* (1996). Efficacy of pamidronate in reducing skeletal events in patients with advanced multiple myeloma. *New Engl. J. Med.* **334**, 488–93.

Berger, L. and Sinkoff, M. (1957). Systemic manifestations of hypernephroma. *Am. J. Med.* **22**, 791–6.

Blay, J.-Y., Rossi, J.-F., Wijdenes, J., *et al.* (1997). Role of interleukin-6 in the paraneoplastic inflammatory syndrome associated with renal-cell carcinoma. *Int. J. Cancer* **72**, 424–30.

Blum, A., Wehner-Caroli, J., Scherwitz, C., *et al.* (1997). Bullous pemphigoid as a paraneoplastic syndrome. A case report in renal-cell carcinoma. *Hautartz.* **48**, 834–7.

Bowman, P. and Hogan, D. (1999). Pemphigus foliaceus and renal cell carcinoma. *Cutis* **63**, 271–4.

Chasan, S., Pthel, R. and Huthen, R. (1989). Management and prognostic significance of hypercalcemia in renal cell carcinoma. *Urology* **33**, 167–70.

Cronin, R., Kaehny, W., Miller, P., *et al.* (1976). Renal cell carcinoma: unusual systemic manifestations. *Medicine*, **55**, 291–331.

Darnell, R.B. (1996). Onconeural antigens and the paraneoplastic neurologic disorders: at the intersection of cancer, immunity, and the brain. *Proc. Natl. Acad. Sci. USA* **93**, 4529–36.

Dawson, N., Barr, C., and Alving, B. (1985). Acquired dysfibrinogenemia: paraneoplastic syndrome in renal cell carcinoma. *Am. J. Med.* **78**, 682.

de Kernion, J., Lowitz, B., and Casciato, D. *et al.* (1995). Urinary tract cancer. In *Manual of clinical oncology*, 2nd edn, eds D.A. Casciato and B.B. Lowitz (Little Brown and Company: Boston MA, 237–42.) pp. 198–219.

Enia, G., Maringhini, S., L'Abbate, A., *et al.* (1981). Light-chain nephropathy in a patient with renal carcinoma. *Br. Med. J. Clin. Res. Educ.* **283**, 339–40.

Evans, B., Fagan, C., Arnold, T., *et al.* (1990). Paraneoplastic motor neuron disease and renal cell carcinoma: improvement after nephrectomy. *Neurology* **40**, 960–2.

Fahn, H., Ying, H., Ming, T., *et al.* (1991). The incidence and prognostic significance of humoral hypercalcemia in renal cell carcinoma. *J. Urol.* **145**, 248–50.

Goldberg, M., Tashjian, A., Order, S., *et al.* (1964). Renal adenocarcinoma containing parathyroid hormone-like substance and associated with marked hypercalcemia. *Am. J. Med.* **36**, 805–14.

Golde, D., Schambelan, M., Weintraub, B., *et al.* (1974). Gonadotropin-secreting renal carcinoma. *Cancer* **33**, 1048–53.

Gotoh, A., Kitazawa, S., Mizuno, Y., *et al.* (1993). Common expression of parathyroid hormone-related protein and no correlation of calcium level in renal cell carcinomas. *Cancer* **71**, 2803–6.

Green, J.R., Muller, K., and Jaegi, K.A. (1994). Preclinical pharmacology of CGP 42′446, a new potent heterocyclic bisphosphonate compound. *J. Bone Miner. Res.* **9**, 745–51.

Gross, A., Wolff, M., Fandrey, J., *et al.* (1994). Prevalence of paraneoplastic erythropoietin production by renal cell carcinomas. *Clin. Investig.* **72**, 337–40.

Hanash, K. (1982). The nonmetastatic hepatic dysfunction syndrome associated with renal cell carcinoma (hypernephroma): Stauffer's syndrome. *Prog. Clin. Biol. Res.* **100**, 301–16.

Handforth, A., Nag, S., Sharp, D., *et al.* (1994). Paraneoplastic subacute necrotic myelopathy. *Can. J. Neurol. Sci.* **10**, 204–7.

Hoag, G. (1987). Renal cell carcinoma and vasculitis: report of two cases. *J. Surg. Oncol.* **35**, 35–8.

Hollifield, J., Page, D., Smith, C., *et al.* (1975). Renin-secreting clear cell carcinoma of the kidney. *Arch. Intern. Med.* **135**, 859–64.

Jobe, B., Bierman, M., and Mezzacappa, F. (1993). Hypercalcemia as a paraneoplastic endocrinopathy in renal cell carcinoma: a case report and review of the literature. *Nebr. Med. J.* **78**, 348–51.

Kazal, L. and Erslev, A. (1975). Erythropoietin production in renal tumors. *Ann. Clin. Lab. Sci.* **5**, 98–109.

Kirkali, Z., Esen, A., Kirkali, G., *et al.* (1995). Ferritin a tumor marker expressed by renal cell carcinoma. *Eur. Urol.* **28**, 131–4.

Laski, M. and Vugrin, D. (1987). Paraneoplastic syndromes in hypernephroma. *Sem. Nephrol.* **7**, 123–30.

Lazarov, A., Lalkin, A., Cordoba, M., *et al.* (1999). Paraneoplastic lichenoides chronica. *Eur. Acad. Dermatol. Venereol.* **12**, 189–90.

Lindop, G. and Fleming, S. (1984). Renin in renal cell carcinoma—an immuno-cytochemical study using an antibody to pure human renin. *J. Clin. Pathol.* **37**, 27–31.

Magyarlaki, T., Kiss, B., Buzogany, I., *et al.* (1999). Renal cell carcinoma and paraneoplastic IgA nephropathy. *Nephron* **82**, 127–30.

Mautner, G., Roth, J., and Grossman, M. (1993). Leukocytoclastic vasculitis in association with cryoglobulinemia and renal cell carcinoma. *Nephron* **63**, 356–7.

McClellan, M.W., Johnson, B., Culley, D., *et al.* (1998). Serum interleukin-6 levels in metastatic renal cell carcinoma before treatment with interleukin-2 correlate with paraneoplastic syndromes but not patient survival. *J. Urol.* **159**, 718–22.

McDougal, W. and Garnick, M. (1995). Clinical signs and symptoms of renal cell carcinoma. In *Comprehensive textbook of genitourinary oncology*, eds. N.J. Vogelzang, P.T. Scardino, W.U. Shipley, D.S. Coffey (William and Wilkins: Media Pennsylvania), 1996, pp. 154–9.

Muggia, F. (1990). Overview of cancer-related hypercalcemia: epidemiology and etiology. *Sem. Oncol.* **17**, 3–9.

Muggia, F. and Heinemann, H. (1970). Hypercalcemia associated with neoplastic disease. *Ann. Intern. Med.* **73**, 281–90.

Mundy, G. (1990). Pathophysiology of cancer-associated hypercalcemia. *Sem. Oncol.* **17**, 10–15.

Mundy, G., Ibbotson, K., and D'Souza, S. (1985). Tumor products and the hypercalcemia of malignancy. *J. Clin. Invest.* **76**, 391–4.

Mundy, G.R., Guise, T.A. (1997). Hypercalcemia of malignancy. *Am. J. Med.* **2**, 134–45.

Myers, W. (1997). Differential diagnosis of hypercalcemia and cancer. *CA Cancer J. Clin.* **27**, 258–72.

Ninet, J., Naouri, A., Colon, S., *et al.* (1994). Triple association: extramembranous glomerulonephritis, renal adenocarcinoma, and splenic hamartoma. Apropos of a case. *Rev. Med. Intern.* **15**, 546–54.

Palgon, N., Greenstein, F., Novetsky, A., *et al.* (1986). Hypercalcemia associated with renal cell carcinoma. *Urology* **28**, 516–17.

Riggs, B. and Sprague, R. (1961). Association of Cushing's syndrome and neoplastic disease. *Arch. Intern. Med.* **108**, 841–9.

Ritch, P. (1990). Treatment of cancer-related hypercalcemia. *Sem. Oncol.* **17**, 26–33.

Rosenblum, S. (1987). Paraneoplastic syndromes associated with renal cell carcinoma. *J.S.C. Med. Assoc.* **83**, 375–8.

Schultz, H., Krenn, V., and Tony, H. (1999). Oligoarthritis mediated by tumor-specific T lymphocytes in renal cell carcinoma. *New Engl. J. Med.* **341**, 290–1.

Singer, F. (1990). Role of the bisphosphonate etidronate in the therapy of cancer-related hypercalcemia. *Sem. Oncol.* **17**, 34–9.

Solon, A., Gilbert, C., and Meyer, C. (1994). Myopathy as a paraneoplastic manifestation of renal cell carcinoma. *Am. J. Med.* **97**, 491–2.

Stauffer, M. (1961). Nephrogenic hepatosplenomegaly [abstract]. *Gastroenterology* **40**, 694.

Strewler, G., Stern, P., Jacobs, J., *et al.* (1987). Parathyroid hormone-like protein from human renal cell carcinoma cells. *J. Clin. Invest.* **80**, 1803–7.

Sufrin, F., Mirand, E., Moore, R., *et al.* (1977). Hormones in renal cancer, *J. Urol.* **117**, 433–8.

Suva, L., Winslow, R., Wettenhall, R., *et al.* (1987). A parathyroid hormone-related protein implicated in malignant hypercalcemia: cloning and expression. *Science* **237**, 893–6.

Torgerson, E., Khalili, R., Dobkin, B., *et al.* (1999). Myasthenia gravis as a paraneoplastic syndrome associated with renal cell carcinoma. *J. Urol.* **152**, 154.

Tsukamoto, T., Kumamoto, Y., Miyao, N., *et al.* (1992). Interleukin-7 in renal cell carcinoma. *J. Urol.* **148**, 1778–82.

Turkington, R. (1971). Ectopic production of prolactin. *New Engl. J. Med.* **285**, 1455-61.

Wallach, P., Flannery, M., and Stewart, J. (1992). Paraneoplastic syndromes for the primary care physician. *Primary Care* **19**, 727–42.

Warrell, R. and Bockman, R. (1989). Metabolic emergencies. In *Cancer principles and practices of oncology*, eds. V.T. DeVita, S. Hellman, S.A. Rosenberg (Lippincott, Philadelphia. pp. 1986–2000.

6. Staging of renal cell carcinoma

J. Stuart Wolf, Jr

Intimately related to the staging of renal cell carcinoma (RCC) is its diagnosis. Both rely heavily upon radiographic imaging. Since subsequent chapters focus on various aspects of diagnosis and staging, including 'tumor markers', 'paraneoplastic syndromes', 'prognostic factors', 'evaluation of a renal mass', and 'radiologic imaging', this overview chapter will serve as an outline for the principles of the diagnosis and staging of RCC.

Diagnosis

Signs and symptoms

Although RCC is increasingly detected incidentally with cross-sectional radiographic imaging, clinical clues to the presence of RCC are still useful. Additionally, aspects of the history and physical examination may lead to the consideration of advanced disease. The most common presenting symptom of RCC is hematuria, noted in 35 per cent of patients in a review of patients presenting with RCC between 1970 and 1986 (Dinney *et al.* 1992). In this series, in which only 10 per cent of tumors were found incidentally, 27 per cent of patients reported flank pain. Pain is thought to be due to compression or infiltration of surrounding tissue, obstruction of the collecting system or ureter, or acute expansion of the renal mass to hemorrhage. Owing to the tumor's propensity for hemorrhage, RCC is found in approximately 50 per cent of cases of spontaneous renal hemorrhage (McClennan 1991; Pode and Caine 1992). The classic triad of hematuria, flank pain, and a palpable mass is now noted in very few cases of RCC, and is often indicative of advanced disease.

Some systemic findings, such as hypertension, erythrocytosis, and elevation of liver function tests, may be attributed to paraneoplastic syndromes of otherwise localized RCC. As with many tumors, unexplained weight loss, malaise, and fever may be associated with metastatic RCC. Features of advanced disease that may be suggested by specific findings include: venous tumor thrombus suggested by lower extremity edema, deep venous thrombosis, caput medusa, or new-onset varicocele; bone metastases suggested by extremity, hip, back, or rib pain; brain metastases suggested by neurologic symptoms or headache; and lung metastases suggested by respiratory symptoms.

Radiography

The interpretation of an incidentally detected solid renal mass with radiography is usually straightforward, as the lesion is considered to be RCC unless specific radiographic characteristics or aspects of the history and physical examination suggest another diagnosis such as angiomyolipoma or xanthogranulomatous pyelonephritis. The detection of a cystic renal mass, which is much more commonly encountered, presents a greater degree of diagnostic uncertainty. Renal cysts are noted in 25 to 33 per cent of computed tomograms obtained in individuals over 50 years of age (Laucks and McLachlan 1981; Tada *et al.* 1983). The four-part Bosniak classification for renal cystic masses has been useful in the assignment of risk of malignancy to these lesions (Bosniak 1986). Bosniak category I cystic renal masses have a thin wall, do not contain septations or calcifications, and have an initial density on computerized tomography (CT) without intravenous (IV) contrast material of 0 to 20 Hounsfield units. Most importantly, Bosniak category I cystic renal masses do not enhance following the administration of IV contrast material. The vast majority of cystic renal masses fall into this category. Bosniak category II cystic masses are often referred to as 'minimally complicated renal cysts'. Their walls are also thin, but a few thin septations and/or calcifications may be present. As with the Bosniak category I cystic renal masses, Bosniak category II lesions have a density of 0 to 20 Hounsfield units on CT without intravenous contrast material, and do not enhance following administration of contrast material. The risk of malignancy developing in a Bosniak category II cystic renal mass was initially thought to be very low, but subsequent studies have suggested that a significant minority of these lesion may harbor RCC (Wolf 1998). Most clinicians recommend serial radiography to assess these lesions, with growth or worrisome change of the lesion being an indication for surgical intervention. A special type of Bosniak category II cystic renal mass is the hyperdense cyst. This lesion fulfills all the criteria of a Bosniak category I cystic renal mass except that the density before contrast administration is greater than 20 Hounsfield units. The increased density prior to IV administration of contrast material is due to protein or blood in the cyst fluid.

Bosniak category III cystic renal masses are considered to be 'truly indeterminate cysts'. For this category the risk of malignancy has been found to approach 50 per cent (Wolf 1998), and surgical intervention is considered more strongly. Bosniak category III cystic renal masses have a slightly thickened wall and more numerous or thicker septations and/or calcifications. As in the previous two categories, the initial CT density before contrast administration is low, and there is no enhancement following IV administration of contrast material. Bosniak category IV cystic renal masses are considered cystic RCC unless proven otherwise, with a malignancy rate of 90 per cent suggested in the published literature (Wolf 1998). These lesions may have thick or nodular walls, numerous or thick septations, coarse or chunky calcifications, and a density without contrast material in excess of 20 Hounsfield units and/or enhancement following IV administration of contrast material.

For cystic renal masses detected initially with IV urography, ultrasonography is usually the best follow-up imaging, especially if the linear tomography performed in association with IV urography suggests a completely cystic lesion. Simple renal cysts (Bosniak category I) are the most common finding. As such, ultrasonography—which can definitively distinguish a simple cyst (imperceptible wall with completely anechoic interior) from more complicated ones in most cases—is the most cost-effective follow-up imaging modality. If the lesion is thought to contain some solid components because of characteristics on the linear tomography portion of the IV urography, or if it is not a clearly definable simple renal cyst on ultrasound, then CT is the next step in evaluation. Here, CT is useful for both the diagnosis of likely RCC (that is, Bosniak category III or IV versus Bosniak category I or II) and also provides the most important first step in the staging evaluation. In some situations, such as renal insufficiency, adverse reaction to IV contrast, or contraindication to ionizing radiation, magnetic resonance imaging (MRI) offers alternative cross-sectional imaging. MRI, while more expensive, less standardized, and less widely available than CT, occasionally provides advantages over CT for diagnosis, especially when the presence of hemorrhage interferes with assessment of the wall of a cystic renal mass by CT.

A combination of standard ultrasonography, CT, and MRI can provide accurate differentiation of RCC from other lesions of the kidney in most cases. For specific uses, other radiographic modalities may be of assistance. Angiography can provide combined diagnostic and therapeutic capacity if embolization of a suspected RCC is indicated because of tumor size, serious hemorrhage, or patient condition. Although scintigrams with dimercaptosuccinic acid (DMSA) have been largely replaced by CT for the differentiation of parenchymal lobulations from space-occupying lesions, single-photon emission computed tomography (SPECT) techniques enhance resolution with this radionuclide and may be clinically useful for problematic cases. Positron emission tomography (PET) with 2-deoxy-2[18F]fluoro-D-glucose (FDG) or carbon-11 acetate is a promising modality for the differentiation of malignant from benign renal tumors, but clinical experience for this indication is still limited. Finally, percutaneous biopsy of the kidney is useful if there is suspicion for lymphoma, infection, or metastases to the kidney rather than primary RCC, or if tissue confirmation of a renal lesion in a patient with poor surgical risk is thought necessary.

Clinical staging

The most common sites of metastases from RCC include the adrenal glands, lung, liver, bone, and brain. The adrenal glands may be involved by direct extension of the tumor or hematogenous spread, which may portend a different prognosis. Additionally, lymphatic metastases, venous tumor thrombus, and involvement of adjacent tissues or organs by direct extension must be considered.

The critical distinctions that need to be made in the clinical staging of RCC are:

- Is there any direct tumor extension beyond that of microscopic perinephric involvement? Microscopic perinephric fat invasion does not alter intended surgical therapy, except in the case of elective partial nephrectomy in which a greater local recurrence

Table 6.1 Staging of suspected renal cell carcinoma

Mandatory
- CT scan or MRI of abdomen
- Anterior–posterior and lateral chest radiographs

Preferred
- Mandatory, plus …
- Complete blood count
- Serum creatinine
- Serum calcium
- Liver function tests
- Sedimentation rate

Optional
- Mandatory and preferred, plus…
- Venous imaging if tumor thrombus suspected
- Bone scintigraphy if serum alkaline phosphatase is elevated, if musculoskeletal symptoms are present, or if other metastases have been detected (patient at greater risk)
- MRI or coned-down radiographs of any suspicious sites on bone scintigraphy
- CT scan of head if neurological symptoms are present or if other metastases have been detected (patient at greater risk)
- CT scan of chest if abnormalities are present on anterior–posterior or lateral chest radiographs
- Percutaneous biopsy/aspiration if lymphadenopathy or sites suspicious for metastatic involvement (liver, adrenal, etc.) require preoperative confirmation, or to confirm primary tumor histology in patients with evidence of systemic metastases

rate may be evident. Substantial perinephric fat involvement might preclude elective nephron-sparing surgery, however. Additionally, suspicion of even greater tumor extension, that is, infiltration of adjacent organs, would prompt preparation for possible *en bloc* resection of involved organs.

- Is there any tumor thrombus above the infrahepatic vena cava? If open surgical radical nephrectomy is the intended treatment, then tumor thrombus with maximal cephalad extent below the liver likely will not alter the incision and approach to the lesion, but demonstration of tumor above this level would mandate changes in the operative planning.
- Is there lymphatic involvement? Depending on other aspects of the clinical evaluation, preoperative needle aspiration of enlarged lymph nodes or aggressive regional lymphadenectomy might be indicated if lymphadenopathy is detected.
- Is there any metastatic disease? Evidence of metastatic disease suggests the need for systemic therapy.

Table 6.1 lists an outline for the clinical staging of suspected RCC. 'Mandatory' staging modalities are the minimum necessary to guide appropriate treatment of RCC. This includes a CT or, in some cases, MRI for assessment of local tumor stage. Standard posterior-anterior and lateral chest radiograph are sufficient to assess for pulmonary metastases in most patients.

The CT should be tailored for the assessment of a renal mass. At the University of Michigan, the dedicated renal mass protocol CT consists of images of 5 mm intervals and thickness obtained before IV administration of contrast material. A helical CT scanner is preferred, since it allows imaging of the entire abdomen in one breath hold. This minimizes motion artifact, provides exact duplication of cuts before and after contrast administration, and provides a volume of data sufficient to reconstruct images retrospectively at any level or plane. Following the pre-contrast imaging, a series of images is obtained during the nephrographic phase following IV administration of contrast material. Some investigators have found that addition of a third series of images obtained during the (earlier) corticomedullallary enhancement phase improves staging accuracy (Kopka *et al.* 1997). Despite advances in helical CT, a large series evaluating its performance for specific aspects of clinical staging has not been presented, such that the figures in the following paragraphs represent the performance of older CT scanners. It might be expected that some aspects of tumor staging might be improved with the new scanners.

On CT, perinephric stranding or the presence of abnormal soft tissue density within the perinephric space suggest involvement of the perinephric fat. Unfortunately, since perinephric spread is often microscopic, the sensitivity of CT for perinephric fat involvement is less than 50 per cent (Johnson *et al.* 1987). While the finding of abnormal soft tissue density within the perinephric space is very specific for involvement of the perinephric fat (98 per cent), perinephric stranding is not. Fortunately, these deficiencies are of little clinical concern in most cases, since the radical or partial nephrectomy that is usually indicated for the management of RCC without evidence of systemic metastases will include resection of the overlying perinephric fat to which microscopic extension would be limited. Similarly, although the sensitivity of CT for adjacent organ involvement is limited

(approximately 60 per cent), the specificity is excellent. Although suspicion of adjacent organ involvement might alter the surgical preparation somewhat, radical nephrectomy would still be the initial management in most cases regardless of the need for *en bloc* resection of involved organs. As such, limited sensitivity for microscopic involvement of adjacent organs is not a significant clinical concern. It has not yet been determined that MRI is superior to CT for the detection of subtle tumor extension into the perinephric fat or adjacent organs, although the capacity of MRI to clearly delineate fat planes with image reconstruction along any axis would suggest that it might prove useful in this regard.

Preoperative detection of lymphadenopathy might alter the therapeutic approach significantly. In general, enlarged lymph nodes in the presence of RCC strongly suggest metastatic lymphatic involvement, although nodes less than 2 cm in diameter are not infrequently inflammatory in origin. Fortunately, the accuracy of CT for the detection of metastatic lymphadenopathy is greater than for detection of perinephric fat or adjacent organ involvement, with a sensitivity of 83 per cent and a specificity of 88 per cent. Here, MRI does have one clear advantage in that it can distinguish between small clusters of blood vessels and lymphadenopathy (Fein *et al.* 1987). Surgical exploration or percutaneous aspiration of the lymph node should be entertained if retroperitoneal adenopathy is noted in the presence of a renal mass suspicious for RCC. CT may yield findings suggestive of venous tumor thrombus, including venous enlargement, abrupt changes in the caliber of the vein, and intraluminal variations in contrast enhancement. These are insensitive and nonspecific findings, however, and MRI is recognized as the optimal study for the staging of a caval tumor thrombus in association with RCC (Horan *et al.* 1989). Magnetic resonance imaging also has the advantage of not requiring administration of potentially nephrotoxic contrast agents. In expert hands, transcutaneous Doppler ultrasonography can provide valuable information about the primary tumor and especially venous tumor thrombus (Bos and Mensink 1998), but this technique is extremely operator-dependent and the anatomical detail generally is inferior to that provided by MRI.

In addition to the required tests of CT or MRI of the abdomen, plus chest radiography, preferred tests in the staging of RCC include a complete blood count, sedimentation rate, serum creatinine, serum calcium, and liver function tests (Table 6.1). Although these tests are not necessary in a patient with a small peripheral renal mass at low risk for metastatic disease, they are indicated in most patients. The complete blood count is useful in screening for polycythemia or anemia, and the serum creatinine provides an assessment of renal function. The sedimentation rate, serum calcium, and liver function tests screen for paraneoplastic syndromes associated with RCC, or may suggest radiographically undetected metastatic disease.

The tests listed under the heading 'Optional' in Table 6.1 are performed in specific situations. Venous imaging, preferably with magnetic resonance imaging, is advised if tumor thrombus is suspected on the basis of CT findings in the vein or the size or the location of the tumor. Bone scintigraphy is necessary only if the serum alkaline phosphatase is elevated, if musculoskeletal symptoms are present, or if other metastases have been detected (patient at greater risk). If bone scintigraphy suggests the presence of metastases, then MRI or coned-down radiographs of the suspicious site are indicated. CT of the head is reserved for evaluation of patients with neurologic symptoms or with other metastases, and CT of the chest is necessary only to investigate abnormalities on routine chest radiography. Finally, percutaneous biopsy can be used to confirm histology of the primary tumor in patients with radiographic evidence of systemic metastases, to assess enlarged lymph nodes, or to sample suspected metastatic lesions.

Pathologic staging

Pathologic staging is important for the determination of prognosis, for analysis and comparison of results, and for the application of adjunctive therapies. The use of the TNM ('tumor–node–metastasis') system for pathologic staging of RCC is strongly recommended. The TNM classification for RCC was updated in 1997 (Table 6.2) (Fleming *et al.* 1997). This system incorporates several changes from the 1992 system, most notably the increase in the cut-off for T1 versus T2 tumors from 2.5 to 7.0 cm. Several studies had shown no prognostic significance of this 2.5 cm cut-off, and analysis of the US National Cancer Institute's Surveillance, Epidemiology, and End Results (SEER) database suggested that a cut-off of 7.0 cm would provide better prognostic information. Independent reports support the utility of the updated TNM classification. Javidan *et al.* (1999), in an analysis of 381 cases of radical nephrectomy for RCC, found that 170 cases were downstaged from T2 to T1 when the cut-off for T1 versus T2 was increased to 7.0 cm. This provided improved separation of the survival curves. In a similar analysis, Gettman *et al.* (1999) evaluated a total of 1371 cases of RCC and downstaged 571 of them using the new system. Again, this provided superior differentiation of the survival curves associated with the two tumor categories. Bryant *et al.* (1999) evaluated 933 cases of T1–T2 RCC, with a 5 cm median tumor size, comparing the survival curves using the 1992 and the 1997 TNM systems. They found a better separation of the survival curves between T1 and T2 lesions with the 1997 system.

In the clinical setting of nephron-sparing surgery, however, this new 7.0 cm cut-off may not be as clinically useful. Belldegrun *et al.* (1999) evaluated 146 patients undergoing nephron-sparing surgery, with a 3.6 cm mean tumor size, and found that the survival of patients with T1 disease as defined by the new 1997 size cut-off did not differ from that of T1 disease as defined in the 1992 system. Additionally, Hafez and Novick (1999), in analysing 485 cases of nephron-sparing surgery in which 64 per cent had a tumor size less than 4 cm, found a significant difference between

Table 6.2 Tumor–nodes–metastases (TNM) classification of renal cell carcinoma (1997)

Primary tumor (T)

TX	Primary tumor cannot be assessed	
T0	No evidence of primary tumor	
T1	Tumor 7 cm or less in greatest dimension limited to the kidney	
T2	Tumor more than 7 cm in greatest dimension limited to the kidney	
T3	Tumor extends into major veins or invades the adrenal gland or perinephric tissues, but not beyond Gerota's fascia	
	T3a	Tumor invades the adrenal gland or perinephric tissues, but not beyond Gerota's fascia
	T3b	Tumor grossly extends into the renal vein(s) or vena cava below the diaphragm
	T3c	Tumor grossly extends into the renal vein(s) or vena cava above the diaphragm
T4	Tumor invades beyond Gerota's fascia	

Regional lymph nodes (N)*

NX	Regional lymph nodes cannot be assessed
N0	No regional lymph node metastases
N1	Metastasis in a single regional lymph node
N2	Metastases in more than one regional lymph node

Distant metastases (M)

MX	Distant metastases cannot be assessed
M0	No distant metastases
M1	Distant metastases

Stage grouping

Stage	T	N	M
I	T1	N0	M0
II	T2	N0	M0
III	T1-2	N1	M0
	T3	N0–1	M0
IV	T4	N0–1	M0
	Any	N2	M0
	Any	Any	M1

* Not affected by laterality. Regional lymph nodes include: renal hilar, paracaval, aortic (para-aortic, periaortic, lateral aortic), and not otherwise specified retroperitoneal.

the survival curves using a 4 cm cut-off. These authors proposed that the T1 category in the TNM system be subdivided into T1a (less than 4 cm) and T1b (4 to 7 cm). Overall then, the 1997 TNM system does appear to be an improvement over the 1992 system, particularly in providing better prognostic information for patients undergoing radical nephrectomy for tumor masses without associated venous tumor thrombus. Refinements of the staging system might be helpful in the setting of nephron-sparing surgery. Additionally, a 4 cm cut-off (that is, lower than the 7.0 cm cut-off in the 1997 system) appears to lend itself well to some of the emerging technologies involving minimally invasive excisional or energy-based ablation modalities, such as laparoscopic nephron-sparing surgery, cryotherapy, microwave, or radiofrequency ablation.

Summary

Most renal lesions can be diagnosed and staged radiographically with clinically acceptable accuracy. A well-performed CT scan is the mainstay of accurate diagnosis and staging. Although some of the refinements in the 1997 TNM staging system are controversial, the new 7.0 cm cut-off between T1 and T2 tumors appears to be prognostically useful in the setting of radical nephrectomy. Finally, the importance of staging will probably increase in the future as new minimally invasive surgical procedures, new energy-based ablative technologies, and new adjunctive treatments are introduced.

References

Belldegrun, A., Tsui, K.-H., deKernion, J., and Smith, R. (1999). Efficacy of nephron-sparing surgery for renal cell carcinoma: analysis based on the new 1997 tumor–node–metastasis staging system. *J. Clin. Oncol.* 17, 2868–75.

Bos, S. and Mensink, H. (1998). Can duplex Doppler ultrasound replace computed tomography in staging patients with renal cell carcinoma? *Scand. J. Urol. Nephrol.* 32, 87–91.

Bosniak, M.A. (1986). The current radiographic approach to renal cysts. *Radiology* 158, 1–10.

Bryant, S., Iocca, A., Gettman, M., Blute, M., and Zincke, H. (1999). Staging of T1 versus T2 renal cell carcinoma: the issue of tumor size cutoff [abstract 741]. *J. Urol.* 161 (suppl.), 194.

Dinney, C.P.N., Awad, S.A., Gajewski, J.B., Belitsky, P., Lannon, S.G., Mack, F.G., *et al.* (1992). Analysis of imaging modalities, staging systems, and prognostic indicators for renal cell carcinoma. *Urology* 39, 122–9.

Fein, A., Lee, J., Balfe, D., Heiken, J., Ling, D., Glazer, H., *et al.* (1987). Diagnosis and staging of renal cell carcinoma: a comparison of MR imaging and CT. *Am. J. Roentgenol.* 148, 749–53.

Fleming, I.D., Cooper, J.S., Henson, D.E., Hutter, R.V.P., Kennedy, B.J., Murphy, G.P., *et al.* (ed.) (1997). *American Joint Committee on Cancer cancer staging manual.* Lippincott–Raven, Philadelphia.

Gettman, M., Blute, N., Iocca, A., and Zincke, H. (1999). Significance of 1997 TNM staging system for pathologic classification of renal cell carcinoma [abstract 735]. *J. Urol.* 161 (suppl.), 193.

Hafez, K. and Novick, A. (1999). Nephron-sparing surgery for localized renal cell carcinoma: impact of tumor size on patient suvival, tumor recurrence, and TNM staging [abstract 732]. *J. Urol.* 161 (suppl.), 192.

Horan, J.J., Robertson, C.N., Choyke, P.L., Frank, J.A., Miller, D.L., Pass, H.I., *et al.* (1989). The detection of renal carcinoma extension into the renal vein and inferior vena cava: a prospective comparison of venacavography and magnetic resonance imaging. *J Urol.* 142, 943–8.

Javidan, J., Stricker, H., Tamboli, P., Amin, M., Peabody, J., Deshpande, A., *et al.* (1999). Prognostic significance of the 1997 TNM classification of renal cell carcinoma. *J. Urol.* 162, 1277–81.

Johnson, C., Dunnick, N., Cohan, R., and Illecas, F. (1987). Renal adenocarcinoma: CT staging of 100 tumors. *Am. J. Roentgenol.* 148, 59–63.

Kopka, L., Fischer, U., Zoeller, G., Schmidt, C., Ringert, R., and Grabbe, E. (1997). Dual phase helical CT of the kidney: value of the corticomedullary and nephrographic phase for evaluation of renal lesions and preoperative staging of renal cell carcinoma. *Am. J. Roentgenol.* 169, 1573–8.

Laucks, S.P., Jr and McLachlan, M.S.F. (1981). Aging and simple cysts of the kidney. *Br. J. Radiol.* 54, 12–14.

McClennan, B. (1991). Oncologic imaging. Staging and follow-up or renal and adrenal carcinoma. *Cancer* 67 (suppl. 4), 1199–208.

Pode, D. and Caine, M. (1992). Spontaneous retroperitoneal hemorrhage. *J. Urol.* 147, 311–18.

Tada, S., Yamagishi, J., Kobayashi, H., Hata, Y., and Kobari, T. (1983). The incidence of simple renal cyst by computed tomography. *Clin. Radiol.* 34, 437–9.

Wolf, J.S., Jr (1998). Evaluation and management of solid and cystic renal masses. *J. Urol.* 159, 1120–33.

7.   **Tumor markers**

Peter Mulders

Introduction

One of the questions most frequently asked of physicians by patients concerns prognosis. Markers of solid tumors are the best prognosticators of the course of these tumors. The effect of these markers on the host will have a substantial impact on prognosis by affecting the performance status of the patient. The last decade has seen an explosion of research into the use of molecular markers as potential prognosticators in various malignancies. Several studies have focused on the evaluation of new molecular markers. Nevertheless, many tumors still lack adequate markers and more research is needed. Tumor markers may indicate the necessity for a certain treatment but may also make it possible to avoid useless toxic treatment strategies.

Tumor markers are usually proteins associated with a malignancy and might be clinically useful in patients with cancer. Tumor markers can be categorized according to where they are detected:

- in a tumor tissue itself;
- in circulating tumor cells in peripheral blood;
- in lymph nodes;
- in bone marrow;
- in other body fluids (ascites, urine, and stool).

A tumor marker may be used to define a particular disease entity, in which case it may be used for diagnosis, staging, or population screening. Markers may also be used to detect the presence of occult metastatic disease, to monitor response to treatment, or to detect recurrence. Recently, they have even been used as targets for therapeutic intervention in clinical trials.

The use of tumor markers in renal cell carcinoma

It becomes clear that tumor markers can be useful in treating renal cell carcinoma (RCC) when we put the variable clinical course of the disease into perspective. RCC is the most common tumor of the adult kidney. Approximately 80–90 per cent of all primary renal neoplasms are RCC. The disease affects approximately 30 000 Americans each year (Boring *et al.* 1995). The natural course of the disease is unpredictable. Currently, the treatment for RCC patients with no clinical sign of distant disease is radical nephrectomy. However, approximately 30 per cent of these patients develop metastases, usually within 1 year. Moreover,

30 per cent of the patients already have metastases at the time of diagnosis and the prognosis is very poor with a 1-year survival of 26 per cent (Stenzl and deKernion 1989). There have been new developments in the therapeutic approach to metastatic RCC. Although a change in the natural history can be obtained by immunotherapy, for example, interleukin-2 administration or adoptive cellular infusion, the durable response rate does not exceed 30 per cent (Pierce *et al.* 1994; Figlin *et al.* 1993; Rosenberg *et al.* 1988). This is most probably due to the lack of specificity and the associated toxicity (Mulders *et al.* 1997). Therefore innovative treatment options are needed. (Mulders *et al.* 1999) In order to select appropriate patients for new treatment options it is of the utmost importance to use adequate tumor markers. Tumor markers may indicate the neccessity for adjuvant therapy but may also indicate the avoidance of these treatments with their associated toxicity. Authors have evaluated the use of various prognostic factors in RCC, such as tumor size, histologic pattern, nuclear morphometry, and DNA content, but none of these factors have been proven to supply information independent of stage and grade (Fuhrman *et al.* 1982; Trasher and Paulson 1993; Medeiros *et al.* 1988; Helpap 1992; Tsui *et al.* 2000).

In other solid tumors tumor markers have already been implemented in clinical decision-making. In the context of tumor markers in RCC a short overview of the use of tumor markers in other tumors follows.

Tumor markers in various diseases: translation to RCC markers?

The cancer-specific marker carcinoembryonic antigen (CEA) has been used for a long time during follow-up to detect early relapse in colorectal cancer. Its use is still controversial, however, and the benefit of the use of this marker in the clinic is therefore unclear (Macdonald 1999). It has recently been shown that detecting CEA by using reversed transcriptase and the polymerase chain reaction (RT–PCR) on lymph nodes at surgery for colorectal cancer is a prognostic factor in stage II of the disease, and it is hoped that this method can be used to identify a subgroup of patients who will benefit from adjuvant treatment. In breast cancer a new cancer antigen, CA15.3, is used to monitor the treatment of patients with the disease, as well as to detect recurrent disease, and another new marker, CA27.29, may predict relapse of disease and can be used to detect whether treatment has failed (European Group on Tumor Markers 1999). The only tumor marker routinely used clinically is the estrogen receptor, the status of which is useful when deciding on adjuvant hormone treatment. Many other markers are currently being studied experimentally, but no consensus has been reached for clinical use. To optimize treatment in breast cancer, a marker is still needed to identify the 30 per cent of patients in the lymph-node-negative group who will have a relapse. Overexpression of the HER-2/neu oncogene has been discussed as being related to poor prognosis in breast cancer (Dowsett *et al.* 2000), and, recently, antibodies directed against this protein have been used in clinical trials. In ovarian cancer the cancer antigen marker CA125 is used for follow-up, and an increase in serum concentrations may predict recurrent disease or serous adenocarcinoma (Rosenthal and Jacobs 1998). The CA19.9 (or CA72.4) marker has been used experimentally in a similar way to follow patients with ovarian mucinous adenocarcinoma. The data are still not sufficient for recommendation of routine use of any of the breast or ovarian cancer markers. Prostate-specific antigen and prostate-specific membrane antigen, diagnosed with immunohistochemistry, have long been used as serum tumor markers for relapse in prostate cancer (Gregorakis *et al.* 1998); they have even been used for population screening and diagnosis. Recently, the detection of circulating prostate cancer cells in the bloodstream by using a RT–PCR assay for prostate-specific antigen has been investigated as a predictor of surgical failure, and further development and use of this technique could give clinically relevant information (Su *et al.* 2000). Tyrosinase is used in the diagnosis of melanoma (Proebstle *et al.* 2000). The use of RT–PCR to detect circulating melanoma cells was described in 1991 as the first example of detecting the hematogenous spread of melanoma cells from a solid tumor in peripheral blood.

Tumor-specific proteins as markers in RCC

A tumor-specific tumor marker is expressed only in tumor cells. The best example is that of the so-called fusion proteins associated with malignant processes in which an oncogene is translocated and fused to an active promoter of another gene. The result is a constantly active production of the fusion protein, leading to the development of a malignant clone. DNA sequences can be recombined not only through translocations but also through inversions and insertions. By recombining DNA in this manner, fusion genes may be created or destroyed, or the regulatory control of genes may be interfered with. These mechanisms frequently occur in hematological malignancies but also in some solid tumors of mesodermal origin. Some of these tumor-specific proteins for RCC have been investigated.

p53, bcl-2, Bax, Ki-67 (MIB1)

At the Department of Cancer Biology of the Cleveland Clinic in Ohio a study has been performed to investigate the impact of p53, bcl-2, and Bax onco/suppressor genes and apoptotic regulators in RCC (Vasavada *et al.* 1998). RCC often show a high degree of resistance to chemotherapy and radiation despite expressing normal function of the protein p53 (Tomasino *et al.* 1994). The

loss of control of apoptosis may contribute to progression and resistance to treatment modalities and can be attributed to an interaction between p53 and the apoptotic regulators, bcl-2 and Bax. To determine whether the expression of p53, bcl-2, or Bax could be correlated with outcome, the expression patterns of these proteins in renal cell tumor samples were analysed. In 28 patients with clear cell RCC along with seven patients with papillary RCC and four with renal oncocytomas, the proteins were quantified. Immunohistochemistry was performed on all samples and correlated with markers of outcome, including tumor grade, metastasis, recurrence, and overall survival rate. In all clear cell tumors, the detection level of p53 expression was below the sensitivity of the assay, consistent with the reported infrequent incidence of p53 mutations in RCC. Bcl-2 expression showed a significant correlation ($p = 0.018$) with higher tumor grade but could not be significantly correlated with other parameters examined including tumor recurrence, metastasis, or survival rate. The expression of Bax could similarly be correlated with higher tumor grade but with none of the other parameters. Therefore it was concluded that, at the present time, the combination of both tumor grade and stage represents the best prognostic markers available. Adjunctive use of bcl-2 and Bax staining currently plays a minimal role in helping to further stratify patients at high risk for disease progression or recurrence.

Another study was performed to evaluate the immunologic markers, Ki-67 (MIB1) and p53, in 73 cases of conventional (clear cell) RCC (Rioux-Leclerq *et al.* 2000). These markers were compared with the accepted prognostic features of grade, stage, and tumor size in predicting outcome. Specimens of 73 RCC of different nuclear grade (20 Furhman I/II, 32 Fuhrman III, and 21 Furhman IV) and different stage (10 pT1, 23 pT2, 36 pT3, and 4 pT4) were immunostained with monoclonal antibodies (mAb) against Ki-67 and p53. Univariate statistical analysis showed that tumor size ($p < 0.001$), nuclear grade ($p < 0.01$), tumor stage ($p < 0.01$), Ki-67 index ($p < 0.001$), and p53 immunostaining ($p < 0.03$) correlated significantly with a poor prognosis. A Ki-67 index of 20 per cent was a powerful predictor of survival in all patients ($p < 0.00001$). On multivariate analysis, the Ki-67 index and metastases were significant independent prognostic factors ($p < 0.02$ and $p < 0.01$, respectively). In this study it can be concluded that Ki-67 immunostaining is an additional prognostic indicator of biologic aggressiveness in RCC. Immunohistochemical assessment of tumor antigens could be used to identify patients at high risk of tumor progression in addition to conventional prognostic factors.

G250/MN/CA9

The mAb G250 raised against a human RCC has been shown to react with a large number of RCC. Recently, G250 antigen was isolated and found to be homologous to the MN/CA9 gene originally identified in HeLa cells (Grabmaier *et al.* 2000). This protein is one of the best markers for clear cell RCC. All clear cell RCC express this protein, whereas no expression can be detected in normal kidney and most other normal tissue. In Fig. 7.1 the RNA expression of G250 is compared between tumor and nontumor tissue. Antibody studies have indicated that this molecule might also serve as a therapeutic target. By fluorescence

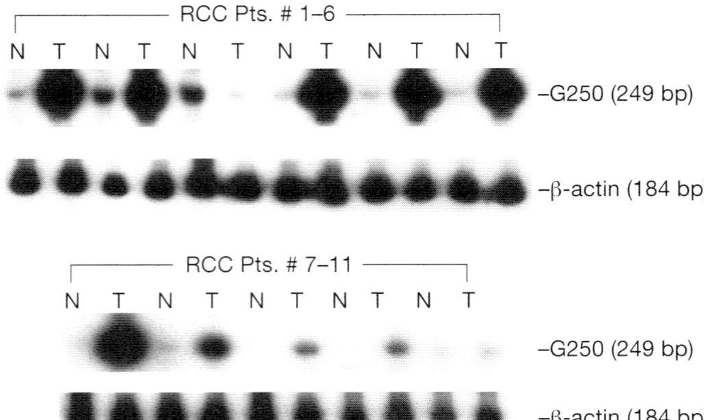

Fig. 7.1 Expression of G250 mRNA in RCC tumors obtained by RT–PCR.

in situ hybridization (FISH) analysis it was determined that the G250/MN/CA9 gene is located on chromosome 9p12–13. To determine whether G250 antigen (MN/CA IX/G250) could be a potential therapeutic target and a tumor marker, a total of 147 cases of RCC were investigated immunohistochemically as well as by RT–PCR analysis. In addition, total RNA samples extracted from patients' peripheral blood samples were analysed for MN/CA9/G250 mRNA signals. Immunohistochemistry demonstrated strong expression in 128/147 (87.1 per cent) of RCC, in contrast to the lack of expression observed in normal tissues. RT–PCR analyses of frozen specimens resulted in the clear detection of MN/CA9/G250 mRNA signals in 137/147 (93.2 per cent) and, despite subtle differences, the results were almost identical to those for immunohistochemistry. Although high-grade and -stage tumors exhibited significantly lower expression than low-grade and -stage tumors, a large proportion of tumors expressed MN/G250 protein as well as mRNA. RT–PCR analysis of patients' blood samples revealed the presence of circulating MN/CA9/G250-expressing cells. These findings suggest that this antigen may be a potential therapeutic target as well as diagnostic marker for RCC. In view of the relative immunogenicity of RCC, it was also investigated whether the G250 antigen can be recognized by tumor-infiltrating lymphocytes (TIL) derived from RCC patients. The initial characterization of 18 different TIL cultures suggests that anti-G250 reactivity is rare.

Another group, from Japan, also compared the levels of MN/CA9 expression with clinicopathological variables in RCC, and thus evaluated MN/CA9 expression as a possible biomarker for RCC (Murakami *et al.* 1999). The level of expression of MN/CA9 was evaluated in 76 surgically obtained tissue samples (49 from RCC, 22 from normal kidney, and five from oncocytoma) using semiquantitative RT–PCR analysis. In RCC, MN/CA9 expression was compared with stage, grade, and cell type. MN/CA9 was expressed in 42 of 49 (86 per cent) RCC samples, but in only two of 22 (9 per cent) normal kidney and none of five oncocytoma samples. Levels of MN/CA9 expression were significantly higher in tumors consisting only of clear cells than in those containing other cell types (p = 0.0189), and MN/CA9 was expressed in 34 of 37 (92 per cent) RCC samples consisting only of clear cells. Tumors of low clinical

stage showed a striking increase in MN/CA9 expression, and high MN/CA9 expression was associated with a good patient outcome. The results suggest that MN/CA9 expression is a potential diagnostic biomarker of RCC, especially the clear-cell type, and can be targeted using molecular biological techniques.

Nonspecific proteins or markers related to malignant cells in RCC

Oncofetal antigens are another kind of marker, less stringent but still very useful. These are expressed in cells during embryological development and in cancer cells. The most commonly used oncofetal antigen, CEA, is expressed in all gastrointestinal tumors as well as in many other tumors. Fetoprotein is used to diagnose hepatocellular cancer but is also expressed in testicular and ovarian cancer.

Adhesion molecules (complex cadherin)

For RCC the so-called cell adhesion molecule (CAM) markers have been investigated. Cancer metastasis is a complex multistage process. Decreased intercellular adhesion enables detachment of tumor cells and can play a role in the early steps of the metastatic process. Although cell adhesion can be mediated through at least four families of adhesion molecules (intergrin, immunoglobulin, selectin, and cadherin), E-cadherin, a Ca^{2+}-dependent epithelial cadherin, is considered to be a critical molecule for epithelial integrity (Nose *et al.* 1988). However, most RCC do not express E-cadherin because renal proximal tubular epithelium from which RCC orginate does not express E-cadherin. In contrast, recent studies have shown that in normal kidney tubular epithelium N-cadherin is expressed (Nouwen *et al.* 1993; Shimazui *et al.* 1996) as well as cadherin 6. Thus, cadherin expression in RCC is more complex than in other carcinomas of the genitourinary tract. On the other hand, cadherin function is modulated through cytoplasmic proteins termed catenins. Immunohistochemical staining revealed that catenins are expressed in all the segments of the nephron including proximal tubules. The catenin family seems to be less divergent than the cadherin family. Therefore, it was thought that there might be a correlation between the aggressiveness of RCC and a decreased expression of alpha-catenin, which is a member of the catenins that link cadherin to the cytoskeleton. Immunohistochemical staining on RCC using antibodies against E-cadherin and alpha-catenin have revealed that the ratios of abnormal staining for E-cadherin and alpha-catenin were 77 and

Table 7.1 Expression pattern* for E-cadherin and α-catenin in RCC

	E-cadherin		α-catenin	
	N	**A**	**N**	**A**
pT1–3N0M0	18	40	45	13
pT4/N1–3/M1	3	29	12	20
p value (χ^2 test)		0.28		0.002
Total	21	69	57	33

* N, normal expression; A, abnormal expression.

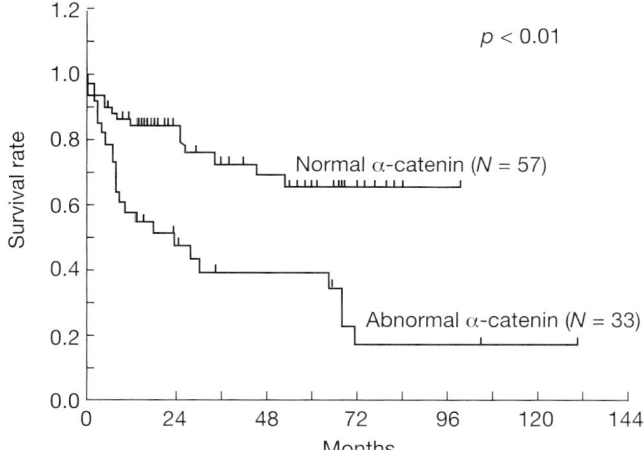

Fig. 7.2 Survival curves constructed by the Kaplan–Maier method show that α-catenin expression significantly correlates with the survival of the patients with RCC (p < 0.01).

37 per cent, respectively. In Table 7.1 the differences in cadherin expression are shown. The prognostic value of E-cadherin is controversial. However, a significant correlation between survival and decreased expression of alpha-catenin was observed. Figure 7.2 shows the correlation with survival. Whether alpha-catenin immunohistochemistry provides additional prognostic information remains to be established.

sICAM-1, sVCAM-1, and sELAM-1

These molecules involved in cell to cell interactions were investigated along with other clinical parameters in patients with metastatic RCC (Tanabe *et al.* 1997). sICAM-1, sVCAM-1, and sELAM-1 serum levels were determined by enzyme-linked immunosorbent assay (ELISA) assays in sera from 99 patients with histologically confirmed progressive metastatic RCC (mRCC) prior to initiation of systemic therapy (Hoffmann *et al.* 1999). Kaplan–Meier survival analysis, log-rank statistics, and two-proportional Cox regression analyses were employed to identify risk factors and to demonstrate statistical independence. In univariate analyses, the following pretreatment risk factors could be identified: serum sICAM-1 level > 360 ng ml^{-1}, erythrocyte sedimentation rate (ESR) > 70 mm h^{-1}, serum C-reactive protein (CRP) level > 8 mg l^{-1}, serum lactic dehydrogenase level > 240 U/l, and neutrophil count > 6000 μl^{-1}. Multivariate analyses demonstrated statistical independence for serum sICAM-1 level, ESR, and serum CRP level as pretreatment predictors of overall patient survival. The prognostic significance of sICAM-1 might indicate a role for this molecule in tumor progression, potentially in association with the abrogation of antitumor immune responses. The possibility of defining a pretreatment risk model based on sICAM-1 level, ESR, and CRP also warrants further investigation, with regard to a possible linkage between acute phase proteins and sICAM-1 levels.

Cyclins A and D1 and p21(waf1/cip1)

The Department of Urology of the Kuopio University Hospital, Finland studied 118 RCC to analyse the expressions of cyclins A and D1 as well as p21 and their relationship to clinical and histopathological parameters as well as to clinical outcome (Aaltomaa *et al.* 1999). Cyclins A and D1 and cyclin-dependent kinase inhibitor p21(waf1/cip1) were not expressed in normal renal tissue. Staining signals of cyclin D1 and p21(waf1/cip1) were always nuclear but cyclin A was also expressed in the cytoplasm of the tumor cells. The mean (range) fractions of cyclin A-, cyclin D1-, and p21(waf1/cip1)-positive tumor cells were 2.2 per cent (range 0–20 per cent), 23.3 per cent (range 0–90 per cent), and 6.8 per cent (range 0–70 per cent), respectively. The expression of cyclin A was related to venous invasion, high nuclear grade, high mitotic rate, high Ki-67 expression, and high proliferating cell nuclear antigen (PCNA) expression (p ≤ 0.006 for all). The expression of cyclin D1 was linked with age over 65 years, low nuclear grade, and high p53 expression (p ≤ 0.05 for all). An inverse correlation was present between p21(waf1/cip1) and cyclin D1 (p = 0.011). Cyclin A predicted survival in the entire study group (p = 0.0014), in T1–4/N0–2/M0 (p = 0.0007), and in T1–2/N0/M0 tumors (p = 0.0007). Cyclin A was also a powerful predictor of disease-free survival in T1–4/N0/M0 (p = 0.0027) and in T1–2/N0/M0 tumors (p = 0.0007). Cyclin D1 and p21(waf1/cip1) were not significantly related to survival or disease-free survival in any of the groups. In the entire sample the independent prognostic factors were the presence of distant metastases (relative risk (RR) 5.16, p < 0.001), T category (RR 2.68, p < 0.001), Ki-67 expression (RR 1.02, p = 0.026), and cyclin A expression (RR 1.12, p = 0.001). The independent predictors in T1–4/N0/M0 tumors were T-category (RR 2.67, p = 0.001) and cyclin A (RR 1.21, p < 0.001), and in T1–2/N0/M0 tumors the only significant predictor was cyclin A (RR 1.19, p = 0.0002). In this study it was concluded that cyclin A is a powerful and independent prognostic factor in all clinical stages of RCC, whereas cyclin D1 and p21(waf1/cip1) have no prognostic value.

nm23-H1 and nm23-H2 proteins

Increasing evidence suggests that the nm23 genes, initially documented as suppressors of the invasive phenotype in some cancer types, are involved in the control of normal development and differentiation (Lombardi *et al.* 2000). A study peformed at the Department of Pathology, Nara Medical University, Kashihara, Japan analysed whether expression of nm23-H1 and nm23-H2 proteins has prognostic significance (Nakagawa *et al.* 1998). A series of 95 RCC was analysed for nuclear grade, tumor size (larger than 50 mm or not), staging in the Robson system, and expression of nm23-H1 and nm23-H2, as well as patient survival. Immunohistochemical staining of nm23-H1 and nm23-H2 was found in 68.4 and 50.5 per cent of the cases, respectively. Significant differences in nm23-H1, but not nm23-H2 expression were noted with regard to nuclear grade and tumor size. The patients with nm23-H1-expression-negative tumors sized ≤ 50 mm had a significantly poorer prognosis than their positive counterparts. Multivariate analysis using the Cox proportional hazards regression model indicated that the staging in the Robson system and expression of nm23-H1 were significant and independent prognostic factors for survival. However, no significant correlation between the incidence of metastasis and expression of nm23-H1 or nm23-H2 was found. The results imply that reduced expression of nm23-H1 influences the prognosis of patients with RCC, but not the likelihood of metastasis. In small tumors sized ≤ 50 mm, reduced expression of nm23-H1 protein was suggested to be an especially strong predictor of a poor prognosis. Other investigators, however, could not confirm the results (Theisinger *et al.* 1998).

Cell-specific proteins overexpressed in malignant cells in RCC

Some proteins are expressed normally by differentiated cells but are expressed at higher rates in the corresponding tumor cells, which is why a relative increase in serum concentrations can be used as a tumor marker; this is the case with prostate-specific antigen concentrations in prostate cancer. Cell-specific proteins are used for diagnostic purposes, for example, the tyrosinase protein expressed in melanocytes. For RCC some of these proteins appear to be useful as markers.

TuM2-PK

At the University of Frankfurt, Germany, various isoforms of the glycolytic enzyme pyruvate kinase (PK) are expressed in different cell-types (Oremek *et al.* 1999). One of these isoforms, the type TuM2-PK, is strongly overexpressed by tumor cells and released into body fluids. The concentration of TuM2-PK in body fluids can be quantitatively determined by a commercially available ELISA kit. Using this kit, the TuM2-PK concentration was measured in EDTA–plasma of 64 patients with RCC and 10 patients suffering from nephritis. The ranges of the TuM2-PK concentrations of the two groups did not overlap, indicating a highly significant discrimination of RCC and benign renal diseases. Furthermore, the TuM2-PK-concentration in EDTA–plasma correlates strongly with the Robson tumor stage of the 64 patients. This indicates that the TuM2-PK might be the first tumor marker to be added as an excellent complement to the diagnostic program for RCC. In addition, in the Department of Urology at the Eberhard-Karls-University, Tübingen, Germany this marker was evaluated as a potential tumor marker for RCC (Wechsel *et al.* 1999). The following were studied:

(1) the expression of TuM2-PK in RCC by immunohisto-chemistry using an mAb recognizing only the mono- or dimeric form of pyruvate kinase;

(2) the stability of TuM2-PK in serum by measuring TuM2-PK in three patients at different times after taking blood with a two-site immunometric assay;

(3) the circadian rhythm of TuM2-PK in blood by measuring levels every 4 hours in five patients;

(4) TuM2-PK-expression in serum in five patients by taking blood from tumor-side vena renalis compared to peripheral blood;

(5) TuM2-PK in 40 RCC patients comparing the results with 39 healthy persons and clinical data of RCC;

(6) the influence of wound healing on TuM2-PK by measuring serum-levels during a period of more than 12 weeks in six patients;

(7) the individual follow-up of four patients with RCC stage Robson III for more than 2 years, comparing TuM2-PK-levels to findings of staging by computed tomography.

In this study the isoenzyme TuM2-PK could be demonstrated in RCC and their metastases by immunohistochemistry with an mAb specific for pyruvate kinase type M2. In normal kidney cells pyruvate kinase type M2 is not detectable. The stability of TuM2-PK was studied in the serum within 30 minutes. No circadian rhythm was found. Most serum TuM2-PK comes from tumor. Serum evaluation in 39 healthy persons was used to determine normal values, with an upper concentration of 28 U/ml of TuM2-PK (95 per cent percentile of normal healthy persons). Serum evaluation in 40 RCC showed a significant difference to that in healthy persons and a positive correlation with Robson stage and grading. No correlation of TuM2-PK was found with histopathological cell type of tumor diameter. After radical nephrectomy normalization of TuM2-PK level was found within 11 weeks in all localized RCC. Continuously elevated serum levels were seen in metastatic RCC. Individual follow-up seems to be possible. Initial discrimination is not possible between localized and metastasized RCC using TuM2-PK; however, it is possible to differentiate between benign and malignant renal processes. The specificity under these circumstances is 75 per cent. After successful surgery of localized RCC, an elevated TuM2-PK will be normalized within 11 weeks, and will remain elevated or will increase again in case of RCC relapse or metastasis. Thus, in this study TuM2-PK would appear to be a useful marker for RCC detection and follow-up. These data still have to be reconfirmed.

MUC1

MUC1 is a glycoprotein that in its hypoglycosolated form is expressed on cancer cells.

In a study from Tokyo surgical specimens of the normal kidney and of RCC tissues at different stages of progression and of various histological grades were examined for the expression of MUC1 mucins with sialylated carbohydrates (sialylated MUC1 mucins) with an mAb MY.1E12 (Fujita *et al.* 1999). Immuno-histochemical studies revealed that the binding sites for this antibody were localized to the apical side of the epithelial cells of the distal convoluted tubules, Henle's loops, and collecting ducts. However, proximal convoluted tubules, where RCC is considered to originate, were not stained. This antibody also bound strongly to RCC at advanced stages of progression and at metastatic sites, and to RCC of histologically high grades (undifferentiated). The epitope, presumably sialylated MUC1 mucin, was detected not only along the surface of the cell membranes but also in the cytoplasm. The level of expression of sialylated MUC1 mucins was inversely correlated with the survival of the patients with RCC and the disease-free survival period after curative surgery. Western blot analysis demonstrated that the electrophoretic mobility of sialylated MUC1 mucins of RCC was greater than that from the normal kidney. It is suggested that high levels of expression of sialylated MUC1 mucins in certain human RCC populations correlate with the aggressiveness of the disease, such as the tendency to form metastases.

CD44

CD44 is a transmembrane glycoprotein involved in cell–cell and cell–matrix interactions. *De novo* expression of CD44 and its variant isoforms has been associated with aggressive behavior in various tumors (Gilcrease *et al.*1999; Heider *et al.*1996). Since few data are available concerning the role of CD44 in the biological behavior of locally confined renal tumors, a group from Paris analysed the expression of CD44 in a large set of conventional RCC to determine its prognostic value in association with other clinicopathologic variables (Paradis *et al.* 1999). Ninety-one patients with locally confined conventional RCC were studied. CD44 standard form (CD44H) and v6 isoform expressions were semiquantitatively evaluated on paraffin-embedded tumor tissue by immunohistochemistry. The prognostic value of the usual clinicopathological variables and CD44 expression was tested using Kaplan–Meier plots by the log rank test and Cox multiple hazard regression analysis. No immunostaining was observed in normal renal tissue. Thirty-two of the 66 conventional RCC (48 per cent) showed CD44H membranous staining of the tumor cells. Only two cancers displayed CD44v6 immunostaining. Among the different clinicopathological variables analysed, tumor stage ($p = 0.001$), nuclear grade ($p = 0.01$), size ($p = 0.02$), vascular ($p = 0.05$) and perirenal adipose tissue invasion ($p = 0.005$), and CD44H expression ($p = 0.01$) were found to be significant prognostic parameters for survival using univariate analysis. Moreover, multivariate analysis indicated stage, nuclear grade, and CD44 expression as independent prognostic factors both for overall and disease-free survival.

In this study it was concluded that CD44 can be a useful prognostic parameter in conventional RCC and may be used in evaluation of the outcome of these tumors.

PCNA

PCNA (proliferating cell nuclear antigen), originally characterized as a DNA polymerase accessory protein, functions as a DNA sliding clamp for DNA polymerase delta and is an essential component for eukaryotic chromosomal DNA replication.

A study from Spain showed in a retrospective study on patients with RCC that the tumoral PCNA is a predictive factor (Morell-Quadreny *et al.* 1998). Immunohistochemical PCNA expression with pc10 mAb in 109 renal tumor paraffin sections was performed. These tumors were previously classified according to cellular type by Thoenes, Fuhrman's grading, and Robson's staging. Moreover, the number of mitoses in 10 high power fields (HPF) was counted and the tumoral necrosis percentage was also evaluated. The 10-year survival curve of Kaplan and Meier was obtained for 90 patients. Nuclear immunostaining for PCNA showed a statistical correlation with Robson's stage, cellular type, and nuclear grade. Moreover, the number of positive nuclei was higher in tumors presenting an elevated mitosis count and higher in degree of necrosis. Survival was significantly poorer in patients whose PCNA index was greater than 5 per cent. Nuclear PCNA immunostaining was shown to be an independent prognostic factor in patients with Robson stage I and also in those who had high cytological grading. These results show PCNA to be a prognostic marker for RCC.

Karyometric markers

Nuclear morphometric analysis has been used successfully to predict the outcome of patients with cancer when classical pathologic grading systems failed. Indeed several investigations showed a significant correlation between morphometric parameters and survival of patients with RCC (Murphy *et al.* 1990; Bibbo *et al.* 1987; Gilchrist *et al.* 1984). We have developed an objective nuclear 'grading' system for RCC using automated image analysis (van der Poel *et al.* 1993). Thus, karyometric features including nuclear profile area, nuclear profile perimeter, elongation factor, nuclear roundness factor, maximal nuclear diameter, and optical density were measured. Cox's regression analyses revealed that karyometric features could provide independent predictive values for tumor stage and, moreover, clinical characteristics. Notably, karyometric parameters associated with tumor heterogeneity (for example, differences in nuclear size and chromatin texture between tumor subpopulations) were of value in predicting prognosis. In addition, heterogeneity of chromatin patterns within the tumors quantified in karyometric analyses appeared to be the karyometric feature most strongly correlated with tumor progression in patients with localized (T1–3N0M0) RCC (van der Poel *et al.* 1994). In contrast, comparative study with DNA flow cytometry has revealed that flow cytometry did not correlate with survival. Another study using flow cytometry showed that DNA contents correlated with the presence of metastasis but not with survival (Ljungberg *et al.* 1986). Recently, it has become widely accepted that genetic alterations play an important role in the development of many cancers. The relationship of abnormal nuclear morphology to molecular genetic alterations in RCC is unknown. In colorectal carcinoma, it was shown that nuclear morphology seemed not to be directly influenced by the individual genetic alterations but was influenced by fractional allelic loss (that is, a global measure of genetic changes; Mulder *et al.* 1992). Thus, it might be suggested that complex tumor properties such as pathologic appearance and metastatic potential cannot be understood unless most of the underlying genetic factors are taken into consideration.

Conclusion

Tumor markers are mainly used to diagnose specific malignancies. The methods commonly involve immunohistochemistry and cytogenetics, including fluorescent *in situ* hybridization (FISH), and reversed transcriptase and polymerase chain reaction (RT–PCR). Markers to be used in population-based screening for early diagnosis such as screening for early colorectal cancer in stool are needed. The only marker that is sometimes used for screening is prostate-specific antigen. Markers used for staging are also needed to optimize treatment; the oestrogen receptor is an important marker for this purpose in breast cancer, and the carcinoembryonic antigen marker looks similarly promising for improved staging of colorectal cancer. The sentinel node technique can improve staging, but more and better markers and techniques are needed in screening, staging, and follow-up of malignant disease.

Table 7.2 Tumor markers in RCC and references

Tumor marker	References
Tumor-specific proteins	
p53, bcl-2, Bax	Vasavada *et al.* 1998; Tomasino *et al.* 1994
Ki-67 (Mib-1)	Rioux-Leclercq *et al.* 2000
G250/MNCa9	Grabmaier *et al.* 2000; Murakami *et al.* 1999
Non-specific proteins	
E-cadherin	Nose *et al.* 1988
N-cadherin, cadherin-6, α-catenin	Nouwen *et al.* 1993; Shimazui *et al.* 1996
sICAM, sVCam-1, sECam-1	Tanabe *et al.* 1997; Hoffmann *et al.* 1999
cyclin A and D1, p21 (waf1/cip-1)	Aaltomaa *et al.* 2000
nm23-H1, H2	Lombardi *et al.* 2000; Theisinger *et al.* 1998
Cell-specific proteins overexpressed in malignant cells	
TuM2-PK	Oremek *et al.* 1999; Wechsel *et al.* 1999
MUC-1	Fujita *et al.* 1999
CD44	Paradis *et al.* 1996; Gilcrease *et al.* 1999; Heider *et al.* (1996)
PCNA	Morell-Quadreny *et al.* 1998
Karyometry	van der Poel *et al.* 1994; Ljungberg *et al.* 1986

In RCC some of the investigated tumor markers seem to be promising (summarized in Table 7.2). They may show additional prognostic value over classical prognostic factors like stage and grade. However, the definitive value of these tumor markers still has to be reconfirmed in larger groups of patients. Ultimately, these factors should show their value in a prospective well-controlled manner.

To summarize:

- Tumor markers are commonly proteins associated with malignancy, offering a putative clinical use in cancer.
- A tumor marker can be detected in a solid tumor, in circulating tumor cells in peripheral blood, in lymph nodes, in bone marrow, or in other body fluids (urine or stool).
- A tumor marker can be used for population screening and for detection, diagnosis, staging, prognosis, or follow-up of malignant diseases.
- A specific tumor marker is a fusion protein associated with a malignant process in which an oncogene is translocated and fused to an active promoter of another gene.
- Unspecific markers include the oncofetal proteins (such as the carcinoembryonic antigen or fetoprotein) expressed by many different types of cancer.
- RCC tumor markers exist and seem promising, but still have to prove their definitive value in well-controlled prospective studies.

References

Aaltomaa, S., Lipponen, P., Ala-Opas, M., Eskelinen, M., Syrjanen, K., and Kosma, V.M. (1999). Expression of cyclins A and D and p21(waf1/cip1) proteins in renal cell cancer and their relation to clinicopathological variables and patient survival. *Br. J. Cancer* **80** (12), 2001–7.

Bibbo, M., Galera-Davidson, H., Dytch, H.E., Gonzalez de Chaves, J., Lopez-Garrido, J., and Bartels, P.H. (1987). *Kaeyometry* and histometry of renal-cell carcinoma. *Anal. Quant. Cytol. Histol.* **9** (2), 182–7.

Boring, C.C., Squires, T.S., Tong, T., *et al.* (1995). Cancer statistics. *CA Cancer J. Clin.* **44**, 7–26.

Dowsett, M., Cooke, T., Ellis, I., Gullick, W.J., Gusterson, B., Mallon, E., and Walker. R. (2000). Assessment of HER2 status in breast cancer: why, when and how? *Eur. J. Cancer* **36** (2), 170–6.

European Group on Tumor Markers (1999). Tumor markers in breast cancer—EGTM recommendations. *Anticancer Res.* **19** (4A), 2803–5.

Figlin, R.A., Pierce, W.C., deKernion, J., and Belldegrun, A. (1993). The biology and clinical activity of CD8+ tumor infiltrating lymphocytes (CD8+ TIL) in patients with metastatic renal cell carcinoma (RCC). *Proc. Am. Soc. Clin. Oncol.* **12**, 288.

Fuhrman, S.A., Lasky, L.C., Limas, C. (1982) Prognostic significance of morphologic parameters in renal cell carcinoma. *Am. J. Surg. Pathol.* 1982 Oct; 6(7), 655–63.

Fujita, K., Denda, K., Yamamoto, M., Matsumoto, T., Fujime, M., and Irimura, T. (1999). Expression of MUC1 mucins inversely correlated with post-surgical survival of renal cell carcinoma patients. *Br. J. Cancer* **80** (1–2), 301–8.

Gilchrist, K.W., Hogan, T.F., Harberg, J., and Sonneland, P.R. (1984). Prognostic significance of nuclear sizing in renal cell carcinoma. *Urology* **24** (2), 122–4.

Gilcrease, M.Z., Guzman-Paz, M., Niehans, G., Cherwitz, D., McCarthy, J.B., and Albores-Saavedra, J. (1999). Correlation of CD44S expression in renal clear cell carcinomas with subsequent tumor progression or recurrence. *Cancer* **86**, 2320–6.

Grabmaier, K., Vissers, J.L., De Weijert, M.C., Oosterwijk-Wakka, J.C., Van Bokhoven, A., Brakenhoff, R.H., Noessner, E., Mulders, P.A., Merkx, G., Figdor, C.G., Adema, G.J., and Oosterwijk. E. (2000). Molecular cloning and immunogenicity of renal cell carcinoma-associated antigen G250. *Int. J. Cancer* **85** (6), 865–70.

Gregorakis, A.K., Holmes, E.H., and Murphy, G.P. (1998). Prostate-specific membrane antigen: current and future utility. *Sem. Urol. Oncol.* **16** (1), 2–12.

Heider, K.H., Ratschek, M., Zatloukal, K., and Adolf, G.R. (1996). Expression of CD44 isoforms in human renal cell carcinomas. *Virch. Arch.* **428**, 267–73.

Helpap, B. (1992) Grading and prognostic significance of urologic carcinomas. *Urol. Int.* **48**(3), 245–57.

Hoffmann, R., Franzke, A., Buer, J., Sel, S., Oevermann, K., Duensing, A., Probst, M., Duensing, S., Kirchner, H., Ganser, A., and Atzpodien, J. (1999). Prognostic impact of *in vivo* soluble cell adhesion molecules in metastatic renal cell carcinoma. *Br. J. Cancer* **79** (11–12),1742–5.

Lombardi, D., Lacombe, M.L., and Paggi, M.G. (2000). nm23: unraveling its biological function in cell differentiation. *J. Cell Physiol.* **182** (2), 144–9.

Ljungberg, B., Forsslund, G., Stenling, R., and Zetterberg, A. (1986). Prognostic significance of the DNA content in renal cell carcinoma. *J. Urol.* **135** (2), 422–6.

Macdonald, J. (1999). Carcinoembryonic antigen screening: pros and cons. *Sem. Oncol.* **26** (5), 556–60.

Medeiros, L.J., Michie, S.A., Johnson, D.E., Warnke, R.A., Weiss, L.M. (1988). An immunoperoxidase study of renal cell carcinomas: correlation with nuclear grade, cell type, and histologic pattern. *Hum. Pathol.* **19**(8), 980–7.

Morell-Quadreny, L., Clar-Blanch, F., Fenollosa-Enterna, B., Perez-Bacete, M., Martinez-Lorente, A., and Llombart-Bosch, A. (1998). Proliferating cell nuclear antigen (PCNA) as a prognostic factor in renal cell carcinoma. *Anticancer Res.* **18** (1B), 677–82.

Mulder, J.W., Offerhaus, G.J., de Feyter, E.P., Floyd, J.J., Kern, S.E., Vogelstein, B., and Hamilton, S.R. (1992). The relationship of quantitative nuclear morphology to molecular genetic alterations in the adenoma–carcinoma sequence of the large bowel. *Am. J. Pathol.* **141** (4), 797–804.

Mulders, P., Figlin, R., deKernion, J.B., Wiltrout, R., Linehan, M., Parkinson, D., deWolf, W., and Belldegrun, A. (1997). Renal cell carcinoma: recent progress and future directions. *Cancer Res.* **57** (22), 5189–95.

Mulders, P., Tso, C.L., Gitlitz, B., Kaboo, R., Hinkel, A., Frand, S, Kiertscher, S., Roth, M.D., deKernion, J., Figlin, R., and Belldegrun, A. (1999). Presentation of renal tumor antigens by human dendritic cells activates tumor-infiltrating lymphocytes against autologous tumor: implications for live kidney cancer vaccines. *Clin. Cancer Res.* **5** (2), 445–54.

Murakami, Y., Kanda, K., Tsuji, M., Kanayama, H., and Kagawa, S. (1999). MN/CA9 gene expression as a potential biomarker in renal cell carcinoma. *BJU Int.* **83** (7), 743–7.

Murphy, G.F., Partin, A.W., Maygarden, S.J., and Mohler, J.L. (1990). Nuclear shape analysis for assessment of prognosis in renal cell carcinoma. *J. Urol.* **143** (6), 1103–7.

Nakagawa, Y., Tsumatani, K., Kurumatani, N., Cho, M., Kitahori, Y., Konishi, N., Ozono, S., Okajima, E., Hirao, Y., and Hiasa, Y. (1998). Prognostic value of nm23 protein expression in renal cell carcinomas. *Oncology* **55** (4), 370–6.

Nose, A., Nagafuchi, A., and Takeichi, M. (1988). Expressed recombinant cadherins mediate cell sorting in model systems. *Cell* **54** (7), 993–1001.

Nouwen, E.J., Dauwe, S., van der Biest, I., and De Broe, M.E. (1993). Stage- and segment-specific expression of cell-adhesion molecules N-CAM, A-CAM, and L-CAM in the kidney. *Kidney Int.* **44** (1), 147–58.

Oremek, G.M., Teigelkamp, S., Kramer, W., Eigenbrodt, E., and Usadel, K.H. (1999). The pyruvate kinase isoenzyme tumor M2 (Tu M2-PK) as a tumor marker for renal carcinoma. *Anticancer Res.* **19** (4A), 2599–601.

Paradis, V., Ferlicot, S., Ghannam, E., Zeimoura, L., Blanchet, P., Eschwege, P., Jardin, A., Benoit, G., and Bedossa, P. (1999). CD44 is an independent prognostic factor in conventional renal cell carcinomas. *J. Urol.* **161** (6), 1984–7.

Pierce, W.C., Belldegrun, A., deKernion, J., *et al.* (1994). Immunotherapy of patients with metastatic renal cell carcinoma (RCCa) using tumor infiltrating lymphocytes (TIL) in combination with outpatient regimen of interleukin-2 (IL2) with or without interferon-alpha (IFN-alpha): UCLA Kidney Program. *Proc. Am. Soc. Clin. Oncol.* **13** (A736), 238.

Proebstle, T.M., Jiang, W., Hogel, J., Keilholz, U., Weber, L., and Voit, C. (2000). Correlation of positive RT–PCR for tyrosinase in peripheral blood of malignant melanoma patients with clinical stage, survival and other risk factors. *Br. J. Cancer* **82** (1), 118–23.

Rioux-Leclercq, N., Turlin, B., Bansard, J., Patard, J., Manunta, A., Moulinoux, J., Guille, F., Ramee, M., and Lobel, B. (2000). Value of immuno-histochemical Ki-67 and p53 determinations as predictive factors of outcome in renal cell carcinoma. *Urology* **55** (4), 501–5.

Rosenberg, S.A., Pachard, B.S., Aebersold, P., *et al.* (1988). Use of tumor infiltrating lymphocytes and interleukin-2 in the immunotherapy of patients with metastatic melanoma. *New Engl. J. Med.* **318**, 1676–80.

Rosenthal, A.N. and Jacobs, I.J. (1998). The role of CA 125 in screening for ovarian cancer. *Int. J. Biol. Markers* **13** (4), 216–20.

Shimazui, T., Schalken, J.A., Giroldi, L.A., Jansen, C.F., Akaza, H., Koiso, K., Debruyne, F.M., and Bringuier, P.P. (1996). Prognostic value of cadherin-associated molecules (alpha-, beta-, and gamma-catenins and p120cas) in bladder tumors. *Cancer Res.* **56** (18), 4154–8.

Stenzl, A. and deKernion, J.B. (1989). Pathology, biology, and clinical staging of renal cell carcinoma. *Sem. Oncol.* **16**, 3–21.

Su, S.L., Boynton, A.L., Holmes, E.H., Elgamal, A.A., and Murphy, G.P. (2000). Detection of extraprostatic prostate cells utilizing reverse transcription–polymerase chain reaction. *Sem. Surg. Oncol.* **18** (1), 17–28.

Tanabe, K., Campbell, S.C., Alexander, J.P., Steinbach, F., Edinger, M.G., Tubbs, R.R., Novick, A.C., and Klein, E.A. (1997). Molecular regulation of inter-cellular adhesion molecule 1 (ICAM-1) expression in renal cell carcinoma. *Urol. Res.* **25** (4), 231–8.

Theisinger, B., Engel, M., Seifert, M., Seitz, G., and Welter, C. (1998). NM23-H1 and NM23-H2 gene expression in human renal tumors. *Anticancer Res.* **18** (2A), 1185–9.

Thrasher, J.B., Paulson, D.F. (1993). Prognostic factors in renal cancer. *Urol. Clin. North Am.* **20**(2), 247–62.

Tomasino, R.M., Morello, V., Tralongo, V., Nagar, C., Nuara, R., Daniele, E., Curti, M., and Orestano, F. (1994). p53 expression in human renal cell carcinoma: an immunohistochemical study and a literature outline of the cytogenetic characterization. *Pathologica* **86** (3), 227–33.

Tsui, K.H., Shvarts, O., Smith, R.B., Figlin, R.A., deKernion, J.B., Belldegrun, A. (2000). Prognostic indicators for renal cell carcinoma: a multivariate analysis of 643 patients using the revised 1997 TNM staging criteria. *J. Urol.* **163**(4), 1090–5.

van der Poel, H.G., Mulders, P.F., Oosterhof, G.O., Schaafsma, H.E., Hendriks, J.C., Schalken, J.A., and Debruyne, F.M. (1993). Prognostic value of karyometric and clinical characteristics in renal cell carcinoma. Quantitative assessment of tumor heterogeneity. *Cancer* **72** (9), 2667–74.

van der Poel, H.G., Mulders, P.F., Oosterhof, G.O., Schaafsma, H.E., Hendriks, J.C., Schalken, J.A., and Debruyne, F.M. (1994). Tumor heterogeneity as prognostic factor in patients with low-stage (T1–3N0M0) renal-cell carcinoma. *Investig. Urol.* (*Berlin*) **5**, 60–5.

Vasavada, S.P., Novick, A.C., and Williams, B.R. (1998). P53, bcl-2, and Bax expression in renal cell carcinoma. *Urology* **51** (6), 1057–61.

Wechsel, H.W., Petri, E., Bichler, K.H., and Feil, G. (1999). Marker for renal cell carcinoma (RCC): the dimeric form of pyruvate kinase type M2 (Tu M2-PK). *Anticancer Res.* **19** (4A), 2583–90.

8. Renal cell carcinoma in dialysis and transplantation

Neyssan Tebyani and H. Albin Gritsch

Since the 1960s the number of patients with end-stage renal disease treated with renal replacement therapy has increased steadily. According to the 2001 United States Renal Data system (USRS) annual report, approximately 340 000 patients were being treated for end-stage renal disease (ESRD) at the end of 1999 and 88 000 new patients started treatment in 1999 (http://www.usrds.org). The estimated rate of growth of new ESRD patients is 7.3 per cent per year for 1995–1999. Renal replacement therapy is comprised of hemodialysis, peritoneal dialysis, and kidney transplantation.

Complications of renal replacement therapy include acquired cystic kidney disease (ACKD) and the development of neoplasms in the nonfunctioning native kidney. The majority of these neoplastic masses are adenomas; however, a significant number of these masses are renal cell carcinoma (RCC), and require special consideration in the surgical and medical management of the disease. Thus, patients with ESRD are at greater risk of developing RCC.

Incidence and epidemiology

The incidence of RCC in the ESRD population is much higher than in the general population. On ultrasound screening of large apparently healthy populations with normal renal function, 0.04–0.10 per cent were found to have RCC (Filipas *et al.* 1998; Terasawa *et al.* 1994). In contrast, RCC has been detected in 0.5–3.8 per cent with ESRD. The prevalence of renal cancer seems to be markedly increased in patients with acquired cystic disease of the kidney (see Table 8.1).

Dunhill and colleagues (1977) described cystic changes in the kidney of hemodialysis patients, and a high incidence of kidney tumors. This study described a 1 per cent incidence of renal cancer. This landmark report stimulated a number of additional studies. An autopsy series of 155 ESRD patients (Miller *et al.* 1989) revealed adenoma in 25 subjects (16 per cent) and RCC in three subjects (2 per cent). A questionnaire-based study (Ishikawa 1993) surveyed dialysis units covering 57 000 patients and

Table 8.1 Incidence of RCC in various studies

Study	Number of cases	Incidence of RCC (%)	Type of study
Sasagawa *et al.* 1992	611	3.85[*], 1.19[†]	Screening of hemodialysis patients
Kliem *et al.* 1997	2372	0.50	Screening of transplant patients
Terasawa *et al.* 1994	1603	2.60	Screening of hemodialysis patients
Ishikawa 1991	425[‡], 1103[§]	0.40[‡], 1.50[§]	Review of reported cases
Doublet *et al.* 1997	129	3	Screening of transplant patients
Ishikawa *et al.* 1997	96	6.20 (0.4[¶])	Longitudinal study of hemodialysis patients
Gulinkar *et al.* 1998	206	3.80	Screening of transplant candidates
Mattoo *et al.* 1997	24	8.30	Screening of young (8–24 years old) hemodialysis patients
Lien *et al.* 1993	v32	6.20	Screening of hemodialysis patients
Hughson *et al.* 1986		5.80	Review of reported cases in dialysis patients with ACKD
MacDougall *et al.* 1987	1000[‖]	0.27[¶]	Longitudinal study of hemodialysis patients
Levine *et al.* 1991	30	7	Longitudinal study of hemodialysis patients
Miller *et al.* 1989	155	2	Autopsy of hemodialysis patients
Takahashi *et al.* 1993	50	8	Autopsy of hemodialysis patients

[*] Incidence rate among patients with ACKD.
[†] Incidence rate among patients without ACKD.
[‡] Patients with CAPD.
[§] Patients with HD.
[¶] Incidence per patient per year.
[‖] Number of patients per year.

130 cases of RCC were reported. This same Japanese group also performed a 20-year longitudinal study of 96 patients on hemodialysis and found six cases of RCC, which gives an incidence of approximately 6 per cent (Ishikawa *et al.* 1997). A smaller American longitudinal study of 30 dialysis patients over 7 years revealed a 7 per cent incidence of RCC (Levine *et al.* 1991).

Studies that screen patients are probably the most useful in establishing the true incidence, and several such studies have been performed. Screening of 206 prospective kidney transplant recipients with ultrasound showed a 3.8 per cent incidence of RCC (Gulanikar *et al.* 1998). Screening of asymptomatic dialysis patients is common in Japan, and two large series are available. Sasagawa *et al.* (1992) reported on 661 dialysis patients who were screened by ultrasonography. In this group 23.6 per cent had ACKD and of these patients, 3.9 per cent were noted to have RCC. The incidence of RCC in patients without ACKD was 1.2 per cent. Terasawa and colleagues (1994) published the results of screening of 1603 hemodialysis patients and 27 933 healthy controls also with ultrasonography. In this series, they noted a 2.6 per cent incidence of RCC in the dialysis patients, and 0.07 per cent incidence of RCC in normal controls.

In addition to dialysis patients, studies of kidney transplant recipients have shown a 0.5–3.7 per cent incidence of RCC (Levine *et al.* 1991; Kliem *et al.* 1997; Doublet *et al.* 1997). RCC has also been described in pediatric dialysis patients and chronic renal failure patients not yet on dialysis; however, the number of such reported cases is small and an accurate incidence is not available (Gentle *et al.* 1996; Boileau *et al.* 1987). The available recent literature suggests that patients with chronic renal failure have an approximately 2–4 per cent risk of developing RCC in their native kidneys, but we have not seen this incidence of renal tumors in patients referred to our center for renal transplantation.

To better understand RCC in chronic failure patients, certain epidemiological factors should be addressed. In some smaller series there appear to be equal numbers of men and women with RCC; however, based on the larger series and meta-analysis, men with chronic renal failure are at higher risk for the development of RCC. Men are approximately 3–5 times more likely to be diagnosed with RCC, when compared to women (Ishikawa 1993; Matson and Cohen 1990; Pope *et al.* 1994). There is no clear explanation for this finding; however, some long-term studies show that, in the first 10 years after the initiation of dialysis, the native kidneys in male patients grow significantly larger than those of their female counterparts. Some authors postulate that there is a substance produced in male patients that is not cleared by dialysis and that leads to this growth. There is some evidence that black patients may have a higher incidence of ACKD and RCC (Matson and Cohen 1990).

In chronic renal failure patients, RCC usually occurs in the third or fourth decade of life, which is younger than the median age of RCC patients in the general population. The association between the cause of renal failure and the development of RCC is week. One report states that patients who have not yet required dialysis and have developed RCC are more likely to have renal failure due to hypertension (Chung-Park *et al.* 1989). Also, some have suggested that patients with diabetic nephropathy are less likely to develop ACKD; however, this is not universally accepted and the significance of this finding with regard to RCC is not clear (Miller *et al.* 1989; Matson and Cohen 1990). One group of patients that does require special attention are those with analgesic nephropathy. These patients are at high risk for the development of transitional cell carcinoma (TCC) of the upper and lower urinary tract (Swindle *et al.* 1998). They should be monitored closely with regular urinary cytology, cystoscopy, and retrograde pyelograms. Even those who are followed closely can present with advanced TCC, and some advocate prophylactic bilateral nephro-reterectomy for patients with chronic renal failure due to analgesic nephropathy (Kliem *et al.* 1996).

Tumor characteristics

The pathology of renal cancers in patients with chronic renal failure appears to be similar to that of RCC seen in the general population, and the tumors are most commonly grade I–II, granular, or clear cell varieties (Sasagawa *et al.* 1994). However, there is a higher incidence of papillary growth pattern noted in patients with chronic renal failure (Ishikawa and Kovacs 1993). Papillary epithelial proliferation is a common finding is cysts associated with renal failure (Hughson *et al.* 1986). Atypical epithelial hyperplasia arising from cystic areas can be seen intermingling with carcinoma (Lin *et al.* 1992). These findings, in addition to the high incidence of cysts and adenomas, support the concept that in patients with chronic renal failure there is extensive epithelial hyperplasia in the native kidneys (Mc Manus *et al.* 1980). Biochemical analysis has shown that C-erb B-2, and epithelial growth factor, is increased (Herrera 1991). Furthermore, serum obtained from dialysis patients acts as a growth factor in some kidney cancer cell lines. The serum of normal controls did not have this property. This substance is most likely a 20 kiloDalton (kDa) glycoprotein (Klotz *et al.* 1991).

Renal cell carcinoma in transplantation

It is well known that patients with kidney transplantation on immunosuppression have an increased risk of some malignancies including skin cancer, oral cancer, vulvar cancer, perineal cancer, and lymphomas (Penn 1995*a*; Birkland *et al.* 1995). However, it is not clear whether renal transplantation changes the risk of RCC for the transplant recipient. RCC in transplant patients can occur in three settings. First, a renal carcinoma may be inadvertently transplanted with the donor organ; second, the recipient may have pre-existing malignancy; third, the patient may develop a *de novo* renal tumor. The most extensive review of this subject has been provided by the late Dr Israel Pen (1995 *b*) who previously maintained the Cincinnati Transplant Tumor Registry (CTTR).

Primary renal carcinomas in the donor

In 47 cases reported to the CTTR from 1968 to 1994, the donor kidney contained RCC at the time of transplantation. In 28 of the donors, the tumor was noted at harvesting. In 14 of these 28 patients a small primary renal carcinoma or oncocytoma was found at harvesting. In 8 of these cases the lesion was widely excised and the kidney was transplanted. Five of these cases had an initial frozen section that was nondiagnostic; however, the permanent sections showed RCC and the renal allograft was subsequently removed. In one patient the initial diagnosis was pleomorphic adenoma; however, the lesion grew rapidly after transplant and a partial nephrectomy revealed carcinoma after 3 months. There have been no recurrences in these 14 patients. Therefore, small tumors identified at the time of harvest should be completely excised and the kidney may be transplanted. However, since renal transplantation is not an immediate life-saving procedure, kidneys with a macroscopic lesion greater than one centimeter in diameter probably should not be transplanted with a pathologic diagnosis of RCC (Jordan 1997). In an additional 14 patients, the grossly normal contralateral kidney from a donor with a renal carcinoma was transplanted. There was no evidence of tumor in the allograft on follow-up imaging from 0.5 to 153 months.

Pre-existing renal carcinoma in the recipient

Four hundred and three kidney transplant recipients with pre-existing renal carcinoma were reported to the CTTR. This group included 71 with incidentally discovered tumors, which were discovered either before or after renal transplantation. Pathologic examination revealed 67 RCC, two Wilms' tumors, and two carcinomas of the renal pelvis. Tumor recurrence has not been noted in these patients one to 223 months, mean 69 months, after nephrectomy. This suggests that it is safe to proceed with renal transplantation immediately after removal of asymptomatic incidental renal carcinomas. Seventy-six patients with known Wilms' tumor and ESRD were treated with renal transplantation. Recurrences occurred in 11. Ten patients with recurrence had been treated 24 months or less pretransplantation and one had been treated 28 months pretransplantation. Based on this data the current recommendation is to wait at least 2 years after treatment of Wilms' tumor before proceeding with renal transplantation. 233 patients with symptomatic renal carcinomas were treated with renal transplantation. Of 59 patients who developed recurrences, 58 per cent had been treated 2 years or less, 31 per cent had been treated 2 to 5 years, and 8 per cent been treated more than 5 years prior to renal transplantation. This data has led to the recommendation that patients with treated symptomatic RCC wait at least 2 years before renal transplantation. A longer waiting period may be required in patients with large tumors or evidence of infiltration outside the kidney.

A study of von Hippel–Lindau (VHL) patients with RCC, who have been surgically rendered anephric, suggests that renal transplantation is an effective option with limited risk of recurrence (Reinberg *et al.* 1992).

De novo renal carcinomas

Two hundred fifty-six primary renal carcinomas, in renal transplant recipients, were reported to the CTTR. Of these, 222 occurred in the native kidneys, 24 in the allograft, and 10 were unspecified. Of the 256 carcinomas, 196 were RCC, 29 were transitional cell carcinoma, and 31 were other. Forty-one per cent died of their malignancies, while 13 per cent died of other causes while clinically free of cancer. At least 11 per cent survived longer than 5 years and 3 per cent survived 10 years or more after the diagnosis of cancer. It is not known if RCC behaves differently in immunosuppressed patients; however, there is *in vitro* data to suggest that RCC cell lines develop a more aggressive phenotype when exposed to cyclosporine (Hojo *et al.* 1999). Transplant patients also tend to present with higher-stage RCC when compared to dialysis patients (Reinberg *et al.* 1992; Pope *et al.* 1994). RCC accounts for approximately 2 per cent of deaths in kidney transplant patients (Bretan *et al.* 1989).

Detection and treatment of renal carcinoma in patients with end-stage renal disease

A controversial issue in the management of patients with chronic renal failure, is the role of screening for renal carcinoma. The various parameters that must be addressed are the availability and cost of an effective screening tool, the incidence of the disease process in the population to be screened, and the natural history of the disease in that population with its associated impact on survival.

Ultrasonography appears to be the most appropriate tool for screening. In institutions where screening is common, expert use of ultrasound can detect virtually all cases of RCC (Terasawa *et al.* 1994). This technique is non-invasive and very well tolerated. However, one drawback of ultrasonography is cost. Considering the large number of patients with chronic renal failure under treatment, the cost of routine screening of asymptomatic patients would be a tremendous financial burden.

Three ways to reduce overall cost would be to reduce the cost of each procedure, screen less frequently, and screen fewer patients. In most institutions the cost of ultrasonography is fixed; however, in some dialysis centers and transplant clinics it may be possible that nephrologist and transplant surgeons can perform office ultrasound at a lower cost. There is no clear consensus as to the recommended frequency of screening; however, based on the theoretical tumor growth rate, screening should be at least once every 3 years. The concept of screening fewer patients leads to the practice of selective screening. At one end of the spectrum is the practice of screening all patients. This has the advantage of detecting the most number of renal cancers. However, as stated earlier, the overall incidence of RCC in patients with chronic renal failure is approximately 2 to 4 per cent. The annual incidence is not well established, but most probably approaches 0.27 per cent (Mac Dougall *et al.* 1989). Therefore, screening of all patients would result in the unnecessary imaging of the vast majority of patients. At the other end of the spectrum is not screening any asymptomatic patient. Only those with symptoms such as flank pain or hematuria would be evaluated for possible RCC. This protocol would undoubtedly give the highest yield; however, the ability to detect early-stage and more curable tumors is greatly limited. Therefore, the answer most probably lies somewhere between these two extremes.

To justify the cost of screening, early detection of asymptomatic renal tumors must improve survival. Based on the review of reported cases, approximately one-fifth of patients with RCC and chronic renal failure present with metastasis (Ishikawa 1991). Furthermore, based on a meta-analysis, it has been calculated that the 5-year survival of chronic renal failure patients with RCC is 35 per cent (Matson and Cohen 1990). The goal of patient selection is to identify high-risk patients, and detect any cancer at a curable stage. High-risk patients include patients with ACKD, male patients, and patients with native kidneys greater than 150 grams (Takahashi *et al.* 1993). Also, Black patients have a slightly higher risk of RCC. Finally, transplant patients do no appear to have a higher incidence of RCC, but they appear to present with more advanced disease (Kliem *et al.* 1997). In the large dialysis patient screening study of Terasawa *et. al.* 1994), of the 40 RCC that were detected, none were metastatic.

In conclusion, selective screening is justified in institutions where expert ultrasound is readily available. The choice of who is screened will be greatly influenced by the clinicians' experience and resources. One reasonable protocol is to screen all renal transplant candidates at the time of evaluation, and patients with acceptable surgical risk factors who have been on hemodialysis for over 5 years. A reasonable frequency of screening is once every 3 years in patients with ACKD.

When a mass lesion is detected in the native kidneys, a confirmatory computerized tomography (CT) or magnetic resonance imaging (MRI) scan with and without contrast should be obtained to confirm the diagnosis and develop a treatment plan (Fig. 8.1). A metastatic evaluation should include a chest X-ray, liver function tests, and possibly a bone scan. Patients with an organ-confined tumor should be treated with radical nephrectomy of the native kidney. Partial nephrectomy of a solid lesion confined to a transplant kidney should be considered. In most cases, a percutaneous biopsy of a solid mass within the transplant kidney should be obtained to exclude the possibility of a post-transplant lymphoproliferative disease.

These tumors may respond to reduction or withdrawal of immunosuppression. The most difficult treatment decisions occur when metastatic RCC is identified in a patient with a functioning renal allogragft. Since many RCC respond to immunotherapy, immunosuppression should be significantly reduced or discontinued completely. This runs the risk of rejection of the renal transplant, and the patient should be informed of the possible need for dialysis. The new immunosuppressive agent, sirolimus, inhibits the cell cycle in the G_0 and early G_1 phase and may have some beneficial antitumor effects (Seufferlein and Rozengurt 1996). Immunosuppression must be discontinued if immunotheraphy is considered. Based on patients who have been treated for hepatitis C after renal transplantation, the administration of interferon alpha, will almost certainly lead to renal transplant rejection. Remarkably, patients who have combined liver and kidney transplantation have a smaller risk of rejection (Chan *et al.* 1993; Magnone *et al.* 1995).

Summary

RCC can be up to 24 times more common in patients with renal failure than in the general population. It is usually associated with ACKD, appears at a younger age, and tends to affect more men than women. It can be seen in patients treated with hemodialysis, peritoneal dialysis, kidney transplantation, and even in those who do not yet require renal replacement therapy. The increased risk of RCC is most probably due to the generalized epithelial proliferation noted in end-stage kidneys, which results in cysts and adenomas. RCC tends to be slightly more aggressive in kidney transplant patients.

Acknowledgement

The authors would like to thank Dr. Gabriel Danovitch for his careful review of this manuscript.

References

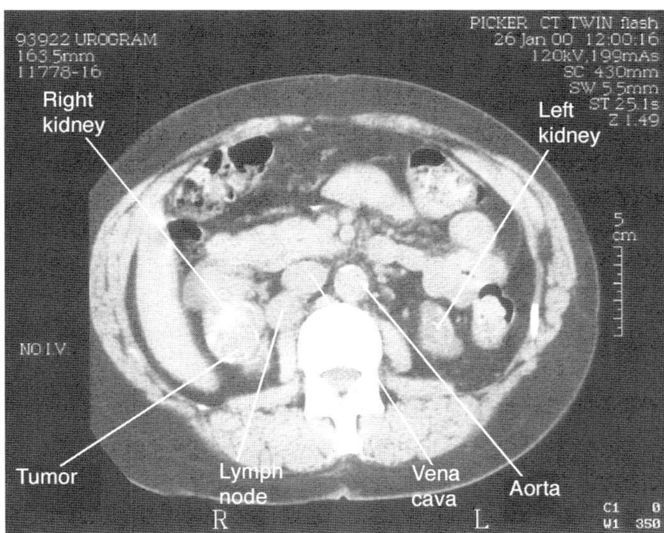

Fig. 8.1 Computed tomography image of RCC with metastasis to the paracaval lymph nodes. Forty-eight year old anuric African American female with ESRD of Unknown etiology for over 10 years, who presented with right flank pain and bloody vaginal discharge. She had a renal transplant 4 years prior which failed after 1 year. Her native kidneys are atrophic with multiple small cysts. The right kidney demonstrates a calcified renal tumor with metastasis to the regional lymph node.

Birkland, S., Storm, H., Lamm, L., Barlow, L., Blohme, I., *et al.* (1995). Cancer risk after renal transplantation in the Nordic countries. *Int. J. Cancer* 60, 183–9.

Boileau, M., Foley, R., Flechner, S., and Weinman, E. (1987). Renal adenocarcinoma and end stage kidney disease. *J. Urol.* **138** (3), 603–6.

Bretan, P.N. Jr, Novick, A.C., Steinmuller, D.R., Dlugosz, B.A., Graneto, D.E., Badhwar, K., Swift, C.L., and Streem, S.B. (1989). Ultrasonographic prospective pretransplant screening in 100 patients for acquired renal cysts and renal cell carcinoma. *Transplant. Proc.* **21** (1, Pt 2), 1974–5.

Chan, T., Lok, A.S.F., Cheng, I.K.P., and Ng, I.O.L. (1993). Chronic hepatitis C after renal transplantation treatment with α-interferon. *Transplantation* **56**, 1095–8.

Chung-Park, M., Parveen, T., and Lam, M. (1989). Acquired cystic disease of the kidneys and renal cell carcinoma in chronic renal insufficiency without dialysis treatment. *Nephron* **53** (2), 157–61.

Doublet, J.D., Peraldi, M.N., Gattegno, B., Thibault, P., and Sraer, J.D. (1997). Renal cell carcinoma of native kidneys: prospective study of 129 renal transplant patients. *J. Urol.* **158** (1), 42–4.

Dunhill, M.S., Millard, P.R., and Oliver, D. (1977). Acquired cystic disease of the kidney: a hazard of long term intermittent hemodialysis. *J. Clin. Pathol.* **30**, 868–77.

Filipas, D., Westermier, T., and Michaelis, J. (1998). Screening of renal cell carcinoma by ultrasound. *J. Urol.* **159**, 168.

Gentle, D.L., Mandell, J., and Jennings, T. (1996). Renal cortical neoplasm in a child with dialysis-acquired cystic kidney disease. *Urology* **47** (2), 254–5.

Gulanikar, A.C., Daily, P.P., Kilambi, N.K., Hamrick-Turner, J.E., and Butkus, D.E. (1998). Prospective pretransplant ultrasonic screening in 206 patients for acquired renal cysts and renal cell carcinoma. *Transplantation* **66**, 1669–72.

Herrara, G.A. (1991). C-erb B-2 amplification in cystic renal disease. *Kidney Int.* **40** (3), 509–13.

Hojo, M., Morimoto, T., Maluccio, M., Asano, T., Morimoto, K., Milagros, L., Shimbo, T., and Suthanthiran, M. (1999). Cyclosporin induces cancer progression by a cell-autonomous mechanism. *Nature* **397** (6719), 530–4.

Hughson, M.D., Buchwald, D., and Fox, M. (1986). Renal neoplasia and acquired cystic kidney disease in patients receiving long-term dialysis. *Arch. Pathol. Lab. Med.* **110** (7), 592–601.

Ishikawa, I. (1991). Acquired cystic disease: mechanisms and manifestations. *Sem. Nephrol.* **11** (6), 671–84.

Ishikawa, I. (1993). Renal cell carcinoma in chronic hemodialysis patients—a 1990 questionnaire study in Japan. *Kidney Int.* **41** (suppl.), 167–9.

Ishikawa, I. and Kovacs, G. (1993). High incidence of papillary renal cell tumours in patients on chronic haemodialysis. *Histopathology* **22** (2), 135–9.

Ishikawa, I., Saito, Y., Nakamura, M., Takeda, K., Ishii, H., Nakazawa, T., Fukuda, Y., Asuka, M., Tamosuji, N., and Yuir, T. (1997). Fifteen year follow up of acquired renal cystic disease—a gender difference. *Nephron* **3**, 315–20.

Jordan, M.L. (1997). Complications of renal transplantation, malignancy after renal transplantation. In *Renal transplantation* (ed. R. Shapiro, R.L. Simmons, and T.E. Starzl), Chapter 11, pp. 353–8. Appleton and Lange, Stamford, Connecticut.

Kliem, V., Thon, W., Krautzig, S., Kolditz, M., Behrend, M., Pichlmayr, R., Koch, K.M., Frei, U., and Brunkhorst, R. (1996). High mortality from urothelial carcinoma despite regular tumor screening in patients with analgesic nephropathy after renal transplantation. *Transplant. Int.* **9** (3), 231–5.

Kliem, V., Kolditz, M., Behrend, M., Ehlerding, G., Pichlmayr, R., Koch, K.M., and Brunkhorst, R. (1997). Risk of renal cell carcinoma after kidney transplantation. *Clin. Transplant.* **11** (4), 255–8.

Klotz, L.H., Kulkarni, C., and Mills, G. (1991). End stage renal disease serum contains a specific renal cell growth factor. *J. Urol.* **145** (1), 156–60.

Levine, E., Slusher, S.L., Grantham, J.J., and Wetzel, H. (1991). Natural history of acquired renal cystic disease in dialysis patients: a prospective longitudinal CT study. *Am. J. Roentgenol.* **156**, 501–6.

Lien, Y.H., Hunt, K.R., Siskind, M.S., and Zukoski, C. (1993). Association of cyclosporin A with acquired cystic kidney disease of the native kidneys in renal transplant recipients. *Kidney Int.* **44** (3), 613–16.

Lin, J.I., Saklayen, M., Ehrenpreis, M., and Hillman, N.M. (1992). Acquired cystic disease of kidney associated with renal cell carcinoma in chronic dialysis patients. *Urology* **39** (2), 190–3.

MacDougall, M.L., Welling, L.W., and Wiegmann, T.B. (1987). Renal adenocarcinoma and acquired cystic disease in chronic hemodialysis patients. *Am. J. Kidney Dis.* **9** (2), 166–71.

Magnone, M., Holley, J.L., Shapiro, R., Scantlebury, V., McCauley, J., Jordan, M.L., Vivas, C., Starzl, T., and Johnson, J.P. (1995). Interferon-α-induced acute renal allograft rejection. *Transplantation* **59**, 1068–70.

Matson, M.A. and Cohen, E.P. (1990). Acquired cystic kidney disease: occurrence, prevalence, and renal cancers. *Medicine* (*Baltimore*) **69** (4), 217–26.

Mattoo, T.K., Greifer, I., Geva, P., and Spitzer, A. (1997). Acquired renal cystic disease in children and young adults on maintenance dialysis. *Pediatr. Nephrol.* **11** (4) 447–50.

McManus, J.F., Hughson, M.D., Hennigar, G.R., Fitts, C.T., Rajagopalan, P.R., and Williams, A.V. (1980). Dialysis enhances renal epithelial proliferations. *Arch. Pathol. Lab. Med.* **104** (4), 192–5.

Miller, L.R., Soffer, O., Nassar, V.H., and Kutner, M.H. (1989). Acquired renal cystic disease in end-stage renal disease: an autopsy study of 155 cases. *Am. J. Nephrol.* **9**, 322–8.

Penn, I. (1995*a*). Occurrence of cancers in immunosuppressed organ transplant recipients. In *Clinical transplants 1994* (ed. P.I. Terasaki and J.M. Cecka), Chapter 7, pp. 99–109. UCLA Tissue Typing Laboratory, Los Angeles, California.

Penn, I. (1995*b*). Primary kidney tumors before and after renal transplantation. *Transplantation* **59** (4), 480–5.

Pope, J.C., Koch, M.O., and Bluth, R.F. (1994). Renal cell carcinoma in patients with end-stage renal disease: a comparison of clinical significance in patients receiving hemodialysis and those with renal transplants. *Urology* **44** (4), 497–501.

Reinberg, Y., Matas, A., Manivel, C., Gonzalez, R., Gillingham, K.J., and Pryor, J.L. (1992). Outcome of renal transplantation or dialysis in patients with a history of renal cancer. *Cancer* **70** (6), 1564–7.

Sasagawa, I., Terasawa, Y., Imai, K., Sekino, H., and Takahashi, H. (1992). Acquired cystic disease of the kidney and renal carcinoma in haemodialysis patients: ultrasonic evaluation. *Br. J. Urol.* **70**, 236–9.

Sasagawa, I., Nakada, T., Kubota, Y., Suzuki, Y., Ishigooka, M., and Terasawa, Y. (1994). Renal cell carcinoma in dialysis patients. *Urol. Int.* **53** (2), 79–81.

Seufferlein, T. and Rozengurt, E. (1996). Rapamycin inhibits constitutive p70s6k phosphorylation, cell proliferation, and colony formation in small cell lung cancer cells. *Cancer Res.* **270**, 815–22.

Swindle, P., Flak, M., Rigby, R., Petie, J., Hawley, C., and Nicol, D. (1998). Transitional cell carcinoma in renal transplant recipients: the influence of compound analgesics. *Br. J. Urol.* **81** (2), 229–33.

Takahashi, S., Shirai, T., Ogawa, K., Imaida, K., Yamazaki, C., Ito, A., Masuko, K., and Ito, N. (1993). Renal cell adenomas and carcinomas in hemodialysis patients: relationship between hemodialysis period and development of lesions. *Acta Pathol. Jpn* **43** (11), 674–82.

Terasawa, Y., Suzuki, Y., Morita, M., Kato, M., Suauki, K., and Sekino, H. (1994). Ultrasonic diagnosis of renal cell carcinoma in haemodialysis patients. *J. Urol.* **152**, 846–51.

Part 1, Section 2

Renal cell carcinoma: molecular genetics and immunobiology

9. Basic biology and clinical behavior of renal cell carcinoma

Allan J. Pantuck, Amnon Zisman, and Arie Belldegrun

Introduction

The clinical behavior of a tumor reflects its underlying genetic abnormalities, which lead to molecular changes that ultimately result in microscopic and macroscopic pathology. A comprehensive understanding and appreciation for the factors that impact upon the biologic behavior of renal cell carcinoma (RCC) is essential for understanding the natural history of the disease in patients. This is important not only for planning therapy, but also for prediction of disease outcome. Useful prognostic factors should be clinically relevant, should correlate with outcome, and should provide independent significance that is not available from other factors already in use. For RCC, tumor grade and stage remain the most useful, available predictors of clinical outcome. However, other important clinical, radiographic, and pathologic features contribute to our understanding of RCC's often unpredictable behavior. Finally, with progress in the understanding of the molecular biology and genetics of RCC, newer biomolecular markers are becoming available and are being rigorously investigated for their ability to enhance our ability to predict outcome and prognosis for patients with RCC.

Presentation: incidental versus symptomatic

RCC can grow to varying sizes before becoming clinically apparent. In fact, the first clinical manifestation may be secondary to the effects of metastatic disease in as many as 30 per cent of patients. RCC has long been known as the 'internist's tumor' because of its propensity to present with a wide variety of signs and symptoms. The classic triad of hematuria, pain, and flank mass occurs in only 10 per cent of patients. The number of patients being diagnosed with incidentally detected tumors is rising (Chow *et al.* 1999); however, it is still more common for patients to present with one or two symptoms, such as hematuria or pain. The location of the kidneys deep in the retroperitoneum tends to delay presentation of symptoms until the tumor involves adjacent structures or involves the kidney's collecting system resulting in hematuria. Patients with advanced disease often present with vague, nonspecific symptoms such as malaise, anorexia, fever, or cough. Finally, symptoms associated with RCC occur as a result of the elaboration of humoral factors as part of a paraneoplastic syndrome. Classic examples of paraneoplastic complexes associated with RCC include abnormal liver function tests (Stauffer's syndrome), hypertension, hypercalcemia, and polycythemia. Resolution of these syndromes often occurs with removal of the primary tumor.

With the advent and mainstream use of abdominal computerized tomography (CT) and ultrasound, an increase in the incidental detection of RCC in asymptomatic patients has been noted (Ueda and Mihara 1987; Smith *et al.* 1989; Homma *et al.* 1995). Because of this increased proportion of incidental RCC lesions, many studies have attempted to ascertain whether the detection of these tumors prior to the onset of symptoms had any clinical significance. Early studies demonstrated that incidental RCC tended to be smaller, lower-stage lesions that yielded better survival outcomes than RCC tumors detected in symptomatic patients (Konnak and Grossman 1985; Thompson and Peek 1998). Such encouraging data led to the belief that incidentally discovered RCC had a better prognosis and inspired many to subsequently even consider routine ultrasound screening of the general population (Tosaka *et al.* 1990). Recent studies, however, have demonstrated that incidental and symptomatic RCC consist of equal proportions of early-stage lesions and thus share similar prognoses (Mevorach *et al.* 1992; Jayson and Sanders 1998). Presented with such conflicting data, we reviewed our experience at UCLA with both incidental and symptomatic RCC to determine any differences in the natural course of these lesions.

The records of 633 consecutive patients undergoing either radical or partial nephrectomy for RCC at the UCLA Medical Center between 1987 and 1998 were reviewed (Tsui *et al.* 2000). The patients were divided into two groups: (1) asymptomatic patients in whom a tumor was diagnosed incidentally; (2) patients diagnosed after presenting with any of the classic symptoms of RCC or subsequent metastasis. Of the 633 patients, 95 (15 per cent) were treated for incidentally discovered RCC and 538 (85 per cent) presented with symptoms secondary to RCC at diagnosis. Patient age and sex distributions were similar in the two groups. This review revealed that, at presentation, incidental tumors were significantly lower in both stage and grade than tumors that produced symptoms. Furthermore, these clinically and histologically less aggressive lesions led to better survival rates and decreased recurrence rates. The 5-year cancer-specific survival rate was found to be significantly higher for incidental tumors (85.3 per cent) than for symptomatic lesions (62.5 per cent) (Fig. 9.1). When adjusted for stage, no difference in survival was

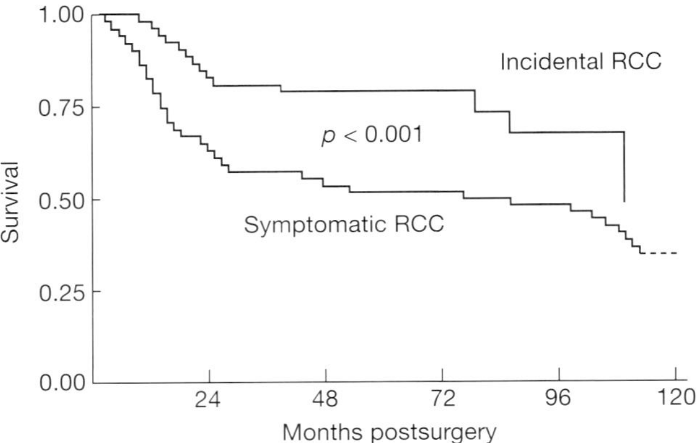

Fig. 9.1 Kaplan–Meier survival estimates for 661 patients undergoing nephrectomy at UCLA based on symptoms at presentation.

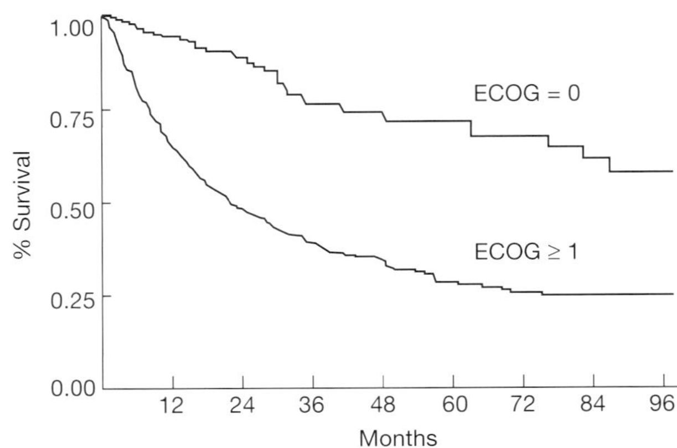

Fig. 9.2 Kaplan–Meier survival estimates for 661 patients undergoing nephrectomy at UCLA (metastatic and non-metastatic) based on performance status at presentation.

noted in the two groups for stages I–III and a minimally significant difference was noted for stage IV. A multivariate analysis of stage and grade attributed the survival difference for stage IV lesions to the significantly higher grade of the symptomatic lesions (Tsui *et al.* 2000). However, the number of symptoms at the time of initial diagnosis was found to be an independent predictor of both time to recurrence and time to death for both non-metastatic and metastatic patients with patients having at least two symptoms experiencing a worse prognosis than those having one or no symptoms (unpublished data).

Other patient-related factors

A number of clinical characteristics have been identified as having an impact on the clinical behavior and subsequent survival in patients with advanced RCC. These include initial performance status, time from diagnosis to metastasis, location and number of metastatic sites, as well as weight loss and whether the patient has been nephrectomized or still has the primary tumor in place (Elson *et al.* 1988; Maldazys and deKernion 1986; deKernion *et al.* 1978; Klugo *et al.* 1977; Belldegrun *et al.* 2000). Elson *et al.* (1988) developed a scoring system to determine prognosis for patients with advanced RCC, stratifying patients into five groups based on Eastern Cooperative Oncology Group (ECOG) performance status, time from diagnosis to metastasis, weight loss, prior chemotherapy, and number of metastatic sites. Expected median survival ranged from 2.1 to 12.8 depending on number of risk points and prognostic group. Droz *et al.* (1993), using a similar approach, identified prognostic subgroups based on performance status, presence or absence of liver metastasis, weight loss, and serum erythrocyte sedimentation rate (ESR). Most recently, Motzer *et al.* (1999) have developed a model based on the study of 670 patients with advanced RCC treated at Memorial Sloan–Kettering Cancer Center defining the relationship between pretreatment clinical features and survival. Median overall survival was 10 months, and five pretreatment features were identified to be associated with a shorter survival as determined

by multivariate analysis. These included low Karnofsky performance status, high serum lactate dehydrogenase (LDH; > 1.5 times normal), low hemoglobin (< lower limit of normal), hypercalcemia (> 10 mg/dl), and absence of prior nephrectomy. Poor-risk patients with three or more risk factors had a median survival time of only 4 months, whereas median survival improved to 20 months in patients with zero risk factors.

At UCLA, we analysed the records of 643 consecutive patients undergoing either partial or radical nephrectomy between 1987 and 1998 (Tsui *et al.* in press). This study identified tumor (T) stage as an effective predictor of survival (see further discussion of stage below); however, T stage did not demonstrate an independent impact on RCC prognosis under multivariate analysis. Instead, other factors such as ECOG score (Fig. 9.2) and, more importantly, grade appeared to significantly affect survival as independent elements.

Tumor-related determinants of clinical behavior

Tumor histology

Histologically, RCC are composed of a remarkable variety of various cell types and morphological patterns. Historically, RCC

Table 9.1 UICC/AJCC classification of renal cell carcinoma

Benign neoplasms
Papillary adenoma
Renal oncocytoma
Metanephric adenoma

Malignant neoplasms
Clear cell carcinoma
Papillary renal carcinoma
Chromophobe renal carcinoma
Collecting duct carcinoma
Renal cell carcinoma, unclassified

was regarded as a single entity that expressed many possible histologic appearances. Today, RCC is more accurately recognized as a family of cancers that result from distinct genetic abnormalities with unique morphologic features, but are all derived from renal tubular epithelium. The variety in appearance has led to a confusion of classification and terminology. In 1997, progress was made in standardization when the Union Internationale Contre le Cancer (UICC) and the American Joint Commission on Cancer (AJCC) released their combined workgroup classification of RCC (Storkel *et al.* 1997). This proposed classification was based on the Mainz classification (Thoenes *et al.* 1986), but took into account subsequent genetic studies as well as practical concerns such as simplicity and consistency with historical usage. Their proposed classification is summarized in Table 9.1.

Clear cell carcinomas are the most common type of renal tumor with malignant potential, accounting for approximately 70 per cent of cases in surgical series. The clear cells have a round or polygonal appearance and have an abundant cytoplasm, which contains cholesterol, glycogen, and lipids, making the cytoplasm clear in routine sections. Cytogenetics of clear cell RCC have demonstrated that loss of the von Hippel–Lindau (VHL) gene on the short arm of chromosome 3 (3p) is the most frequent abnormality expressed (Kovacs *et al.* 1988). There is a variant of clear cell RCC with a predominantly cystic pattern that is called multilocular cystic RCC (Taxy and Marshall 1983). Cystic RCC is thought to have a low potential for recurrence or metastasis (Sherman *et al.* 1987). In a recent review (Bielsa *et al.* 1998), 96 per cent of cases occurred in male patients, and nuclear grade and stage were lower than in patients with other types of RCC. In addition, cystic RCC had a slower growth rate and was associated with improved prognosis and longer survival than conventional RCC.

Papillary RCC is the second most common histologic type, accounting for approximately 10 per cent of surgical series (Mancilla-Jimenez *et al.* 1976). Previously known as chromophil carcinoma in the Mainz classification, the cells covering the papillae in papillary RCC are pleiomorphic with variable cytoplasmic staining. Papillary RCC occurs more commonly in end-stage kidneys (Ishikawa and Kovacs 1993) and is more frequently multifocal and associated with tubular dysplasia. The characteristic cytogenetic finding for papillary RCC is chromosomal trisomy of, most commonly, chromosomes 7, 16, and 17 (Kovacs *et al.* 1991). It is uncertain whether the prognosis for papillary RCC is better or worse than for clear cell RCC (Medeiros and Weiss 1990). However, it seems that, for low-grade, low-stage papillary RCC, the prognosis is better than for similarly graded and staged clear cell tumors (Amin *et al.* 1997). However, a recent analysis comparing subtypes of RCC found that, at Brigham and Women's Hospital, papillary RCC were more likely than clear cell RCC to be Fuhrman grade 3 or 4, to be metastatic at the time of resection, and more likely to metastasize to lymph nodes (Renshaw and Richie 1999).

Chromophobe RCC is the third most common carcinoma arising from renal tubular epithelium, accounting for approximately 5 per cent of cases of RCC in surgical series (Crotty *et al.* 1995). There are two histologic variants within chromophobe: typical and eosinophilic. Morphologically, these tumors have cells that are large with finely reticulated cytoplasm that stain lightly with routine hematoxylin and eosin processing. A positive reaction with Hale's colloidal iron technique is a characteristic histologic finding and helps to differentiate chromophobe tumors from oncocytomas. Genetically, chromophobe RCC is characterized by monosomy of multiple chromosomes and hypodiploidy (Kovacs and Kovacs 1992). Several large, recent studies demonstrated that patients with chromophobe RCC have an excellent prognosis, especially for patients with tumors less than 8 cm in diameter (Akhtar *et al.* 1995; Hamad *et al.* 1996). While the overall survival of patients with chromophobe RCC appears to be better than that of patients with other RCC, no survival difference could be appreciated when adjustment was made for stage, and the benefit may merely be the result of a high proportion of low-stage tumors at the time of diagnosis (Akhtar *et al.* 1995; Hamad *et al.* 1996). In a series of 768 nephrectomies from Japan, survival for papillary and clear cell RCC was equivalent, whereas the prognosis for patients with chromophobe RCC was better than in those with papillary RCC (Onishi *et al.* 1999). Although metastases arising from chromophobe RCC are rare, they may have a propensity for spread to the liver when metastases do occur (Renshaw and Richie 1999).

Collecting duct carcinoma, or medullary carcinoma of the kidney, is an aggressive RCC variant, accounting for fewer than 1 per cent of surgical cases. Little information is available concerning the genetics of collecting duct carcinoma. Microscopically, these tumors appear to arise in the medulla and consist of irregular, duct-like structures, nests, and cords of cells that sometimes have a hobnail appearance in an abundant, loose stroma (Eble 1997). Collecting duct carcinomas are aggressive and tend to develop systemic metastases rapidly (Kennedy *et al.* 1990). Renal medullary carcinoma (RMC) is a newly described tumor almost exclusively diagnosed in African-American men with sickle cell trait or sickle cell disease (Davis *et al.* 1995). RMC tend to occur in young patients with a mean age of 22 to 24 years (Davis *et al.* 1995; Avery *et al.* 1996). Davis *et al.* (1995) report an average survival from the time of surgery of only 15 weeks (range 3–52 weeks) in a series of 34 patients. Survival does not seem to be improved despite a variety of chemotherapy or immunotherapy regimens that have been attempted (Davis *et al.* 1995).

Sarcomatoid change has been noted to occur in all histologic types of RCC, with less than 5 per cent of RCC containing areas resembling sarcoma (Tomera *et al.* 1993). Undeniably associated with poor clinical outcome, sarcomatoid change is no longer viewed as arising *de novo* as a unique type, but rather it is now viewed as a manifestation of high-grade carcinoma (Storkel *et al.* 1997) and will be discussed further under 'tumor grade'.

Tumor grade

Numerous histopathologic, tumor-grading systems have been proposed for RCC. The histologic grading of cells in RCC has been used to interpret the clinical behavior of these tumors and to serve as a prognostic factor. Microscopic grading has provided no additional prognostic value when related to tumor stage. On the other hand, nuclear grading has shown to be a valuable prognostic indicator of patient survival. Second in importance only to stage, nearly all grading systems have shown independent prognostic value in studies in which grade was included as a variable (Thrasher and Paulson 1993; Medeiros *et al.* 1988; Fuhrman *et al.* 1982). Skinner *et al.* (1971) directed attention to the correlation between nuclear features and survival. These observations were later expanded into a four-tier scheme based on nuclear size, shape, and content as proposed by Fuhrman *et al.* (1982), which remains the most commonly used system in North America. Fewer than 10 per cent of cases are grade 1, grade 2 and 3 each represent approximately 35 per cent of cases, and about 20 per cent are grade 4 (Medeiros *et al.* 1988).

Analysis of the kidney cancer database at UCLA (Tsui *et al.* in press) revealed that 20 per cent were grade 1, 42 per cent were grade 2, and 38 per cent were grades 3 and 4. When tumor grade was evaluated on a stage by stage basis, stage I tumors were 49 per cent grade 1, 42 per cent grade 2, and 9 per cent grade 3 and 4. In contrast, stage IV tumors were 3 per cent grade 1, 36 per cent grade 2, and 61 per cent grade 3 and 4. When survival was analysed in terms of overall grade, 5-year cancer-specific survival for patients with stage I, II, III, and IV tumors was 91, 74, 67, and 32 per cent, respectively (Fig. 9.3). When these survival rates were further classified according to T stage, the 5-year cancer-specific survival was found to be 83 per cent for Stage T1, 57 per cent for Stage T2, 42 per cent for stage T3, and 28 per cent for stage T4. Five-year cancer-specific survival rates for patients based on tumor grade were determined to be 88.7 per cent for grade 1, 65.3 per cent for grade 2, and 46.1 per cent for grades 3 and 4. T stage survival rates were then adjusted for grade. For patients with stage T1 lesions, 5-year cancer-specific patient survival rates were 91 per cent for grade 1, 83 per cent for grade 2, 60 per cent for grade 3, and 0 per cent for grade 4. For patients with stage T4 lesions, 5-year cancer-specific survival rates were 46 per cent for grade 2, 38 per cent for grade 3, and 0 per cent for grade 4. There were no grade 1 lesions within the T4 stage. For all T stages analysed, lesions with lower grade (grade 1 or 2) demonstrated better survival than higher-grade lesions (grade 3 or 4).

Unfortunately, controversy still exists concerning interobserver reproducibility of grading as well as disagreement regarding relevant breakpoints between the different grades and survival. The recent UICC/AJCC international consensus conference on RCC also took up the issue of grading (Medeiros *et al.* 1997). The conference proposed the development of a new grading scheme that is easier to apply and is based on patient outcome, suggesting the combination of the first two grades in Fuhrman's system to convert it into a three-grade system. Such a system has not yet been developed.

Sarcomatoid change represents a relatively rare, high-grade form of RCC typified by a spindle cell growth pattern that is seen in less than 5 per cent of RCC and that bodes for a generally poor outcome (Tomera *et al.* 1983). Clinically, sarcomatoid RCC is characterized by its locally aggressive nature, metastatic potential, and poor prognosis (Tomera *et al.* 1983; Sella *et al.* 1987; Oda and Machinami 1993). Surgical resection alone does not appear to significantly affect the clinical course since these tumors are usually metastatic or locally advanced at the time of diagnosis. The reported median survival of these patients from the time of diagnosis is 3.8 to 6.8 months with no treatment (Sella *et al.* 1987; Farrow *et al.* 1968). Ro and colleagues (1987) found two factors to independently predict poorer prognosis. These were amount of tumor necrosis and the proportion of sarcomatoid tumor, but only in low-stage tumors. When stratified by T stage, sarcomatoid variant patients were found to have a mean survival of 49.7 months for stage I and 6.8 months for stages II–IV (Ro *et al.* 1987; Selli *et al.* 1983).

We retrospectively analysed 31 consecutive patients from the UCLA Kidney Cancer Program who had a diagnosis of sarcomatoid variant made between 1990 and 1997 (Cangiano *et al.* 1999). All 31 patients were treated with aggressive surgical management and 25/31 patients (80.7 per cent) were treated with postoperative adjuvant immunotherapy, making it the largest series of sarcomatoid RCC treated with immunotherapy. Twenty-eight of the patients (84 per cent) had known metastases at the time of radical nephrectomy (67 per cent lung, 40 per cent bone, 21 per cent liver, 33 per cent lymphatic, and 15 per cent brain). Various forms of immunotherapy were used, including low-dose interleukin-2 (IL-2; 5 patients), tumor-infiltrating lymphocytes (TIL) based plus IL-2 (9 patients), high-dose IL-2 based (9 patients), and dendritic cell therapy (1 patient). Overall, two patients (6 per cent) achieved a complete response with a median duration of 46+ months. Five patients (15 per cent) achieved a partial response with a median duration of 36 months. One- and 2-year overall survival were 48 and 37 per cent, respectively. Using a multivariate analysis, age, gender, and per cent sarcomatoid tumor (greater or less than 50 per cent) did not significantly correlate with survival. Instead, improved survival was found only in those patients receiving immunotherapy. When adjusted for age, gender, and per cent sarcomatoid, the relative risk of death was 10.4 times higher in patients not receiving high-dose IL-2.

Other tumor-related factors

Numerous biomolecular factors are currently under investigation to determine their utility and correlation with diagnosis, stage, and prognosis for patients with RCC. These molecular markers include measures of tumor cell proliferation, growth factors, cell

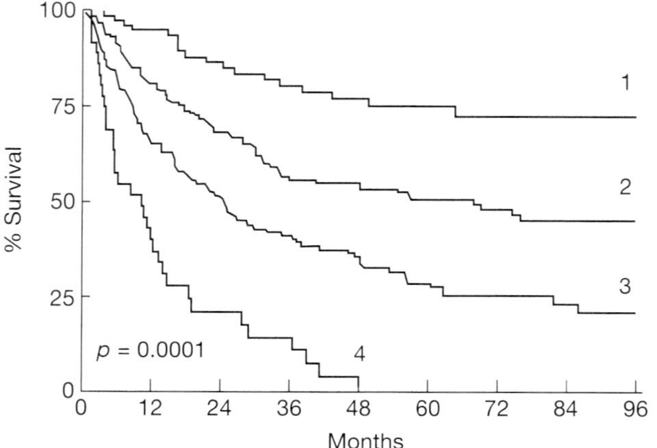

Fig. 9.3 Kaplan–Meier survival estimates for 661 patients undergoing nephrectomy at UCLA based on Fuhrman grade.

Table 9.2 Classification of molecular markers for RCC*

I	Well supported by the literature, generally used in patient management
II	Extensively studied biologically and or clinically
	IIA Tested in clinical trials
	IIB Biologic and correlative studies performed; few clinical outcome studies
III	Currently do not meet criteria for category I or any II

* College of American Pathologists' working classification for prognostic markers (Henson *et al.* 1995). In 1997 at the joint meeting of UICC and AJCC, only Ki-67 and argyrophilic nucleolar proteins qualified for IIB. No molecular marker qualified as I or IIA. All the others are classified III.

adhesion, apoptosis, telomerase activity, and angiogenesis. A wide variety of markers have been examined in small studies, and some have shown enough promise to legitimize further research to prove their value as prognostic tools. Some of the markers that currently hold the most promise are listed in Tables 9.2 and 9.3. However, at this point these markers, which will be covered in greater depth in a separate chapter, must still be considered investigational in nature.

Tumor stage

Tumor stage, which reflects the anatomic spread and involvement of disease, is recognized as the most important prognosticator for the clinical behavior and outcome for RCC (Thrasher and Paulson 1993). Currently, there are several staging systems in use. The two most commonly used staging systems are Robson's modification of the system described by Flocks and Kadesky (Robson *et al.*

1969) and the TNM (tumor–node–metastasis) staging system proposed by the International Union Against Cancer. The TNM system is notable for its systematic emphasis on local spread, nodal spread, and distant metastasis. At UCLA, 5-year cancer-specific survival rates were found to be 91, 74, 67, and 32 per cent for stage I, II, III, and IV lesions, respectively, when analysed according to the revised 1997 TNM system (Fig. 9.4; Tsui *et al.* in press). Analysis of survival rates in terms of T stage demonstrated a survival rate of 83 per cent for stage T1, 57 per cent for stage T2, 42 per cent for stage T3, and 28 per cent for stage T4. Multivariate

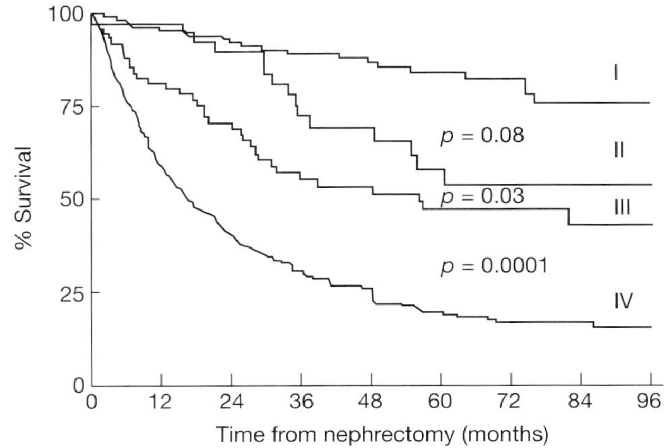

Fig. 9.4 Kaplan–Meier survival estimates for 661 patients undergoing nephrectomy at UCLA based on TNM tumor stage.

Table 9.3 Molecular markers shown to be associated with different aspects of survival

Molecular marker	Reference	Incidence	Expression correlates with
Globo-series gangliosides	Saito *et al.* 1997	55 cases were checked	Metastatic propensity
Heat shock protein 72	Santarosa *et al.* 1997	33% RCC, 6% normal renal epithelium	Favorable prognosis
Human mutT homologue gene	Okamoto *et al.* 1996		Advanced stage
Ki-67 (MIB-1)	Aaltomaa *et al.* 1997	Cancer in general	Independent prognostic factor
Ratio of matrix metalloproteinases to their inhibitors (MMP/TIMP ratio): MMP-1/TIMP-1 MMP-9/TIMP-2	Kugler *et al.* 1998		Aggressiveness: Normal = 1 Locally confined = 2.43 Advanced = 4.86
MMP-2	Gohji *et al.* 1998		Survival (?)
Metallothionein (MT)	Izawa *et al.* 1998		Grade (?)
Multidrug resistance-associated protein 2 (MRP2)	Kartenbeck *et al.* 1998	95% of clear cell RCC; expressed in normal kidney	Lack of expression correlates with high grade
FHIT	Hadaczek *et al.* 1998	50% (associated with Chr 3p14.2 familial RCC)	Expression correlates with low grade
PCNA (proliferating cell nuclear antigen)	Sejima *et al.* 1999		High grade, venous invasion
Plasminogen activator inhibitor (PAI)-1	Hofman *et al.* 1996		Independently predict relapse
Fas/APO-1	Cardi *et al.* 1998	33% express (6/18) 5/5 cell lines express	Tumor volume

analysis demonstrated that overall TNM stage and grade serve as the two most important prognostic indicators for RCC. ECOG classification was found to be a less significant predictor of survival.

Both the Robson and TNM systems include tumors confined to the renal capsule as the lowest stage category, although the Robson system does not take primary tumor size into account. Recognition of a size-dependent survival difference (Gelb *et al.* 1993), perhaps due to microscopic local or distant metastasis, favors the use of the TNM system, which currently distinguishes between tumors greater and less than 7 cm in diameter. Further dividing TNM's T1 category based on a cut point of 4 cm has also been suggested by some investigators to mark off this commonly accepted cut-off for renal-sparing surgery (Licht *et al.* 1994). The issue of tumor size remains somewhat controversial with different groups recommending different size breakpoints to stratify the stages. Based on classic autopsy studies, Bell (1938) first reported an association between tumor size and prognosis for patients with RCC, noting an increased propensity for the development of metastasis for tumors greater than 3 cm. Grignon *et al.* (1989) have further demonstrated that tumor size is an independent, significant predictor of patient outcome. T1 in the TNM system was increased in 1997 from 2.5 cm to 7 cm when it was noted that the lower size cut-off did not provide for statistically significant survival differences (Hermanek and Schrott 1990; Guinan *et al.* 1994). Others have suggested that alternative cut-offs be used, including 5 (Gelb *et al.* 1993), 5.5 (Kinouchi *et al.* 1999), 8 (Green *et al.* 1989), and 10 cm (Medeiros *et al.* 1988).

The TNM system subdivides the T3 category to differentiate perinephric fat extension from renal vein as well as level of vena caval extension, whereas the Robson system does not make these distinctions. Patients with disease that extends through the capsule of the kidney into the perinephric fat, while having a better prognosis than patients with nodal involvement, experience a reduction in 5-year survival rates as compared to those associated with organ-confined disease of up to 20 per cent (Skinner *et al.* 1971; Selli *et al.* 1983). The issue of the prognostic significance of extension into the venous system also remains controversial. RCC has a unique propensity for extension in the venous system and, at the time of diagnosis, 4–10 per cent of patients will present with evidence of extension into the inferior vena cava (IVC) (Marshall *et al.* 1988). RCC is notably a hyper vascular tumor, and tumor propagation into the renal veins and vena cava occurs by direct extension. Because of the relative shortness of the right renal vein, extension into the vena cava occurs more frequently with right-sided tumors (Ney 1946). Extension of the tumor thrombus into the vena cava occurs in a cephalad direction, following the normal direction of the venous return to the heart. The intraluminal growth and development of vena caval obstruction by these tumor thrombi is usually gradual enough to permit the development of extensive venous collateralization to allow for sufficient venous return to the heart from the lower torso to prevent symptoms referable to caval obstruction. Kaufman *et al.* (1956) noted that 50 per cent of patients with complete caval obstruction on inferior cavagrams were asymptomatic.

Surgical extirpation remains the mainstay in the treatment of RCC with intraluminal venous extension. Aggressive surgical therapy for patients using hypothermia, temporary cardiac arrest with exsanguination, and cardiopulmonary bypass, when necessary, has been shown to be feasible with an operative mortality rate of 5 to 10 per cent (Montie *et al.* 1991). Five-year survival rates of 47 to 68 per cent have been reported following complete excision of localized RCC with concurrent caval extension (Libertino *et al.* 1987; Neves and Zincke 1987). Although, the presence of lymph node involvement and distant metastasis is known to significantly diminish survival, the prognostic significance of the cephalad extent of an inferior vena caval tumor thrombus continues to cause controversy. Some reports have suggested an increased risk of metastasis and early death with more cephalad propagation (Skinner *et al.* 1989; Sosa *et al.* 1984), whereas others have questioned whether the level of extension poses an adverse prognosis (Cherrie *et al.* 1982; Hatcher *et al.* 1991). Still others have suggested that microscopic extension with local tumor infiltration may adversely impact survival to a greater extent than macroscopic thrombus (Novick *et al.* 1990). Novick reported his long-term follow-up of patients with tumor thrombus into the right atrium and, in his series, there was no difference in the incidence of lymph node or distant metastasis at initial presentation between these patients and those with intra- or infrahepatic involvement (Mrstik *et al.* 1992). Furthermore, there was no difference in the risk of early metastasis or death following surgical extirpation in patients with atrial involvement when compared to lower level involvement (Glazer and Novick 1996). Novick's report of 60 per cent cancer-specific 5-year survival is similar to that of other contemporary series.

Given the markedly worse prognosis seen for patients whose primary tumor extended into the IVC and who had distant metastasis at the time of presentation, it has been widely reported in the literature that metastatic disease should be a contraindication to surgical resection (Neves and Zincke 1987; Hatcher *et al.* 1991). We recently reported our experience using aggressive, multimodality therapy for a high-risk group of patients who have metastatic RCC and concurrent IVC extension (Naitoh *et al.* 1999). Patients were included in the study if they underwent radical nephrectomy and IVC thombectomy, with immunotherapy planned for the postoperative period. Thirty-one cases of metastatic RCC with extensive disease and caval extension were identified. Twenty-three per cent of the patients had isolated lung metastasis, 53 per cent had lung metastasis along with other sites, while the remainder had involvement primarily at non-pulmonary metastatic sites (38 per cent lymph node, 13 per cent soft tissue, 29 per cent liver, and 10 per cent bone). Eighty per cent of the patients received the full course of surgery and postoperative immunotherapy. With a mean follow-up of 18 months (34 months for the survivors), 26 per cent of patients were alive. Actuarial overall 5-year survival for the entire group was 17 per cent. Level of tumor thrombus did not correlate to overall survival. On the other hand, immunotherapy, tumor grade, and site of metastasis did provide significant prognostic information. Patients with isolated pulmonary metastasis had a 5-year survival rate of 43 per cent, while patients with low-grade tumors had a 5-year survival rate of 52 per cent.

Approximately 23 per cent of patients will have metastatic disease at the time of presentation, and a further 25 per cent of patients with disease apparently localized to the kidney will develop metastasis within 5 years after nephrectomy (Richie and deKernion 1987). Patients with metastatic RCC generally have a poor prognosis with 5-year survival rates of 5 to 10 per cent and 10-year survival rates of 0 to 7 per cent (Skinner *et al.* 1971; Maldazys and deKernion 1986; McNichols *et al.* 1981). The clinical course of RCC is often unpredictable, and recurrence can occur 10 years after nephrectomy in as many as 10 per cent of patients who survive that long (McNichols *et al.* 1981). It has been possible, however, to select subgroups of patients who have a more favorable survival, including good performance status, long disease-free interval after nephrectomy, metastases limited in number and to the lungs only, and removal of the primary tumor (Maldazys and deKernion 1986). Dernevik *et al.* (1985) reported an increase in survival for patients who had more than one metastatic pulmonary lesion who were treated with nephrectomy and complete excision of metastatic disease.

There is some evidence accumulating that indicates that aggressive management of patients with metastasis can alter the clinical course of the disease. DeKernion *et al.* (1978) demonstrated that nephrectomy alone had a minimal impact on survival in patients with metastatic RCC in the pre-immunotherapy era. However, recent advances in molecular medicine have enhanced the understanding of the biology of RCC tumors, demonstrating the possibility that RCC tumors may produce immunosuppresive factors such as transforming growth factor beta (TGFβ) that can reduce the efficacy of immunotherapy (Belldegrun and deKernion 1998). Such findings suggest that, while nephrectomy alone may not be effective, a possible benefit can be achieved using aggressive multimodality treatment with aggressive surgical resection and combination with immunotherapy.

At UCLA, we sought to determine the impact of surgery and immunotherapy on the outcome of patients with metastatic RCC (Belldegrun *et al.* 2000) by examining the survival of 353 consecutive patients with metastatic RCC treated with IL-2 based immunotherapy. Patients were divided into five groups based on whether or not nephrectomy was performed, and the relationship between the timing of nephrectomy, timing of immunotherapy, and the onset of metastasis. Patients with metastatic RCC treated with IL-2 based immunotherapy and their primary tumor in place demonstrated 1- and 2-year survival rates of 29 and 4 per cent, respectively, versus 1- and 2-year survival rates of 67 and 44 per cent for those patients undergoing immunotherapy and adjunctive nephrectomy. The best survival was attained with adoptive immunotherapy using IL-2 and TIL, which yielded 1- and 2-year survival rates of 73 and 55 per cent, respectively. Patients inititially presenting with metastasis and undergoing IL-2 immunotherapy and nephrectomy demonstrated 1- and 2-year survival rates of 53 and 25 per cent, respectively. For those patients initially undergoing nephrectomy for localized disease, patients receiving IL-2 based immunotherapy for subsequent metastasis more than 6 months following nephrectomy yielded 1- and 2-year survival rates of 64 and 40 per cent, respectively. Those patients developing metastasis less than 6 months following nephrectomy yielded 1- and 3-year survival rates of 45 and 15 per cent, respectively, following IL-2 based immunotherapy.

The UCLA integrated staging system (UISS)

At UCLA, we have sought to combine pathological staging information with some of these additional prognostic variables in order to better stratify patients into prognostic categories using statistical tools that can accurately define an individual patient's probability of survival (Zisman *et al.* in press). We evaluated these factors in 661 patients, including age, sex, Fuhrman grade, TNM stage, tumor size alone, ECOG performance status, laterality, bilaterality, smoking, number of presenting symptoms, weight loss alone, tumor histologic type, administration of immunotherapy, IVC involvement, number of metastatic sites, lung metastasis as opposed to other metastasis, and time interval between nephrectomy and metastasis, to determine which factors were having the greatest impact on RCC patients' survival. Ultimately, we constructed a model with five groups based on the most significant explanatory variables, namely TNM stage, grade, and ECOG performance status. The projected 2- and 5-year survival for patients in UISS group I are 96 and 94 per cent, respectively; for group II, 89 and 67 per cent; for group III, 66 and 39 per cent; for group IV, 42 and 23 per cent; and for group V, 9 and 0 per cent, respectively (Fig. 9.5). Subsequently, we have developed separate mathematical formulas based on Nadas' (1970) principles for localized and metastatic patients that are capable of predicting the survival for individual patients with RCC. These novel tools for staging and predicting survival for patients with RCC are simple to use, superior to stage alone in differentiating patients' survival, and may prove to be important prognostic tools for counseling patients with various stages of kidney cancer and for interpreting the results of experimental protocols.

On the horizon

Despite considerable progress in understanding the basic biology of RCC, many questions remain unanswered. The long-term safety and efficacy of renal ablative surgery needs to be clarified.

UISS	TNM stage	ECOG PS	Grade	Survival (%)	
				2 yr	5 yr
I	I	0	1,2	96	94
II	I	0	3,4	89	67
	II	any	any		
	III	0	any		
	III	1+	1		
III	III	1+	2–4	66	39
	IV	0	1,2		
IV	IV	0	3,4	42	23
		1+	1–3		
V	IV	1+	4	9	0

Fig. 9.5 The UCLA Integrated Staging System (UISS) uses TNM stage, grade, and ECOG performance status to divide patients into five prognostic categories.

The role of adjuvant cytokine therapy for high-risk patients with locally advanced disease needs further exploration. The mechanisms underlying the host immune response need greater definition. Furthermore, the events that dictate which tumors will progress despite local therapy, which tumors possess invasive capacities, and which tumors are sensitive to radiation or chemotherapy need to be better understood. While answers to some of these questions have been generalized based solely on histologic data, the advent of new molecular markers and chromosomal analyses provides a much more precise and effective means to fingerprint individual tumors and, in turn, provide more specific information regarding their biology. In order to be able to test specific tumors with new molecular and chromosomal markers, researchers need to determine which markers are of clinical significance for given types of tumors. To determine the efficacy and clinical utility of each marker in question, many tumors need to be screened. The use of new pathologic tools such as micro and tissue arrays (Moch *et al.* 1999), which allow us to evaluate hundreds of tumors simultaneously, will increase the efficiency of such proposed studies. Furthermore, being able to correlate histologic and chromosomal findings with accurate survival data is necessary in order to determine their potential utility.

References

Aaltomaa, S. *et al.* (1997). *Eur. Urol.* **31**, 350–5.

Akhtar, M., Kardar, H., Linjawi, T., *et al.* (1995). Chromophobe cell carcinoma of the kidney: a clinicopathologic study of 21 cases. *Am. J. Surg. Pathol.* **19**, 1245–56.

Amin, M.B., Corless, C.L., Renshaw, A.A., *et al.* (1997). Papillary (chromophil) renal cell carcinoma: histomorphologic characteristics and evaluation of conventional pathologic prognostic parameters in 62 cases. *Am. J. Surg. Pathol.* **21**, 621–35.

Avery, R.A., Harris, J.E., Davis, C.J., *et al.* (1996). Renal medullary carcinoma: clinical and therapeutic aspects of a newly described tumor. *Cancer* **78**, 128–32.

Bell, E.T. (1938). A classification of renal tumors with observation on the frequency of various types. *J. Urol.* **39**, 238.

Belldegrun, A. and deKernion, J.B. (1998). Renal tumors. In *Campbell's urology*, 7th edn (ed. P.C. Walsh, A.B. Retik, E.D. Vaughan, Jr, and A.J. Wein), p. 2283. W.B. Saunders, Philadelphia.

Belldegrun, A., Shvarts, O., and Figlin, R.A. (2000). Expanding the indications for surgery and adjuvant IL-2-based immunotherapy in patients with advanced renal cell carcinoma. *Cancer J. Sci. Am.* **6**, S88–92.

Bielsa, O., Lloreta, J., and Gelabert-Mas, A. (1998). Cystic renal cell carcinoma: pathologic features, survival, and prognostic implications for treatment. *Br. J. Urol.* **82**, 16–20.

Cangiano, T., Liao, J., Naitoh, J., *et al.* (1999). Sarcomatoid variant renal cell carcinoma: biologic behavior, prognosis and response to combined surgical resection and immunotherapy. *J. Clin. Oncol.* **17**, 523–8.

Cardi, G., Heaney, J.A., Schned, A.R., *et al.* Expression of FAS (AP01/CD95) in tumor infiltrating and peripheral blood lymphocytes in patients with renal cell carcinoma. *Cancer Res.* **15**, 2078–80.

Cherrie, R.J., Goldman, D.G., Linder, A., *et al.* (1982). Prognostic implications of vena caval extension of renal cell carcinoma. *J. Urol.* **128**, 910–12.

Chow, W.H., Devesa, S.S., Warren, J.L., *et al.* (1999). Rising incidence of renal cell cancer in the United States. *J. Am. Med. Assoc.* **281**, 1628–31.

Crotty, T.B., Farrow, G.M., and Lieber, M.M. (1995). Chromophobe renal cell carcinoma: clinicopathologic features of 50 cases. *J. Urol.* **154**, 964–7.

Davis, C.J., Mostofi, F.K., and Sesterhenn, I.A. (1995). Renal medullary carcinoma: the seventh sickle cell nephropathy. *Am. J. Surg. Pathol.* **19**, 1–11.

deKernion, J.B., Ramming, K.P., and Smith, R.B. (1978). The natural history of metastatic renal cell carcinoma: a computer analysis. *J. Urol.* **120**, 148–52.

Dernevik, L., Berggren, H., Larsson, S., *et al.* (1985). Surgical removal of pulmonary metastasis from renal cell carcinoma. *Scand. J. Urol. Nephrol.* **19**, 133–7.

Droz, J., Rey, A., Mahjoub, M., *et al.* (1993). Prognostic factors in renal cell carcinoma. In *Renal cell carcinoma: immunotherapy and cellular biology* (ed. E. Klein, R. Bukowski, and J. Finke). Marcel Decker Inc, New York.

Eble, J.N. (1997). Neoplasms of the kidney. In *Urologic surgical pathology* (ed. D.G. Bostwick and J.N. Eble). Mosby, St. Louis.

Elson, P.J., Witte, R.S., and Trump, D.L. (1988). Prognostic factors for survival in patients with recurrent or metastatic renal cell carcinoma. *Cancer Res.* **48**, 7310–13.

Farrow, G., Harrison, E., and Utz, D. (1968). Sarcomas and sarcomatoid and mixed malignant tumors of the kidney in adults. *Cancer* **22**, 556.

Fuhrman, S.A., Lasky, L.C., and Limas, C. (1982). Prognostic significance of morphologic parameters in renal cell carcinoma. *Am. J. Surg. Pathol.* **6**, 655–63.

Gelb, A.B., Shibuya, R.B., Weiss, L.M., *et al.* (1993). Stage I renal cell carcinoma. A clinicopathologic study of 82 cases. *Am. J. Surg. Pathol.* **17**, 275–86.

Glazer, A.A. and Novick, A.C. (1996). Long-term follow up after surgical treatment for renal cell carcinoma extending into the right atrium. *J. Urol.* **155**, 448–50.

Gohji, K., Nomi, M., Hara, I., Arakawa, S., and Kamidono, S. (1998). Influence of cytokines and growth factors on matrix metalloproteinase-2 production and invasion of human renal cancer. *Urol. Res.* **26** (1), 33–7.

Green, L.K., Ayala, A.G., Ro, J.Y., *et al.* (1989). Role of nuclear grading in stage I renal cell carcinoma. *Urology* **34**, 310–15.

Grignon, D.J., El-Naggar, A., Green, L.K., *et al.* (1989). DNA flow cytometry as a predictor of outcome of stage I renal cell carcinoma. *Cancer* **63**, 1161–5.

Guinan, P., Frank, W., Saffrin, R., *et al.* (1994). Staging and survival of patients with renal cell carcinoma. *Sem. Surg. Oncol.* **10**, 47–50.

Hadaczek, P, Kovatich, A, Gronwald, J. *et al.* (1998). Absence or reduction of FHIT expression in most clean cell renal carcinomas. *Cancer Res.* **58**, 2946–51.

Hamad, G., Perez-Ordonez, B., Russo, P., *et al.* (1996). Chromophobe renal cell carcinoma: a clinicopathologic study of 51 cases. *Mod. Pathol.* **9**, 74A.

Hatcher, P.A., Anderson, E.E., Paulson, D.F., *et al.* (1991). Surgical management and prognosis of renal cell carcinoma involving the vena cava. *J. Urol.* **145**, 20–4.

Henson, D.E., Fielding, L.P., Grinon, D.J., *et al.* (1995). College of American Pathologists Conference XXVI on clinical relevance of prognostic markers in solid tumors. *Arch. Pathol. Lab. Med.* **119**, 1109–12.

Hermanek, P. and Schrott, K.M. (1990). Evaluation of the new tumor, nodes, and metastases classification of renal cell carcinoma. *J. Urol.* **144**, 238–42.

Hofman, R., Lehmer, A, Harting, R., *et al.* (1996). Prognostic value of urokinase plasminogen activator and plasminogen activator inhibitor-1 in renal cell cancer. *J. Urol.* **155** (3), 858–62.

Homma, Y., Kawabe, K., and Kitamura, T. (1995). Increased incidental detection and reduced mortality in renal cell cancer: recent retrospective analysis at eight institutions. *Int. J. Urol.* **2**, 77.

Ishikawa, I. and Kovacs, G. (1993). High incidence of papillary renal cell carcinoma in patients on chronic hemodialysis. *Histopathology* **22**, 135–9.

Izawa, J.I., Moussa, M., Cherian, M.B., *et al.* (1998). Metallothionein expression in renal cancer. *Urology* **52**, 767–72.

Jayson, M. and Sanders, H. (1998). Increased incidence of serendipitously discovered renal cell carcinoma. *Urology* **51**, 2.

Kartenbeck *et al.* (1998). ACCR98 Abstract 1148, p. 168.

Kaufman, J.J., Burke, D.E., and Goodwin, W.E. (1956). Abdominal venography in urological disease. *J. Urol.* **75**, 160–5.

Kennedy, S.M., Merino, M.J., Linehan, W.M., *et al.* (1990). Collecting duct carcinoma of the kidney. *Hum. Pathol.* **21**, 449–56.

Kinouchi, T., Saiki, S., Meguro, N., *et al.* (1999). Impact of tumor size on the clinical outcomes of patients with Robson stage I renal cell carcinoma. *Cancer* **85**, 689–95.

Klugo, M.D., Stilos, R.E., Talley, R.W., *et al.* (1977. Aggressive versus conservative management of stage IV renal cell carcinoma. *J. Urol.* **118**, 244–6.

Konnak, J.W. and Grossman, H.B. (1985). Renal cell carcinoma as an incidental finding. *J. Urol.* **134**, 1094.

Kovacs, A. and Kovacs, G. (1992). Low chromosome number in chromophobe renal cell carcinomas. *Genes Chromosom. Cancer* **4**, 267–8.

Kovacs, G., Erlandsson, R., Boldog, F., *et al.* (1988). Consistent chromosome 3p deletion and loss of heterozygosity in renal cell carcinoma. *Proc. Natl Acad. Sci., USA* **85**, 1571–5.

Kovacs, G., Fuzesi, L., Emanuel, A., *et al.* (1991).Cytogenetics of papillary renal cell tumors. *Genes Chromosom. Cancer* **3**, 249–55.

Kugler, A., Hemmerlein, B., Thelen, P., Kallerhoff, M., Radzun, H.J., and Ringert, R.H. (1998). Expression of metalloproteinase 2 and 9 and their inhibitors in renal cell carcinoma. *J. Urol.* **160**, 1914–18.

Libertino, J.A., Zinman, L., and Watkins, E., Jr (1987). Long-term results of resection of renal cell carcinoma with extension into inferior vena cava. *J. Urol.* **137**, 21–4.

Licht, M., Novick, A., and Goormastic, M. (1994). Nephron sparing surgery in incidental vs suspected renal cell carcinoma. *J. Urol.* **152**, 39–43.

Maldazys, J.D., and deKernion, J.B. (1986). Prognostic factors in metastatic renal cell carcinoma. *J. Urol.* **136**, 376–9.

Mancilla-Jimenez, R., Stanley, R.J., and Blath, R.A. (1976). Papillary renal cell carcinoma: a clinical, radiologic, and pathologic study of 34 cases. *Cancer* **38**, 2469–80.

Marshall, F.F., Dietrick, D.D., Baumgartner, W.A., *et al.* (1988). Surgical management of renal cell carcinoma with intracaval neoplastic extension above the hepatic veins. *J. Urol.* **139**, 1166–72.

McNichols, D.W., Segura, J.W., and DeWeerd, J.H. (1981). Renal cell carcinoma: long term survival and late recurrence. *J. Urol.* **126**, 17–23.

Medeiros, L.J. and Weiss, L.M. (1990). Renal adenocarcinoma. In *Tumors and tumor-like conditions of the kidneys and ureter* (ed. J.N. Eble). Churchill Livingston, New York.

Medeiros, L.J., Gelb, A.B., and Weiss, L.M. (1988). Renal cell carcinoma. Prognostic significance of morphologic parameters in 121 cases. *Cancer* **61**, 1639–51

Medeiros, L.J., Jones, E.C., Aizawa, S., *et al.* (1997). Grading of renal cell carcinoma. *Cancer* **80**, 988–9.

Mevorach, R.A., Segal, A.J., Tersegno, M.E., and Frank, I.N. (1992). Renal cell carcinoma: incidental diagnosis and natural history: review of 235 cases. *Urology* **39**, 512.

Moch, H., Schraml, P., Bubendorf, L., *et al.* (1999). High-throughput tissue microarray analysis to evaluate genes uncovered by cDNA microarray screening in renal cell carcinoma [see comments]. *Am. J. Pathol.* **154**, 981.

Montie, J.E., Pontes, J.E., Novick, A.C., *et al.* (1991). Resection of inferior vena cava tumor thrombi from renal cell carcinoma. *Am. Surg.* **57**, 56–61.

Motzer, R., Mazumbar, M., Bacik, J., Berg, W., *et al.* (1999). Survival and prognostic stratification of 670 patients with advanced renal cell carcinoma. *J. Clin. Oncol.* **17**, 2530–40.

Mrstik, C., Salamon, J., Weber, R., *et al.* (1992). Microscopic venous infiltration as predictor of relapse in renal cell carcinoma. *J. Urol.* **148**, 271–4.

Nadas, A. (1970). On proportional hazard functions. *Technometrics* **12**, 413.

Naitoh, J., Kaplan, A., Dorey, F., *et al.* (1999). Metastatic renal cell carcinoma with concurrent inferior vena caval invasion: long-term survival after combination therapy with radical nephrectomy, vena caval thrombectomy and postoperative immunotherapy. *J. Urol.* **162**, 46–50.

Neves, R.J. and Zincke, H. (1987). Surgical treatment of renal cancer with vena cava extension. *Br. J. Urol.* **59**, 390–5.

Ney, C. (1946). Thrombosis of the inferior vena cava associated with malignant renal tumors. *J. Urol.* **55**, 583–90.

Novick, A.C., Kaye, M.C., Cosgrove, D.M., *et al.* (1990). Experience with cardiopulmonary bypass and deep hypothermic arrest in the management of retroperitoneal tumors with large vena cava thrombi. *Ann. Surg.* **212**, 472–7

Oda, H. and Machinami, R. (1993). Sarcomatoid renal cell carcinoma. A study of its proliferative activity. *Cancer* **71**, 2292.

Okamoto, K., Toyokuni, S, Kim, W.J., *et al.* (1996). Overexpression of human multi homologue gene messenger RNA in renal cell carcinoma: evidence of persistent oxidarine stress in cancer. *Int. J. Cancer* **65**, 437–41.

Onishi, T., Onishi, Y., Goto, H., *et al.* (1999). Papillary renal cell carcinoma: clinicopathologic characteristics and evaluation of prognosis in 42 patients. *BJU International* **83**, 937–43.

Renshaw, A.A. and Richie, J.P. (1999). Subtypes of renal cell carcinoma. Different onset and sites of metastatic disease. *Am. J. Clin. Pathol.* **111**, 539–43.

Richie, A.W.S. and deKernion, J.B. (1987). The natural history and clinical features of renal carcinoma. *Sem. Nephrol.* **7**, 131–9.

Ro, J., Ayala, A., Sella, A., *et al.* (1987). Sarcomatoid renal cell carcinoma: clincopathologic. *Cancer* **59**, 516.

Robson, C.J., Churchill, B.M., and Andreson, W. (1969). The results of radical nephrectomy for renal cell carcinoma. *J. Urol.* **101**, 297–302.

Saito, S., Orikasa, S., Sato, H.M., *et al.* (1997). Expression of globo-series gangliosides in human renal cell carcinoma. *Jpn J. Cancer Res.* **88**, 652–9.

Santarosa, M., Favaro, D., Qvaia, M., *et al.* (1997). Expression of heart shock protein 72 in renal cell carcinoma: possible role and prognostic implications in cancer patients. *Eur. J. Cancer* **33**, 873–7.

Sejima T. and Miyagawa, I. (1999). Expression of bcl-2, p53 oncoprotein, and proliferating cell nuclear antigen in renal cell carcinoma. *Eur. Urol.* **35**, 242–8.

Sella, A., Logothetis, C.J., Ro, J., *et al.* (1987). Sarcomatoid renal cell carcinoma. A treatable entity. *Cancer* **60**, 1313.

Selli, C., Hinshaw, W., Woodard, B., *et al.* (1983). Stratification of risk factors in renal cell carcinoma. *Cancer* **52**, 899.

Sherman, M.E., Silverman, M.L., Balogh, K., *et al.* (1987). Multilocular renal cyst. *Arch. Pathol. Lab. Med.* **111**, 732–6.

Skinner, D.G., Colvin, R.B., Vermillion, C.D., *et al.* (1971). Diagnosis and management of renal cell carcinoma, a clinical and pathological study of 309 cases. *Cancer* **28**, 1165–77.

Skinner, D.G., Pritchett, T.R., Lieskovsky, G., *et al.* (1989). Vena caval involvement by renal cell carcinoma. Surgical resection provided meaningful long-term survival. *Ann. Surg.* **210**, 387–93.

Smith, S.J., Bosniak, M.A., Megibow, A.J., Hulnick, D.H., Horii, S.C., and Raghavendra, B.N. (1989). Renal cell carcinoma: earlier discovery and increased detection. *Radiology* **170**, 699.

Sosa, R.E., Muecke, E.C., Vaughan, E.D., *et al.* (1984). Renal cell carcinoma extending into the inferior vena cava: the prognostic significance of the level of vena caval involvement. *J. Urol.* **132**, 1097–100.

Storkel, S., Eble, J.N., Adlakha, K., Amin, M., *et al.* (1997). Classification of renal cell carcinoma. *Cancer* **80**, 987–9.

Taxy, J.B. and Marshall, F.F. (1983). Multilocular renal cysts in adults, possible relationship to renal adenocarcinoma. *Arch. Pathol. Lab. Med.* **107**, 633–7.

Thoenes, W., Storkel, S., and Rumpelt, H.J. (1986). Histopathology and classification of renal cell tumors (adenomas, oncocytomas and carcinomas) the basic cytological and histopathological elements and their use for diagnostics. *Pathol. Res. Pract.* **181**, 125–43.

Thompson, I.M. and Peek, M. (1998). Improvement in survival of patients with renal cell carcinoma—the role of serendipitously detected tumor. *J. Urol.* **140**, 487.

Thrasher, J.B. and Paulson, D.F. (1993). Prognostic factors in renal cancer. *Urol. Clin. North Am.* **20**, 247–62.

Tomera, K.M., Farrow, G.M., and Lieber, M.M. (1983). Sarcomatoid renal carcinoma. *J. Urol.* **130**, 657–9.

Tosaka, A., Ohya, K., Yamada, K., Ohashi, H., Kitahara, S., Sekine, H., Takehara, Y., and Oka, K. (1990). Incidence and properties of renal masses and asymptomatic renal cell carcinoma detected by abdominal ultrasonography. *J. Urol.* **144**, 1097.

Tsui, K.H., Shvarts, O., Smith, R.B., Figlin, A., deKernion, J.B., and Belldegrun, A. (2000). Renal cell carcinoma: prognostic significance of incidentally detected tumors. *J. Urol.* **163**, 426–30.

Tsui, K.H., Shvarts, O., Smith, R.B., *et al.* (2000). Prognostic indicators in renal cell carcinoma: a multivariate analysis of 643 patients implementing the revised 1997 TNM staging criteria. *J. Urol.* **163**, 1090–95.

Ueda, T. and Mihara, Y. (1987). Incidental detection of renal cell carcinoma during radiological imaging. *Br. J. Urol.* **59**, 513.

Zisman, A., Pantuck, A., Dorey, F., *et al.* (2001). Improved prognostication of RCC using an integrated staging system (UISS). *J. Clin. Oncol.* **19**, 1649–57.

10. Molecular cytogenetics of renal cell tumors

Gyula Kovacs

Diagnostic and classification systems at any time reflect our technical abilities in the analysis of tumors and our actual theories on tumor development. For many years, renal cell tumors (RCT) were divided into clear and granular cell types on the basis of their cytoplasmic staining characteristics. Bannasch *et al.* (1974) worked out a cytomorphologically oriented classification of experimental kidney tumors of the rat, which later was 'translated' for human kidney cancers (Thoenes *et al.* 1989). RCT were then divided into clear, chromophilic, chromophobe, and oncocytic as well as spindle cell type. Rarely occurring tumors such as collecting duct carcinoma (CDC), renal medullary carcinoma (RMC), and metanephric adenoma (MA) have been recognized in recent years (Jones *et al.* 1995; Fleming and Lewi 1986; Jones *et al.* 1995).

Advances in our understanding of the genetics of renal cancer have led to the recognition of genetically distinct types of tumors (Kovacs 1993). The central idea of the novel classification system is that specific genetic changes affect tumor-related genes that determine the biology of tumor cells, in respect to proliferation, cell death, differentiation, and cell adhesion. The Heidelberg Classification of RCT is based on the existence of specific genetic alterations in tumors and on the morphological pattern characteristic of each genetic subtype (Kovacs *et al.* 1997).

Type of tumor

Conventional renal cell carcinoma

Conventional renal cell carcinoma (RCC) accounts for about 75–80 per cent of renal cell neoplasms and is composed of clear, granular/eosinophilic or sometimes large pale reticular cells arranged in a solid, trabecular, tubular, papillary, or cystic growth pattern. Mixed cytological and growth characteristics within the same tumor occur frequently. The 5-year survival rate after surgery is about 45 per cent with steadily increasing tendency due to early detection and surgical treatment. The overwhelming majority of conventional RCC occur in sporadic form, but families with inherited tumors have been described. Sporadic conventional RCC is usually a solitary tumor, whereas multiple/bilateral tumors develop in familial cases.

Inherited conventional renal cell carcinoma
Von Hippel–Lindau (VHL) disease is an autosomally inherited phacomatosis. The VHL gene was cloned from the chromosome

3p25 region (Latif *et al.* 1993). Germline mutations in the VHL gene are associated with a high risk of developing renal cysts and conventional RCC as well as pancreatic and epididymal cysts, hemangioblastomas of the central nervous system, and pheochromocytomas at early onset. Missense mutations in the VHL gene are associated with the manifestation of conventional RCC and hemangioblastomas (VHL type 1), while truncation mutations are associated with development of pheochromocytomas (VHL type 2A) (Zbar and Lerman 1998). Patients with VHL type 2B may develop all lesions occurring in type 1 and type 2A. Nearly all individuals carrying a missense mutation of the VHL gene in their germ line develop multiple bilateral renal cysts and conventional RCC if they live long enough. VHL-associated RCC represent less than 2 per cent of conventional RCC diagnosed in the general population.

Three families with a constitutional translocation 2;3, 3;6, and 3;8 associated with development of conventional RCC have been published (Li *et al.* 1993; Kovacs *et al.* 1989; Bodmer *et al.* 1999). As the breakpoints at chromosome 3p are located 10 Mb apart in these cases, disruption of a tumor suppressor gene could be excluded. Loss of the derivative chromosomes with chromosome 3p in a large number of cells during forced cell division during embryonal kidney development may explain the development of conventional RCC in such families. Some small nuclear families without VHL mutation and constitutional translocation have also been recognized (Teh *et al.* 1997).

Sporadic conventional renal cell carcinoma
Inactivation of tumor suppressor gene(s) at chromosome 3p, which is deleted in 97 per cent of the cases, is a critical event in the pathogenesis of most common conventional RCC (Chudek *et al.* 1997). Somatic mutations of the VHL gene occur in approximately 40–50 per cent and methylation in approximately 10–15 per cent of sporadic conventional RCC (Gnarra *et al.* 1994; Herman *et al.* 1994) Somatic mutations, in contrast to germline mutations, are distributed along the three exons of the VHL gene. There is no difference in biological behavior between sporadic conventional RCC with and without VHL mutations.

The smallest overlapping deletion in conventional RCC encompasses an approximately 55 cM interval between chromosomal bands 3p14.2 and 3p25 including one allele of the VHL gene (Chudek *et al.* 1997). The deletion of chromosome 3p occurs in 97 per cent of conventional RCC while the remaining allele of the VHL gene is mutated in half of the cases. The consequent deletion of a large chromosomal region proximal to the VHL locus suggests the existence of another tumor suppressor gene. Several genes are cloned from the chromosome 3p21 region, but none of them proved to be a tumor suppressor gene. The fragile histidine triad (*FHIT*) gene at the fragile site FRA3B is localized centromeric to the common overlapping deletion at chromosome 3p. Although the breakpoint in the familial translocation 3;8 disrupts the *FHIT* gene between exons 3 and 4, its role in the development of conventional RCC can be excluded with all certainty (Bugert *et al.* 1997*b*). Recently, a small hemizygous deletion of approximately 100 kb has been detected in a conventional RCC showing two normal appearing chromosome 3. This region may mark the RCC tumor suppressor gene locus (Hanke *et al.* 2001).

Trisomy of the long arm of chromosome 5 is the second most frequent alteration (50 per cent) in conventional RCC. Frequently, a nonhomologous mitotic recombination between chromosomes 3p and 5q results in deletion of chromosome 3p and duplication of chromosome 5q regions (Kovacs and Kung 1991). The breakpoints at chromosome 3p are distributed along an approximately 25 cM interval, whereas the breakpoints at chromosome 5q22 are clustered between the APC and MCC genes (Chudek *et al.* 1997; Kenck *et al.* 1997). Neither the APC nor the MCC genes are mutated in conventional RCC. High-density microsatellite analysis identified two target regions of duplication of approximately 1 Mb each, one at chromosome 5q22 including the a-catenin gene and another at chromosome 5q31.1 (Bugert *et al.* 1998). No mutation or abnormal expression of the a-catenin gene have been found in conventional RCC. Recently, a transcription factor RBCC728 (RING-finger/B-box/coiled-coil) has been cloned from the chromosome 5q22 region (Kovacs, unpublished data).

Loss of heterozygosity (LOH) at chromosome 6q, 8p, 9p, and 14q occurs in 23, 33, 33, and 45 per cent of conventional RCC, respectively (Schullerus *et al.* 1997). These genetic alterations do not correlate with the size of tumors but are associated with tumor grade and stage. The strongest correlation was found between LOH at chromosome 14q and nuclear grade. Loss of the Y chromosome has been observed in 26 per cent of conventional RCC of males, which corresponds to the frequency of Y chromosome loss in normal somatic cells.

Papillary renal cell tumor

Papillary RCT account for approximately 10 per cent of renal cancers in surgical series, but the number of small papillary lesions accompanying clinically recognized tumors or being detected by autopsy is much higher than that of all other types of renal tumors together. Papillary RCT were defined first by the characteristic papillary growth pattern and later by specific genetic alterations (Kovacs 1989). Some authors suggest that papillary RCT may be divided into basophilic small cell and eosinophilic large cell types. However, the vast majority of tumors display cells of medium size with finely granulated pale cytoplasm and a mixture of small basophilic and large eosinophilic cells within the same tumor. A papillary growth pattern predominates in almost all of these tumors, although tubulopapillary or solid architecture may be seen. It was estimated that about 82–90 per cent of patients with papillary RCT are alive 5 years after surgery (Amin *et al.* 1997). As differentiation between papillary renal cell adenomas (RCA) and papillary RCC based on the histological characteristics is not always possible, these series included benign papillary RCA with all certainty. Both sporadic and familial papillary RCT are characterized by development of multiple/bilateral tumors as well as by a high number of microscopic nephrogenic rest-like lesions, the number of lesions being higher in hereditary cases (Kovacs and Kovacs 1993; Ornstein *et al.* 2000). It was suggested that papillary RCT develop from not fully differentiated nephrogenic rest-like lesions, which persist during life (Fig. 10.1).

Inherited papillary renal cell tumor

Until now, 18 families with hereditary papillary RCT (HPRCT) have been published (Zbar and Lerman 1998). Missense mutations in the tyrosine kinase domain of the MET oncogene in the germline is associated with the development of multiple papillary RCT at earlier age of onset (Schmidt *et al.* 1997; Fischer *et al.*

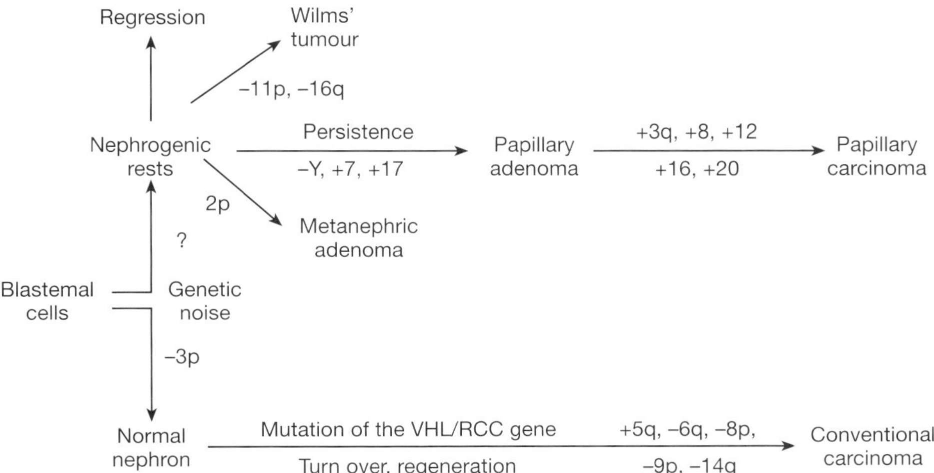

Fig. 10.1 Model of development of renal cell tumors.

1998). Most of these mutations affect the activation loop causing a constitutive phosphorylation of c-MET without ligand binding or receptor dimerization. These mutations have been shown to be tumorigenic *in vitro* (Williams *et al.* 1999). Since family members carrying the c-MET mutation in the germline develop normally functioning nephrons, the mutation of one allele itself seems to be insufficient for tumor initiation. Indeed, the mutant allele is subsequently duplicated and overexpressed in tumor cells (Fischer et al. 1998; Zhuang et al. 1998). A possible explanation for multiple tumor development in these families may come from cytogenetic studies, which detected an organ-specific trisomy of chromosome 7 in up to 10 per cent of normal kidney cells (Emanuel *et al.* 1992). As a duplication of the mutant MET allele is necessary before cells enter the tumorigenic pathway, the chromosomal instability during embryonal development and the number of cells with duplication of the mutant allele have a strong impact on the penetrance of the disease phenotype in HPRCT families. The duplication of the same parental allele of chromosome 7 in multiple tumors of members from HPRCT families that do not carry the germline mutation of the MET tyrosine kinase suggests that a germline event other than mutation of MET might have occurred (Fischer *et al.* 1998).

Small papillary RCT in both sporadic and inherited forms consequently display a combined trisomy of chromosome 7 and 17 (Kovacs *et al.* 1991; Fischer *et al.* 1998). Duplication of different parental alleles in multiple tumors excludes a germline mutation at chromosome 17q. These findings suggest that even the over-representation of MET tyrosine kinase in precursor cells is not enough for tumor development. Probably, the inherited constitutional activation of the MET through mutation or other events leads to a delayed differentiation and/or continuous proliferation of blastemal cells carrying a duplication of the mutant chromosome 7. These cells proliferate slowly forming embryonal rest-like lesions and, after acquiring trisomy of chromosome 17, they develop a papillary RCT.

Sporadic papillary renal cell tumor
Both inherited and sporadic papillary RCT display unique genetic alterations in the form of consequent duplications at specific genomic sites (Kovacs 1993). Combined trisomy of chromosome 7 and 17 (and loss of the Y chromosome in males) are considered to be the primary genetic changes in papillary renal cell adenomas, whereas trisomies at chromosome 3q, 8p, 12q, 16q, and 20q are suggested to be markers for tumor progression in both sporadic and hereditary cases (Fig. 10.1).

Trisomy or tetrasomy of chromosome 7 occurs in approximately 85 per cent of sporadic papillary RCT but mutation of the *MET* tyrosine kinase has been seen in only 5–13 per cent of cases (Kovacs 1993; Lubensky *et al.* 1999; Schmidt *et al.* 1997). This finding arises the question about possible mechanisms of MET activation other than mutation in sporadic papillary RCT. The hepatocyte growth factor/scatter factor HGF/SF (mapped to chromosome 7q21) mediates via *MET* morphogenic, mitogenic, and motogenic signals (Montesano *et al.* 1991) and plays a crucial role in the development of the normal kidney through inductive signaling (Davies *et al.* 1999). The MET gene is ubiquitously expressed in renal parenchymal cells and, therefore, a concomitant

overexpression of the MET tyrosine kinase and its ligand HGF/SF may activate the MET signal pathway in precursor cells (Rong *et al.* 1993). A critical threshold in MET expression has to be reached for cell proliferation (Glukhova *et al.* 2000). The MET gene can also be activated even in the absence of this normal ligand HGF, apart from mutation and overexpression, through a cross-talk with epidermal growth factor receptor (EGFR) activated constitutively by transforming growth factor (TGF) (Jo *et al.* 2000). A selective duplication of chromosomal regions 7q21.1 with the SF/HGF gene and 7p12–13 with the EGFR genes in some of the papillary RCT suggests a complex genetic mechanims of the initial step (Kovacs, unpublished).

Polysomy of chromosome 7 is accompanied by duplication of chromosome 17 in the vast majority of papillary RCT (Kovacs *et al.* 1991; Palmedo *et al.* 1997). A detailed allelotyping study localized the smallest overlapping duplication to an approx. 300 kb genomic segment at chromosome 17q21.32, which is only 3 cM apart from the familial Wilms' tumor gene 1 (FWT1) locus (Balint *et al.* 1999). Alteration of this region has been seen in 92 per cent of sporadic and hereditary papillary RCT as well.

Selective duplication of chromosome 16q22 and 16q24 regions occurs in approximately 55 per cent of papillary RCT (Palmedo *et al.* 1997). Chromosome 16q harbors several genes that are involved in epithelial cell–cell adhesion. The E-cadherin is mapped to chromosome 16q22, whereas the cell adhesion regulator, M- and H-cadherins are localized to chromosome 16q24 region. How the increased copy number of several genes at chromosome 16q contributes to the progression of papillary RCT is not yet known. Duplication of the chromosomal regions 3q, 8q, 12q12–14, 3q22–24, 20q11.2, and 20q13.2 occurs in 24–67 per cent of papillary RCC (Palmedo *et al.* 1997, 1999). The development of papillary RCT shows a strong male preponderance (8:1) and loss of the Y chromosome occurs in 80 per cent of the tumors arising in male patients.

A small subset of RCT occurring in younger patients is characterized by translocation between Xp11.2 and other chromosomes either as the sole genetic alteration or in combination with trisomies of chromosomes 7 and 17. The most frequently described rearrangement leads to the fusion of the transcription factor *TFE3* on chromosome Xp11.2 with the *PRCC* gene on chromosome 1q21 (Sidhar *et al.* 1996). In tumor cells both chimeric genes, the *PRCC/TEF3* and the *TFE3/PRCC* as well as the normal *PRCC* but not the *TFE3* are expressed. The transactivation efficiency of the PRCC/TFE3 transcript is at least threefold when compared to TFE3 itself (Weterman *et al.* 2000). In the translocation (X;1)(p11.2;p34) the TFE3 is fused to the splicing factor gene PSF, but in this case TFE3 is still expressed (Clark *et al.* 1997). The Xp11.2 region is involved in some other rare translocations such as t(X;17)(p11.2:q25) or t(X;10)(p11.2;q23).

Metanephric adenoma

Metanephric adenoma (MA) is a rare benign neoplasm composed of a diffuse array of discrete, round tubules with occasional tubulopapillary structures and glomeruloid bodies lined by small dark cuboidal cells with minimal cytoplasma, reminiscent of embryonal metanephric tissue (Jones *et al.* 1995). Only few and controversial data are available on the genetics of MA. Chromosome and fluorescence *in situ* hybridization (FISH) analysis revealed a normal karyotype and/or two copies of chromosome 7 and 17 in some cases (Jones *et al.* 1995), whereas another study showed a consequent duplication of chromosomes 7 and 17 in 8 of 11 tumors diagnosed as MA (Brown *et al.* 1997). A recent allelotyping study detected allelic changes at chromosome 2p13 in 56 per cent of MA as well as allelic changes at chromosomes 7, 8p, 12q, 16q, and 20q in 33, 43, 22, 18, and 40 per cent of the cases, respectively (Pesti *et al.* 2001). None of the tumors showed genetic alterations at chromosome 17q21.32 region or at the WT1 locus on chromosome 11p13. region.

Chromophobe renal cell carcinoma

Chromophobe RCC accounts for approximately 3–5 per cent of renal cell neoplasms in surgical series. Chromophobe RCC displays a compact growth of large polygonal cells with fine reticular cytoplasm and prominent cell membranes. The characteristic 'chromophobe' staining results from the large number of intra cytoplasmic vesicles. Most chromophobe RCC are confined to the kidney at the time of diagnosis which suggests a good prognosis (Crotty *et al.* 1995). A sarcomatous transformation with rapid progression may occur in some cases. Chromophobe RCC display LOH in different combinations at chromosome 1p, 2, 6, 10, 13, 17, and 21 in 100, 95, 88, 95, 95, 76, and 88 per cent, respectively (Speicher *et al.* 1994; Bugert *et al.* 1997*a*). Loss of several specific and also of some randomly involved chromosomes leads to chromosome number between 35 and 40 and to a low DNA index between 0.7 and 0.9 in chromophobe RCC. Mutation of the p53 tumor suppressor gene has been detected in 27 per cent of chromophobe RCC (Contractor *et al.* 1997). Although LOH at chromosome 10 occurs in 95 per cent of the tumors, no mutation of the PTEN suppressor gene has been found (Kovacs, unpublished). Gross rearrangements of the mitochondrial DNA were seen in some cases (Kovacs *et al.* 1992).

Renal oncocytoma

Renal oncocytoma (RO) is a benign tumor that comprises about 3–5 per cent of renal cell neoplasms in surgical series. Even cases showing infiltration into the perirenal fat or renal vein invasion have a benign clinical course (Davis *et al.* 1991). RO are composed of cells with abundant eosinophilic cytoplasm filled with mitochondria showing acinar growth pattern, but solid, trabecular or even cystic growth may occur. RO show heterogeneous genetic alterations. The largest group has no visible genetic alteration by karyotyping. A subgroup of RO displays LOH at chromosome 1 and 14 and another group balanced translocations between chromosome 11q13 and other chromosomes (Herbers *et al.* 1998; Sinke *et al.* 1997). Interestingly, nearly all translocation sites encode mitochondrial genes, which are involved in the oxidative phosphorylation (OXPHOS). These data suggest that possible disfunction in the OXPHOS system leads to compensatory proliferation of mitochondria/mitochondrial DNA in RO. Recently, some exceptional families with development of RO have been identified (Zbar and Lerman 1998).

Collecting duct carcinoma

Collecting duct carcinoma (CDC) accounts for less than 1 per cent of renal cell neoplasms in surgical series. CDC is a term that has been applied to carcinomas with differing appearances (Fleming and Lewi 1986). CDC is a highly malignant tumor occurring in younger patients. Controversial results have been obtained by karyotyping, microsatellite, and comparative genomic hybridization (CGH) analyses in small series of tumors that were diagnosed as CDC. A detailed allelotyping study revealed recurrent LOH at chromosomes 1q (57 per cent), 6p (45 per cent), 8p (40 per cent), and 21q (40 per cent) (Polascik *et al.* 1996), whereas another study showed LOH at chromosome 9p, 13q, 17p (Fogt *et al.* 1998). Because an appropriate definition of CDC based on morphological pattern has not yet been established and the tumors in these series show a variety of genetic alterations, a specific pattern of DNA alterations for CDC cannot be suggested.

Renal medullary carcinoma

Renal medullary carcinoma (RMC) is an extremely rare tumor occurring preferentially in Black patients with sickle cell trait in the second and third decade of life. RMC is a highly malignant tumor; the mean survival is approximately 3–5 months after diagnosis. Usually, RMC is detected in an advanced stage with venous and lymphatic invasion. Karyotyping of four RMC revealed monosomy of chromosome 11 in each case and monosomy 3 as well as a t(3;8)(p21;q24) each in one case (Avery *et al.* 1996). This finding is intriguing as the beta globulin gene is mapped to chromosome 11p.

Unclassified renal cell tumors

Approximately 3 per cent of RCT cannot be assigned to any of the types of tumors mentioned above even after genetic analysis. Several combinations of chromosomal alteration or single genetic changes have been mentioned at the case report level.

Renal cell tumors in end-stage renal disease

An increased incidence of RCT has been described in patients with end-stage renal disease (ESRD), especially with aquired cystic kidney disease (ACKD). The observation that about 20 per cent of the cases develop a metastatic tumor suggests that RCC may be a life-threatening complication for patients undergoing long-term renal replacement therapy. The incidence of papillary RCT in ESRD/ACKD is five times higher than in the general population (Ishikawa and Kovacs 1993). Tumors in ESRD may display genetic alterations similar to those seen in conventional, papillary, or chromophobe RCC arising in the general population. Some papillary RCT, however, lack the initial alterations at chromosome 7 and 17 (Chudek *et al.* 1997). Mutation of the MET oncogene has also been excluded as an initial genetic event (Kovacs, unpublished). Interestingly, a high rate of cell division has been found among cells of atropic tubuli in ESRD kidneys and an increased expression of renal cyst growth factor, EGFR, PDGF, and ERBB-2 were also documented (for review see Chudek *et al.* 1997). Probably, an increased expression of growth factors replaces the dosage effect of trisomy of chromosomes 7 during remodeling of the end-stage kidney and leads to monoclonal growth of some cells. Only a few conventional RCC arising in ESRD showed LOH at chromosome 3p and none of them had mutation of the VHL gene (Hughson *et al.* 1999; Chudek *et al.* 1997).

Model of development of renal cell tumors

Thoenes *et al.* (1989) extrapolated the presumed cellular origin of RCT by comparing the tumor phenotypes with their possible counterparts in the renal tubular system. However, lectin and immunohistochemical studies using markers for different parts of the adult renal tubular system yielded conflicting results regarding the proximal versus distal origin of RCT. Kovacs (1993) suggested two main developmental pathways for RCT (Fig. 10.1). Tumors may arise from not fully differentiated embryonal cells or from fully differentiated but potential stem cells of the tubular system. The two most common types of RCT, the conventional and papillary RCC, have basically distinct natural histories.

There is a strong association between the persistence of embryonal rest-like structures and development of sporadic as well as hereditary papillary RCT in the same kidney (Kovacs and Kovacs 1993; Ornstein *et al.* 2000). The link between embryonal rests and Wilms' tumor is well documented (Beckwith *et al.* 1990). It was suggested that both Wilms' tumor and papillary RCT arise from blastemal cells persisting after cessation of the kidney development in the 36th week of gestation (Kovacs 1993). If one such lesion aquires an alteration at the WT1 gene or at another yet unknown WT gene, a Wilms' tumor may develop. If such lesions persist and aquire alteration at chromosome 2p13 and/or at other genes, an MA may arise. Alteration in the MET signaling pathway or in the function of another yet unknown gene at chromosome 7 may initiate the development of papillary RCT. Duplication of multiple chromosomal regions is a hallmark of embryonal tumors, which arise from cells retaining the proliferative capacity. Therefore, an increased dosage of mutant or normal gene products seems to be sufficient for triggering neoplastic cell proliferation. Trisomies of chromosomes 7, 8, 12, 17, and 20, which are specific genetic alterations in papillary RCT, occur in 13 to

38 per cent of Wilms' tumors as well as in 18 to 43 per cent of MA (Kaneko *et al.* 1991; Pesti *et al.* 2001).

Conventional RCC display consequently a loss of heterozygosity at several chromosomal regions as do most cancers developing from differentiated adult tissues. Most chromosomal alterations arise during forced mitotic activity of cells, whereas gene mutations occur independently from cell proliferation and their rate is time-dependent. Probably, most chromosomal aberrations occurring in mosaic form in adult tissues arise during embryonal development (Emanuel *et al.* 1992). During life, mutation of the RCC tumor suppressor gene may occur in some of the phenotypically normal kidney cells carrying chromosome 3p deletion. When these cells undergo cellular turnover, the lack of tumor suppressor gene protein may lead to a lack of growth control of potential stem cells in renal tubuli, for example, 'overproliferation', and finally to the development of conventional RCC. In VHL disease each renal cell carries a mutation of the VHL gene. Therefore, cells acquiring random chromosome 3p deletions due to 'genetic noise' may develop renal cysts increasing enormously the number of cells with such alterations. Mutation of the RCC tumor suppressor gene located on the remaining chromosome 3p21 allele may lead to the development of conventional RCC in some of the cystic changes.

Clinical application

Because the incidence of hereditary RCC in the general population is extremely low, screening for germline mutation of the *VHL* and *MET* genes should include only individuals at high risk. This includes those suspected of having VHL disease and members of the VHL families. Familial occurrence of papillary RCT or occurrence of multiple bilateral papillary RCT in young patients indicates a search for mutation in the MET tyrosine kinase. An early diagnosis of VHL disease and HPRCT facilitates timely treatment and continued surveillance for disease manifestations.

The genetic classification system allows a quick, accurate, and reproducible diagnosis. The morphologic heterogeneity and overlapping cytologic and growth characteristics of RCT result in inter- and intraobserver variations in the histological diagnosis (Fig. 10.2). Granular or chromophilic cell type may occur in

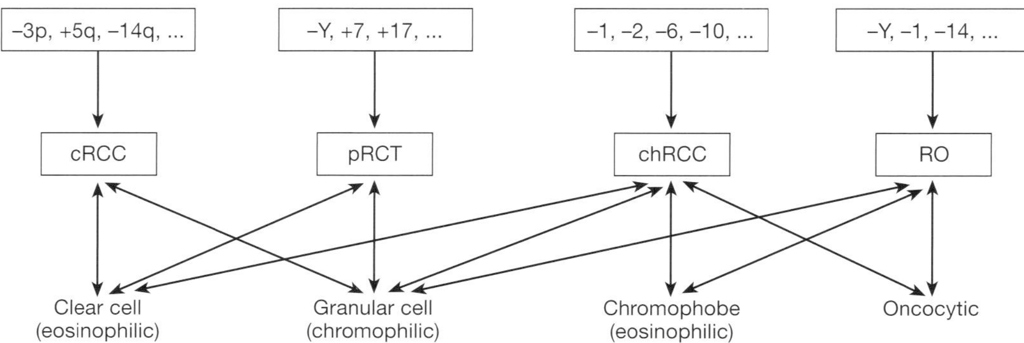

Fig. 10.2 Genetic versus phenotypical markers for diagnosis of renal cell tumors

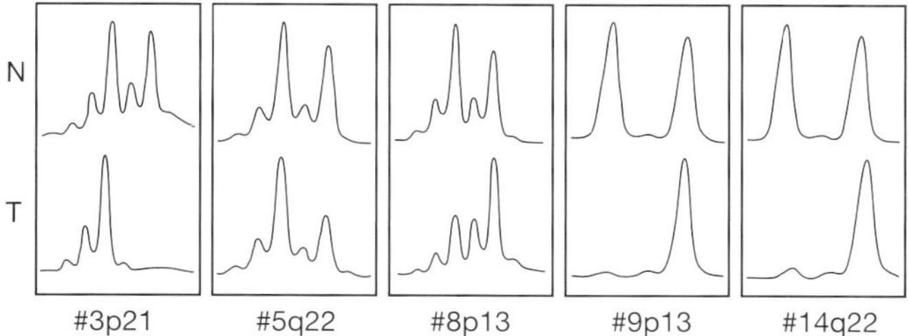

Fig. 10.3 Microsatellite analysis of a conventional RCC. Note the loss of one allele at chromosomes 3p21, 8p13, 9p13, and 14q22 and allelic imbalance corresponding to duplication at chromosome 5q22.

genetically distinct types of tumors including conventional, papillary and chromophobe RCC and RO. Although a clear cell phenotype is said to be the hallmark of conventional RCC, it may appear in some areas of papillary and chromophobe RCC and, on rare occasions, the entire chromophobe or papillary RCC may be composed of 'clear' cells.

Chromosomal and/or gene mutations occurring in progenitor cells mark all descendant cells during their entire life span regardless of intratumoral morphological variations. Therefore, the constant genetic markers are superior in the diagnosis of RCT (Fig. 10.2). Although the molecular basis for most of the genetic changes is not yet established, they are marked by loss of heterozygosity (LOH) or by duplication of DNA fragments, which may efficiently be used in diagnosis. For example, a differentiation between renal oncocytomas with atypical cytological and growth characteristics and chromophobe, papillary, and sometimes conventional RCC based on phenotype may be difficult. LOH at multiple regions including chromosome 1, 2, 6, 10, 13, 17, and 21 corresponds to the diagnosis of a chromophobe RCC, LOH at chromosome 3p, 6q, 8p, 9p, and 14q confirms the diagnosis of conventional RCC, whereas allelic duplication at chromosomes 3q, 7, 8p, 12q, 16q, 17, and 20 suggests the diagnosis of a papillary

RCC. The lack of these genetic changes or LOH only at chromosome 1 or in combination with 14 will confirm the diagnosis of a renal oncocytoma.

There are different methods to detect genetic alterations in tumor cells. Chromosome analysis and spectral karyotyping are time-consuming techniques and require dividing cells in short-term cultures. Comparative genomic hybridization (CGH) has a strong limitation in detecting small deletions or duplications and also uniparental isodisomy, which occurs frequently at some chromosomal regions. The large number of probes necessary for diagnosis sets a limitation on the use of fluorescence *in situ* hybridization (FISH) in routine work. A computer-controled, automated fragment-length analysis by applying microsatellites from the specific chromosomal regions offers a high diagnostic throughput, easy material handling, and a quick analysis of distinct types of renal cell tumors (Bugert and Kovacs 1996) (Fig. 10.3). Recent progress in the microarray technology resulted in the development of matrix CGH, that is, analysis of DNA samples with high resolution in a single hybridization. It is now possible to diagnose the main types of RCT by hybridizing genomic DNA to arrayed BAC or cosmid clones obtained from specific chromosomal regions (Wilhelm *et al.* 2000) (Fig. 10.4).

Summary

A new genetic classification of renal cell tumors as well as the morphologic hallmarks for the diagnosis of biologically distinct types is now available. Allelic losses and duplications as well as translocations at specific genomic sites for the most common RCT are identified. However, the substantial part of our knowledge on the molecular genetics of RCT comes from studies of rare hereditary cases. The *VHL* gene responsible for the manifestation of von Hippel–Lindau disease is cloned and ongoing studies should explain the role of the VHL protein in certain biological processes.

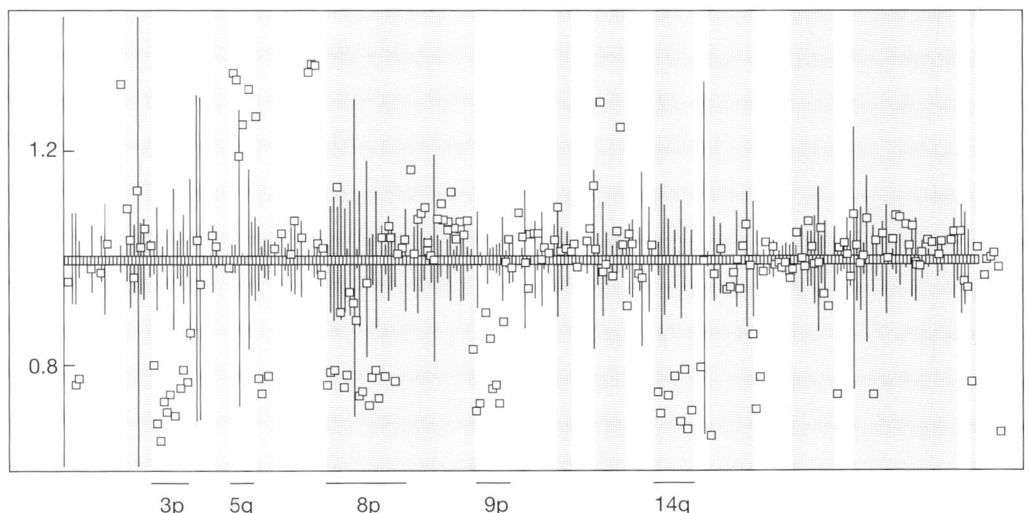

Fig. 10.4 Result of microarray analysis of a conventional RCC. Note the decrease in signal intensity at chromosome 3p, 8p, 9p, and 14q and increase in signal at chromosome 5q (from Wilhelm *et al.* 2000)

A correlation between germline mutation in the tyrosine kinase domain of the *MET* oncogene and familial papillary RCC has been established. A fusion of transcription factor TFE3 at Xp11.2 and other genes has also been identified. These tumors make up less than 1 per cent of all RCT and the genes involved in the development of sporadic conventional, papillary, and chromophobe RCC and RO are not yet known. Much more effort should be made to understand the genetic changes underlying the development and progression of sporadic tumors, which may allow an early detection, improve the outcome, and lead to novel therapeutic approaches.

References

Amin, M.B., Corless, C.L., Renshaw, A.A., Ticko, S.K., Kubus, J., and Schultz, D.S. (1997). Papillary (chromophil) renal cell carcinoma: histomorphologic characteristics and evaluation of conventional pathologic prognostic parameters in 62 cases. *Am. J. Surg. Pathol.* **21**, 621–35.

Avery, R.A., Harris, J.E., Davis, C.J., Borgaonkar, D.S., Byrd, J.C., and Weiss, R.B. (1996). Renal medullary carcinoma: clinical and therapeutic aspects of a newly described tumor. *Cancer* **78**, 128–32.

Balint, I., Fischer, J., Ljungberg, B., and Kovacs, G. (1999). Mapping the papillary renal cell carcinoma gene between loci D17S787 and D17S1799 on chromosome 17q21.32. *Lab. Invest.* **79**, 1713–18.

Bannasch, P., Schacht, U., and Storch, E. (1974). Morphogenesis and micromorphology of epithelial tumors of the kidney of nitrosomorpholine intoxicated rats. I. Induction and histology. *Cancer Res. Clin. Oncol.* **81**, 311–31.

Beckwith, J.B., Kiviat, N.B., and Bonadio, J.F. (1990). Nephrogenic rests, nephroblastomatosis, and the pathogenesis of Wilms' tumor. *Pediatr. Pathol.* **10**, 1–36.

Bodmer, D., Eleveld, M.J., Ligtenberg, M.J.L., Weterman, M.A.J., Janssen, B.A.P., Smeets, D.F.C.M., de Wit, P.R.J., van den Berg, A., van den Berg, E., Kooeln, M.I., and van Kessel, A.G. (1999). An alternative route for multistep tumorigenesis in a novel vase of hereditary renal cell cancer and a t(2;3)(q35;q21) chromosome translocation. *Am. J. Hum. Genet.* **62**, 1475–83.

Brown, J.A., Anderl, K.L., Borell, T.J., Qian, J., Bostwick, D.G., and Jenkins, R.B. (1997). Simultaneous chromosome 7 and 17 gain and sex chromosome loss provide evidence that renal metanephric adenoma is related to papillary renal cell carcinoma. *J. Urol.* **158**, 370–4.

Bugert, P. and Kovacs, G. (1996). Molecular differential diagnosis of renal cell carcinomas by microsatellite analysis. *Am. J. Pathol.* **149**, 2081–8.

Bugert, P., Gaul, C., Weber, K., Akhtar, M., Ljungberg, B., and Kovacs, G. (1997*a*). Specific genetic changes of diagnostic importance in chromophobe renal cell carcinomas. *Lab. Invest.* **76**, 203–8.

Bugert, P., Wilhelm, M., and Kovacs, G. (1997*b*). The FHIT gene and FRA3B region are not involved in genetics of hereditary and sporadic renal cell carcinomas. *Genes Chromosom. Cancer* **20**, 9–15.

Bugert, P., von Knobloch, R., and Kovacs, G. (1998). Duplication of two distinct regions on chromosome 5q in nonpapillary renal cell carcinomas. *Int. J. Cancer* **76**, 337–40.

Chudek, J., Wilhelm, M., Bugert, P., Herbers, J., and Kovacs, G. (1997). Detailed microsatellite analysis of chromosome 3p region in nonpapillary renal cell carcinomas. *Int. J. Cancer* **73**, 225–9.

Chudek, J., Herbers, J., Kenck, C., Wilhelm, M., Bugert, P., Ritz, E., Waldman, F., and Kovacs, G. (1998). The genetics and morphology of renal cell tumors in end stage renal failure may differ from those occurring in the general population. *J. Am. Soc. Nephrol.* **9**, 1045–51.

Clark, J., Lu, Y.J., Sidhar, S.K., Parker, C., Gill, S., Smedley, D., Hamoudi, R, Linehan, W.M., Shipley, J., and Cooper, C.S. (1997). Fusion of splicing factor genes PSF and NonO (p54nrb) to the TFE3 gene in papillary renal cell carcinoma. *Oncogene* **15**, 2233–9.

Contractor, H., Zariwala, M., Bugert, P., Zeisler, J., and Kovacs , G. (1997). Mutation of the p53 tumor suppressor gene occurs preferentially in the chromophobe type of renal cell tumor. *J. Pathol.* **181**, 136–9.

Crotty, T.B., Farrow, G.M., and Lieber, M.M. (1995). Chromophobe cell renal carcinoma: clinicopathological feature of 50 cases. *J. Urol.* **154**, 964–7.

Davies, J.A., Perera, A.D., and Walker, C.L. (1999). Mechanisms of epithelial development and neoplasia in the metanephric kidney. *Int. J. Develop. Biol.* **43**, 473–8.

Davis, C.J., Sesterhenn, I.A., Mostofi, F.K., and Ho, C.K. (1991). Renal oncocytoma. Clinicopathological study of 166 patients. *J. Urogen. Pathol.* **1**, 41–52.

Emanuel, A., Szücs, S., Weier, H.U.G., and Kovacs, G. (1992). Clonal aberrations of the X and Y chromosomes and chromosomes 7 and 10 in normal kidney tissue of patients with renal cell tumors. *Genes Chromosom. Cancer* **4**, 75–7.

Fischer, J., Palmedo, G., von Knobloch, R., Bugert, P., Prayer-Galetti, T., Pagano, F., and Kovacs, G. (1998). Duplication and overexpression of the mutated allele of the MET proto-oncogene in multiple hereditary papillary renal cell tumors. *Oncogene* **17**, 733–9.

Fleming, S. and Lewi, H. (1986). Collecting duct carcinoma of the kidney. *Histopathology* **10**, 1131–41.

Fogt, F., Zhuang, Z., Linehan, W.M., and Merino, M.J. (1998). Collecting duct carcinomas of the kidney: a comparative loss of heterozygosity study with clear cell carcinoma. *Oncol. Rep.* **5**, 923–6.

Glukhova, L., Lavialle, C., Fauvet, D., Chudoba, I., Danglot, G., Angevin, E., Bernheim, A., and Goguel, A.F. (2000). Mapping of the 7q31 subregion common to the small chromosome 7 derivatives from two sporadic papillary renal cell carcinomas: increased copy number and overexpression of the MET proto-oncogene. *Oncogene* **19**, 754–61.

Gnarra, J.R., Tory, K., Weng, Y., Schmidt, L., Wei, M.H., Li, H., Latif, F., Liu, S., Chen, F., Duh, F-M., Lubensky, I., Duan, D.R., Florence, C., Pozzatti, R., Walther, M.M., Bander, N.H., Grossman, H.B., Brauch, H., Pomer, S., Brooks, J.D., Isaacs, W.B., Lerman, M.I., Zbar, B., and Linehan, W.M. (1994). Mutation of the VHL tumor suppressor gene in renal carcinoma. *Nature Genet.* **7**, 8580–4.

Hanke, S., Bugert, P., Chudek, J., and Kovacs, G. (2001). Cloning a calcium channel $\alpha 2\delta$-3 subunit gene from a putative tumor suppressor gene region at chromosome 3p21.1 in conventional renal cell carcinoma. *Gene* **264(1)**, 69–75.

Herbers, J., Schullerus, D., Bugert, P., Kanamaru, H., Zeisler, J., Ljungberg, B., Akhtar, M., and Kovacs, G. (1998). Lack of genetic changes separates renal oncocytoma from renal cell carcinomas. *J. Pathol.* **184**, 58–62.

Herman, J.G., Latif, F., Weng, Y., Lerman, M.I., Zbar, B., Liu, S., Samid, D., Duan, D.S., Gnarra, J.R., and Linehan W.M. (1994). Silencing of the *VHL* tumor-suppressor gene by DNA methylation in renal carcinoma. *Proc. Natl Acad. Sci., USA* **91**, 9700–4.

Hughson, M.D., Bigler, S., Dickman, K., and Kovacs, G. (1999). Renal cell carcinoma of end stage renal disease: an analysis of chromosomes 3, 7, and 17 abnormalities by microsatellite amplification. *Mod. Pathol.* **12**, 301–9.

Ishikawa, I. and Kovacs, G. (1993). High incidence of papillary renal cell tumors in patients with chronic haemodialysis. *Histopathology* **22**, 135–9.

Jo, M., Stolz, D.B., Esplen, J.E., Dorko, K., Michalopoulos, G.K., and Strom, S.C. (2000). Crosstalk between epidermal growth factor receptor and c-Met signal pathways in transformed cells. *J. Biochem. Chem.* **275**, 8806–11.

Jones, E.C., Pins, M., Dickersin, R., and Young, R.H. (1995). Metanephric adenoma of the kidney. A clinicopathological, immunohistochemical, flow cytometric, cytogenetic, and electron microscopic study of seven cases. *Am. J. Surg. Pathol.* **19**, 615–26.

Kaneko, Y., Homma, C., Maseki, N., Sakurai, M., and Hata, J. (1991). Correlation of chromosome abnormalities with histological and clinical feature in Wilms' and other childhood renal tumors. *Cancer Res.* **51**, 5937–42.

Kenck, C., Bugert, P., Wilhelm, M., and Kovacs, G. (1997). Duplication of an approximately 1.5 Mb DNA segment at chromosome 5q22 indicates the locus of a new tumor gene in nonpapillary renal cell carcinomas. *Oncogene* 14, 1093–8.

Kovacs, A., Störkel, S., Thoenes, W., and Kovacs, G. (1992). Mitochondrial and chromosomal DNA alterations in human chromophobe renal cell carcinomas. *J. Pathol.* 167, 273–7.

Kovacs, G. (1989). Papillary renal cell carcinoma: a morphologic and cytogenetic tudy of 11 cases. *Am. J. Pathol.* 134, 27–34.

Kovacs, G. (1993). Molecular cytogenetics of renal cell tumors. *Advan. Cancer Res.* 62, 89–124.

Kovacs, G. and Kovacs, A. (1993). Parenchymal abnormalities associated with papillary renal cell tumors: a morphologic study. *J. Urol. Pathol.* 1, 301–12.

Kovacs, G. and Kung, H. (1991). Non-homologous chromatid exchange in hereditary and sporadic renal cell carcinomas. *Proc. Natl Acad. Sci., USA* 88, 184–98.

Kovacs, G., Brusa, P., and DeRiese, W. (1989). Tissue specific expression of a constitutional 3;6 translocation: development of multiple bilateral renal cell carcinomas. *Int. J. Cancer* 43, 422–7.

Kovacs, G., Füzesi, L., Emanuel, A., and Kung, H. (1991). Cytogenetics of papillary renal cell tumors. *Genes Chromosom. Cancer* 3, 249–55.

Kovacs, G., Akhtar, M., Beckwith, B.J., Bugert, P., Cooper, C.S., Delahunt, B., Eble, J.N., Fleming, S., Ljungberg, B., Medeiros, L.J., Moch, H., Reuter, V.E., Ritz, E., Roos, G., Schmidt, D., Srigley, J.R., Störkel, S., van den Berg, E., and Zbar, B. (1997). The Heidelberg classification of renal cell tumors. *J. Pathol.* 183, 131–3.

Latif, F., Tory, K., Gnarra, J., Yao, M., Duh, F-M., Orcutt, M.L., Stackhouse, T., Kuzmin, I., Modi, W., Geil, L., Schmidt, L., Zhou, F., Li, H., Wei, M.H., Chen, F., Glenn, G., Choyke, P., Walther, M.M., Weng, Y., Duan, D.R., Dean, M., Glavac, D., Richards, F.M., Crossey, P.A., Ferguson-Smith, M.A., Le Paslier, D., Chumakov, I., Cohen, D., Chinault, A.C., Maher, E.R., Linehan, W.M., Zbar, B., and Lerman, M.I. (1993). Identification of the von Hippel–Lindau disease tumor suppressor gene. *Science* 260, 1317–20.

Li, F.P., Decker, H.J.H., Zbar, B., Stanton, V.P., Kovacs, G., Seizinger, B.R., Aburatani, H., Sandberg, A.A., Berg, S., Hosoe, S., and Brown, R.S. (1993). Clinical and genetic studies of renal cell carcinomas in a family with constitutional chromosome 3;8 translocation. *Ann. Intern. Med.* 118, 106–11.

Lubensky, I.A., Schmidt, L., Zhuang, Z., Weirich, G., Pack, S., Zambrano, N., Walther, M.M., Choyke, P., Linehan, W.M., and Zbar, B. (1999). Hereditary and sporadic papillary renal carcinomas with c-met mutations share a distinct morphological phenotype. *Am. J. Pathol.* 155, 517–26.

Montesano, R., Matsumoto, K., Nakamura, T., and Orci, L. (1991). Identification of a fibroblast-derived epithelial morphogen as hepatocyte growth factor. *Cell* 67, 901–8.

Ornstein, D.K., Lubensky, I.A., Venzon, D., Zbar, B., Linehan, W.M., and Walther, M.M. (2000). Prevalence of microscopic tumors in normal appearing renal parenchyma of patients with hereditary papillary renal cancer. *J. Urol.* 163, 431–3.

Palmedo, G., Fischer, J., and Kovacs, G. (1997). Fluorescent microsatellite analysis reveals duplication of specific chromosomal regions in papillary renal cell tumors. *Lab. Invest.* 77, 633–8.

Palmedo, G., Fischer, J., and Kovacs, G. (1999). DNA sequences between loci D20S478 and D20S206 at 20q11.2 and between loci D20S902 and D20S480 at 20q13.2 are duplicated in papillary renal cell carcinoma. *Lab. Invest.* 79, 311–16.

Pesti, T., Jones, T., Sükösd, F., and Kovacs, G. (2001). Mapping a tumor suppressor gene to chromosome 2p13 in metanephric adenoma by microsatellie allelotyping. *Hum. Pathol.* 32(1), 101–4.

Polascik, T.J., Cairns, P., Epstein, J.I., Füzesi, L., Ro, J.Y., Marschall, F.F., Sidransky, D., and Schoenberg, M. (1996). Distal nephron renal tumors: microsatellite allelotype. *Cancer Res.* 56, 1892–5.

Rong, S., Oskarsson, M., Faletto, D., Tsarfaty, I., Resau, J.H., Nakamura, T., Rosen, E., Hopkins, R.F., and Vande Woude, G.F. (1993). Tumorigenesis induced by coexpression of human hepatocyte growth factor and the human met protooncogene leads to high levels of expression of the ligand and receptor. *Cell Growth Differentiat.* 4, 563–9.

Schmidt, L., Duh, F.M., Chen, F., Kishida, T., Glenn, G., Choyke, P., Scherer, S., Zhuang, Z., Lubensky, I., Dean, M., Allikmets, R., Chidambaram, A., Bergerheim, U.R., Feltis, J.T., Casadevall, C., Zamarron, A., Bernues, M., Richard, S., Lips, C.J.M., Walther, M.M., Tsui, L-C., Geil, L., Orcutt, M.L., Stackhouse, T., Lipan, J., Slife, L., Brauch, H., Decker, J., Niehans, G., Hughson, M.D., Moch, H., Störkel, S., Lerman, M.I., Linehan, W.M., and Zbar, B. (1997). Germline and somatic mutations in the tyrosine kinase domain of the MET proto-oncogene in papillary renal carcinomas. *Nature Genet.* 16, 68–73.

Schullerus, D., Herbers, J., Chudek, J., Kanamaru, H., and Kovacs, G. (1997). Loss of heterozygosity at chromosomes 8p, 9p and 14q is associated with stage and grade of nonpapillary renal cell carcinomas. *J. Pathol.* 183, 151–5.

Sidhar, S.K., Clark, J., Gill, S., Hamoudi, R., Crew, A.J., Gwillin, R., Ross, M., Linehan, W.M., Birdsall, S., Shipley, J., and Cooper, C.S. (1996). The t(X;1)(p11.2;q21.2) translocation in papillary renal cell carcinoma fuses a novel gene PRCC to the TFE3 transcription factor gene. *Hum. Mol. Genet.* 5, 1333–8.

Sinke, R.J., Dijkhuizen, T., Janssen, B., Olde Weghuis, D, Merkx, G., van den Berg, E., Schuuring, E., Meloni, A.M., de Jong, B., and Geurts van Kessel, A. (1997). Fine mapping of the human renal oncocytoma-associated translocation(5;11)(q35;q13) breakpoint. *Cancer Genet. Cytogenet.* 96, 95–101.

Speicher, M., Schoel, B., duManoir, S., Ried, T., Kovacs, A., Störkel, S., Cremer, T., and Kovacs, G. (1994). Loss of chromosomes 1, 2, 6, 10, 13, 17 and 21 in chromophobe renal cell carcinomas revealed by comparative genomic hybridisation. *Am. J. Pathol.* 145, 356–64.

Teh, B.T., Giraud, S., Sari, N.F., Hii, S.I., Bergerat, J.P., Larsson, C., Limarcher, J.M., and Nicol, D. (1997). *Lancet* 349, 848–9.

Thoenes, W., Störkel, S., and Rumpelt, H.F. (1989). Histopathology and classification of renal cell tumors (adenomas, oncocytomas and carcinomas). *Pathol. Res. Pract.* 181, 125–43.

Weterman, M.J., van Groningen, J.J., Jansen, A., and van Kessel, A.G. (2000). Nuclear localization and transactivating capacities of the papillary renal cell carcinoma-associated TFE3 and PRCC (fusion) proteins. *Oncogene* 19, 69–74.

Wilhelm, M., Presti, J., Kovacs, G., and Waldman, F. (2000). Array-based CGH for the differential diagnosis of renal cell carcinoma. *Proceedings of the 91th Annual Meeting of AACR*, Vol. 41, Abstract 2000.

Williams, T.A., Longati, P., Pugliese, L., Gual, P., Bardelli, A., and Michieli, P. (1999). MET (PRC) mutations in the Ron receptor result in up-regulation of tyrosine kinase activity and acquisition of oncogenic potential. *J. Cell Physiol.* 181, 507–14.

Zbar, B. and Lerman, M. (1998). Inherited carcinomas of the kidney. *Advan. Cancer Res.* 75, 163–201.

Zhuang, Z., Park, W.S., Pack, S., Schmidt, L., Vortmeyer, A.O., Pak, E., Pham, T., Weil, R.J., Candidus, S., Lubensky, I.A., Linehan, W.M., Zbar, B., and Weirich, G. (1998). Trisomy 7-harbouring non-random duplication of the mutant MET allele in hereditary papillary renal carcinomas. *Nature Genet.* 20, 66–9.

11. Hereditary renal cell carcinoma and the von Hippel–Lindau gene

Jodie K. Maranchie and W. Marston Linehan

Introduction

Renal cell carcinoma (RCC) represents 3 per cent of adult cancers and occurs most commonly in the sixth and seventh decades of life. It is responsible for over 12 000 deaths per year in America (Boring *et al.* 1994). For nearly two decades, investigators have attempted to unravel the mysteries of renal cell carcinoma (RCC) by examining families that carry a predisposition for kidney tumors. Families have been identified that carry a predilection for each of the common histologic subtypes of RCC. Large lineages have permitted identification of precise defects that lead to malignant transformation in both familial and sporadic kidney cancer. Through a better understanding of the genetics and biochemistry of renal malignancy we hope to develop new therapeutic strategies for RCC prevention, treatment, and cure.

Hereditary papillary renal cell carcinoma (HPRCC)

Ten per cent of sporadic renal cell cancers have a tubulo-papillar architecture (Fig. 11.1) and tend to be less vascular, lower-grade, and more indolent than the more common clear cell type. Several large families have been described who develop multiple and

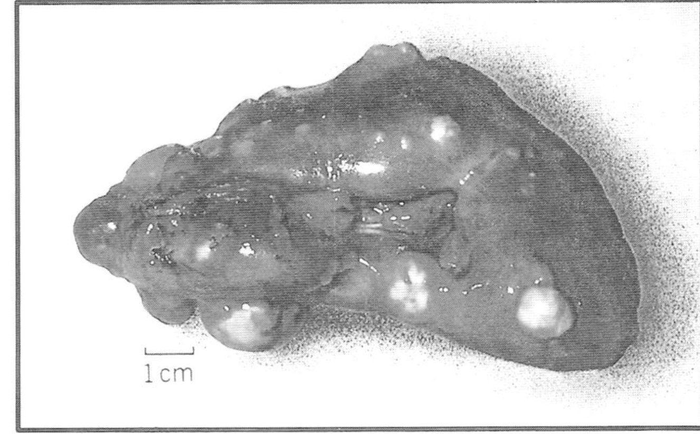

Fig. 11.2 Photograph of a kidney from a patient with hereditary papillary RCC demonstrating multifocal papillary tumors. (From Zbar *et al.* (1994).)

bilateral renal tumors of exclusively papillary histology (Figs. 11.2, 11.3) (Zbar *et al.* 1994). Because of frequent reports of trisomy of chromosome 7 in sporadic papillary RCC, this chromosome was subjected to genetic linkage analysis resulting in the identification

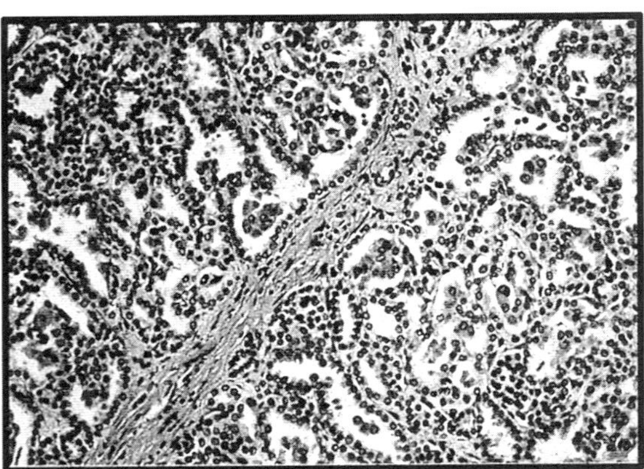

Fig. 11.1 High-power view of a renal tumor from a patient with hereditary papillary RCC demonstrating tubulopapillary architecture.

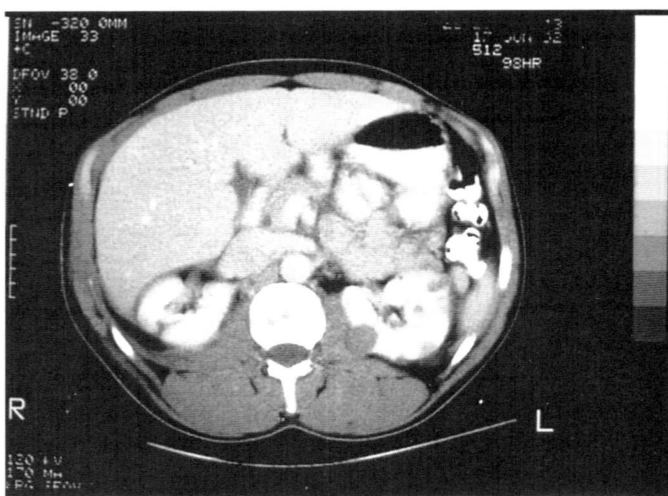

Fig. 11.3 CT scan from a patient with hereditary papillary RCC showing multiple bilateral solid tumors.

of missense mutations in the tyrosine kinase domain of the met proto-oncogene (MET). One of these mutations was homologous to a mutation commonly seen in the tyrosine kinase domain of RET, a proto-oncogene responsible for multiple endocrine neoplasia type 2B and sporadic medullary carcinoma of the thyroid gland (Schmidt *et al.* 1997). Other members of this oncogene superfamily include c-kit, mutated in patients with malignant hematologic disorders and C-erbB, an avian proto-oncogene.

MET is active in the development of muscle and liver during normal embryogenesis. It transduces motility, proliferation, and morphogenic signals of hepatocyte growth factor/scatter factor (HGF/SF) in epithelial cells. Increased expression of wild-type MET has been described in tumors derived from multiple tissues. Overexpression is believed to confer a growth and invasion advantage. Cell lines bearing MET mutants demonstrate higher levels of tyrosine phosphorylation than their wild-type counterparts and only the MET mutant cells were tumorigenic in nude mice (Fischen *et al.*1998).

Sequence and fluorescence *in situ* hybridization (FISH) data reveal nonrandom duplication of the mutated MET allele in tumor cells (Zhuang *et al.* 1998). Different tumors from the same patient contain clonally unique karyotypic errors in addition to trisomy 7, including trisomy of 17, 16, or 20 or deletion of chromosome Y. This suggests that mutations of MET render cells more susceptible to errors in chromosomal replication resulting in nonrandom chromosomal duplication. Duplication of the mutant MET allele serves as a 'second hit' for tumor formation by conferring a growth advantage (Fig. 11.4) (Zhuang).

Hereditary oncocytoma

A small number of families have a predisposition to develop multiple bilateral oncocytomas (Weirich *et al.* 1998). Sporadic oncocytic RCC and its more malignant counterpart, the chromophobe tumor, represent 3–5 per cent of renal neoplasms (Figs 11.5 and 11.6). They are believed to arise from the intercalated cells of the renal collecting duct (Kovacs *et al.* 1992); Storkel *et al.* 1988). These tumors demonstrated neither chromosome 7 nor 3p abnor-

malities and the genetic defects responsible have not yet been identified.

Interestingly, the majority of these families also carry the dermatologic diagnosis of Birt–Hogg–Dube syndrome (BHD). In these families, BHD and RCC segregate together in an autosomal dominant fashion. It is not clear if these tumors represent different manifestations of the same familial syndrome with differential penetrance of individual lesions (Toro *et al.* 1999). Of note, one family with BHD developed a non-MET papillary RCC variant rather than oncytoma (Toro *et al.* 1999). Further definition of this unique hereditary syndrome is in progress.

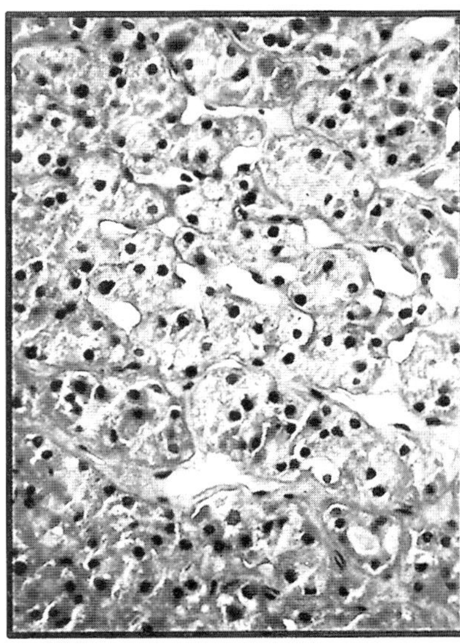

Fig. 11.5 High-power view of an oncocytoma from a patient with bilateral multifocal tumors.

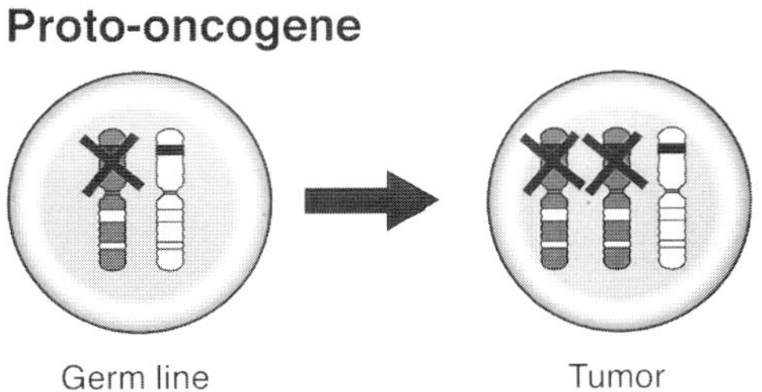

Fig. 11.4 Cartoon depicting tumor formation due to a proto-oncogene mutation and duplication. The proto-oncogene is mutated in the germ line. The mutated allele is nonrandomly duplicated in tumors providing a growth advantage.

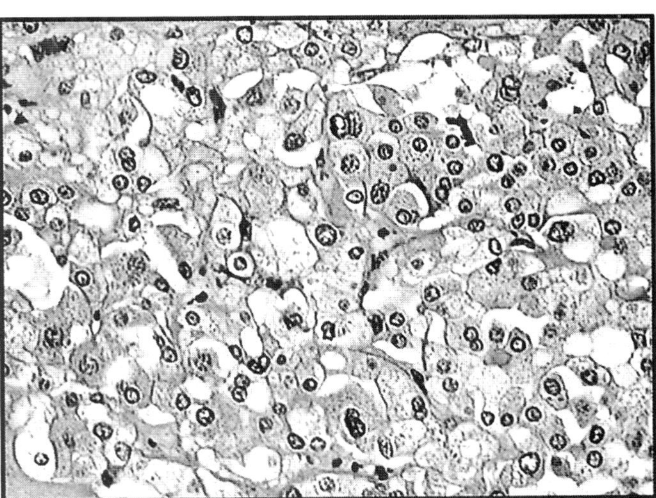

Fig. 11.6 Chromophobe RCC [high-power view.]

Hereditary clear cell renal cell carcinoma

Balanced translocations

Familial multifocal bilateral clear cell RCC (Fig. 11.7) is seen in some families with none of the classic nonrenal manifestations of the von Hippel–Lindau syndrome (Cohen *et al.* 1979, Kovacs *et al.* 1989). These families carry a balanced translocation between the short arm of chromosome 3 (3p) and another chromosome, commonly 6 or 8, meaning that, despite rearrangement, all genetic material is present in the germline. Tumors in these patients uniformly demonstrate loss of the derivative chromosome bearing

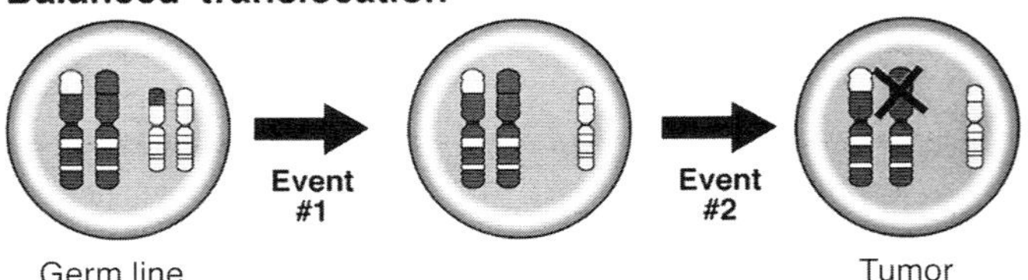

Fig. 11.8 Cartoon depicting tumor formation due to a germ line balanced translocation. In the germ line all DNA is present but rearranged. Tumors occur when the derivative chromosome is lost.

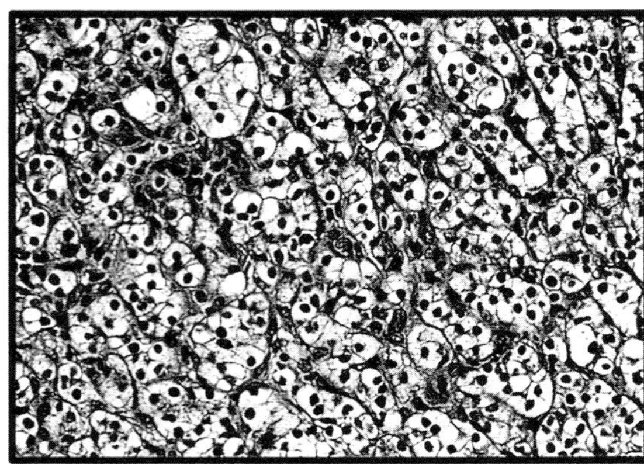

Fig. 11.7 High-power view of clear cell RCC.

the relocated 3p (Schmidt *et al.* 1995). The majority of tumors also reveal a mutation in the remaining allele of the von Hippel–Lindau gene. It is not clear why this syndrome is phenotypically different from von Hippel–Lindau syndrome (Fig. 11.8) (Li *et al.* 1993).

The von Hippel–Lindau syndrome

The best described condition that causes bilateral multifocal clear cell RCC is the von Hippel–Lindau syndrome (VHL). VHL occurs in 1 out of 36 000 live births in the USA and follows an autosomal dominant pattern of inheritance with nearly 100 per cent penetrance by the age of 65 years. Life expectancy for affected family members has been reported as 49 years with renal cancer the leading cause of death (Maher *et al.* 1991). Although VHL patients represent fewer than 2 per cent of RCC patients, they carry a 70 per cent probability of developing RCC by the age of 60 years. The full VHL phenotype includes benign and malignant tumors

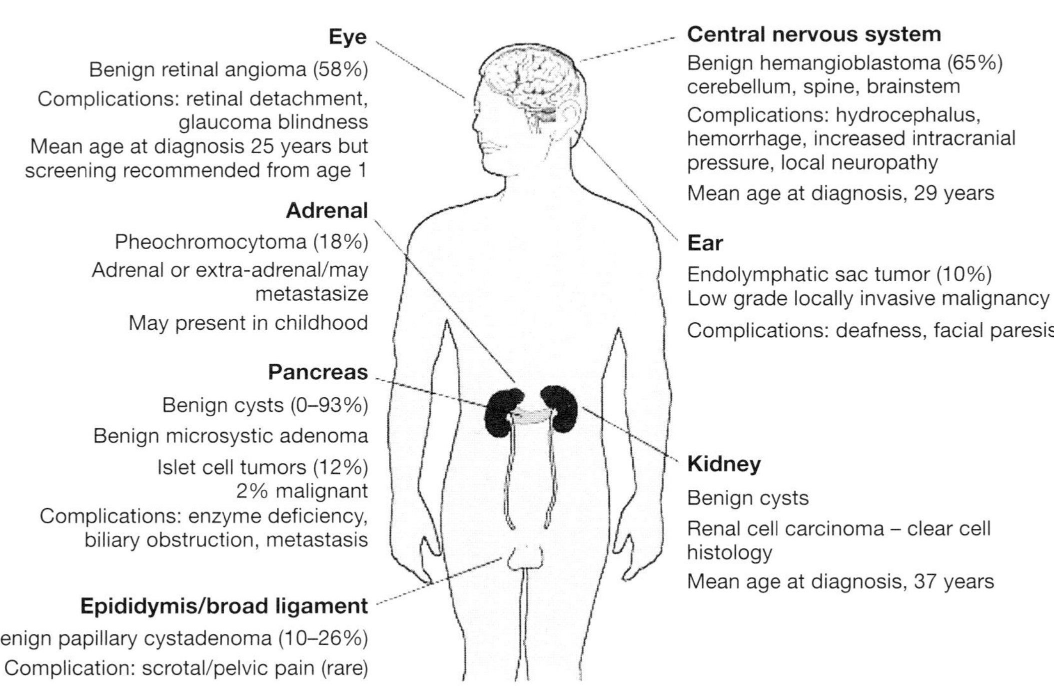

Fig. 11.9 von Hippel-Lindau syndrome manifestations.

of multiple organs. The urologist should maintain an awareness of the entire syndrome because the occasional patient will present with bilateral multifocal RCC as their first manifestation.

Nonrenal manifestations of VHL (Fig. 11.9)

Retinal angiomas are the earliest lesions to manifest. Ophthalmologic screening is recommended as early as 1 year of age for patients at risk (Choyke *et al.* 1995). Although benign, angiomas may cause glaucoma or retinal detachment and blindness. Vigilant screening and laser resection can help to maintain vision.

Endolymphatic sac tumors of the inner ear are seen in up to 10 per cent of VHL patients. These low-grade malignancies invade locally and can cause rapid irreversible hearing loss or facial paresis.

Hemangioblastomas are benign vascular proliferations that occur throughout the central nervous system. Although most common in the spine and cerebellum, they are seen in the brainstem and at the cranio-cervical angle. Rarely, they have been reported in the cerebral cortex or pituitary. Neurologic symptoms are due to mass effect, obstructive hydrocephalus, or hemorrhage. Lesions can be demonstrated by magnetic resonance imaging (MRI), and small asymptomatic tumors may be followed radiographically. It is not uncommon for affected patients to require multiple neurosurgical resections.

Diffuse **pancreative cysts** are present in up to 93 per cent of affected members of certain VHL lineages. Complete cystic replacement of functioning tissue may result in pancreatic insufficiency requiring enzyme replacement therapy. **Microcystic adenomas** are clusters of thick-walled cysts around a central calcified nidus. Symptoms occur when compression of the bile duct results in biliary obstruction. Pancreatic **islet cell tumors** are seen in 12 per cent of affected VHL patients independent of pancreatic cysts. These neural tumors can be locally invasive and 2 per cent metastasize (Zbar *et al.* 1999).

Pheochromocytomas can be either adrenal or extra-adrenal and may possess metastatic potential. Paroxysmal or sustained hypertension may cause fatal myocardial infarction or cerebral hemorrhage. Occult pheochromocytoma can be a life-threatening intraoperative complication and it is essential to rule out coexistent pheochromocytoma before contemplating renal surgery. Adrenal lesions are identified on abdominal computerized tomography (CT) or MRI (Choyke *et al.* 1990) and confirmed by catecholamine levels in the blood or urine. It is not uncommon for radiographic detection to precede the elevation of catecholamine levels by a number of years. I[131] metaiodobenzylguanidine scintigraphy (MIBG) is helpful for identifying suspected extra-adrenal pheochromocytomas. VHL syndrome has been subdivided clinically based on the propensity for developing pheochromocytoma. Type 1 VHL has a low rate of pheochromocytoma while type 2 carries a high risk. Type 2 families have been further subdivided into 2A with low risk of RCC, 2B with high risk of RCC, and 2C with no RCC (Table 11.1) (Maher and Kaelin 1997; Glenn *et al.* 1991).

Benign **papillary cystadenomas of the epididymis** are seen in 10–26 per cent of affected males, ranging in size from 2 to 5 cm. Analogous **broad ligament** papillary cystadenomas arise from mesonephric remnants near the lateral uterine wall (Choyke *et al.* 1997; Karsdorp *et al.* 1994).

Renal manifestations of VHL

VHL patients develop both cystic and solid renal lesions. RCC tends to be the latest VHL lesion with a mean age of diagnosis of 35 years. Simple cysts are frequently numerous bilaterally and should be followed closely for any sign of malignant transformation. Solid cancers can be multifocal and bilateral (Fig. 11.10). Examination of grossly normal renal parenchyma from 16 VHL patients revealed multiple microscopic foci of clear cell RCC and

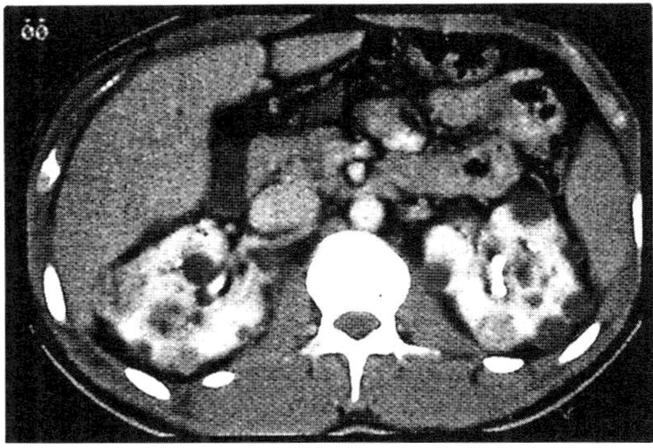

Fig. 11.10 CT scan from a patient with von Hippel-Lindau syndrome demonstrating multiple bilateral solid and cystic tumors.

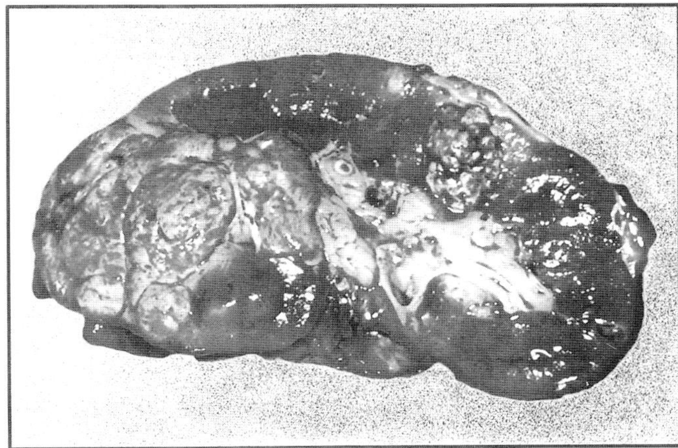

Fig. 11.11 Photograph of a kidney from a patient with von Hippel-Lindau syndrome.

Table 11.1 Phenotypic subclassification of von Hippel–Lindau syndrome

Type 1	Low risk of pheochromocytoma	
Type 2	High risk of pheochromocytoma	
	2A	Low risk of concurrent RCC
	2B	High risk of concurrent RCC
	2C	Pheochromocytoma only

cysts. By extrapolation, an estimated 600 independent solid neoplasms and 1100 cysts reside in the kidney of a 37-year-old VHL patient (Walther *et al.* 1995).

Because these patients carry a life-long risk of developing new RCC, treatment strategies aim to minimize the number of surgical procedures and preserve renal parenchyma. Multiple studies have demonstrated a low rate of metastasis from small tumors. The US National Cancer Institute documented no metastases in 54 patients followed with renal tumors smaller than 3 cm in diameter, resulting in the '3-cm rule' (Zbar *et al.* 1999). Tumors are followed radiographically, often for years, until they approach 3 cm in diameter. At that time, open exploration of the kidney is recommended with enucleation of all identifiable solid tumors (Fig. 11.11). Intraoperative ultrasound is indispensable for identification of small intraparenchymal tumors not appreciated on CT. Excision of all large tumors and cysts effectively 'resets the clock' for a given kidney, but regular CT screening should continue for life.

History

The ophthalmologist, Treacher Collins, first reported multiple retinal angiomata in two related patients in 1894. Ten years later Dr Ernst von Hippel (1904) described the rare familial ocular disease, angiomatosis retinae. Dr Arvid Lindau (1926) recognized the relationship between familiar retinal angiomata and central nervous system (CNS) lesions. The term von Hippel–Lindau syndrome was coined by Cushing and Bailey (1928) in their landmark paper that described the full familial syndrome.

In 1988, sporadic RCC was mapped to the short arm of chromosome 3(3p) (Seizinger *et al.* 1988). Examination of renal, pancreatic, and CNS tumors from VHL patients showed a consistent loss of DNA from the 3p inherited from the unaffected parent suggesting that this region contained a classic tumor suppressor gene as described by Knudsen (Fig. 11.12) (Tory *et al.* 1989).

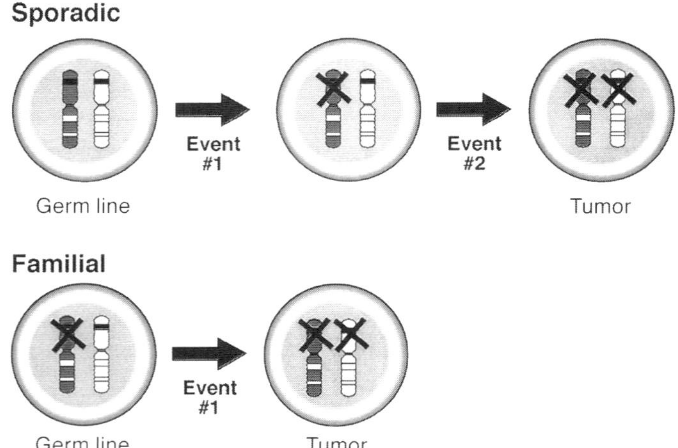

Fig. 11.12 Cartoon depicting tumor formation due to sequential loss of both alleles of a tumor suppressor gene. If the first mutation is present in the germ line only one event is required, leading to early presentation and higher frequency of tumor formation.

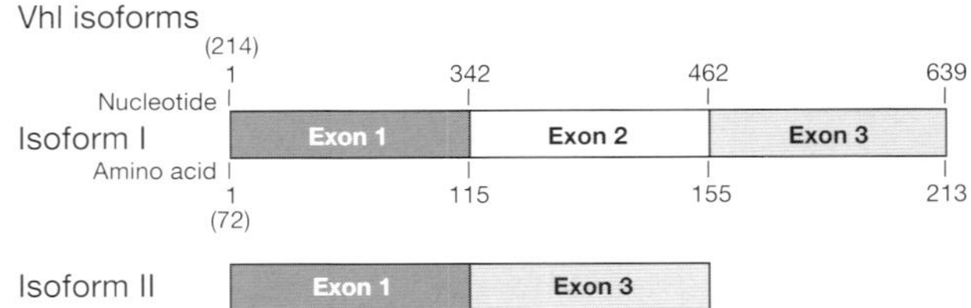

Fig. 11.13 Linkage analysis showing co-segregation of the A1 allele of a chromosome 3p marker with clinical expression of von Hippel-Lindau syndrome, indicating that this marker and the vhl gene are located near each other on chromosome 3p. Squares represent males and circles, females. Darkened members are affected. (From Hosoe *et al.* (1990).)

Genetic linkage analysis using germline 3p deletions detected by pulsed-field electrophoresis further localized the defect to 3p25–26 and ultimately resulted in the cloning of the von Hippel–Lindau gene (vhl) in 1993 (Fig. 11.13) (Hosoe *et al.* 1990; Latif *et al.* 1993).

The normal von Hippel–Lindau gene

The gene

The VHL gene (vhl) contains three exons and has a full mRNA transcript of 4.7 kilobases (kb). Alternative splicing results in a smaller transcript lacking the second exon but, because several naturally occurring germline mutations in VHL patients lead to the exclusive production of this isoform, it is not thought to produce a functional tumor supressor (Fig. 11.14). The full mRNA bears no homology to any known gene with the exception of five acidic repeats near the amino terminus that are reminiscent of a membrane-associated protein in *T. cruzi*. Although there is no hint of its action, vhl is highly conserved between mammals, *Drosophila*, and even sea urchin suggesting a crucial function in multicellular organisms (Latif *et al.* 1993). Only two intragenic polymorphisms have been described, 1149 A/G and 19 A/G (Chen *et al.* 1995*a*). The vhl promotor contains a binding site for the

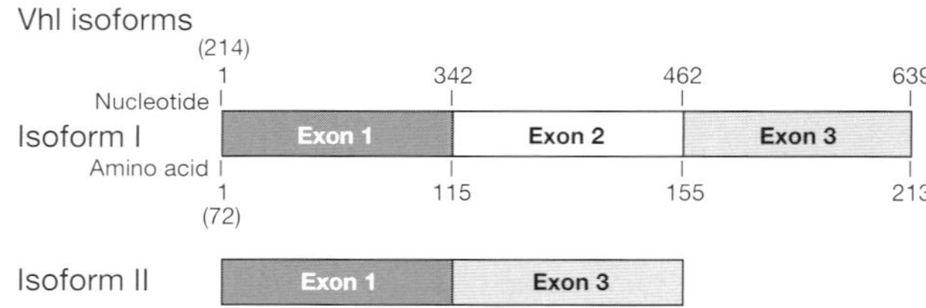

Fig. 11.14 Schematic map of the isoforms of the von Hippel-Lindau gene transcript indicating nucleotide number (above) and amino acid residue number (below). The second isoform results from alternative splicing of exons one and three. It was initially thought that a large section of the *N*-terminal gene was missing from the cloned vhl. However, subsequent identification of the actual transcription start site (Kuzmin *et al.* 1995) resulted in the removal of the first 71 amino acid residues (Kaelin *et al.* 1998). The original numbering system is provided in parentheses.

pax transcription activator, known to coordinate transcription of genes involved in organogenesis. This promotor lies within a CpG island that is subject to methylation (Fig. 11.14) (Kuzmin *et al.* 1995).

Localization

In situ hybridization of whole human embryo and fetal kidney sections demonstrates ubiquitous mesodermal expression of vhl mRNA, predominantly in the genital ridge and nephrogenic cord and not limited to the organs commonly affected by VHL. Expression is also high in the endodermal lining of the lung and vestibular apparatus of the inner ear while minimal expression is seen in the pancreas or lining of the gut. By 23 weeks of gestation, vhl is present throughout the kidney (Richards *et al.* 1996) in a pattern consistent with normal renal development (Maher and Kaelin 1997). Similar studies of murine embryogenesis revealed vhl mRNA levels to be most prominent in the lung, adrenal, and renal tubular epithelium (Kessler *et al.* 1995)/

vhl knock-out studies

Knock-out mice bearing only one wild-type vhl allele (analogous to the VHL syndrome patients) developed normally and did not demonstrate a predisposition to form tumors of any type (Gnarra *et al.* 1997). It is possible that the short mouse life span does not allow adequate time for tumors to form. Mice homozygous for the vhl deletion died *in utero* at 9.5–10.5 days of gestation. Histologic examination of the embryos revealed the absence of placental embryonal vasculogenesis resulting in placental hemorrhage and necrosis. A marked reduction in vascular endothelial growth factor (VEGF) expression in labyrinth trophoblasts correlated with the failure of vasculogenesis. VEGF knock-out mice have also been examined. Interestingly, both heterozygotes and homozygotes for the VEGF deletion, die at day of gestation 9.5–11.5 due to defects in both vasculogenesis and hematopoiesis (Gnarra *et al.* 1997).

Germline vhl mutations

Detection

Over the past 10 years, improvement in detection techniques have improved identification of vhl mutations to the current rate of 100 per cent. Sequencing of single-stranded restriction fragments will identify 50 per cent of vhl mutations. Southern blotting for individual exons, examination of flanking polymorphic markers, and intragenic vhl polymorphisms identify an additional 30 per cent. Finally, the addition of quantitative Southern analysis and FISH has permitted detection of complete vhl gene deletions (Stolle *et al.* 1998; Pack *et al.* 1999).

Germline mutations

Germline vhl mutations are widely distributed throughout the coding sequences with the notable exception of the region encoding the first 54 amino acids (Fig. 11.15) (Maher and Kaelin 1997). Approximately 20 per cent are deletions, 27 per cent are missense mutations altering only one amino acid residue, and 27 per cent result in a frameshift or internal stop codon. Several mutations occur repeatedly in unrelated families and are believed to represent mutational 'hotspots'. Consistent with this hypothesis, four of the most common mutations, C550T, C694T, C712T and G713A, occur at CpG dinucleotides known to be highly mutable because

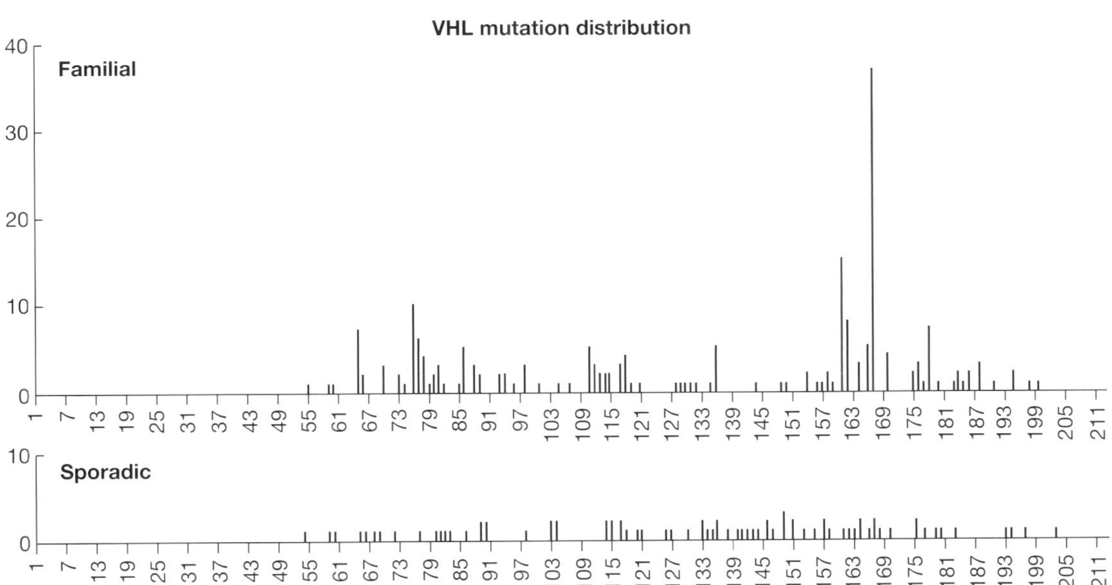

Fig. 11.15 Graphic depiction of the site of vhl mutation in 211 different von Hippel-Lindau syndrome families and in 80 sporadic clear cell carcinomas demonstrating broad distribution after residue 54. Note that residue 167 is the most common site of germ line mutation, represented in almost 40 separate lineages.

of inefficient repair of the deamination product of 5-methylcyto-sine (Richards *et al.* 1995). Haplotyping was used to rule out the possibility of common ancestry (founder effect) between unrelated families with identical mutations. Only one such founder effect was reported, the 'Black Forest' mutation. This missense mutation of nucleotide 505, known for its mild phenotype and low rate of RCC, is present in families in Germany and in descendants of the Pennsylvania Dutch (Branch *et al.* 1995).

De novo mutations

Several European groups examined the rate of formation of new germline mutations at the vhl locus. Rates ranged from 0.18×10^{-6} gametes/generation in Germany to 4.4×10^{-6} gametes/generation in England (Richards *et al.* 1995). Several well described genetic syndromes, including MEN2b and achondroplasia, are known to carry a paternal bias for new mutation. In these syndromes, the correlation between paternal age and *de novo* mutations is thought to occur because male gametes have gone through 15 times the number of divisions as female by the age of 30, with opportunity for DNA damage at each division. In 13 documented new mutations for whom the parent of origin for the mutated allele could be established, 7 were paternal and 6 maternal indicating no paternal bias for vhl mutation (Richards *et al.* 1995).

Differential phenotype

As mentioned above, there appear to be two distinct subclasses of von Hippel–Lindau syndrome: with or without a predominance of pheochromocytoma. Maher examined the germline mutations in these families and found that risk of pheochromocytoma was 59 per cent by age 50 in patients with missense mutations but only 9 per cent in those with vhl deletions or truncations. Missense mutations at nucleotide 712 or 713 (residue 167) resulted in the highest risk of pheochromocytoma with 82 per cent penetrance by age 50 (Maher *et al.* 1996; Chen *et al.* 1995*a*). It is thought that some residual function of the mutant vhl must be contributing to the development of pheochromocytoma. Ongoing studies to correlate phenotypic differences in tumor type or severity with the genotypic mutations may further elucidate the function of vhl.

The second hit

Examination of tumors of vhl patients reveals inactivation of the wild-type vhl allele in every tissue type, either by loss of heterozygosity (LOH), second mutation, or silencing of the vhl promotor by hypermethylation (Prowse *et al.* 1997). Loss of the wild-type copy of vhl was seen even in pre-malignant simple renal cysts (Kaelin and Maher 1998), indicating that this is a very early step in malignant transformation and suggesting that subsequent mutations are necessary for tumor formation. Requisite loss of the second allele is consistent with the classic model of tumor suppressor genes as described by Knudson's two-hit hypothesis (Fig. 11.12) (Knudson 1995). VHL patients are essentially born with the first hit, dramatically increasing the statistical chance of tumor development. Clinically, this translates to an earlier age of presentation, and an increased frequently of tumor formation.

Correlation with sporadic tumors

Examination of the sporadic forms of tumors frequently seen in VHL has been enlightening. In two independent studies of sporadic RCC, 50–65 per cent of clear cell tumors contained mutations at the vhl locus. No tumors of papillary or chromophobe histology had vhl mutations. Further 85 per cent of these tumors have loss of heterozygosity for the vhl allele (Gnarra *et al.* 1994; Foster *et al.* 1994*a, b*), and an additional 19 per cent had complete silencing of the wild-type allele by hypermethylation of the vhl promotor (Herman *et al.* 1994). Thus, nearly two-thirds of sporadic RCC of clear cell histology demonstrates loss of both copies of the vhl gene (Fig. 11.15).

Similarly, the majority of sporadic hemagioblastomas carried vhl mutations (Kanno *et al.* 1994). However, sporadic tumors from 20 other tissue including pheochromocytoma revealed no further vhl mutations (Foster *et al.* 1995; Gnarra *et al.* 1994).

Wild-type vhl suppresses tumor formation

Cell lines derived from renal carcinomas are known to form tumors when injected subcutaneously in nude mice. Reintroduction of a wild-type copy of the vhl gene into these cell lines before injection the prevents growth of tumors (Iliopoulos *et al.* 1995). Truncated vhl constructs or those bearing naturally occurring vhl mutations did not prevent tumor formation (Chen *et al.* 1995*b*). The presence of wild-type vhl had no noticeable effect on growth of the cells in culture suggesting that its function is dependent upon three-dimensional cell–cell interactions.

Biochemistry of vhl

The vhl protein (pvhl)

The full-length mRNA produces a 213 amino acid protein detected by polyacrylamide gel electrophoresis (PAGE) at approximately 30 kDa ($pvhl_{30}$) with no homology to any known protein. A second translation product of about 19 kDa ($pvhl_{19}$) corresponds to an internal start codon at residue 54. Both products are recovered from cells in culture in different ratios depending on the cell line and growth conditions. It is not clear what role the two translation products play endogenously. Interestingly, only one naturally occurring germline vhl mutation to date has involved the first 54 amino acids, suggesting that the tumor suppressor function is satisfied by the shorter product alone. Consistent with this, constructs created to exclusively express $pvhl_{19}$ are capable of preventing tumor growth in nude mice (Iliopoulos *et al.* 1998).

Localization

Immunohistochemical studies demonstrate diffuse pvhl expression in multiple tissue types including organs not known to be involved in the VHL syndrome. Expression is particularly abundant in the renal tubular system, exocrine pancreas, and in the epithelial linings of the bronchioli, intestines, and bile ducts. It is primarily cytoplasmic in every tissue except the adrenal gland where it consistently demonstrates a perinuclear pattern (Los *et al.* 1996). The greatest pvhl expression is in the proximal renal tubule (Corless *et al.* 1997).

phvl shutting

In cell culture, pvhl$_{30}$ localizes to the nucleus in sparsely plated cells. As cells reach confluence, the protein is transported ('shuttled') to the cytoplasm. pvhl constructs lacking the first exon demonstrate persistent cytosolic localization regardless of growth conditions and exon 3 deletions cause persistent nuclear localization (Lee *et al.* 1996). Cell trafficking is transcription-dependent and abolished by the transcription inhibitor actinomycin D. However, deletion of exon 2 eliminates this transcription dependence (Lee *et al.* 1999). pvhl$_{19}$ localizes equally to the nucleus and cytosol in all growth conditions and does not appear to shuttle (Iliopoulos *et al.* 1996).

The vhl cellular phenotype

Differential gene expression

Some important clues to the function of vhl are derived from comparison of the relative phenotype of matched cell lines with (pvhl$^+$) and without (pvhl$^-$) normal functioning vhl protein. Vascular endothelial growth factor (VEGF), glucose transporter 1 (Glut1), and platelet-derived growth factor-beta (PDGFβ) are all upregulated in pvhl$^-$ cells. Normally, these proteins are maintained at low intracellular levels but expression increase rapidly on exposure to hypoxia. pvhl$^-$ cell lines demonstrate hypoxic levels of these transcripts under both normoxic and hypoxic conditions (Iliopoulos *et al.* 1996; Siemeister *et al.* 1996). Up-regulation of TGFα, carbonic anhydrases 12 and 9, NOTCH2, tyrosine hydroxylase, and DECI have all been described for pvhl$^-$ cells (Ivanor *et al.* 1998); Kroll *et al.* 1999). The mechanism by which wild-type pvhl maintains low levels of gene expression is unclear. Evidence exists to support models of decreased gene transcription, posttranscriptional destabilization of mRNA products, or a combination of the two (Gnarra *et al.* 1996; Mukhopadhyay *et al.* 1997; Maxwell *et al.* 1999).

Cell cycle exit

pvhl is required for exit from the cell cycle on exposure to serum deprivation. pvhl$^-$ cells continue to divide despite the lack of nutrients. Ultimately, resources are exhausted and the cells undergo apoptotic death. pvhl$^+$ cells exit the cell cycle and become quiescent. No further cell division occurs until environmental conditions to improve. This protective ability to 'hibernate' correlates with changes in the levels of p27/kip1 (Pause *et al.* 1998).

Fibronectin matrix assembly

Fibronectin is an extracellular glycoprotein that binds cell surface integrins to form an intricate three-dimensional matrix between neighboring cells. Loss of this matrix is a common sign of malig-

nant transformation. pvhl$^-$ cells exhibit grossly defective matrix assembly, which is corrected by reintroduction of wild-type pvhl. The normal vhl protein interacts with intracellular fibronectin at the endoplasmic reticulum where fibronectin is folded and processed prior to secretion. A proposed model suggests that pvhl serves to eliminate malfolded fibronectin that would otherwise disrupt matrix assembly (Ohh *et al.* 1998).

Branching morphogenesis

Three-dimensional branching assays have been developed to assess the 'invasive' potential of tumor cell lines. The MET oncogene product is responsible for branching morphogenesis and motility in response to stimulation by the hepatocyte growth factor (HGF). pvhl$^-$ cells branch and migrate in response to HGF, while pvhl$^+$ cells do not. The differential branching correlates with levels of tissue inhibitor of metalloproteinase 2 (TIMP-2) (Koochekpour *et al.* 1999).

VHL-associated proteins

Elongins B and C

Several proteins consistently co-immunoprecipitate (Fig. 11.16) from detergent extracts with pvhl suggesting a noncovalent interaction (Table 11.2). The first two of these blinding partners to be identified were elongin B and elongin C (BC). *In vitro* translation studies did not demonstrate any interaction between pvhl and elongin B alone but detected some binding to elongin C. When the two elongins were translated together, the binding of both was enhanced (Kibel *et al.* 1995; Duan *et al.* 1995a). These proteins are already well described as regulatory subunits of the SIII heterotrimeric elongin binding complex, which is known to increase the transcription rate of certain genes by suppressing transient pauses of polymerase II. The active submit of SIII,

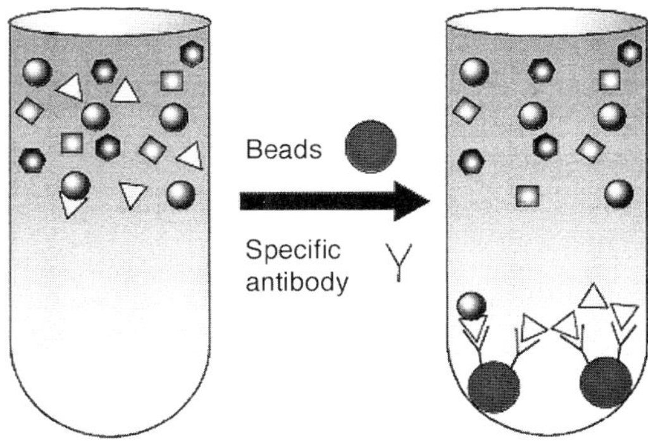

Fig. 11.16 Co-immunoprecipitation assay. Suspended cell lysates contain all of the proteins present within the cell. Antibody specific to the protein of interest (triangle) is added along with large beads that nonspecifically bind antibody. The large beads fall to the bottom of the suspension by gravity or centrifugation, and unbound proteins can then be washed away. Any proteins normally bound to the desired protein (small sphere) will co-immunoprecipitate.

Table 11.2 Binding partners of the von Hippel–Lindau protein

	Reference
Elongin C	Duan *et al.* 1995*b*; Kibel *et al.* 1995
Elongin B	Duan *et al.* 1995*b*; Kibel *et al.* 1995
Cul-2	Pause *et al.* 1997
Rbx1/ROC	Kamura *et al.* 1999
NEDD8	Liakopoulos *et al.* 1999
Hif 1-alpha	Maxwell *et al.* 1999
Hif 2-alpha	Maxwell *et al.* 1999
VBP 1	Tsuchiya *et al.* 1996
Sp1	Mukhopadhyay *et al.* 1997
Protein kinase C (isoforms delta and zeta)	Pal *et al.* 1997
Fibronectin	Ohh *et al.* 1998

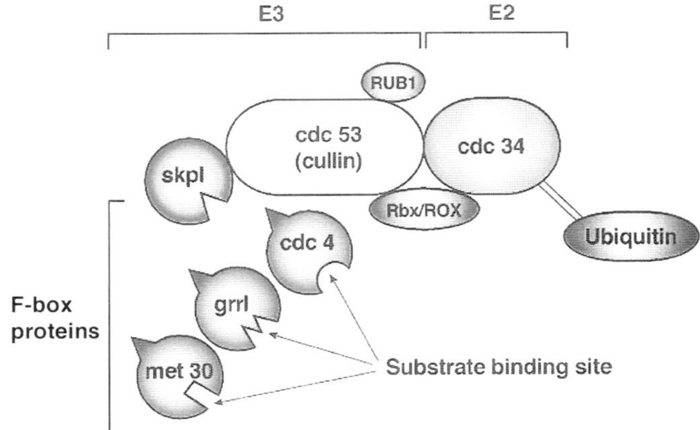

Fig. 11.17 Cartoon depicting the SCF (skpl/cdc53/f-box) E3 complex in yeast. Cdc53 binds the ubiquitin conjugating protein cdc 34. The f-box protein is an adapter subunit that confers substrate specificity. Various f-box proteins are used at different points in the cell cycle to target the appropriate substrate for degradation. Skp1 links cdc53 to the fbox protein and is essential for E3 function.

elongin A, does not interact with pvhl but competes for binding of BC *in vitro*. This caused by early speculation that pvhl might downregulate transcription by sequestration of BC. However, this is now felt to be unlikely given that BC is 100–1000-fold more abundant than elongin A or pvhl *in vivo* (Shilatifard 1998). The minimal pvhl peptide required for BC binding *in vitro* corresponds to residues 157–171. This is also the only region that pvhl shares in common with elongin A (Kibel *et al.* 1995). Despite this, more than 70 per cent of all naturally occurring vhl mutations have been shown to disrupt binding of BC (Conaway *et al.* 1998) including many that map outside of this short binding domain. Presumably, the tertiary structure of pvhl contributes to BC binding.

In addition to pvhl and elongin A, BC also binds proteins bearing the SOCS-box motif. Initially named for the SOCS (suppressors of cytokine signaling) family of proteins, this 50 amino acid domain has been identified in a large number of additional proteins. Embedded within the SOCS-box is the BC binding motif found in both elongin A and pvhl. Degradation of the SOCS-1 protein was inhibited by BC binding. Thus, it appears that BC may serve as a regulatory complex capable of controlling multiple intracellular pathways (Kamura *et al.* 1998).

Cul-2

Protein binding studies using the entire pvhl–BC complex (VBC) demonstrate an interaction with Cul-2, a member of the cullin family. Cul-2 does not co-precipitate with pvhl in the absence of BC and does not complex with BC alone. Thus, binding of Cul-2 is dependent upon the integrity of the entire VBC complex. Elongin C serves as a bridge between Cul-2 and pvhl. The yeast Cul-2 homolog, cdc53, is a component of a ubiquitin protein ligase complex (SCF) that targets cell cycle proteins for degradation by the ubiquitin proteolytic pathway. This provided the first major hint of a potential function for pvhl (Pause *et al.* 1997).

SCF and the E3 hypothesis

Rapid unidirectional control is essential for many cellular functions, particularly the cell cycle. Progression through DNA replication and cell division requires efficient elimination of sequential

phase specific proteins. Targeting of proteins for degradation is achieved by the ubiquitination cascade. First, a ubiquitin-activating enzyme (E1) consumes adenosine triphosphate (ATP) to create a ubiquitin thiol ester. This activated ubiquitin is then transferred to a conjugating enzyme (E2) capable of cross-linking the ubiquitin to a lysine residue on the target protein. Repeated conjugation forms a polyubiquitin chain recognized by the 26S proteosome as a signal for destruction. Target specificity is conferred by an E3 specificity factor that bears a binding site for both the E2 and the substrate (Scheffner *et al.* 1995); Hershko *et al.* 1983).

Although E3 is frequently a single protein, several multiunit E3 complexes have been described. SCF is a prototypic E3 complex in yeast comprised of three core subunits, skp1, cdc53, and an f-box protein. Cdc53, a member of the cullin family, binds an E2 while the f-box protein specifically recognizes the target. Skp1 serves as a bridge between the two. F-box proteins are interchangeable adapter subunits that allow the SCF to bind a variety of substrates depending on the needs of the cell (Fig. 11.17) (Patton *et al.*

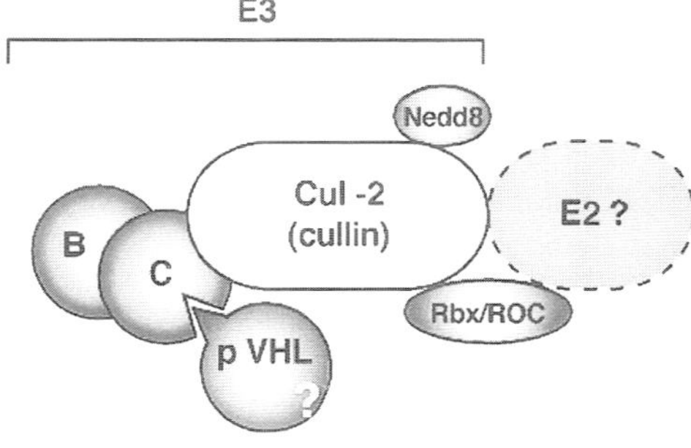

Fig. 11.18 The proposed VBCC E3 complex. Cul-2 is a cdc53 homolog, presumably able to bind an as yet unidentified E2 ubiquitin-conjugating enzyme. Elongin C is skp1-like and serves as a bridge between pvhl and cul-2. By analogy, pvhl may be a substrate-specific adaptor subunit in this complex to target an unknown substrate for ubiquitin-mediated degradation.

1998). Two minor SCF subunits have recently been described. Rbx1/ROC binds cdc53 and is essential for E2 recruitment (Kamura *et al.* 1999) and Rubl is a regulatory subunit that modifies E3 activity (Liakopoulos *et al.* 1999).

Striking similarities between human VBC–Cul-2 (VBCC) and the SCF complex have prompted speculation that pvhl may be involved in the process of ubiquitination (Fig. 11.18). Cul-2 shares significant identity with cdc53, and elongin C is a skpl homolog (Kaelin *et al.* 1998). Further, human homologs of the yeast Rbx1 and Rub1 (Rbx1 and NEDD8) have both been shown to bind VBCC (Liakopoulos *et al.* 1999; Kamura *et al.* 1999). If VBCC is indeed an SCF-like E3, is pvhl the substrate specific subunit? If so, what substrates does it recognize?

Recently, several investigators demonstrated that VBCC does function as an E3 in *in vitro* assays only when E1, E2, ATP, and ubiquitin are provided (Iwai *et al.* 1999; Lisztwan *et al* 1999). Efforts are underway to identify the ubiquitinated substrates.

Three-dimensional modeling

The crystal structure of VBC using pvhl$_{19}$ was determined in 1999 (Fig. 11.19). It suggests two potential binding domains in the tertiary structure of pvhl, alpha, and beta. The alpha domain (residues 155–189) is in contact with BC. The beta domain comprised of exon 1 is exposed to solvent and believed to represent a possible substrate binding site. Interestingly, the majority of germline vhl mutations are now known either to be in the BC binding site or to affect the binding of BC. However, many missense mutations map to the beta domain and may function by preventing substrate binding. Of the six major mutational hotspots, three are in each domain. Finally, although there is no sequence homology, the pattern of hydrophobic residues in the

Table 11.3 Hypoxia-inducible genes regulated by Hif-alpha transcription activation

	References
Vascular endothelial growth factor (VEGF)	—
Erythropoietin (Epo)	Bunn *et al.* 1998
Glucose transporter 1 (Glut-1)	Ouiddir *et al.* 1999
Platelet-derived growth factor (PDGF)	—
Transferrin receptor (TfR)	Bianchi *et al.* 1999
Adrenomedullin	Nguyen and Claycomb 1999
Endothelin	Hu *et al.* 1998
Phosphoglycerate kinase 1 (PGK 1)	—
Pyruvate kinase M2 (PKM2)	Kress *et al.* 1998
Phosphoglycerate mutase B	Takahashi *et al.* 1998
Atrial natriuretic peptide (ANP)	Chen *et al.* 1997
Nitric oxide (NO)	Palmer and Johns 1998

alpha domain resembles that of both the SOCS-box and the F-box (Stebbins *et al.* 1999).

Hypoxia-inducible factors

pvhl also associates with the hypoxia-inducible factors Hif 1-alpha and Hif 2-alpha (Hif-α) (Maxwell *et al.* 1999). Hypoxic conditions result in increased expression of a number of genes including erythropoietin, VEGF, PDGF, and Glut1 (Table 11.3). Each of these genes contains a specific DNA sequence termed the hypoxia regulation element (HRE) that is recognized by the Hif-α/ARNT dimer transcription factor. Binding of the dimer results in increased transcripton. Hif-α is the hypoxia-sensitive subunit (Iyer *et al.* 1998). Normally, Hif-α protein levels are negligible due to rapid ubiquitin-mediated degradation (Salceda and Caro 1997; Kallio *et al.* 1999). Under hypoxic conditions, the protein is stabilized and leads to increased transcription within hours. In pvhl$^-$ cells, Hif-α is stable even in normoxic conditions. Restoration of wild-type pvhl restores oxygen-dependent instability (Maxwell *et al.* 1999). It is tempting to speculate that Hif-α might be a VBCC substrate. The exact nature of the Hif-α interaction is under investigation.

Fibronectin

As mentioned above, fibronectin is another binding partner identified by immunoprecipitation. Interestingly, all known vhl mutations interrupt fibronectin binding, including those that do no affect the BC binding site. The interaction occurs exclusively in the membrane subfraction of the cells (Ohh *et al.* 1998). Pvhl$_{19}$ does not bind fibronectin (Iliopoulos *et al.* 1998), suggesting that the first 54 residues are essential to this particular function. Recall that these *N*-terminal residues of pvhl resemble a *T. cruzi* membrane protein. Perhaps this region is required for pvhl monitoring of endoplasmic reticular processing of fibronectin.

Sp 1

Sp 1 is another transcription factor known to upregulate VEGF expression that interacts with pvhl. In pvhl$^-$ cells, increased transcription is measured from the VEGF promotor. Reintroduction

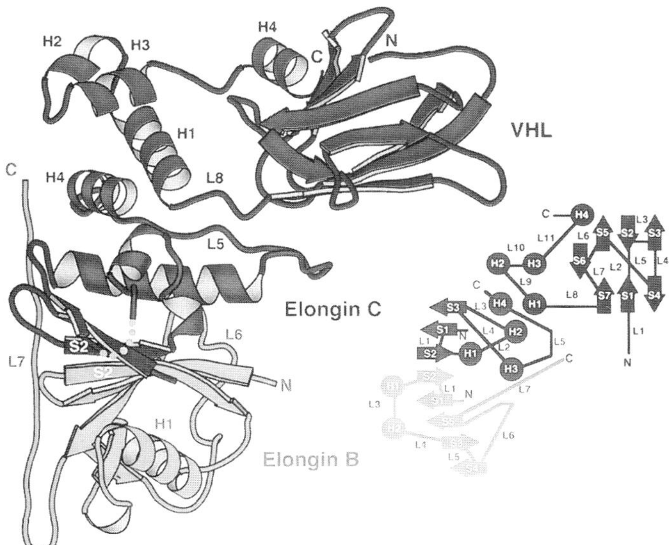

Fig. 11.19 Crystal structure of VBC. On the left is a ribbon diagram illustrating the secondary structure of the VCB complex. On the right is a topology diagram in which circles indicate helices and wide arrows indicate strands. C, COOH-terminus; N, NH2-terminus. (Taken with permission from Stebbins *et al.* (1999).)

of wild-type pvhl decreases this transcription by 90 per cent. Interestingly, introduction of a truncated protein consisting of the first 116 amino acid residues of pvhl actually upregulated VEGF transcription twofold (Mukhopadhyay *et al.* 1997).

Protein kinase C

pvhl also forms complexes with protein kinase C isoforms delta and zeta. Phosphorylation of sp1 is essential for its activity as a transcription activator for VEGF. Binding by pvhl prevents phosphorylation of sp1 and other targets resulting in further downregulation of VEGF expression (Pal *et al.* 1997).

VBP-1 is another protein that interacts with pvhl. No function has yet been determined for this association (Tsuchiya *et al.* 1996).

Summary

Von Hippel–Lindau tumor suppressor gene function is lost in the majority of sporadic clear cell RCC and pre-malignant cysts. Cells from these highly vascular tumors demonstrate increased expression of VEGF and other proteins normally present during development and under hypoxic conditions. At least four independent pathways have been identified for direct downregulation of VEGF expression by pvhl. Interestingly, proliferations of vessels resembling hemangioblastomas can be induced in mouse brains by simple overexpression of VEGF (Benjamin and Keshet 1997). Ongoing efforts to further elucidate the function of pvhl may highlight specific strategies for tumor prevention and treatment in both familial and sporadic clear cell renal cell carcinoma.

Conclusion

Familial syndromes exist for each of the histologic subtypes of RCC. Comparison of DNA from affected and unaffected individuals from large families has facilitated the identification of precise genetic defects responsible for malignant transformation.

References

Benjamin, L.E. and Keshet, E. (1997). Conditional switching of vascular endothelial growth factor (VEGF) expression in tumors: induction of endothelial cell shedding and regression of hemangioblastoma-like vessels by VEGF withdrawal. *Proc. Natl Acad. Sci., USA* **94**, 8761–6.

Bianchi, L., Tacchini, L., and Cairo, G. (1999). HIF-1-mediated activation of transferrin receptor gene transcription by iron chelation [in process citation]. *Nucl. Acids Res.* **27**, 4223–7.

Boring, C.C., Squires, T.S., Tong, T., and Montgomery, S. (1994). Cancer statistics, 1994. *CA Cancer J. Clin.* **44**, 7–26.

Brauch, H. *et al.* (1995). Von Hippel–Lindau (VHL) disease with pheochromocytoma in the Black Forest region of Germany: evidence for a founder effect. *Hum. Genet.* **95**, 551–6.

Bunn, H.F., Gu, J., Huang, L.E., Park, J.W., and Zhu, H. (1998). Erythropoietin: a model system for studying oxygen-dependent gene regulation. *J. Exp. Biol.* **201**, 1197–201.

Chen, F. *et al.* (1995*a*). Germline mutations in the von Hippel–Lindau disease tumor suppressor gene: correlations with phenotype. *Hum. Mutat.* **5**, 66–75.

Chen, F. *et al.* (1995*b*). Suppression of growth of renal carcinoma cells by the von Hippel–Lindau tumor suppressor gene. *Cancer Res.* **55**, 4804–7.

Chen, Y.F., Durand, J., and Claycomb, W.C. (1997). Hypoxia stimulates atrial natriuretic peptide gene expression in cultured atrial cardiocytes. *Hypertension* **29**, 75–82.

Choyke, P.L. *et al.* (1990). von Hippel–Lindau disease: radiologic screening for visceral manifestations. *Radiology* **174**, 815–20.

Choyke, P.L. *et al.* (1995). von Hippel–Lindau disease: genetic, clinical, and imaging features [published erratum appears in *Radiology* (1995) **196** (2), 582]. *Radiology* **194**, 629–42.

Choyke, P.L. *et al.* (1997). Epididymal cystadenomas in von Hippel–Lindau disease. *Urology* **49**, 926–31.

Cohen, A.J. *et al.* (1979). Hereditary renal-cell carcinoma associated with a chromosomal translocation. *New Engl. J. Med.* **301**, 592–5.

Collins, E. (1894). Two cases, brother and sister, with peculiar vascular new growth, probably primarily retinal, affecting both eyes. *Trans. Ophthalmol. Soc., UK* **14**, 141–9.

Conaway, J.W., Kamura, T., and Conaway, R.C. (1998). The Elongin BC complex and the von Hippel–Lindau tumor suppressor protein. *Biochim. Biophys. Acta* **1377**, M49–54.

Corless, C.L., Kibel, A.S., Iliopoulos, O., and Kaelin, W.G., Jr (1997). Immunostaining of the von Hippel–Lindau gene product in normal and neoplastic human tissues. *Hum. Pathol.* **28**, 459–64.

Cushing, H. and Bailey, P. (1928). Hemangiomas of cerebellum and retina (Lindau's disease), with a report of a case. *Arch. Ophthalmol.* **57**, 447–63.

Duan, D.R. *et al.* (1995*a*). Characterization of the VHL tumor suppressor gene product: localization, complex formation, and the effect of natural inactivating mutations. *Proc. Natl Acad. Sci., USA* **92**, 6459–63.

Duan, D.R. *et al.* (1995*b*). Inhibition of transcription elongation by the VHL tumor suppressor protein [see comments]. *Science* **269**, 1402–6.

Fischer, J. *et al.* (1998). Duplication and overexpression of the mutant allele of the MET proto-oncogene in multiple hereditary papillary renal cell tumours. *Oncogene* **17**, 733–9.

Foster, K. *et al.* (1994*a*). Somatic mutations of the von Hippel–Lindau disease tumour suppressor gene in non-familial clear cell renal carcinoma. *Hum. Mol. Genet.* **3**, 2169–73.

Foster, K. *et al.* (1994*b*). Molecular genetic investigation of sporadic renal cell carcinoma: analysis of allele loss on chromosomes 3p, 5q, 11p, 17 and 22. *Br. J. Cancer* **69**, 230–4.

Foster, K. *et al.* (1995). Molecular genetic analysis of the von Hippel–Lindau disease (VHL) tumor suppressor gene in gonadal tumors. *Eur. J. Cancer* **31A**, 2392–5.

Glenn, G.M. *et al.* (1991). Von Hippel–Lindau (VHL) disease: distinct phenotypes suggest more than one mutant allele at the VHL locus. *Hum. Genet.* **87**, 207–10.

Gnarra, J.R. *et al.* (1994). Mutations of the VHL tumour suppressor gene in renal carcinoma. *Nat. Genet.* **7**, 85–90.

Gnarra, J.R. *et al.* (1996). Post-transcriptional regulation of vascular endothelial growth factor mRNA by the product of the VHL tumor suppressor gene. *Proc. Natl Acad. Sci., USA* **93**, 10589–94.

Gnarra, J.R. *et al.* (1997). Defective placental vasculogenesis causes embryonic lethality in VHL-deficient mice. *Proc. Natl Acad. Sci., USA* **94**, 9102–7.

Herman, J.G. *et al.* (1994). Silencing of the VHL tumor-suppressor gene by DNA methylation in renal carcinoma. *Proc. Natl Acad. Sci., USA* **91**, 9700–4.

Hershko, A., Heller, H., Elias, S., and Ciechanover, A. (1983). Components of ubiquitin–protein ligase system. Resolution, affinity purification, and role in protein breakdown. *J. Biol. Chem.* **258**, 8206–14.

Hosoe, S. *et al.* (1990). Localization of the von Hippel–Lindau disease gene to a small region of chromosome 3. *Genomics* **8**, 634–40.

Hu, J., Discher, D.J., Bishopric, N.H., and Webster, K.A. (1998). Hypoxia regulates expression of the endothelin-1 gene through a proximal hypoxia-inducible factor-1 binding site on the antisense strand. *Biochem. Biophys. Res. Comun.* **245**, 894–9.

Iliopoulos, O., Kibel, A., Gray, S., and Kaelin, W.G., Jr (1995). Tumor suppression by the human von Hippel–Lindau gene product. *Nat. Med.* **1**, 822–6.

Iliopoulos, O., Levy, A.P., Jiang, C., Kaelin, W.G., Jr, and Goldberg, M.A. (1996). Negative regulation of hypoxia-inducible genes by the von Hippel–Lindau protein. *Proc. Natl Acad. Sci., USA* **93**, 10595–9.

Iliopoulos, O., Ohh, M., and Kaelin, W.G., Jr (1998). pVhl19 is a biologically active product of the von Hippel–Lindau gene arising from internal translation initiation. *Proc. Natl Acad. Sci., USA* **95**, 11661–6.

Ivanov, S.V. *et al.* (1998). Down-regulation of transmembrane carbonic anhydrases in renal cell carcinoma cell lines by wild-type von Hippel–Lindau transgenes. *Proc. Natl Acad. Sci., USA* **95**, 12596–601.

Iwai, K. *et al.* (1999). Identification of the von Hippel–Lindau tumor-suppressor protein as part of an active E3 ubiquitin ligase complex [in process citation]. *Proc. Natl Acad. Sci., USA* **96**, 12436–41.

Iyer, N.V. *et al.* (1998). Cellular and developmental control of O2 homeostasis by hypoxia-inducible factor 1 alpha. *Genes Dev.* **12**, 149–62.

Kaelin, W.G., Jr and Maher, E.R. (1998). The VHL tumor-suppressor gene paradigm. *Trends Genet.* **14**, 423–6.

Kaelin, W.G., Iliopoulos, O., Lonergan, K.M., and Ohh, M. (1998). Functions of the von Hippel–Lindau tumour suppressor protein. *J. Intern. Med.* **243**, 535–9.

Kallio, P.J., Wilson, W.J., S, O.B., Makino, Y., and Poellinger, L. (1999). Regulation of the hypoxia-inducible transcription factor 1 alpha by the ubiquitin–proteasome pathway. *J. Biol. Chem.* **274**, 6519–25.

Kamura, T. *et al.* (1998). The Elongin BC complex interacts with the conserved SOCS-box motif present in members of the SOCS, ras, WD-40 repeat, and ankyrin repeat families. *Genes Dev.* **12**, 3872–81.

Kamura, T. *et al.* (1999). Rbx1, a component of the VHL tumor suppressor complex and SCF ubiquitin ligase [see comments]. *Science* **284**, 657–61.

Kanno, H. *et al.* (1994). Somatic mutations of the von Hippel–Lindau tumor suppressor gene in sporadic central nervous system hemangioblastomas. *Cancer Res.* **54**, 4845–7.

Karsdorp, N. *et al.* (1994). Von Hippel–Lindau disease: new strategies in early detection and treatment. *Am. J. Med.* **97**, 158–68.

Kessler, P.M. *et al.* (1995). Expression of the von Hippel–Lindau tumor suppressor gene, VHL, in human fetal kidney and during mouse embryogenesis. *Mol. Med.* **1**, 457–66.

Kibel, A., Iliopoulos, O., DeCaprio, J.A., and Kaelin, W.G., Jr (1995). Binding of the von Hippel–Lindau tumor suppressor protein to Elongin B and C [see comments]. *Science* **269**, 1444–6.

Knudson, A.G. (1995). VHL gene mutation and clear-cell renal carcinomas. *Cancer J. Sci. Am.* **1**, 180.

Koochekpour, S. *et al.* (1999). The von Hippel–Lindau tumor suppressor gene inhibits hepatocyte growth factor/scatter factor-induced invasion and branching morphogenesis in renal carcinoma cells. *Mol. Cell Biol.* **19**, 5902–12.

Kovacs, A., Storkel, S., Thoenes, W., and Kovacs, G. (1992). Mitochondrial and chromosomal DNA alterations in human chromophobe renal cell carcinomas. *J. Pathol.* **167**, 273–7.

Kovacs, G., Brusa, P., and De Riese, W. (1989). Tissue-specific expression of a constitutional 3;6 translocation: development of multiple bilateral renal-cell carcinomas. *Int. J. Cancer* **43**, 422–7.

Kress, S. *et al.* (1998). Expression of hypoxia-inducible genes in tumor cells. *J. Cancer Res. Clin. Oncol.* **124**, 315–20.

Kroll, S.L. *et al.* (1999). von Hippel–Lindau protein induces hypoxia-regulated arrest of tyrosine hydroxylase transcript elongation in pheochromocytoma cells. *J. Biol. Chem.* **274**, 30109–14.

Kuzmin, I. *et al.* (1995). Identification of the promoter of the human von Hippel–Lindau disease tumor suppressor gene. *Oncogene* **10**, 2185–94.

Latif, F. *et al.* (1993). Identification of the von Hippel–Lindau disease tumor suppressor gene [see comments]. *Science* **260**, 1317–20.

Lee, S. *et al.* (1996). Nuclear/cytoplasmic localization of the von Hippel–Lindau tumor suppressor gene product is determined by cell density. *Proc. Natl Acad. Sci., USA* **93**, 1770–5.

Lee, S. *et al.* (1999). Transcription-dependent nuclear-cytoplasmic trafficking is required for the function of the von Hippel–Lindau tumor suppressor protein. *Mol. Cell. Biol.* **19**, 1486–97.

Li, F.P. *et al.* (1993). Clinical and genetic studies of renal cell carcinomas in a family with a constitutional chromosome 3;8 translocation. Genetics of familial renal carcinoma. *Ann. Intern. Med.* **118**, 106–11.

Liakopoulos, D., Busgen, T., Brychzy, A., Jentsch, S., and Pause, A. (1999). Conjugation of the ubiquitin-like protein NEDD8 to cullin-2 is linked to von Hippel–Lindau tumor suppressor function. *Proc. Natl Acad. Sci., USA* **96**, 5510–15.

Lindau, A. (1926). Studien über kleinhirncysten Bau: Pathogenese und Beziehungen zur angiomatous Retinae. *Acta Pathol. Microbiol. Scand.* **Suppl. 1**, 1–128.

Lisztwan, J., Imbert, G., Wirbelauer, C., Gstaiger, M., and Krek, W. (1999). The von Hippel–Lindau tumor suppressor protein is a component of an E3 ubiquitin–protein ligase activity. *Genes Dev.* **13**, 1822–33.

Los, M. *et al.* (1996). Expression pattern of the von Hippel–Lindau protein in human tissues. *Lab. Invest.* **75**, 231–8.

Maher, E.R. and Kaelin, W.G., Jr (1997). von Hippel–Lindau disease. *Medicine* (*Baltimore*) **76**, 381–91.

Maher, E.R. *et al.* (1991). Von Hippel–Lindau disease: a genetic study. *J. Med. Genet.* **28**, 443–7.

Maher, E.R. *et al.* (1996). Phenotypic expression in von Hippel–Lindau disease: correlations with germline VHL gene mutations. *J. Med. Genet.* **33**, 328–32.

Maxwell, P.H. *et al.* (1999). The tumour suppressor protein VHL targets hypoxia-inducible factors for oxygen-dependent proteolysis [see comments]. *Nature* **399**, 271–5.

Mukhopadhyay, D., Knebelmann, B., Cohen, H.T., Ananth, S., and Sukhatme, V.P. (1997). The von Hippel–Lindau tumor suppressor gene product interacts with Sp1 to repress vascular endothelial growth factor promoter activity. *Mol. Cell Biol.* **17**, 5629–39.

Nguyen, S.V. and Claycomb, W.C. (1999). Hypoxia regulates the expression of the adrenomedullin and HIF-1 genes in cultured HL-1 cardiomyocytes [in process citation]. *Biochem. Biophys. Res. Commun.* **265**, 382–6.

Ohh, M. *et al.* (1998). The von Hippel–Lindau tumor suppressor protein is required for proper assembly of an extracellular fibronectin matrix. *Mol. Cell* **1**, 959–68.

Ouiddir, A., Planes, C., Fernandes, I., Van Hesse, A., and Clerici, C. (1999). Hypoxia upregulates activity and expression of the glucose transporter GLUT1 in alveolar epithelial cells. *Am. J. Resp. Cell Mol. Biol.* **21**, 710–18.

Pack, S.D. *et al.* (1999). Constitutional von Hippel–Lindau (VHL) gene deletions detected in VHL families by fluorescence *in situ* hybridization [in process citation]. *Cancer Res.* **59**, 5560–4.

Pal, S., Claffey, K.P., Dvorak, H.F., and Mukhopadhyay, D. (1997). The von Hippel–Lindau gene product inhibits vascular permeability factor/vascular endothelial growth factor expression in renal cell carcinoma by blocking protein kinase C pathways. *J. Biol. Chem.* **272**, 27590–12.

Palmer, L.A. and Johns, R.A. (1998). Hypoxia upregulates inducible (type II) nitric oxide synthase in an HIF-1 dependent manner in rat pulmonary microvascular but not aortic smooth muscle cells. *Chest* **114**, 33S–34S.

Patton, E.E., Willems, A.R., and Tyers, M. (1998). Combinatorial control in ubiquitin-dependent proteolysis: don't Skp the F-box hypothesis. *Trends Genet.* **14**, 236-43.

Pause, A. *et al.* (1997). The von Hippel–Lindau tumor-suppressor gene product forms a stable complex with human CUL-2, a member of the Cdc53 family of proteins. *Proc. Natl Acad. Sci., USA* **94**, 2156–61.

Pause, A., Lee, S., Lonergan, K.M., and Klausner, R.D. (1998). The von Hippel–Lindau tumor suppressor gene is required for cell cycle exit upon serum withdrawal. *Proc. Natl Acad. Sci., USA* **95**, 993–8.

Prowse, A.H. *et al.* (1997). Somatic inactivation of the VHL gene in von Hippel–Lindau disease tumors [see comments]. *Am. J. Hum. Genet.* **60**, 765–71.

Richards, F.M. *et al.* (1995). Molecular analysis of *de novo* germline mutations in the von Hippel–Lindau disease gene. *Hum. Mol. Genet.* **4**, 2139–43.

Richards, F.M., Schofield, P.N., Fleming, S., and Maher, E.R. (1996). Expression of the von Hippel–Lindau disease tumor suppressor gene during human embryogenesis. *Hum. Mol. Genet.* **5**, 639–44.

Salceda, S. and Caro, J. (1997). Hypoxia-inducible factor 1 alpha (HIF-1alpha) protein is rapidly degraded by the ubiquitin–proteasome system under normoxic conditions. Its stabilization by hypoxia depends on redox-induced changes. *J. Biol. Chem.* **272**, 22642–7.

Scheffner, M., Nuber, U., and Huibregtse, J.M. (1995). Protein ubiquitination involving an E1–E2–E3 enzyme ubiquitin thioester cascade. *Nature* **373**, 81–3.

Schmidt, L. *et al.* (1995). Mechanism of tumorigenesis of renal carcinomas associated with the constitutional chromosome 3;8 translocation. *Cancer J. Sci. Am.* **1**, 191.

Schmidt, L. *et al.* (1997). Germline and somatic mutations in the tyrosine kinase domain of the MET proto-oncogene in papillary renal carcinomas. *Nat. Genet.* **16**, 68–73.

Seizinger, B.R. *et al.* (1988). Von Hippel–Lindau disease maps to the region of chromosome 3 associated with renal cell carcinoma. *Nature* **332**, 268–9.

Shilatifard, A. (1998). Factors regulating the transcriptional elongation activity of RNA polymerase II. *Fed. Am. Soc. Exp. Biol. J.* **12**, 1437–46.

Siemeister, G. *et al.* (1996). Reversion of deregulated expression of vascular endothelial growth factor in human renal carcinoma cells by von Hippel–Lindau tumor suppressor protein. *Cancer Res.* **56**, 2299–301.

Stebbins, C.E., Kaelin, W.G., Jr, and Pavletich, N.P. (1999). Structure of the VHL–elongin C–elongin B complex: implications for VHL tumor suppressor function. *Science* **284**, 455–61.

Stolle, C. *et al.* (1998). Improved detection of germline mutations in the von Hippel–Lindau disease tumor suppressor gene. *Hum. Mutat.* **12**, 417–23.

Storkel, S. *et al.* (1988). Intercalated cells as a probable source for the development of renal oncocytoma. *Virch. Arch. B, Cell Pathol. Mol. Pathol.* **56**, 185–9.

Takahashi, Y., Takahashi, S., Yoshimi, T., and Miura, T. (1998). Hypoxia-induced expression of phosphoglycerate mutase B in fibroblasts. *Eur. J. Biochem.* **254**, 497–504.

Toro, J.R. *et al.* (1999). Birt–Hogg–Dube syndrome: a novel marker of kidney neoplasia. *Arch. Dermatol.* **135**, 1195–202.

Tory, K. *et al.* (1989). Specific genetic change in tumors associated with von Hippel–Lindau disease. *J. Natl Cancer Inst.* **81**, 1097–101.

Tsuchiya, H., Iseda, T., and Hino, O. (1996). Identification of a novel protein (VBP-1) binding to the von Hippel–Lindau (VHL) tumor suppressor gene product. *Cancer Res.* **56**, 2881–5.

von Hippel, E. (1904). Über eine sehr seltene Erkrankrung der Netzhaut. *Klin. Beobacht. Arch. Ophthalmol.* **59**, 83–106.

Walther, M.M., Lubensky, I.A., Venzon, D., Zbar, B., and Linehan, W.M. (1995). Prevalence of microscopic lesions in grossly normal renal parenchyma from patients with von Hippel–Lindau disease, sporadic renal cell carcinoma and no renal disease: clinical implications. *J. Urol.* **154**, 2010–14 [discussion, 2014–15].

Weirich, G. *et al.* (1998). Familial renal oncocytoma: clinicopathological study of 5 families. *J. Urol.* **160**, 335–40.

Zbar, B. *et al.* (1994). Hereditary papillary renal cell carcinoma [see comments]. *J. Urol.* **151**, 561–6.

Zbar, B., Kaelin, W., Maher, E., and Richard, S. (1999). Third International Meeting on von Hippel–Lindau disease. *Cancer Res.* **59**, 2251–3.

Zhuang, Z. *et al.* (1998). Trisomy 7-harbouring non-random duplication of the mutant MET allele in hereditary papillary renal carcinomas. *Nat. Genet.* **20**, 66–9.

12. Antigens recognized by T lymphocytes on renal cell carcinoma

Benoît J. Van den Eynde and Michael Probst-Kepper

Introduction: the melanoma paradigm

The study of tumor antigens recognized by T cells was made possible about 15 years ago when cytolytic T lymphocytes (CTL) capable of killing the autologous tumor cells were isolated from the lymphocytes of cancer patients. Human melanoma cells can be grown relatively easily *in vitro*, and the first CTL were obtained from blood lymphocytes of melanoma patients. Melanoma therefore has become the paradigmatic tumor for human tumor immunology (Boon *et al.* 1994). Anti-melanoma CTL have also been isolated from tumor-infiltrating lymphocytes (TIL), and in some cases homogeneous CTL clones were obtained by limiting dilution cloning of CTL lines. In a few cases it has been possible to test the recognition of some normal cells by the CTL clones, and thereby determine the specificity with which they are able to kill the tumor cells. However, the definitive assessment of their specificity has required the molecular identification of the target antigen recognized by the CTL at the surface of the tumor cells. This has been achieved for a number of melanoma antigens via a genetic approach aimed at cloning the gene encoding the antigen (De Plaen *et al.* 1997). This approach is based on the transfection of recombinant libraries into recipient cells which are then screened for their ability to stimulate the CTL. The antigens usually correspond to peptides that are derived from intracellular proteins and presented at the cell surface by human leukocyte antigen (HLA) class I molecules. Antigens recognized by CTL on melanoma can be categorized according to their expression profiles (Van den Eynde and van der Bruggen 1997). A first distinction can be made between shared and unique antigens.

The unique antigens result from point mutations in genes that are expressed ubiquitously. The mutation affects the coding region of the gene; and the peptide recognized by the CTL contains the mutated residue. These mutations are usually unique to the tumor of an individual patient, and some of them may play a role in tumoral transformation. Such antigens, which are strictly tumor-specific, may play an important role in the natural antitumor immune response of individual patients, but they cannot easily be used as immunotherapeutic targets because they are not shared by tumors from different patients.

The shared antigens, on the other hand, are present on many tumors. They can be further divided into three groups (Van den Eynde and van der Bruggen 1997). One group corresponds to peptides encoded by genes such as *MAGE*, which are expressed in many tumors but not in normal tissues. The only normal cells expressing such genes are male germ cells, which do not have HLA molecules and therefore cannot present the peptides at their surface. It follows that these antigens are strictly tumor-specific, and represent ideal targets for specific immunotherapeutic strategies. Genes of the *MAGE* family are expressed not only in 40–70 per cent of melanomas, but also in many other tumor types, including lung carcinomas and bladder carcinomas (Boon and Van den Eynde 2000). However, they are not or very rarely expressed in renal cell carcinoma (RCC). A second group of shared antigens are derived from proteins such as tyrosinase, which are expressed in most melanomas but also in normal melanocytes. Tyrosinase is an enzyme involved in the synthesis of melanin, which is a hallmark of the melanocytic differentiation lineage. This second group of antigens, sometimes referred to as differentiation antigens, are not tumor-specific, and their use as targets for cancer immunotherapy may result in autoimmunity towards normal melanocytes, which are located in the skin and the retina. However, the risk of inducing severe side-effects appears minimal, and could be limited to the appearance of vitiligo, which is considered a good prognosis factor in melanoma patients and has already been observed in melanoma patients responding to interleukin 2 (IL-2)-based nonspecific immunotherapy (Rosenberg and White 1996). It is much more difficult to make predictions regarding the safety of targeting the third group of shared antigens, which are expressed in a wide variety of normal tissues and overexpressed in many tumors. These include peptides derived from genes such as *p53*, *HER2-neu*, and *telomerase*. Because a minimal amount of peptide is required for CTL recognition, a low level of expression in normal tissues may mean that autoimmune damage is not incurred. However, this threshold is difficult to define, as is the normal level of expression of those genes for each cell type.

With the exception of a few overexpressed antigens, which will be considered in more detail below, the antigens identified on melanomas are not expressed on RCC. Circumstantial evidence suggests that RCC is sensitive to immunological control, however, as indicated by the occasional reports of spontaneous tumor regression, and by the results of non-specific immunotherapy based on interferon alpha (IFN-α) and IL-2, with a response rate in the 10–20 per cent range (Atkins *et al.* 1993; Fyfe *et al.* 1995; Figlin *et al.* 1999; Franzke *et al.* 1999; Ritchie *et al.* 1999). These considerations have prompted efforts by various groups to isolate

CTL against RCC in order to characterize the putative RCC antigens.

Isolation of CTL against renal cell carcinoma

Once the first RCC cultures were established *in vitro*, cells of these tumor lines were used to stimulate autologous blood lymphocytes in the presence of IL-2, following the classical protocol of mixed lymphocytes–tumor cell culture (MLTC) that has proved successful with melanoma. In this way, CTL clones were obtained with the cells from a few patients, but with other patients the T cells either did not proliferate or did not exert specific lytic activity (Brändle *et al.* 1996; Brouwenstijn *et al.* 1996; Gaugler *et al.* 1996; Van den Eynde *et al.* 1999). In those cases, the transfection of costimulatory molecule B7 into the tumor cells used for stimulating the lymphocytes, and the addition of IL-12 and IL-6 to the MLTC improved the efficiency of the stimulation (Morel *et al.* 2000). Specific CTL were then obtained using this modified MLTC protocol, which may result in the *in vitro* activation of CTL that have not been primed *in vivo*. Another successful approach uses TIL instead of blood lymphocytes as responder cells. Such TIL can sometimes be expanded from the primary tumor sample in the presence of IL-2 (Belldegrun *et al.* 1988; Schendel *et al.* 1993; Brouwenstijn *et al.* 1996, 1998; Gaudin *et al.* 1999; Ronsin *et al.* 1999). The advantage of TIL is that they are enriched in T cells that have been recruited at the tumor site and therefore presumably primed against relevant tumor antigens *in vivo*. This can be documented by the analysis of TCR usage by TIL, a clear enrichment of a given TCR indicating *in situ* expansion of the corresponding T lymphocyte clone (Gaudin *et al.* 1995; Caignard *et al.* 1996; Ronsin *et al.* 1999). When a CTL line has been obtained, it is essential to clone it, so as to obtain monoclonal CTL cultures. This can be done by limiting dilution. This cloning step is essential because it is almost impossible to establish the fine specificity of CTL recognition using a polyclonal line. Once stable CTL clones have been obtained, they can be used as screening reagents to identify the target antigen, using the genetic approach mentioned above.

A different approach to obtain CTL starts from the analysis of the sequence of a protein known to be (over)expressed in RCC. The sequence is searched for peptides bearing a binding motif for a common HLA molecule (Rammensee *et al.* 1997). Binding to the HLA molecule can be confirmed using synthetic peptides, which can then be used to stimulate T cells from a blood donor with peptide-pulsed dendritic cells (Brossart *et al.* 1998, 1999; Vissers *et al.* 1999; Vonderheide *et al.* 1999). Peptide-specific CTL can be derived after such a primary *in vitro* immunization, and the ability of those CTL to recognize target cells expressing the parent protein endogenously needs to be tested thoroughly, as all the predicted peptides are not necessarily processed and presented by the cellular machinery (Van den Eynde and van der Bruggen 1997).

In all cases, a crucial step is the definition of the specificity of the CTL. At this point, the unique or shared character of the antigen can be examined. If the CTL can be shown to recognize not only the autologous, but also one or several allogeneic tumor lines, it can be considered as recognizing a shared antigen. If HLA-matched allogeneic RCC lines are not available, the presenting HLA molecule can be introduced by transfection of an appropriate plasmid construct before the CTL assay. If the CTL recognizes a shared antigen, the next question is to know whether its antigen is tumor-specific. This is more difficult to test, as normal cells are not easy to obtain and maintain in culture *in vitro*. Fortunately, the epithelial cells of the kidney tubules, which are the putative cells of origin of RCC, can be maintained *in vitro* for a few passages in the presence of epithelial growth factor (Detrisac *et al.* 1984). They can then be used as targets in CTL assays, and they can even be transfected with HLA plasmid constructs before testing CTL recognition (Fig. 12.1) (Brouwenstijn *et al.* 1996; Van den Eynde *et al.* 1999).

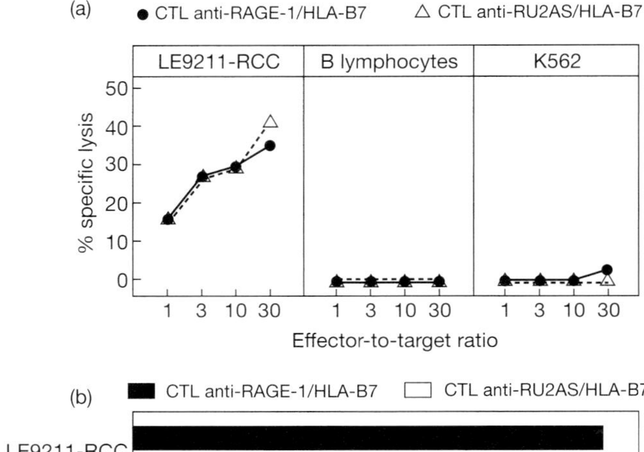

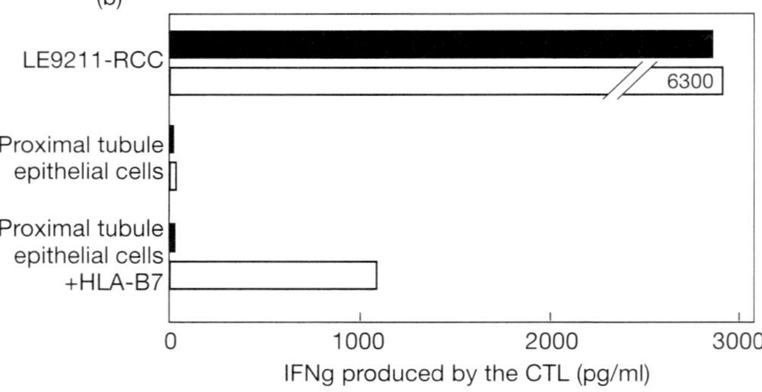

Fig. 12.1 Activity of two CTL clones raised against RCC line LE9211-RCC. (a) CTL activity can be tested in a chromium release assay, which measures the ability to lyse chromium-labeled target cells after 4 hours of incubation at various CTL-to-target ratios. (b) It can also be assessed by testing the production of a cytokine such as gamma-interferon (IFNγ) by the CTL after an overnight incubation with different target cells. Both CTL recognize a peptide presented by HLA-B7. One peptide is encoded by *RAGE-1*, the other by *RU2AS* (see text). The different targets used were: LE9211-RCC, the autologous tumor cells; B lymphocytes, autologous B lymphocytes immortalized with the Epstein–Barr virus; K562, a natural killer target cell line; and proximal tubule epithelial cells, a short-term cell line derived from the proximal kidney tubules. As the latter cell line does not express HLA-B7, it was previously transfected with a plasmid construct encoding HLA-B7. The results show that the anti-RAGE-1 CTL does not recognize normal kidney cells, whereas the anti-RU2AS CTL does.

Antigens recognized by CTL on renal cell carcinoma

Unique antigens

The first antigen to be defined on RCC happened to result from a point mutation, which was responsible for the expression of the antigen in a very unusual way. Instead of changing the sequence of an antigenic peptide presented by a HLA class I molecule, the mutation affects the gene encoding the HLA molecule itself, namely HLA-A2. This mutation results in an amino acid exchange in the alpha-2 domain that borders the peptide-binding cleft of the molecule (Brändle *et al.* 1996). The mutated HLA-A2 molecule is apparently recognized by the CTL independently of a specific antigenic peptide bound to the HLA. The mutation, which was initially found *in vitro* in the tumor line, was also detected in a fresh tumor sample from the patient, indicating that it is not an artifact of *in vitro* culture. However, the mutation was not found in any HLA-A2$^+$ tumor samples from the 34 other patients who were screened, indicating that it is unique to this patient. Despite the presence of this highly immunogenic tumor antigen, however, this patient died from regionally invasive disease.

A similar uniqueness applies to the hsp70–2 mutation, which was found to create a peptide that is presented by HLA-A2 to TIL that recognize the autologous RCC tumor line (Table 12.1) (Gaudin *et al.* 1999).

Shared antigens

The ideal target for cancer immunotherapy is an antigen that is both shared by many tumors and tumor-specific, meaning that it is not expressed in any normal tissue. Although this was the case for the MAGE-type antigens, these are not expressed in kidney tumors, and an RCC antigen with those features has now become something of a Holy Grail for tumor immunologists. Indeed, a

Table 12.1 Renal cell carcinoma antigens resulting from mutations

Gene	HLA presenting molecule	Peptide	Position	Reference
HLA-A2	—	—	170	Brändle *et al.* 1996
Hsp70–2	A2	SLFEGID/YT*	286–295	Gaudin *et al.* 1999

*The residue modified by the mutation is italicized.

variety of shared antigens have been defined in recent years, but none of them has proved to be strictly tumor-specific. Most are also expressed in a limited number of normal tissues—not necessarily in the kidney—and usually at a lower level. Therefore, if these antigens are contemplated as targets for RCC immunotherapy, the potential risk of inducing autoimmune damage is not negligible, and has to be considered separately for every antigen according to its expression pattern.

RAGE-1

The first shared RCC antigen to be identified was found to be encoded by a new gene, termed *RAGE-1*, which is silent in normal tissues except in the retina. The *RAGE*-encoded peptide is presented by HLA-B7 to CTL that recognize different RCC cell lines (Table 12.2). Although *RAGE-1* is expressed in a high fraction of RCC cell lines (37 per cent), it is only rarely expressed in fresh samples (2 per cent). *In vitro* culture therefore appears to result in the activation of the gene. *RAGE-1* is also expressed in small fractions of samples of other tumor types, such as sarcomas (12 per cent), infiltrating bladder carcinomas (8 per cent), and melanoma (3 per cent). It is not known which cell type expresses *RAGE* in the retina, but these cells might benefit from the immunological privilege of the eye. This notion is corroborated by the early results of vaccination trials of melanoma patients with melanocyte differentiation antigens, which are also expressed in the retina: no

Table 12.2 Shared antigens recognized by CTL on renal cell carcinoma

Gene	Normal tissue expression	HLA	Peptide	Position	Reference
RAGE	Retina	B7	SPSSNRIRNT	11–20	Gaugler *et al.* 1996
*iCE (alt.ORF)**	Kidney, liver, intestine, heart	B7	SPRWWPTCL	124–132	Ronsin *et al.* 1999
G250/MN/CA9	Stomach, liver, pancreas	A2	HLSTAFARV	254–262	Vissers *et al.* 1999
RU2AS†	Kidney, liver	B7	LPRWPPPQL	38–46	Van den Eynde *et al.* 1999
HER2-Neu	Ubiquitous (low level)	A2	KIFGSLAFL	369–377	Brossart *et al.* 1998
		A2	IISAVVGIL	654–662	
Telomerase	Hematopoietic stem cells, activated B lymphocytes, gonadal cells, basal keratinocytes	A2	ILAKFLHWL	540–548	Vonderheide *et al.* 1999
		A2	RLVDDFLLV	865–873	Minev *et al.* 2000
MUC-1	Epithelial cells	A2	STAPPVHNV	950–958	Brossart *et al.* 1999
		A2	LLLLTVLTV	leader	
*M-CSF (alt.ORF)**	Kidney, liver	B35	LPAVVGLSPGEQEY	4–17	‡

* Alternative open reading frame.
† Peptide translated from an antisense transcript of the *RU2* gene.
‡ Probst-Kepper *et al.*, manuscript in preparation.

ophthalmic toxicity was observed, even in the patients who developed vitiligo (Rosenberg and White 1996). The major obstacle to the use of the *RAGE-1* antigen for immunotherapy of RCC is rather its low frequency of expression in tumor samples. Although a higher frequency of *RAGE-1* expression in RCC samples was reported recently, this was based on expression studies performed by reverse transcriptase polymerase chain reaction (RT–PCR) followed by Southern blotting and hybridization (Neumann *et al.* 1998). As compared to the usual RT–PCR evaluated by ethidium bromide visualization of the PCR product, Southern blotting can detect extremely low expression levels that are below the threshold of expression required for CTL recognition (Lethé *et al.* 1997); Van den Eynde, unpublished results). A recent reassessment of the expression of *RAGE-1* in RCC samples based on ethidium bromide staining confirmed the earlier data (2/44 positive samples; Van den Eynde, unpublished results). A second RAGE peptide was recently identified by mass spectrometry after biochemical purification of peptides eluted from the HLA of RCC cells (Flad *et al.* 1998). CTL obtained by stimulating T cells *in vitro* with this peptide appear to recognize HLA-B8-positive RCC cells.

A cDNA coding for a new member of the MAP kinase family, named MOK, was recently isolated, and its 3' end was found to be identical to the 3'-terminal sequence of the RAGE cDNA (Miyata *et al.* 1999). The analysis of the partial structure of this gene showed that the RAGE and the MOK transcript indeed arise from the same gene and share the same exons at their 3' end, but use different promoters and 5' exons (Van den Eynde, unpublished results). The first exon of *RAGE* is located within a *MOK* intron, which therefore also contains the *RAGE* promoter. It is unclear why this intronic promoter is active in tumors and not in normal tissues, whereas the MOK transcript is widely expressed in normal tissues. Although it contains the exons coding for the RAGE-1/HLA-B7 peptide, the MOK cDNA cannot actually code for this peptide because the relevant sequence is interrupted by an intronic sequence that is not spliced in the MOK cDNA. In addition, the phase of the MOK open reading frame (ORF) is different from that of the ORF encoding the RAGE-1 peptide.

Intestinal carboxyl esterase (iCE)

Another shared antigen recognized by TIL on various RCC cell lines is encoded by the intestinal carboxyl esterase (*iCE*) gene, which is expressed in normal tissues such as liver, kidney, small intestine, colon, and heart (Ronsin *et al.* 1999). Despite its wide expression pattern, this antigen is interesting in two respects. First, because a PCR analysis of TCR usage showed that the CTL clone recognizing this peptide was strongly expanded among the lymphocytes infiltrating the tumor of this patient. This indicates that a strong CTL response had appeared spontaneously against this antigen *in vivo*, and that this response did not cause obvious autoimmune damage to iCE-expressing tissues. The second interesting feature lies in the fact that the antigenic peptide does not derive from degradation of the iCE protein, but is translated from an alternative ORF of the iCE mRNA (Table 12.2). This alternative ORF is located in another reading phase, and codes for a polypeptide that is different from the iCE polypeptide and contains the antigenic peptide. Interestingly, the translation of this ORF is not initiated on the classical AUG codon, but rather on an ACG triplet. In another system, the translation of ORF initiated at non-AUG codons was found to be activated in stressed or transformed cells (Vagner *et al.* 1996; Galy *et al.* 1999). This raises the possibility that the alternative ORF of iCE is translated efficiently in tumor cells but not in normal cells. This idea, however, is not supported by the fact the CTL can kill untransformed renal cell lines (Ronsin *et al.* 1999).

RU2AS

Other CTL raised against an RCC cell line were found to recognize a peptide whose expression also results from a very unusual genetic mechanism (Van den Eynde *et al.* 1999). The antigenic peptide, which is presented by HLA-B7, is encoded by a new gene, termed *RU2* (Table 12.2). This gene is transcribed in both directions. The antigenic peptide is not encoded by the sense transcript, called RU2S, which is expressed ubiquitously. It is encoded by an antisense transcript named RU2AS, which starts from a cryptic promoter located on the reverse strand of the first intron and ends up on the reverse strand of the RU2S promoter, which contains a polyadenylation signal. Antisense transcript RU2AS is expressed in a high proportion of tumors of various histological types. It is absent in most normal tissues, but it is expressed in testis, normal kidney, and, at lower levels, in urinary bladder and liver. The CTL can kill untransformed renal proximal tubular epithelial cells, which express significant levels of the RU2AS message (Fig. 12.1(b)). This antigen is therefore not tumor-specific.

G250

G250 is a monoclonal antibody that was raised more than 10 years ago by immunization of mice with human RCC homogenates (Oosterwijk *et al.* 1986). When the specificity of this antibody was tested by immunohistochemistry, it was found to stain the majority of RCC, but not any normal kidney cell. Staining was observed, however, in normal gastric mucosa and in liver bile ducts. The antigen recognized by this antibody was defined recently by cloning the encoding gene (Grabmaier *et al.* 2000). This gene is identical to the *MN/CA9* gene, which codes for an enzyme of the carbonic anhydrase family and is also frequently expressed in cervical carcinoma. The expression of this gene was then further tested by RT–PCR (McKiernan *et al.* 1997). This sensitive technique confirmed the frequent expression of G250/MN/CA9 in most RCC, and its lack of expression in normal kidney. In agreement with the immunohistochemistry data, expression of G250/MN/CA9 was also detected in normal tissues of the upper gastrointestinal tract, such as stomach, liver, and pancreas. Because of its frequent expression in kidney tumors and its absence from normal kidney, G250/MN/CA9 was considered a good potential target for CTL against RCC. *In vitro* immunization was therefore used to generate CTL-recognizing peptides selected from the G250 sequence for their ability to bind to HLA-A2. The peptides were pulsed on to dendritic cells and used to stimulate CD8 T cells from healthy donors (Vissers *et al.* 1999). One of the peptides made it possible to derive a CTL line that recognized melanoma cells transfected with G250 (Table 12.2). Although recognition of RCC lines by this CTL was not tested, this result indicated that this G250 peptide is naturally processed and should therefore be presented by a majority of RCC, since most of them express G250 and roughly half of them bear the HLA-A2 specificity. However, no significant G250-specific reactivity was detected in a screening of 18 different TIL cultures from RCC patients, indicating the absence or very infrequent occurrence of a spontaneous CTL response to G250 *in vivo* (Grabmaier *et al.* 2000). Vaccination trials could be performed to try to stimulate such a CTL response, although it would be necessary to balance the potential benefits of such a procedure against the risk of inducing autoimmunity in the upper gastrointestinal tract, including the liver.

Her-2/neu

HER2-neu/erbB2 is a tyrosine kinase receptor belonging to the epidermal growth factor receptor (EGFR) erbB1 family. It is expressed at moderate levels in many normal tissues and over-expressed in a number of human cancers of various types, including breast, ovarian, and renal cell carcinomas. CTL were raised against two distinct HLA-A2-binding peptides of HER2-neu by *in vitro* stimulation of CD8 lymphocytes with peptide-pulsed dendritic cells (Table 12.2) (Brossart *et al.* 1998). These CTL were capable of killing HLA-A2$^+$ RCC cell lines expressing HER2-neu, indicating that these peptides are naturally processed and presented by the tumor cells, and could represent attractive targets for immunotherapy. However, significant expression of HER2-neu was observed in normal kidney, particularly in tubular and collecting duct cells (Stumm *et al.* 1996). Recognition of normal kidney cell lines by the CTL was not tested, so that it is difficult to determine whether this expression in normal kidney represents a serious risk of autoimmune side-effects.

Telomerase

A similar protocol of *in vitro* stimulation was used to generate CTL against peptides derived from telomerase, an enzyme required for preventing the shortening of chromosome ends that occurs at each cellular division as a result of DNA replication (Vonderheide *et al.* 1999). Beyond a certain threshold of telomere length, cell viability decreases dramatically. It is therefore not surprising that telomerase is absent in most normal cells, which have a limited lifespan, but is expressed in cell types with an unlimited proliferation potential, such as hematopoietic progenitor cells, gonadal germ cells, basal keratinocytes, and activated lymphocytes (Greider 1996). Telomerase is also expressed in the majority of tumors of most histological types—including RCC—and probably contributes to the unlimited lifespan that is also the hallmark of tumor cells (Fujioka *et al.* 2000). CTL were obtained against two HLA-A2-binding telomerase peptides using responder lymphocytes from different donors and cancer patients (Table 12.2) (Vonderheide *et al.* 1999; Minev *et al.* 2000). These CTL were able to lyse HLA-A2$^+$ tumor lines expressing telomerase. These peptides might therefore represent widely expressed tumor antigens. However, the expression of telomerase in normal cells such as hematopoietic stem cells might represent a major obstacle to the use of those peptides as imunotherapeutic targets. Recognition of telomerase-positive normal cells by the CTL has been tested: although CD34$^+$ progenitor cells were apparently resistant to lysis by telomerase-specific CTL, activated B lymphocytes were clearly recognized and killed by the CTL (Vonderheide *et al.* 1999).

Mucin

The *MUC-1* gene codes for a large heavily glycosylated membrane mucin that is expressed in most epithelial cells, such as the breast ductal cells, gastric and pancreatic mucosa cells, and kidney tubular cells (Ho *et al.* 1995; Fujita *et al.* 1999). The expression of the molecule is usually restricted to the apical surface of the cells, which is not accesible to T cells. In many carcinomas, the mucin appears to be overexpressed, underglycosylated, and redistributed to the entire cellular membrane. This results in the unmasking of peptide epitopes, which can be recognized in a major histocompatibility complex (MHC)-unrestricted manner by CTL isolated from TIL of breast, ovarian, and pancreatic carcinomas (Barratt-Boyes 1996). The peptide epitope is part of a highly repeated peptide motif, which is normally masked as a result of both the high glycosylation status of the molecule and its sequestration at the apical surface of the epithelial cells. The recognition of this epitope without presentation by HLA molecules appears to result from its repetition, which could allow a direct cross-linking of the TCR. Because of this peculiar mechanism, these MHC-unrestricted epitopes appear to be tumor-specific. Since MUC1 is also overexpressed—and presumably underglycosylated—in RCC, these epitopes should be present on RCC cells. However the recognition of RCC cells by unrestricted MUC1-specific CTL has not been tested. More recently, another type of MUC-1-specific CTL has been isolated by stimulating T cells *in vitro* with peptides selected for their capacity to bind HLA-A2 (Table 12.2). Those CTL were able to lyse, in an HLA-A2-restricted manner, cells of an RCC line expressing MUC-1 and HLA-A2 (Brossart *et al.* 1999). In theory, as opposed to the MHC-unrestricted MUC-1 epitopes, the class I-restricted epitopes should not be tumor-specific, since their presentation should not be sensitive to the glycosylation status, and since the peptide/HLA complexes should be distributed over the whole cell surface rather than be confined to the apical surface. However, it is possible that a lower level of *MUC-1* expression in normal epithelial cells will allow those cells to escape CTL recognition. This issue cannot be solved without a quantitative estimation of the different expression levels and a direct testing of the recognition of untransformed epithelial cells by the MUC-1-specific CTL.

M-CSF

A CTL clone isolated from the TIL of an HLA-B35 RCC patient was recently studied in detail, and its target antigen was found to be encoded by the gene of the macrophage-colony stimulating factor (M-CSF or CSF1) (Probst-Kepper *et al.*, manuscript in preparation). Like the iCE antigen, the peptide here does not come from the M-CSF protein itself, but from the product of an alternative ORF which is located in another reading phase (Table 12.2). The M-CSF transcript is present in most normal tissues, but the translation of the major ORF is normally repressed, and only induced by inflammatory conditions. Translation of the alternative ORF appears to be regulated differently, as its product has been detected constitutively in kidney tubular cells and hepatocytes. Accordingly, the CTL was found to recognize untransformed kidney tubular cells, confirming the lack of tumor-specificity of this antigen (Probst-Kepper *et al.*, manuscript in preparation).

Conclusion and perspectives

It is impossible at this stage to predict whether the use of one of these shared RCC antigens as a target for immunotherapy will cause autoimmune side-effects. Several authors have addressed this issue in preclinical models, and conflicting data were obtained, ranging from a total lack of autoimmunity to the induction of severe autoimmune toxicity in essential organs after immunization against model tumor antigens also expressed in those tissues (Hu *et al.* 1993; Morgan 1998; Ludewig *et al.* 2000). These differences most probably result from the different model systems used, but also from differences in the efficiency of immunization. It is reasonable to consider that, the more efficient the induction of CTL will be, the more severe the autoimmune toxicity will be. Since strong CTL responses are presumably required also for tumor rejection, the therapeutic window may be very small. A wise strategy might be to wait until more complete results are available from the clinical trials currently being performed in melanoma with truly tumor-specific antigens (Nestle *et al.* 1998; Rosenberg *et al.* 1998; Marchand *et al.* 1999). In this case, trials with less specific tumor antigens could begin only if a clear tumor benefit can be reasonably expected.

For the immunologist, it might seem paradoxical to find CTL directed against self-antigens among circulating blood lymphocytes. Why do those CTL escape negative selection in the thymus? Why do they not normally cause autoimmunity? A possible explanation is that these cells remain 'ignorant' of their antigen because it is never presented in a proper way to trigger their response. This is supported by a recent observation we made using another CTL raised against a RCC line. This CTL recognizes normal cells such as fibroblasts and kidney tubular cells. Its target antigen is a peptide derived from an ubiquitous protein, termed RU1 (Morel *et al.* 2000). This peptide can be processed by cells bearing standard proteasomes, but not by cells carrying immunoproteasomes, such as gamma-interferon-treated cells, Epstein–Barr virus (EBV)-transformed B cells, and dendritic cells. Therefore, dendritic cells are not recognized by the anti-RU1 CTL, although they express RU1. As dendritic cells are responsible both for the presentation of antigens to self-reactive thymocytes and for the triggering of naive T cells in the periphery, this might explain how certain autoreactive CTL can escape negative selection in the thymus and fail to be activated in the periphery.

References

Atkins, M.B., Sparano, J., Fisher, R.I., Weiss, G.R., Margolin, K.A., Fink, K.I., *et al.* (1993). Randomized phase II trial of high-dose interleukin-2 either alone or in combination with interferon alfa-2b in advanced renal cell carcinoma. *J. Clin. Oncol.* **11**, 661–70.

Barratt-Boyes, S.M. (1996). Making the most of mucin: a novel target for tumor immunotherapy. *Cancer Immunol. Immunother.* **43**, 142–51.

Belldegrun, A., Muul, L.M., and Rosenberg, S.A. (1988). Interleukin-2 expanded tumor-infiltrating lymphocytes in human renal cell cancer: isolation, characterization, and antitumor activity. *Cancer Res.* **48**, 206–14.

Boon, T., Cerottini, J.-C., Van den Eynde, B., van der Bruggen, P., and Van Pel, A. (1994). Tumor antigens recognized by T lymphocytes. *Ann. Rev. Immunol.* **12**, 337–65.

Boon, T. and Van den Eynde, B. (2000). Shared tumor-specific antigens. In: *Principles and Practice of the biologic therapy of cancer*, 3rd edn (ed. S.A. Rosenberg). Lippincott Williams & Wilkins Philadelphia, p. 493–504

Brändle, D., Brasseur, F., Weynants, P., Boon, T., and Van den Eynde, B. (1996). A mutated HLA-A2 molecule recognized by autologous cytotoxic T lymphocytes on a human renal cell carcinoma. *J. Exp. Med.* **183**, 2501–8.

Brossart, P., Stuhler, G., Flad, T., Stevanovic, S., Rammensee, H.-G., Kanz, L., *et al.* (1998). Her-2/neu-derived peptides are tumor-associated antigens expressed by human renal cell and colon carcinoma lines and are recognized by *in vitro* induced specific cytotoxic T lymphocytes. *Cancer Res.* **58**, 732–6.

Brossart, P., Heinrich, K.S., Stuhler, G., Behnke, L., Reichardt, V.L., Stevanovic, S., *et al.* (1999). Identification of HLA-A2-restricted T-cell epitopes derived from the MUC1 tumor antigen for broadly applicable vaccine therapies. *Blood* **93**, 4309–17.

Brouwenstijn, N., Gaugler, B., Krüse, K.M., Van der Spek, C.W., Mulder, A., Osanto, S., *et al.* (1996). Renal cell carcinoma-specific lysis by cytotoxic T lymphocyte clones isolated from peripheral blood lymphocytes and tumor-infiltrating lymphocytes. *Int. J. Cancer* **68**, 177–82.

Brouwenstijn, N., Hoogstraten, C., Verdegaal, E.M.E., Van der Spek, C.W., Deckers, J.G., Mulder, A., *et al.* (1998). Definition of unique and shared T-cell defined tumor antigens in human renal cell carcinoma. *J. Immunother.* **21**, 427–34.

Caignard, A., Guillard, M., Gaudin, C., Escudier, B., Triebel, F., and Dietrich, P.-Y. (1996). *In situ* demonstration of renal-cell-carcinoma-specific T-cell clones. *Int. J. Cancer* **66**, 564–70.

De Plaen, E., Lurquin, C., Brichard, V., van der Bruggen, P., Renauld, J.-C., Coulie, P., *et al.* (1997). Cloning of genes coding for antigens recognized by cytolytic T lymphocytes. In *The immunology methods manual, MHC ligands and peptide binding* (ed. I. Lefkovits). Academic Press San Diego, p. 691–718.

Detrisac, C.J., Sens, M.A., Garvin, J., Spicer, S.S., and Sens, D.A. (1984). Tissue culture of human kidney epithelial cells of proximal tubule origin. *Kidney Int.* **25**, 383–90.

Figlin, R.A., Thompson, J.A., Bukowski, R.M., Vogelzang, N., Novick, A.C., Lange, P., *et al.* (1999). Multicenter, randomized, phase III trial of CD8[+] tumor-infiltrating lymphocytes in combination with recombinant interleukin-2 in metastatic renal cell carcinoma. *J. Clin. Oncol.* **17**, 2521–9.

Flad, T., Spengler, B., Kalbacher, H., Brossart, P., Baier, D., Kaufmann, R., *et al.* (1998). Direct identification of major histocompatibility complex class I-bound tumor-associated peptide antigens of a renal carcinoma cell line by a novel mass spectrometric method. *Cancer Res.* **58**, 5803–11.

Franzke, A., Peest, D., Probst-Kepper, M., Buer, J., Kirchner, G.I., Brabant, G., *et al.* (1999). Autoimmunity resulting from cytokine treatment predicts long-term survival in patients with metastatic renal cell cancer. *J. Clin. Oncol.* **17**, 529–33.

Fujioka, T., Hasegawa, M., Suzuki, Y., Suzuki, T., Sugimura, J., Tanji, S., *et al.* (2000). Telomerase activity in human renal cell carcinoma. *Int. J. Urol.* **7**, 16–21.

Fujita, K., Denda, K., Yamamoto, M., Matsumoto, T., Fujime, M., and Irimura, T. (1999). Expression of MUC1 mucins inversely correlated with post-surgical survival of renal cell carcinoma patients. *Br. J. Cancer* **80**, 301–8.

Fyfe, G., Fisher, R.I., Rosenberg, S.A., Sznol, M., Parkinson, D.R., and Louie, A.C. (1995). Results of treatment of 255 patients with metastatic renal cell carcinoma who received high-dose recombinant interleukin-2 therapy. *J. Clin. Oncol.* **13**, 688–96.

Galy, B., Maret, A., Prats, A.-C., and Prats, H. (1999). Cell transformation results in the loss of the density-dependent translational regulation of the expression of fibroblast growth factor 2 isoforms. *Cancer Res.* **59**, 165–71.

Gaudin, C., Dietrich, P.-Y., Robache, S., Guillard, M., Escudier, B., Terrier Lacombe, M.-J., *et al.* (1995). *In vivo* local expansion of clonal T cell subpopulations in renal cell carcinoma. *Cancer Res.* **55**, 685–90.

Gaudin, C., Kremer, F., Angevin, E., Scott, V., and Triebel, F. (1999). A hsp70–2 mutation recognized by CTL on a human renal cell carcinoma. *J. Immunol.* **162**, 1730–8.

Gaugler, B., Brouwenstijn, N., Vantomme, V., Szikora, J.-P., Van der Spek, C.W., Patard, J.-J., *et al.* (1996). A new gene coding for an antigen recognized by autologous cytolytic T lymphocytes on a human renal carcinoma. *Immunogenetics* **44**, 323–30.

Grabmaier, K., Vissers, J.L.M., De Weijert, M.C.A., Oosterwijk-Wakka, J.C., Van Bokhoven, A., Brakenhoff, R.H., *et al.* (2000). Molecular cloning and immunogenicity of renal cell carcinoma-associated antigen G250. *Int. J. Cancer* **85**, 865–70.

Greider, C.W. (1996). Telomere length regulation. *Ann. Rev. Biochem.* **65**, 337–65.

Ho, S.B., Shekels, L.L., Toribara, N.W., Kim, Y.S., Lyftogt, C., Cherwitz, D.L., *et al.* (1995). Mucin gene expression in normal, preneoplastic, and neoplastic human gastric epithelium. *Cancer Res.* **55**, 2681–90.

Hu, J., Kindsvogel, W., Busby, S., Bailey, M.C., Shi, Y.-Y., and Greenberg, P.D. (1993). An evaluation of the potential to use tumor-associated antigens as targets for antitumor T cell therapy using transgenic mice expressing a retroviral tumor antigen in normal lymphoid tissues. *J. Exp. Med.* **177**, 1681–90.

Lethé, B., van der Bruggen, P., Brasseur, F., and Boon, T. (1997). MAGE-1 expression threshold for the lysis of melanoma cell lines by a specific CTL. *Melanoma Res.* **7**, S83–S88.

Ludewig, B., Ochsenbein, A.F., Odermatt, B., Paulin, D., Hengartner, H., and Zinkernagel, R.M. (2000). Immunotherapy with dendritic cells directed against tumor antigens shared with normal host cells results in severe autoimmune disease. *J. Exp. Med.* **191**, 795–803.

Marchand, M., van Baren, N., Weynants, P., Brichard, V., Dréno, B., Tessier, M.-H., *et al.* (1999). Tumor regressions observed in patients with metastatic melanoma treated with an antigenic peptide encoded by gene *MAGE-3* and presented by HLA-A1. *Int. J. Cancer* **80**, 219–30.

McKiernan, J.M., Buttyan, R., Bander, N.H., Stifelman, M.D., Katz, A.E., Chen, M.-W., *et al.* (1997). Expression of the tumor-associated gene MN: a potential biomarker for human renal cell carcinoma. *Cancer Res.* **57**, 2362–5.

Minev, B., Hipp, J., Firat, H., Schmidt, J.D., Langlade-Demoyen, P., and Zanetti, M. (2000). Cytotoxic T cell immunity against telomerase reverse transcriptase in humans. *Proc. Natl Acad. Sci., USA* **97**, 4796–801.

Miyata, Y., Akashi, M., and Nishida, E. (1999). Molecular cloning and characterization of a novel member of the MAP kinase superfamily. *Genes Cells* **4**, 299–309.

Morel, S., Lévy, F., Burlet-Schiltz, O., Brasseur, F., Probst-Kepper, M., Peitrequin, A.-L., *et al.* (2000). Processing of some antigens by the standard proetasome but not by the immunoproteasome results in poor presentation by dendritic cells. *Immunity* **12**, 107–17.

Morgan, D.J. (1998). Activation of low avidity CTL specific for a self epitope results in tumor rejection but not autoimmunity. *J. Immunol.* **160**, 643–51.

Nestle, F.O., Alijagic, S., Gilliet, M., Sun, Y., Grabbe, S., Dummer, R., *et al.* (1998). Vaccination of melanoma patients with peptide- or tumor lysate-pulsed dendritic cells. *Nature Med.* **4**, 328–32.

Neumann, E., Engelsberg, A., Decker, J., Störkel, S., Jaeger, E., Huber, C., *et al.* (1998). Heterogeneous expression of the tumor-asociated antigens RAGE-1, PRAME, and glycoprotein 75 in human renal cell carcinoma: candidates for T-cell-based immunotherapies. *Cancer Res.* **58**, 4090–5.

Oosterwijk, E., Ruiter, D.J., Hoedemaeker, P.J., Pauwels, E.K.J., Jonas, U., Zwartendijk, J., *et al.* (1986). Monoclonal antibody G250 recognizes a determinant present in renal-cell carcinoma and absent from normal kidney. *Int. J. Cancer* **38**, 489–94.

Rammensee, H.-G., Bachmann, J., and Stevanovic, S. (1997). *MHC ligands and peptide motifs.* Molecular Biology Intelligence Unit, Springer, New York.

Ritchie, A., Griffiths, G., Parmar, M., Fossa, S.D., Selby, P.J., Combleet, M.A., *et al.* (1999). Interferon-alpha and survival in metastatic renal carcinoma: early results of a randomised controlled trial. *Lancet* **353**, 14–17.

Ronsin, C., Chung-Scott, V., Poullion, I., Aknouche, N., Gaudin, C., and Triebel, F. (1999). A non-AUG-defined alternative open reading frame of the intestinal carboxyl esterase mRNA generates an epitope recognized by renal cell carcinoma-reactive tumor-infiltrating lymphocytes *in situ*. *J. Immunol.* **163**, 483–90.

Rosenberg, S.A. and White, D.E. (1996). Vitiligo in patients with melanoma: normal tissue antigens can be target for cancer immunotherapy. *J. Immunother.* **19**, 81–4.

Rosenberg, S.A., Yang, J.C., Schwartzentruber, D.J., Hwu, P., Marincola, F.M., Topalian, S.L., *et al.* (1998). Immunologic and therapeutic evaluation of a synthetic peptide vaccine for the treatment of patients with metastatic melanoma. *Nature Med.* **4**, 321–7.

Schendel, D.J., Gansbacher, B., Oberneder, R., Kriegmair, M., Hofstetter, A., Riethmüller, G., *et al.* (1993). Tumor-specific lysis of human renal cell carcinomas by tumor-infiltrating lymphocytes. I. HLA-A2-restricted recognition of autologous and allogeneic tumor lines. *J. Immunol.* **151**, 4209–20.

Stumm, G., Eberwein, S., Rostock-Wolf, S., Stein, H., Pomer, S., Schlegel, J., *et al.* (1996). Concomitant overexpression of the *EGFR* and *erb*B-2 genes in renal cell carcinoma (RCC) is correlated with dedifferentiation and metastasis. *Int. J. Cancer* **69**, 17–22.

Vagner, S., Touriol, C., Galy, B., Audigier, S., Gensac, M.-C., Amalric, F., *et al.* (1996). Translation of CUG- but not AUG-initiated forms of human fibroblast growth factor 2 is activated in transformed and stressed cells. *J. Cell Biol.* **135**, 1391–402.

Van den Eynde, B. and van der Bruggen, P. (1997). T cell-defined tumor antigens. *Curr. Opin. Immunol.* **9**, 684–93.

Van den Eynde, B.J., Gaugler, B., Probst-Kepper, M., Michaux, L., Devuyst, O., Lorge, F., *et al.* (1999). A new antigen recognized by cytolytic T lymphocytes on a human kidney results from reverse strand transcription. *J. Exp. Med.* **190**, 1793–9.

Vissers, J.L.M., De Vries, I.J.M., Schreurs, M.W.J., Engelen, L.P.H., Oosterwijk, E., Figdor, C.G., *et al.* (1999). The renal cell carcinoma-associated antigen G250 encodes a human leukocyte antigen (HLA)-A2.1-restricted epitope recognized by cytotoxic T lymphocytes. *Cancer Res.* **59**, 5554–9.

Vonderheide, R.H., Hahn, W.C., Schultze, J.L., and Nadler, L.M. (1999). The telomerase catalytic subunit is a widely expressed tumor-associated antigen recognized by cytolytic T lymphocytes. *Immunity* **10**, 673–9.

13. Monoclonal antibodies to renal cancer antigens

C. Divgi, E. Oosterwijk, M. Steffens, and N. Bander

Role of the immune system in renal cancer

Ludwig Gross's (1943) observation that inbred mice could be immunized against tumor transplants from syngeneic animals signaled the start of the modern era of cancer immunology. Prehn and Main (1957) demonstrated, subsequently, that cancers possessed tumor-related antigens, responsible for inducing the protective effect. Burnet (1970) proposed that cancers expressed aberrant antigens, which would allow their detection and elimination by the host's immune system, and coined the expression 'immune surveillance'.

Cancer immunologists continued to attempt to define recognized tumor antigens and discern the reasons why immune surveillance sometimes fails and allows cancer development. The occasional spontaneous regression in renal cancer (Everson and Cole 1966; Freed *et al.* 1977; Snow and Schellhammer 1982; Vogelzang *et al.* 1992) provides indirect evidence implying a role of the immune system in the natural history of renal cancer. Oliver *et al.* (1989) observed a series of 73 patients with metastatic renal cancer without therapy until disease progression. This study provided data on the natural history of metastatic renal cancer as well as a baseline for comparison to therapy trials. Oliver *et al.* (1989) found that, without treatment, 4 per cent of patients had a complete response and 3 per cent at partial response. Tellingly, 5 per cent of patients had progression-free intervals of more than 12 months; these data suggest that some of the 'responses' in the absence of treatment reflect the immune system at work.

There are, moreover, many cases where metastases develop 10, 20, or even more years after resection of an apparently localized cancer, providing presumptive evidence that metastatic foci, 'seeded' prior to resection, had been kept in check by the immune system. Finally, dramatic regressions are occasionally seen in patients treated with immunotherapy such as interleukin 2 (IL-2) (Rosenberg *et al.* 1993). This anti tumor ability of an agent that physiologically activates lymphocytes is certainly consistent with an immune mechanism in the natural history of renal cancer.

Normal and neoplastic kidney antigens defined by monoclonal antibodies

The development of hybridoma technology (Kohler and Milstein 1975) gave new impetus to the search for tumor-related antigens. The impact of this technology, which resulted in the discoverers

Table 13.1 Monoclonal antibodies and defined antigens in normal kidney and renal cancer.

Monoclonal antibody	Defined antigen	Site of antigen expression
T138	gp25	Vascular endothelium
J143 (URO-1)	gp140, 120, 30	Glomerular epithelium
C5H	p115	Glomerulus
S22	gp115	Bowman's capsule
D5D	Not defined	Bowman's capsule
AJ8 or J5	Neutral endopeptidase (NEP)	Glomerulus, proximal tubule
S4 (URO-2)	Aminopeptidase A (APA)	Glomerulus, proximal tubule
F23 (URO-3)	Aminopeptidase N (APN)	Proximal tubule
T43 (URO-10)	gp85	Proximal tubule—convoluted segment
F31 (URO-8)	Acidic lipid	Proximal tubule—straight segment
S27 (URO-4)	Dipeptidyl peptidase (DPP) IV	Proximal tubule, loop of Henle
A6H	Not defined	Proximal tubule
10.32	gp90, Tamm–Horsfall protein	Loop of Henle, distal tubule
C26	gp40	Distal tubule, collecting duct
T16 (URO-5)	gp48, 42	Distal tubule, collecting duct
anti-A, B, O(H)	Blood group antigens	Collecting duct
G250	Carbonic anhydrase (CA) IX	Clear cell RCC only

being awarded the Nobel Prize, is reflected in the development of diagnostic immunoassays (of which 'prostrate-specific antigen' is but one of many examples) and in almost all aspects of immunological investigation. Hybridoma technology has provided many useful antibody probes, new insight into cancer biology, and the promise of developing diagnostic and therapeutic advances, manifest by the approval by the US Food and Drug Administration (FDA) of monoclonal antibodies (mAb) for in vivo diagnostic and therapeutic applications in cancer.

Various laboratories have developed numerous mAb probes specific for kidney-related antigens, useful for the definition of their respective antigens either in fresh tissue specimens or *in vitro*, and, in many cases, the cloning, sequencing, and identification of the detected gene. Some of the important mAb in the study of renal cancer and the antigens they helped define are listed in Table 13.1.

Expression of these antigens is, in most cases, quite specific for particular segments of the nephron; this allows development of an 'antigen map' of the kidney (Fig. 13.1). This provides the antigenic or molecular phenotype of the normal kidney cells, analogous to red blood cell (for example, A, B, O(H), Rh, etc.) typing based on antigenic expression. mAb may also be used to subclassify histologically indistinguishable lymphocytes into T- (CD3 antigen-positive) or B-cells (CD3$^-$) and further subclassify T cells into functional subcategories (helper CD3$^+$/CD4$^+$/CD8$^-$) or cytotoxic (CD3$^+$/CD4$^-$/CD8$^+$) T-cells). Proximal convoluted tubular cells, for example, have the molecular phenotype URO-10$^+$/ aminopeptidase A$^+$/ aminopeptidase N$^+$/neutral endopeptidase$^+$/dipeptidyl peptidase IV$^+$/Lewis x$^+$/URO-8$^-$/ABH$^-$, while cells of the collecting duct express virtually the reciprocal pattern of expression, URO-10$^-$/ aminopeptidase A$^-$/ aminopeptidase N$^-$/ neutral endopeptidase$^-$/ dipeptidyl peptidase IV$^-$/Lewis x$^-$/URO-8$^-$/ABH$^+$ (Bander *et al.* 1985, 1989; Cordon-Caro *et al.* 1986, 1987).

Definition of normal adult nephron antigenic or molecular phenotype allows determination of aberrant cell types, for example, the phenotype of fetal kidney cells to study renal development. Fetal proximal tubule cells express both URO-8 and URO-10 antigens. These antigens are reciprocally expressed in the mature proximal tubule (Bander *et al.* 1989): convoluted proximal tubule cells are URO-10$^+$/URO-8$^-$, while cells of the straight segment of the proximal tubule are URO-10$^-$/URO-8$^+$. Antigenic differences, therefore, permit determination of the maturity and origin of these cells.

One can also use these probes to study renal cancer histogenesis. Analysis of the molecular phenotype of renal cancers has shown that the vast majority of renal cancers derive from the proximal tubule (Bander *et al.* 1989). This work confirms earlier ultrastructural and conventional immunological data. Antibody probes allow this classification to be taken a step further, because of the ability of mAb to distinguish cells from the convoluted or the straight portion of the proximal tubule. In 200 renal cancers studied (Bander *et al.* 1989), approximately 30 per cent had a molecular phenotype consistent with derivation from the convoluted proximal tubule and 20 per cent from the straight segment; 50 per cent had the phenotype of less well-differentiated, fetal proximal tubular cells. The clinical significance of this finding remains to be determined.

The defined antigenic phenotypes of normal kidney cells may be applied to tissue-cultured normal and neoplastic renal epithelium. The molecular phenotyping of normal renal epithelial cultures reveals that these cells are derived from the proximal tubule—the same cell type that transforms to cancer. The ability to readily grow short-term cultures of normal kidney cells, and to establish renal cancer lines, both from the same patient, is a unique experimental advantage in the study of human cancers (Ebert *et al.* 1990). This ability provides an unparalleled opportunity for the study of neoplastic transformation at a molecular level.

Virtually every clear cell renal cancer studied with mAb probes demonstrates a pattern consistent with proximal tubular derivation. It is, however, not uncommon for one or more proximal tubular antigens to be deleted, creating a series of molecular subtypes of renal cancer. The direct correlation between the number of antigenic markers expressed and the degree of differentiation of the cancer suggests that scoring the antigenic expression of a patient's cancer may provide an objective grading for renal cancer. Furthermore, we have seen that the number of antigens deleted is related to disease progression and thus prognosis. It is currently unresolved whether antigen loss represents an independent prognostic variable or whether these observations are merely a reflection of tumor grade. Follow-up of a larger number of patients will be necessary to clarify this point.

Advances in molecular biology herald an era of molecular pathology. Molecular probes (mAb, oligonucleotides) can discriminate multiple, molecular subtypes of renal cancer that have clinical relevance. An example where molecular differences resolve different clinical findings is the previously recognized morphological entities of papillary (chromophilic) and non-papillary clear cell renal cancers. The differences go beyond their morphology. It has long been recognized that the substantial majority (80 per cent) of renal cancers have a clear or granular cell histology and are hypervascular, while a minority (10–15 per cent)

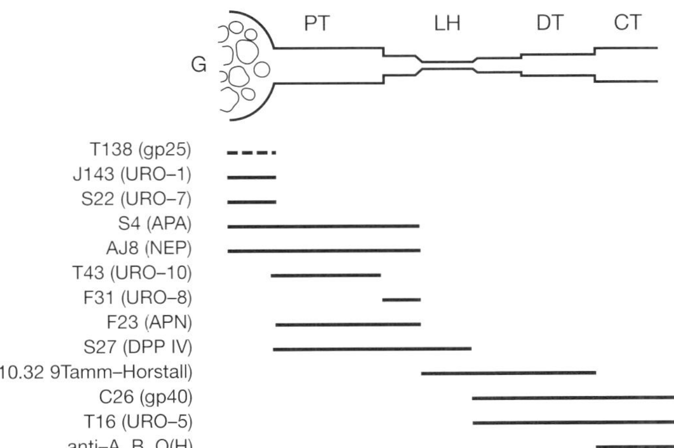

Fig. 13.1 Antigenic map of the human nephron. The nephron is schematically represented below; the sites of antigen expression are indicated by the solid bars. G, glomerulus; PT, proximal tubule; LH, Loop of Henle; DT, distal tubule; CT, collecting duct. The definitions of the antigens are found in Table 13.1.

have a papillary growth pattern and are typically hypovascular. Elucidation of the molecular genetics of renal cancer reveals that different genetic defects underlie these subtypes. Non-papillary clear cell renal cancers have a defective von Hippel–Lindau (VHL) gene (Gnarra *et al.* 1994), while papillary (chromophilic) renal cancers have normal VHL genes but overexpress the c-MET oncogene (Schmidt *et al.* 1997). At least one mAb, G250, can distinguish these cell types: the 'G250' antigen (carbonic anhydrase IX (CA IX); see below) is expressed by the clear/granular cell type but by neither normal kidney epithelia nor by papillary renal cell carcinoma (RCC) (Dosterwijk *et al.* 1993). Ivanov *et al.* (1998) found that synthesis of CA IX is suppressed by the normal VHL gene product (pVHL). Therefore, in normal proximal tubule cells and in papillary RCC, both with normal pVHL, CA IX is undetectable. In clear cell RCC, however, the mutated VHL gene product does not suppress CA IX, resulting in its expression. CA IX expression by RCC cells, detectable with the G250 mAb, may therefore serve as a surrogate marker of VHL mutation. Loss of pVHL function (in clear cell RCC) leads to vascular endothelial growth factor (VEGF) expression and consequent hypervascularity, accounting for the differential vascularity of clear cell and papillary RCC. With normal pVHL in papillary RCC, hypervascularity is not seen.

Cloning the G250 antigen

In view of the restricted tissue expression and the induction/upregulation of G250 antigen in clear cell RCC and therefore its potential as a therapeutic target, we set out to molecularly identify the cDNA encoding the G250 antigen. Immunohistochemical screening of a cDNA expression library (Brakenhoff *et al.* 1994) resulted in the isolation of pMW1, a cDNA clone of 1534 bp. This cDNA was used as a probe for Northern analysis of mRNA isolated from mAbG250$^+$ and mAbG250$^-$ RCC cell lines, RCC and normal kidney surgical specimens obtained from the same patients, and a variety of normal human organs. After hybridization under stringent conditions, a single 1.5 kb transcript was detected in mAbG250-positive cell lines and RCC specimens. Complete correlation with respect to G250 mRNA and protein expression, as detected by mAbG250 immunohistochemistry, was observed. G250 mRNA expression levels in fresh RCC were comparable to the highest mRNA levels observed in RCC cell lines. Conversely, no transcript was detected in mAb250-negative cell lines, normal kidney specimens, or any normal human organ investigated. Transfection of mAbG250-negative cell lines resulted in a conversion to the G250-positive phenotype, confirming that the cDNA encoded for G250 protein.

The gene encoding for G250 was shown by human chromosomal DNA Southern blot analysis to be present in the human genome as a single copy gene of approximately 7.2 kb. Fluorescent *in situ* hybridization (FISH) assigned the G250 gene to chromosome 9p12–13. There was no amplification of G250-encoding DNA in any of the RCC cell lines or surgically obtained specimens.

The proposed open reading frame encodes for a protein of 459 amino acids (aa), with a predicted molecular weight of approximately 49.7 kDa. Homology analysis showed that the protein

could be divided into regions containing a signal peptide (aa 1–37), a carbonic anhydrase domain (aa 134–391) and a hydrophobic transmembrane region of 20 aa and a *C* terminus of 25 aa. Computer-assisted comparison with the EMBL database revealed partial homology with MN, a recently cloned human tumor-associated protein, originally identified in HeLa cells using mAb M75 (Pastorek *et al.* 1994), and complete homology with a revised MN version (Opavsky *et al.* 1996). The G250 sequence has been deposited under accession number DS 35472.

Western blots probed with M75 mAb after mAb G250 affinity purification revealed reactivity with a protein of 63 kDa molecular weight, compared to the predicted molecular weight of 49 kDa. After correction for the introduced his–myc tag modifications, this points to posttranslational modification of 10 kDa. In RCC, three proteins of 49, 52, and 59 kDa, most probably representing the unmodified, intermediate modified, and final product, respectively, were detected by M75.

Characterization of the genomic organization of the G250 gene revealed that the gene consists of 11 exons and 10 exons, identical to the MN gene structure (Opavsky *et al.* 1996). With the exception of the first exon, all exons are small. Splice donor and acceptor sequences conformed to consensus splice sequences. No differences were observed between the cDNA and genomic sequence, with the exception of an A–G transition in codon 33 in exon 1 (nucleotide 106), leading to the change of methionine to valine. The sequence surrounding this ATG does not conform to a Kozak consensus sequence and it is unlikely that this methionine functions as an alternative start site. Single-strand conformation polymorphism (SSCP) analysis of exon 1 showed no differences between RCC and corresponding normal kidney tissue in 10 cases examined. Thus, this transition seems to represent a naturally occurring polymorphism. Both alleles are functional since homozygous cell lines showed G250 expression, irrespective of codon 33 use.

Northern analysis or reverse transcriptase polymerase chain reaction (RT–PCR) failed to detect G250 transcripts in normal kidney specimens (adult and fetal). Hybridization of G250 cDNA with a cDNA library constructed from normal kidney did not identify any clone with G250 sequence homology. These observations indicate that G250 transcription is not involved in renal organogenesis but is induced or dramatically upregulated upon malignant transformation of proximal tubular cells. Furthermore, mAb G250 does not recognize a unique epitope on a (kidney) differentiation-antigen, but reacts with an aberrant expressed protein. Studies by Ivanov *et al.* (1998) showed a direct correlation between G250 expression and loss of functional VHL product, explaining the cause of universal G250 expression in all clear cell RCC.

Potential use of monoclonal antibodies in vivo for diagnosis and therapy

mAb are being studied extensively in clinical trials in numerous tumor types. They have been shown to specifically target to tumor sites while sparing normal tissues. Radiolabeled mAb are now FDA-approved for the detection of colon, ovary, prostate, and small cell lung cancer. Chimeric and humanized antibodies with

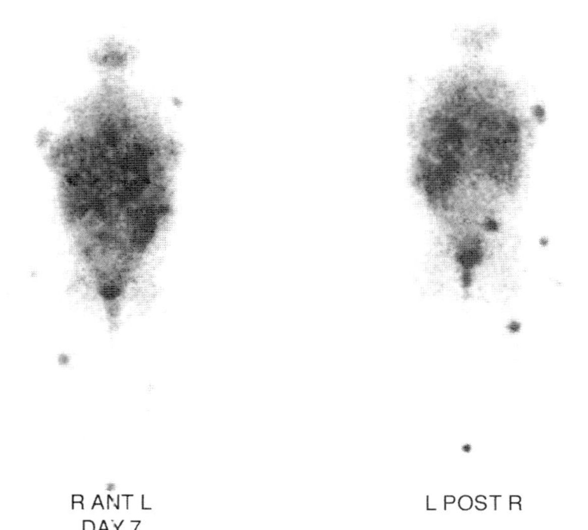

Fig. 13.2 Anterior and posterior whole-body I-131 image obtained 3 days after 45 mCi/m^2 ^{131}I-labelled mG250 in a patient with metastatic clear cell renal cancer. Targeting to disease in nodes, liver, lung, bone, and skin metastases is clear.

potential cytotoxic activity and less immunogenic potential than their murine counterparts have been FDA-approved for the treatment of non-Hodgkin's lymphoma (NHL) and breast cancer, and antibodies conjugated with radioactivity or other cytotoxic agents are nearing FDA approval for the treatment of NHL and acute myelogenous leukemia.

mAb G250, initially developed by Oosterwijk *et al.* (1986), has been most extensively studied in RCC. CA IX, the antigen recognized by mAb G250, is suppressed in normal renal epithelium by pVHL. In clear cell RCC, loss of pVHL function leads to expression of CA IX and, therefore, reactivity with mAb G250. G250 is not tumor-specific: the antibody demonstrates some reactivity with normal gastric mucosal cells and with biliary ductules.

Clinical trials with murine G250
Clinical trials with radiolabeled mAb G250 in patients with RCC (Oosterwijk *et al.* 1993; Divgi *et al.* 1998; Steffens *et al.* 1997; Bander *et al.* 1996) have demonstrated selective and specific delivery of mAb to renal cancer sites. Both primary and metastatic RCC, including both bone and soft tissue metastasis, are targeted and imaged (Fig. 13.2). Tissue biopsies of approximately 30 imaged lesions were taken from 23 patients receiving murine G250; all lesions were pathologically documented to represent site of renal cancer. There were no false-positive scans. Antibody localization to tumor was selective and specific, with quantitative analysis of tissue samples demonstrating peak ratios of tumor: serum of 178:1, tumor:normal kidney of 285:1 and tumor: liver of 92:1 one week after mAb administration (Oosterwijk *et al.*1993). In addition, previously unsuspected (that is, undetectable by computerized tomography (CT), magnetic resonance imaging (MRI), or bone scan) lesions were detected by antibody imaging in 10 of 43 (21 per cent patients (Oosterwijk *et al.* 1993;

Bander *et al.* 1996). In many cases, these sites were pathologically confirmed, with a consequent change in clinical management in many cases. For example, two patients with presumed solitary bone metastasis referred for surgery were found to have additional lesions, thereby avoiding needless surgery. In at least two other cases, unsuspected sites imaged by the mAb were resected and proven to be metastatic RCC, thereby completing surgical resection of tumor.

Phase I/II radioimmunotherapy

Thirty-three patients with measurable metastatic RCC were studied to determine the maximum tolerated dose (MTD) and therapeutic potential of ^{131}I-G250 (Divgi *et al.* 1998). Groups of at least three patients received escalating amounts of ^{131}I (30, 45, 60, 75, 90 mCi/m^2 ^{131}I) labeled to 10 mg murine G250 (mG250), administered as a single intravenous infusion. Fifteen patients were studied at the maximum tolerated dose of activity (MTD$_A$), defined as that dose at which not more than a third of patients had grade 3 or greater hematopoietic toxicity.

Transient hyperbilirubinemia lasting less than 2 weeks occurred at all dose levels. After the first dose level (30 mCi/m^2 ^{131}I), therefore, a protocol modification was approved by the IRB and the FDA considering hepatic toxicity dose-limiting only when it persisted for 2 or more weeks. No patient had prolonged hepatic toxicity, an this transient toxicity was therefore not considered dose-limiting. Transient reversible liver function test abnormalities were observed in the majority of patients (27/33). There was no correlation between the amount of ^{131}I administered, or hepatic absorbed radiation dose (median: 0.073 Gy/mCi), and the extent or nature of hepatic toxicity.

Two of the first six patients at 90 mCi/m^2 had $\geq$ grade 3 thrombocytopenia; the MTD was determined to be 90 mCi/m^2 ^{131}I, and a total of 15 patients were studied at this dose level. Figure 13.3 details the platelet counts over time in the

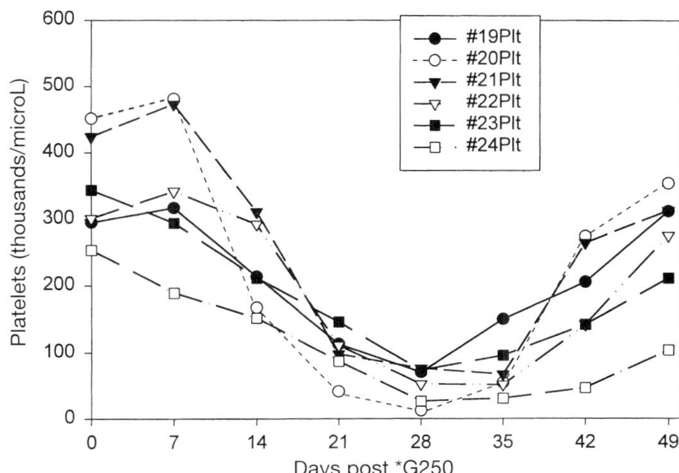

Fig. 13.3 Platelet counts over time in the first six patients treated at the MTD$_A$ of 90 MCi/m^2 ^{131}I-labelled mG250.

first six patients treated at the MTD$_A$. Severe toxicity did not last more than a week in any patient. No patient required platelet transfusion. Red blood cell counts were unchanged after therapy. Hematopoietic toxicity in this study was comparable to that seen in other studies with ^{131}I-labeled antibodies, confirming that dose-limiting toxicity was radionuclide-dependent.

There was targeting of radioactivity to all known tumor sites ≥ 2 cm, confirming the high fraction of G250-antigen-expressing tumors in patients with the clear cell subtype of RCC. Lesions ≥ 2 cm in size independent of location were visualized by scintigraphy by the first imaging scan, between 2 and 4 days after administration of ^{131}I-labeled G250. Targeting was comparable to the primary tumor (in those patients who had not had nephrectomy), as well as to bone, liver, lung, nodal, and subcutaneous metastases.

All patients developed human antimouse antibodies (HAMA) within 4 weeks posttherapy; re-treatment was therefore not possible. Seventeen of 33 evaluable patients had stable disease. There were no major responses.

Clinical trials with chimeric (human/mouse) G250

In order to reduce immunogenicity and permit multiple administrations, a chimeric version of G250 (cG250), where a human Fc region has replaced the murine Fc (crystallizable fragment) region, was engineered. This genetic manipulation maintains the murine Fab (antigen-binding fragment) region and, therefore, the specificity of CA IX binding while eliminating many potentially immunogenic murine peptide sequences.

Phase I protein dose escalation study

This study, similar in design to the initial study with murine G250 (Oosterwijk *et al.* 1993), was carried out to determine the pharmacokinetics, toxicity, immunogenicity, and imaging characteristics of ^{131}I-labeled chimeric mAb G250 in patients with RCC (Steffens *et al.* 1997).

The *in vitro* binding characteristics of cG250 were similar to those of mG250, demonstrating that chimerization of the antibody did not affect specificity, affinity, or avidity. In general, the *in vivo* behaviour, including the half-life ($t_{1/2}\beta$), of cG250 was comparable to mG250 ($t_{1/2}\beta$ cGT250 68.5 h versus $t_{1/2}\beta$ mG250 47 h).

Saturable, antigen-mediated liver uptake was observed with cG250, similar to that with mG250. This liver uptake is in accordance with the known antigen expression on the larger bile ducts, and comparable to mG250 uptake.

Tumor uptake exceeding 0.1 per cent infectious dose (ID)/g was observed only at the 2, 5, and 10 mg dose levels, while maximum uptake at the 25 and 50 mg dose level was 0.0170 and 0.0120 per cent ID/g, respectively, suggesting saturation of accessible G250 epitopes in the tumor at the higher protein doses. In the study

with mG250 a similar relative decrease in tumor uptake with increasing protein dose was observed. These observations are similar to those made in myelogenous leukemia with antibody M195, against the CD33 receptor (Scheinberg *et al.* 1991). In contrast, in investigations with other antitumor antibodies, doses of 10 mg/kg or more have been administered without any indication of tumor saturation.

Antigen-mediated tumor uptake of ^{131}I-labeled cG250 was demonstrated by the difference in uptake between antigen-positive versus antigen-negative tumors: uptake in samples of antigen-negative tumors (7 days post-intake) did not exceed 0.0040 per cent ID/g (blood 7 days post-intake: 0.0042 per cent ID/g), while uptake in antigen-positive tumors was as high as 0.5233 per cent ID/g (blood: 0.0028 per cent ID/g). Extensive sampling of the primary tumors showed that regional differences in tumor uptake were as high as two orders of magnitude.

A weak human anti-chimeric antibody (HACA) response was observed in two of 16 patients, illustrating the reduced immunogenicity of cG250 compared to its murine progenitor. Therefore, multiple treatments with cG250 seemed feasible. These observations are in accordance with the results of numerous other studies; Meredith *et al.*(1993) showed that chimerization of mAb 17-1A reduced immunogenicity, and Buist *et al.* (1993) found similar results with chimeric mAb MOv18. Chimeric G250 was able to localize to clear cell RCC in a manner comparable to the parent murine vesion. Dosimetry analysis indicated that lymph node and bone metastases received approximately 0.20–0.23 Gy/mCi. Assuming a 2 Gy maximum tolerated dose to bone marrow (the dose-limiting organ), 200 mCi should be tolerable. This would yield radiation absorbed doses to tumor close to sterilizing levels.

All antigen-positive primary tumors as well as all metastatic lesions, as identified by conventional imaging techniques, were visualized. No additional lesions were detected. Bander *et al.* (1996) reported 90 per cent successful imaging of primary RCC sites with ^{131}I-labeled mG250. Additionally, occult lesions, confirmed at surgery were visualized. Larger, prospective studies are needed to evaluate the diagnostic potential of mAb G250 as an imaging agent. This study demonstrated that radiation-absorbed doses close to tumor-sterilizing levels seemed achievable, whereas the highly reduced immunogenicity opened the possibility of multiple treatment therapy.

Phase I ^{131}I-labeled cG250 radioimmunotherapy

Based on the cG250 protein dose escalation study, a dose escalation with ^{131}I-labeled cG250 study was performed (Steffens *et al.* 1999). Patients initially received a scout dose of 5 mg ^{131}I-labeled cG250 (6 mCi) to demonstrate tumor targeting, followed a week later with 5 mg labeled with increasing amounts of ^{131}I, provided the scout dose had demonstrated targeting to tumor.

Twelve patients with metastatic RCC were studied. All patients had undergone nephrectomy and had measurable, progressing disease at the time of treatment. The scout ^{131}I-labeled cG250 images demonstrated tumor targeting in nine of 12 patients. As with murine G250, metastatic tumors were visualized from 1 to 2 days after injection, with improving image quality over time due to the background clearance of ^{131}I-labeled cG250 and, presumably, the lack of shedding or modulation of antibody/antigen. One patient progressed precluding therapy. Eight patients therefore received a second injection.

Immunoscintigrams obtained after injection were almost identical to one another, confirming that the distribution of the therapeutic injection could be accurately predicted on the basis of the scans obtained after the administration of the tracer dose. Again, as with the murine studies, hematopoietic toxicity was dose-limiting, with a nadir between 4 and 6 weeks. Based on the observations in these eight patients, MTD was determined to be 60 mCi/m^2 [131]I.

In contrast to radioimmunotherapy with murine mAb G250, no hepatic toxicity was seen in any of the patients treated. The only difference in trial design was the administration of a diagnostc, scout dose of 5 mg cG250 (labeled with 6 mCi ^{131}I). The absence of live-toxicity may be explained by saturation of the hepatic compartment by the first dose (Steffens *et al.* 1999; Divgi *et al.* 1998), or the lower hepatic uptake of chimeric mAb cG250. At equal doses, liver uptake of murine mAb G250 (Divgi *et al.* 1998) was 2–3 times higher than the liver uptake of chimeric mAb cG250 (Steffens *et al.* 1997).

Another difference between the murine ^{131}I-labeled G250 and the chimeric ^{131}I-labeled cG250 is the lower MTD of ^{131}I-labeled cG250. The MTD with murine ^{131}I-labeled G250 was 90 mCi/m^2 [131]I (Divgi *et al.* 1998), whereas that of a single therapeutic dose of ^{131}I-labeled cG250 MTD was 60 mCi/m^2 [131]I. This lower MTD can be explained by the longer circulation time of chimeric mAb cG250 compared to murine mAb G250 ($t_{1/2}$*gb: 69 h versus 47 h, respectively), with consequently higher bone marrow radiation absorbed dose.

For both chimeric and murine G250 radioimmunotherapy, bone marrow dose was a better predictor of hematopoietic toxicity than administratered activity. Sgouros *et al.* (1997) reported that determination of whole-body radiation absorbed dose was the best predictor for bone marrow toxicity.

One patient treated at the MTD had a partial response (> 50 per cent reduction in size of tumor lesions) lasting for 9 months. One patient who had already received cG250 had a positive HACA response. No HACA responses were detected in the sera of any other patients collected up to 10 weeks after the second ^{131}I-labeled cG250 administration. These results warrant further study in a phase II setting at MTD. Despite the reported radioresistance of RCC, the radiation-absorbed doses to tumor seen in these trials offer the potential for significant tumoricidal effects. cG250 is a very suitable candidate for radioimmunotherapy of RCC. Several strategies—necessary to increase the radiation dose to tumors—are available and future studies will focus on optimization of this therapeutic approach for patients with metastasized RCC.

Fractionated cG250 therapy

Tumor uptake of cG250 in patients with primary RCC is among the highest reported in solid tumors. However, as in other tumor types, heterogeneous intratumoral antibody distribution may limit the efficacy of radioimmunotherapy. In a subsequent study we showed that this heterogeneous mAb cG250 distribution could not be attributed solely to: (1) antigen expression; (2) blood vessel density; (3) reactive stromal tissue; or (4) necrosis (Steffens *et al.* 1999*b*).

To further analyse the heterogeneous tumor uptake of mAb cG250, a study was performed (Steffens *et al.* 1999*c*) to investigate whether tumor uptake is influenced by dynamic factors, for example, heterogeneous blood supply, elevated interstitial pressure, or large transport distances in the interstitium. If these factors play a major role in the intratumoral distribution of antibodies, mAb cG250 distribution in RCC is likely to change with time. Repetitive injections would then target different areas within a tumor.

Ten patients with a clinical diagnosis of primary RCC were studied. Nine days before surgery patients received ^{125}I-cG250 (5 mg cG250, 50 μCi ^{125}I) followed by a second injection of ^{131}I-cG250 (5 mg cG250, 3.5 mCi ^{131}I) 4 days later. Tumor obtained at surgery was sliced, mapped, and cut into 1 cm^3 cubes. Each cube was analyzed for ^{125}I-cG250 and ^{131}I-cG250 uptake and the ^{131}I/^{125}I ratio determined. For each tumor slice, the distribution patterns of both isotopes were reconstructed and compared with each other.

There was heterogeneous distribution of both isotopes throughout all tumor slices, with focal uptake varying from high (up to 0.19 per cent ID/g) to relatively low (as low as 0.0047 per cent ID/g) uptake. Surprisingly, without any exception, the uptake of ^{125}I-cG250 was similar to ^{131}I-cG250 uptake in all samples analyzed ($n = 692$). Overall, the [131]I / ^{125}I-ratio was 1.72 ± 0.45 (mean ± SD), while regional differences (that is, different samples) in uptake of the same antibody injection sometimes exceeded a factor of 40 or more. This is an unexpected finding in view of temporal and spatial blood flow heterogeneity. The constant [131]I / ^{125}I-ratios, observed in all tumor smaples investigated, suggest that parameters governing mAb cG250 uptake in tumor do not alter significantly within the time period studied. This observation has implications for timing of fractionated immunotherapy: the separate fractions must be sufficiently spaced to allow targeting of different tumor areas, possibly accessible by radiation-induced alterations in the tumor. Additionally, heterogeneous tumor uptake may be less prominent in smaller tumors, circumventing insufficient cG250 uptake in particular areas.

Fractionated radioimmunotherapy with ^{131}I-labeled cG250

Experimental data suggests that multiple administrations of radiolabeled antibody may have greater therapeutic effect than a single infusion (Schlom *et al.* 1990). A phase I radioimmunotherapy trial to evaluate the utility of multiple, out-patient administrations of ^{131}I-labeled cG250 in patients with measurable metastatic RCC has just been concluded. The lack of immunogenicity permitted a design whereby whole-body and serum clearance characteristics of an initial dose of ^{131}I-labeled cG250 were used, using a two-compartment model, to calculate fractionated radio-immunotherapy with multiple doses of ^{131}I-labeled cG250 that would deliver a specified whole-body radiation dose.

Starting with an initial dose of 30 mCi/5 mg ^{131}I-labeled cG250, varying amounts of ^{131}I-labeled cG250 were administered at 2–3 day intervals such that the total amount of radioactivity in the body did not exceed 30 mCi [131]I. Patients with no evidence of disease progression were retreated at intervals of between 8 and 12 weeks, after recovery from any toxicity.

A total of 15 patients were treated. The maximum tolerated whole-body radiation absorbed dose was determined to be 0.75 Gy. Again, in contrast to the radioimmunotherapy trial with ^{131}I-labeled murine G250, there was no hepatic toxicity, presumably due to saturation of hepatic receptors by the scout doses of cG250. Moreover, an anti-antibody response, manifest by altered serum and whole body clearance of radioactivity, and (subsequently) by detection of serum HACA, was seen in only one of 15 patients. Three patients completed two treatment courses (five, eight, and four infusions each, respectively); one patient could not complete the third course because of altered serum and whole-body clearance of radioactivity. Interestingly, his serum HACA titers were negative at the time of initiation of the third course of therapy. Two other patients completed three treatment courses (five and eight infusions each, respectively). There has been close correlation between actual and predicted clearance of all treaments, except in the one patient who developed HACA. Targeting to tumor has been excellent in all patients, and targeting of each treatment has been comparable. Figure 13.4 shows whole-body images obtained at comparable time points in a patient treated at the 50 cGy whole-body dose. There have been no major responses.

Summary

In summary, there is strong indirect evidence that the host immune system is intimately involved in the natural history of renal cancer. Immunological studies are providing information on tumor-related differentiation antigens of the kidney and beginning to allow molecular subclassification of renal cancer subtypes. Initial indications are that these subtypes have practical clinical relevance. Lastly, mAb probes, which have clearly proven their value as *in vitro* diagnostics, are now demonstrating a role as *in vivo* imaging agents and therapeutics in nonneoplastic and neoplastic diseases. Efforts continue to develop such an approach in RCC.

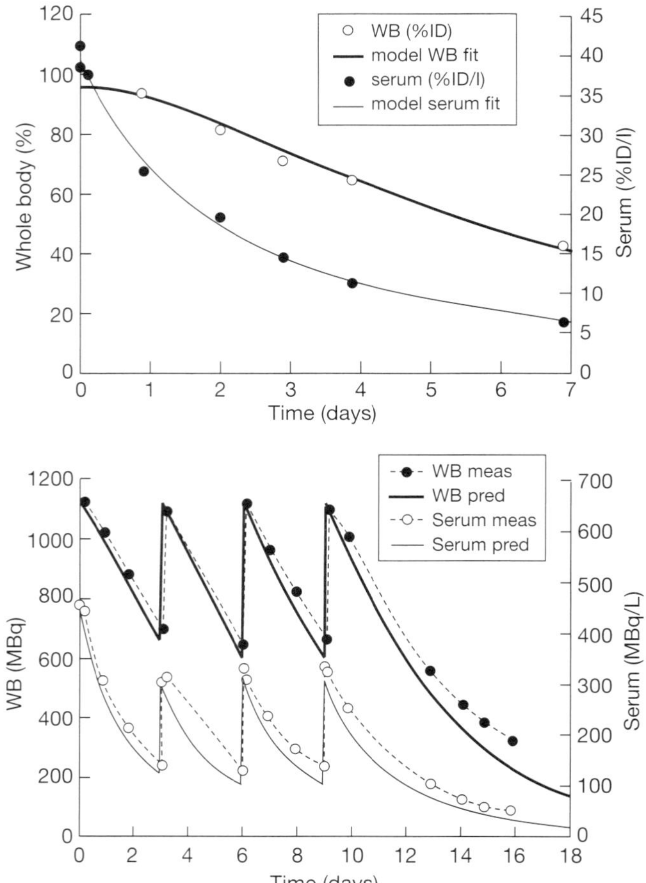

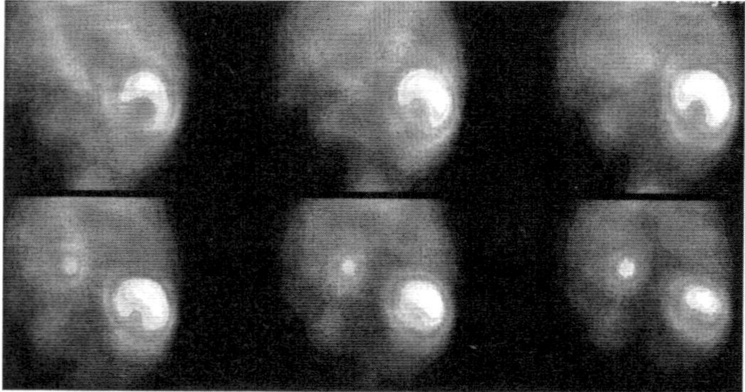

Fig. 13.4 Fractionated radioimmunotherapy with ^{131}I-labelled cG250. Upper left figure demonstrates 2compartmental model fitted on whole-body and serum radioactivity clearance data, obtained over a week. Upper right figure demonstrates actual (broken curves) and predicted (solid curves) clearances in the same patient. The images represent coronal slices (posterior to anterior, upper left to lower right) obtained 3 days after 30 mCi/5 mg ^{131}I-labelled cG250 in a patient with RCC (with its photopenic center, solid arrow) and liver (broken arrow) metastases.

References

Bander, N.H., Cordon-Cardo, C., Finstad, C.L., *et al.* (1985). Immuno-histologic dissection of the human kidney using monoclonal antibodies. *J. Immunol.* **133**, 502–5.

Bander, N.H., Finstad, C.L., Cordon-Cardo, C., *et al.* (1989). Analysis of a mouse monoclonal antibody that reacts with a specific region of the human proximal tubule and subsets of renal cell carcinomas. *Cancer Res.* **49**, 6774–80.

Bander, N.H., Divgi, C., Finn, R.D., Larson, S., and Old, L.J. (1996). Renal cancer imaging with monoclonal antibody (mAb) G250. *J. Urol.* **155** (Suppl.;abstract 1088), 583A.

Brakenhoff, R.H., Knippels, E.M., and van Dongen, G.A. (1994). Optimization and simplification of expression cloning in eukaryotic vector/host systems. *Anal. Biochem.* **218**, 460–63. [Published erratum in *Anal. Biochem.* **221** (1994), 434.]

Buist, M.R., Kenemans, P., Den Hollander, W., *et al.* (1993). Kinetics and tissue distribution of the radiolabeled monoclonal antibody Mov18 IgG and F(ab')$_2$ fragments in ovarian carcinoma patients. *Cancer Res.* **53**, 5413–18.

Burnet, M. (1970). *Immunological surveillance.* Pergamon Press, Oxford.

Cordon-Cardo, C., Lloyd, K.O., Finstad, C.L., *et al.* (1986). Immunoanatomic distribution of blood group antigens in the human urinary tract. *Lab. Invest.* **55**, 444–54.

Cordon-Cardo, C., Finstad, C.L., Bander, N.H., and Melamed, M.R. (1987). Immunoanatomic distribution of cytostructural and tissue-associated antigens in the human urinary tract. *Am. J. Pathol.* **126**, 269–84.

Divgi, C.R., Bander, N.H., Scott, A.M., *et al.* (1998). Phase I/II radio-immunotherapy trial with iodine-131-labeled monoclonal antibody G250 in metastatic renal cell carcinoma. *Clin. Cancer Res.* **4**, 2729–39.

Ebert, T., Bander, N.H., Finstad, C.L., Ramsawak, R.D., and Old. L.J. (1990). Establishment and characterization of human renal cancer and normal kidney cell lines. *Cancer Res.* **50**, 5531–6.

Everson, T.C. and Cole, W.H. (1966). *Spontaneous regression of cancer.* Saunders, Philadelphia.

Freed, S.Z., Halperin, J.P., and Gordon, M. (1977). Idiopathic regression of metastases from renal cell carcinoma. *J. Urol.* **118**, 538–42.

Gnarra, J.R., Tory, K., Weng, Y., *et al.* (1994). Mutations of the VHL tumor suppressor gene in renal carcinoma. *Nature Genet.* **7**, 85–90.

Gross, L. (1943). Intradermal immunization of C33H mice against a sarcoma that originated in an animal of the same line. *Cancer Res.* **3**, 326–33.

Ivanov, S.V., Kuzmin, I., Wei, M.H., Pack,S., Geil, L., Johnson, B.E., Stanbridge, E.J., and Lerman, M.I. (1998). Down-regulation of transmembrane carbonic anhydrases in renal cell carcinoma cell lines by wild-type von Hippel–Lindau transgenes. *Proc. Natl Acad. Sci., USA* **95**, 12596–601.

Kohler, G. and Milstein, C. (1975). Continuous cultures of fused cells secreting antibody of predefined specificity. *Nature* **256**, 495–7.

Meredith, R.F., Khazaeli, M.B., Grizzle, W.E., *et al.* (1993). Direct localization comparison of murine and chimeric B72.3 antibodies in patients with colon cancer. *Human Antibodies Hybridomas* **4**, 190–7.

Oliver, R.T., Nethersell, A.B., and Bottomley, J.M. (1989), Unexplained spontaneous regression and alpha-interferon as treatment for metastatic renal carcinoma. *Br. J. Urol.* **63**, 128–31.

Oosterwijk, E., Ruiter, D.J., Hoedemaeker, P.J., *et al.* (1986). Monoclonal antibody G250 recognizes a determinant present in renal-cell carcinoma and absent from normal kidney. *Int. J. Cancer* **38**, 489–94.

Oosterwijk, E., Bander, N.H., Divgi, C.R., *et al.* (1993). Antibody localization in human renal cell carcinoma: a phase I study of monoclonal antibody G250. *J. Clin. Oncol.* **11**, 738–50.

Opavsky, R., Pastorekova, S., Zelnik, V., Gibadulinova, A., Stanbridge, E.J., Zavada, J., Kettmann, R., and Pastorek, J. (1996). Human MN/CA9 gene, a novel member of the carbonic anhydrase family: structure and exon to protein domain relationships. *Genomics* **33**, 480–7.

Pastorek, J., Pastorekova, S., Callebaut, I., Mornon, J.P., Zelnik, V., Opavsky, R., Zat'ovicova, M., Liao, S., Portetelle, D., and Stanbridge, E.J. (1994). Cloning and characterization of MN, a human tumor-associated protein with a domain homologous to carbonic anhydrase and a putative helix-loop-helix DNA binding segment. *Oncogene* **9**, 2877–88.

Prehn, R.T. and Main, J.M. (1957). Immunity to methylocholanthrene-induced sarcomas. *J. Natl Cancer Inst.* **18**, 769–78.

Rosenberg, S.A., Lotze, M.T., Yang, J.C., *et al.* (1993). Prospective randomized trial of high-dose interleukin-2 alone or in conjunction with lymphokine-activated killer cells for the treatment of patients with advanced cancer. *J. Natl. Cancer Inst.* **85**, 622–32.

Scheinberg, D.A., Lovett, D., Divgi, C.R., Graham, M.C., Berman, E., Pentlow, K., Feirt, N., Finn, R.D., Clarkson, B.D., Gee, T.S., *et al.* (1991). A phase I trial of monoclonal antibody M195 in acute myelogenous leukemia: specific bone marrow targeting and internalization of radionuclide. *J. Clin. Oncol.* **9**, 478–90.

Schlom, J., Molinolo, A., Simpson, J.F., *et al.* (1990). Advantage of dose fractionation in monoclonal antibody-targeted radioimmunotherapy. *J. Natl Cancer Inst.* **82**, 763–71.

Schmidt, L., Duh, F.M., Chen, F., *et al.* (1997). Germline and somatic mutations in the tyrosine kinase domain of the MET proto-oncogene in papillary renal carcinomas. *Nature Genet.* **16**, 68–73.

Sgouros, G., Deland, D., Loh, A.C., *et al.* (1997). Marrow and whole-body absorbed dose vs marrow toxicity following ^{131}I-G250 antibody therapy in patients with renal-cell carcinoma. *J. Nucl. Med.* **1997**, 252P.

Snow, R.M. and Schellhammer, P.F. (1982). Spontaneous regression of metastatic renal cell carcinoma. *J. Urol.* **20**, 177–81.

Steffens, M.G., Boerman, O.C., Oosterwijk-Wakka, J.C., Oosterhof, G.O., Witjes, J.A., Koenders, E.B., Oyen, W.J., Buijs, W.C., Debruyne, F.M., Corstens, F.H., and Oosterwijk, E. (1997). Targeting of renal cell carcinoma with iodine-131-labeled chimeric monoclonal antibody G250. *J. Clin. Oncol.* **15**, 1529–37.

Steffens, M.G., Boerman, O.C., de Mulder, P.H., Oyen, W.J., Buijs, W.C., Witjes, J.A., van den Broek, W.J., Oosterwijk-Wakka, J.C., Debruyne, F.M., Corstens, F.H., and Oosterwijk, E. (1999*a*). Phase I radioimmunotherapy of metastatic renal cell carcinoma with ^{131}I-labeled chimeric monoclonal antibody G250. *Clin. Cancer Res.* **5** (10 Suppl.), 3268s–3274s.

Steffens, M.G., Oosterwijk, Wakka, J.C., Zegwaart-Hagemeier, N.E., Boerman, O.C., Debruyne, F.M., Corstens, F.H., and Oosterwijk, E. (1999*b*). Immunohistochemical analysis of tumor antigen saturation following injection of monoclonal antibody G250. *Anticancer Res.* **19**, 1197–200.

Steffens, M.G., Boerman, O.C., Oyen, W.J., Krst, P.H., Witjes, J.A., Oosterhof, G.O., van Leenders, G.J., Debruyne, F.M., Corstens, F.H., and Oosterwijk, E. (1999*c*). Intratumoral distribution of two consecutive injections of chimeric antibody G250 in primary renal cell carcinoma: implications for fractionated dose radioimmunotherapy. *Cancer Res.* **59**, 1615–19.

Vogelzang, N.J., Priest, E.R., and Borden, L. (1992). Spontaneous regression of histologically proven pulmonary metastases from renal cell carcinoma: a case with five-year follow-up. *J. Urol.* **148**, 1247–8.

14. Tumor vaccines

Stephen J. Freedland, Amnon Zisman, and Arie S. Belldegrun

Introduction and background

The concept of vaccines dates back thousands of years, but until recently vaccines were used primarily to prevent infectious diseases. With recent advances in cellular biology, molecular biology, and immunology there has been an interest in the use of vaccines not only to prevent infectious diseases, but also to treat a wide variety of human diseases. This has given hope that vaccines can be developed that will treat cancer.

History of vaccines

The first recorded attempts at vaccination occurred in China as early as 1014 C.E. (Plotkin and Plotkin 1994). Scabs from patients infected with smallpox were used to vaccinate healthy patients. Edward Jenner carried out the first scientific attempts at vaccination in 1798, using cowpox to vaccinate people against smallpox. The next milestone in the history of vaccines occurred in 1885, when Louis Pasteur developed a live attenuated vaccine against rabies. By the early 1900s several vaccines had been developed that relied on the use of whole killed organisms. It was during this period that the bacille Calmette–Guérin (BCG) vaccine for tuberculosis was developed in 1909. However, the golden age of vaccine development began in the late 1940s with the discovery by a group of researchers from Boston Children's Hospital of how to grow human viruses outside a living host. This development allowed Jonas Salk to develop his vaccine for poliomyelitis in 1954. Public concern about the safety of vaccines led scientists to investigate new methods of vaccination that did not rely on whole killed, or attenuated organisms. The search for safer vaccines and the rise of molecular biology led to the development of a recombinant DNA vaccine for hepatitis B in 1986. The ultimate dream of vaccination became a reality in 1980, when the World Health Organization declared smallpox eradicated. With the hope of similar achievements scientists are beginning to investigate the use of vaccines for the treatment of cancer.

Results of cytokine-based immunotherapy

Renal cell carcinoma (RCC) metastasis has been shown on rare occasion to regress following removal of the primary tumor. The incidence in the literature ranges from 0 to 6 per cent, with the true incidence probably less than 1 per cent (Myers *et al.* 1968; Montie *et al.* 1977; Oliver 1989). Those patients with large primary tumors and small metastases and those with isolated pulmonary nodules are most likely to have spontaneous regression following removal of the primary tumor. This suggests that the host immune system is capable of eradicating metastatic disease and that the primary tumor has an immunosuppressive effect.

The results of chemotherapy for RCC have been very disappointing with a total response rate of around 6 per cent (Yagoda *et al.* 1995). The fact that RCC on rare occasions undergoes spontaneous regression suggesting it can be an immunogenic tumor and the poor response rates with chemotherapy led investigators to use immunotherapy utilizing various cytokines such as interleukin-2 (IL-2) and interferon-alpha (IFNα). Early studies of IFNα as single agent for metastatic RCC showed promising results with total response rates of around 40 per cent (deKernion and Lindner 1982; Quesada *et al.* 1983). However, larger studies showed that the response is 15–20 per cent (deKernion *et al.* 1983; Kirkwood *et al.* 1985; Figlin *et al.* 1988).

High-dose IL-2 has been shown to stimulate an antitumor response against RCC when given as a single agent with total response rates around 15–20 per cent (Fisher *et al.* 1988, 2000; Rosenberg *et al.* 1994; Fisher *et al.* 2000). Based upon these results, the US Food and Drug Administration (FDA) has approved high-dose IL-2 for the therapy of good performance status patients with metastatic RCC. It is currently the only FDA-approved treatment for metastatic RCC. However, high-dose IL-2 is associated with significant toxicity including the development of a capillary leak syndrome with associated hypotension, prerenal azotemia, and respiratory distress (Belldegrun and deKernion 1998). In attempts to minimize the toxicity of high-dose IL-2, it has been given at low dose or combined with other cytokines such as IFNα (Belldegrun and deKernion 1998). The combination of IL-2 and IFNα has been shown to result in around 25–30 per cent total response with markedly decreased toxicity relative to high-dose IL-2 (Figlin *et al.* 1995; Locatelli *et al.* 1999).

Passive versus active immunotherapy

Passive or adoptive immunotherapy involves the transfer to the tumor-bearing host of active immunologic reagents, such as cells with antitumor reactivity that can mediate either directly or indirectly antitumor effects. Rosenberg and colleagues (1985) first reported on this type of immunotherapy for RCC from the National Cancer Institute. Patients were treated with lymphokine-activated killer (LAK) cells and recombinant IL-2. Subsequent studies showed a total response rate of 33 per cent (Rosenberg 1988). Whereas LAK cells are mainly activated natural killer (NK) cells, tumor-infiltrating lymphocytes (TIL) are activated cytotoxic T cells. In experimental systems, TIL are 50–100 times more powerful than LAK cells. Despite early exciting results from the use of TIL for adoptive immunotherapy protocols (Pierce *et al.* 1995), a recent large multicenter trial showed no benefit relative to IL-2 alone (Figlin *et al.* 1999).

Active immunotherapy refers to the immunization of the tumor-bearing host with materials that attempt to induce in the host a state of immune responsiveness to the tumor. Most attempts at active immunotherapy in the last several decades have involved active immunotherapy using nonspecific immune stimulators with the hope that a nonspecific increase in human reactivity would lead to an augmented antitumor response. The nonspecific immune stimulators used have included BCG (Morales and Eidinger 1976; Morales *et al.* 1982; Oliver *et al.* 1988), *Corynebacterium parvum* (McCune *et al.* 1981), and transfer factor (Montie *et al.* 1977).

Besides nonspecific immune stimulators, active immunotherapy can be carried out using specific immune stimulators. Examples include irradiated tumor cells with or without adjuvant immune stimulators, irradiated tumor cells genetically engineered to secrete specific cytokines, soluble tumor cell antigens or irradiated tumor cells along with specific cytokines, dendritic cell therapy, and antibody-based tumor vaccines. It is this active specific immunotherapy that is most often referred to as 'tumor vaccines'.

Designing human tumor vaccines

Unfortunately, there are relatively few answers to the many questions that need to be answered when designing a tumor vaccine trial. Questions include the following:

- Which anatomic location of vaccine inoculation provides the greatest response?
- How many inoculations are needed to provide a sustained immune response?
- How many tumor cells are needed in each inoculation to elicit an immune response?
- What level of cytokine expression from genetically engineered cells is required to promote an antitumor response?

While answers to some of these questions have been suggested, no definitive answers exist. Moreover, what works best in animal models may not be ideal in human trials. Thus, though the field contains many examples of human clinical trials, much more understanding of the basic biology of tumor vaccines is required in order to design the 'ideal' tumor vaccine.

Unmodified tumor cells as vaccines

Allogeneic tumor vaccines

Allogeneic tumor vaccines have the advantage of ease of use. A separate cell line does not need to be created for each individual patient. This obviates the need to expand individual patient's tumor cells *in vitro* with the associated difficulties and cost thereof. Moreover, the propagation of human tumor cells is difficult and often results in a single (or few) clone(s) that might not express all the associated antigens of the parental heterogeneous tumor. Therefore, the use of an allogeneic tumor could potentially supply a greater diversity of antigens.

In animal studies, treatment with an allogeneic, but not autologous cell line resulted in an antitumor effect against the autologous tumor (Knight *et al.* 1996). However, Aruga *et al.* (1997) found that syngeneic cells are more potent as a tumor vaccine adjuvant than allogeneic cells. Kugler *et al.* (1998) compared the vaccination of patients with a hybrid of irradiated allogeneic tumor cells and allogeneic activated lymphocytes to unmodified autologous tumor cells. Six of the 13 patients receiving the hybrid vaccine responded to the treatment compared to only three of the 13 who received autologous tumor. However, it is difficult to draw any conclusions from this small sample size. A recently suggested approach is to fuse allogeneic cells with tumor cells for use as a vaccine (Gong *et al.* 1997). Gong and colleagues fused autologous tumor cells with allogeneic dendritic cells (see below) and used the fusion cells as a tumor vaccine. In preclinical studies, this was shown to inhibit tumorigenicity, protect against tumor challenge, and induce rejection of established metastasis (Gong *et al.* 1997).

Autologous tumor

Autologous tumor has the theoretical advantage of being able to generate a more specific antitumor response. Allogeneic tumor vaccines rely on the fact that common antigens exist between the host tumor and the allogeneic tumor. However, until these common antigens are identified and their prevalence among RCC tumors is known, autologous tumor vaccines will predominate. One such tumor-specific antigen, G250, has been identified and studies on how to use this antigen to design more specific tumor vaccines are ongoing (see below).

Repmann *et al.* (1997) treated 116 patients with autologous tumor vaccine. All patients had undergone a radical nephrectomy with curative intent. They compared these patients to a retrospectively collected cohort of 106 patients treated by nephrectomy alone. With a mean observation of 15 months, those patients who received adjuvant tumor vaccine had a clear survival advantage ($p = 0.0007$). The 2-year survival for the treated group was 92 per cent compared to 75 per cent for the control group. Treatment was associated with minimal toxicity in less than 2 per cent of patients. Though this study is retrospective and suffers from potential selection bias with a short follow-up, the results are exciting.

BCG as adjuvant

BCG was originally developed as a vaccine for tuberculosis in the early 1900s. With the discovery of its antitumor effect in bladder cancer (Morales *et al.* 1976), there has been interest in using BCG for immunotherapy on other types of cancer. BCG has been used as a single-agent treatment for patients with RCC with modest success (Morales and Eidinger 1976; Morales *et al.* 1982, Oliver *et al.* 1988). Hara *et al.* (1996) vaccinated animals with tumor cells modified to secrete IL-2, and found that co-vaccination with BCG led to an enhanced antitumor response.

Several investigators have treated patients with a combination of either irradiated autologous tumor cells or soluble tumor antigens and BCG (Neidhart *et al.* 1980; Adler *et al.* 1987; Galligioni *et al.* 1996; Logan *et al.* 1998; Li *et al.* 2000). One of the early studies, using soluble tumor antigens and BCG, suggested a prolonged disease-free survival and overall survival relative to no treatment in 43 evaluable patients (Adler *et al.* 1987). While the majority of the studies since have demonstrated induction of a delayed type hypersensitivity to autologous tumor, none has shown any survival benefit from treatment (Neidhart *et al.* 1980; Galligioni *et al.* 1996; Logan *et al.* 1998; Li *et al.* 2000).

Cytokine-based tumor cell vaccines

In vitro and *in vivo* tumor models have largely focused on the use of autologous tumor vaccines rather than on allogeneic tumors. Theoretically, autologous tumors provide more specific antitumor response. *In vivo* models rely upon *ex vivo* expanded autologous tumor cells, which are then irradiated to prevent tumorigenicity and injected into the patient. Tumor vaccination studies have utilized either unmodified tumor cells, the co-application of unmodified tumor cells and systemic cytokine therapy, or tumor cells modified to express a wide array of cytokines. The cytokines examined in human and animal studies have included IL-2, IL-4, IL-12, IFNγ, tumor necrosis factor alpha (TNFα), and granulocyte–macrophage colony stimulating factor (GM-CSF). There are currently no prospective randomized clinical trials involving cytokine-based tumor cell vaccines in RCC showing a survival benefit. No phase III or even phase II trials have been completed. Therefore, what follows is a discussion of preclinical studies, non-randomized retrospective studies, and early phase I studies.

IL-2

IL-2 is a 15.5 kDa glycoprotein produced by activated T cells. It was first identified in 1975 as a growth-stimulating molecule for T cells (Morgan *et al.* 1976), and is produced by T helper cells upon antigen-induced activation of resting T cells. The list of actions of IL-2 is long, but it primarily appears to be involved in the growth and differentiation of T cells, B cells, NK cells, LAK cells, monocytes, macrophages, and oligodendrocytes. It is also important in the production of lymphokines from T helper cells.

On the basis of the results of using IL-2 as single-agent treatment for RCC (see above), several investigators have examined using tumor cells modified to express IL-2 as a tumor vaccine for RCC (Gansbacher *et al.* 1990*b*; Gastl *et al.* 1992; Hock *et al.* 1993). *In vitro* work has shown that the addition of RCC tumor cells transfected with the IL-2 gene to cultured TIL resulted in an augmented human leukocyte antigen (HLA)-restricted tumor-specific cytotoxicity (Itoh *et al.* 1994; Mulders *et al.* 1998). The use of control parental RCC cells failed to induce antitumor cytotoxicity (Itoh *et al.* 1994).

Animal studies have shown that vaccination with autologous tumor cells modified to secrete IL-2 prevented tumorigenicity and produced longlasting immunity to further challenges to the parental cell line in several different tumor models (Gansbacher *et al.* 1990*b*; Fearon *et al.* 1990; Hara *et al.* 1996). Human RCC cells modified to secrete IL-2 but not IFNγ prevented tumor formation by an allogeneic RCC cell line (Gastl *et al.* 1992). However, other studies showed tumor cells engineered to secrete IL-2 provided no advantage as potential immunogens to induce immunity relative to parental cells engineered to secrete GM-CSF (Dranoff *et al.* 1993) or adjuvant *Corynebacterium parvum* (Hock *et al.* 1993). Several studies have looked at the use of adjuvant treatment in addition to vaccination with autologous tumor cells modified to secrete IL-2. Various models tested include the co-transfection of B7–1, a co-stimulatory molecule for T cells; co-vaccination with BCG; and radiation therapy (Salvadori *et al.* 1995; Hara *et al.* 1996; Nishisaka *et al.* 1999). All of these studies showed that adjuvant treatment resulted in an augmented immune response and/or decreased tumorigenicity. Krup *et al.* (1999) looked at the use of unmodified autologous tumor given as a mixture with liposomal encapsulated IL-2. They found that, within a narrow IL-2 dose window, they were able to demonstrate longlasting immunity with a single vaccination.

Based upon the preclinical success with IL-2 based tumor vaccines, many clinical trials have focused on the use of IL-2. Human studies have generally used unmodified autologous tumor cells along with subcutaneous IL-2 injections (Williams *et al.* 1992; Pomer *et al.* 1995; Kirchner *et al.* 1995; Fenton *et al.* 1996). Another study used a mixture of autologous tumor cells and allogeneic fibroblasts modified to secrete IL-2 to vaccinate RCC patients (Veelken *et al.* 1997). While the results of these studies demonstrated establishment of delayed-type hypersensitivity to the vaccination, no clear treatment response or survival benefit was identified relative to IL-2 alone. Since several studies have shown that delayed-type hypersensitivity is associated with clinical response (Adler *et al.* 1987; McCune *et al.* 1990; Simons *et al.* 1997; Chang *et al.* 1997), it is possible that, with the inclusion of more patients, differences in treatment responses and survival will be identified.

IL-4

IL-4, first identified in 1982, is a 19 kDa glycoprotein that bears a close structural resemblance to GM-CSF. It is produced predominantly by T helper-2 cells and acts upon many different cell types, with the results often depending on the surrounding cells and other cytokines present. In general though, it is a growth stimulator for B cells.

Golumbek *et al.* (1991) modified a spontaneously arising murine RCC to secrete high levels of IL-4. Vaccination with the modified tumor cells resulted in rejection of the tumor cells in a T-cell-independent fashion and provided specific immunity to challenge with the parental line in a T-cell-dependent fashion. Moreover, inoculation with the modified tumor cells resulted in eradication of established parental tumors. Other studies have shown that tumor cells engineered to secrete IL-4 lost their tumorigenicity (Tepper *et al.* 1989; Li *et al.* 1990), which was found to mediated by an eosinophil-dependent pathway (Tepper *et al.* 1992) and could be blocked by antibodies against IFNγ

(Platzer *et al.* 1992). Dranoff *et al.* (1993) found that vaccination with IL-4-modified tumor cells provided specific immunity to further tumor challenges.

Currently, only one phase I trial of IL-4-directed tumor vaccines has been published (Suminami *et al.* 1995). Patients were given irradiated autologous tumor along with autologous fibroblasts modified to secrete IL-4. IL-4 expression was detectable at the biopsy site 14 days after vaccination. However, no clinical results have been published yet.

IL-12

IL-12 is a 75 kDa heterodimer that is produced primarily by activated macrophages. It modulates the cytolytic and proliferative activities of NK and LAK cells and helps direct naive T helper cells to a T helper-1 cytokine production profile.

IL-12 has been used as single-agent immunotherapy of metastatic RCC (Atkins *et al.* 1997). The intradermal injection of cDNA encoding the IL-12 gene has been shown to provide a continuous source of *in situ* IL-12 production, which inhibits tumor growth following the injection of unmodified murine renal carcinoma cells (Tan *et al.* 1996). Hara *et al.* (2000) transduced mouse RCC cells to secrete IL-12 and showed that this abrogated their tumorigenicity and prevented tumor growth from simultaneously injected unmodified tumor cells.

IFNγ

IFNγ is produced by activated T helper cells. It stimulates the increased production of class II major histocompatibility complex (MHC) molecules on antigen-presenting cells. This results in increased antigen presentation, which, in turn, stimulates cytotoxic T cells (CD8+) and results in an augmented immune response. Indeed, the modification of melanoma and RCC to express IFNγ resulted in increased expression of HLA class II molecules and augmented cytokine expression from co-cultured TIL (Ogasawara and Rosenberg 1993). Moreover, the modification of tumor cells to express IFNγ abrogated their tumorigenicity and created longlasting immunity to further challenges with the parental line (Gansbacher *et al.* 1990*a*). Similar findings have been obtained in other non-RCC tumor models (Watanabe *et al.* 1989; Esumi *et al.* 1991; el-Shami *et al.* 1999). Tumor cells modified to express IFNγ are protected from NK-cell-mediated death, which prolongs *in vivo* vaccine tumor cell half-life, allowing more time for T-cell priming (Zier and Gansbacher 1996). However, other studies found that IFNγ-directed tumor vaccines are inferior at abrogating tumorigenicity relative to other cytokines, such as IL-2 (Gastl *et al.* 1992) and GM-CSF (Dranoff *et al.* 1993).

TNFα

TNFα is a 17 kDa molecule produced predominantly by macrophages though a large variety of cells can produce TNFα. It was co-discovered by two separate groups, one who demonstrated its potent antitumor effects and thus named it TNF and by another group who demonstrated its significant systemic toxicity and named it cachectin. Later, these two molecules were found to be identical. The concept of tumor cells modified to secrete TNFα

as a tumor vaccine is attractive in that this would potentially avoid the systemic toxicity associated with high serum levels of TNFα.

Tumor cells engineered to secrete TNFα have resulted in decreased or abrogated tumorigenicity in several tumor models (Asher *et al.* 1991; Blankenstein *et al.* 1991; Teng *et al.* 1991). However, concerns about the use of TNFα have been raised by studies that showed that the injection of cells engineered to secrete TNFα resulted in cachexia and more rapid death, particularly when cells secreting high levels of TNFα were used (Oliff *et al.* 1987; Teng *et al.* 1991). Moreover, in animal experiments, TNFα-transfected tumor cells were less immunogenic than cells transfected with other cytokines, namely, GM-CSF (Dranoff *et al.* 1993). In the future, it is possible that new members of the TNF superfamily may show promising results in the development of tumor vaccines. Work is currently ongoing at UCLA to test the applicability of TNF-related apoptosis-inducing ligand (TRAIL) as a tumor vaccine to induce programmed cell death.

GM-CSF

GM-CSF is a 23 kDa glycoprotein that is secreted by a wide array of cells. GM-CSF, as its name implies, is a potent stimulator for the formation of granulocytes and macrophages. It has been used systematically in combination with IL-2 (Ryan *et al.* 2000). The results appear to present no additional benefit over IL-2 monotherapy for metastatic RCC. Using modified autologous tumor cells, Dranoff *et al.* (1993) directly compared several different cytokines for their ability to induce tumor immunity. Melanoma cells were engineered to express 10 different cytokines. Dranoff and colleagues found that, among animals vaccinated with tumor cells modified to express the various cytokines, those tumor cells expressing GM-CSF resulted in the most potent and longest lasting immunity to future tumor challenges. Moreover, they were able to show similar results in several different tumor models. Similarly, Nishisaka *et al.* (1999) showed that autologous tumor cells modified to express GM-CSF provided a comparable if not a greater reduction in tumorigenicity than cells modified to secrete IL-2 or IFNγ.

Despite the interest in GM-CSF based upon preclinical studies there have only been two phase I prospective randomized clinical trails published using GM-CSF tumor vaccines for RCC (Mahvi *et al.* 1997; Simons *et al.* 1997). While no follow-up data is available on the patients in these series, Simons *et al.* (1997) showed no dose-limiting toxicity in the first 16 patients, and that the toxicity of the GM-CSF arm was comparable to that of the unmodified autologous tumor vaccine arm. Hopefully, these ongoing clinical trials and others like them will shed light on the role of GM-CSF modified autologous tumor cell vaccines for patients with RCC.

Dendritic-cell-based tumor vaccines

Dendritic-cell-based immunization is an emerging new field in cancer immunotherapy research (Cella *et al.* 1997) (Fig. 14.1). Dendritic cells are the most potent antigen-presenting cells having the unique ability to take up, process, and present antigens including tumor epitopes (Steinman 1991). Dendritic-cell-based anticancer immunotherapy regimens seem appealing because well-characterized pathways of uptake, processing, and presentation have to be exploited. In general, dendritic cells can be generated by stimulation of bone-marrow-derived stem cells (CD34+) with GM-CSF and TNF (Caux *et al.* 1992) or by stimulation of circulating CD14+ monocytes with GM-CSF and IL-4 (Romani *et al.* 1994). Several strategies for introducing clinically relevant antigens to dendritic cells have been used in order to give a bottom line result of tumor epitope presentation in association with HLA class I or class II molecules: fusion of autologous (Gong *et al.* 1997) or allogeneic dendritic cells (Kugler *et al.* 2000) with tumor cells; pulsing dendritic cells with tumor lysate (Tuly) (Nestle *et al.* 1998), whole proteins (Paglia *et al.* 1996), peptides (van Elsas *et al.* 1996), or tumor-derived RNA (Boczkowski *et al.* 1996); and viral-mediated transfection of dendritic cells with genes encoding known tumor-associated antigens (Dietz and Vuk-Pavlovic 1998; Brossart *et al.* 1997). The practical advantages of these therapeutically outlined strategies are obvious. Dendritic cells can be isolated from patients' blood, armed with tumor antigens, and subsequently used to induce specific cytotoxic T cells (CD8+) (Romani *et al.* 1994; Celluzzi *et al.* 1996). A number of human phase I clinical trials have been launched using peptide/protein-loaded dendritic cells in different human cancers. Promising results were obtained, with no apparent side-effects after vaccination (Hsu *et al.* 1996; Murphy *et al.* 1996; Mukherji *et al.* 1995).

Antibody-based tumor vaccines

As for RCC, tumor antigens may be immunogenic and interact with components of the immune system to generate an antitumor effect (Boon *et al.* 1997; Rosenberg 1997) through binding to HLA-molecules (Rosenberg 1997; Van den Eynde and van der Bruggen 1997). Along with colon cancer, malignant melanoma, and other malignancies, RCC is believed to be immunogenic (Yannelli *et al.* 1996). The rare clinical phenomenon of spontaneous regression of metastases of RCC after nephrectomy is believed to result from an immune-mediated antitumor effect, endogenously generated by a yet unknown trigger (Papac 1996). RCC tumors have been shown to contain both CD4+ T helper TIL and anti-autologous RCC cytotoxic T lymphocytes (CTL) with specific antitumor reactivity (Yannelli *et al.* 1996). This supports the concept of interaction between RCC tumor antigens and cellular effectors of the immune system (Freed *et al.* 1977; Marcus *et al.* 1993; Gleave *et al.* 1998).

In order to launch a cellular anti-RCC attack using tumor-derived antigens, the antigen should be tissue-specific, expressed only in RCC cells, and found in all the tumors of the same histological type. Moreover, targeted antigens should not be subjected to fast mutations leading to changes in their antigenic epitopes. Lacking a distinctive tumor marker for RCC, CTL lines raised against autologous RCC Tuly were established and were found to have specific antitumor activity (Koo *et al.* 1991; Finke *et al.* 1992; Schendel *et al.* 1993; Gaugler *et al.* 1996; Mulders *et al.* 1998; Hinkel *et al.* 2000). Several clinical trials using dendritic cells loaded with Tuly alone and in combination with systemic IL-2 administration are under evaluation at UCLA and other centers.

Efforts to isolate antigens that are expressed in a majority of tumor lysates led to the identification and characterization of a mouse monoclonal antibody (mAb) against G250. Approximately 95 per cent of primary and 86 per cent of metastatic clear cell RCC are recognized by mouse mAb against G250, but normal renal or other cells are not, which is consistent with overexpression of G250 in RCC (Oosterwijk *et al.* 1986). Recent studies showed that G250 antigen is a transmembrane protein identical to the cervical cancer antigen NN/CA IX (Opavsky *et al.* 1996; Grabmaier 2000). The peptide sequence corresponding to amino acids 254 to 262 from G250 (BLSTAFARV) has been established as one possible epitope involved in the stimulation of CTL capable of HLA-A2.1-restricted lysis of cells expressing G250 (Vissers *et al.* 1999). To date, G250 is the only abundant and characterized RCC tumor antigen and may be a candidate for the development of anti-RCC cancer vaccines. To generate specific cytotoxic T cells against the G250 tumor antigen, dendritic cells can be exposed to either the full-length G250 protein or an immunogenic peptide within the protein sequence. Another novel approach is to combine a tumor antigen or anti-idiotype antibody of a specific tumor antigen to a cytokine, such as GM-CSF, capable of promoting the maturation of monocytes into dendritic cells (Tripathi *et al.* 1999). Such a fusion protein was constructed in UCLA using G250 and GM-CSF. By joining the RCC 'common denominator' antigen G250 with GM-CSF an enhanced antitumor activity was achieved *in vitro*, combining specifically targeted antigenicity and improved antigen presentation in an immune stimulated environment.

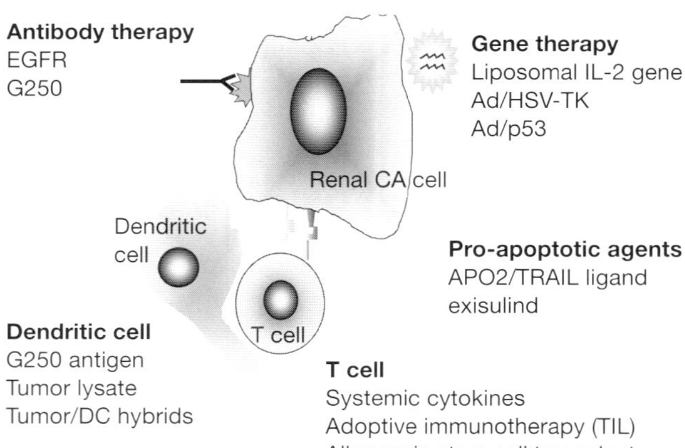

Fig. 14.1 New therapeutic approaches for the treatment of renal cell carcinoma.

References

Adler, A., Gillon, G., Lurie, H., Shaham, J., Loven, D., Shachter, Y., Shani, A., Servadio, C., and Stein, J.A. (1987). Active specific immunotherapy of renal cell carcinoma patients: a prospective randomized study of hormono-immuno-versus hormonotherapy. Preliminary report of immunological and clinical aspects. *J. Biol. Response Mod.* **6** (6), 610–24.

Aruga, A., Aruga, E., and Chang, A.E. (1997). Reduced efficacy of allogeneic versus syngeneic fibroblasts modified to secrete cytokines as a tumor vaccine adjuvant. *Cancer Res.* **57** (15), 3230–7.

Asher, A.L., Mule, J.J., Kasid, A., Restifo, N.P., Salo, J.C., Reichert, C.M., Jaffe, G., Fendly, B., Kriegler, M., and Rosenberg, S.A. (1991). Murine tumor cells transduced with the gene for tumor necrosis factor-alpha. Evidence for paracrine immune effects of tumor necrosis factor against tumors. *J. Immunol.* **146** (9), 3227–34.

Atkins, M.B., Robertson, M.J., Gordon, M., Lotze, M.T., DeCoste, M., DuBois, J.S., Ritz, J., Sandler, A.B., Edington, H.D., Garzone, P.D., Mier, J.W., Canning, C.M., Battiato, L., Tahara, H., and Sherman, M.L. (1997). Phase I evaluation of intravenous recombinant human interleukin 12 in patients with advanced malignancies. *Clin. Cancer Res.* **3** (3), 409–17.

Belldegrun. A.B. and deKernion, J.B. (1998). Renal tumors. In *Campbell's urology*, 7th edn (ed. P.C. Walsh, A.B. Retik, E.D. Vaughan, and A.J. Wein), pp. 2283–326. W.B. Saunders, Philadelphia.

Blankenstein, T., Qin, Z.H., Uberla, K., Muller, W., Rosen, H., Volk, H.D., and Diamantstein, T. (1991). Tumor suppression after tumor cell-targeted tumor necrosis factor alpha gene transfer. *J. Exp. Med.* **173** (5), 1047–52.

Boczkowski, D., Nair, S.K., Snyder, D., and Gilboa, E. (1996). Dendritic cells pulsed with RNA are potent antigen-presenting cells *in vitro* and *in vivo*. *J. Exp. Med.* **184** (2), 465–72.

Boon, T., Coulie, P.G., and Van den Eynde, B. (1997). Tumor antigens recognized by T cells. *Immunol. Today* **18** (6), 267–8.

Brossart, P., Goldrath, A.W., Butz, E.A., Martin, S., and Bevan, M.J. (1997). Virus-mediated delivery of antigenic epitopes into dendritic cells as a means to induce CTL. *J. Immunol.* **158** (7), 3270–6.

Caux, C., Dezutter-Dambuyant, C., Schmitt, D., and Banchereau, J. (1992). GM-CSF and TNF-alpha cooperate in the generation of dendritic Langerhans cells. *Nature* **360** (6401), 258–61.

Cella, M., Sallusto, F., and Lanzavecchia. A. (1997). Origin, maturation and antigen presenting function of dendritic cells. *Curr. Opin. Immunol.* **9** (1), 10–16.

Celluzzi, C.M., Mayordomo, J.I., Storkus, W.J., Lotze, M.T., and Falo, L.D.J. (1996). Peptide-pulsed dendritic cells induce antigen-specific CTL-mediated protective tumor immunity. *J. Exp. Med.* **183** (1), 283–7.

Chang, A.E., Aruga, A., Cameron, M.J., Sondak, V.K., Normolle, D.P., Fox, B.A., and Shu, S. (1997). Adoptive immunotherapy with vaccine-primed lymph node cells secondarily activated with anti-CD3 and interleukin-2. *J. Clin. Oncol.* **15** (2), 796–807.

deKernion, J.B. and Lindner, A. (1982). Treatment of advanced renal cell carcinoma. In *Proceedings of the First International Symposium on Kidney Tumors* (ed. R. Kuss, G. Murphy, S. Khoury, and J. Karr), p. 614. Alan R. Liss, New York.

deKernion, J.B., Sarna, G., Figlin, R., Lindner, A., and Smith, RB. (1983). The treatment of renal cell carcinoma with human leukocyte alpha-interferon. *J. Urol.* **130** (6), 1063–6.

Dietz, A.B. and Vuk-Pavlovic, S. (1998). High efficiency adenovirus-mediated gene transfer to human dendritic cells. *Blood* **91** (2), 392–8.

Dranoff, G., Jaffee, E., Lazenby, A., Golumbek, P., Levitsky, H., Brose, K., Jackson, V., Hamada, H., Pardoll, D., and Mulligan, R.C. (1993). Vaccination with irradiated tumor cells engineered to secrete murine granulocyte–macrophage colony-stimulating factor stimulates potent, specific, and long-lasting anti-tumor immunity. *Proc. Natl Acad. Sci., USA* **90** (8), 3539–43.

el-Shami, K.M., Tzehoval, E., Vadai, E., Feldman, M., and Eisenbach, L. (1999). Induction of antitumor immunity with modified autologous cells expressing membrane-bound murine cytokines. *J. Interferon Cytokine Res.* **19** (12), 1391–401.

Esumi, N., Hunt, B., Itaya, T., and Frost, P. (1991). Reduced tumorigenicity of murine tumor cells secreting gamma-interferon is due to nonspecific host responses and is unrelated to class I major histocompatibility complex expression. *Cancer Res.* **51** (4), 1185–9.

Fearon, E.R., Pardoll, D.M., Itaya, T., Golumbek, P., Levitsky, H.I., Simons, J.W., Karasuyama, H., Vogelstein, B., and Frost, P. (1990). Interleukin-2 pro-duction by tumor cells bypasses T helper function in the generation of an antitumor response. *Cell* **60** (3), 397–403.

Fenton, R.G., Steis, R.G., Madara, K., Zea, A.H., Ochoa, A.C., Janik, J.E., Smith, J.W. 2nd, Gause, B.L., Sharfman, W.H., Urba, W.J., Hanna, M.G., DeJager, R.L., Coyne, M.X., Crouch, R.D., Gray, P., Beveridge, J., Creekmore, S.P., Holmlund, J., Curti, B.D., Sznol, M., and Longo, D.L. (1996). A phase I randomized study of subcutaneous adjuvant IL-2 in combination with an autologous tumor vaccine in patients with advanced renal cell carcinoma. *J. Immunother. Emphasis Tumor Immunol.* **19** (5), 364–74.

Figlin, R.A., deKernion, J.B., Mukamel, E., Palleroni, A.V., Itri, L.M., and Sarna, G.P. (1988). Recombinant interferon alfa-2a in metastatic renal cell carcinoma: assessment of antitumor activity and anti-interferon antibody formation. *J. Clin. Oncol.* **6** (10), 1604–10.

Figlin, R.A., Gitlitz, B.J., and Belldegrun, A. (1995). Immunologic approaches to the treatment of cancer. *Cancer Invest.* **13** (3), 339–40.

Figlin, R.A., Thompson, J.A., Bukowski, R.M., Vogelzang, N.J., Novick, A.C., Lange, P., Steinberg, G.D., and Belldegrun, A.S. (1999). Multicenter, randomized, phase III trial of CD8 (+) tumor-infiltrating lymphocytes in combination with recombinant interleukin-2 in metastatic renal cell carcinoma. *J. Clin. Oncol.* **17** (8), 2521–9.

Finke, J.H., Rayman, P., Edinger, M., Tubbs, R.R., Stanley, J., Klein, E., and Bukowski, R. (1992). Characterization of a human renal cell carcinoma specific cytotoxic CD8+ T cell line. *J. Immunother.* **11** (1), 1–11.

Fisher, R.I., Coltman, C.A. Jr, Doroshow, J.H., Rayner, A.A., Hawkins, M.J., Mier, J.W., Wiernik, P., McMannis, J.D., Weiss, G.R., Margolin, K.A., *et al.* (1988). Metastatic renal cancer treated with interleukin-2 and lym-phokine-activated killer cells. A phase II clinical trial. *Ann. Intern. Med.* **108** (4), 518–23.

Fisher, R.I., Rosenberg, S.A., and Fyfe, G. (2000). Long-term survival update for high-dose recombinant interleukin-2 in patients with renal cell carci-noma. *Cancer J. Sci. Am.* **6** (suppl. 1), S55–7.

Freed, S.Z., Halperin, J.P., and Gordon, M. (1977). Idiopathic regression of metastases from renal cell carcinoma. *J. Urol.* **118** (4), 538–42.

Galligioni, E., Quaia, M., Merlo, A., Carbone, A., Spada, A., Favaro, D., Santarosa, M., Sacco, C., and Talamini, R. (1996). Adjuvant immuno-therapy treatment of renal carcinoma patients with autologous tumor cells and bacillus Calmette–Guerin: five-year results of a prospective randomized study. *Cancer* **77** (12), 2560–6.

Gansbacher, B., Bannerji, R., Daniels, B., Zier, K., Cronin, K., and Gilboa, E. (1990*a*). Retroviral vector-mediated gamma-interferon gene transfer into tumor cells generates potent and long lasting antitumor immunity. *Cancer Res.* **50** (24), 7820–5.

Gansbacher, B., Zier, K., Daniels, B., Cronin, K., Bannerji, R., and Gilboa, E. (1990*b*). Interleukin 2 gene transfer into tumor cells abrogates tumori-genicity and induces protective immunity. *J. Exp. Med.* **172** (4), 1217–24.

Gastl, G., Finstad, C.L., Guarini, A., Bosl, G., Gilboa, E., Bander, N.H., and Gansbacher, B. (1992). Retroviral vector-mediated lymphokine gene transfer into human renal cancer cells. *Cancer Res.* **52** (22), 6229–36.

Gaugler, B., Brouwenstijn, N., Vantomme, V., Szikora, J.P., Van der Spek, C.W., Patard, J.J., Boon, T., Schrier, P., and Van den Eynde, B.J. (1996). A new gene coding for an antigen recognized by autologous cytolytic T lympho-cytes on a human renal carcinoma. *Immunogenetics* **44** (5), 323–30.

Gleave, M.E., Elhilali, M., Fradet, Y., Davis, I., Venner, P., Saad, F., Klotz, L.H., Moore, M.J., Paton, V., and Bajamonde, A. (1998). Interferon gamma-1b compared with placebo in metastatic renal-cell carcinoma. Canadian Urologic Oncology Group. *New Engl. J. Med.* **338** (18), 1265–71.

Golumbek, P.T., Lazenby, A.J., Levitsky, H.I., Jaffee, L.M., Karasuyama, H., Baker, M., and Pardoll, D.M. (1991). Treatment of established renal cancer by tumor cells engineered to secrete interleukin-4. *Science* **254** (5032), 713–16.

Gong, J., Chen, D., Kashiwaba, M., and Kufe, D. (1997). Induction of antitu-mor activity by immunization with fusions of dendritic and carcinoma cells. *Nat. Med.* **3** (5), 558–61.

Grabmaier, K. (2000). Molecular cloning and immunogenicity of renal cell carcinoma-associated antigen G250. *Int J. Cancer* **85** (6), 865–70.

Hara, I., Hotta, H., Sato, N., Eto, H., Arakawa, S., and Kamidono, S. (1996). Rejection of mouse renal cell carcinoma elicited by local secretion of interleukin-2. *Jpn J. Cancer Res.* **87** (7), 724–9.

Hara, I., Nagai, H., Miyake, H., Yamanaka, K., Hara, S., Micallef, M.J., Kurimoto, M., Gohji, K., Arakawa, S., Ichihashi, M., and Kamidono, S. (2000). Effectiveness of cancer vaccine therapy using cells transduced with the interleukin-12 gene combined with systemic interleukin-18 administration. *Cancer Gene Ther.* **7** (1), 83–90.

Hinkel, A., Tso, C.L., Gitlitz, B.J., Neagos, N., Schmid, I., Paik, S.H., deKernion, J., Figlin, R., and Belldegrun, A. (2000). Immunomodulatory dendritic cells generated from nonfractionated bulk peripheral blood mononuclear cell cultures induce growth of cytotoxic T cells against renal cell carcinoma. *J. Immunother.* **23** (1), 83–93.

Hock, H., Dorsch, M., Kunzendorf, U., Uberla, K., Qin, Z., Diamantstein, T., and Blankenstein, T. (1993). Vaccinations with tumor cells genetically engineered to produce different cytokines: effectivity not superior to a classical adjuvant. *Cancer Res.* **53** (4), 714–16.

Hsu, F.J., Benike, C., Fagnoni, F., Liles, T.M., Czerwinski, D., Taidi, B., Engleman, E.G., and Levy, R. (1996). Vaccination of patients with B-cell lymphoma using autologous antigen-pulsed dendritic cells. *Nat. Med.* **2** (1), 52–8.

Itoh, K., Umezu, Y., Morita, T., Saya, H., Seito, D., Augustus, L.B., Nakao, M., Sakata, M., Miyajima, J., Masuoka, K., *et al.* (1994). Increase in the capability of interleukin 2 gene-transduced renal cell carcinoma cells to induce cytotoxic lymphocytes. *Kurume Med. J.* **41** (2), 53–63.

Kirchner, H.H., Anton, P., and Atzpodien, J. (1995). Adjuvant treatment of locally advanced renal cancer with autologous virus-modified tumor vaccines. *World J. Urol.* **13** (3), 171–3.

Kirkwood, J.M., Harris, J.E., Vera, R., Sandler, S., Fischer, D.S., Khandekar, J., Ernstoff, M.S., Gordon, L., Lutes, R., Bonomi, P., *et al.* (1985). A randomized study of low and high doses of leukocyte alpha-interferon in metastatic renal cell carcinoma: the American Cancer Society collaborative trial. *Cancer Res.* **45** (2), 863–71.

Knight, B.C., Souberbielle, B.E., Rizzardi, G.P., Ball, S.E., and Dalgleish, A.G. (1996). Allogeneic murine melanoma cell vaccine: a model for the development of human allogeneic cancer vaccine. *Melanoma Res.* **6** (4), 299–306.

Koo, A.S., Tso, C.L., Shimabukuro, T., Peyret, C., deKernion, J.B., and Belldegrun, A. (1991). Autologous tumor-specific cytotoxicity of tumor-infiltrating lymphocytes derived from human renal cell carcinoma. *J. Immunother.* **10** (5), 347–54.

Krup, O.C., Kroll, I., Bose, G., and Falkenberg, F.W. (1999). Cytokine depot formulations as adjuvants for tumor vaccines. I. Liposome-encapsulated IL-2 as a depot formulation. *J. Immunother.* **22** (6), 525–38.

Kugler, A., Seseke, F., Thelen, P., Kallerhoff, M., Muller, G.A., Stuhler, G., Muller, C., and Ringert, R.H. (1998). Autologous and allogenic hybrid cell vaccine in patients with metastatic renal cell carcinoma. *Br J. Urol.* **82** (4), 487–93.

Kugler, A., Stuhler, G., Walden, P., Zoller, G., Zobywalski, A., Brossart, P., Trefzer, U., Ullrich, S., Muller, C.A., Becker, V., Gross, A.J., Hemmerlein, B., Kanz, L., Muller, G.A., and Ringert, R.H. (2000). Regression of human metastatic renal cell carcinoma after vaccination with tumor cell-dendritic cell hybrids. *Nat. Med.* **6** (3), 332–6.

Li, Q., Normolle, D.P., Sayre, D.M., Zeng, X., Sun, R., Jiang, G., Redman, B.D., and Chang, A.E. (2000). Immunological effects of BCG as an adjuvant in autologous tumor vaccines. *Clin. Immunol.* **94** (1), 64–72.

Li, W.Q., Diamantstein, T., and Blankenstein, T. (1990). Lack of tumorigenicity of interleukin 4 autocrine growing cells seems related to the anti-tumor function of interleukin 4. *Mol. Immunol.* **27** (12), 1331–7.

Locatelli, M.C., Facendola, G., Pizzocaro, G., Piva, L., Pegoraro, C., Pallavicini, E.B., Signaroldi, A., Meregalli, M., Lombardi, F., Beretta, G.D., Scanzi, F., Labianca, R., Dallavalle, G., and Luporini, G. (1999). Subcutaneous administration of interleukin-2 and interferon-alpha 2b in advanced renal cell carcinoma: long-term results. *Cancer Detect. Prevent.* **23** (2), 172–6.

Logan, T.F., Banner, B., Rao, U., Ernstoff, M.S., Wolmark, N., Whiteside, T.L., Miketic, L., and Kirkwood, J.M. (1998). Inflammatory cell infiltrate in a responding metastatic nodule after vaccine-based immunotherapy. *Clin. Exp. Immunol.* **114** (3), 347–54.

Mahvi, D.M., Sondel, P.M., Yang, N.S., Albertini, M.R., Schiller, J.H., Hank, J., Heiner, J., Gan, J., Swain, W., and Logrono, R. (1997). Phase I/IB study of immunization with autologous tumor cells transfected with the GM-CSF gene by particle-mediated transfer in patients with melanoma or sarcoma. *Hum. Gene Ther.* **8** (7), 875–91.

Marcus, S.G., Choyke, P.L., Reiter, R., Jaffe, G.S., Alexander, R.B., Linehan, W.M., Rosenberg, S.A., and Walther, M.M. (1993). Regression of meta static renal cell carcinoma after cytoreductive nephrectomy. *J. Urol.* **150** (2, Pt 1), 463–6.

McCune, C.S., Schapira, D.V., and Henshaw, E.C. (1981). Specific immunotherapy of advanced renal carcinoma: evidence for the poly-clonality of metastases. *Cancer* **47** (8), 1984–7.

McCune, C.S., O'Donnell, R.W., Marquis, D.M., and Sahasrabudhe, D.M. (1990). Renal cell carcinoma treated by vaccines for active specific immunotherapy: correlation of survival with skin testing by autologous tumor cells. *Cancer Immunol. Immunother.* **32** (1), 62–6.

Montie, J.E., Stewart, B.H., Straffon, R.A., Banowsky, L.H., Hewitt, C.B., and Montague, D.K. (1977). The role of adjunctive nephrectomy in patients with metastatic renal cell carcinoma. *J. Urol.* **117** (3), 272–5.

Morales, A. and Eidinger, D. (1976). Bacillus Calmette–Guerin in the treatment of adenocarcinoma of the kidney. *J. Urol.* **115** (4), 377–80.

Morales, A., Eidinger, D., and Bruce, A.W. (1976). Intracavitary bacillus Calmette–Guerin in the treatment of superficial bladder tumors. *J. Urol.* **116** (2), 180–3.

Morales, A., Wilson, J.L., Pater, J.L., and Loeb, M. (1982). Cytoreductive surgery and systemic bacillus Calmette–Guerin therapy in metastatic renal cancer: a phase II trial. *J. Urol.* **127** (2), 230–5.

Morgan, D.A., Ruscetti, F.W., and Gallo, R. (1976). Selective *in vitro* growth of T lymphocytes from normal human bone marrows. *Science* **193** (4257), 1007–8.

Mukherji, B., Chakraborty, N.G., Yamasaki, S., Okino, T., Yamase, H., Sporn, J.R., Kurtzman, S.K., Ergin, M.T., Ozols, J., Meehan, J., *et al.* (1995). Induction of antigen-specific cytolytic T cells *in situ* in human melanoma by immunization with synthetic peptide-pulsed autologous antigen presenting cells. *Proc. Natl Acad. Sci., USA* **92** (17), 8078–82.

Mulders, P., Tso, C.L., Pang, S., Kaboo, R., McBride, W.H., Hinkel, A., Gitlitz, B., Dannull, J., Figlin, R., and Belldegrun, A. (1998). Adenovirus-mediated interleukin-2 production by tumors induces growth of cytotoxic tumor-infiltrating lymphocytes against human renal cell carcinoma. *J. Immunother.* **21** (3), 170–80.

Murphy, G., Tjoa, B., Ragde, H., Kenny, G., and Boynton, A. (1996). Phase I clinical trial: T-cell therapy for prostate cancer using autologous dendritic cells pulsed with HLA-A0201-specific peptides from prostate-specific membrane antigen. *Prostate* **29** (6), 371–80.

Myers, G.H. Jr, Fehrenbaker, L.G., and Kelalis, P.P. (1968). Prognostic significance of renal vein invasion by hypernephroma. *J. Urol.* **100** (4), 420–3.

Neidhart, J.A., Murphy, S.G., Hennick, L.A., and Wise, H.A. (1980). Active specific immunotherapy of stage IV renal carcinoma with aggregated tumor antigen adjuvant. *Cancer* **46** (5), 1128–34.

Nestle, F.O., Alijagic, S., Gilliet, M., Sun, Y., Grabbe, S., Dummer, R., Burg, G., and Schadendorf, D. (1998). Vaccination of melanoma patients with peptide- or tumor lysate-pulsed dendritic cells. *Nat. Med.* **4** (3), 328–32.

Nishisaka, N., Maini, A., Kinoshita, Y., Yasumoto, R., Kishimoto, T., Jones, R.F., Morse, P., Hillman, G.G., Wang, C.Y., and Haas, G.P. (1999). Immuno-therapy for lung metastases of murine renal cell carcinoma: synergy between radiation and cytokine-producing tumor vaccines. *J. Immunother.* **22** (4), 308–14.

Ogasawara, M. and Rosenberg, S.A. (1993). Enhanced expression of HLA molecules and stimulation of autologous human tumor infiltrating lymphocytes following transduction of melanoma cells with gamma-interferon genes. *Cancer Res.* **53** (15), 3561–8.

Oliff, A., Defeo-Jones, D., Boyer, M., Martinez, D., Kiefer, D., Vuocolo, G., Wolfe, A., and Socher, S.H. (1987). Tumors secreting human TNF/cachectin induce cachexia in mice. *Cell* **50** (4), 555–63.

Oliver, R.T. (1989). Surveillance as a possible option for management of metastatic renal cell carcinoma. *Sem. Urol.* **7** (3), 149–52.

Oliver, R.T., Miller, R.M., Mehta, A., and Barnett, M.J. (1988). A phase 2 study of surveillance in patients with metastatic renal cell carcinoma and assessment of response of such patients to therapy on progression. *Mol. Biother.* **1** (1), 14–20.

Oosterwijk, E., Ruiter, D., Hoedemaeker, P., Pauwels, E., Jonas, U., Zwartendijk, J., and Warnaar, S. (1986). Monoclonal antibody G 250 recognizes a determinant present in renal-cell carcinoma and absent from normal kidney. *Int. J. Cancer* **38** (4), 489–94.

Opavsky, R., Pastorekova, S., Zelnik, V., Gibadulinova, A., Stanbridge, E., Zavada, J., Kettmann, R., and Pastorek, J. (1996). Human MN/CA9 gene, a novel member of the carbonic anhydrase family: structure and exon to protein domain relationships. *Genomics* **33** (3), 480–7.

Paglia, P., Chiodoni, C., Rodolfo, M., and Colombo, M.P. (1996). Murine dendritic cells loaded *in vitro* with soluble protein prime cytotoxic T lymphocytes against tumor antigen *in vivo*. *J. Exp. Med.* **183** (1), 317–22.

Papac, R. (1996). Spontaneous regression of cancer. *Cancer Treat. Rev.* **22** (6), 395–423.

Pierce, W.C., Belldegrun, A., and Figlin, R.A. (1995). Cellular therapy: scientific rationale and clinical results in the treatment of metastatic renal-cell carcinoma. *Sem. Oncol.* **22** (1), 74–80.

Platzer, C., Richter, G., Uberla, K., Hock, H., Diamantstein, T., and Blankenstein, T. (1992). Interleukin-4-mediated tumor suppression in nude mice involves interferon-gamma. *Eur. J. Immunol.* **22** (7), 1729–33.

Plotkin, S.L. and Plotkin, S.A. (1994). A short history of vaccination. In *Vaccines*, 2nd edn (ed. S.A. Plotkin and E.A. Mortimer), pp. 1–11. W.B. Saunders, Philadelphia.

Pomer, S., Thiele, R., Staehler, G., Drehmer, I., Lohrke, H., and Schirrmacher V. (1995). [Tumor vaccination in renal cell carcinoma with and without interleukin-2 (IL-2) as adjuvant. A clinical contribution to the development of effective active specific immunization]. *Urologe A* **34** (3), 215–20.

Quesada, J.R., Swanson, D.A., Trindade, A., and Gutterman, J.U. (1983). Renal cell carcinoma: antitumor effects of leukocyte interferon. *Cancer Res.* **43** (2), 940–7.

Repmann, R., Wagner, S., and Richter, A. (1997). Adjuvant therapy of renal cell carcinoma with active-specific-immunotherapy (ASI) using autologous tumor vaccine. *Anticancer Res.* **17** (4B), 2879–82.

Romani, N., Gruner, S., Brang, D., Kämpgen, E., Lenz, A., Trockenbacher, B., Konwalinka, G., Fritsch, P.O., Steinman, R.M., and Schuler, G. (1994). Proliferating dendritic cell progenitors in human blood. *J. Exp. Med.* **180** (1), 83–93.

Rosenberg, S.A. (1988). Immunotherapy of cancer using interleukin-2: current status and future prospects. *Immunol. Today* **9**, 58.

Rosenberg, S.A. (1997). Cancer vaccines based on the identification of genes encoding cancer regression antigens. *Immunol. Today* **18** (4), 175–82.

Rosenberg, S.A., Lotze, M.T., Muul, L.M., Leitman, S., Chang, A.E., Ettinghausen, S.E., Matory, Y.L., Skibber, J.M., Shiloni, E., Vetto, J.T., *et al.* (1985). Observations on the systemic administration of autologous lymphokine-activated killer cells and recombinant interleukin-2 to patients with metastatic cancer. *New Engl. J. Med.* **313** (23), 1485–92.

Rosenberg, S.A., Yang, J.C., Topalian, S.L., Schwartzentruber, D.J., Weber, J.S., Parkinson, D.R., Seipp, C.A., Einhorn, J.H., and White, D.E. (1994). Treatment of 283 consecutive patients with metastatic melanoma or renal cell cancer using high-dose bolus interleukin 2. *J. Am. Med. Assoc.* **271** (12), 907–13.

Ryan, C.W., Vogelzang, N.J., Dumas, M.C., Kuzel, T., and Stadler, W.M. (2000). Granulocyte–macrophage-colony stimulating factor in combination immunotherapy for patients with metastatic renal cell carcinoma: results of two phase II clinical trials. *Cancer* **88** (6), 1317–24.

Salvadori, S., Gansbacher, B., Wernick, I., Tirelli, S., and Zier, K. (1995). B7–1 amplifies the response to interleukin-2-secreting tumor vaccines *in vivo*, but fails to induce a response by naive cells *in vitro*. *Hum. Gene Ther.* **6** (10), 1299–306.

Schendel, D.J., Gansbacher, B., Oberneder, R., Kriegmair, M., Hofstetter, A., Riethmüller, G., and Segurado, O.G. (1993). Tumor-specific lysis of human renal cell carcinomas by tumor-infiltrating lymphocytes. I. HLA-A2-restricted recognition of autologous and allogeneic tumor lines. *J. Immunol.* **151** (8), 4209–20.

Simons, J.W., Jaffee, E.M., Weber, C.E., Levitsky, H.I., Nelson, W.G., Carducci, M.A., Lazenby, A.J., Cohen, L.K., Finn, C.C., Clift, S.M., Hauda, K.M., Beck, L.A., Leiferman, K.M., Owens, A.H. Jr, Piantadosi, S., Dranoff, G., Mulligan, R.C., Pardoll, D.M., and Marshall, F.F. (1997). Bioactivity of autologous irradiated renal cell carcinoma vaccines generated by *ex vivo* granulocyte–macrophage colony-stimulating factor gene transfer. *Cancer Res.* **57** (8), 1537–46.

Steinman, R. (1991). The dendritic cell system and its role in immunogenicity. *Ann. Rev. Immunol.* **9**, 271–96.

Suminami, Y., Elder, E.M., Lotze, M.T., and Whiteside, T.L. (1995). *In situ* interleukin-4 gene expression in cancer patients treated with genetically modified tumor vaccine. *J. Immunother. Emphasis Tumor Immunol.* **17** (4), 238–48.

Tan, J., Newton, C.A., Djeu, J.Y., Gutsch, D.E., Chang, A.E., Yang, N.S., Klein, T.W., and Hua, Y. (1996). Injection of complementary DNA encoding interleukin-12 inhibits tumor establishment at a distant site in a murine renal carcinoma model. *Cancer Res.* **56** (15), 3399–403.

Teng, M.N., Park, B.H., Koeppen, H.K., Tracey, K.J., Fendly, B.M., and Schreiber, H. (1991). Long-term inhibition of tumor growth by tumor necrosis factor in the absence of cachexia or T-cell immunity. *Proc. Natl Acad. Sci., USA* **88** (9), 3535–9.

Tepper, R.I., Pattengale, P.K., and Leder, P. (1989). Murine interleukin-4 displays potent anti-tumor activity *in vivo*. *Cell* **57** (3), 503–12.

Tepper, R.I., Coffman, R.L., and Leder, P. (1992). An eosinophil-dependent mechanism for the antitumor effect of interleukin-4. *Science* **257** (5069), 548–51.

Tripathi, P., Qin, H., Bhattacharya-Chatterjee, M., Ceriani, R., Foon, K., and Chatterjee, S. (1999). Construction and characterization of a chimeric fusion protein consisting of an anti-idiotype antibody mimicking a breast cancer-associated antigen and the cytokine GM-CSF. *Hybridoma* **18** (2), 193–202.

Van den Eynde, B.J. and van der Bruggen, P. (1997). T cell defined tumor antigens. *Curr. Opin. Immunol.* **9** (5), 684–93.

van Elsas, A., van der Burg, S.H., van der Minne, C.E., Borghi, M., Mourer, J.S., Melief, C.J., and Schrier, P.I. (1996). Peptide-pulsed dendritic cells induce tumoricidal cytotoxic T lymphocytes from healthy donors against stably HLA-A*0201-binding peptides from the Melan-A/MART-1 self antigen. *Eur. J. Immunol.* **26** (8), 1683–9.

Veelken, H., Mackensen, A., Lahn, M., Kohler, G., Becker, D., Franke, B., Brennscheidt, U., Kulmburg, P., Rosenthal, F.M., Keller, H., Hasse, J., Schultze-Seemann, W., Farthmann, E.H., Mertelsmann, R., and Lindemann, A. (1997). A phase-I clinical study of autologous tumor cells plus interleukin-2-gene-transfected allogeneic fibroblasts as a vaccine in patients with cancer. *Int. J. Cancer* **70** (3), 269–77.

Vissers, J., De, V.I., Schreurs, M., Engelen, L., Oosterwijk, E., Figdor, C., and Adema, G. (1999). The renal cell carcinoma-associated antigen G250 encodes a human leukocyte antigen (HLA)-A2.1-restricted epitope recognized by cytotoxic T lymphocytes. *Cancer Res.* **59** (21), 5554–9.

Watanabe, Y., Kuribayashi, K., Miyatake, S., Nishihara, K., Nakayama, E., Taniyama, T., and Sakata, T. (1989). Exogenous expression of mouse interferon gamma cDNA in mouse neuroblastoma C1300 cells results in reduced tumorigenicity by augmented anti-tumor immunity. *Proc. Natl Acad. Sci., USA* **86** (23), 9456–60.

Williams, T.W., Yanagimoto, J.M., Mazumder, A., and Wiseman, C.L. (1992). Interleukin-2 increases the antibody response in patients receiving autologous intralymphatic tumor cell vaccine immunotherapy. *Mol. Biother.* **4** (2), 66–9.

Yagoda, A., Abi-Rached, B., and Petrylak, D. (1995). Chemotherapy for advanced renal-cell carcinoma: 1983–1993. *Sem. Oncol.* **22** (1), 42–60.

Yannelli, J.R., Hyatt, C., McConnell, S., Hines, K., Jacknin, L., Parker, L., Sanders, M., and Rosenberg, S.A. (1996). Growth of tumor-infiltrating lymphocytes from human solid cancers: summary of a 5-year experience. *Int. J. Cancer* **65** (4), 413–21.

Zier, K.S. and Gansbacher, B. (1996). Tumour cell vaccines that secrete interleukin-2 (IL-2) and interferon gamma (IFN gamma) are recognised by T cells while resisting destruction by natural killer (NK) cells. *Eur. J. Cancer* **32A** (8), 1408–12.

15. New approaches for biological therapy of kidney tumors: preclinical models and perspectives

Robert H. Wiltrout and Jon M. Wigginton

Summary

Tumors of the kidney are generally refractory to conventional forms of cancer therapy. However, there are some encouraging indications that these tumors may be successfully targeted by appropriately designed biological therapies. In particular, interferon α (IFNα) and interleukin-2 (IL-2) have shown some effectiveness for the treatment of renal cell carcinoma (RCC) in humans. The mechanisms by which biological therapies may induce tumor regression in humans remain unclear, and there are relatively few preclinical orthotopic models of kidney cancer available for performing such studies. The available rodent models fall into several broad categories: spontaneous tumors of unknown etiology; spontaneous tumors of defined genetic etiology; carcinogen-induced tumors; or human tumor xenografts in immunodeficient mice. In general, orthotopic models, where the appropriate physiological interplay between tumor cells and their relevant organ environment occurs, are desirable since therapeutic approaches must be active in the context of the actual host–tumor environment. The most widely used mouse RCC model has been the Renca renal adenocarcinoma of spontaneous origin in BALB/c mice. In this review we will discuss the attributes of these different models and the past and prospective contributions they have made or may make for the development of new biologic strategies to treat RCC. We will also discuss our extensive experience with the Renca RCC model, and describe a new orthotopic transplantable model of RCC recently derived from a streptozotocin-induced kidney tumor in BALB/c mice.

Background

Approximately 30 000 new cases of RCC are diagnosed each year in the US and about 12 000 patients die of their disease annually (Figlin 1999; Godfrey and Stinchcombe 1999). Up to 20–30 per cent of patients present with metastatic disease at the time of initial diagnosis (Cohen 1999; Vogelzang and Stadler 1998). The classification of RCC can be complicated because diagnosis often depends on a combination of histologic and cytologic criteria. The predominant histologic subtypes of RCC include the clear cell and papillary forms, accounting for 70–80 and 10–15 per cent of all kidney cancers, respectively (Zambrano *et al.* 1999). The molecular basis for most inherited and sporadic clear cell RCC is inactivation of the von Hippel–Lindau (VHL) tumor suppressor gene on chromosome 3p25 (Gnarra *et al.* 1994; Vogelzang and Stadler 1998), while mutations in the c-met proto-oncogene have been associated with the hereditary form of papillary renal cell cancer (Schmidt *et al.* 1997).

Although, the prognosis for patients presenting with metastatic kidney cancer remains unfavorable, biological approaches using IL-2 have proved to be as good or better than conventional chemotherapy (Fyfe *et al.* 1995; Vogelzang and Stadler 1998),

Table 15.1 Preclinical rodent tumor models of RCC

Tumor model	Etiology	Species	Strain	References
Renca renal adenocarcinoma	Spontaneous	Mouse	BALB/c	Murphy and Hrushesky 1973; Salup *et al.* 1987; Wiltrout 1993
RKC rat kidney carcinoma	Spontaneous	Rat	Wistar–Lewis	de Vere White and Olsson 1980; deVere White *et al.* 1983
Streptozotocin-induced	Carcinogen	Mouse	CBA/T6J	Hard 1985
	Carcinogen	Mouse	BALB/c	Gruys *et al.*, in preparation
N-nitrosodimethylamine (NDMA)-induced	Carcinogen	Rat	Wistar	Hard 1984; Shiao *et al.* 1998
Eker rat RCC	Mutation in Tsc2 gene	Rat	Eker	Everitt *et al.* 1995
Human RCC xenograft	Spontaneous	Human	Athymic or SCID	Ebert *et al.* 1990; Fidler *et al.* 1990

suggesting that a better understanding of the interaction between the immune system and renal cancer cells may yield additional therapeutic benefits. Unfortunately, there are relatively few preclinical tumor models of renal carcinoma ((Hillman *et al.* 1994; Table 15.1). The desired attributes of an appropriate histopathologically characterized experimental model for kidney cancer would include spontaneous origin, slow growth rate, predictable spontaneous metastatic progression to regional lymph nodes and lungs, a well developed neovasculature, and a defined genetic etiology. The available syngeneic rodent models of spontaneous RCC origin include the Renca adenocarcinoma of BALB/c mice (Murphy and Hrushesky 1973; Salup *et al.* 1987; Vogelzang and Stadler 1998; Williams *et al.* 1981), a rat kidney carcinoma (RKC) (White and Olsson 1980), and the hereditary RCC model in Eker rats, which derives from a defect in the tuberous sclerosis (TSC2) gene (Everitt *et al.* 1995). Several carcinogens, including streptozotocin in mice (Hard 1985) and *N*-nitrosodimethylamine in rats (NDMA; Hard 1984), induce renal tumors in rodents with relatively high frequency. These carcinogen-dependent models have been used to only a limited degree to date in the preclinical evaluation of new therapeutic modalities. Several human tumor xenograft models have been well characterized in athymic mice (Kozlowski *et al.* 1984; Naito *et al.* 1987). The perceived usefulness of various models has been re-emphasized by the growing awareness that the organ microenvironment can exert a pronounced influence on the growth and metastasis of tumors by providing appropriate growth factors, tissue degradative enzymes that favor metastatic spread, enhanced expression of drug resistance mechanisms, and favorable disposition for neovascularization (reviewed in Fidler 1995; Fidler *et al.* 1990). Such orthotopic models have also been reported to favor the development of heterogeneous subpopulations of tumor cells as are often observed in human cancers (Killion *et al.* 1998), and to be most suitable for the assessment of new gene therapy approaches (Kerbel *et al.* 1991). These findings have re-emphasized the need for orthotopic preclinical tumor models that may provide unique insight into critical biological events, and important tissue-specific events during the use of biological therapy (An *et al.* 1999; Fidler 1999; Gohji *et al.* 1990; Nakajima *et al.* 1990; Tepper and Mule 1994; Wilmanns *et al.* 1992). This review will therefore focus on the attributes and contributions of the available preclinical models in the context of their use for the study of different experimental biologic approaches to the treatment of RCC.

Transplantable rodent models for RCC

The Renca renal adenocarcinoma model

Background and biology
The Renca renal adenocarcinoma arose spontaneously in syngeneic BALB/c mouse and was originally isolated by Dr Sarah Stewart at the National Cancer Institute, and characterized by Murphy and Hrushesky (1973) as well as by Williams *et al.* (1981). After orthotopic implantation into the kidney, the primary tumor grows progressively, invades locally, and then metastasizes predictably to local lymph nodes, lungs, and later to the liver (Salup *et al.* 1987; Wiltrout 1993). A novel aspect of this model is that a unilateral nephrectomy can be performed after the development of spontaneous pulmonary and/or hepatic metastases (Wiltrout 1993), providing a setting in which the immune system of the mouse has been conditioned by the process of primary tumor development and metastasis before the start of various immunotherapeutic approaches.

Use of the Renca model for the study of cytokine-based approaches to cancer treatment
The Renca renal tumor model has provided useful preclinical information for the design of a variety of early clinical trials where new approaches using biological therapy have been applied to the treatment of RCC. In the mid- and late-1980s, our laboratory pioneered the use of this model for preclinical biologic therapy studies by demonstrating that several IL-2-based strategies had activity against well-established, metastatic Renca. Using this model, we have shown that IL-2 alone or in combination with adoptive immunotherapy (AIT) (Salup *et al.* 1987), or cytokine-inducing flavanoid compounds (Hornung *et al.* 1988; Mace *et al.* 1990; Wiltrout *et al.* 1988) possesses substantial therapeutic activity. These results suggest that, as a single agent, IL-2 can induce consistent but incomplete tumor regression. Subsequent clinical trials of IL-2 have shown that it is active against metastatic RCC, with most induced responses being partial, and a minority being complete (Dutcher *et al.* 1997; Fyfe *et al.* 1995). At this time IL-2 is the treatment of choice for human metastatic RCC, although combinations of IL-2 with other cytokines continue to be explored (Dutcher *et al.* 1997; Vogelzang and Stadler 1998). IFNa also has the ability to induce partial regression of Renca (Sayers *et al.* 1990), findings similar to those reported in the clinical setting among patients with RCC (Godfrey and Stinchcombe 1999; Negrier *et al.* 1998; Vogelzang and Stadler 1998).

More recently, we and others have found that IL-12 can also induce partial regression of primary and/or metastatic Renca tumors (Tannenbaum *et al.* 1998; Wigginton *et al.* 1996), and that synergistic antitumor effects are achieved by combined systemic administration of IL-12 and intermittent pulse IL-2 (Wigginton *et al.* 1996). As a single agent, IL-12 has induced infrequent responses and an appreciable incidence of stable disease in early phase clinical studies to date (Atkins *et al.* 1997; Motzer *et al.* 1998). Phase I trials of IL-2 and IL-12 will begin in early 2000 at the National Cancer Institute, and a number of experimental clinical endpoints will be investigated based on mechanistic insights derived from preclinical evaluation of this combination in the Renca model. Specifically, we have noted that the orthotopically-implanted Renca tumors are rapidly and extensively neovascularized, and treatment with IL-12/pulse IL-2 has a rapid antineovascular effect that can be observed grossly by an overall reduction in tumor-associated vasculature as defined by the injection of liquid latex and quantitated by incorporation of radioisotope into the infused latex, (Wigginton *et al.*, submitted for publication). Electron micrographs reveal apoptosis of tumor-associated endothelial cells very early in the course of therapy (Wigginton *et al.*, submitted for publication). These findings demonstrate that discrete anti-neovascular effects precede the actual reduction in tumor burden that follows administration of IL-12/pulse IL-2, and suggest that this anti-angiogenic response may be an important part of the mechanism by which this cytokine combination induces the complete regression of metastatic Renca. Other critical mediators of the antitumor activity engaged by IL-12/pulse IL-2 in Renca-bearing mice include IFNγ, the FAS/FAS-L pathway, and and CD8$^+$ T cells (Wigginton *et al.*, submitted for publication). The potential involvement of Fas-mediated killing in host responses against Renca has also been further highlighted by the findings of Lee *et al.* (2000) who demonstrated that stable overexpression of Fas in Renca cells resulted in an IFNγ-dependent inhibition of growth *in vivo*. These defined biological endpoints are closely associated with therapeutic efficacy and there are a number of genes whose induction also coincides with, or immediately precedes, the initiation of tumor regression. The therapeutic effects of IL-12 alone against established subcutaneous Renca primary tumors are dependent on induction of the production of IFNγ-inducible, antiangiogenic CXC chemokines Mig and IP-10 (Tannenbaum *et al.* 1998), and there is also an increased upregulation of the IFNγ-inducible Mig and Crg-2/IP-10 CXC chemokine genes in the tumor bed of mice treated with IL-12/pulse IL-2 (Wigginton *et al.*, submitted for publication). In addition, the localization of CD8$^+$ T cells to established primary tumors has been shown to be vital for the effects of IL-12 (Tannenbaum *et al.* 1998) alone or the IL-12/pulse IL-2 combination (Wigginton *et al.*, submitted for publication), while the administration of IL-12/pulse IL-2 induces enhanced expression of the Fas and FasL genes in the local tumor bed and cell surface expression of FAS-L on lymph-node-derived CD8$^+$ T cells (Wigginton *et al.*, submitted for publication). These findings provide a number of biological endpoints that can be evaluated coincident with toxicity and tumor status in the initial phase I trials.

Use of the Renca model to study cytokine gene therapeutic approaches to cancer treatment

Early studies from our laboratory demonstrated that Renca cells could be readily transfected with a variety of cytokine genes and that cells transfected with IL-2, but not IFNγ, regressed after implantation (Wiltrout *et al.* 1995). More recently, several investigators have used the Renca model to study the delivery of cytokine genes into established tumors. Siders *et al.* (1998) have shown that adenoviruses modified to express the IL-12 gene have potent antitumor effects against established Renca hepatic metastases, while Fenton *et al.* (1997) demonstrated antitumor effects of IL-12 gene-modified pox viruses. DNA plasmids containing the IL-2 or IL-12 genes can be introduced into established primary tumors by the use of gene gun technology (Rakhmilevich *et al.* 1996; Sun *et al.* 1995) or by other chemical approaches that facilitate the incorporation of DNA plasmids into normal host or tumor cells. Mendiratta *et al.* (1999) have reported that the intratumoral injection of IL-12/polyvinyl pyrrolidone complex (PVP) resulted in efficient *in vivo* translation of IL-12 protein and the induction of CD8$^+$ T cell-dependent tumor regression. Similar effects were also achieved using this technology against a small localized Renca primary tumor when the IFNα gene was delivered intratumorally

in a complex with PVP (Coleman *et al.* 1998). Saffran *et al.* (1998) have employed a similar approach to show that intratumoral injection of a plasmid DNA vector encoding the IL-2 gene and complexed to a cationic lipid could cause the rejection of established Renca primary tumors. Intradermal injection of naked DNA plasmids encoding the IL-12 gene can result in high levels of IL-12 gene expression (Tan *et al.* 1996; Watanabe *et al.* 1999) and can protect against subsequent tumor challenge (Tan *et al.* 1996). More recently, Watanabe *et al.* (manuscript submitted for publication) have shown that expression of IL-12 protein and systemic induction of natural killer (NK) activity can be enhanced by the use of a novel fusion gene construct in which the p35 and p40 genes that code for the two chains of the IL-12 heterodimer are linked using the same technology as that previously described for the construction of single-chain antibodies. The resulting IL-12 fusion gene encodes equal amounts of both p35 and p40, thereby avoiding the antagonization of IL-12's biological effects by excess plasmid expression of the p40 monomer or homodimer.

The Renca tumor model has also been used to develop novel non-cytokine-based gene therapeutic strategies for cancer treatment. Yamamoto *et al.* (1997) has reported that the transfer of the herpes simplex virus thymidine kinase (HSV-TK) gene into Renca cells followed by their implantation and subsequent exposure to gancyclovir *in vivo* induced tumor cell suicide conferred resistance to rechallenge by wild-type Renca cells. Overall, the results summarized above show that this model has been useful for establishing technology and providing initial proof-of-principle for a variety of novel gene therapeutic strategies.

Use of the Renca model to evaluate the antitumor effects of anti-angiogenic agents

Because the Renca tumor, like human RCC (Strohmeyer 1999), is highly vascularized, it provides a useful *in vivo* model with which to study novel approaches that target neovasculature as a cancer treatment strategy. Stable transfection with a construct encoding the angiostatic mouse endostatin sequence slows the growth of primary Renca implants and prevents the formation of experimentally established Renca metastases in the lung and liver (Yoon *et al.* 1999). Yonekura *et al.* (1999) have used a model where Renca cells were placed in a diffusion chamber that was then implanted in mice and used as an angiogenic stimulus in a dorsal air sac assay where it was used to identify antiangiogenic activity of a tegafur/uracil chemotherapy. More recently, as outlined above, our laboratory has used the highly vascularized Renca model to investigate the anti-angiogenic effects of IL-12 and IL-12/pulse IL-2 (Wigginton *et al.*, submitted for publication). These studies have shown that tumor-associated endothelial cells exhibit an early (within 4 days of the initiation of therapy) increase in apoptotic index that is then followed by an ability to detect a decrease in the overall tumor-associated vascular supply. These anti-angiogenic effects precede, or occur coincident with, obvious reductions in total tumor volume, suggesting that the anti-neovascular effects may be important early components of an overall antitumor mechanism that is dependent on the presence of CD8$^+$ T cells and functional IFNγ and FasL. Studies are now in process to investigate the degree to which the initiation of an anti-neovascular effect is linked to the overall antitumor effect, and to elucidate the

Table 15.2 Characteristics of Renca renal adenocarcinoma model

Spontaneous origin in BALB/c mice
Adapted to serial orthotopic transplant
Grows progressively after intrarenal implant
    Highly vascularized
    Metastasizes spontaneously to lungs and liver
    Unilateral nephrectomy can be performed up to 2 weeks post tumor implantation into the kidney
Responsive to IL-2 in combination with
    Interferon-inducing flavonoid compounds
    Interferons
    IL-12
Induces alteration in some T-cell signal transduction events
Successfully applied to several approaches for cytokine-gene therapy
Used as a model for development of anti-neovascular therapies

cellular and molecular mechanisms by which IL-12/pulse IL-2 induces these events.

Use of the Renca model for studying mechanisms of immune escape
There is general agreement that the immune system of tumor-bearing mice and cancer patients is either actively dysregulated and/or unable to effectively recognize and respond productively to tumor-associated epitopes. There are some reports that mice bearing the Renca tumor do exhibit some functional deficits in their ability to mount T- and NK-cell-mediated immune responses *in vitro* (Gregorian and Battisto 1990*a*,*b*). Deficits in critical immune-related signal transduction pathways have also been reported and it has been proposed that they contribute to functional immune defects in tumor-bearing hosts (Li *et al.* 1994; Mizoguchi *et al.* 1992; Whiteside 1999). However, there has been some controversy about the degree to which these deficits occur in mice bearing rapidly growing transplantable tumors (Franco *et al.* 1995; Levey and Srivastava 1995). We have shown alterations in the FKB family of transcription factors in mouse T lymphocytes from mice bearing advanced Renca tumors (Ghosh *et al.* 1994). Finke and colleagues (Uzzo *et al.* 1999*a*) subsequently reported a similar finding for T lymphocytes obtained from human renal cancer patients and associated this suppression of NFKB activation in T cells with effects induced by RCC-derived gangliosides (Uzzo *et al.* 1999*b*). Another proposed mechanism for tumor-mediated immune suppression has been described as the Fas counterattack (O'Connell *et al.* 1996; Walker *et al.* 1997). In this setting, tumor cells that express functional FasL may eliminate Fas+ T cells that localize to the tumor. Renca does not express FasL either constitutively or in response to various cytokine stimuli (Wiltrout, unpublished observation). Therefore, it is unlikely that this mechanism contributes to tumor progression in this model. However, it has recently been reported that the transfection of FasL into Renca cells resulted in an acceleration of growth in euthymic, but not athymic BALB/c mice (Nishimatsu *et al.* 1999), suggesting that the enhancement of growth was dependent on the circumvention of an endogenous T-cell-mediated immune response. Overall, the Renca tumor is probably the most widely used rodent model for the study of new biological therapy approaches to RCC (Table 15.2). It shares some biological characteristics with human RCC, but its use is somewhat restricted because of its relatively rapid growth rate, a trait it shares with many other transplantable rodent tumors.

Transplantable rat kidney carcinoma (RKC) model

The RKC model, first described by de Vere White, is a clear cell renal adenocarcinoma that metastasizes to the lungs after orthotopic intrarenal implantation, and is unresponsive to hormonal and/or chemotherapeutic intervention (deVere White *et al.* 1983; deVere White and Olsson 1980). In Lewis rats, 67 per cent present with lung metastases after orthotopic renal tumor transplantation, and primary renal tumors grow appreciably faster in rats depleted of NK cells (Winter *et al.* 1992). These tumors are sensitive to NK-cell-mediated cytotoxicity *in vitro* and offer the advantage of a relatively slow growth rate with survival up to about 11 weeks after intrarenal tumor implantation (Winter *et al.* 1992). Limitations in the availability of immunological reagents and the dose requirements imposed by the larger size of rats compared to mice limit the overall utility of this model for the evaluation of new biological therapies and the requisite approaches for delineating antitumor mechanisms.

Carcinogen-induced models of rodent renal carcinoma

Induction of renal carcinomas by streptozotocin in BALB/c and C57BL/6 mice

Although the transplantable renal cancer models outlined above have proven useful for a number of novel approaches to cancer treatment, most are somewhat limited by a relatively rapid growth rate *in vivo*. In this characteristic they differ substantively from human renal cancers, which may often progress over a period of months or years. From a practical perspective, this rapid growth results in a relatively small window of opportunity in which to apply new therapeutic strategies against well-established tumors in the preclinical setting. This is a particular limitation for the study of approaches that attempt to engage adaptive antitumor immune responses, which often require about 2 weeks to evolve to maximum effect. Also, widely used transplantable tumors were often initially isolated many years ago and may have been passaged hundreds of times, usually *in vitro* or, in non-orthotopic sites *in vivo*. This can mean that the phenotype and physiology of current lines may differ dramatically from the original isolate.

Given these considerations and our focus on the development of new approaches to the biological therapy of renal cancer, we have induced and characterized several novel transplantable murine RCC lines, which have been conditioned in orthotopic sites of implantation *in vivo*. These new tumor isolates have been induced by the nitrosamine compound, streptozotocin, an antibiotic and diabetogenic agent produced by *Streptomyces achromogenes* (Herr *et al.* 1967) that has been reported to induce a high frequency of renal carcinomas in CBA/T6J mice (Hard 1985) following a single intravenous (IV) dose. Tumors induced in CBA mice by this method have been reported to share some ultrastructural features with human RCC (Delahunt *et al.* 1997).

Many of the available mouse tumor models are syngeneic to BALB/c or C57BL/6 mice, and numerous immunological reagents specific for the histocompatibility profile of these two strains are available for characterization of innate and adaptive immune response components. Therefore, our studies were performed to: (1) determine whether streptozotocin could induce renal carcinomas in BALB/c and C57BL/6 mice; (2) determine whether these arising tumors could be adapted to reproducible regrowth as orthotopic transplants; (3) determine the heterogeneity of growth and progression within the new tumors; (4) characterize the new isolates by histopathological and molecular analyses. Two separate experiments were performed to determine the ability of streptozotocin to induce RCC in BALB/c and C57BL/6 mice (Gruys *et al.*, manuscript in preparation). In the first study a total of 180 mice were injected with 200 mg/kg streptozotocin and mice were euthanized when moribund, between 51 and 92 weeks later. Six per cent of these mice presented with renal adenomas and 18 per cent with renal carcinomas. Only one renal carcinoma and one renal adenoma were detected in C57BL/6 mice. Although this experiment clearly demonstrated the feasibility of using streptozotocin to induce primary renal cancers in BALB/c mice, no transplantable isolates were obtained. Therefore, a second experiment was initiated to reproduce these findings and obtain low-passage, transplantable isolates of mouse renal cancer for subsequent molecular and/or immunophysiologic studies. In these studies we injected 30 BALB/c and C57BL/6 mice with streptozotocin delivered IV or intrarenally (IR). Histologically confirmed renal carcinomas arose in 10 per cent of BALB/c mice after IV induction and in 3 per cent of mice that received a single IR injection of strepto-

zotocin. This latter tumor, designated streptozotocin-induced renal cell carcinoma-1 (SIRCC-1), was adapted to serial orthotopic transplant and was frozen after the second passage. Only one RCC was detected in the C57BL/6 mice(in the IV group), and it was not successfully adapted to *in vivo* passage. Overall, these results demonstrate that streptozotocin can reproducibly induce RCC in BALB/c mice, but that these are difficult to successfully adapt to serial orthotopic transplant. The ability of streptozotocin to induce renal tumors in C57BL/6 mice is very limited, at least using the same protocol that was successful for BALB/c mice.

Heterogeneity of primary tumor growth and metastasis formation by cloned sublines from SIRCC-1

The use of currently available transplantable mouse renal carcinomas is limited by their rapid growth rate *in vivo* and the brief time interval between the establishment of well developed primary tumors and the subsequent death of the mouse. These rapidly growing mouse tumors may thus be of limited practical value for the study of some types of biological therapy, such as therapeutic vaccines, because the interval available for development of beneficial adaptive immune responses is inadequate. These mice may be close to death or harbor an insurmountable tumor burden before any meaningful host immune response can be engaged by such approaches. In contrast, the SIRCC-1 isolate grows relatively slowly and metastasizes spontaneously after orthotopic (IR) implantation of 1×10^5 tumor cells, with a mean survival time of about 3 months. Because tumors are often heterogeneous due to inherent genetic instability and can contain subpopulations of cells with differing biological characteristics (Fidler 1999), the SIRCC-1 tumor was cloned *in vitro* and the isolates were compared for differences in *in vivo* growth rates and propensity for metastasis. These sublines demonstrated considerable heterogeneity in growth and metastasis after orthotopic implantation into syngeneic BALB/c mice. Mean survival times of mice bearing these tumors may range from as little as 60 days to as much as 100 days. The metastatic potential of these different cell lines was also heterogeneous. Overall, these results demonstrate that streptozotocin can reproducibly induce RCC in BALB/c mice and that these tumors can be successfully adapted to serial intrarenal transplant *in vivo*. The data further demonstrate that the parental SIRCC-1 tumor line is composed of subpopulations of cells that differ in their aggressiveness *in vivo*, and may therefore also differ with regard to other biological properties such as the expression of genes that may regulate their own growth and function, or functions of other host cells. These biological differ-

Table 15.3 Characteristics of streptozotocin-induced tumors

Induced with high frequency in CBA mice and moderate frequency in BALB/c mice
C57BL/6 mice are relatively resistant to induction
BALB/c isolates are adaptable to serial orthotopic transplant
    Primary tumors grow relatively slowly
    Transplants metastasize spontaneously to lungs
    Highly vascularized
    Sublines exhibit different *in vivo* growth kinetics and gene expression profiles
Mutation analyses, oncogene expression, and responsiveness to biological therapy are currently in progress

ences might also reflect inherent variability in the genetic profiles of these sublines. These tumor isolates are now being studied for variations in physiology, molecular etiology, and responsiveness to cytokine and gene therapies. Overall, these newly-derived, streptozotocin-induced tumors exhibit a number of biological features similar to those exhibited by human RCC, including a much slower *in vivo* growth rate than that of many older transplant models (Table 15.3). Further effort will be required to delineate the genetic basis for the origin of these tumors and their overall suitability as models for biologic therapy.

Induction of renal carcinomas in rats by NDMA or methyl (methoxymethyl) nitrosamine

There is evidence that cigarette-smoking is linked to the induction of sporadic human RCC (Coughlin *et al.* 1997), and NDMA, (a component of cigarette smoke) is a kidney carcinogen in rodents (Muscat *et al.* 1995). Recently, Shiao *et al.* (1998) reported that some NDMA-induced kidney tumors of the clear or mixed clear/granular type in Wistar rats expressed four different (three G:C to A:T and one A:T to G:C) VHL gene mutations. Thirty to 70 per cent of base substitutions in the VHL gene mutations observed in human sporadic renal cell cancers are G:C to A:T or A:T to G:C (Foster *et al.* 1994; Gnarra *et al.* 1994). Thus, these NDMA-induced tumors may be genetically analogous to a large subset of human renal cell tumors and could prove very useful in the investigation of biological functions of the VHL gene during the evolution of renal tumors.

Another model of nitrosamine-induced RCC is provided by the administration of methyl (methoxymethyl) nitrosamine to newborn F344 rats (Sukumar *et al.* 1986). A single intraparenteral (IP) injection of this compound to rats induces an increased incidence of RCC and these tumors overexpress both K-ras and N-ras oncogenes. This finding provides another nitrosamine-based preclinical model in which the etiology of RCC is associated with expression of known oncogenes. The possible involvement of VHL mutations in this model is unclear.

Preclinical models where the development of RCC is associated with defined genetic mutations

Although several mutations have been clearly associated with RCC etiology in humans, appropriate preclinical models with similar defined etiology are limited. An exception is the development of hereditary RCC in the Eker rat (Everitt *et al.* 1992, 1995), with a germline mutation in the rat homolog of the human tuberous sclerosis 2 (Tsc2) gene (Hino *et al.* 1994; Kobayashi *et al.* 1995; Yeung *et al.* 1994). This model may provide some unique opportunities to understand the genetic etiology of oncogenesis of RCC. It shares some important physiological characteristics with human RCC, including overexpression of transforming growth factor alpha (TGFα) and an absence of p53 and ras mutations; but differs with regard to a lack of mutations in the VHL gene (Everitt *et al.* 1995). Thus, the model may provide unique insight into the

molecular mechanisms underlying tubular epithelial carcinogenesis (Hino *et al.* 1999), but to date the Eker model has not been widely used as a preclinical model for biologic therapy of RCC.

Induction of RCC-associated genetic mutations in appropriate murine genetic homologs

An attractive approach to the development of preclinical models of RCC with a defined genetic etiology is the introduction of oncogenic mutations into the appropriate rodent homolog genes, based on mutations that have been associated with etiology of RCC in humans. In this regard, Gnarra *et al.* (1997) have induced targeted disruption of the VHL gene in C57BL/6 mice. Heterozygous VHL (+/–) mice appear phenotypically normal while VHL (–/–) mice die *in utero* at 10.5 to 12.5 days of gestation as a result of failed placental vasculogenesis. The embryonic lethality associated with homozygosity of the VHL mutation occurs in conjunction with decreased vascular endothelial growth factor (VEGF) levels in the embryo, suggesting that dysregulation of VEGF expression may contribute to the mechanisms accounting for the observed embryonic lethality. Unfortunately, the disruption of the VHL gene in all cells and tissues in this (–/–) mouse does not allow for an analysis of kidney-specific events. Thus, it is likely that new approaches to disrupt one or both alleles of the VHL gene selectively in the kidney will be required to determine whether appropriately targeted mutations in the rodent VHL gene will result in the development of RCC. Successful induction of renal-targeted mutations of the VHL gene, or other genes associated with human RCC (for example, HGF/met; Horie *et al.* 1999; Schmidt *et al.* 1997) might also provide novel models for genetically induced murine RCC. Such models could prove very useful for the development of biological gene therapeutic approaches to the treatment of RCC because the etiology and physiology of tumor development in this setting would be more analogous than currently available transplantable models to the events contributing to development of human cancer.

Orthotopic xenografts of human RCC in athymic mice

Implantation of various human tumor xenografts in immunodeficient mice has also been reported (Ebert *et al.* 1990; Fidler *et al.* 1990). Fidler *et al.* (1990) have demonstrated that human RCC (HRCC) obtained from surgical specimens have different growth and metastatic characteristics depending on the organ site into which they are transplanted. In general, orthotopic implantation of HRCC into the kidney results in a higher incidence of pulmonary metastases compared to other sites of implantation. More recently, it has been reported that the orthotopic surgical implantation of histologically intact tumor tissue results in more aggressive primary tumor growth and increased metastasis than orthotopic injection of a disaggregated cell suspension (An *et al.* 1999). This approach of solid tumor implantation was then subsequently exploited to investigate the process of angiogenesis and metastasis by HRCC through the use of transfectants stably expressing green fluorescent protein (GFP) (Hoffman 1998). Thus, these models offer the advantage of being able to study some aspects of the behavior of actual human tumors *in vivo*. Nonetheless, the interpretation of immune responses induced by biologic agents in these models is limited by the fact that any responses are likely due to xenogeneic recognition.

Prospects

At present there are no perfect preclinical models for human RCC. The best models for the development of new experimental biological treatments for renal cell cancer and its faithful translation to application against human RCC would probably have several defined characteristics. First, the tumors should consistently develop spontaneously as a result of a defined genetic mutation(s) consistent with those identified in human RCC. This would allow the immune system of the host to be appropriately conditioned by the entire process of oncogenesis, in contrast to many transplantable tumor models where neoplastic cells are injected into an otherwise healthy adult mouse with an unmodified immune system. Such approaches may eventually become feasible when defined mutations may be more readily targeted specifically to the kidney, or where dysregulated gene expression may be introduced in a controled manner by the use of targeted, tissue-specific gene expression technology. In addition to such defined etiology, tumor growth and metastasis should proceed consistently but slowly, with reliable formation of pulmonary metastases. This protracted growth pattern is more generally characteristic of human solid tumors than many widely used, rapidly growing mouse transplantable tumors, and such growth characteristics would make the experimental models more amenable to the testing of biologic or gene therapies, which may require an extended period of time to achieve maximum impact.

The available transplantable mouse models do offer some of these attributes. After orthotopic implantation Renca cells grow progressively, potently expresses VEGF, develop an extensive neovasculature, metastasize reproducibly to the lungs, are moderately immunogenic, and respond to some cytokines (for example, IL-2, IFNα, and IL-12). The newly derived streptozotocin-induced transplantable tumor and its subline variants offer most of the same advantages as the Renca model, but also possess growth characteristics that are slower and thus more consistent with human RCC. The responsiveness of this new primary tumor and its sublines to biologic therapy remains unknown, as does its genetic etiology. However, its slower growth rate could make this model particularly attractive for the investigation of biologic approaches seeking to disrupt antiangiogenic mechanisms or induce adaptive immune responses. Both of these models are syngeneic to BALB/c mice and therefore offer the advantage for biologic studies in the context of a defined MHC in a model system for which an extensive array of immunologic reagents are available.

Overall, while these currently available transplantable rodent models of RCC are not perfect, they do offer useful attributes for developing at least some forms of experimental biological therapy. Their use will probably be superseded as the technology to reproduce the genetic etiology of human RCC in mice becomes available.

References

An, Z., Jiang, P., Wang, X., Moossa, A.R., and Hoffman, R.M. (1999). Development of a high metastatic orthotopic model of human renal cell carcinoma in nude mice: benefits of fragment implantation compared to cell-suspension injection. *Clin. Exp. Metastas.* **17**, 265–70.

Atkins, M.B., Robertson, M.J., Gordon, M., Lotze, M.T., DeCoste, M., DuBois, J.S., *et al.* (1997). Phase I evaluation of intravenous recombinant human interleukin 12 in patients with advanced malignancies. *Clin. Cancer Res.* **3**, 409–17.

Cohen, H.T. (1999). Advances in the molecular. basis of renal neoplasia. *Curr. Opin. Nephrol. Hypertension*, **8**, 325–31.

Coleman, M., Muller, S., Quezada, A., Mendiratta, S.K., Wang, J., Thull, N.M., *et al.* (1998). Nonviral interferon alpha gene therapy inhibits growth of established tumors by eliciting a systemic immune response. *Hum. Gene Ther.* **9**, 2223–30.

Coughlin, S.S., Neaton, J.D., Randall, B., and Sengupta, A. (1997). Predictors of mortality from kidney cancer in 332 547 men screened for the Multiple Risk Factor Intervention Trial. *Cancer* **79**, 2171–7.

Delahunt, B. and Wakefield, J.S. (1997). Ultrastructure of streptozotocin-induced renal tumours in mice. *Virch. Arch.* **430**, 173–80.

deVere White, R. and Olsson, C.A. (1980). Renal adenocarcinoma in the rat, a new tumor model. *Invest. Urol.* **17**, 405–12.

deVere White, R., Deitch, A.D., and Olsson, C.A. (1983). Limitations of DNA histogram analysis by flow cytometry as a method of predicting chemosensitivity in a rat renal cancer model. *Cancer Res.* **43**, 604–10.

Dutcher, J.P., Atkins, M., Fisher, R., Weiss, G., Margolin, K., Aronson, F., *et al.* (1997). Interleukin-2-based therapy for metastatic renal cell cancer: the cytokine working group experience: 1989–1997. *Cancer J. Am. Sci.* **3**, 573–8.

Ebert, T., Bander, N.H., Finstad, C.L., Ramsawak, R.D., and Old, L.J. (1990). Establishment and characterization of human renal cancer and normal kidney cell lines. *Cancer Res.* **50**, 5531–6.

Everitt, J.I., Goldsworthy, T.L., Wolf, D.C., and Walker, C.L. (1992). Hereditary renal cell carcinoma in the Eker rat: a rodent familial cancer syndrome. *J. Urol.* **148**, 1932–6.

Everitt, J.I., Goldsworthy, T.L., Wolf, D.C., and Walker, C.L. (1995). Hereditary renal cell carcinoma in the Eker rat: a unique animal model for the study of cancer susceptibility. *Toxicol. Lett.* **82–83**, 621–5.

Fenton, R.G., Back, T.C., Wigginton, J.M., Siders, W.M., Tartagalia, J., and Wiltrout, R.H. (1997). IL-12-expressing recombinant viruses mediate antitumor effects in murine tumor models. In *Program from the Keystone Symposium on Molecular and Cellular Biology: Cellular immunology and the immunotherapy of cancer—III*, p. 57.

Fidler, I.J. (1995). Modulation of the organ microenvironment for treatment of cancer metastasis. *J. Natl Cancer Inst.* **87**, 1588–92.

Fidler, I.J. (1999). Critical determinants of cancer metastasis: rationale for therapy. *Cancer Chemother. Pharmacol.* **43** (suppl.), S3–10.

Fidler, I.J., Naito, S., and Pathak, S. (1990). Orthotopic implantation is essential for the selection, growth and metastasis of human renal cell cancer in nude mice [corrected; published erratum appears in *Cancer Metastas. Rev.* 1991 May;**10** (1), 79]. *Cancer Metastas. Rev.* **9**, 149–65.

Figlin, R.A. (1999). Renal cell carcinoma: management of advanced disease. *J. Urol.* **161**, 381–6.

Foster, K., Prowse, A., van den, Berg, A., Fleming, S., Hulsbeek, M.M., Crossey, P.A., *et al.* (1994). Somatic mutations of the von Hippel–Lindau disease tumour suppressor gene in non-familial clear cell renal carcinoma. *Hum. Mol. Genet.* **3**, 2169–73.

Franco, J.L., Ghosh, P., Wiltrout, R.H., Carter, C.R., Zea, A.H., Momozaki, N., *et al.* (1995). Partial degradation of T-cell signal transduction molecules by contaminating granulocytes during protein extraction of splenic T cells from tumor-bearing mice. *Cancer Res.* **55**, 3840–6.

Fyfe, G., Fisher, R.I., Rosenberg, S.A., Sznol, M., Parkinson, D.R., and Louie, A.C. (1995). Results of treatment of 255 patients with metastatic renal cell carcinoma who received high-dose recombinant interleukin-2 therapy. *J. Clin. Oncol.* **13**, 688–96.

Ghosh, P., Sica, A., Young, H.A., Ye, J., Franco, J.L., Wiltrout, R.H., *et al.* (1994). Alterations in NF kappa B/Rel family proteins in splenic T-cells from tumor-bearing mice and reversal following therapy. *Cancer Res.* **54**, 2969–72.

Gnarra, J.R., Tory, K., Weng, Y., Schmidt, L., Wei, M.H., Li, H., *et al.* (1994). Mutations of the VHL tumour suppressor gene in renal carcinoma. *Nature Genet.* **7**, 85–90.

Gnarra, J.R., Ward, J.M., Porter, F.D., Wagner, J.R., Devor, D.E., Grinberg, A., *et al.* (1997). Defective placental vasculogenesis causes embryonic lethality in VHL-deficient mice. *Proc. Natl Acad. Sci., USA* **94**, 9102–7.

Godfrey, P.A. and Stinchcombe, T.E. (1999). Renal cell carcinoma. *Curr. Opin. Oncol.* **11**, 213–17.

Gohji, K., Nakajima, M., Dinney, C.P., Fan, D., Pathak, S., Killion, J.J., *et al.* (1990). The importance of orthotopic implantation to the isolation and biological characterization of a metastatic human clear cell renal carcinoma in nude mice. *Int. J. Oncol.* **2**, 23–32.

Gregorian, S.K. and Battisto, J.R. (1990*a*). Immunosuppression in murine renal cell carcinoma. I. Characterization of extent, severity and sources. *Cancer Immunol. Immunother.* **31**, 325–34.

Gregorian, S.K. and Battisto, J.R. (1990*b*). Immunosuppression in murine renal cell carcinoma. II. Identification of responsible lymphoid cell phenotypes and examination of elimination of suppression. *Cancer Immunol, Immunother.* **31**, 335–41.

Hard, G.C. (1984). High frequency, single-dose model of renal adenoma/carcinoma induction using dimethylnitrosamine in Crl:(W)BR rats. *Carcinogenesis* **5**, 1047–50.

Hard, G.C. (1985). Identification of a high-frequency model for renal carcinoma by the induction of renal tumors in the mouse with a single dose of streptozotocin. *Cancer Res.* **45**, 703–8.

Herr, R.R., Jahnke, J.K., and Argoudelis, A.D. (1967). The structure of streptozotocin. *J. Am. Chem. Soc.* **89**, 4808–9.

Hillman, G.G., Droz, J.P., and Haas, G.P. (1994). Experimental. animal models for the study of therapeutic approaches in renal cell carcinoma. *In Vivo* **8**, 77–80.

Hino, O., Kobayashi, T., Tsuchiya, H., Kikuchi, Y., Kobayashi, E., Mitani, H., *et al.* (1994). The predisposing gene of the Eker rat inherited cancer syndrome is tightly linked to the tuberous sclerosis (TSC2) gene. *Biochem. Biophys. Res. Commun.* **203**, 1302–8.

Hino, O., Fukuda, T., Satake, N., Kobayashi, T., Honda, S., Orimoto, K., *et al.* (1999). TSC2 gene mutant (Eker) rat model of a Mendelian dominantly inherited cancer. *Prog. Exp. Tumor Res.* **35**, 95–108.

Hoffman, R.M. (1998). Orthotopic transplant mouse models with green fluorescent protein- expressing cancer cells to visualize metastasis and angiogenesis. *Cancer Metastas. Rev.* **17**, 271–7.

Horie, S., Aruga, S., Kawamata, H., Okui, N., Kakizoe, T., and Kitamura, T. (1999). Biological role of HGF/MET pathway in renal cell carcinoma. *J. Urol.* **161**, 990–7.

Hornung, R.L., Back, T.C., Zaharko, D.S., Urba, W.J., Longo, D.L., and Wiltrout, R.H. (1988). Augmentation of natural killer activity, induction of IFN and development tumor immunity during the successful treatment of established murine renal cancer using flavone acetic acid and IL-2. *J. Immunol.* **141**, 3671–9.

Kerbel, R.S., Cornil, I., and Theodorescu, D. (1991). Importance of orthotopic transplantation procedures in assessing the effects of transfected genes on human tumor growth and metastasis. *Cancer Metastas. Rev.* **10**, 201–15.

Killion, J. J., Radinsky, R., and Fidler, I. J. (1998). Orthotopic models are necessary to predict therapy of transplantable tumors in mice. *Cancer Metastasis Rev.* **17**, 279–84.

Kobayashi, T., Hirayama, Y., Kobayashi, E., Kubo, Y., and Hino, O. (1995). A germline insertion in the tuberous sclerosis (Tsc2) gene gives rise to the Eker rat model of dominantly inherited cancer [published erratum appears in *Nature Genet.* 1995 Feb; **9** (2), 218]. *Nature Genet.* **9**, 70–4.

Kozlowski, J.M., Fidler, I.J., Campbell, D., Xu, Z.L., Kaighn, M.E., and Hart, I.R. (1984). Metastatic behavior of human tumor cell lines grown in the nude mouse. *Cancer Res.* **44**, 3522–9.

Lee, J.K., Sayers, T.J., Brooks, A.D., Back, T.C., Young, H.A., Komschlies, K.L., *et al.* (2000). IFN-gamma-dependent delay of *in vivo* tumor progression by Fas overexpression on murine renal cancer cells. *J. Immunol.* **164**, 231–9.

Levey, D.L. and Srivastava, P.K. (1995). T cells from late tumor-bearing mice express normal levels of p56lck, p59fyn, ZAP-70, and CD3 zeta despite suppressed cytolytic activity. *J. Exp. Med.* **182**, 1029–36.

Li, X., Liu, J., Park, J.K., Hamilton, T.A., Rayman, P., Klein, E., *et al.* (1994). T cells from renal cell carcinoma patients exhibit an abnormal pattern of kappa B-specific DNA-binding activity: a preliminary report. *Cancer Res.* **54**, 5424–9.

Mace, K.F., Hornung, R.L., Wiltrout, R.H., and Young, H.A. (1990). Correlation between *in vivo* induction of cytokine gene expression by flavone acetic acid and strict dose dependency and therapeutic efficacy against murine renal cancer. *Cancer Res.* **50**, 1742–7.

Mendiratta, S.K., Quezada, A., Matar, M., Wang, J., Hebel, H.L., Long, S., *et al.* (1999). Intratumoral delivery of IL-12 gene by polyvinyl polymeric vector system to murine renal and colon carcinoma results in potent antitumor immunity. *Gene Ther.* **6**, 833–9.

Mizoguchi, H., O'Shea, J.J., Longo, D.L., Loeffler, C.M., McVicar, D.W., and Ochoa, A.C. (1992). Alterations in signal transduction molecules in T lymphocytes from tumor-bearing mice. *Science* **258**, 1795–8.

Motzer, R.J., Rakhit, A., Schwartz, L.H., Olencki, T., Malone, T.M., Sandstrom, K., *et al.* (1998). Phase I trial of subcutaneous recombinant human interleukin-12 in patients with advanced renal cell carcinoma. *Clin. Cancer Res.* **4**, 1183–91.

Murphy, G.P. and Hrushesky, W.J. (1973). A murine renal cell carcinoma. *J. Natl Cancer Inst.* **50**, 1013–25.

Muscat, J.E., Hoffmann, D., and Wynder, E.L. (1995). The epidemiology of renal cell carcinoma. A second look. *Cancer* **75**, 2552–7.

Naito, S., Giavazzi, R., Walker, S.M., Itoh, K., Mayo, J., and Fidler, I.J. (1987). Growth and metastatic behavior of human tumor cells implanted into nude and beige nude mice. *Clin. Exp. Metastas.* **5**, 135–46.

Nakajima, M., Morikawa, K., Fabra, A., Bucana, C.D., and Fidler, I.J. (1990). Influence of organ environment on extracellular matrix degradative activity and metastasis of human colon carcinoma cells. *J. Natl Cancer Inst.* **82**, 1890–8.

Negrier, S., Escudier, B., Lasset, C., Douillard, J.Y., Savary, J., Chevreau, C., *et al.* (1998). Recombinant human interleukin-2, recombinant human interferon alfa-2a, or both in metastatic renal-cell carcinoma. Groupe Francais d'Immunotherapie. *New Engl. J. Med.* **338**, 1272–8.

Nishimatsu, H., Takeuchi, T., Ueki, T., Kajiwara, T., Moriyama, N., Ishida, T., *et al.* (1999). CD95 ligand expression enhances growth of murine renal cell carcinoma *in vivo. Cancer Immunol. Immunother.* **48**, 56–61.

O'Connell, J., O'Sullivan, G.C., Collins, J.K., and Shanahan, F. (1996). The Fas counterattack: Fas-mediated T cell killing by colon cancer cells expressing Fas ligand. *J. Exp. Med.* **184**, 1075–82.

Rakhmilevich, A.L., Turner, J., Ford, M.J., McCabe, D., Sun, W.H., Sondel, P.M., *et al.* (1996). Gene gun-mediated skin transfection with interleukin 12 gene results in regression of established primary and metastatic murine tumors. *Proc. Natl Acad. Sci., USA* **93**, 6291–6.

Saffran, D.C., Horton, H.M., Yankauckas, M.A., Anderson, D., Barnhart, K.M., Abai, A.M., *et al.* (1998). Immunotherapy of established tumors in mice by intratumoral injection of interleukin-2 plasmid DNA: induction of CD8+ T-cell immunity. *Cancer Gene Ther.* **5**, 321–30.

Salup, R.R., Back, T.C., and Wiltrout, R.H. (1987). Successful treatment of advanced murine renal cell cancer by bicompartmental adoptive chemoimmunotherapy. *J. Immunol.* **138**, 641–7.

Sayers, T.J., Wiltrout, T.A., McCormick, K., Husted, C., and Wiltrout, R.H. (1990). Antitumor effects of alpha-interferon and gamma-interferon on a murine renal cancer (Renca) *in vitro* and *in vivo. Cancer Res.* **50**, 5414–20.

Schmidt, L., Duh, F.M., Chen, F., Kishida, T., Glenn, G., Choyke, P., *et al.* (1997). Germline and somatic mutations in the tyrosine kinase domain of the MET proto-oncogene in papillary renal carcinomas. *Nature Genet.* **16**, 68–73.

Shiao, Y.H., Rice, J.M., Anderson, L.M., Diwan, B.A., and Hard, G.C. (1998). von Hippel–Lindau gene mutations in *N*-nitrosodimethylamine-induced rat renal epithelial tumors. *J. Natl Cancer Inst.* **90**, 1720–3.

Siders, W.M., Wright, P.W., Hixon, J.A., Alvord, W.G., Back, T.C., Wiltrout, R.H., *et al.* (1998). T-cell and NK cell-independent inhibition of hepatic metastases by systemic administration of an IL-12 expressing recombinant adenovirus. *J. Immunol.* **160**, 5465–74.

Strohmeyer, D. (1999). Pathophysiology of tumor angiogenesis and its relevance in renal cell cancer. *Anticancer Res.* **19**, 1557–61.

Sukumar, S., Perantoni, A., Reed, C., Rice, J.M., and Wenk, M.L. (1986). Activated K-ras and N-ras oncogenes in primary renal mesenchymal tumors induced in F344 rats by methyl(methoxymethyl)nitrosamine. *Mol. Cell. Biol.* **6**, 2716–20.

Sun, W.H., Burkholder, J.K., Sun, J., Culp, J., Turner, J., Lu, X.G., *et al.* (1995). *In vivo* cytokine gene transfer by gene gun reduces tumor growth in mice. *Proc. Natl Acad. Sci., USA* **92**, 2889–93.

Tan, J., Newton, C.A., Djeu, J.Y., Gutsch, D.E., Chang, A.E., Yang, N.S., *et al.* (1996). Injection of complementary DNA encoding interleukin-12 inhibits tumor establishment at a distant site in a murine renal carcinoma model. *Cancer Res.* **56**, 3399–403.

Tannenbaum, C.S., Tubbs, R., Armstrong, D., Finke, J.H., Bukowski, R.M., and Hamilton, T.A. (1998). The CXC chemokines IP-10 and Mig are necessary for IL-12-mediated regression of the mouse RENCA tumor. *J. Immunol.* **161**, 927–32.

Tepper, R.I. and Mule, J.J. (1994). Experimental and clinical studies of cytokine gene-modified tumor cells. *Hum. Gene Ther.* **5**, 153–64.

Uzzo, R.G., Clark, P.E., Rayman, P., Bloom, T., Rybicki, L., Novick, A.C., *et al.* (1999*a*). Alterations in NFkappaB activation in T lymphocytes of patients with renal cell carcinoma. *J. Natl Cancer Inst.* **91**, 718–21.

Uzzo, R.G., Rayman, P., Kolenko, V., Clark, P.E., Cathcart, M.K., Bloom, T., *et al.* (1999*b*). Renal cell carcinoma-derived gangliosides suppress nuclear factor- kappaB activation in T cells. *J. Clin. Invest.* **104**, 769–76.

Vogelzang, N.J. and Stadler, W.M. (1998). Kidney cancer. *Lancet* **352**, 1691–6.

Walker, P.R., Saas, P., and Dietrich, P.Y. (1997). Role of Fas ligand (CD95L) in immune escape: the tumor cell strikes back. *J. Immunol.* **158**, 4521–4.

Watanabe, M., Fenton, R.G., Wigginton, J.M., McCormick, K.L., Volker, K.M., Fogler, W.E., *et al.* (1999). Intradermal delivery of IL-12 naked DNA induces systemic NK cell activation and Th1 response *in vivo* that is independent of endogenous IL-12 production. *J. Immunol.* **163**, 1943–50.

White, R.V. and Olsson, D.A. (1980). Renal adenocarcinoma in the rat: a new tumor model. *Invest. Urol.* **17**, 405–12.

Whiteside, T.L. (1999). Signaling defects in T lymphocytes of patients with malignancy. *Cancer Immunol. Immunother.* **48**, 346–52.

Wigginton, J.M., Komschlies, K.L., Back, T.C., Franco, J.L., Brunda, M.J., and Wiltrout, R.H. (1996). Administration of interleukin 12 with pulse interleukin 2 and the rapid and complete eradication of murine renal carcinoma. *J. Natl Cancer Inst.* **88**, 38–43.

Williams, P.D., Pontes, E.J., and Murphy, G.P. (1981). Studies of the growth of a murine renal cell carcinoma and its metastatic patterns. *Res. Commun. Chem. Pathol. Pharmacol.* **34**, 345–9.

Wilmanns, C., Fan, D., O'Brian, C.A., Bucana, C.D., and Fidler, I.J. (1992). Orthotopic and ectopic organ environments differentially influence the sensitivity of murine colon carcinoma cells to doxorubicin and 5- fluorouracil. *Int. J. Cancer* **52**, 98–104.

Wiltrout, R.H. (1993). The use of preclinical rodent models for cancer immunotherapy. In G. Gallagher, R.C. Rees, and C.W. Reynolds (eds.) *Tumor immunobiology: a practical approach*, Oxford University Press, pp. 369–82.

Wiltrout, R.H., Boyd, M.R., Back, T.C., Salup, R.R., Arthur, J.A., and Hornung, R.L. (1988). Flavone-8-acetic acid augments systemic natural killer cell activity and synergizes with IL-2 for treatment of murine renal cancer. *J. Immunol.* **140**, 3261–5.

Wiltrout, R.H., Gregorio, T.A., Fenton, R.G., Longo, D.L., Ghosh, P., Murphy, W.J., *et al.* (1995). Cellular and molecular studies in the treatment of murine renal cancer. *Sem. Oncol.* **22**, 9–16.

Winter, B.K., Wu, S., Nelson, A.C., and Pollack, S.B. (1992). Renal cell carcinoma and natural killer cells: studies in a novel rat model *in vitro* and *in vivo*. *Cancer Res.* **52**, 6279–86.

Yamamoto, S., Suzuki, S., Hoshino, A., Akimoto, M., and Shimada, T. (1997). Herpes simplex virus thymidine kinase/ganciclovir-mediated killing of tumor cell induces tumor-specific cytotoxic T cells in mice. *Cancer Gene Ther.* **4**, 91–6.

Yeung, R.S., Xiao, G.H., Jin, F., Lee, W.C., Testa, J.R., and Knudson, A.G. (1994). Predisposition to renal carcinoma in the Eker rat is determined by germ-line mutation of the tuberous sclerosis 2 (TSC2) gene. *Proc. Natl Acad. Sci., USA* **91**, 11413–16.

Yonekura, K., Basaki, Y., Chikahisa, L., Okabe, S., Hashimoto, A., Miyadera, K., *et al.* (1999). UFT and its metabolites inhibit the angiogenesis induced by murine renal cell carcinoma, as determined by a dorsal air sac assay in mice. *Clin. Cancer Res.* **5**, 2185–91.

Yoon, S.S., Eto, H., Lin, C.M., Nakamura, H., Pawlik, T.M., Song, S.U., *et al.* (1999). Mouse endostatin inhibits the formation of lung and liver metastases. *Cancer Res.* **59**, 6251–6.

Zambrano, N.R., Lubensky, I.A., Merino, M.J., Linehan, W.M., and Walther, M.M. (1999). Histopathology and molecular genetics of renal tumors toward unification of a classification system. *J. Urol.* **162**, 1246–58.

16. Preclinical animal models for the investigation of biological approaches to the therapy of neuroblastoma

Jon M. Wigginton

Introduction

Neuroblastoma (NBL) is the most common extracranial solid tumor among children (Young and Miller 1975) and the most common neoplasm overall among infants less than 1 year of age. It accounts for approximately 8–10 per cent of all childhood cancers. Several aspects of the biology and/or clinical presentation of neuroblastoma are predictive of patient outcome, and have facilitated the development of risk-based strategies for patient management. Although age and stage are among the most important prognostic indicators (Breslow and McCann 1971, Evans *et al.* 1987), other factors that have been reported to be associated with adverse prognosis in patients with neuroblastoma include elevation of serum ferritin concentrations, presence of unfavorable histology, amplification of the N-myc oncogene, diploid DNA content, deletions of the short arm of chromosome 1, overexpression of the multidrug resistance-associated protein (MRP), low expression of the cellular adhesion molecule CD44, low-level expression of TrkA, and increased tumor vascularity (Castleberry 1997, Katzenstein and Cohn 1998; Matthay 1997). Despite the favorable prognosis of patients with low-risk disease (that is, low stage and favorable biologic features), those with advanced disease continue to do extremely poorly despite therapy, which may include surgery, radiotherapy, and intensive chemotherapy with or without hematologic reconstitution (Castleberry 1997; Katzenstein and Cohn 1998; Matthay 1997). There remains an urgent need then to develop new therapeutic strategies for these patients. Two modalities that are under active investigation include biologically targeted strategies to enhance the host immune response against neuroblastoma and/or methods directed at inhibition of tumor neovascularization (angiogenesis).

To facilitate preclinical investigation of the *in vivo* biology of neuroblastoma, and the evaluation of new therapeutic strategies, rodent models utilizing both human and murine transplantable neuroblastoma cell lines have been developed. The most commonly used murine cell lines include C-1300 and its subclones Neuro-2a and TBJ implanted into syngeneic mice, as well as the hybrid cell line, NXS2. Numerous human cell lines have been utilized in rodent xenograft models, although these models have been used primarily for the investigation of chemotherapeutic agents. Although some murine neuroblastoma cell lines (for example, TBJ, NXS2) are spontaneously metastatic, human cells are poorly metastatic in rodent models, and thus lack an important feature of the clinical behavior of neuroblastoma tumors. Although many preclinical studies have used heterotopic subcutaneous tumor cell implantation, models that more closely reflect the biology of neuroblastoma tumors in humans have recently been established as well. These include induced models of hepatic and/or bone marrow metastasis, retroperitoneal or orthotopic intra-adrenal neuroblastoma models characterized by progressive tumor growth with spontaneous metastasis, and transgenic models of spontaneous murine neuroblastoma based on tissue-specific targeted overexpression of the N-myc oncogene. The present discussion will review the biology of existing preclinical neuroblastoma models, their relative strengths and limitations, and the results of studies in these models that have investigated biologically targeted treatment strategies. Further, the experience in our laboratory and future prospects for both new model development and the application of these models to the investigation of novel biological treatment strategies will be presented.

Transplantable models of murine neuroblastoma

The most commonly used transplantable murine neuroblastoma cell lines include C-1300 and its subclones, Neuro-2a and TBJ, implanted in syngeneic A/J mice, as well as the C57BL/6xA/J hybrid cell line, NXS2. C-1300 arose spontaneously as a paraspinal mass in A/J mice (Dunham and Stewart 1953; Pons *et al.* 1982), and possesses many of the characteristic features of human neuroblastoma, including aggressive growth, catecholamine production, overexpression of the N-myc oncogene, and rare spontaneous regression (Ziegler *et al.* 1986). Although TBJ is a clone derived from the original C-1300 cell line, it demonstrates significant differences in biology. Subcutaneous C-1300 tumors grow progressively and are poorly metastatic, while TBJ has both aggressive local growth characteristics, and a strong propensity for lymph node and/or visceral (liver, lungs, adrenals) metastasis (Fowler *et al.* 1995; Ziegler *et al.* 1997). In contrast to C-1300, TBJ overexpresses matrix metalloproteinases-2 and -9, two important mediators of tumor metastasis (Fowler *et al.* 1995).

Several model systems using the C-1300/Neuro-2a and/or TBJ cell lines have now been characterized including subcutaneous or retroperitoneal (Katsanis *et al.* 1994*a*) tumor cell implantation as well as intrasplenic or intravenous injection to experimentally induce hepatic (Naito *et al.* 1992) or systemic (hepatic, bone, bone marrow) (Iwakawa *et al.* 1994; Yoshino *et al.* 1996) metastases, respectively. The impact of therapeutic intervention on metastatic tumor establishment or the progression of established metastatic disease may be investigated in mice after intrasplenic/intravenous tumor cell injection. Nonetheless, the induced nature of metastases formed in these models may not fully reflect the dynamic interactions between host physiology and the complex mechanisms mediating tumor progression and metastasis. Retroperitoneal Neuro-2a implants grow progressively and metastasize spontaneously (Katsanis *et al.* 1994*a*), as confirmed by subcutaneous implantation of cell suspensions from the liver, spleen, and bone marrow into normal hosts (Katsanis *et al.* 1994*a*). Further, retroperitoneal tumor cell implants grow more aggressively than either subcutaneous or intraperitoneal neuroblastoma tumors.

Although the biology of TBJ more closely reflects the clinical behavior of human neuroblastoma than C-1300/Neuro-2a, its responsiveness to various therapeutic modalities (including biologics) remains to be defined. We have now characterized a novel model of established *in vivo*-conditioned TBJ (as well as Neuro-2a) murine neuroblastoma, based on direct visualization and orthotopic implantation of tumor cells into the adrenal gland, a common site of origin for neuroblastoma in humans. The median survival time of mice after orthotopic intraadrenal implantation of 5.0×10^4 TBJ or Neuro-2a cells is approximately 25 days versus 40–45 days among mice receiving 1.0–0.5×10^5 cells via intrasplenic injection and 25–35 days among mice receiving a subcutaneous implant of 1.0–2.0×10^6 tumor cells (Wigginton, unpublished observations). Despite receiving one to two log-fold fewer tumor cells, mice with orthotopic intraadrenal tumor cell implants demonstrate comparable or even diminished survival compared to mice with subcutaneous or intrahepatic tumors, demonstrating the important influence of implantation site (that is, heterotopic vesus orthotopic) on the *in vivo* biology of transplantable tumor cell lines. In this unique model, tumors grow progressively to form hemorrhagic, highly vascularized tumors, which in the case of TBJ (but not Neuro-2a) metastasize spontaneously to the lungs and livers (Wigginton, unpublished observations). We have also devised a novel *in vivo* method for direct visualization and quantitation of tumor neovascularization utilizing the infusion of latex with or without radioisotope (Wigginton *et al.*, 2001).This technique enables assessment of the vascularization of orthotopic adrenal primary tumors, enhanced visualization of the formation and vascularization of spontaneous or induced hepatic and pulmonary tumor metastases, and semiquantitative evaluation of the impact of therapeutic interventions on these processes. Thus, these methods collectively provide a novel, therapeutically challenging model system that closely reflects the biology of human neuroblastoma, and may provide a more directly relevant setting for the preclinical evaluation of the antitumor and/or antivascular activity of new biological approaches for the treatment of neuroblastoma.

Transgenic models of murine neuroblastoma

Although transgenic models of spontaneous tumor may present some practical difficulties in the implementation of therapeutic studies, they may offer unique advantage over transplantable syngeneic or xenograft tumor models, particularly for the investigation of new therapeutic modalities based on promotion of the host antitumor immune response. In contrast to transplantable tumor models, in which the host is presented simultaneously with a substantial burden of implanted tumor cells, spontaneous tumors in transgenic mice evolve in a host conditioned by the complete dynamic process of neoplastic progression and tumorigenesis. Transgenic models with complete tumor penetrance also provide an opportunity for the investigation of preventative strategies directed at blockade of the spontaneous neoplastic progression and tumorigenesis induced by various oncogenic transgenes. Several transgenic models have now been described in which neuroblastoma tumors may develop spontaneously as a consequence of the overexpression of transforming genes including H-Ras (Sweetser *et al.* 1997), simian virus 40 (SV40) large T antigen (Giraldi *et al.* 1994; Servenius *et al.* 1994; Skalnik *et al.* 1991), polyoma virus middle T antigen (Aguzzi *et al.* 1990), a metallothionein/ret fusion gene (Iwamoto *et al.* 1993), and N-myc (Weiss *et al.* 1997). Targeted overexpression of activated H-Ras induces the formation of ganglioneuromas and in some instances neuroblastoma in the adrenal glands and sympathetic ganglia of transgenic mice (Sweetser *et al.* 1997), while overexpression of the oncogenic SV40 large T antigen gene induces the formation of highly metastatic neuroblastoma tumors in these sites (Servenius *et al.* 1994). Transgenic mice engineered to overexpress the SV40 T antigen under the control of promoter sequences from the gp-91 phox or growth hormone releasing hormone genes develop neuroblastomas in the prostate (Skalnik *et al.* 1991) or adrenal glands (Giraldi *et al.* 1994), respectively, while overexpression of the polyoma virus middle T antigen induces hyperplastic lesions and ultimately neuroblastoma tumors that overexpress N-myc in the sympathetic ganglia and adrenal glands (Aguzzi *et al.* 1990).

Perhaps the most extensively characterized system is a recently reported model in which the human N-myc oncogene is overexpressed in a targeted, tissue-specific fashion via an expression vector driven by the promoter sequence from the tyrosine bydroxylase gene (Weiss *et al.* 1997), a gene characteristically expressed in neural crest tissue. As a consequence of N-myc overexpression in neural-crest-derived tissues such as the adrenal glands, mice develop neuroblastoma tumors that manifest as abdominal/adrenal masses or thoracic or abdominal paraspinous tumors (Weiss *et al.* 1997). These tumors can metastasize spontaneously to the liver, lungs, ovaries, lymphatics, kidney, brain, or muscle and reveal a spectrum of concurrent genetic lesions that closely mirror those observed in human neuroblastoma (Weiss *et al.* 1997). The tumorigenicity of N-myc overexpression is further potentiated in the offspring of N-myc transgenic mice that have been crossed with mice with targeted disruption of either the nuerofibromatosis-1 (NF-1) or retinoblastoma-1 (RB-1) tumor suppressor genes (Weiss *et al.* 1997).

Transgenic tumor models also provide an opportunity for the derivation of new transplantable cell lines arising from orthotopic sites of origin. Utilizing the N-myc transgenic mouse described by Weiss *et al.* (1997), we have recently established several novel cell lines derived from spontaneous neuroblastoma tumors that have arisen in the adrenal glands or paraspinal sympathetic ganglia. All of these cell lines overexpress the N-myc oncogene and form large, highly vascularized tumors that grow progressively and invade locally after subcutaneous or intraadrenal implantation. Although little or no information has been generated regarding the efficacy of therapeutic interventions in these systems, transgenic models of spontaneous neuroblastoma may provide information that complements that obtained utilizing transplantable cell lines and, along with derivative autochthonous cell lines, proved excellent new model systems for the investigation of biologically targeted treatment strategies. As described by Weiss *et al.* (1997). N-myc transgenic mice can also be bred with other strains such as those with targeted disruption (knock-out) of various relevant tumor suppressor genes (for example, Rb, NF-1, p53) to attempt to enhance the tumorigenicity of N-myc overexpression and provide models for investigation of the interaction of these genes *in vivo*. We are currently deriving N-myc transgenic mice and cell lines with concurrent disruption of the interferon gamma (IFNγ) receptor gene. This system will provide an important new model for dissection of the role of host versus tumor cell responses to IFNγ-mediated antitumor mechanisms. Similar approaches are planned for other genes relevant tomechanisms mediating the antitumor effects of various biologics, such as anti-angiogenic agents and the potent antitumor cytokines interleukin 12 (IL-12) and IL-18.

Xenograft models of human neuroblastoma

A number of preclinical xenograft models have been reported in which human neuroblastoma cells are implanted into immuno-deficient rodents including severe combined immunodeficiency (SCID) mice and/or athymic nude mice or rats. A broad range of human neuroblastoma cell lines have been used in these models in which tumor cells have been implanted subcutaneously (Cinatl *et al.* 1999; Zamboni *et al.* 1998), intravascularly to induce disseminated metastases (Bogenmann 1996; Martinez *et al.* 1996), or within the eye (Yoshida *et al.* 1994), leptomeninges/epidural space (Bergman *et al.* 1993, 1999), central nervous system (CNS) (Morton *et al.* 1995, Taghian *et al.* 1993), peritoneum (Helson *et al.* 1975), or adrenal glands (Flickinger *et al.* 1994). Xenograft models have been used primarily to investigate cytotoxic agents, inhibitors of tumor neovascularization, or modulators of intracellular signal transduction. Although xenograft models utilizing tumor cells implanted into immunodeficient mice may be well suited to the investigation of non protein, small-molecule agents that act directly on tumor cells themselves, they have significant disadvantages when used to evaluate biologies, such as immunoregulatory agents or anti-angiogenic/antivascular drugs that may act on the host endothelium. For protein-based therapeutics, limitations imposed by species specificity may result in altered or even nonresponsiveness to agents whose activity is dependent on the engagement of host antitumor mechanisms. In light of these considerations, it appears that syngeneic tumor models, particularly those based on orthotopic sites of tumor implantation, or transgenic models of spontaneous neuro-

blastoma may be the most directly relevant for the preclinical investigation of biologics.

Utilization of preclinical models for evaluation of the biological therapy of neuroblastoma

Several different transplantable models have been utilized for the evaluation of biologically targeted treatment strategies for neuroblastoma, including subcutaneous, retroperitoneal, or direct intraadrenal implantation of C-1300/Neuro-2a or TBJ tumor cells in syngeneic mice, spontaneous or experimentally induced hepatic and/or bone metastases of the hybrid NXS2 cell line as well as human neuroblastoma xenograft models in immunodeficient mice. Collectively, these model systems provide a framework for the investigation of therapies directed at disrupting the establishment of primary and/or metastatic tumors, as well as more recent efforts to induce the regression of even well-established primary and/or metastatic disease. Two approaches that are under active investigation are potentiation of the host antitumor immune response and inhibition of tumor neovascularization.

Immunotherapy

Background
Substantial effort has focused on preclinical investigation of the host immune response to neuroblastoma and the definition of methods to therapeutically augment this response and induce tumor regression. Both human and murine neuroblastoma cells constitutively express relatively low levels of class I human leukocyte antigen/major histocompatibility complex (HLA/MHC) antigen on their surface, and this expression correlates inversely with N-myc amplification (Cheng *et al.* 1996; Sugio *et al.* 1991). Nonetheless, IFNγ may potently enhance HLA/MHC class I antigen expression by cells *in vitro* and *in vivo* (Lode *et al.* 1998*a*; Ponzoni *et al.* 1993, Sigal *et al.* 1991; Ucar *et al.* 1995; Watanabe *et al.* 1989). Further, neuroblastomas may express the tumor antigens MART-1, MAGE-1, and MAGE-3 (Corrias *et al.* 1996), and specific T-cell-mediated responses and immunologic memory may be induced in mice experiencing tumor regression in response to immunotherapy (Hock *et al.* 1995; Katsanis *et al.* 1994*b*, 1995, 1996, Lode *et al.* 1998*a*). It would appear then that a specific host immune response against neuroblastoma tumors probably does occur *in vivo*, suggesting that enhancement of this response may be a reasonable target for the therapeutic induction of tumor regression.

In vitro studies

Modulation of tumor cell physiology
Cytokines not only enhance the host immune response against human or murine neuroblastoma cells, but also may directly modulates the physiology of tumor cells themselves. Treatment with IFNγ enhances the cell surface expression of HLA/MHC class I (Lode *et al.* 1998*b*; Ponzoni *et al.* 1993; Sigal *et al.* 1991; Ucar *et al.* 1995; Watanabe *et al.* 1989) and class II (Ponzoni *et al.*

1993; Ucar *et al.* 1995) molecules and promotes the differentiation of neuroblastoma cells *in vitro* (Montaldo *et al.* 1993). Further IFNγ enhances cell surface FAS expression on neuroblastoma cells engineered to overexpress N-myc (Bernassola *et al.* 1999; Lutz *et al.* 1998), sensitizes them to FAS-induced killing (Bernassola *et al.* 1999), and can inhibit DNA synthesis and the expression of insulin-like growth factor II (IGFII) (Martin *et al.* 1993), a mediator that can prevent stress-induced apoptosis and enhances the tumorigenicity of neuroblastoma cells *in vivo* (Singleton *et al.* 1996). IFNγ alone also enhances TrkA but not TrkB expression *in vitro* (Lucarelli *et al.* 1995). Neuroblastoma cells engineered to overexpress N-myc are also sensitized to programme cell death upon subsequent *in vitro* exposure to TNF-related apoptosis-inducing ligand (TRAIL) or tumor necrosis factor alpha (TNFα) (Lutz *et al.* 1998). In combination with retinoic acid, another agent that can induce the differentiation of neuroblastoma cells, IFNγ downregulates expression of the N-myc oncogene (Wada *et al.* 1997) and additively enhances expression of intercellular adhesion molecule 1 (ICAM-1) (Bouillon and Audette 1993). IFNγ and TNFα synergistically promote the terminal differentiation of human neuroblastoma cells into mature neurons *in vitro* (Montaldo *et al.* 1994, Munoz-Fernandez *et al.* 1994), and appear to do so via a mechanism dependent on the induction of tumor cell nitric oxide production (Munoz-Fernandez *et al.* 1994). Combined treatment of neuroblastoma cells with IFNγ and nerve growth factor (NGF) can inhibit proliferation and induce terminal differentiation of these cells *in vitro* (Ridge *et al.* 1996). Thus, although they are important modulators of the antitumor immune response, cytokines such as IFNγ may also act directly on tumor cells themselves to engage mechanisms that may ultimately facilitate tumor regression.

Modulation of leukocyte effector cell function

The cytolytic activity of various leukocyte populations against neuroblastoma cell lines *in vitro* may be potently enhanced by cytokines. Natural killer (NK)/lymphokine-activated killer (LAK) cell-mediated killing of human and/or murine neuroblastoma cells may be enhanced by IL-2 alone (Atzpodien *et al.* 1988; Handgretinger *et al.* 1989*a*), or in combination with anti-CD3 (Anderson *et al.* 1988), IFNα (Alvarado *et al.* 1989), or IL-12 (Rossi *et al.* 1994). Prior treatment of human neuroblastoma cells with IFNγ enhances their sensitivity to killing by untreated or

IL-2 activated NK cells (Handgretinger *et al.* 1989*b*), and combined treatment with IFNγ or IL-2 inhibits the establishment of C-1300 neuroblastoma implants and enhances NK/LAK-mediated killing of C-1300 *in vitro* (Reynolds *et al.* 1989; Sigal *et al.* 1991). Culture of neuroblastoma-derived tumor-infiltrating lymphocytes (TIL) in IL-2 induces increases in cytolytic CD56[+] and CD8[+] lymphocytes capable of lysing NK- and LAK-sensitive cell lines (Facchetti *et al.* 1996), and CD8[+] T cells isolated from TIL treated with IL-12 plus IL-2 reveal much greater cytolytic activity against autologous neuroblastoma tumor cells, than those from TIL treated with IL-2 alone (Kuge *et al.* 1995). Collectively, these findings demonstrate that both T-cell and NK/LAK-cell reactivity against neuroblastoma cells may be potently enhanced by cytokine treatment *in vitro* and provide a framework for the design of *in vivo* studies to investigate immunotherapeutic treatment strategies.

In vivo studies

Systemic cytokine-based strategies

Several cytokine-based approaches for the therapy of murine neuroblastoma have been reported, including systemic administration of IL-2 alone (Ishizu *et al.* 1994), or in combination with perioperative administration of low-dose cyclophosphamide and retinyl palmitate in conjunction with resection of established subcutaneous primary tumors (Fowler *et al.* 1991, 1993) (Table 16.1) Systemic administration of continuous-infusion IL-2 significantly prolongs the survival of mice bearing day 3 established neuroblastoma metastases, and induces complete responses in 50 per cent of treated mice (Ishizu *et al.* 1994). Combined therapy with IL-2/retinyl palmitate/low-dose cyclophosphamide in the perioperative setting enhances tumor cell MHC class I antigen expression, delays tumor growth, prolongs the survival of treated mice, and markedly reduces rates of local recurrence after resection of established subcutaneous primary C-1300 tumors (Fowler *et al.* 1991, 1993). Systemic administration of a fusion protein consisting of IL-2 linked to a tumor-targeted anti-GD2 ganglioside antibody (ch14.18-IL-2) in conjunction with adoptive transfer of IL-2-activated LAK cells derived from normal human peripheral blood mononuclear cells (PBMC) inhibits the establishment of experimentally induced human neuroblastoma hepatic metastases in immunodeficient SCID mice (Sabzevari *et al.* 1994), and can

Table 16.1 Preclinical investigations of systemic cytokine-based therapy of neuroblastoma

Agent	Reference
IL-2	Ishizu *et al.* 1994
IL-2/retinylpalmitate/cyclophosphamide + surgery	Fowler *et al.* 1991, 1993
IL-2/anti-GD2 antibody fusion protein (ch14.18-IL-2)	Lode *et al.* 1997, 1998*b*; Sabzevari *et al.* 1994
ch14.18–IL-2 + adoptive LAK cell transfer	Pancook *et al.* 1996
ch14.18–IL-2 + IFNγ	Lode *et al.* 1998*b*
IFNγ	Reynolds *et al.* 1989
IL-4–Pseudomonas exotoxin chimera	Puri *et al.* 1994
TNFα	Sohmura *et al.* 1986
TNFα + radiotherapy	Leonard *et al.* 1992
TNFα + chemotherapy	Leonard *et al.* 1991

also induce the regression of day 8 established hepatic metastases (Pancook *et al.* 1996).

To facilitate evaluation of local tumor-targeted immuno-therapeutic strategies in immunocompetent mice, a cell line has been established by the fusion of C-1300 cells (A/J background) and dorsal root ganglion cells (C57BL/6J background) to create the hybrid NX31T28 cell line, which was subsequently subcloned to establish the high-level GD2 expressor, NXS2 (Lode *et al.* 1997). Models of induced and/or spontaneous hepatic and bone marrow metastasis have now been characterized utilizing the NXS2 cell line (Lode *et al.* 1997, 1999*a*). Early systemic administration of ch14. 18-IL-2 inhibits the establishment of day 1 hepatic and bone marrow NXS2 metastases (Lode *et al.* 1997), and induces the regression of day 5 established hepatic and bone marrow metastases via a mechanism that is dependent on NK cells, but not CD8$^+$ T cells (Lode *et al.* 1998*b*). Administration of ch14.18-IL-2 also significantly limits the development of spontaneous hepatic and bone marrow metastases after the resection of established subcutaneous NXS2 tumors (Lode *et al.* 1997) and ch14.18-IL-2 enhances cytolytic activity of murine splenocytes *in vitro* (Lode *et al.* 1998*b*). Continuous infusion of IFNγ induces local MHC class I antigen expression within established NXS2 tumors, potentiates the therapeutic activity of ch14.18-IL-2 against established hepatic and bone marrow NXS2 metastases, and enhances the *ex vivo* cytolytic activity of splenocytes compared to those from mice treated with IFNγ or ch14.18-IL-2 alone (Lode *et al.* 1998*b*). Other systemic cytokine-based approaches that have demonstrated some therapeutic activity in preclinical neuroblastoma models include IFNγ (Reynolds *et al.* 1989), an IL-4 *Pseudomonas* exotoxin chimera targeted to the IL-4 receptor (Puri *et al.* 1994), and TNFα delivered alone (Sohmura *et al.* 1986), or in conjunction with radiotherapy (Leonard *et al.* 1992) or chemotherapy (Leonard *et al.* 1991).

Gene therapy/tumor vaccines

In an effort to limit the toxicities that have been observed in conjunction with systemic delivery of some cytokines in the clinical setting, a large number of studies have investigated gene therapy approaches to achieve local cytokine delivery in preclinical

Table 16.2 Tumor cells engineered to overexpress various cytokines for the gene therapy of neuroblastoma

Agent	Reference
IFNγ	Ucar *et al.* 1995; Watanabe *et al.* 1989
IL-2	Corrias *et al.* 1998; Katsanis *et al.* 1994*b*; Yoshida *et al.* 1998*a,b*, 1999
IL-4	Yoshida *et al.* 1998*c*
IL-12	Davidoff *et al.* 1999; Lode *et al.* 1998*a*
IL-18	Heuer *et al.* 1999
GM-CSF	Bausero *et al.* 1996; Yoshida *et al.* 1998*a,b*, 1999
CD40L	Grossmann *et al.* 1997
B7.1	Katsanis *et al.* 1995
B7.2	Enomoto *et al.* 1997
Class II	Hock *et al.* 1995, 1996
ICAM-1	Katsanis *et al.* 1994*c*
B7.1 + IFNγ	Katsanis *et al.* 1996
B7.1 + class II	Heuer *et al.* 1996
IFNγ + GM-CSF	Bausero *et al.* 1996

neuroblastoma models (Table 16.2). Among the most extensively studied factors are the co-stimulatory molecules B7.1 (Katsanis *et al.* 1995) and B7.2 (Enomoto *et al.* 1997), MHC class II antigens (Hock *et al.* 1995, 1996), and cytokines such as IFNγ (Ucar *et al.* 1995; Watanabe *et al.* 1989), IL-2 (Corrias *et al.* 1998; Katsanis *et al.* 1994*b* Yoshida *et al.* 1998*a, b*, 1999), IL-12 (Davidoff *et al.* 1999; Lode *et al.* 1998*a*), and IL-18 (Heuer *et al.* 1999). Transduction of Neuro-2a cells with the B7.1 gene reduces their tumorigenicity after retroperitoneal implantation and, although a CD8$^+$ T-cell-dependent immune response is generated in treated mice, vaccination with Neuro-2a-B7.1 does not appear to confer resistance to a subsequent challenge with wild-type tumor cells (Katsanis *et al.* 1995). Co-expression of B7.1 and IFNγ almost completely abrogates the tumorgenicity of retroperitoneal Neuro-2a, and improves the survival of tumor-bearing mice compared to that of those that receive tumor cells transduced with either B7.1 or IFNγ alone (Katsanis *et al.* 1996). Although reduced by B7.1, the tumorigenicity of subcutaneous Neuro-2a implants is completely abrogated by concurrent overexpression of MHC class II molecules (Heuer *et al.* 1996). Further, this effect is dependent on both CD4$^+$ and CD8$^+$ T cells, and vaccination of mice with Neuro-2a-B7.1/class II induces the generation of specific cytolytic splenic T cells *in vivo* (Heuer *et al.* 1996). C-1300 cells engineered to overexpress B7.2 are nontumorigenic after subcutaneous implantation, and *in vitro* restimulation of splenocytes from treated mice potently enhances cytolytic T lymphocyte (CTL) activity (Enomoto *et al.* 1997). This CTL activity is further enhanced by IL-2, can very effectively limit the establishment of induced systemic metastases when splenocytes are adoptively transferred 2 days after the implantation of wild-type tumor cells, and is accounted for primarily by CD8$^+$ T cells (Enomoto *et al.* 1997). Collectively, these findings demonstrate that transduction of tumor cells with the co-stimulatory molecules B7.1 or B7.2 alone or in combination with class II molecules or IFNγ can induce T-cell-dependent antitumor immune responses *in vitro* and *in vivo*. Nonetheless, although these interventions can engage the host immune response and induce specific cytolytic T-cell responses, as well as abrogate the tumorigenicity and limit the establishment of primary and/or metastatic tumors, there is little evidence to date in preclinical models that such strategies may be utilized to induce the regression of well-established tumors as one would attempt to accomplish in the clinical setting.

Transduction with the genes encoding IL-2 and/or granulo-cyte–macrophage colony-stimulating factor (GM-CSF) abrogates the tumorigenicity of retroperitoneal (Katsanis *et al.* 1994*b*), subcutaneous (Yoshida *et al.* 1998*a*), or intravenous (Yoshida *et al.* 1998*a*) C-1300/Neuro-2a implants in syngenic mice and, in the case of Neuro-2a, does so via a CD8$^+$ T-cell-dependent and NK-cell-independent mechanism. Vaccination of mice with C-1300/Neuro-2a-IL-2 or C-1300-GM-CSF cells confers resistance to a subsequent challenge with wild-type tumor cells (Katsanis *et al.* 1994*b*; Yoshida *et al.* 1998*a,b*) and, in mice bearing established wild-type C-1300 or Neuro-2a tumor implants, prolongs survival (Katsanis *et al.* 1994*b*) and induces tumor regression (Yoshida *et al.* 1999). Although CD8$^+$ T cells appear to be important mediators of the immunoregulatory/antitumor effects of IL-2 transduced murine neuroblastoma cells implanted in syngeneic mice (Katsanis *et al.* 1994*b*), transduction of human neuroblastoma cells with IL-2 abrogates their tumorigenicity even in a host that lacks functional T cells (for example, nude mice), and this effect is lost after depletion of NK cells (Corrias *et al.* 1998). Thus, contrasting mechanims appear to be engaged in immunodeficient versus syngeneic mice bearing IL-2 gene-transduced neuroblastoma tumors. Concurrent overexpression of IFNγ and GM-CSF abrogates the tumorigenicity of Neuro-2a, and prior vaccination of mice with Neuro-2a-GMCSF or Neuro-2a-GM-CSF/IFNγ prolongs the survival of mice bearing established wild-type retroperitoneal tumors (Bausero *et al.* 1996).

IL-12 and IL-18 are two recently described cytokines that potently enhance IFNγ production (Chan *et al.* 1991; Nakamura *et al.* 1989), and possess striking therapeutic activity in various non-neuroblastoma tumor models (Brunda *et al.* 1993; Hashimoto *et al.* 1999; Micallef *et al.* 1997; Nastala *et al.* 1994). Transfection of hybrid NXS2 neuroblastoma cells to overexpress a single-chain IL-12 p35/p40 fusion protein abrogates the tumorigenicity of subcutaneous tumor implants and induced bone marrow or liver metastases (Lode *et al.* 1998*a*). Vaccination of mice with NXS2-IL-12 cells prevents the establishment of wild-type hepatic or bone marrow metastases, and induces substantial reductions or even eradication of early established bone marrow and hepatic metastases (Lode *et al.* 1998*a*).The tumorigenicity of NXS2-IL-12 cells is restored in immunoeficient SCID mice or in A/J mice depleted of CD8$^+$ T cells (Lode *et al.* 1998*a*), thus demonstrating an important role for T cells in the therapeutic activity of IL-12 in these models. *In situ* transduction of Neuro-2a tumors via intratumoral injection of adenovirus engineered to overexpress IL-12 promotes the regression of established tumors, and confers immunologic memory and resistance to subsequent challenge with wild-type Neuro-2a tumor cells (Davidoff *et al.* 1999). IL-18 transduction abrogates the tumorigenicity of subcutaneous Neuro-2a tumor implants via a CD4$^+$/CD8$^+$ T-cell-dependent mechanism, and vaccination of mice with Neuro-2a-IL-18 confers resistance to a subsequent wild-type tumor challenge (Heuer *et al.* 1999). Thus, overexpression of IL-12 or IL-18 in the local tumor site via gene therapy can induce T-cell-dependent antitumor immune responses, confer resistance to subsequent wild-type tumor challenge, and even induce the regression of early established tumors. We have shown that combined systemic administration of IL-2 and IL-12 synergistically enhances the host antitumor immune response and induces the complete regression of even well-established primary and/or metastatic tumor (Wigginton *et al.* 1996; Wigginton *et. al.* 2001). Administration of ch14.18-KL-2 in conjunction with vaccination of mice with NXS2-IL-12 synergistically inhibits the establishment of wild-type NXS2 bone marrow and hepatic metastases (Lode *et al.* 1999*b*). It does so via a mechanism that is dependent primarily on CD8$^+$ T cells, and is observed even when the wild-type tumor challenge occurs as long as 90 days after the initial vaccination with NXS2-IL-12 (Lode *et al.* 1999*b*).

Immunotherapy in novel models of advanced orthotopic neuroblastoma

Despite the positive therapeutic effects of a wide range of cytokine-based strategies in existing preclinical neuroblastoma models, relatively limited information is available regarding the efficacy of such approaches in more challenging models of well-established primary and/or metastatic orthotopic tumor, or in transgenic models of autochthonous neuroblastoma, where the host immune system has been conditioned by the complete process of neoplastic progression and tumorigenesis. This may account in part for the observation that positive therapeutic results obtained with agents such as IL-2 in existing preclinical neuroblastoma models have not generally translated to comparable efficacy in IL-2-based clinical studies to date (Bauer *et al.* 1995; Bowman *et al.* 1998; Frost *et al.* 1997; Ribeiro *et al.* 1993; Roper *et al.* 1992). Assessment of new agents in models of primary and/or metastatic tumor establishment or in the setting of very early established disease, particularly in heterotopic sites of implantation, may not adequately reflect the spectrum of barriers to successful induction of tumor regression in the clinical setting. Patients often come to clinical attention with advanced primary and/or metastatic tumor, with alterations in host immune-responsiveness, as well as significant perturbations in physiology and/or organ dysfunction. More advanced and therapeutically challenging models of neuroblastoma may provide several advantages in the preclinal evaluation of immune-based treatment strategies, and better facilitate the identification of those approaches that offer the most potential for efficacy in the clinical setting.

In light of these considerations, we have begun to investigate several therapeutic approaches including systemic administration of cytokines alone or in combination with other cytokines, chemotherapy or targeted antagonists of tumor neovascularization in novel transplantable models of advanced orthotopic, intradrenal TBJ or Neuro-2a neuroblastoma, and in N-myc transgenic mice bearing spontaneous neuroblastoma tumors (Table 16.3). Systemic administration of IL-12 or IL-18 alone or in combination with IL-2 can induce complete and durable regression of well-established intraadrenal or subcutaneous TBJ or Neuro-2a tumors in the majority of treated mice (Wigginton, J.M., unpublished observations). Similar responses to IL-12 with or without IL-2 are noted in mice bearing well-established subcutaneous TBJ or Neuro-2a tumors (Wigginton, J.M., unpub-

Table 16.3 Characteristics of orthotopic intraadrenal murine neuroblastoma tumors and responsiveness to various therapeutic interventions

- Progressive local growth with spontaneous metastasis (TBJ) to the liver and/or lung
- Form highly vascularized, hemorrhagic tumors consistent with clinical neuroblastoma
- Treatment of well-established tumors with IL-12 ± IL-2 induces complete tumor regression, induces resistance to tumor rechallenge, enhances infiltration of CD3+ T cells into the local tumor site, and inhibits tumor neovascularization
- Treatment of well-established tumors with IL-18 ± IL-2 induces complete tumor regression
- Growth of established tumor may be inhibited by anti-angiogenic compounds
- Regression of established tumor induced by chemotherapeutic agents such as cyclophosphamide

lished observations). Treatment with IL-12 with or without IL-2 potently enhances local CD3[+] T cell infiltration and inhibits the vascularization of established subcutaneous TBJ tumors. Further, the majority of mice cured of their original TBJ neuroblastoma tumors by IL-12 with or without IL-2 are resistant to tumor rechallenge, suggesting that T-cell-mediated immunologic memory responses are generated in these mice. The resistance of these mice to induced-relapse (that is, tumor rechallenge) is further enhanced by retreatment with low-dose IL-12. This suggests that immunologic memory responses may be potentiated by IL-12 administration and that, unlike chemotherapy where the subsequent clinical responsiveness to retreatment with an agent may be limited due to the emergence of mechanisms of multidrug resistance, IL-12 might ultimately retain therapeutic efficacy, even in the setting of retreatment of relapse.

Angiogenesis in preclinical models of neuroblastoma

Background

Given the general interest in angiogenesis as a therapeutic target in the management of patients with solid tumors, and the recognition that human neuroblastoma tumors are often highly vascularized and/or hemorrhagic, recent efforts have focused on the modulation of tumor neovascularization as a strategy for the treatment of neuroblastoma. Although a retrospective review of neuroblastoma biopsy specimens identified a significant correlation between increased tumor vascularity and the presence of N-myc amplification, concurrent metastatic disease, and poor outcome (Meitar *et al.* 1996), a more recent study failed to support a relationship between tumor vascularity and the incidence of relapse or survival (Canete *et al.* 2000). Still others have reported that neuroblastoma cells produce three molecules *in vitro* that are capable of inhibiting endothelial cell growth, and that overexpression of N-myc downregulates the production of these molecules, thus implicating N-myc amplification in the

engagement of mechanisms favoring the vascularization of neuroblastoma tumors *in vivo* (Fotsis *et al.* 1999).

Profile of the angiogenic phenotype of neuroblastoma

As previous reports have described in detail, the process of tumor neovascularization is regulated by a complex range of molecular signals (Brem 1999; Hanahan and Folkman 1996; Pluda 1997). According to the 'angiogenic switch' hypothesis proposed by Hanahan and Folkman (1996), tumor neovascularization is regulated by a relative balance between the production/expression of various proangiogenic versus anti-angiogenic mediators and their receptors acting within the local tumor site (Table 16.4; Brem 1999; Hanahan and Folkman 1996; Pluda 1997). These factors may be produced by tumor cells or endothelium, as well as stromal elements and/or infiltrating leukocytes within the local tumor site. Despite the above observations, and the general recognition that neuroblastomas are highly vascularized tumors, relatively little information has been reported regarding mechanisms regulating the vascularization of these tumors. Such information will likely prove to be essential in the rational design of targeted antivascular strategies for the treatment of neuroblastoma, and for the combination of such approaches with other therapeutic modalities such as chemotherapy, immunotherapy, and/or specific inhibitors of tumor cell signal transduction. High-level constitutive expression of vascular endothelial growth factor (VEGF), and its receptors FLT-1 and FLK-1, is noted in a variety of human neuroblastoma cell lines *in vitro*, as well as in primary tumor specimens (Meister *et al.* 1999). Still others have reported that human neuroblastoma cell lines produce VEGF, but do not express FLT-1 and FLK-1 (Rossler *et al.* 1999; Wigginton, J.M. *et al.*, unpublished observations), and that VEGF production is inducible by hypoxia *in vitro* (Rossler *et al.* 1999). Both human and murine neuroblastoma cell lines as well as primary human neuroblastoma tumors constitutively express the matrix metalloproteinases, MMP-2 and MMP-9 (Fowler *et al.* 1995; Ribatti *et al.* 1998; Sugiura *et al.* 1998).

Table 16.4 Genes that have demonstrated a role in the regulation of angiogenesis

Proangiogenic mediators/receptors	Anti-angiogenic mediators/receptors
$\alpha_v\beta_3$-integrin	Angiopoietin-2
Angiogenin	Angiostatin
Angiopoietin-1	Endostatin
fibroblast growth factor (aFGF, bFGF)	Interferon-α,β,γ
flT-1/flK-1	Interferon-inducible protein-10 (IP-10)
Hepatocyte growth factor (HGF)	Interleukin-12 (IL-12)
Hypoxia-inducible factor-1α (HIF-1α)	Monokine-induced by interferon-gamma (MIG)
Matrix metalloproteinases-2 and -9 (MMP-2/MMP-9)	Plasminogen activator-inhibitor 1 (PAI-1)
Placental growth factor	Platelet factor-4 (PF-4)
Pigment epithelium-derived factor (PEDF)	Stromal-derived factor (SDF-1β)
Platelet-derived growth factor (PDGF)	Thrombospondin-1 (TSP-1)
Thymidine phosphorylase	Tissue inhibitors of metalloproteinases (TIMP-1,2,3)
TIE-2	
Transforming growth factor-α,β (TGFα,β)	
Vascular endothelial growth factor (VEGF)	

To provide more comprehensive background information for the investigation of mechanisms regulating the vascularization of neuroblastoma tumors, and to facilitate the design of targeted anti-angiogenic treatment strategies, we have characterized the expression of genes encoding various proangiogenic and anti-angiogenic mediators (that is, angiogenic phenotype) by murine and human neuroblastoma cell lines *in vitro* and *in vivo* utilizing reverse transcriptase polymerase chain reaction (RT-PCR) and/or ribonuclease protection assays (RPA). Murine neuroblastoma cell lines (Neuro-A, TBJ, and NB41A3) produce substantial quantities of VEGF protein in a time-dependent fashion *in vitro*. Further, intense expression of genes encoding the proangiogenic mediators VEGF; FLT-1 and FLK-1 (VEGF receptors); angiopoietin-1; TIE-2 (angiopoietin receptor); MMP-2 and MMP-9, as well as anti-angiogenic mediators such as IP-10, MIG, angiopoietin-2, and thrombospondin-1 is noted within orthotopic intraadrenal TBJ or Neuro-2a neuroblastoma tumors (Wigginton, J.M., unpublished observations). Constitutive expression of the genes encoding VEGF, FLT-1, FLK-1, angiopoietin-1, and TIE-2 is also noted within spontaneous neuroblastoma tumors from N-myc transgenic mice (Wigginton, J.M., unpublished observations). The relative role of these and other mediators in regulation of the vascularization of neuroblastoma tumors remains to be defined, and is a focus of active investigation within our laboratory.

Therapeutic inhibition of tumor neovascularization
Currently reported investigations of anti-angiogenic agents in preclinical neuroblastoma models have been limited to non-specific first-generation agents such as TNP-470. TNP-470 can significantly delay the growth of heterotropic subcutaneous neuroblastoma tumors in syngeneic mice (Nagabuchi *et al.* 1997) and human neurolastoma xenografts in immunodeficient mice (Katzenstein *et al.* 1999; Wassberg *et al.* 1997). In mice bearing human neuroblastoma xenografts, administration of TNP-470 not only delays tumor growth, but also induces chromaffin differentiation and induces tumor and apoptosis (Wassberg *et al.* 1999). Administration of an anti-endothelial immunotoxicin induces complete regression of C-1300 tumors engineered to overexpress the IFNγ gene (Burrows *et al.* 1994; Huang *et al.* 1997). Available nonspecific and targeted agents with apparent anti-angiogenic activity and, ultimately, potential utility in the treatment of neuroblastoma and other solid tumors are shown in Table 16.5. Collectively, our studies directed at characterization of the angiogenic phenotype of neuroblastoma tumors suggest that efforts directed at disruption of the production and/or function of VEGF, angiopoietin-1, or the matrix metalloproteinases may offer particular promise as anti-angiogenic strategies for the treatment of neuroblastoma.

Future prospects for the biological therapy of neuroblastoma

The prognosis of patients with advanced neuroblastoma remains relatively poor despite the application of conventional modalities of therapy, which may include surgery, external or targeted radiotherapy, chemotherapy with or without hematologic reconstitu-

Table 16.5 Anti-angiogenic drugs currently undergoing preclinical and/or clinical investigation

ABT-627 (Abbott)
Angiostatin (Entremed)
Capecitabine (Roche)
Carboxyamidoimidazole (CAI)
CM101 (Carbomed/Zeneca)
Combretastatin (Oxigene)
Endostatin (Entremed)
Farnesyl transferase inhibitors
    L-778, 123 (Merck)
    SCH66336 (Schering-Plough)
IMR862 (Cytran)
Integrin antagonists
    EMD121974 (Merck)
    Vitaxin (Ixsys)
Interferon-α,β
Interleukine-12, 18 (Genetics Institute, SmithKline-Beecham)
Matrix metalloproteinase inhibitors
    AE-941 (Neovastat)
    AG3340 (Agouron)
    BAY 12-9566 (Bayer)
    BMS-275291 (Bristol-Myers Squibb)
    CGS27023A (Novartis)
    COL-3 (Collagenex)
    Marimastat (British Biotech)
2-Metoxyestradiol (2-ME) (Entremed)
MM1270B (Novartis)
Penicillamine
PNU-145156E (Pharmacia-UpJohn)
Squalamine (Magainin)
Suramin
Thalidomide (Celgene)
TNP-470 (TAP)
VEGF Antagonists
    Angiozyme (Ribozyme)
    Monoclonal anti-VEGF antibody (RhuMAb) (Genentech)
    PKC412 (Novartis)
    PTK787/ZK222584 (Novartis)
    SU5402 (Sugen)
    SU5416 (Sugen)
    SU6668 (Sugen)

tion, or differentiation therapy with retinoids among others. New biological strategies for the treatment of neuroblastoma seek to exploit therapeutic targets mediating novel aspects of the biology of neuroblastoma. Such approaches include efforts directed at the inhibition of neovascularization or intracellular signal transduction in tumors, or therapeutic potentiation of the host anti-tumor immune response. Although IL-2 is approved for use and has demonstrated efficacy in the treatment of patients with advanced RCC and melanoma, clinical studies to investigate the use of agents such as IL-2 alone for the treatment of patients with neuroblastoma or other pediatric tumors have produced relatively disappointing results to date (Bauer *et al.* 1995; Ribeiro *et al.* 1993; Roper *et al.* 1992). Nonetheless, more recent studies both in non-neuroblastoma tumor models and in preclinical systems including advanced orthotopic models of neuroblastoma suggest that there may be reason for optimism that new approaches combining various biologics can ultimately provide meaningful therapeutic benefit in the clinical setting. Systemic administration of IL-12 or IL-18 alone or in combination with IL-2 can induce complete and durable tumor regression in several models of well-established primary and/or metastatic disease, including even well-established neuroblastoma tumors (Wigginton *et al.* 1996; Wigginton, J.M., unpublished observations). We have also found that, although systemic administration of IL-12 with or without IL-2 induces complete tumor regression in a substantial portion of treated mice in preclinical models of RCC and neuroblastoma, and potently inhibits tumor neovascularization, it appears to do so without appreciably altering the otherwise constitutive expression of various proangiogenic mediators such as VEGF and angiopoietin-1, or their respective receptors FLT-1/FLK-1 and TIE-2 (Wigginton *et al.* 1996; Wigginton, J.M., unpublished observations). This suggests that biological approaches combining potent immunoregulatory cytokines such as IL-12 or IL-18 with or without IL-2 and targeted small-molecule antagonists of tumor vascularization may achieve greater therapeutic efficacy than either agent alone—a proposed immunoangiostatic approach.

Combined administration of tumor-targeted ch14.18-Il-2 in conjunction with an antivascular alpha-v integrin antagonist delays the growth of early established subcutaneous NXS2 tumors, and does so more effectively than either single agent alone (Lode *et al.* 1999*a*). Although no information is provided regarding the expression of integrins in NXS2 tumors *in vivo*, and the specificity of the observed effects of administration of the alpha-v integrin antagonist are unclear, the authors do report that mice treated with the antagonist reveal reduced tumor vascularity as evidenced by immunohistochemical staining for the vascular marker CD31 (Lode *et al.* 1999*a*). Combined administration of these agents also inhibits the establishment of hepatic metastases that develop spontaneously after subcutaneous implantation of NXS2 tumor cells (Lode *et al.* 1999*a*). Still others have reported enhanced therapeutic efficacy by combined administration of IL-12 in conjunction with radiotherapy (Seetharam *et al.* 1999; Teicher *et al.* 1996), and/or chemotherapy (Teicher *et al.* 1997) in non-neuroblastoma preclinical tumor models. Thus, a number of strategies combining various biologics have demonstrated promise in the preclinical setting. It remains to be established whether biologically targeted therapeutic treatment regimens such as those described here will ultimately stand alone, or whether their role in the treatment of neuroblastoma will be restricted to adjunctive use in conjunction with conventional therapeutic modalities. Nonetheless, much as occurred with the evolution of combination chemotherapy itself, it appears most likely that optimal therapeutic responses to biological therapy will ultimately be achieved by rationally designed combinations of agents with complementary mechanisms of action including chemotherapy, immunomodulators, and inhibitors of tumor neovascularization and signal transduction among others.

References

Aguzzi, A., Wagner, E.F., Williams, R.L., and Courtneidge, S.A.(1990). Sympathetic hyperplasia and neuroblastomas in transgenic mice expressing polyoma middle T antigen. *New Biol.* **2**, 533–43.

Alvarado, C.S., Findley, H.W., Chan, W.C., Hnath, R.S., Abdel-Mageed, A., Pais, R.C., *et al.* (1989). Natural killer cells in children with malignant solid tumors. Effect of recombinant interferon-alpha and interleukin-2 on natural killer cell function against tumor cell lines. *Cancer* **63**, 83–9.

Anderson, P.M., Bach, F.H., and Ochoa, A.C. (1988). Augmentation of cell number and LAK activity in peripheral blood mononuclear cells activated with anti-CD3 and interleukin-2. Preliminary results in children with acute lymphocytic leukemia and neuroblastoma. *Cancer Immunol. Immunother.* **27**, 82–8.

Atzpodien, J., Gulati, S.C., Kwon, J.H., Kushner, B.H., Shimazaki, C., Buhrer, C., *et al.* (1988). Anti-tumor efficacy of interleukin-2 activated killer cells in human neuroblastoma *ex vivo*. *Exp. Cell Biol.* **56**, 236–44.

Bauer, M., Reaman, G.H., Hank, J.A., Cairo, M.S., Anderson, P., Blazar, B.R. *et al.* (1995). A phase II trial of human recombinant interleukin-2 administered as a 4-day continuous infusion for children with refractory neuroblastoma, non-Hodgkin's lymphoma, sarcoma, renal cell carcinoma, and malignant melanoma. A Children's Cancer Group study. *Cancer* **75**, 2959–65.

Bausero, M.A., Panoskaltsis-Mortari, A., Blazar, B.R., and Katsanis, E. (1996). Effective immunization against neuroblastoma using double-transduced tumor cells secreting GM-CSF and interferon-gamma. *J. Immunother. Emphasis Tumor Immunol.* **19**, 113–24.

Bergman, I., Arbit, E., Rosenblum, M., Larson, S.M., Heller, G., and Cheung, N.K. (1993). Treatment of spinal epidural neuroblastoma xenografts in rats using anti-GD2 monoclonal antibody 3F8. *J. Neurooncol.* **15**, 235–42.

Bergman, I., Pohl, C.R., Venkataramanan, R., Burckart, G.J., Stabin, M., Barmada, M.A., *et al.* (1999). Intrathecal administration of an anti-ganglioside antibody results in specific accumulation within meningeal neoplastic xenografts in nude rats. *J. Immunother.* **22**, 114–23.

Bernassola, F., Scheuerpflug, C., Herr, I., Krammer, P.H., Debatin, K.M., and Melino, G. (1999). Induction of apoptosis by IFN gamma in human neuroblastoma cell lines through the CD95/CD95L autocrine circuit. *Cell Death Differentiat.* **6**, 652–60.

Bogenmann, E. (1996). A metastatic neuroblastoma model in SCID mice. *Int. J Cancer* **67**, 379–85.

Bouillon, M. and Audette, M. (1993). Transduction of retinoic acid and gamma-interferon signal for intercellular adhesion molecule-1 expression on human tumor cell lines: evidence for the late-acting involvement of proteinkinase C inactivation. *Cancer Res.* **53**, 826–32.

Bowman, L., Grossmann, M., Rill, D., Brown, M., Zhong, W.Y., Alexander, B., *et al.* (1998). IL-2 adenovector-transduced autologous tumor cells induce antitumor immune responses in patients with neuroblastoma. *Blood* **92**, 1941–9.

Brem, S. (1999). Angiogenesis and cancer control: from concept to therapeutic trial. *J. Mol. Cell. Cardiol.* **6**, 436–58.

Brewslow, N. and McCann, B. (1971). Statistical estimation of prognosis for children with neuroblastoma. *Cancer Res.* **31**, 2098–103.

Brunda, M.J., Luistro, L., Warrier, R.R., Wright, R.B., Hubbard, B.R., Murphy, M., *et al.* (1993). Antitumor and antimetastatic activity of interleukin 12 against murine tumors. *J. Exp. Med.* **178**, 1223–30.

Burrows, F.J., Overholser, J.P., and Thorpe, P.E. (1994). Potent antitumor effects of an antitumor endothelial cell immunotoxin in a murine vascular targeting model. *Cell Biophys.* **24–25**, 15–25.

Canete, A., Navarro, S., Bermudez, J., Pellin, A., Castel, V., and Llombart-Bosch, A. (2000). Angiogenesis in neuroblastoma: relationship to survival and other prognostic factors in a cohort of neuroblastoma patients [in process citation]. *J. Clin. Oncol.* **18**, 27.

Castleberry, R.P. (1997). Biology and treatment of neuroblastoma. *Pediatr. Clin. N. Am.* **44**, 919–37.

Chan, S.H., Perussia, B., Gupta, J.W., Kobayashi, M., Pospisil, M., Young, H.A., *et al.* (1991). Induction of interferon gamma production by natural killer cell stimulatory factor: characterization of the responder cells and synergy with other inducers. *J. Exp. Med.* **173**, 869–79.

Cheng, N.C., Beitsma, M., Chan, A., OpdenCamp, I. Westerveld, A., Pronk, J., *et al.* (1996). Lack of class I HLA expression in neuroblastoma is associated with high N-myc expression and hypomethylation due to loss of the MEMO-1 locus. *Oncogene* **13**, 1737–44.

Cinatl, J. Jr, Cinatl, J., Kotchetkov, R., Vogel, J.U., Woodcock, B.G., Matousek, J., *et al.* (1999). Bovine seminal ribonuclease selectively kills human multidrug-resistant neuroblastoma cells via induction of apoptosis. *Int. J. Oncol.* **15**, 1001–9.

Corrias, M.V., Basso, S., Meazza, R., Musiani, P., Santi, L., Bocca, P., *et al.* (1998). Characterization and tumorigenicity of human neuroblastoma cells transfected with the IL-2 gene. *Cancer Gene Ther.* **5**, 38–44.

Corrias, M.V., Scaruffi, P., Occhino, M., De Bernardi, B., Tonini, G.P., and Pistoia, V. (1996). Expression of MAGE-1, MAGE-3 and MART-1 genes in neuroblastoma. *Int. J. Cancer* **69**, 1–5.

Davidoff, A.M., Kimbrough, S.A., Ng, C.Y., Shochat, S.J., and Vanin, E.F. (1999). Neuroblastoma regression and immunity induced by transgenic expression of interleukin-12. *J. Pediatr. Surg.* **34**, 902–6.

Dunham, L.C. and Stewart, H.L. (1953). A survey of transplantable and transmissable animal tumors. *J. Cancer Inst.* **13**, 1299–377.

Enomoto, A., Kato, K., Yagita, H., and Okumura, K. (1997). Adoptive transfer of cytotoxic T lymphocytes induced by CD86-transfected tumor cells suppresses multi-organ metastases of C1300 neuroblastoma in mice. *Cancer Immunol. Immunother.* **44**, 204–10.

Evans, A.E., D'Angio, G.J., Propert, K., Anderson, J., and Hann, H.W. (1987). Prognostic factor in neuroblastoma. *Cancer* **59**, 1853–9.

Facchetti, P., Prigione, I., Ghiotto, F., Tasso, P., Garaventa, A., and Pistoia, V. (1996). Functional and molecular characterization of tumour-infiltrating lymphocytes and clones thereof from a major-histocompatibility-complex-negative human tumour: neuroblastoma. *Cancer Immunol. Immunother.* **42**, 170–8.

Flickinger, K.S., Judware, R., Lechner, R., Carter, W.G., and Culp, L.A. (1994). Integrin expression in human neuroblastoma cells with or without N-myc amplification and in ectopic/orthotopic nude mouse tumors. *Exp. Cell Res.* **213**, 156–63.

Fotsis, T., Breit, S., Lutz, W., Rossler, J., Hatzi, E., Schwab, M., *et al.* (1999). Down-regulation of endothelial cell growth inhibitors by enhanced MYCN oncogene expression in human neuroblastoma cells. *Eur. J. Biochem.* **263**, 757–64.

Fowler, C., Zimmer, C., Boghaert, E., Thomas, M., and Zimmer, S. (1995). Metastasis of C1300 and TBJ murine neuroblastomas correlates with expression of matrix metalloproteinases. *Cancer Lett.* **93**, 171–7.

Fowler, C.L., Brooks, S.P., Squire, R., Rich, G.A., Rossman, J.E., Finegold, M.J., *et al.* (1991). Enhanced resection and improved survival in murine neuroblastoma (C1300-NB) after preoperative immunotherapy. *J Pediatr. Surg.* **26**, 381–7.

Fowler, C.L., Brooks, S.P., Rossman, J.E., and Cooney, D.R. (1993). Combined preoperative and postoperative immunotherapy for murine C1300 neuroblastoma. *J. Pediatr. Surg.* **28**, 420–6.

Frost, J.D., Hank, J.A., Reaman, G.H., Frierdich, S., Seeger, R.C., Gan, J. *et al.* (1997). A phase I/IB trial of murine monoclonal anti-GD2 antibody 14.G2a plus interleukin-2 in children with refractory neuroblastoma: a report of the Children's Cancer Group. *Cancer* **80**, 317–33.

Giraldi, F.P., Mizobuchi, M., Horowitz, Z.D., Downs, T.R., Aleppo,g., Kier, A., *et al.* (1994). Development of neuroepithelial tumors of the adrenal medulla in transgenic mice expressing a mouse hypothalamic growth hormone–releasing hormone promoter–simian virus-40 T-antigen fusion gene. *Endocrinology* **134**, 1219–24.

Grossmann, M.E., Brown, M.P., and Brenner, M.K. (1997). Antitumor responses induced by transgenic expression of CD40 ligand. *Hum. Gene Ther.* **8**, 1935–43.

Hanahan, D. and Folkman, J. (1996). Patterns and emerging mechanisms of the angiogenic switch during tumorigenesis. *Cell* **86**, 353–64.

Handgretinger, R., Bruchelt, G., Kimmig, A., Dopfer, r., Niethammer, D., and Treuner, J. (1989*a*). *In vitro* induction of lymphokine-activated killer (LAK) activity in patients with neuroblastoma. *Pediatr. Hematol. Oncol.* **6**, 307–17.

Handgretinger, R., Kimmig, A., Lang, P., Daurer, B., Kuci, S., Bruchelt, G., *et al.* (1989*b*). Interferon-gamma upregulates the susceptibility of human neuroblastoma cells to interleukin-2-activated natural killer cells. *Nat. Immuni. Cell Growth Reg.* **8**, 189–96.

Hashimoto, W., Osaki, T., Okamura, H., Robbins, P.D., Kurimoto, M., Nagata, S., *et al.* (1999). Differential antitumor effects of administration of recombinant IL-18 or recombinant IL-12 are mediated primarily by Fas–Fas ligand. *J. Immunol.* **163**, 583–9.

Helson, L., Das, S.K., and Hajdu, S.I. (1975). Human neuroblastoma in nude mice. *Cancer Res.* **35**, 2594–9.

Heuer, J.G., Tucker-McClung, C., Gonin, R., and Hock, R.A. (1996). Retrovirus-mediated gene transfer of B7-1 and MHC class II converts a poorly immunogenic neuroblastoma into a highly immunogenic one. *Hum. Gene Ther.* **7**, 2059–68.

Heuer, J.G., Tucker-McClung, C., and Hock, R.A. (1999). Neuroblastoma cells expressing mature IL-18, but not proIL-18, induce a strong and immediate antitumor immune response. *J. Immunother.* **22**, 324–35.

Hock, R.A., Reynolds, B.D., Tucker-McClung, C.L., and Kwok, W.W. (1995). Human class II major histocompatibility complex gene transfer into murine neuroblastoma leads to loss of tumorigenicity, immunity against subsequent tumor challenge, and elimination of microscopic preestablished tumors. *J. Immunother. Emphasis Tumor Immunol.* **17**, 12–18.

Hock, R.A., Reynolds, B.D., Tucker-McClung, C.L. and Heuer, J.G. (1996). Murine neuroblastoma vaccines produced by retroviral transfer of MHC class II genes. *Cancer Gene Ther.* **3**, 314–20.

Huang, X., Molema, G., King, S., Watkins, L., Edgington, T.S., and Thorpe, P.E. (1997). Tumor infarction in mice by antibody-directed targeting of tissue factor to tumor vasculature [see comments]. *Science* **275**, 547–50.

Ishizu, H., Bove, K.E., Ziegler, M.M., and Arya, G. (1994). Immune-mediated regression of 'metastatic' neuroblastoma in the liver. *J. Pediatr. Surg.* **29**, 155–9.

Iwakawa, M., Ando, K., Ohkawa, H., Koike, S., and Chen, Y.J. (1994). A murine model for bone marrow metastasis established by an i.v. injection of C-1300 neuroblastoma in A/J mice. *Clin. Exp. Metastas.* **12**, 231–7.

Iwamoto, T., Taniguchi, M., Wajjwalku, W., Nakashima, I., and Takahashi, M. (1993). Neuroblastoma in a transgenic mouse carrying a metallothionein/ret fusion gene. *Br. J. Cancer* **67**, 504–7.

Katsanis, E., Orchard, P.J., Bausero, M.A., Gorden, K.B., McIvor, R.S., and Blazar, B.R. (1994*b*). Interleukin-2 gene transfer into murine neuroblastoma decreases tumorigenicity and enhances systemic immunity causing regression of preestablished retroperitoneal tumors. *J. Immunother. Emphasis Tumor Immunol.* **15**, 81–90.

Katsanis, E., Bausero, M.A., Panoskaltsis-Mortari, A., Dancisak, B.B., Xu, Z., Orchard, P.J. *et al.* (1996). Irradiation of singly and doubly transduced murine neuroblastoma cells expressing B7-1 and producing interferon-gamma reduces their capacity to induce systemic immunity. *Cancer Gene Ther.* **3**, 75–82.

Katsanis, E., Bausero, M.A., Xu, H., Orchard, P.J., Xu, Z., McIvor, R.S. *et al.* (1994*c*). Transfection of the mouse ICAM-1 gene into murine neuroblastoma enhances susceptibility to lysis, reduces *in vivo* tumorigenicity and decreases ICAM-2-dependent killing. *Cancer Immunol. Immunother.* **38**, 135–41.

Katsanis, E., Xu, Z., Bausero, M.A., Dancisak, B.B., Gorden, K.B., Davis, G. *et al.* (1995). B7-1 expression decreases tumorigenicity and induces partial systemic immunity to murine neuroblastoma deficient in major histocompatibility complex with costimulatory molecules. *Cancer Gene Ther.* **2**, 39–46.

Katsanis, E., Blazar, B.R., Bausero, M.A., Gunther,R., and Anderson, P.M. (1994*a*). Retroperitoneal inoculation of murine neuroblastoma results in a reliable model for evaluation of the antitumor immune response. *J. Pediatr. Surg.* **29**, 538–42.

Katzenstein, H.M. and Cohn, S.L. (1998). Advances in the diagnosis and treatment of neuroblastoma. *Curr. Opin. Oncol.* **10**, 43–51.

Katzenstein, H.M., Rademaker, A.W., Senger, C., Salwen, H.R., Nguyen, N.N., Thorner, P.S. *et al.* (1999). Effectiveness of the angiogenesis inhibitor TNP-470 in reducing the growth of human neuroblastoma in nude mice inversely correlates with tumor burden [in process citation]. *Clin. Cancer Res.* **5**, 4273–8.

Kuge, S., Watanabe, K., Makino, K., Tokuda, Y., Mitomi, t., Kawamura, N., *et al.* (1995). Interleukin-12 augments the generation of autologous tumor-reactive CD8+ cytotoxic T lymphocytes from tumor-infiltrating lymphocytes. *Jpn. J. Cancer Res.* **86**, 135–9.

Leonard, M.P., Gearhart, J.P., and Jeffs, R.D. (1991). Chemoimmunotherapy in conjunction with surgery: strategies for management of murine neuroblastoma. *J. Pediatr. Surg.* **26**, 1224–9.

Leonard, M.P., Jeffs, R.D., Gearhart, J.P., and Coffey, D.S. (1992). Recombinant human tumor necrosis factor enhances radiosensitivity and improves animal survival in murine neuroblastoma. *J. Urol.* **148**, 743–6.

Lode, H.N., Xiang,R., Varki, N.M., Dolman, C.S., Gillies, S.D., and Reisfeld, R.A. (1997). Targeted interleukin-2 therapy for spontaneous neuroblastoma metastases to bone marrow. *J. Natl. Cancer Inst.* **89**, 1586–94.

Lode, H.N., Dreier, T., Xiang, R., Varki, N.M., Kang, A.S., and Reisfeld, R.A. (1998*a*). Gene therapy with a single chain interleukin 12 fusion protein induces T cell-dependent protective immunity in a syngeneic model of murine neuroblastoma. *Proc. Nat. Acad. Sci. USA* **95**, 2475–80.

Lode,H.N., Xiang, R., Dreier, T., Varki, N.M., Gillies, S.D., and Reisfeld, R.A. (1998*b*). Natural killer cell-mediated eradication of neuroblastoma metastases to bone marrow by targeted interleukin-2 therapy. *Blood* **91**, 1706–15.

Lode, H.N., Moehler, T., Xiang, R., Joncyzke, A., Gillies, S.D., Cheresh, D.A. *et al.* (1999*a*). Synergy between an antiangiogenic integrin alpha v antagonist and an antibody-cytokine fusion protein eradicates spontaneous tumor metastases. *Proc. Nat. Acad. Sci. USA* **96**, 1591–6.

Lode, H.N., Xiang, R., Duncan, S.R., Theofilopoulos, A.N., Gillies, S.D., and Reisfeld, R.A. (1999*b*). Tumor-targeted IL-2 amplifies T cell-mediated immune response induced by gene therapy with single-chain IL-12. *Proc. Nat. Acad. Sci. USA* **96**, 8591–6.

Lucarelli, E., Kaplan, D.R., and Thiele, C.J. (1995). Selective regulation of TrkA and TrkB receptors by retinoic acid and interferon-gamma in human neuroblastoma cell lines. *J. Biol. Chem.* **270**, 24725–31.

Lutz, W., Fulda, S., Jeremias, I., Debatin, K.M., and Schwab, M. (1998). MycN and IFN gamma cooperate in apoptosis of human neuroblastoma cells. *Oncogene* **17**, 339–46.

Martin, D.M., Carlson, R.O., and Feldman, E.L. (1993). Interferon-gamma inhibits DNA synthesis and insulin-like growth factor-II expression in human neuroblastoma cells. *J. Neurosci. Res.* **34**, 489–501.

Martinez, D.A., Kahwash, S., O'Dorisio, M.S., Lloyd, T.V., McGhee, R.B. Jr, and Qualman, S.J. (1996). Disseminated neuroblastoma in the nude rat. A xenograft model of human malignancy. *Cancer* **77**, 409–19.

Matthay, K.K. (1997). Neuroblastoma: biology and therapy. *Oncology (Hunting)* **11**, 1857–66.

Meister, B., Grunebach, F., Bautz, F., Brugger, W., Fink, F.M., Kanz, L., *et al.* (1999). Expression of vascular endothelial growth factor (VEGF) and its receptors in human neuroblastoma. *Eur. J. Cancer* **35**, 445–9.

Meitar, D., Crawford, S.E., Rademaker, A.W., and Cohn, S.L. (1996). Tumor angiogenesis correlates with metastatic disease. N-myc amplification, and poor outcome in human neuroblastoma. *J. Clin Oncol.* **14**, 405–14.

Micallef, M.J., Yoshida, K., Kawai, S., Hanaya, T., Kohno, K., Arai, S., *et al.* (1997). *In vivo* antitumor effects of murine interferon-gamma-inducing factor/inerleukin-18 in mice bearing syngeneic Meth A sarcoma malignant ascites. *Cancer Immunol. Immunother.* **43**, 361–7.

Montaldo, P.G., Carbone, R., Cornaglia, F.P., and Ponzoni, M. (1993). Interferon-gamma-induced differentiation of human neuroblastoma cells increases cellular uptake and half life of metaiodobenzylguanidine. *Cytotechnology* **11** (suppl. 1), S140–S143.

Montaldo, P.G., Carbone, R., Corrias, M.V., Ferraris, P.C., and Ponzoni, M. (1994). Synergistic differentiation-promoting activity of interferon gamma and tumor necrosis factor-alpha: role of receptor regulation on human neuroblasts. *J. Nat. Cancer Inst.* **86**, 1694–701.

Morton, A.J., Williams, M.N., Emson, P.C., and Faull, R.L. (1995). The morphology of human neuroblastoma cell grafts in the kainic acid-lesioned basal ganglia of the rat. *J. Neurocytol.* **24**, 568–84.

Munoz-Fernandez, M.A., Cano, E., O'Donnell, C.A., Doyle, J., Liew, F.Y., and Fresno, M. (1994). Tumor necrosis factor-alpha (TNF-alpha), interferon-gamma, and interleukin-6 but not TNF-beta induce differentiation of neuroblastoma cells: the role of nitric oxide. *J. Neurochem.* **62**, 1330–6.

Nagabuchi, E., VanderKolk, W.E., Une, Y., and Ziegler, M.M. (1997). TNP-470 antiangiogenic therapy for advanced murine neuroblastoma. *J. Pediatr. Surg.* **32**, 287–93.

Naito, H., Ziegler, M.M., Miyakawa, A., Tokunaga, O., and Sasaki, M. (1992). Establishment of animal liver metastatic model for C-1300 murine neuroblastoma and immunotherapy for it using OK-432, streptococcus preparation. *J. Surg. Res.* **52**, 79–84.

Nakamura, K., Okamura, H., Wada, M., Nagata, K., and Tamura, T. (1989). Endotoxin-induced serum factor that stimulates gamma interferon production. *Infection Immunol.* **57**, 590–5.

Nastala, C.L., Edington, H.D., McKinney, T.G., Tahara, H., Nalesnik, M.A., Brunda, M.J. *et al.* (1994). Recombinant IL-12 administration induces tumor regression in association with IFN-gamma production. *J. Immunol.* **153**, 1697–706.

Pancook, J.D., Becker, J.C., Gillies, S.D., and Reisfeld, R.A. (1996). Eradication of established hepatic human neuroblastoma metastases in mice with severe combined immunodeficiency by antibody-targeted interleukin-2. *Cancer Immunol. Immunother.* **42**, 88–92.

Pluda, J.M. (1997). Tumor-associated angiogenesis: mechanisms, clinical implications, and therapeutic strategies. *Sem. Oncol.* **24**, 203–18.

Pons, G., O'Dea, R.F., and Mirkin, B.L. (1982). Biological characterization of the C-1300 murine neuroblastoma: an *in vivo* neural crest tumor model. *Cancer Res.* **42**, 3719–23.

Ponzoni, M., Guarnaccia, F., Corrias, M.V., and Cornaglia-Ferraris, P. (1993). Uncoordinate induction and differential regulation of HLA class-I and class-II expression by gamma-interferon in differentiating human neuroblastoma cells. *Int. J. Cancer* **55**, 817–23.

Puri, R.K., Leland, P., Kreitman, R.J., and Pastan, I. (1994) Human neurological cancer cells express interleukin-4 (IL-4) receptors which are targets for the toxic effects of IL-4–*Pseudomonas* exotoxin chimeric protein. *Int. J. Cancer* **58**, 574–81.

Reynolds, J.V., Shou, J., Choi, H., Sigal, R., Ziegler, M.M., and Daly, J.M. (1989). The influence of natural killer cells in neuroblastoma. *Arch. Surg.* **124**, 235–9.

Ribatti, D., Alessandri, G., Vacca, A., Iurlaro, M., and Ponzoni, M. (1998). Human neuroblastoma cells produces extracellular matrix-degrading enzymes, induce endothelial cell proliferation and are angiogenic *in vivo*. *Int. J. Cancer* **77**, 449–54.

Ribeiro, R.C., Rill, D., Roberson, P.K., Furman, W.L., Pratt, C.B., Brenner, M., *et al.* (1993). Continuous infusion of interleukin-2 in children with refractory malignancies. *Cancer* **72**, 623–8.

Ridge, J., Terle, D.A., Dragunsky, E., and Levenbook, I. (1996). Effcts of gamma-IFN and NGF on subpopulations in a human neuroblastoma cell line: flow cytometric and morphological analysis. *In Vitro Cell. Dev. Biol. Animal* **32**, 238–48.

Roper, M., Smith, M.A., Sondel, P.M., Gillespie, A., Reaman, G.H., Hammond, G.D., *et al.* (1992). A phase I study of interleukin-2 in children with cancer. *Am. J. Pediatr. Hematol. Oncol.* **14**, 305–11.

Rossi, A.R., Pericle, F., Rashleigh, S., Janiec, J., and Djeu, J.Y. (1994). Lysis of neuroblastoma cell lines by human natural killer cells activated by interleukin-2 and interleukin-12. *Blood* **83**, 1323–8.

Rossler, J., Breit, S., Havers, W., and Schweigerer, L. (1999). Vascular endothelial growth factor expression in human neuroblastoma: up-regulation by hypoxia. *Int. J. Cancer* **81**, 113–17.

Sabzevari, H., Gillies, S.D., Mueller, B.M., Pancook, J.D., and Reisfeld, R.A. (1994). A recombinant antibody–interleukin 2 fusion protein suppresses growth of hepatic human neuroblastoma metastases in severe combined immunodeficiency mice. *Proc. Nat. Acad. Sci. USA* **91**, 9626–30.

Seetharam, S., Staba, M.J., Schumm, L.P., Schreiber, K., Schreiber, H., and Kufe, D.W. (1999). Enhanced eradication of local and distant tumors by genetically produced interleukin-12 and irradiation. *Int. J. Oncol.* **15**, 743–59.

Servenius, B., Vernachio, J., Price, J., Andersson, L.C., and Peterson, P.A. (1994). Metastasizing neuroblastomas in mice transgenic for simian virus 40 large T (SV40T) under the olfactory marker protein gene promoter. *Cancer Res.* **54**, 5198–205.

Sigal, R.K., Lieberman, M.D., Reynolds, J.V., Shou, J., Ziegler, M.M., and Daly, J.M. (1991). Low-dose interferon gamma renders neuroblastoma more susceptible to interleukin-2 immunotherapy. *J. Pediatr. Surg.* **26**, 389–95.

Singleton, J.R., Randolph, A.E., and Feldman, E.L. (1996). Insulin-like growth factor I receptor prevents apoptosis and enhances neuroblastoma tumorigenesis. *Cancer Res.* **56**, 4522–9.

Skalnik, D.G., Dorfman, D.M., Williams, D.A., and Orkin, S.H. (1991). Restriction of neuroblastoma to the prostate gland in transgenic mice. *Mol. Cell. Biol.* **11**, 4518–27.

Sohmura, Y., Nakata, K., Yoshida, H., Kashimoto, S., Matsui, Y., and Furuichi, H. (1986). Recombinant human tumor necrosis factor–II. Antitumor effect on murine and human tumors transplanted in mice. *Int. J. Immunopharmacol.* **8**, 357–68.

Sugio, K., Nakagawara, A., and Sasazuki, T. (1991). Association of expression between N-myc gene and major histocompatibility complex class I gene in surgically resected human neuroblastoma. *Cancer* **67**, 1384–8.

Sugiura, Y., Shimada, H., Seeger, R.C., Laug, W.E., and DeClerck, Y.A. (1998). Matrix metalloproteinases-2 and -9 are expressed in human neuroblastoma: contribution of stromal cells to their production and correlation with metastasis. *Cancer Res.* **58**, 2209–16.

Sweetser, D.A., Kapur, R.P., Froelick, G.J., Kafer, K.E., and Palmiter, R.D. (1997). Oncogenesis and altered differentiation induced by activated Ras in neuroblasts of transgenic mice. *Oncogene* **15**, 2783–94.

Taghian, A., Budach, W., Zietman, A., Freeman, J., Gioioso, D., and Suit, H.D. (1993). Quantitative comparison between the transplantability of human and murine tumors into the brain of NCr/Sed-nu/nu nude and severe combined immunodeficient mice. *Cancer Res.* **53**, 5018–21.

Teicher, B.A., Ara, G., Menon, K., and Schaub, R.G. (1996). *In vivo* studies with interleukin-12 alone and in combination with monocyte colony-stimulating factor and/or fractionated radiation treatment. *Int. J. Cancer* **65**, 80–4.

Teicher, B.A., Ara, G., Buxton, D., Leonard, J., and Schaub, R.G. (1997). Optimal scheduling of interleukin 12 and chemotherapy in the murine MB-49 bladder carcinoma and B16 melanoma. *Clin Cancer Res.* **3**, 1661–7.

Ucar, K., Seeger, R.C., Challita, P.M., Watanabe, C.T., Yen, T.L., Morgan, J.P., *et al.* (1995). Sustained cytokine production and immunophenotypic changes in human neuroblastoma cell lines transduced with a human gamma interferon vector. *Cancer Gene Therapy* **2**, 171–81.

Wada, R.K., Pai, D.S., Huang, J., Yamashiro, J.M., and Sidell, N. (1997). Interferon-gamma and retinoic acid down-regulate N-myc in neuroblastoma through complementary mechanisms of action. *Cancer Lett.* **121**, 181–8.

Wassberg, E., Pahlman, S., Westlin, J.E., and Christoffeson, R. (1997). The angiogenesis inhibitor TNP-470 reduces the growth rate of human neuroblastoma in nude rats. *Pediatr. Res.* **41**, 327–33.

Wassberg, E., Hedborg, F., Skoldenberg, E., Stridsberg, M., and Christofferson, R. (1999). Inhibition of angiogenesis induces chromaffin differentiation and apoptosis in neuroblastoma. *Am. J. Pathol.* **154**, 395–403.

Watanabe, Y., Kuribayashi, K., Miyatake, S., Nishihara, K., Nakayama, E., Taniyama, T., *et al.* (1989). Exogenous expression of mouse interferon gamma cDNA in mouse neuroblastoma C1300 cells results in reduced tumorigenicity by augmented anti-tumor immunity. *Proc. Nat. Acad. Sci. USA* **86**, 9456–60.

Weiss, W.A., Aldape, K., Mohapatra, G., Feuerstein, B.G., and Bishop, J.M. (1997). Targeted expression of MYCN causes neuroblastoma in transgenic mice. *EMBO J.* **16**, 2985–95.

Wigginton, J.M., Komschlies, K.L., Back, T.C., Franco, J.L., Brunda, M.J., and Wiltrout, R.H. (1996). Administration of interleukin 12 with pulse interleukin 2 and the rapid and complete eradication of murine renal carcinoma. *J. Nat. Cancer Inst.* **88**, 38–43.

Wigginton, I.M., Gruys, E., Gieselhart, L., Subleski, J., Komschlies, K.L., Park, I.W., Wiltrout, T.A., Nagashima, K., Back, T.C., and Wiltrout, R.H. (2001). IFN-γ and Fas/FasL are required for the antitumor and antiangiogenic effects of IL-12/pulse IL-2 therapy. *J. Clin. Invest.* **108**, 51–62.

Yoshida, H., Enomoto, H., Tagawa, M., Takenaga, K., Tasaki, K., Nakagawara, A., *et al.* (1998a). Impaired tumorigenicity and decreased liver metastasis of murine neuroblastoma cells engineered to secrete interleukin-2 or granulocyte macrophage colony-stimulating factor. *Cancer Gene Ther.* **5**, 67–73.

Yoshida, H., Enomoto, H., Kawamura, K., Takenaga, K., Tanabe, M., Ohnuma, N., *et al.* (1998b). Antitumor vaccine effect of irradiated murine neuroblastoma cells producing interleukin-2 or granulocyte macrophage-colony stimulating factor. *Int. J. Oncol.* **13**, 73–8.

Yoshida, H., Enomoto, H., Miyauchi, M., Takenaga, K., Tanabe, M., Ohnuma, N., *et al.* (1998c). Impaired tumorigenicity of IL-4-producing murine-neuroblastoma cells in immunodeficient nude mice. *Int. J. Oncol.* **12**, 1067–71.

Yoshida, H., Tanabe, M., Miyauchi, M., Kawamura, K., Takenaga, K., Ohnuma, N., *et al.* (1999). Induced immunity by expression of interleukin-2 or GM-CSF gene in murine neuroblastoma cells can generate antitumor response to established tumors. *Cancer Gene Ther.* **6**, 395–401.

Yoshida, K., Yoshizawa, g., Yamazaki, Y., Fujikawa, T., Tanabe, A., and Sakurai, K. (1994). A cranial invasion model of human neuroblastoma using congenitally athymic mice. *Surg. Today* **24**, 526–9.

Yoshino, K., Tanabe, M., Ohnuma, N., and Takahashi, H. (1996). Histopathologic analysis of bone marrow and bone metastasis in murine neuroblastoma. *Clin. Exp. Metastas.* **14**, 459–65.

Young, J.L. Jr and Miller, R.W. (1975). Incidence of malignant tumors in U.S. children. *J. Pediatr.* **86**, 254–8.

Zamboni, W.C., Stewart, C.F., Thompson, J., Santana, V.M., Cheshire, P.J., Richmond, L.B., *et al.* (1998). Relationship between topotecan systemic exposure and tumor response in human neuroblastoma xenografts [see comments]. *J. Nat Cancer Inst.* **90**, 505–11.

Ziegler, M.M., Naito, H., McCarrick, J.W. III, *et al.* (1986). C-1300 murine neuroblastoma: a suitable animal model of human disease. In: Brooks, B.F. *Malignant Tumors of Childhood*. Austin: University of Texas Press, 1986: 114–26.

Ziegler, M.M., Ishizu, H., Nagabuchi, E., Takada, N., and Arya, G. (1997). A comparative review of the immunobiology of murine neuroblastoma and human neuroblastoma. *Cancer* **79**, 1757–66.

17.   Angiogenesis in renal cell carcinomas

Jeff A. Wieder and Arie Belldegrun

Angiogenesis is the formation of new capillaries by outgrowth of endothelial cells from pre-existing blood vessels. The role of angiogenesis in tumor growth and metastasis was first described by Folkman and co-workers (Folkman 1971, 1972; Folkman *et al.* 1971). They demonstrated that a tumor can grow up to 1.75 mm when it obtains nutrients only by diffusion. Growth beyond this size requires angiogenesis (Folkman 1972). They concluded that tumors need new blood vessels to supply nutrients for growth and spread. Folkman suggested that cancer could be treated by inhibiting angiogenesis (Folkman 1971, 1972; Folkman *et al.* 1971). Tumors that are highly vascular, such as renal cell carcinoma (RCC), appear to be fertile targets for this type of therapy. Modern research seeks to elucidate the role of angiogenesis in the biology and treatment of kidney cancer.

Overview of angiogenesis

Angiogenesis is regulated by a delicate equilibrium between numerous inhibitory and stimulatory molecules and is dependent on a complex cascade of interactions between components of the local environment, such as endothelial cells, the basement membrane, the extracellular matrix (ECM), leukocytes, and macrophages (Carmeliet and Jain 2000; Bussolino *et al.* 1996; O'Brien and Harris 1995; Liotta *et al.* 1991; Ellis and Fidler 1996; Brooks 1996; Polverini 1996). The role of each of these components in angiogenesis is beyond the scope of this chapter and the reader is referred to several recent review articles (Carmeliet and Jain 2000; Bussolino *et al.* 1996; O'Brien and Harris 1995; Liotta *et al.* 1991; Ellis and Fidler 1996; Brooks 1996; Polverini 1996).

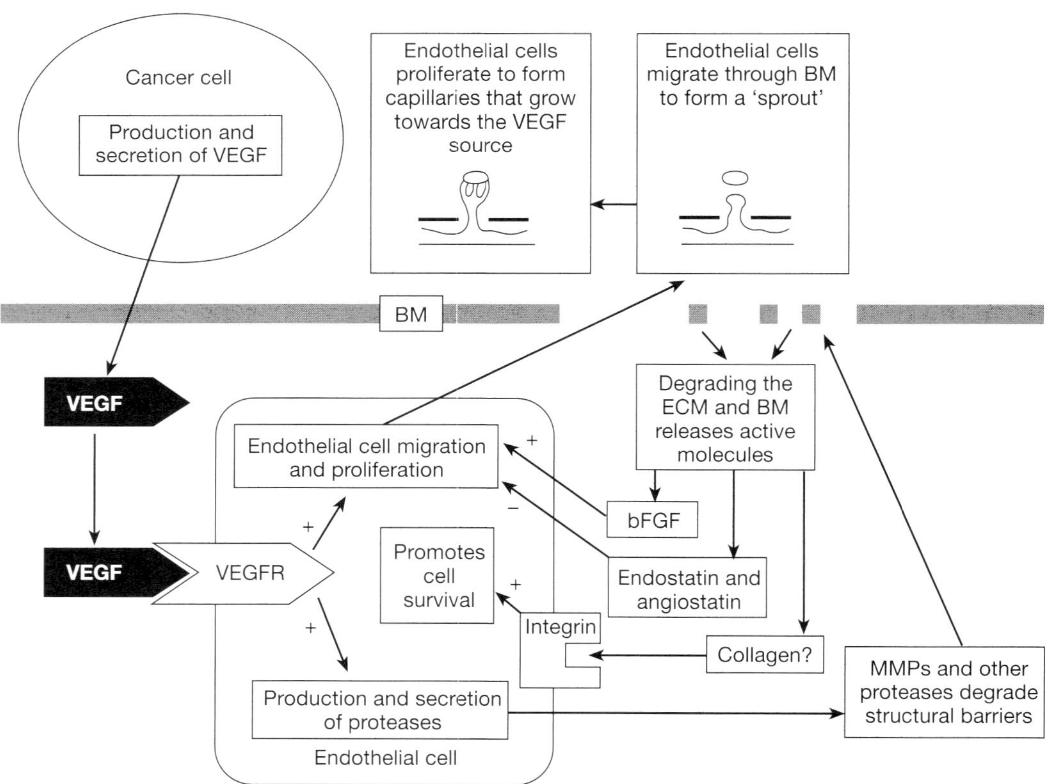

Fig. 17.1 Critical steps in angiogenesis. BM, basement membrane; ECM, extracellular matrix; VEGF, vascular endothelial growth factor; VEGFR, VEGF receptor; MMP, matrix metalloproteinases; bFGF, basic fibroblast growth factor.

To form new blood vessels, the equilibrium in the extracellular milieu must shift toward activation of angiogenesis. Once this process is activated, three critical steps are required for successful completion of angiogenesis (Liotta *et al.* 1991). The first step is local degradation of the basement membrane, ECM, and other structural barriers that impede ingrowth of new blood vessels. The second step is migration of the endothelial cells toward the angiogenic stimulus to form a 'sprout'. The final step is proliferation of endothelial cells to form new capillaries. Figure 17.1 outlines several of the pathways by which these steps are accomplished. It is important to remember that some of these pathways are speculative and that only the most relevant factors that regulate angiogenesis are shown.

Vascular endothelial growth factor (VEGF) is an endothelial cell mitogen that can induce all of the steps required to achieve angiogenesis (Ferrara 1996). Hypoxia stimulates release of VEGF (Carmeliet and Jain 2000; Fleming 1999). However, tumor cells can produce VEGF (Thelen *et al.* 1999; Brown *et al.* 1993; Takahashi *et al.* 1994; Tricarico *et al.* 1999; Berse *et al.* 1992; Sato *et al.* 1994; Tomisawa *et al.* 1999), often in the absence of hypoxia (Levy *et al.* 1997). Once released into the extracellular environment, VEGF binds to surface receptors on endothelial cells (Ferrara 1996; Brown *et al.* 1993; Nicol *et al.* 1997). Two VEGF receptors have been identified: VEGFR1 (flt-1) (Ferrara 1996; de Vries *et al.* 1992) and VEGFR2 (flk-1 or KDR) (Ferrara 1996; Quinn *et al.* 1993; Terman *et al.* 1992). VEGFR1 regulates structural organization and stability of new vessels, whereas VEGFR2 regulates proliferation of endothelial cells (Ferrara 1996; Bigelow *et al.* 2000) and appears to have a more prominent role in promoting angiogenesis (Ferrara 1996). When VEGF stimulates these receptors, endothelial cells release proteases, such as matrix metalloproteinases (MMP), which degrade the ECM and basement membrane, creating a window through which new blood vessels can grow (Polverini 1996). VEGF induces endothelial cell migration and proliferation through this window, ultimately leading to capillary formation toward the source of the VEGF stimulus (Ferrara 1996).

Molecules that modulate angiogenesis, such as endostatin, angiostatin, collagen, and basic fibroblast growth factor, may be released by degradation of the basement membrane and ECM (Brooks 1996; Polverini 1996; Jones and Harris 2000; Cirri *et al.* 1999). Basic fibroblast growth factor (bFGF) is produced by tumor cells, endothelial cells, fibroblasts, and macrophages (Bussolino *et al.* 1996; O'Brien and Harris 1995). These cells secrete bFGF into the ECM (Bussolino *et al.* 1996) where it is sequestered in extracellular 'storage' (Bussolino *et al.* 1996; O'Brien and Harris 1995; Polverini 1996; Folkman *et al.* 1988). When enzymes degrade the ECM, active bFGF is released (Bussolino *et al.* 1996; O'Brien and Harris 1995; Polverini 1996). bFGF can promote all steps in angiogenesis, including release of proteases and migration and proliferation of endothelial cells (Bussolino *et al.* 1996; Yoshida *et al.* 1996; Pepper *et al.* 1992). bFGF stimulates endothelial cell proliferation more profoundly than VEGF (Yoshida *et al.* 1996). However, bFGF is not as potent as VEGF in stimulating migration of endothelial cells (Yoshida *et al.* 1996). There is evidence that VEGF and bFGF act synergistically to promote angiogenesis (Pepper *et al.* 1992). Endostatin

and angiostatin are natural endogenous substances that inhibit angiogenesis and endothelial cell proliferation through an unknown mechanism (Cirri *et al.* 1999). They may serve as 'feedback inhibitors'. Collagen probably binds to and stimulates integrins (Brooks 1996). Integrins are surface receptors on endothelial cells that are involved in multiple cellular processes including adhesion, invasion, migration, proliferation, apoptosis, and cell survival (Brooks 1996; Jones and Harris 2000). When the integrins are inhibited, endothelial cells undergo apoptosis and angiogenesis is interrupted (Brooks 1996). Therefore, the role of integrins in angiogenesis is most probably a permissive one. In other words, stimulation of integrins may promote endothelial cell survival (Brooks 1996). During angiogenesis, upregulation of integrins and stimulation of integrins by collagen probably enhance this function (Brooks 1996).

The role of angiogenesis in metastases

Angiogenesis is required for the growth of established tumors (Folkman 1972). For a new hematogenous metastasis to develop, a tumor must 'shed' neoplastic cells into the circulation (Liotta *et al.* 1974). However, shedding of cancer cells can only occur when a vascular supply exists. Thus, angiogenesis is required for hematogenous metastasis to develop (Liotta *et al.* 1974; Singh *et al.* 1994). In fact, highly vascular tumors are more likely to shed cells into the circulation (Liotta *et al.* 1974; McCulloch *et al.* 1995). VEGF, also known as vascular permeability factor, increases the permeability of blood vessels (Ferrara 1996). These 'leaky' vessels may permit tumor cells to escape more easily into the circulation. Not all cells that escape into the circulation become metastases. A complex sequence of events must occur in order for the cell to attach and invade (Liotta *et al.* 1991; Ellis and Fidler 1996). Once a metastasis is established, its ability to continue to grow depends on angiogenesis (Ellis and Fidler 1996). The environment in which a metastasis establishes itself probably influences the tumor's ability to induce angiogenesis. This concept is supported by Singh *et al.* (1994) who found a higher level of bFGF, greater vascularity, and a higher metastatic rate in a human RCC cell line injected into murine kidney compared to those injected subcutaneously. Thus, angiogenesis is required for the development and growth of hematogenous metastases. In addition, the environment in which a metastasis develops influences local angiogenesis.

Measuring angiogenesis and angiogenic potential

Angiogenesis can be indirectly measured by determining tumor microvessel density (Vermeulen *et al.* 1996). A standard method for quantifying microvessel density has been proposed (Vermeulen *et al.* 1996). This method begins with immunostaining of the specimen to permit identification of endothelial cells using light microscopy. 'Hot spots', which are areas of highly vascular viable tumor, are analyzed to determine microvessel density. The presence of a lumen and blood cells is not necessary to identify a microvessel (Vermeulen *et al.* 1996; Delahunt *et al.* 1997; Nativ *et al.* 1998). The use of this method as a measure of angiogenesis is supported by studies that correlate expression of angiogenic factors with higher microvessel density (Vermeulen *et al.* 1996). For example, high microvessel density is associated with high VEGF expression in RCC (Thelen *et al.* 1999; Paradis *et al.* 2000).

Since angiogenesis is intimately related to tumor growth and metastasis, defining the angiogenic potential of a tumor may be important in assessing the tumor's aggressiveness. In addition, angiogenic potential may be utilized as a 'tumor marker' to predict prognosis and to help direct therapy. Determining the angiogenic potential of a tumor may be accomplished by several methods, including calculating microvessel density, quantifying angiogenic molecules within the tumor, determining the expression of angiogenic factors by measuring their mRNA within the neoplastic cells, assessing the presence of angiogenic receptors within the tumor tissue, and by measuring angiogenic factors in the serum and urine of cancer patients (Vermeulen *et al.* 1996; Ziche *et al.* 1999; Wechsel *et al.* 1999). At present, it is not possible to measure the balance between the stimulatory and inhibitory processes (Ziche *et al.* 1999). Nonetheless, researchers are utilizing angiogenic potential to investigate therapeutic and prognostic factors. Studies examining the angiogenic potential of RCC are described later in this chapter.

Evidence for angiogenesis in renal cell carcinoma

Most of the evidence for angiogenesis in RCC derives from studies on VEGF. Recent data supports the concept that VEGF is produced by RCC cells, released into the ECM, and bound by VEGF receptors on the endothelial cells (Ferrara 1996; Brown *et al.* 1993; Nicol *et al.* 1997). In fact, RCC usually overexpresses VEGF. In other words, RCC cells produce more VEGF than normal renal tissue (Thelen *et al.* 1999; Brown *et al.* 1993; Takahashi *et al.* 1994; Tricarico *et al.* 1999; Berse *et al.* 1992; Sato *et al.* 1994; Tomisawa *et al.* 1999; Nicol *et al.* 1997; Nakagawa *et al.* 1997; Siemeister *et al.* 1996). When all histologic types of RCC are included, VEGF mRNA is overexpressed in 60–100 per cent of tumors compared to normal renal tissue (Takahashi *et al.* 1994; Sato *et al.* 1994; Tomisawa *et al.* 1999; Nicol *et al.* 1997; Nakagawa *et al.* 1997). When only hypervascular RCC (based on angiography or computerized tomography (CT)) were examined, 96 per cent expressed VEGF mRNA (Takahashi *et al.* 1994). In clear cell RCC, VEGF mRNA overexpression ranges from 92 (Brown *et al.* 1993) to 100 per cent (Takahashi *et al.* 1994; Tricarico *et al.* 1999). Lower levels of VEGF mRNA have been reported in hypovascular (Takahashi *et al.* 1994) and papillary RCC (Brown *et al.* 1993; Berse *et al.* 1992). Nonetheless, VEGF mRNA expression has been described in clear cell (Brown *et al.* 1993; Takahashi *et al.* 1994; Tricarico *et al.* 1999; Sato *et al.* 1994; Paradis *et al.* 2000), sarcomatoid (Brown *et al.* 1993; Takahashi *et al.* 1994; Tricarico *et al.*

1999), and papillary RCC (Tricarico *et al.* 1999; Sato *et al.* 1994; Paradis *et al.* 2000). In addition, serum VEGF is significantly higher in patients with RCC compared to patients without tumors (Wechsel *et al.* 1999).Only one study has investigated VEGF expression in oncocytomas. This study examined two oncocytomas and found that neither overexpressed VEGF (Nicol *et al.* 1997). It is unknown if angiomyolipomas produce VEGF. Since there is minimal data regarding VEGF in benign renal masses, it is unclear whether VEGF can be used as a marker of malignancy.

At least four isoforms of VEGF (121,165,189, and 206) have been described (Ferrara 1996). There are limited data regarding the role of these isoforms in the angiogensis of RCC. VEGF121 (Thelen *et al.* 1999; Takahashi *et al.* 1994; Sato *et al.* 1994; Tomisawa *et al.* 1999; Nicol *et al.* 1997; Nakagawa *et al.* 1997), VEGF165 (Thelen *et al.* 1999; Takahashi *et al.* 1994; Sato *et al.* 1994; Tomisawa *et al.* 1999; Nicol *et al.* 1997; Nakagawa *et al.* 1997), and VEGF189 (Sato *et al.* 1994; Tomisawa *et al.* 1999; Nicol *et al.* 1997) have been detected in RCC. So far, VEGF206 has not been detected in RCC (Tomisawa *et al.* 1999; Nicol *et al.* 1997; Nakagawa *et al.* 1997). Recent evidence suggests that VEGF189 may be the primary isoform responsible for angiogenesis. Expression of VEGF189 is higher in RCC than in normal renal tissue and is associated with a significantly higher microvessel density than the other isoforms (Tomisawa *et al.* 1999). Furthermore, VEGF189 overexpression occurred with pathologic tumor stage T3–T4 RCC significantly more often than with stage T0–T2 (Tomisawa *et al.* 1999). However, VEGF189 levels did not correlate with tumor grade, tumor cell type, renal vein invasion, or prognosis (Tomisawa *et al.* 1999).

Increased production and release of VEGF by RCC cells is accompanied by a corresponding increase in the expression of VEGF receptors on endothelial cells. In fact, several studies demonstrate higher VEGF receptor mRNA in endothelial cells of RCC compared to endothelial cells of normal kidney (Ferrara 1996; Brown *et al.* 1993; Tomisawa *et al.* 1999). The mechanism of this receptor upregulation is unknown. Nonetheless, increased VEGF receptor expression probably contributes to enhanced tumor angiogenesis.

Recent data also implicate bFGF in RCC angiogenesis. bFGF induces endothelial cell microvessel tube formation in human renal cell cancer cell lines (Emoto *et al.* 1997) and is present in 80–97 per cent of RCC (Emoto *et al.* 1997; Nanus *et al.* 1993). RCC cells can secrete bFGF (Fujimoto *et al.* 1995); however, they do not overexpress bFGF compared to normal renal tissue (Takahashi *et al.* 1994). In RCC, higher tumor cell density inhibits bFGF expression (Singh *et al.* 1996). Nanus *et al.* (1993) showed that bFGF is present in 97 per cent of RCC, but that most of it is localized to the blood vessels or ECM. However, in a small number of cases (16 per cent), tumor cells contained bFGF. This supports the assumption that bFGF is produced and released by local cells and stored in the ECM. Serum bFGF is often significantly higher in patients with RCC compared to patients without tumors (Wechsel *et al.* 1999; Fujimoto *et al.* 1991; Duensing *et al.* 1995). Urinary bFGF is not elevated with renal malignancy (Fujimoto *et al.* 1991).

In summary, RCC angiogenesis is enhanced by increased VEGF production from malignant cells and by upregulation of VEGF receptors on endothelial cells. VEGF189 may be the most potent isoform. bFGF is present in most RCC and is located primarily in the ECM. After bFGF is released by degradation of the ECM it stimulates angiogenesis.

Angiogenesis and the von Hippel–Lindau gene

The wild-type von Hippel–Lindau (VHL) gene encodes a tumor suppressor that also appears to inhibit angiogenesis by preventing VEGF expression (Fleming 1999). Deletion or mutation of the wild-type VHL gene interferes with tumor suppression, resulting in the development of multiple vascular neoplasms, including RCC (Fleming 1999). Recent evidence suggests that loss of this tumor suppressor also enhances angiogenesis.

Loss of the wild-type VHL gene prolongs the life span of VEGF mRNA, resulting in greater production of VEGF (Levy *et al.* 1997). As expected, VEGF levels are higher in RCC with the VHL mutation/deletion compared to RCC with the wild-type VHL gene (Levy *et al.* 1997; Siemeister *et al.* 1996; Pal *et al.* 1997; Iliopoulos *et al.* 1996). Loss of the wild-type VHL gene also induces RCC cells to become less responsive to hypoxia as a stimulus for VEGF release (Levy *et al.* 1997). This evidence suggests that angiogenesis is more pronounced in tumors with the VHL mutation (Fleming 1999). bFGF expression was not influenced by the VHL gene; therefore, it may not be a prominent angiogenic factor in RCC with the VHL mutation (Siemeister *et al.* 1996). In summary, the VHL deletion/mutation results in longer VEGF mRNA survival, greater VEGF production, and reduced dependence on hypoxia for VEGF stimulation. These changes ultimately lead to greater angiogenesis and vascularity in RCC with the VHL mutation/deletion.

Prognostic significance of angiogenic potential

Since angiogenesis is intimately related to tumor growth and metastasis, defining the angiogenic potential of RCC may provide important prognostic information. The impact of microvessel density on the prognosis of RCC is unclear. In patients with clear cell RCC, Delahunt *et al.* (1997) reported longer 5-year survival in patients with a high microvessel density compared to those with low microvessel density. This datum implies that highly vascular tumors actually had a better prognosis. However, these investigators recognized that vascular cancers with large vessels may not have a high microvessel density because they have few microscopic vessels. These cancers would not be categorized as 'vascular' using microvessel density. Therefore, they developed the concept of microvessel area, which is independent of vessel size and may more accurately reflect the vascular nature of a tumor. They demonstrated no association between microvessel area and survival. Yoshino *et al.* (1998) found a shorter survival and a higher incidence of metastasis in patients with tumors having a higher mean microvessel density. Multivariate analysis revealed that

microvessel density was the only statistically significant predictor of prognosis in 45 patients with stage T1–2M0 RCC (Yoshino *et al.* 1998). Others have reported that the microvessel density of RCC did not correlate with stage (Ou *et al.* 1998; Kohler *et al.* 1996), tumor size (Kohler *et al.* 1996), presence of metastasis (Ou *et al.* 1998), or survival (Ou *et al.* 1998). Microvessel density has been reported to decrease as tumor grade increases (Delahunt *et al.* 1997; Kohler *et al.* 1996).

Serum VEGF is significantly higher in patients with RCC compared to patients without tumors; however, serum levels are not related to tumor stage, tumor grade, or patient survival (Wechsel *et al.* 1999). Some investigators have reported that *tumor* VEGF levels do not correlate with pathologic stage, grade, cell type, or size of the tumor (Sato *et al.* 1994; Nicol *et al.* 1997). However, others found that increased levels of tumor VEGF were associated with higher grade, larger tumor size, and shorter survival (Paradis *et al.* 2000).

Serum bFGF is often significantly higher in patients with RCC compared to patients without tumors (Wechsel *et al.* 1999; Fujimoto *et al.* 1991; Duensing *et al.* 1995). However, it is unclear if these elevated levels are related to tumor stage, tumor grade, or patient survival (Wechsel *et al.* 1999; Fujimoto *et al.* 1991). Duensing *et al.* (1995) showed that increased serum bFGF may be associated with a higher frequency of progressive pulmonary metastasis. *Tumor* bFGF levels are not related to tumor grade, tumor stage, or survival (Nanus *etal.* 1993). In summary, patients with RCC may have higher serum levels of VEGF and bFGF. In addition, VEGF is overexpressed by the tumor compared to normal renal tissue. However, these observations have not translated into consistent prognostic information. Furthermore, it is unclear if tumor microvessel density predicts prognosis.

Anti-angiogenesis therapy for RCC

Inhibition of angiogenesis, or anti-angiogenesis, was defined by Folkman (1971) as '…prevention of new vessel sprouts from penetrating into an early tumor implant'. It does not include '…vasoconstriction or infarction of vessels already connected to the tumor'. Several steps are required to complete angiogenesis (Fig. 17.1). Any of these steps are possible targets for anti-angiogenesis therapy.

An ideal anti-angiogenic agent should have all of the following characteristics (Ziche *et al.* 1999). First, the agent should inhibit tumor angiogenesis without affecting other tissues. Angiogenesis is rare in humans, but does occur under normal circumstances (such as wound healing and certain types of inflammation (Carmeliet and Jain 2000; Senger *et al.* 1993)) and under other pathologic conditions (such as myocardial ischemia (Hojo *et al.* 2000; Lee *et al.* 2000; Huwer *et al.* 1999)). Obviously, an anti-angiogenic agent would not be ideal if it severely impaired wound healing or inhibited revascularization after myocardial infarction. Second, the tumor should not become resistant to this agent. It is possible that a tumor could develop a way of directly counteracting the inhibitor (such as through inhibitor degradation) or by recruiting other angiogenic pathways. If this type of resistance is seen, multiple agents may be required to prevent angiogenesis. Third, the agent should cause minimal toxicity. Other ideal characteristics include low cost and ease of administration.

It is important to recognize that this type of therapy is not targeted at the tumor, but at the processes that permit the cancer to grow. Therefore, these treatments are not expected to be cytotoxic. By halting the development of new blood vessels, these agents will inhibit the growth of tumors (Morita *et al*. 1994). Thus, response to anti-angiogenesis treatment should be considered successful if a patient's tumor burden is stable. Response to therapy may be assessed by measuring angiogenic factors in the patients serum or urine or by assessing tumor blood flow using magnetic resonance imaging (MRI), positron emission tomography (PET) scanning, or other imaging modalities (Jones and Harris 2000). When anti-angiogenic agents are stopped, angiogenesis and tumor growth is expected to resume (Rowe *et al*. 2000). Thus, anti-angiogenesis therapy may need to be administered indefinitely. In addition, utilizing a single anti-angiogenesis agent may be unrealistic because angiogenesis depends upon many soluble factors. If one pathway of angiogenesis is inhibited, the tumor may recruit alternate pathways. Thus, several angiogenesis inhibitors may be required. In addition, angiogenesis inhibitors may be administered with other anticancer treatments. A multifaceted approach may ultimately prove to be the treatment of choice.

Treatment of RCC with anti-angiogenesis agents is still under investigation and data are limited because clinical research on these drugs is still in its infancy. Nonetheless, an overview of the current anti-angiogenic approaches to RCC may provide insight into these therapies. The angiogenesis inhibitors listed below are classified according to their mechanism of action (http://cancertrials.nci.nih.gov; updated on 11/06/00).

Matrix metalloproteinase inhibitors (MMPI)

Matrix metalloproteinases (MMP) are a family of enzymes that can degrade the ECM and basement membrane. They can be classified according to their substrate (Belotti *et al*. 1999): collagenases (which degrade fibrillar collagen); gelatinases (which degrade denatured and basement membrane collagen); and stromelysins (which degrade proteoglycans and glycoproteins). During angiogenesis, certain MMP degrade the ECM and basement membrane, creating a window in these structural barriers through which new capillaries can grow. The MMP involved in angiogenesis must degrade type IV collagen, a major component of the vascular basement membrane. In fact, MMP-2 (gelatinase A) and MMP-9 (gelatinase B), which both degrade type IV collagen (Talbot and Brown 1996), are the most important MMP in angiogenesis (Jones and Harris 2000). MMP-2 and MMP-9 activity have been reported in several different tumor types (Belotti *et al*. 1999) including RCC (Gohji *et al*. 1998; Kugler *et al*. 1998; Miyake *et al*. 1999; Walther *et al*. 1997; Lein *et al*. 2000). Most research has been conducted on MMP-2. A high-level RCC MMP-2 (often in comparison to its naturally occurring inhibitor) has been linked with tumor invasion (Miyake *et al*. 1999), development of metastasis (Miyake *et al*. 1999), and decreased survival (Walther *et al*. 1997).

In animal models, matrix metalloproteinase inhibitors (MMPI) have been shown to inhibit primary and metastatic tumor growth, prevent metastasis, and prolong survival (Belotti *et al*. 1999). Batimastat (BB-94) is one of the most widely studied MMPI. However, human trials were halted because intraperitoneal administration often resulted in peritonitis and an orally administered analog, Marimastat, became available (Belotti *et al*. 1999). MMPI such as Marimastat (BB-2516), Neovastat (AE-94), CGS 27023A, AG-3340, BAY12–9566, and COL-3 are undergoing clinical trials for cancer treatment (http://cancertrials.nci.nih.gov; updated on 11/06/00). At present, Neovastat is the only MMPI in clinical trials (phase III) for kidney cancer (http://cancertrials.nci. nih.gov; updated on 11/06/00).

Inhibitors of endothelial cell proliferation

The replication rate of endothelial cells that are undergoing angiogenesis is much higher than that of resting endothelial cells. This increased rate of replication may make these cells easier to target with anti-proliferative therapy (Albini *et al*. 1999). One of the most studied inhibitors of endothelial cell proliferation is TNP-470 (also known as AGM-1470). TNP-470 is a synthetic analog of fumagillin, a natural molecule derived from fungi (Yoshida *et al*. 1996; Minischetti *et al*. 2000). In animal models of RCC, TNP-470 reduces tumor angiogenesis, inhibits primary tumor growth, decreases development of metastasis, and increases survival (Morita *et al*. 1994; Fujioka *et al*. 1996). In humans, a single phase II study (Stadler *et al*. 1999) involving 33 patients with previously treated metastatic RCC demonstrated one partial response. However, six patients had stable disease for 6 or more months. At present, there are no known ongoing clinical trials of TNP-470 in renal cancer.

Endostatin is a naturally occurring inhibitor of endothelial cell proliferation and angiogenesis (Cirri *et al*. 1999). Endostatin has been shown to inhibit growth of RCC in mice (Dhanabal *et al*. 1999). Phase I clinical trials are underway for solid neoplasms (http://cancertrials.nci.nih.gov; updated on 11/06/00). Angiostatin in also a naturally occurring inhibitor of endothelial cell proliferation and angiogenesis. Currently, its use in clinical trials is limited by inability to develop enough biologically active protein (Bigelow *et al*. 2000). Thalidomide appears to inhibit endothelial cell proliferation through an unknown mechanism (http://cancertrials.nci.nih.gov; updated on 11/06/00). In a recent phase II trial in 18 patients with advanced renal cancer, 100 mg oral thalidomide each night resulted in three partial responses and three patients with stable disease for 6 or more months (Eisen *et al*. 2000). Phase III trials using thalidomide to treat RCC are currently being conducted (http://cancertrials.nci.nih.gov; updated on 11/06/00).

Inhibitors of angiogenic factors and receptors

PTK787/ZK222584 is an oral inhibitor of both VEGF receptors. In the murine RCC model, this substance reduces microvessel density, tumor growth, and incidence of lung and lymph node metastases (Drevs *et al*. 2000). SU5416 is a selective inhibitor of the VEGF2 (flk-1) receptor (Vajkoczy *et al*. 1999). Recall that the VEGFR2 appears to have a more prominent role in promoting angiogenesis than VEGFR1 (Ferrara 1996). SU5416 inhibits tumor growth, decreases the incidence of metastasis, and reduces microvessel density in several types of malignancies (Vajkoczy *et al.* 1999; Shaheen *et al.* 1999). SU6668, which inhibits VEGF and bFGF receptors, has similar effects (Shaheen *et al.* 1999). SU5416 is currently in phase II trials for VHL disease and in phase III trials for metastatic renal cancer (http://cancertrials.nci.nih.gov; updated on 11/06/00). SU6668 is undergoing phase I trials in advanced cancers (http://cancertrials.nci.nih.gov; updated on 11/06/00).

Anti-VEGF antibodies have been shown to decrease tumor growth and metastasis in many cancers (Vitaliti *et al.* 2000; Schlaeppi and Wood 1999) including Wilms' tumor (Rowe *et al.* 2000). They also decrease endothelial tube formation in RCC (Nakagawa *et al.* 1997). Anti-VEGF antibodies are in phase I trials for refractory solid tumors and phase II trials for metastatic RCC (http://cancertrials.nci.nih.gov; updated on 11/06/00).

Interferon alpha (IFNα) can mediate antitumor activity through many mechanisms (Tretter *et al.* 2000), including inhibition of VEGF and bFGF (Yoshida *et al.* 1996; Minischetti *et al.* 2000; Ruszczak *et al.* 1990). When IFNα is used as a single agent to treat metastatic RCC, response rates are approximately 15 per cent (Tretter *et al.* 2000). However, stable disease has been reported in 6 (Muss *et al.* 1984) to 50 per cent (Kempf *et al.* 1986; Vugrin *et al.* 1986) of patients. IFNα is currently in clinical trials for treatment of RCC, usually in combination with other agents (http://cancertrials.nci.nih.gov; updated on 11/06/00).

Inhibitors of endothelial cell survival

Integrins promote endothelial cell survival (Brooks 1996). When integrins are inhibited, endothelial cells undergo apoptosis and angiogenesis is interrupted (Brooks 1996). Anti-integrin molecules have been used to treat several types of neoplasms, including squamous cell carcinoma, Lehdig cell tumors, and melanoma (Mitjans *et al.* 2000; Van Waes *et al.* 2000; Kerr *et al.* 1999; Carron *et al.* 1998). Anti-integrin compounds such as Vitaxin are currently undergoing phase I trials (http://cancertrials.nci.nih.gov; updated on 11/06/00).

Agents with a nonspecific action

Carboxyamidotriazole (CAI) inhibits angiogenesis by preventing cellular influx of calcium (Kohn *et al.* 1994). When applied to tumors, this agent decreases VEGF expression (Bauer *et al.* 2000), release of MMP (Wu *et al.* 1997), migration and proliferation of endothelial cells (Wu *et al.* 1997), microvessel density (Bauer *et al.* 2000), and malignant cell proliferation (Kohn *et al.* 1994). CAI has been investigated in phase I trials that included patients with advanced RCC (Kohn *et al.* 1997). Phase II trials for metastatic RCC are ongoing (http://cancertrials.nci.nih.gov; updated on 11/06/00).

Interleukin 12 (IL-12) induces release of IFNγ, which in turn disrupts angiogenesis through endothelial apoptosis (Gee *et al.* 1999; Yao *et al.* 1999; Majewski *et al.* 1996; Voest *et al.* 1995). A phase I study using IL-12 to treat metastatic RCC is currently accruing patients (http://cancernet.nci.nih.gov/trialsrch.shtml; as of 12/01/00).

Gene therapy

Systemic administration of anti-angiogenic compounds poses several problems. First, rapid degradation of these agents *in vivo* may require repetitive administration and high doses to maintain adequate levels at the tumor. Second, systemic distribution of these therapies may inhibit angiogenesis in normal tissue, impairing processes such as wound healing. Third, systemic exposure to these agents may increase side-effects. Gene therapy may overcome these problems (Albini *et al.* 1999). By introducing a gene encoding an anti-angiogenic protein into the tumor, continuous local exposure to a high concentration of these inhibitors may be achieved. Furthermore, this mode of administration avoids the toxicity associated with systemic administration. In cell cultures and in animals, gene therapy with IFNα (Albini *et al.* 2000), endostatin (Chen *et al.* 2000; Feldman *et al.* 2000), angiostatin (Tanaka *et al.* 1998), and other anti-angiogenesis agents (Goldman *et al.* 1998; Li *et al.* 1999) has been shown to inhibit angiogenesis, halt tumor growth, prevent metastasis, and prolong survival. A clinical trial using IL-12 gene therapy has recently begun (http://cancernet.nci.nih.gov/trialsrch.shtml; as of 12/01/00). Additional trials of anti-angiogenic gene therapy are expected.

Summary

Angiogenesis is a complex cascade of events that depends on the interaction of several elements in the local environment. Tumors require angiogenesis to grow and to metastasize hematogenously. Cancers promote angiogenesis by producing VEGF. This process is augmented by upregulation of VEGF receptors and release of collagen and bFGF during degradation of the ECM and basement membrane. In RCC, angiogenesis occurs frequently and is more pronounced in tumors with the VHL mutation/deletion. The angiogenic potential of renal neoplasms, regardless of the method of assessment, has not provided conclusive prognostic information. Nonetheless, anti-angiogenic therapy in animals clearly inhibits angiogenesis, tumor growth, and development of metastasis. Clinical trials in humans are currently underway. Gene therapy appears to be a promising method of administering anti-angiogenic agents, but additional research is required.

References

Albini, A., Noonan, D., and Santi, L. (1999). Angiogenesis at the interface between basic and clinical research. *Int. J. Biol. Markers* 14 (4), 202–6.

Albini, A., Marchisone, C., Del Grosso, F., Benelli, R., Masiello, L., Tacchetti, C., Bono, M., Ferrantini, M., Rozera, C., Truini, M., Belardelli, F., Santi, L., and Noonan, D.M. (2000). Inhibition of angiogenesis and vascular tumor growth by interferon-producing cells: a gene therapy approach. *Am. J. Pathol.* 156 (4), 1381–93.

Bauer, K.S., Cude, K.J., Dixon, S.C., Kruger, E.A., and Figg, W.D. (2000). Carboxyamido-triazole inhibits angiogenesis by blocking the calcium-mediated nitric-oxide synthase–vascular endothelial growth factor pathway. *J. Pharmacol. Exp. Ther.* 292 (1), 31–7.

Belotti, D., Paganoni, P., and Giavazzi, R. (1999). MMP inhibitors: experimental and clinical studies. *Int. J. Biol. Markers* 14 (4), 232–8.

Berse, B., Brown, L.F., Van de Water, L., Dvorak, H.F., and Senger, D.R. (1992). Vascular permeability factor (vascular endothelial growth factor) gene is expressed differentially in normal tissues, macrophages, and tumors. *Mol. Biol. Cell* **3** (2), 211–20.

Bigelow, K.R., Spiotto, M.T., and Stadler, W.M. (2000). Antiangiogenic agents and strategies in renal cell carcinoma. In *Current clinical oncology: renal cell carcinoma: molecular biology, immunology, and clinical management* (ed. RM Bukowski and AC Novick), pp. 381–95. Human Press Inc, Totowa, New Jersey.

Brooks, P.C. (1996). Role of integrins in angiogenesis. *Eur. J. Cancer* **32A** (14), 2423–9.

Brown, L.F., Berse, B., Jackman, R.W., Tognazzi, K., Manseau, E.J., Dvorak, H.F., and Senger, D.R. (1993). Increased expression of vascular permeability factor (vascular endothelial growth factor) and its receptors in kidney and bladder carcinomas. *Am. J. Pathol.* **143** (5), 1255–62.

Bussolino, F., Albini, A., Camussi, G., Presta, M., Viglietto, G., Ziche, M., and Persico. G. (1996). Role of soluble mediators in angiogenesis. *Eur. J. Cancer* **32A** (14), 2401–12.

Carmeliet, P. and Jain, R.K. (2000). Angiogenesis in cancer and other diseases. *Nature* **407** (6801), 249–57.

Carron, C.P., Meyer, D.M., Pegg, J.A., Engleman, V.W., Nickols, M.A., Settle, S.L., Westlin, W.F., Ruminski, P.G., and Nickols, G.A. (1998). A peptidomimetic antagonist of the integrin alpha(v)beta3 inhibits Leydig cell tumor growth and the development of hypercalcemia of malignancy. *Cancer Res.* **58** (9), 1930–5.

Chen, C.T., Lin, J., Li, Q., Phipps, S.S., Jakubczak, J.L., Stewart, D.A., Skripchenko, Y., Forry-Schaudies, S., Wood, J., Schnell, C., and Hallenbeck, P.L. (2000). Antiangiogenic gene therapy for cancer via systemic administration of adenoviral vectors expressing secretable endostatin. *Hum. Gene Ther.* **11** (14), 1983–96.

Cirri, L., Donnini, S., Morbidelli, L., Chiarugi, P., Ziche, M., and Ledda, F. (1999). Endostatin: a promising drug for antiangiogenic therapy. *Int. J. Biol. Markers* **14** (4), 263–7.

Delahunt, B., Bethwaite, P.B., and Thornton, A. (1997). Prognostic significance of microscopic vascularity for clear cell renal cell carcinoma. *Br. J. Urol.* **80**(3), 401–4.

de Vries, C., Escobedo, J.A., Ueno, H., Houck, K., Ferrara, N., and Williams, L.T. (1992). The fms-like tyrosine kinase, a receptor for vascular endothelial growth factor. *Science* **255** (5047), 989–91.

Dhanabal, M., Ramchandran, R., Volk, R., Stillman, I.E., Lombardo, M., Iruela-Arispe, M.L., Simons, M., and Sukhatme, V.P. (1999). Endostatin: yeast production, mutants, and antitumor effect in renal cell carcinoma. *Cancer Res.* **59** (1), 189–97.

Drevs, J., Hofmann, I., Hugenschmidt, H., Wittig, C., Madjar, H., Muller, M., Wood, J., Martiny-Baron, G., Unger, C., and Marme, D. (2000). Effects of PTK787/ZK 222584, a specific inhibitor of vascular endothelial growth factor receptor tyrosine kinases, on primary tumor, metastasis, vessel density, and blood flow in a murine renal cell carcinoma model. *Cancer Res.* **60** (17), 4819–24.

Duensing, S., Grosse, J., and Atzpodien, J. (1995). Increased serum levels of basic fibroblast growth factor (bFGF) are associated with progressive lung metastases in advanced renal cell carcinoma patients. *Anticancer Res.* **15** (5B), 2331–3.

Eisen, T., Boshoff, C., Mak, I., Sapunar, F., Vaughan, M.M., Pyle, L., Johnston, S.R., Ahern, R., Smith, I.E., and Gore, M.E. (2000). Continuous low dose thalidomide: a phase II study in advanced melanoma, renal cell, ovarian and breast cancer. *Br. J. Cancer* **82** (4), 812–17.

Ellis, L.M. and Fidler, I.J. (1996). Angiogenesis and metastasis. *Eur. J. Cancer* **32A** (14), 2451–60.

Emoto, A., Nakagawa, M., Wakabayashi, Y., Hanada, T., Naito, S., and Nomura, Y. (1997). Induction of tubulogenesis of microvascular endothelial cells by basic fibroblast growth factor from human SN12C renal cancer cells. *J. Urol.* **157** (2), 699–703.

Feldman, A.L., Restifo, N.P., Alexander, H.R., Bartlett, D.L., Hwu, P., Seth, P., and Libutti, S.K. (2000). Antiangiogenic gene therapy of cancer utilizing a recombinant adenovirus to elevate systemic endostatin levels in mice. *Cancer Res.* **60** (6), 1503–6.

Ferrara, N. (1996). Vascular endothelial growth factor. *Eur. J. Cancer* **32A**, 2413–22.

Fleming, S. (1999). Renal cancer genetics: von Hippel Lindau and other syndromes. *Int. J. Dev. Biol.* **43** (5), 469–71.

Folkman, J. (1971). Tumor angiogenesis: therapeutic implications. *New Engl. J. Med.* **285** (21), 1182–6.

Folkman, J. (1972). Anti-angiogenesis: new concept for therapy of solid tumors. *Ann. Surg.* **175** (3), 409–16.

Folkman, J., Merler, E., Abernathy, C., and Williams, G. (1971). Isolation of a tumor factor responsible for angiogenesis. *J. Exp. Med.* **133** (2), 275–88.

Folkman, J., Klagsbrun, M., Sasse, J., Wadzinski, M., Ingber, D., and Vlodavsky, I. (1988). A heparin-binding angiogenic protein–basic fibroblast growth factor–is stored within basement membrane. *Am. J. Pathol.* **130** (2), 393–400.

Fujimoto, K., Ichimori, Y., Kakizoe, T., Okajima, E., Sakamoto, H., Sugimura, T., and Terada, M. (1991). Increased serum levels of basic fibroblast growth factor in patients with renal cell carcinoma. *Biochem. Biophys. Res. Commun.* **180** (1), 386–92.

Fujimoto, K., Ichimori, Y., Yamaguchi, H., Arai, K., Futami, T., Ozono, S., Hirao, Y., Kakizoe, T., Terada, M., and Okajima, E. (1995). Basic fibroblast growth factor as a candidate tumor marker for renal cell carcinoma. *Jpn J. Cancer Res.* **86** (2), 182–6.

Fujioka, T., Hasegawa, M., Ogiu, K., Matsushita, Y., Sato, M., and Kubo, T. (1996). Antitumor effects of angiogenesis inhibitor 0-(chloroacetyl-carbamoyl) fumagillol (TNP-470) against murine renal cell carcinoma. *J. Urol.* **155** (5), 1775–8.

Gee, M.S., Koch, C.J., Evans, S.M., Jenkins, W.T., Pletcher, C.H. Jr, Moore, J.S., Koblish, H.K., Lee, J., Lord, E.M., Trinchieri, G., and Lee, W.M. (1999). Hypoxia-mediated apoptosis from angiogenesis inhibition underlies tumor control by recombinant interleukin 12. *Cancer Res.* **59** (19), 4882–9.

Gohji, K., Nomi, M., Hara, I., Arakawa, S., and Kamidono, S. (1998). Influence of cytokines and growth factors on matrix metalloproteinase-2 production and invasion of human renal cancer. *Urol. Res.* **26** (1), 33–7.

Goldman, C.K., Kendall, R.L., Cabrera, G., Soroceanu, L., Heike, Y., Gillespie, G.Y., Siegal, G.P., Mao, X., Bett, A.J., Huckle, W.R., Thomas, K.A., and Curiel, D.T. (1998). Paracrine expression of a native soluble vascular endothelial growth factor receptor inhibits tumor growth, metastasis, and mortality rate. *Proc. Natl Acad. Sci., USA* **95** (15), 8795–800.

Hojo, Y., Ikeda, U., Zhu, Y., Okada, M., Ueno, S., Arakawa, H., Fujikawa, H., Katsuki, T., and Shimada, K. (2000). Expression of vascular endothelial growth factor in patients with acute myocardial infarction. *J. Am. Coll. Cardiol.* **35** (4), 968–73.

Huwer, H., Rissland, J., Vollmar, B., Nikoloudakis, N., Welter, C., Menger, M.D., and Schafers, H.J. (1999). Angiogenesis and microvascularization after cryothermia-induced myocardial infarction: a quantitative fluorescence microscopic study in rats. *Basic Res. Cardiol.* **94** (2), 85–93.

Iliopoulos, O., Levy, A.P., Jiang, C., Kaelin, W.G. Jr, and Goldberg, M.A. (1996). Negative regulation of hypoxia-inducible genes by the von Hippel–Lindau protein. *Proc. Natl Acad. Sci., USA* **93** (20), 10595–9.

Jones, P.H. and Harris, A.L. (2000). The current status of clinical trials in antiangiogenesis. *PPO Updates* **14** (1), 1–9.

Kempf, R.A., Grunberg, S.M., Daniels, J.R., Skinner, D.G., Venturi, C.L., Spiegel, R., Neri, R., Greiner, J.M., Rudnick, S., and Mitchell, M.S. (1986). Recombinant interferon alpha-2 (INTRON A) in a phase II study of renal cell carcinoma. *J. Biol. Response Mod.* **5** (1), 27–35.

Kerr, J.S., Wexler, R.S., Mousa, S.A., Robinson, C.S., Wexler, E.J., Mohamed, S., Voss, M.E., Devenny, J.J., Czerniak, P.M., Gudzelak, A. Jr, and Slee, A.M. (1999). Novel small molecule alpha v integrin antagonists: comparative anti-cancer efficacy with known angiogenesis inhibitors. *Anticancer Res.* **19** (2A), 959–68.

Kohler, H.H., Barth, P.J., Siebel, A., Gerharz, E.W., and Bittinger, A. (1996). Quantitative assessment of vascular surface density in renal cell carcinomas. *Br. J. Urol.* **77** (5), 650–4.

Kohn, E.C., Felder, C.C., Jacobs, W., Holmes, K.A., Day, A., Freer, R., and Liotta, L.A. (1994). Structure–function analysis of signal and growth inhibition by carboxyamido-triazole, CAI. *Cancer Res.* **54** (4), 935–42.

Kohn, E.C., Figg, W.D., Sarosy, G.A., Bauer, K.S., Davis, P.A., Soltis, M.J., Thompkins, A., Liotta, L.A., and Reed, E. (1997). Phase 1 trial of micronized formulation carboxyamidotriazole in patients with refractory solid tumors: pharmacokinetics, clinical outcome, and comparison of formulations. *J. Clin. Oncol.* **15** (5), 1985–93.

Kugler, A., Hemmerlein, B., Thelen, P., Kallerhoff, M., Radzun, H.J., and Ringert, R.H. (1998). Expression of metalloproteinase 2 and 9 and their inhibitors in renal cell carcinoma. *J. Urol.* **160** (5), 1914–18.

Lee, S.H., Wolf, P.L., Escudero, R., Deutsch, R., Jamieson, S.W., and Thistlethwaite, P.A. (2000). Early expression of angiogenesis factors in acute myocardial ischemia and infarction. *New Engl. J. Med.* **342** (9), 626–33.

Lein, M., Jung, K., Laube, C., Hubner, T., Winkelmann, B., Stephan, C., Hauptmann, S., Rudolph, B., Schnorr, D., and Loening, S.A. (2000). Matrix-metalloproteinases and their inhibitors in plasma and tumor tissue of patients with renal cell carcinoma. *Int. J. Cancer* **85** (6), 801–4.

Levy, A.P., Levy, N.S., Iliopoulos, O., Jiang, C., Kaplin, W.G. Jr, and Goldberg, M.A. (1997). Regulation of vascular endothelial growth factor by hypoxia and its modulation by the von Hippel–Lindau tumor suppressor gene. *Kidney Int.* **51** (2), 575–8.

Li, H., Griscelli, F., Lindenmeyer, F., Opolon, P., Sun, L.Q., Connault, E., Soria, J., Soria, C., Perricaudet, M., Yeh, P., and Lu, H. (1999). Systemic delivery of antiangiogenic adenovirus AdmATF induces liver resistance to metastasis and prolongs survival of mice. *Hum. Gene Ther.* **10** (18), 3045–53.

Liotta, L.A., Kleinerman, J., and Saidel, G.M. (1974). Quantitative relationships of intravascular tumor cells, tumor vessels, and pulmonary metastases following tumor implantation. *Cancer Res.* **34** (5), 997–1004.

Liotta, L.A., Steeg, P.S., and Stetler-Stevenson, W.G. (1991). Cancer metastasis and angiogenesis: an imbalance of positive and negative regulation. *Cell* **64** (2), 327–36.

Majewski, S., Marczak, M., Szmurlo, A., Jablonska, S., and Bollag, W. (1996). Interleukin-12 inhibits angiogenesis induced by human tumor cell lines *in vivo*. *J. Invest. Dermatol.* **106** (5), 1114–18.

McCulloch, P., Choy, A., and Martin, L. (1995). Association between tumour angiogenesis and tumour cell shedding into effluent venous blood during breast cancer surgery. *Lancet* **346** (8986), 1334–5.

Minischetti, M., Vacca, A., Ribatti, D., Iurlaro, M., Ria, R., Pellegrino, A., Gasparini, G., and Dammacco, A.F. (2000). TNP-470 and recombinant human interferon-alpha2a inhibit angiogenesis synergistically. *Br. J. Haematol.* **109** (4), 829–37.

Mitjans, F., Meyer, T., Fittschen, C., Goodman, S., Jonczyk, A., Marshall, J.F., Reyes, G., and Piulats, J. (2000). *In vivo* therapy of malignant melanoma by means of antagonists of alphav integrins. *Int. J. Cancer* **87** (5), 716–23.

Miyake, H., Hara, I., Gohji, K., Yamanaka, K., Hara, S., Arakawa, S., Nakajima, M., Kamidono, S. (1999). Relative expression of matrix metalloproteinase-2 and tissue inhibitor of metalloproteinase-2 in mouse renal cell carcinoma cells regulates their metastatic potential. *Clin. Cancer Res..* **5** (10), 2824–9.

Morita, T., Shinohara, N., and Tokue, A. (1994). Antitumour effect of a synthetic analogue of fumagillin on murine renal carcinoma. *Br. J. Urol.* **74** (4), 416–21.

Muss, H.B., Kempf, R.A., Martino, S., Rudnick, S.A., Greiner, J., Cooper, M.R., Decker, D., Grunberg, S.M., Jackson, D.V., Richards, F., *et al.* (1984). A phase II study of recombinant alpha interferon in patients with recurrent or metastatic breast cancer. *J. Clin. Oncol.* **2** (9), 1012–16.

Nakagawa, M., Emoto, A., Hanada, T., Nasu, N., and Nomura, Y. (1997). Tubulogenesis by microvascular endothelial cells is mediated by vascular endothelial growth factor (VEGF) in renal cell carcinoma. *Br. J. Urol.* **79** (5), 681–7.

Nanus, D.M., Schmitz-Drager, B.J., Motzer, R.J., Lee, A.C., Vlamis, V., Cordon-Cardo, C., Albino, A.P., and Reuter, V.E. (1993). Expression of basic fibroblast growth factor in primary human renal tumors: correlation with poor survival. *J. Natl Cancer Inst.* **85** (19), 1597–9.

Nativ, O., Sabo, E., Reiss, A., Wald, M., Madjar, S., and Moskovitz, B. (1998). Clinical significance of tumor angiogenesis in patients with localized renal cell carcinoma. *Urology* **51** (5), 693–6.

Nicol, D., Hii, S.I., Walsh, M., The, B., Thompson, L., Kennett, C., and Gotley, D. (1997). Vascular endothelial growth factor expression is increased in renal cell carcinoma. *J. Urol.* **157** (4), 1482–6.

O'Brien, T.S. and Harris, A.L. (1995). Angiogenesis in urological malignancy. *Br. J. Urol.* **76** (6), 675–82.

Ou, Y.C., Chen, J.T., Yang, C.R., Horng, Y.Y., Kao, Y.L., and Cheng, C.L. (1998). Tumor angiogenesis and metastasis: correlation in invasive renal cell carcinoma. *Chung Hua I Hsueh Tsa Chih (Taipei)* **61** (8), 441–7.

Pal, S., Claffey, K.P., Dvorak, H.F., and Mukhopadhyay, D. (1997). The von Hippel–Lindau gene product inhibits vascular permeability factor/vascular endothelial growth factor expression in renal cell carcinoma by blocking protein kinase C pathways. *J. Biol. Chem.* **272** (44), 27509–12.

Paradis, V., Lagha, N.B., Zeimoura, L., Blanchet, P., Eschwege, P., Ba, N., Benoit, G., Jardin, A., and Bedossa. P. (2000).Expression of vascular endothelial growth factor in renal cell carcinomas. *Virch. Arch.* **436** (4), 351–6.

Pepper, M.S., Ferrara, N., Orci, L., and Montesano, R. (1992). Potent synergism between vascular endothelial growth factor and basic fibroblast growth factor in the induction of angiogenesis *in vitro*. *Biochem. Biophys. Res. Commun.* **189** (2), 824–31.

Polverini, P.J. (1996). How the extracellular matrix and macrophages contribute to angiogenesis-dependent diseases. *Eur. J. Cancer* **32A** (14), 2430–7.

Quinn, T.P., Peters, K.G., de Vries, C., Ferrara, N., and Williams, L.T. (1993). Fetal liver kinase 1 is a receptor for vascular endothelial growth factor and is selectively expressed in vascular endothelium. *Proc. Natl Acad. Sci., USA* **90** (16), 7533–7.

Rowe, D.H., Huang, J., Kayton, M.L., Thompson, R., Troxel, A., O'Toole, K.M., Yamashiro, D., Stolar, C.J., and Kandel, J.J. (2000). Anti-VEGF antibody suppresses primary tumor growth and metastasis in an experimental model of Wilms' tumor. *J. Ped. Surg.* **35** (1), 30–2.

Ruszczak, Z., Detmar, M., Imcke, E., and Orfanos, C.E. (1990). Effects of rIFN alpha, beta, and gamma on the morphology, proliferation, and cell surface antigen expression of human dermal microvascular endothelial cells *in vitro*. *J. Invest. Dermatol.* **95** (6), 693–9.

Sato, K., Terada, K., Sugiyama, T., Takahashi, S., Saito, M., Moriyama, M., Kakinuma, H., Suzuki, Y., Kato, M., and Kato, T. (1994). Frequent overexpression of vascular endothelial growth factor gene in human renal cell carcinoma. *Tohoku J. Exp. Med.* **173** (3), 355–60.

Schlaeppi, J.M. and Wood, J.M. (1999). Targeting vascular endothelial growth factor (VEGF) for anti-tumor therapy, by anti-VEGF neutralizing monoclonal antibodies or by VEGF receptor tyrosine-kinase inhibitors. *Cancer Metastas. Rev.* **18** (4), 473–81.

Senger, D.R., Van de Water, L., Brown, L.F., Nagy, J.A., Yeo, K.T., Yeo, T.K., Berse, B., Jackman, R.W., Dvorak, A.M., and Dvorak, H.F. (1993). Vascular permeability factor (VPF, VEGF) in tumor biology. *Cancer Metastas. Rev.* **12** (3–4), 303–24.

Shaheen, R.M., Davis, D.W., Liu, W., Zebrowski, B.K., Wilson, M.R., Bucana, C.D., McConkey, D.J., McMahon, G., and Ellis, L.M. (1999). Antiangiogenic therapy targeting the tyrosine kinase receptor for vascular endothelial growth factor receptor inhibits the growth of colon cancer liver metastasis and induces tumor and endothelial cell apoptosis. *Cancer Res.* **59** (21), 5412–16.

Siemeister, G., Weindel, K., Mohrs, K., Barleon, B., Martiny-Baron, G., and Marme, D. (1996). Reversion of deregulated expression of vascular endothelial growth factor in human renal carcinoma cells by von Hippel–Lindau tumor suppressor protein. *Cancer Res.* **56** (10), 2299–301.

Singh, R.K., Bucana, C.D., Gutman, M., Fan, D., Wilson, M.R., and Fidler, I.J. (1994). Organ site-dependent expression of basic fibroblast growth factor in human renal cell carcinoma cells. *Am. J. Pathol.* **145** (2), 365–74.

Singh, R.K., Llansa, N., Bucana, C.D., Sanchez, R., Koura, A., and Fidler, I.J. (1996). Cell density-dependent regulation of basic fibroblast growth factor expression in human renal cell carcinoma cells. *Cell Growth Different.* 7 (3), 397–404.

Stadler, W.M., Kuzel, T., Shapiro, C., Sosman, J., Clark, J., and Vogelzang, N.J. (1999). Multi-institutional study of the angiogenesis inhibitor TNP-470 in metastatic renal carcinoma. *J. Clin. Oncol.* 17 (8), 2541–5.

Takahashi, A., Sasaki, H., Kim, S.J., Tobisu, K., Kakizoe, T., Tsukamoto, T., Kumamoto, Y., Sugimura, T., and Terada, M. (1994). Markedly increased amounts of messenger RNAs for vascular endothelial growth factor and placenta growth factor in renal cell carcinoma associated with angiogenesis. *Cancer Res.* 54 (15), 4233–7.

Talbot, D.C. and Brown, P.D. (1996). Experimental and clinical studies on the use of matrix metalloproteinase inhibitors for the treatment of cancer. *Eur. J. Cancer* 32A (14), 2528–33.

Tanaka, T., Cao, Y., Folkman, J., and Fine, H.A (1998). Viral vector-targeted antiangiogenic gene therapy utilizing an angiostatin complementary DNA. *Cancer Res.* 58 (15), 3362–9.

Terman, B.I., Dougher-Vermazen, M., Carrion, M.E., Dimitrov, D., Armellino, D.C., Gospodarowicz, D., and Bohlen, P. (1992). Identification of the KDR tyrosine kinase as a receptor for vascular endothelial cell growth factor. *Biochem. Biophys. Res. Commun.* 187 (3), 1579–86.

Thelen, P., Hemmerlein, B., Kugler, A., Seiler, T., Ozisik, R., Kallerhoff, M., and Ringert, R.H. (1999). Quantification by competitive quantitative RT-PCR of VEGF121 and VEGF165 in renal cell carcinoma. *Anticancer Res.* 19 (2C), 1563–5.

Tomisawa, M., Tokunaga, T., Oshika, Y., Tsuchida, T., Fukushima, Y., Sato, H., Kijima, H., Yamazaki, H., Ueyama, Y., Tamaoki, N., and Nakamura, M. (1999). Expression pattern of vascular endothelial growth factor isoform is closely correlated with tumour stage and vascularisation in renal cell carcinoma. *Eur. J. Cancer* 35 (1), 133–7.

Tretter, C.P.G. and Ernstoff, M.S. (2000). Chemotherapy, hormonal therapy, and interferons. In *Comprehensive textbook of genitourinary oncology*, 2nd edn (ed. N.J. Vogelzang, P.T. Scardino, W.U. Shipley, and D.S. Coffey), pp.248–59. Lippincott Williams and Wilkins, Philadelphia.

Tricarico, C., Salvadori, B., Villari, D., Nicita, G., Della Melina, A., Pinzani, P., Ziche, M., and Pazzagli, M. (1999). Quantitative RT-PCR assay for VEGF mRNA in human tumors of the kidney. *Int. J. Biol. Markers* 14 (4), 247–50.

Vajkoczy, P., Menger, M.D., Vollmar, B., Schilling, L., Schmiedek, P., Hirth, K.P., Ullrich, A., and Fong, T.A. (1999). Inhibition of tumor growth, angiogenesis, and microcirculation by the novel Flk-1 inhibitor SU5416 as assessed by intravital multi-fluorescence videomicroscopy. *Neoplasia* 1 (1), 31–41.

Van Waes, C., Enamorado-Ayala, I., Hecht, D., Sulica, L., Chen, Z., Batt, D.G., and Mousa, S. (2000). Effects of the novel alpha integrin antagonist SM256 and cis-platinum on growth of murine squamous cell carcinoma PAM LY8. *Int. J. Oncol.* 16 (6), 1189–95.

Vermeulen, P.B., Gasparini, G., Fox, S.B., Toi, M., Martin, L., McCulloch, P., Pezzella, F., Viale, G., Weidner, N., Harris, A.L., and Dirix, L.Y. (1996). Quantification of angiogenesis in solid human tumours: an international consensus on the methodology and criteria of evaluation. *Eur. J. Cancer* 32A (14), 2474–84.

Vitaliti, A., Wittmer, M., Steiner, R., Wyder, L., Neri, D., and Klemenz, R. (2000). Inhibition of tumor angiogenesis by a single-chain antibody directed against vascular endothelial growth factor. *Cancer Res.* 60 (16), 4311–14.

Voest, E.E., Kenyon, B.M., O'Reilly, M.S., Truitt, G., D'Amato, R.J., and Folkman, J. (1995). Inhibition of angiogenesis *in vivo* by interleukin 12. *J. Natl Cancer Inst.* 87 (8), 581–6.

Vugrin, D., Hood, L., and Laszlo, J. (1986). A phase II trial of high-dose human lymphoblastoid alpha interferon in patients with advanced renal carcinoma. *J. Biol. Response Mod.* 5 (4), 309–12.

Walther, M.M., Kleiner, D.E., Lubensky, I.A., Pozzatti, R., Nyguen, T., Gnarra, J.R., Hurley, K., Venzon, D., Linehan, W.M., and Stetler-Stevenson, W.G. (1997). Progelatinase A mRNA expression in cell lines derived from tumors in patients with metastatic renal cell carcinoma correlates inversely with survival. *Urology* 50 (2), 295–301.

Wechsel, H.W., Bichler, K.H., Feil, G., Loeser, W., Lahme, S., and Petri, E. (1999). Renal cell carcinoma: relevance of angiogenetic factors. *Anticancer Res.* 19 (2C), 1537–40.

Wu, Y., Palad, A.J., Wasilenko, W.J., Blackmore, P.F., Pincus, W.A., Schechter, G.L., Spoonster, J.R., Kohn, E.C., and Somers, K.D. (1997). Inhibition of head and neck squamous cell carcinoma growth and invasion by the calcium influx inhibitor carboxyamido-triazole. *Clin. Cancer Res.*. 3 (11), 1915–21.

Yao, L., Sgadari, C., Furuke, K., Bloom, E.T., Teruya-Feldstein, J., and Tosato, G. (1999). Contribution of natural killer cells to inhibition of angiogenesis by interleukin-12. *Blood* 93 (5), 1612–21.

Yoshida, A., Anand-Apte, B., and Zetter, B.R. (1996). Differential endothelial migration and proliferation to basic fibroblast growth factor and vascular endothelial growth factor. *Growth Factors* 13 (1–2), 57–64.

Yoshino, S., Kato, M., and Okada, K. (1998). Evaluation of the prognostic significance of microvessel count and tumor size in renal cell carcinoma. *Int. J. Urol.* 5 (2), 119–23.

Ziche, M., Sorriso, C., Parenti, A., Brogelli, L., Tricarico, C., Villari, D., and Pazzagli, M. (1999). Biological parameters for the choice of antiangiogenic therapy and efficacy monitoring. *Int. J. Biol. Markers* 14 (4), 214–17.

18. Spontaneous regression and the natural history of renal cell cancer

R.T.D. Oliver

It is now more than 30 years since Everson and Cole (1966) reviewed the occurrence of spontaneous regression of cancer in the world literature. They were the first to draw attention to the fact that renal cell cancer had nearly the highest frequency among such events. It is now 22 years since I first became interested in this phenomenon. This interest developed because of the untoward experience I had with the first renal cancer patient I treated using chemotherapy. He had had a single lung metastasis for nearly 10 years, which had been slowly growing and was beginning to become symptomatic. Three weeks after a single dose of cyclophosphamide he had widespread multiple lung metastases and was dead within 6 weeks.

At that time there was considerable controversy regarding the frequency with which spontaneous regression occurred. Bloom (1973) estimated that it was 0.3 per cent from a literature review, while Werf-Messing (1971) from a personal series of 35 metastatic renal cancer patients observed without treatment reported that 30 per cent showed nonprogression at 6 months. This polarity of view and the increasing recognition of the impact of patient selection on outcome of treatment (deKernion *et al.* 1978) prompted me to set out to investigate prospectively the frequency of spontaneous regression in the setting of the good performance status patients referred to tertiary centers who undertake clinical trials. An increasingly recognized characteristic of trials in renal cell cancer was that initial reports were often double that achieved when the treatment became generally available. Because of this I felt it vital to exclude the possibility that the responses reported for biological treatment simply reflected episodes of spontaneous regression in the highly selected subgroup referred to these specialist centers.

In order to investigate this further, patients with early but asymptomatic metastases underwent a period of surveillance to investigate the frequency of spontaneous regression and whether there was any relation between spontaneous regression and response to cytokine therapy.

An initial report of the first 72 patients observed a 7 per cent spontaneous regression and an additional 7 per cent non-progression at 12 months (Oliver 1989; Oliver *et al.* 1988, 1989). It is the aim of this chapter to give a preliminary overview of an ongoing update of patients entered into this study and to review possible factors involved in the effect of this study on response in subsequent cytokine studies. The chapter will end by focusing on how these new observations may be relevant to increasing interest in the use of cytokines as a preoperative treatment for renal cell cancer patients and how they might have a more generalized application in the therapy of all primary cancers.

Spontaneous tumor regression in renal cancer and possible mechanisms to explain it

In the 30 years since Everson and Cole (1966) first published that spontaneous regression of cancer was a real entity, there have been more than 70 cases reported (Fairlamb 1981) and four major attempts (Bloom 1973; Oliver *et al.* 1988; Possinger *et al.* 1988; Gleave *et al.* 1998) to estimate the frequency (Table 18.1). Bloom's (1973) attempt, though only detecting a frequency of 0.3 per cent in the retrospective literature review, did report 2 of 172 (1.2 per cent) in his own personal series. An update of this retrospective overview was reported by Possinger *et al.* (1988). In that report of 1247 patients, only 0.24 per cent showed spontaneous regression. It was 2.5 × higher in the 50 per cent of patients with sufficiently good performance status to enable nephrectomy to be performed. Both prospective studies (Oliver *et al.* 1988; Gleave *et al.* 1998) report a much higher incidence of spontaneous regression (7.1 and 6.1 per cent, respectively). The latter study (Gleave *et al.* 1998) was the most interesting as these cases were the control arm of a randomized double-blind trial with placebo injections given to the controls who all had a reasonable performance status. Today our own prospective phase II surveillance study has recruited 292 patients with 13 unexplained regressions and an

Table 18.1 'Unexplained' regression in renal cell cancer

Study	No. of cases	'Unexplained' regression (%)
Possinger *et al.* 1988 (all metastases)	1247	0.24
Possinger *et al.* 1988 (postnephrectomy)	663	0.6
Bloom 1973 (personal series)	172	1.0
Oliver *et al.* 1988 (personal series)	72	7.1
Gleave *et al.* 1998 (placebo injections; randomized trial)	99	6.1

Table 18.2 'Spontaneous' regressions and prolonged stable disease in St Bartholomew's and Royal London's renal cell cancer surveillance studies

| | | No. of cases | Response (%) | | Stable disease (%) |
			Complete	Partial	
Retrospective	<1978	55	0	2	NA*
Prospective	1978–85	73	4	3	6
Prospective	1986–93	91	0	4	3
Prospective	1994–98	73	0	4	3
Total		292	1	3	3

* NA, information not available.

Table 18.3 'Spontaneous' regression with response to subsequent therapy in patients with metastatic renal cancer

| | No. of cases | Response (%) | | |
		Complete	Partial	Overall
Total surveillance series	292	1	3	3
Lung metastases only	71	8	5	13
Others	221	0	2	2
Entered into cytokine studies after progression on surveillance	132	3	8	16
Lung metastases only	23	14	30	50
Others	109	0	2	2

additional 9 patients with prolonged stable disease. Although the regression rate in the initial personally treated series was 7 per cent, with increased numbers and a wider range of doctors seeing the patients, the response rate has declined to 4.5 per cent in the more recently treated series (Table 18.2). These latter series also coincided with the advent of interleukin-2 (IL-2) and a trend to delay treatment for less time if there was any suspicion of progression.

Currently the data are being computerized in order to do a formal prognostic factor analysis and are not at present available for review. The limited analysis performed seems to confirm the previously reported association with performance status, site of metastasis (that is, lung versus other) (Table 18.3), and the presence or absence of hypercalcemia (Oliver *et al.* 1988).

As far as mechanisms are concerned, spontaneous regression has been assumed to have some sort of immunological basis, though non-immunological anti-angiogenic effects have by no means been excluded. Two of the eight patients in this department's studies have features that would fit with an immunological mechanism. The first was a patient who had a regression that lasted nearly 4 years. It began after her husband, who was a violent alcoholic, dried out and stopped beating her. Her metastases regrew when his alcoholism returned and then regressed again when she left him but then recurred after 3 years and she ultimately died at 4 years. The concept of chronic stress-related immunosuppression accelerating tumor growth has been well documented in experimental animal models (Temoshok *et al.* 1985) and supported by observations from breast cancer (Spiegel

et al. 1989). The second case was an example of the rarely reported (Ritchie *et al.* 1988) spontaneous regression of liver metastases. The history given by the patient suggested that it may have been caused by *in vivo* viral oncolysis. Eight years prior to presentation the patient had had a nephrectomy and been well until about 4 weeks before he was first seen. He had just returned from Indonesia where he had developed an acute episode of swinging fever, nausea, and vomiting that had continued when he returned home. Because he got so progressively ill, he was investigated and found to have an enlarged liver with elevated enzymes. A computerized tomography (CT) scan showed that nearly one-third of the liver was replaced by metastases and biopsy confirmed clear cell carcinoma. Within 1 week of biopsy he began to feel better, paralleled by a reduction in hepatomegaly and an improvement in liver enzymes, which slowly returned to normal after about 8 weeks. By 3 months his CT scan was nearly normal and remained so for 10 months when he relapsed and died within 12 weeks with an enlarging liver and no other metastases; at this point he was totally unresponsive to cytokines or chemotherapy. Although viral antibody titers to known hepatitis-causing viruses were negative, it was concluded that he had probably been infected with an obscure South East Asian hepatitis virus that had induced viral oncolysis as has been demonstrated using the Newcastle disease virus (Lindenmann and Klein 1967; Schirrmacher *et al.* 1989).

Although these studies of surveillance have proved to be safe, the frequency of response in this highly selected group of tertiary referrals was less than that seen from cytokine treatment. Although the response rate to cytokines after progression on surveillance was little different to that reported by other authors who did not have strict criteria for progression, as it is the same group of good risk patients with small-volume lung metastases developing late or being present at the time of nephrectomy who respond to cytokines and show spontaneous regression (Table 18.3), there remains some degree of anxiety that surveillance could prejudice response. Currently, our policy is to use a brief period of surveillance before entry into cytokine trials to get an assessment of the patient's disease progression rate and assess for psychological factors contributing to tumor progression. Surveillance is only continued in patients obviously improving.

Response to therapy after exclusion of spontaneous regression compared with literature reports

The overall results from our sequential phase II studies undertaken with patients progressing after surveillance (Table 18.4) were somewhat less than reported in the major overviews of published series (Table 18.5). All of our studies have been with subcutaneous IL-2 and some authors have suggested that results have been better after high-dose intravenous (IV) schedules.

Table 18.4 Royal London Hospital phase II studies in metastatic renal cell cancer

Treatment	No. of cases	Response (%)		
		Complete	Partial	Stable disease
BCG	19	10	5	15
IFNα	21	0	13	13
IL-2	25	4	8	12
IL-2/IFNα	24	0	0	2
IL-2/IFNα/5-FU	43	2	12	21
Total	132	3	8	16

Table 18.5 Overview of cytokine phase II studies in metastatic renal cell cancer

Treatment	No. of cases	Response (%)		
		Complete	Partial	Overall
IFNα alone*	1100	2	14	16
IL-2 alone (IV)[†]	848	5	11	16
IL-2 alone (SC)[†]	146	3	21	24
IL-2/IFNα (IV)[†]	121	7	18	25
IL-2/IFNα (SC)[†]	513	6	15	21
IL-2/IFNα/5-FU[†]	313	7	26	33

* Source: Horoszewicz and Murphy (1989).
[†] Source: Jeal and Goa (1997).

Table 18.6 Schedule and response of metastatic renal cancer to IL-2

Schedule	Route	Total dose**	No. of cases	Response (%)	
				Complete	Partial
18/9 × 5/wk/4 wks*	SC	279	116	4	10
3 b.d. × 5/wk/6 wks[†]	SC	180	92	2	19
18/9 × 5/wk/6 wks[†]	SC	315	53	5.5	5.5
5 t.d.s. × 5/wk/1–2 wks[†]	IV	61	55	0	4
50 t.d.s. × 5/wk/1–2 wks[†]	IV	605	56	7	9
36 × 5/wk/2 wks[§]	CIV	342	225	3.5	8.5

* Source: Nieken et al. (1996); Tourani et al. 1997.
[†] Source: Bordin et al. (1999).
[‡] Source: Young and Rosenberg (1997).
[§] Source: Jeal and Goa (1997).
** CIV: continuous intravenous.

Table 18.6 summarizes recent large phase II series and demonstrates that there is no obvious benefit from high-dose IV IL-2 and that more is not necessarily better in terms of total dose. The published response rate of renal cell cancer metastases to alpha interferon (IFNα) is somewhat less than that to IL-2. However, given the degree of selection for good-risk patients in the IL-2 studies because of worry about cardiac risks, it is unlikely that the difference is of any significance as the survival and incidence of long-term disease-free survivors is the same. The lack of any advantage for the higher-dose continuous IV infusion route of administration over the lower-dose subcutaneous regimen has obvious economic benefits, though it will be important to wait for the report on the long-term follow-up of the randomized low-dose versus high-dose IV versus subcutaneous IL-2 study currently being run by the US National Cancer Institute (Table 18.5) before the issue is closed.

The lack of more than an extremely marginal difference between IL-2 and IL-2 plus IFNα (Table 18.5) could be more significant than the lack of difference between IL-2 and IFNα as the selection criteria for the former studies were similar. This issue is of some importance given what appears, at first glance, to be a substantial advantage for the latest combination to be reported, namely, 5-fluorouracil (5-FU) combined with IL-2 and IFNα. However, not all of the centers who have so far reported on this regimen have had such a high response to the three-drug IFNα/IL-2/5-FU regimen (Table 18.7). In the study of Joffe *et al.* (1996), if patients who had not been nephrectomized were excluded, the response rate was similar to that of Atzpodien and colleagues who originated the somewhat complicated regimen (Lopez Hanninen *et al.* 1996). This was not true in our series (Table 18.7) as one of the best responses was in a patient with extensive bone metastases. However, from a clinical point of view there was little doubt that there was more substantial clinical benefit seen in poor-risk patients than in previous series using monotherapy. This translated into the fact that 21 per cent of patients demonstrated major durable (greater than 6 months) clinical benefit with improved performance status off treatment even though they did not achieve adequate shrinkage for this disease to be considered a definite measurable response. Furthermore, there was one other new dimension that emerged from this study that could help in understanding why some centers report a better response than others. There was a higher response rate the farther the patient had to travel and the lowest response rate was observed in our local patients (Table 18.8). There is increasing recognition of the role of poverty in a poor outcome from cancer treatment, most notably in the outcome of breast cancer. In our own center (Oliver 2000) where the same degree of difference in survival is demonstrated if our surgeons operate on people referred in from high cure rate regions as are visible in the cancer registry figures (Table 18.9), it is clear that this difference is not due to poorer provision of surgical care. There is increasing evidence from studies of the effect of poverty on resistance to infectious disease that vitamin A enhances CD4 T-cell immune responses (Semba *et al.* 1993), vitamin D enhances CD8 T-cell and macrophage function (Veldman *et al.* 2000; Koga *et al.* 1999), and zinc enhances general immune response (Umeta *et al.* 2000). There is evidence from several cancers for the importance of vitamin A deficiency in accelerating cancer deaths (though importantly, in respect of cancer prevention trials, no benefit from supplements in individuals with already adequate levels of dietary intake; Hunter *et al.* 1993). There is also evidence from studies of breast and prostate cancer for the importance of vitamin D (Hanchette and Schwartz 1992). In addition, there are data showing that vitamin D suppresses production of metalloproteinases that play major role in tumor invasion (Koli and Keski-Oja 2000). These observations suggest that more attention will need to be paid to the issue of poverty in assessing response to treatments in the future.

Table 18.7 IFNα/IL-2/5-FU in metastatic renal cell cancer

| | | Response (%) | | |
Reference	No. of cases	Complete	Partial	Overall
Lopez Hanninen *et al.* 1996	120	11	28	39
Ellenhorst *et al.* 1997	46	8	35	43
Hofmockel *et al.* 1996	34	9	29	38
Allen *et al.* 2000	55	6	25	31
Joffe *et al.* 1996	55	—	16	16
Oliver *et al.* 1999	43	2	12	14
van Hespen *et al.* 2000	51	0	12	12

Table 18.8 Clinical benefit with IL-2/IFNα/5-FU biotherapy according to source of referral (Oliver, unpublished)

| | | Response (%) | | Major clinical | Disease status (%) | |
	N	Complete	Partial	benefit (%)	Stable	Progressive
All cases	43	2	14	23	14	49
Local district	5	—	—	20	20	60
East London and Essex	12	—	16	8	16	58
Remote referrals	26	4	15	27	12	42

Table 18.9 Impact of district of origin on breast and prostate cancer treatment outcomes at Royal Hospitals Trust (RHT) 1991*

	Breast cancer		Prostate cancer
	RHT 2-year survival (%; N = 384)	Cancer registry 5-year survival (%; N = 2560)	RHT 2-year survival (%; N = 69)
Inner East London	77	62	47
Outer East London	82	69	58
West London	87	72	25
Outside M25	90	83	75

* Source: Oliver (2000).

Survival and randomized cytokine trials

As yet there is less evidence from study of survival than from study of response to suggest a higher survival rate after combination therapy rather than monotherapy. In our own studies, though there is a difference in survival at 12 months between the 46; most recently treated patients receiving IFNα/IL-2/5-FU and the historic series of 58 receiving monotherapy before 1995 (28 versus 16 per cent), the difference narrowed when the survival at 12 months of 22 concurrent patients unfit for the three-drug regimen and treated with IFNα alone was examined (20 per cent). Clearly, only a randomized trial comparing monotherapy to the three-drug regimen will determine whether there is a survival advantage. There are two randomized trials, one of which compared non-cytokine therapy with monotherapy and the other of which compared non-cytokine therapy with the three-drug combination which provide some evidence for a survival advantage from cytokine therapy. Both showed significant relapse-free and overall survival advantage for cytokine therapy (Table 18.10). In addition, the only trial of monotherapy versus dual agent therapy interferon plus IL-2 showed progression-free but no overall survival advantage. In view of these three trials, the proposed UK Medical Research Council's (MRC) trial comparing monotherapy to triple therapy is extremely timely.

Influence of spontaneous regression and lead-time bias on prognostic factor analyses

Since the landmark study (Table 18.11) of de Kernion *et al.* (1978) it is well established that selection can have a powerful effect on outcome . This is equally true of the incidence of spontaneous

Table 18.10 Randomized cytokine trials in renal cancer cells

Trial	Reference	Control (N)	Experimental (N)
MPA* vs. IFNα	Steinbeck *et al.* 1990	28% (30)[†]	28% (30)[†]
MPA* vs. IFNα	Ritchie *et al.* 1999 (MRC study)	31% (168)[†]	43 % (167)[†]
Placebo vs. IFNγ	Gleave *et al.* 1998	7% (90)[‡]	4% (91)[§]
Tamoxifen vs. IFNα/IL-2	Henriksson *et al.* 1997	3% (63)[§]	8% (68)[§]
IFNα vs. IFNα/IL-2	Negrier *et al.* 1998	7% (138)[‡]	19% (140)[‡]
Tamoxifen vs. IFNα/IL-2/5-FU	Atzpodien *et al.* 1997	0% (38)[‡¶]	33% (41)[‡‖]

* MPA, medroxyprogesterone.
[†] 1-year survival.
[‡] Overall response.
[§] Complete response.
[¶] Median survival, 14 months.
[‖] Median survival, > 42 months.

Table 18.11 Prognostic factors and renal cell cancer survival*

	No. of cases	Median survival (months)	Alive at 1 year (%)
Lung only	52	22	81
Other patients	129	9	35
Free of disease > 24 months	22	24	68
Free of disease < 24 months	159	10	44
Karnofski > 80	48	35	79
Karnofski < 80	24	7	37
All cases	181	11	47

* Source: deKernion *et al.* (1978).

Table 18.12 Autopsy as a detector of 'occult' renal cell cancer*

Number of autopsies	16 294
Total renal cell cancers	350 (2%)
Unrecognized renal cell cancers *pre mortem*	235 (67%)
Unrecognized metastatic renal cell cancers	56 (23%)

* Source: Johnsen and Hellsten (1987).

regression (Oliver *et al.* 1988). It is these observations that led me to question the extent to which selection and lead-time bias play a part in the apparent benefit of cytokine therapy.

While it is well recognized that lead-time bias from early diagnosis is a major problem in interpreting the results of radical prostatectomy (Dennis and Resnick 2000), the few people who have considered the impact of early diagnosis (arising from the increased availability of ultrasound, intravenous urograms (IVU), and CT scans) on the prognosis of renal cancer have not as yet demonstrated any evidence for change in survival. There are several anecdotal reports demonstrating that, if renal tumors are diagnosed incidentally at the time of angiography or ultrasound in a non-malignant disease investigation, the prognosis is apparently better in terms of a lower frequency of metastases (Thompson and Peek 1988; Mevorach *et al.* 1992). However, this does not make allowance for two factors. First, such cases are obviously diagnosed long before they would present clinically, that is, there is a lead-time bias. Second, if autopsies are done on people dying of other causes, many more renal cancers are found than are actually detected clinically and a proportion of these even have metastases (Table 18.12).

Access to ultrasound for diagnosis of renal cell cancer is substantially less available in the UK than in Germany where it is available in general practitioner's surgeries. As a result a higher proportion of UK patients have unresectable primary tumors. Given these observations it is easy to understand why the two UK unselected series of cases treated with the IFNα/IL-2/5-FU regimen

(Joffe *et al.* 1996, Oliver *et al.* 1999) and a recently published Dutch study (Herpen *et al.* 2000) demonstrated substantially less obvious advantage for the three-drug regimen (Table 18.7).

It may be concluded that, at present, evidence that treatment actually reduces population-based mortality is still in doubt. It could be clouded by lead-time bias and overdiagnosis of small tumors with small amounts of metastases that could be accelerated by surgery and then be more susceptible to response to treatment thus ending up with a survival neutral effect.

New approaches to prognostic factor analysis using simple peripheral blood parameters

There is increasing evidence that several peripheral blood parameters, such as erythrocyte sedimentation rate (ESR), pretreatment platelet count and granulocyte count, posttreatment lymphocytosis (Table 18.13), and pretreatment hemoglobin (Table 18.14), may predict for overall patient response and survival, though to date no single series has been large enough to do a multivariate analysis to separate these factors out. Nevertheless, clinically these parameters are extremely interesting because they provide an insight into the biology of renal cancer.

For many years ESR was the only way to monitor disease activity in patients with tuberculosis and, as such, probably gave a good indication of the degree of disarray of immune response to the bacterium. Little work has been done on this parameter in recent years and it is certainly worth re-examining in the face of the new data but also because of the observation that the acute phase reactant, c-reactive protein response after treatment can serve as a prognosticator for response (Deehan *et al.* 1994).

Both IL-6 and vascular endothelial growth factor (VEGF)have been identified as tumor products that could be involved in causing increased levels of platelets. With increasing interest and

Table 18.13 Hematological indices and response to low-dose subcutaneous IL-2

ESR*	No. of cases	Response (%)
< 20	11	55
20–50	39	28
> 50	42	10
Response to IL-2*	**No. of cases**	**Degree of lymphocytosis (%)**
Complete + partial response	21	163
Stable disease	37	67
Progressive disease	34	28
Platelets†	**No. of cases**	**1-year survival (%)**
< 338 × 10⁹/l	16	48
> 338 × 10⁹/l	17	11
Platelets‡	**No. of cases**	**Median survival (months)**
< 4 × 10⁵/ml	112	34
> 4 × 10⁵/ml	147	18

* Source: Bordin *et al.* (1999).
† Source: Unfound 82.
‡ Source: Unfound 83.

Table 18.14 RE01 MRC Renal Cancer study: impact of pretreatment hemoglobin on outcome[*]

	Dose (G)		
	< 11 (*N* = 76)	11–13.2[†]; 11–12.7[‡] (*N* = 82)	> 13.2[†]; > 12.7[‡] (*N* =85)
Measurable response (%)	Nil	5	9
Stable disease (%)	8	12	24

[*] Source: Oliver *et al.* (2000).
[†] Male dosage.
[‡] Female dosage.

new clinical trials on compounds that block tumor angiogenesis (Cao *et al.* 1998; Browder *et al.* 2000), the study of the molecular basis of the platelet overproduction could provide important information in the near future.

There is increasing recognition that overproduction of granulocytes and granulocyte–macrophage colony stimulating factor (GM-CSF) is a common oncofetal change detected in tumor cell lines *in vitro* (particularly bladder) and is associated with a poor outcome (Ito *et al.* 1990; Ohigashi *et al.* 1992). A similar effect may explain why a high neutrophil count is a poor prognostic feature in renal cancer patients. Both G-CSF and GM-CSF are the product of mesenchymal cells. In renal cell cancer mesenchymal elements, that is, sarcomatoid change, is associated with a poor prognosis. It will be important to investigate this correlation further as its simplicity makes it easier to measure than serum levels of G-CSF and/or GM-CSF.

In contrast to the association of poor prognosis with a raised neutrophil count is the good prognostic effect of an elevated lymphocytosis induced by IL-2 (Table 18.13). It is surprising that, despite the large number of studies of IL-2, few have commented on this parameter. In the one study that has systematically examined it, this seems to be a powerful predictor that needs to be assessed prospectively in association with induction of autoimmune thyroiditis, another immunological parameter predicting for a good outcome (Franzke *et al.* 1999). It could be worth collecting cases of spontaneous regression worldwide to see how many of them also manifest any of these immune characteristics after rejection of their metastases.

That low hemoglobin was associated with a poorer outcome has been well established for several cancers and in cervical cancer transfusing up to a normal level has been shown to improve survival in one study (Harper *et al.* 1996). In general, it is not thought to add much to the general effect of poor performance status from widespread poorly differentiated malignant tumor. However, in renal cancer, admittedly so far only from one study involving 370 patients, there has emerged an even more interesting observation in relation to elevated hemoglobin level. This study (Table 18.14; Oliver *et al.* 2000) was a randomized trial comparing medroxyprogesterone acetate and IFNα. There was a higher response rate and survival overall for those with hemoglobin in the upper third. In detection only those with hemoglobin levels in the upper third showed significant response and survival benefit from treatment with IFNα. Erythropoietin is a normal differentiation product of renal cells and its production by a proportion of renal cancers is well established. This observation could indicate that more differentiated, less clonally evolved tumors are the ones that respond to immunotherapy, as has been demonstrated by the high response of early bladder cancer to bacille Calmette–Guérin (BCG). A suggestion that the effect may be due to more than differentiation alone comes from an *in vitro* study that demonstrated that transfection of an erythropoietin gene into a non-secreting tumor enhanced susceptibility to immune T lymphocytes (Miyajima *et al.* 1996). The observed association of the clear cell phenotype with erythropoietin production is therefore very interesting as the small pilot study of allo peripheral bloodstem cell grafts (Childs *et al.* 2000) suggested that most of the responding patients had clear cell phenotype (9 of 12 clear cell versus 1 of 7 mixed tumors responded). The final possible factor that might be involved is anoxia as erythropoietin is produced in response to anoxia (Gleadle and Ratcliffe 1997) and such tumors could then be considered to lack adequate vascularization and therefore to be very susceptible to anti-angiogenic drugs.

As all of these parameters can be assessed on a single blood sample, they offer a very simple approach to prognosis. Their mechanisms of action represent a wide perspective of cell biology. However, they fall into two groups: (1) those that increase the chance of response to immune therapy, namely, lymphocytosis, induction of autoimmune response on therapy, or high hemoglobin pretreatment; (2) mainly paraneoplastic inappropriate switches, such as G-CSF, IL-6, VEGF anemia induction, which presumably indicate poorly differentiated cancer. These observations need to be investigated in large databases with multivariate analysis to establish whether they are independently significant or linked prognostic factors. They also need to be compared retrospectively in series of patients who have undergone spontaneous regression.

Prognostic factor analysis and the need for adjuvant and neoadjuvant trials

There is a small amount of data (Tables 18.15 and 18.16), admittedly from serial phase II studies, suggesting that good-prognosis patients have a greater gain from three-drugs therapy (IFNα/IL-2/5-FU) than from the two-drug combination (IFNα/IL-2). If this is real, it could well be that there is even more benefit from use of these drugs in early stages of disease. This is one of the observations justifying the current European Organization for

Table 18.15 Atzpodien prognostic factor analysis*

Variable	χ^2 **Log rank**	p	**Risk score**
ESR > 70	17	0.0001	2
LDH[†] > 280	21	0.0001	2
Neutrophils > 6 × 10⁹	7.6	0.005	1
Metastases			
Extrapulmonary	7.8	0.005	1
Bone	8.2	0.004	1

* Source: Lopez Hanninen et al. (1996).
[†] LDH, lactate dehydrogenase.

Table 18.17 Nephrectomy prior to IFNα for metastatic renal cancer*

	No. of cases	**Median survival (months)**
IFNα alone	123[a]/41[b]	8.2[a]/7[b]
IFNα after nephrectomy	123[a]/41[b]	12.5[a]/17[b]

* Sources: [a] Flanigan et al. 2000; [b] Mickisch et al. 2000. A single-center study (Bennet et al. 1995) found that seven of 30 (23 per cent) nephrectomized patients with metastases proceeded to cytokine therapy.

Table 18.18 Impact of post-IL-2 surgical resection on metastatic renal cell cancer relapse-free survival*

Objective response/ total no. of cases	62/399 (16%)
Relapse-free/complete response	14/18 (76%)
Relapse-free/ partial response: post-surgical resection	11/11 (100%)
Relapse-free/ partial response: no surgery	15/33 (46%)

* Source: Kim and Louie (1992).

Research and Treatment of Cancer (EORTC) adjuvant study in patients with poor risk defined on the basis of the pathological criteria of vascular invasion and tumor size (Ravi and Oliver 1999). This is at present recruiting rather slowly but, given the increasing importance of the question it is asking, there is a clear need to increase focus on this issue as a priority.

The reporting of two studies with a benefit from nephrectomy in the face of metastases prior to starting interferon (Table 18.17) is encouraging (Flanigan et al. 2000; Mickisch et al. 2000). However there have been several reports demonstrating that a sizeable minority varying from 9 to 40 per cent of metastatic disease patients are not suitable for such studies as they are either inoperable or, after undergoing nephrectomy, progress so rapidly after surgery that they receive no treatment (Robertson et al. 1990; Bennett et al. 1995; Fleischmann and Kim 1991; Rackley et al. 1994; Walther et al. 1997; Franklin et al. 1996). This observation raises the question as to whether it might be better to give cytokines as a preoperative neoadjuvant treatment. One phase II study has reported encouraging results from this approach in terms of tumor downstaging and overall survival from surgery (Table 18.18; Kim and Louie 1992). In a second study it was possible to generate tumor-infiltrating lymphocytes (TIL) for therapy (Figlin et al. 1997). A randomized trial comparing pre- versus postsurgery cytokines is needed to clarify the value of this approach. Given the longstanding debate about the value of radical versus limited surgery in cancer this will be an important trial. It has long been accepted that in breast cancer super radical mastectomy does not improve the results over mastectomy (Lacour et al. 1983). That the same may apply to radical prostatectomy remains *sub judice* despite the negative underpowered trial in the US Veterans

Administration hospitals (Iversen et al. 1995). This is because a trial in a Scandinavian hospital has been recruited with an adequate number to answer the question about the impact of radical prostatectomy or survival in men with prostate cancer. However, there are several observations that help explain why radical surgery may accelerate metastatic growth so that the gain from extended surgery is undermined by its acceleration of metastases and local recurrence. Minimizing these factors by tumor downstaging could be the potential gain from the experimental arm of the proposed trial of pre- versus postsurgery cytokines.

The first potentially reversible effect of surgery is the immunosuppressive effect of anesthesia, which has been well established from studies of phytohemagglutinin (PHA)-induced lymphocytes before and after surgery. This effect is at least as immunosuppressive as that of azothiaprine, the principal drug used to immunosuppress transplant recipients; the degree of immunosuppression is proportional to the duration of anesthesia (Riddle and Berenbaum 1967).

The second factor is the effect of handling the tumor at the time of surgery. Studies in patients undergoing radical prostatectomy using reverse transcriptase polymerase chain reaction (RT-PCR) have demonstrated showers of tumor cell activity in the blood

Table 18.16 Risk factors and response in Atzpodien IL-2 studies*

	No. of cases	**Response (%)**		
		Complete	**Partial**	**Total**
Good risk (score 0)				
Three drugs	51	14	45	59
Two drugs	31	19	19	38
Intermediate risk (score 1–3)				
Three drugs	62	8	18	26
Two drugs	44	–	23	23
Poor risk (score 4)				
Three drugs	7	14	0	14
Two drugs	4	0	0	0

* Source: Lopez Hanninen et al. (1996). Three drugs: IFNα + IL-2 + 5-FU; two drugs: IFNα + IL-2.

after surgery (Eschwege *et al.* 1995). Given that renal call cancer is one of the most vascular of all tumors and that there are now markers to detect renal cancer cells in the circulation (Taille *et al.* 2000), the same sort of data could be produced by renal vein sampling at time of nephrectomy. A comparison of results in patients in the proposed pre- versus postsurgery cytokine study could be an interesting surrogate endpoint to justify the study.

The third factor undermining the effect of radical surgery is tissue repair cytokine-induced tumor acceleration. This has been known about since the time of Peyton Rous (Rous and Beard 1935) but there was relatively little attention paid to this issue. This is despite confirmatory data published by Alexander *et al.* (1988) who demonstrated a potential way of preventing its deleterious effects by using anti-EGF (epidermal growth factor) antibody.

The fourth factor is renal-specific growth factors whose existence is demonstrated by the occurrence of compensatory hypertrophy of the contralateral kidney after unilateral nephrectomy.

Despite this myriad of potentially confounding tumor accelerating effects of surgery, there is still uncertainty as to whether they play a sufficiently important role in the actual clinical situation in the cancer patient to justify attention. However, the increasing evidence that immune-related treatments work better on the early stages of clonal evolution is providing a justification for a pre- versus postsurgery cytokine trial; such a trial could enable a prospective investigation of these peri-operative issues.

It may be concluded that, at present, evidence that early treatment of renal cell cancer actually reduces population-based mortality survival is still in doubt. It could be clouded by lead-time bias and overdiagnosis of small tumors with small amounts of metastases that could be accelerated by surgery and then be more susceptible to response to treatment thus ending up with a survival neutral effect. To resolve this there is a need to investigate whether animal data demonstrating that the use of an antibody to block epithelial growth factor receptor prevents tumor implantation at sites of tissue repair apply clinically. If the proposed pre- versus postsurgery cytokine trial is successful, it could be followed by a randomized trial to investigate the use of the anti-EGF approach. Resolving this longstanding issue could be of relevance to the use of surgery at several tumor sites. Another issue that might be of relevance to examine in such trials is the role of laparoscopic surgery (Walther *et al.* 1999) as potentially such surgery might reduce some of the tumor-accelerating factors discussed above.

Mechanism of spontaneous regression and its relative response in cytokine trials

Because most of the early IL-2 trials included lymphokine-activated killer cells (LAK) and most of the studies on TIL in all tumor types except melanoma (Itoh *et al.* 1988) failed to demonstrate a high frequency of specific cytolytic T lymphocytes, it has been assumed that LAK/natural killer (NK) cells rather than specific human leukocyte antigen (HLA)-restricted T-cell-mediated mechanisms are involved. However Uchida's (1993) observation that those patients who presurgery or postimmunotherapy had autologous tumor-specific cytolytic cells (either alone or with NK cells) had a better prognosis than those with only NK-type killer cells suggests that immunologically specific T-lymphocyte-mediated response may be of primary importance. One possible explanation of this association is that these assays are defining individuals with a high immune responder genetic predisposition that easily develop some form of autoimmune response. The multiple reports demonstrating a correlation between induction of autoimmune thyroid response and occurrence of tumor regression would support this view (Franzke *et al.* 1999). Future studies should attempt to resolve this issue, as it is possible that the autoimmune antitumor immune process could produce new insights into the pathogenesis of autoimmune disease. There has been a longstanding contention, originally raised by MacFarlain Burnett, that autoimmune disease was a necessary by-product of genetic selection for effective antitumor immunity. It would be equally interesting to know if any of the targets of anticancer bystander immunity are previously non-immunogenic antigens that are being recognized by autoreactive T-cell clones in patients with autoimmune disease (Zhang and DeGroot 2000; Noort *et al.* 2000).

Over the last decade several experimental studies in animal models have demonstrated that correction of class I defects on tumors produces a vaccine that is capable of inducing bystander immunity to reject uncorrected cells (Nouri *et al.* 1992). Although successful studies have been reported in melanoma (Hersh *et al.* 1994), the studies in renal cancer (Rini *et al.* 1999) were negative despite a higher degree of HLA class I loss in primary tumors (Ohnmacht and Marincola 2000; Brasanac *et al.* 1999). In melanoma the majority of the responders had clonally early disease, that is, in transit skin or nodal metastases rather than blood-borne M+ disease. Such cases were rare in the renal study. With increasing evidence for absent or nonfunctioning HLA class II and adhesion molecules being added to the loss of HLA class I as tumors progress (Oliver and Nouri 1992), it is perhaps not surprising that the renal cell cancer HLA-B7 gene therapy study was negative.

There is clearly a need for more studies on the cellular mechanism of cytokine-induced and spontaneous regressions. This could be helped by the development of experimental models to study the presurgery downstaging approach. The relative ease of access via the renal artery means that it would be possible to do presurgery gene therapy in patients with established metastases and examine bystander immunity. Reports that cultured renal cell cancers regain suppressed adhesion molecules (Jung *et al.* 1999) as has been seen in lymphoma (Pizzoferrato *et al.* 1997) suggest an additional possibility for the development of tumor vaccine.

The significance of tumors arising in immunosuppressed individuals to the natural history of renal cell cancer

Even today there are many who remain skeptical about the importance of immune surveillance in the common cancer. This is partly because the spectrum of tumors that occur after immunosuppression is different from that seen in spontaneous tumors

(Penn 1990). However, it must be remembered that immunosuppression *per se* does not produce mutations of DNA, which are, of course, necessary to determine which individuals and what organ develops malignancy. Equally, patients on immunosuppressive drugs are often under regular medical control and may well have reduced incidence of smoking, one of the major risk factors for cancer, and dialysis patients will often be under major protein restrictions limiting intake of red meat and other forms of burnt fat, which are major risk factors for colorectal and breast cancer. If these provisos are taken into consideration, it is clear that there is a massive increase in cancer on immunosuppression with 25 per cent of patients getting some malignancy by the age of 55 which is 10 years before most common cancers develop (Frezza *et al.* 1997). More critical is the demonstration that tumor development is faster the more successful the immunosuppression (Penn 1988).

A most dramatic demonstration of the critical role of immune surveillance in renal cancer is a recent case report of complete remission of lung metastases (5 cm × 4 cm and 1.2 × 1.2 lesions) and partial remission of liver metastases (10 cm reduced to 2 cm) after anti-HIV treatment without any cytokine therapy (Morris 2000). Were there to be any confirmation of this it might become necessary to investigate the HIV status of all patients with renal cancer.

While academically it is important to establish the effect of major immunosuppressive events, minor but continuous immunosuppression associated with routine treatment may be more critical to the success of everyday cancer treatment.

As discussed in an early section it has long been known that surgical anesthesia is associated with a degree of immunosuppression (Riddle and Berenbaum 1967). This is proportional to duration of anesthesia, which suggests that there may be some increased risk from primary major reconstructive surgery such as breast or bladder reconstructions or complicated cardiothoracic operations to remove vena cava exterior from renal cancer in patients who have not had curative medical treatment before surgery. The second immunosuppressive factor relating to surgery is blood transfusion. It has been clearly established that preoperative blood transfusion can induce prolongation of renal transplants (Glass *et al.* 1985) and there is a considerable body of data suggesting that preoperative transfusion may accelerate tumor recurrence (Amato and Pescatori 1998), although, as clear-cut negative studies do exist, there remains dispute about its relevance. The demonstration that the effect is less marked in patients receiving packed cells as compared to whole blood (Heiss *et al.* 1994) is perhaps the most convincing evidence, though the critical and as yet unresolved issue is whether the data are strong enough to recommend packed cells for all cancer surgery.

There has been much less research undertaken on the effect of the immunosuppression induced by radiotherapy on post-treatment survival. Today radiotherapy is rarely used in renal cancer patients. Multiple trials in the 1960s and 1970s showed no benefit and some actually had worse survival (Bloom and Oliver 1991); it has been well documented since 1972 that there is a 50 per cent reduction in circulating T cells acutely after radiation (Sternswald *et al.* 1978) and more recent reports have demonstrated that this persists for at least 6 years after treatment (Fossa *et al.* 1989). Recent reports of second cancers arising with increased frequency outside the radiation field in patients with

testis germ cell cancer (Travis *et al.* 1997) and breast cancer (Neugut *et al.* 1999) may be a delayed manifestation of this prolonged immunosuppression. Despite this there have been few studies attempting to correct the defect, though there are small studies reporting a positive benefit (Pines 1976). Further research in this area may be beneficial.

Two other more subtle forms of immunosuppression are smoking and ultraviolet radiation. There have been several reports from patients with melanoma, breast, bladder, testis, and head and neck cancer, though none as yet in renal cancer, demonstrating that smokers have a more accelerated progression of their disease though little evidence is given as to the mechanism involved. There is some evidence that an immunosuppressive effect of smoking may be one component of this mechanism (Kalra *et al.* 2000).

Ultraviolet light as well as being involved in causing mutations that lead to the development of skin cancers has been well documented in experimental animals as causing damage to tissue dendritic cells (Azizi *et al.* 1987) that are involved in the presentation of antigen to T lymphocytes.

The final form of immunosuppression, whose influence on tumor growth is much disputed is pregnancy. It has been most clearly documented in melanoma and breast cancer (Mackie *et al.* 1991; Gemignani *et al.* 1999). In both of these tumors there is no evidence for an increased incidence of tumors over that expected, but the disease presents at a more advanced stage, as measured in melanomas by depth of invasion and in breast cancer by frequency of node dissemination, if discovered during pregnancy. Because the impact of pregnancy on survival has not been shown to be independent of these other prognostic variables it has been ignored as being of any clinical significance. One reason for taking these observations seriously might be if tumors arising under situations of immunosuppression responded to different treatments. Although there is no evidence of this at yet, one small study has demonstrated substantially less loss of HLA antigens in a series of lymphomas arising in immunosuppressed individuals (List *et al.* 1993) suggesting that there is a need for more investigation of this issue as such cancers might be more responsive to cytokines or other methods of immune-reconstitution as loss of HLA antigens is clearly established as a factor in nonresponse to tumor vaccines (Ransom *et al.* 1992).

Conclusion

As an increasing number of studies confirm, it is now clear that spontaneous regression of metastatic renal cancer occurs in 4–6 per cent of patients eligible for cytokine trials in which response rates of 12–18 per cent are reported. Furthermore, as with cytokine-induced responses, spontaneous regression is more frequent in good risk patients with small volumes of metastatic disease. There is as yet little formal proof that the same immunological mechanisms are involved in both types of response. However the strongest anecdotal evidence for T cells being involved comes from a single case report of spontaneous regression of established metastases after reversion of immunosuppression following treatment of HIV disease with anti-HIV therapy and, less unequivocally, from reports of regressions occurring after relief of major psychological stress and after an episode of postulated acute nonspecific viral-hepatitis-induced viral oncolysis. With evidence from three sources (namely, a melanoma HLA-B7 gene therapy study, a study of hemoglobin production by renal cancer, and a study of the use of BCG and cytokines in bladder cancer) highlighting the view that immunosurveillance and immune-related therapies function most effectively in clonal early cancer, there is a clear need to develop research trials that examine the role of such treatments in the perioperative setting. A proposal for a pre- versus postnephrectomy cytokine study in patients presenting with already established metastases is one approach to investigate this issue. The evidence that the level of lymphocyte response to cytokines and the degree of autoimmunity induced by therapy are predictors of the likelihood of response to cytokines is increasingly firm. Furthermore, there is increasing recognition of the importance of normal expression of HLA class I antigen expression in tumors responding to immunological treatments. These observations suggest that the currently ongoing attempts to develop vaccines for renal cell cancer could benefit from a study of the immunological basis of autoimmunity and the antigenic determinants that are the targets for the response.

References

Alexander, P., Murphy, P., and Skipper, D. (1988). Preferential growth of blood borne cancer cells at site of trauma—a growth promoting role of macrophages. *Adv. Exp. Med. Biol.* **233**, 245–51.

Amato, A. and Pescatori, M. (1998). Effect of perioperative blood transfusions on recurrence of colorectal cancer: metaanalysis stratified on risk factors. *Dis. Colon Rectum* **41** (5), 570–85.

Atzpodien, J., Kirchner, H., Franzke, A., *et al.* (1997). Results of a randomised clinical trial comparing SC interleukin-2, SC alpha-2a-interferon and IV bolus 5-fluorouracil against oral tamoxifen in progressive metastatic renal cell carcinoma patients. *J. Clin. Oncol.* (supplement) *Proceedings of the American Society of Clinical Oncology*, Vol. 16, Abstr. 1164.

Azizi, E., Bucana, C., Goldberg, L., and Kripke, L. (1987). Perturbation of epidermal Langerhan cells in basal cell carcinomas. *Am. J. Dermatol.* **9**, 6465–73.

Bennett, R., Lerner, S., Taub, H., Dutcher, J., and Fleischmann, J. (1995). Cytoreductive surgery for stage IV renal cell carcinoma. *J. Urol.* **154** (1), 32–4.

Bloom, H.J. (1973). Hormone-induced and spontaneous regression of metastatic renal cancer. *Cancer* **32** (5), 1066–71.

Bloom, H.J.G. and Oliver, R.T.D. (1991). Renal adenocarcinoma: response and resistance to non-surgical treatment—a 30 year perspective. In *Urological oncology—dilemmas and developments*, pp. 49–69.

Bordin, V., Giani, L., Meregalli, S., *et al.* (1999). Five year survival resultsof subcutaneous low dose immunotherapy with interleukin-2 alone in metastatic renal cell cancer patients. *Urologia Internationalis* **64**, 3–8.

Brasanac, D., Muller, C., Muller, G., Hadzi-Dzokic, J., and Markovic-Lipkovski, J. (1999). HLA class I antigen expression in renal cell carcinoma: histopathological and clinical correlation. *J. Exp. Clin. Cancer Res.* **18** (4), 505–10.

Browder, T., Butterfield, C., Kraling, B., *et al.* (2000). Antiangiogenic scheduling of chemotherapy improves efficacy against experimental drug-resistant cancer. *Cancer Res.* **60** (7), 1878–86.

Cao, Y., O'Reilly, M., Marshall, B., Flynn, E., Ji, R., and Folkman, J. (1998). Expression of angiostatin cDNA in a murine fibrosarcoma suppresses primary tumour growth and produces long-term dormancy of metastases. *J. Clin. Invest.* **101** (5), 1055–63.

Childs, R., Chernoff, A., and Contentin, N. (2000). Regression of metastatic renal cell carcinoma after nonmyeloablative allogenic peripheral blood stem cell transplantation. *New Engl. J. Med.* **343**, 750–8.

Deehan, D., Heys, S., Simpson, W., Herriot, R., Broom, J., and Eremin, O. (1994). Correlation of serum cytokine and acute phase reactant levels with alterations in weight and serum albumin in patients receiving immunotherapy with recombinant IL-2. *Clin. Exp. Immunol.* **95** (3), 366–72.

deKernion, J.B., Ramming, K.P., and Smith, R.B. (1978). The natural history of metastatic renal cell carcinoma: a computer analysis. *J. Urol.* **120**, 148–52.

Dennis, L. and Resnick, M. (2000). Analysis of recent trends in prostate cancer incidence and mortality. *Prostate* **42** (4), 247–52.

Ellerhorst, J., Sella, A., Amato, R., *et al.* (1997). Phase II trial of 5-fluorouracil, interferon-alpha and continuous infusion interleukin-2 for patients with metastatic renal cell carcinoma. *Cancer* **80** (11), 2128–32.

Eschwege, P., Dumas, F., Blanchet, P., *et al.* (1995). Haematogenous dissemination of prostatic epithelial cells during radical prostatectomy. *Lancet* **346**, 1528–9.

Everson, T.C. and Cole, W.H. (1966). Spontaneous regression of cancer. 11–87.

Fairlamb, D. (1981). Spontaneous regression of metastases of renal cancer: a report of two cases including the first recorded regression following irradiation of a dominant metastasis and review of the world literature. *Cancer* **47** (8), 2102–6.

Figlin, R.A., Pierce, W.C., Kaboo, R., *et al.* (1997). Treatment of metastatic renal cell carcinoma with nephrectomy, interleukin-2 and cytokine-primed or CD8(+) selected tumor infiltrating lymphocytes from primary tumor. *J. Urol.* **158** (3 Pt 1), 740–5.

Flanigan, R., Blumenstein, B., Salmon, S., and Crawford, E. (2000). Cytoreduction nephrectomy in metastatic renal cancer: The results of Southwest Oncology Group trial 8949. *J. Clin. Oncol.* (supplement) *Proceedings of the American Society of Clinical Oncology*, Vol. 2a, Abstr. 3.

Fleischmann, J. and Kim, B. (1991). Interleukin-2 immunotherapy followed by resection of residual renal cell carcinoma. *J. Urol.* **145**, 938–41.

Fossa, S., Aass, N., and Kaalhus, O. (1989). Long term mobidity after infradiaphragmatic radiotherapy in young men with testicular cancer. *Cancer* **64** (2), 404–8.

Franklin, J., Figlin, R., Rauch, J., Gitlitz, B., and Belldegrun, A. (1996). Cytoreductive surgery in the management of metastatic renal cell carcinoma: the UCLA experience. *Sem. Urol. Oncol.* **14** (4), 230–6.

Franzke, A., Peest, D., Probst-Kepper, M., *et al.* (1999). Autoimmunity resulting from cytokine treatment predicts long-term survival in patients with metastatic renal cell cancer. *J. Clin. Oncol.* **17** (2), 529–33.

Frezza, E., Fung, J., and vanThiel, D. (1997). Non-lymphoid cancer after liver transplantation. *Hepatogastroenterology* **44** (16), 1172–81.

Gemignani, M., Petrek, J., and Borgen, P. (1999). Breast cancer and pregnancy. *Surg. Clin. North Am.* **79** (5), 1157–69.

Glass, N., Miller, D., Sollinger, H., and Belzer, F. (1985). A four year experience with donor blood transfusion protocols for living donor renal transplantation. *Transplantation* **39** (6), 615–19.

Gleadle, J. and Ratcliffe, P. (1997). Induction of hypoxia-inducible factor-1, erythropoietin, vascular endothelial growth factor, and glucose transporter-1 by hypoxia: evidence against a regulatory role for Src kinase. *Blood* **89** (2), 503–9.

Gleave, M.E., Elhilali, M., *et al.* (1998). Interferon gamma-1b compared with placebo in metastatic renal cell carcinoma. *New Engl. J. Med.* **338**, 1265–71.

Hanchette, C. and Schwartz, (1992). Inverse correlation between UV radiation exposure in USA and prostate cancer mortality. *Cancer* **70**, 2861–9.

Harper, P., MacDonald, L., Tong, D., *et al.* (1996). Anglian Germ Cell Group randomized phase two toxicity of one course carboplatin versus radiotherapy for stage one seminoma [abstract PO15]. *Br. J. Cancer* **74** (suppl. XXVIII), 29.

Heiss, M., Mempel, W., Delanoff, C., *et al.* (1994). Blood transfusion—modulated tumour recurrence: first results of a randomised study of autologous versus allogeneic blood transfusion in colorectal cancer surgery. *J. Clin. Oncol.* **12** (9), 1859–67.

Henriksson, R., Nilsson, S., Colleen, S., *et al.* (1997). Survival in renal cell carcinoma—a randomised evaluation of tamoxifen versus interleukin-2, alpha-interferon (leukocyte) and tamoxifen. *Br. J. Cancer.*

Herpen, C.V., Jansen, R., Kruit, W., *et al.* (2000). Immunochemotherapy with interleukin-2, interferon-alpha and 5-fluorouracil for progressive metastatic renal cell carcinoma: a multicentre phase II study. Dutch Immunotherapy Working Party. *Br. J. Cancer* **82** (4), 772–6.

Hersh, E.M., Akporiaye, E., Harris, D., *et al.* (1994). Phase I study of immunotherapy of malignant melanoma by direct gene transfer. *Hum. Gene Ther.* **5** (11), 1371–84.

Hofmockel, G., Langer, W., and Theiss, M. (1996). Immunochemotherapy for metastatic renal cell carcinoma using a regimen of interleukin-2, interferon-α and 5-fluorouracil. *J. Urol.* **156**, 18–21.

Horoszewicz, J.S. and Murphy, G.P. (1989). An assessment of the current use of human interferons in therapy of urological cancers. *J. Urol.* **142** (5), 1173–80.

Hunter, D.J., Manson, J.E., Colditz, G.A., *et al.* (1993). A prospective study of the intake of vitamins C, E and A and the risk of breast cancer. *New Engl J. Med.* **329**, 234–40.

Ito, N., Matsuda, T., Kakchi, Y., Takeuchi, E., Takashi, T., and Yoshida, O. (1990). Bladder cancer producing granulocyte colony stimulating factor. *New Engl. J. Med.* **323**, 1709–10.

Itoh, K., Platsoucas, C.D., and Balch, C.M. (1988). Autologous tumour specificc cytotoxic T lymphocytes in the infiltrate of human metastatic melanomas: activation by interleukin-2 and autologous tumour cells and involvement of the T cell receptor. *J. Exp. Med.* **168**, 1419.

Iversen, P., Madsen, P.O., and Corle, D.K. (1995). Radical prostatectomy versus expectant treatment for early carcinoma of the prostate. Twenty-three year follow-up of a prospective randomized study. *Scand. J. Urol. Nephrol. Suppl.* **172**, 65–72.

Jeal, W. and Goa, K. (1997). Aldesleukin (recombinant interleukin-2). A review of its pharmacological properties, clinical efficacy and tolerability in patients with renal cell carcinoma. *BioDrugs* **7**, 285–317.

Joffe, J., Banks, R., Forbes, M., *et al.* (1996). A phase II study of interferon-alpha, interluekin-2 and 5-fluorouracil in advanced renal carcinoma: clinical data and laboratory evidence of protease activation. *Br. J. Urol.* **77**, 638–49.

Johnsen, J. and Hellsten, S. (1987).Lymphatogenous spread of renal cell carcinoma: an autopsy study. *J. Urol.* **157** (2), 450–3.

Jung, D., Hilmes, C., Knuth, A., Jaegar, E., Huber, C., and Seliger, B. (1999). Gene transfer of the co-stimulatory molecules B7-1 and B7-2 enhances the immunogenicity of human renal cell carcinoma to a different extent. *Scand. J. Immunol.* **50** (3), 242–9.

Kalra, R., Singh, S., Savage, S., Finch, G., and Sopori, M. (2000). Effects of cigarette smoking on immune response: chronic exposure to cigarette smoke impairs antigen-mediated signaling in T cells and depletes IP3-sensitive Ca (2+) stores. *J. Pharmacol. Exp. Ther.* **293** (1), 166–71.

Kim, B. and Louie, A.C. (1992). Surgical resection followng interleukin-2 therapy for metastatic renal cell carcinoma prolongs remission. *Arch. Surg.* **127**, 1343–9.

Koga, Y., Naraparaju, V., and Yamamoto, N. (1999). Antitumour effect of vitamin D-binding protein derived macrophage activating factor on Ehrlich ascites tumour-bearing mice. *Proc. Soc. Exp. Biol. Med.* **220** (1), 20–6.

Koli, K. and Keski-Oja, J. (2000). 1 alpha, 25 dihydroxyvitamin d3 and its analogues down-regulate cell invasion-associated proteases in cultured malignant cells. *Cell Growth Different.* **11** (4), 221–9.

Lacour, J., Le, M., Caceres, E., Koszarowski, T., Veronesi, U., and Hill, C. (1983). Radical mastectomy versus radical mastectomy plus internal mammary dissection. Ten year results of an international cooperative trial in breast cancer. *Cancer* **51** (10), 1941–3.

Lindenmann,, J. and Klein, P.A. (1967). Viral oncolysis: increased immunogenicity of host cell antigen associated with influenza virus. *J. Exp. Med.* **126** (1), 93–108.

List, A.F., S.C., Miller, T.P., and Grogan, T.M. (1993). Deficient tumour infiltrating T lymphocyte response in malignant lymphoma—relationship to HLA expression and host immunocompetence. *Leukemia* **7** (3), 398–403.

Lopez Hanninen, E., Kirchner, H., and Atzpodien, J. (1996). Interleukin-2 based home therapy of metastatic renal cell carcinoma: risks and benefits in 215 consecutive single institution patients. *J. Urol.* **155** (1), 19–25.

Mackie, R.M., Bufalino, R., Morabito, A., Sutherland, C., and Cascinelli, N. (1991). Lack of effect of pregnancy on outcome of melanoma. *Lancet* **337**, 653–5.

Mevorach, R., Segal, A., Tersegno, M., and Frank, I. (1992). Renal cell carcinoma: incidental diagnosis and natural history. Review of 235 cases. *Urology* **39**, 519–22.

Mickisch, G., Garin, A., Madej, M., Prijck, L., and Sylvester, R.D. (2000). Tumour nephrectomy plus interferon alpha is superior to interferon alpha alonein metastatic renal cell carcinoma. *J. Urol.* **163** (suppl.), Abstr. 778.

Miyajima, J., Imai, Y., Nakao, M., Noda, S., and Itoh, K. (1996). Higher susceptibility of erythropoietin-producing renal cell carcinomas to lysis by lymphokine-activated killer cells. *J. Immunother. Emphasis Tumor Immunol.* **19** (6), 399–404.

Morris, D. (2000). Dramatic response of renal cell carcinoma to epivir and viramune in a HIV positive patient. *J. Clin. Oncol.* (supplement) *Proceedings of the American Society of Clinical Oncology,* Abstr. 1390.

Negrier, S., Escudier, B., and Lasset, C. (1998). Recombinant human interleukin-2, recombinant human interferon alpha-2a, or both in metastatic renal cell carcinoma. *New Engl. J. Med.* **338**, 1272–8.

Neugut, A., Weinberg, M., Ahsan, H., and Rescigno, J. (1999). Carcinogenic effects of radiotherapy for breast cancer. *Oncology* **13** (9), 1245–56.

Nieken, J., Sleijfer, D., and Buter, J. (1996). Outpatient based sub cututaneous IL-2 in patients with advanced renal cell carcinoma. *Cancer Biother. Radiopharmacol.* **11**, 289–95.

Noort, J.V., Bajramovic, J., Plomp, A., and Stipdonk, M.V. (2000). Mistaken self, a novel model that links microbial infections with myelin-directed autoimmunity in multiple sclerosis. *J. Neuroimmunol.* **105** (1), 46–57.

Nouri, A.M.E., Hussain, R.F., Santos, A.V.L.D., Gillott, D.J., and Oliver, R.T.D. (1992). Induction of MHC antigens by tumour cell lines in response to interferons. *Eur. J. Cancer* **28**, 1110–15.

Ohigashi, T., Tachibana, M., Tazaki, H., and Nakamura, K. (1992). Bladder cancer cells express functional receptors for granulocyte-colony stimulating factor. *J. Urol.* **147**, 283–6.

Ohnmacht, G. and Marincola, F. (2000). Heterogeneity in expression of human leukocyte antigens and melanoma associated antigens in advanced melanoma. *J. Cell Physiol.* **182** (3), 332–8.

Oliver, R.T.D. (1989).Psychological support for cancer patients. *Lancet* 1989, 1209.

Oliver, R. (2000). Poorer outcome from treatment of breast cancer in poorer areas of Glasgow. *Br. Med. J.* Rapid response submission: www.bmj.com/cgi/eletters/320/7247/1442#EL3.

Oliver, R.T.D. and Nouri, A.M.E. (1992). T cell immune response to cancer in humans and its relevance for immunodiagnosis and therapy. *Cancer Surv.* **13**, 173–204.

Oliver, R.T.D., Miller, R.M., Mehta, A., and Barnett, M.J. (1988). A phase 2 study of surveillance in patients with metastatic renal cell carcinoma and assessment of response of such patients to therapy on progression. *Mol. Biother.* **1**, 14–20.

Oliver, R.T.D., Nethersall, A.B.W., and Bottomley, J.M. (1989). Unexplained spontaneous regression and alpha-interferon as treatment for metastatic renal carcinoma. *Br J. Urol.* **63**, 128–31.

Oliver, R., Steele, J., and Ansell, W. (1999). Should spontaneous regression be excluded before commencing biotherapy in renal cancer? *Br. J. Int.* **83** (Suppl. 4), Abstr. p137.

Oliver, R., Griffiths, G., and Ritchie, A. (2000). Pretreatment haemoglobin level as a predictor of response to subsequent treatment. Brit. J. Urol. (supplement) Proceedings British Association Urological Surgeons Annual Meeting 2000, Birmingham, Abstr. 54.

Penn, I. (1988). Tumours of the immunocompromised patient. *Ann. Rev. Med.* **323**, 1967–8.

Penn, I. (1990). Cancers complicating organ transplantation. *New Engl. J. Med.* **323**, 1967–8.

Pines, A. (1976). A 5 year controlled study of BCG and radiotherapy for inoperable lung cancer. *Lancet* i, 380–5.

Pizzoferrato, E., Chu, N., Hawley, T., *et al.* (1997). Enhanced immunogenecity of B cell lymphoma genetically engineered to express both B7–1 and interleukin-2. *Hum. Gene Ther.* **8** (18), 2217–28.

Possinger, K., Wagner, H., Beck, R., and Staebler, A. (1988). Renal cell carcinoma. *Controvers. Oncol.* **30**, 195–207.

Rackley, R., Novick, A., Klein, E., Bukowski, R., McLain, D., and Goldfarb, D. (1994). The impact of adjuvant nephrectomy on multimodality treatment of metastatic renal cell carcinoma. *J. Urol.* **152** (5, pt 1), 1399–403.

Ransom, J., Pelle, B., and Hanna, M. (1992). Expression of class II major histo-compatability complex molecules correlates with human colon tumour vaccine efficacy. *Cancer Res.* **52** (12), 3460–6.

Ravi, R. and Oliver, R.T.D. (1999). Recent progress in cytokine therapy for renal cell cancer. The case for the EORTC adjuvant cytokine trial in patients with poor risk renal cell cancer after maximum debulking surgery. *Br. J. Urol.* **83**, 219–21.

Riddle, P. and Berenbaum, M. (1967). Postoperative depression of the lymphocyte response to phytohaemagglutinin. *Lancet* 1 (7493), 746–8.

Rini, B., Selk, L., and Vogelzang, N. (1999). Phase I study of direct intralesional gene transfer of HLA-B7 into metastatic renal carcinoma lesions. *Clin. Cancer Res.* **5** (10), 2766–72.

Ritchie, A., Layfield, L., and deKernion, J. (1988). Spontaneous regression of liver metastases from renal carcinoma. *J. Urol.* **140**(3), 596–7.

Ritchie, A.W.S., Griffiths, G., Oliver, R.T.D., Cook, P., Hancock, B., and Parmar, M.K.B. (1999). Alpha interferon improves survival in patients with metastatic renal carcinoma—preliminary results of an MRC randomised contolled study. *Lancet* 17.

Robertson, C., Lineham, W., and Pass, H. (1990). Preparative cytoreductive surgery in patients with metastastic renal cell carcinoma treated with adoptive immunotherapy with interleukin-2 or interleukin-2 plus lymphokine activated killer cells. *J. Urol.* **144**, 614–18.

Rous, P. and Beard, J. (1935). The progression to carcinoma of virus-induced rabbit papillomas (Shope). *J. Exp. Med.* **62**, 523–48.

Schirrmacher, V., Hoegen, P., Schlag, P., Liebrich, W., Lehner, B., and Schumaker, K. (1989). Active specific immunotherapy with autologous tumor cell vaccines modified by Newcastle disease virus: experimental and clinical studies. In *Cancer metastasis*, pp. 157–70. Springer Verlag, Berlin.

Semba, R., Muhilal, Ward, B., *et al.* (1993). Abnormal T cell subset proportions in vitamin A deficient children. *Lancet* **341**, 5–8.

Spiegel, D., Bloom, J., Kraemer, H., and Gottheil, E. (1989). Effect of psycho-social treatment on survival in patients with metastatic breast cancer. *Lancet* **2** (8668), 888–91.

Steinbeck, G., Strander, H., Carbin, B., *et al.* (1990). Recombinant leukocyte interferon alpha-2a and medroxyprogesterone in advanced renal cell carcinoma. *Acta Oncol.* **29**, 155–62.

Sternswald, J., Jondal, M., and Vanky, F. (1978). Lymphopenia and change in distribution of human B and T lymphocyte in periperal blood induced by irradiation for mammary carcinoma. *Lancet* i, 1352–6.

Taille, A.D.L., Cho, Y., Shabsigh, A., *et al.* (2000). Potential diagnostic significance of blood based RT-PCR assays of MN/CA9 and PSMA. *J. Urol.* **163** (suppl. Proc. AUA), Abst. 686.

Temoshok, L., Peeke, H.V.S., Mehard, C.W., Axelsson, K., and Sweet, S.M. (1985). Stress–behaviour interactions in hamster tumor growth. *Neuroimmune Interact.* **496**, 501–9.

Thompson, I. and Peek, M. (1988). Improvement in survival of patients with renal cell carcinoma—the role of the serendipitously detected tumour. *J. Urol.* **140**, 487–90.

Tourani, J., Luas, V., and Mayeur. D. (1996). Subcutaneous recombinant IL-2 (rIL-2) in outpatients with metastastic renal cell carcinoma. Results of a SCAPPI trial. *Ann. Oncol.* **7**, 525–8.

Travis, L., Rochelle, E., Curtis, H., Per, H., Holloway, E. (1997). Risk of second malignant neoplasms among long term survivors of testicular cancer. *J. Natl Cancer Inst.* **89**, 1429–39.

Uchida, A. (1993). Biological significance of autologous tumor-killing activity and its induction therapy. *Cancer Immunol. Immunother.* **37**, 75–83.

Umeta, M., West, C., Haidar, J., Deurenberg, P., and Hautvaset, J. (2000). Zinc supplementation and stunted infants in Ethiopia: a randomised controlled trial. *Lancet* **355** (9220), 2021–6.

Unfound_82. .

Unfound_83. .

Vaughan, M., Johnson, S., and Moore, J. (1997). A phase II study of subcutaneous interleukin-2, alpha interferon and prolonged venous infusional 5 FU in metastatic renal cell cancer. *Br. J. Cancer* **76** (suppl. I), 50.

Veldman, C., Cantorna, M., and DeLuca, H. (2000). Expression of 1,25-dihydroxyvitamin D (3) receptor in the immune system. *Arch. Biochem. Biophys.* **374** (2), 334–8.

Walther, M., Yang, J., Pass, H., Linehan, W., and Rosenberg, S. (1997). Cytoreductive surgery before high dose interleukin-2 based therapy in patients with metastatic renal cell carcinoma. *J. Urol.* **158** (5), 1675–8.

Walther, M., Lyne, J., Libutti, S., and Linehan, W. (1999). Laparoscopic cytoreductive nephrectomy as preparation for administration of systemic interleukin-2 in the treatment of metastatic renal cell carcinoma: a pilot study. *Urology* **53** (3), 496–501.

Werf-Messing, V.D. (1971). Hormonal treatment of metastases of renal carcinoma. *Br. J. Cancer* **25** (3), 423–7.

Young, J. and Rosenberg, S. (1997). *Cancer J. Sci. Am.* **3** (suppl. 1), 579–84.

Zhang, R. and DeGroot, L. (2000). Gene therapy of established medullary thyroid carcinoma with herpes simplex viral thymidine kinase in a rat tumour model: relationship of bystander effect and antitumor efficacy. *Thyroid* **10** (4), 313–19.

19. Prognostic indicators: localized disease

Dieter Bruno and David F. Paulson

Introduction

Although renal cell carcinoma (RCC) comprises only 2 per cent of adult cancers, it is the third most common genitourinary malignancy with an incidence of 28 800 new cases in 1998 and an associated mortality of 11 300 lives (Parker *et al.* 1997). The classic triad of gross hematuria, flank pain, and a palpable mass has been used to describe the presentation of RCC; however, historically only 10 per cent of patients present in this fashion (Jayson and Sanders 1998; Figlin 1999). The modern advent of computerized tomography (CT) and ultrasound has revolutionized the diagnosis of RCC with incidentally detected tumors being the rule rather than the exception (Storkel *et al.* 1989; Engelmann *et al.* 1988). For example, between 1935 and 1965 Skinner *et al.* (1971) reported only a 7 per cent incidental detection rate for RCC. Similarly Konnak and Grossman (1985) reported that only 13 per cent of cases diagnosed between 1961 and 1973 were discovered incidentally. However, more contemporary series report a 61 per cent incidental tumor detection rate with most of these tumors being amenable to curative therapy (Jayson and Sanders1998).

In general, most urologic malignancies have been amenable to multimodal therapy including combinations of cytoreduction, chemotherapy, and radiation. RCC has unfortunately been less responsive to the adjunctive therapies, with surgical extirpation being the mainstay for curative management (Thrasher and Paulson 1993; Van Brussel and Mickisch 1999; Van Poppel *et al.* 1997). With respect to localized RCC, a number of factors have been determined to impact upon patient survival. These can be separated into tumor-specific factors (pathologic stage, nuclear grade, cell type, histologic pattern, tumor size, nuclear morphometry, and DNA content) and patient-specific factors (age, race, gender, and performance status) (Thrasher and Paulson 1993). This chapter will discuss current concepts regarding these factors and their relationship to the prognosis of localized RCC.

Tumor-specific factors

Pathologic stage

A number of both historical and contemporary studies suggest that pathologic staging (that is, tumor extent at surgery) is the single most important factor in the prognosis of localized RCC (Czaplicki *et al.* 1986; Skinner *et al.* 1971; Dinney *et al.* 1992;

Giuliani *et al.* 1990; Golimbu *et al.* 1986; Holland 1973; Robson *et al.* 1969; Medeiros *et al.* 1988; Giberti *et al.* 1997). In series where patients present with organ-confined RCC, 5 year survival rates range from 60 to 90 per cent (Skinner *et al.* 1971; Van Poppel *et al.* 1997; Dinney *et al.* 1992; Golimbu *et al.* 1986; Robson *et al.* 1969; McNichols *et al.* 1981; Selli *et al.* 1983). In series where patients present with metastatic disease, 5-year survival rates approximate 5 to 10 per cent with a median survival of approximately 8 months (Thrasher and Paulson 1993; Van Brussel and Mickisch 1999). The one exception to the poor prognosis observed in patients with metastatic disease is in patients with isolated pulmonary metastases. These patients tend to respond favorably to nephrectomy with pulmonary metastasis resection (Skinner *et al.* 1972), whereas patients with other forms of metastatic disease generally do not benefit from surgical intervention.

Although there are a number of staging systems for RCC, the most commonly employed are the Robson classification (Robson *et al.* 1969) and the Union International Contre le Cancer (UICC) TNM (tumor–node–metastasis) classification (Guinan *et al.* 1997) (see Table 19.1). The predominant difference between these staging systems is manifested by the inability of the Robson system to differentiate between renal vein and inferior vena cava involvement (Thrasher and Paulson 1993), as well as between venous and lymph node involvement (Lanigan 1995; Bassil *et al.* 1985; Siminovitch *et al.* 1983). Despite this theoretical shortcoming, some series indicate that the Robson staging system provides greater prognostic information than the TNM staging system (Storkel *et al.* 1989). One difficulty in comparing outcome data between these two systems is that, whereas the Robson staging system has remained unchanged, the 1978 TNM classification system has undergone two subsequent modifications (1987 and 1997). Consequently, the comparison of data from different series is somewhat problematic. Table 19.2 demonstrates stage-specific survival data utilizing radical nephrectomy to treat RCC. It also suggests the survival advantage associated with organ-confined versus locally extensive RCC.

One dilemma regarding the stage-specific prognosis of RCC includes renal vein and inferior vena cava extension. The important distinction to be made is between vascular extension of the tumor without invasion into the vascular wall and vascular wall invasion. Whereas some series suggest that even microscopic vascular invasion confers an accelerated rate of disease progression (Van Poppel *et al.* 1997; Samma *et al.* 1991), despite extensive debate most studies do not support isolated renal vein

Table 19.1 Comparison of the Robson and TNM (1978 and 1997) staging systems for renal cell carcinoma

	Robson	TNM 1978	1997
Small tumor, minimal caliceal distortion (confined to the renal capsule)	I	T1	T1 (< 7.0 cm)
Large tumor, caliceal distortion (confined to the renal capsule)	I	T2	T2 (> 7.0 cm)
Tumor extension to the perirenal fat or ipsilateral adrenal gland (confined by Gerota's fascia)	II	T3a	T3a
Renal vein involvement	IIIa	T3b	T3b
Renal vein and vena cava involvement	IIIa	T3c	T3b
Vena cava involvement above the diaphragm	IIIa	T4b	T3c
Single ipsilateral node involved	IIIb	N1	N1
Multiple regional, contralateral, or bilateral nodes involved	IIIb	N2	N2
Fixed regional nodes	IIIb	N3	—
Juxtaregional nodes involved	IIIb	N4	—
Combination of IIIa and IIIb	IIIc	T3,4, N1–4	T3b,c N1–2
Spread to contiguous organs except the ipsilateral adrenal gland	IVa	T4a	T4
Distant metastases	IVb	M1	M1

Table 19.2 1987 TNM pathologic stage-specific survival using nephrectomy to treat renal cell carcinoma (Storkel et al. 1989)

1987 TNM stage	5-year survival (%)
pT1	98
T2	83
pT3a	58
pT3b	35

extension as a negative prognostic indicator (Skinner et al. 1971; Golimbu et al. 1986; Selli et al. 1983; Boxer et al. 1979). Selli et al. (1983) performed a multivariate analysis on data from 115 patients who underwent nephrectomy for RCC. Utilizing the TNM classification for stage comparison it was demonstrated that renal vein extension by itself does not affect prognosis. Similarly, Skinner et al. (1971) reported a 65 per cent 5-year survival rate for kidney-confined RCC versus a 66 per cent 5-year survival rate for organ-confined RCC with renal vein extension. Ultimately, the significance in venous extension/invasion may lie in concomitant lymph node status. For example, Guiliani et al. (1990) and Ljungberg et al. (1995) reported positive lymph nodes or distant metastases in 55 and 57 per cent of their patients with vein involvement, respectively. This begs the question of vein involvement being an independent prognostic indicator or just a factor related to 'occult' metastases.

Tumor invasion into the renal pelvis has been the subject of debate with less conclusive data than those of venous involvement. It appears that renal pelvis involvement confers a poorer prognosis than tumors without renal pelvis involvement. It has been suggested that this is so because the studies examining this issue have difficulty identifying patients with renal pelvis invasion as an isolated event as opposed to just a manifestation of patients presenting with higher stage disease (Thrasher and Paulson 1993). Additionally, these studies have been retrospective reviews with their attendant biases.

McNichols et al. (1981) analysed data from patients with stage III lesions with and without renal pelvis invasion. Although similar 15-year survival curves were rendered for each group, other stage comparisons were hampered by the tendency for renal pelvis invasion to be associated with higher stage tumors (McNichols et al. 1981). As a result the conclusion was that, rather than renal pelvis invasion being an independent prognostic indicator, it is a reflection of advanced stage disease with its attendant prognosis (McNichols et al. 1981).

Golimbu and associates (1986) examined patients with collecting system involvement by RCC. Regardless of the stage at presentation, the mortality rate was unfavorable. In this series patients with stage I, II, and III disease experienced mortality rates of 100, 82.5, and 98 per cent respectively. The authors concluded that renal medulla tumor infiltration confers an unfavorable prognosis (Golimbu et al. 1986).

There is a significant amount of data concerning the prognostic significance of inferior vena cava extension by RCC which occurs in 5–10 per cent of cases (Hatcher et al. 1991; Marshall et al. 1970). Siminovitch et al. (1983) reported on a series subset of 11 patients with vena cava involvement managed by nephrectomy with a 5-year survival of 11 per cent and 9 patients with positive regional lymph nodes. The authors concluded that the prognosis was just as dismal in patients with vena cava involvement.

Most other series, however, suggest that, in the absence of metastatic disease, inferior vena cava involvement does not portend a poorer prognosis as long as the complete cava thrombus is removed (Hatcher et al. 1991; Libertino et al. 1987; O'Donohue et al. 1987). In a series containing 44 patients with RCC with extension into the inferior vena cava (16.7 per cent renal vein level, 62.5 per cent infradiaphragmatic, 12.5 per cent supradiaphragmatic, and 8.3 per cent right atrial), Libertino et al. (1987) reported 5- and 10-year survivals of 47.3 ± 9.6 and 41.4 ± 10.0 per cent, respectively. As long as the tumor thrombus burden was completely removed, the authors reported no difference in survival between infradiaphragmatic and supradiaphragmatic vena cava extension.

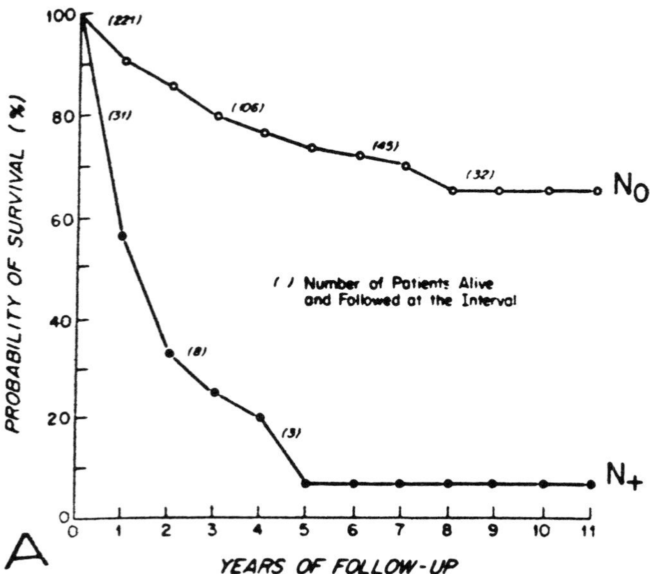

Fig. 19.1 From reference[8], page 252 (figure 4)

Similarly, a series of 44 patients with vena cava thrombi published by Hatcher and associates (1991) suggests that there is no survival difference with respect to the level of vena cava thrombus extension provided that all of the thrombus is removed. In this series patients with organ-confined tumor with no evidence of metastatic disease realized a 69 per cent 5-year survival (9.9 year median survival). Patients with vena cava invasion fared worse with a 25 per cent 5-year survival (1.2 year median survival). Interestingly, the 5-year survival increased to 57 per cent (5.3 year median survival) if the cava side wall was successfully removed (Hatcher et al. 1991).

On the other hand, other researchers have reported slightly different statistics regarding inferior vena cava involvement. Sosa et al. (1984) reviewed a series of 24 patients with vena cava involvement and concluded that the level of inferior vena cava involvement does alter the prognostic significance of the surgical outcome. In this series, 10 patients with infrahepatic thrombi experienced an 80 per cent 2-year survival (mean survival 61.4 months), whereas the 14 patients with suprahepatic thrombi experienced a 21 per cent 2-year survival (mean survival 22.9 months). One must take note however, that 9 of the 14 patients with hepatic or suprahepatic vein extension had either perinephric fat or positive regional lymph nodes (Sosa et al. 1984). As a result, this patient population may be skewed because the latter group cannot be validly compared to the former group without extrarenal tumor.

Historically, locoregional lymph node involvement in patients with RCC has portended an unfavorable prognosis (Skinner et al. 1971, 1972; Golimbu et al. 1986; Bassil et al. 1985; Siminovitch et al. 1983; Libertino et al. 1987; Nurmi 1984) with

the 5- and 10-year survivals being 5–30 per cent and 0–5 per cent, respectively (Fig. 19.1) (Thrasher and Paulson 1993). There is evidence to suggest that retroperitoneal lymphadenectomy prolongs survival in carefully selected patients. Herrlinger et al. (1991) reported on a prospective series of 511 patients that demonstrated that, for Robson stages I–III (pathologic (p)T1–3, N0–3, M0, R0), a 5-year survival increase from 58 to 66 per cent and a 10-year survival increase from 40.9 to 56.1 per cent was observed after extended retroperitoneal lymphadenectomy. Although these statistics are not durable for stage III disease, the survival increases are statistically significant and durable for Robson stage I–II disease past 10 years (Herrlinger et al. 1991).

Similarly to Herrlinger et al. (1991), Schafhauser et al. (1999) realized a survival benefit in 4 per cent of the patients in a retrospective analysis of 1035 patients with clinical (c)T1–4, cM0 RCC who underwent systematic retroperitoneal lymph node dissection.

Golimbu et al. (1986) realized a 5-year survival increase from 65 to 80 per cent in patients with stage II disease who underwent lymphadenectomy. Additionally, patients with stage III disease with concomitant renal vein involvement experienced a 5-year survival increase from 47 to 60 per cent after lymphadenectomy (Golimbu et al. 1986).

As it stands, numerous series addressing the issue of lymphadenectomy in the management of localized RCC suggest a survival benefit from a lymph node dissection. However, more data that include prospectively randomized trials should be designed to more solidly answer this question since the difficulty lies in the inability to accurately stage patients preoperatively for the randomization process.

In general, metastatic RCC portends a dismal prognosis with survival rates being around 11 per cent in patients managed conservatively (Kavolius et al. 1998). Although surgical intervention has been demonstrated to be ineffective in widely metastatic RCC, there is evidence to support resection in patients with solitary metastases. Five-year survival rates have been noted to improve to the 25–35 per cent range after such resections (Miyao et al. 1997; Skinner and Lieskovsky 1988). Barney and Churchill (1939) described the initial experience with nephrectomy and solitary metastases resection. In this landmark case, the patient had a single pulmonary metastasis resected and lived 23 years succumbing to cardiac disease (Barney and Churchill 1939).

Kavolius et al. (1998) reported on a retrospective analysis of 278 patients with recurrent RCC. In this review, 141 patients underwent resection of initial recurrence tumor burden with a 5-year survival rate of 44 per cent (Kavolius et al. 1998). Seventy patients underwent incomplete metastases resection with a 14 per cent 5-year survival rate and 67 patients were managed conservatively with an 11 per cent 5-year survival rate (Kavolius et al. 1998). In this series the authors noted that the most common metastases in decreasing order of frequency were: lung (57 per cent), bone (19 per cent), lymph nodes (11 per cent), and brain (8 per cent) (Kavolius et al. 1998). Interestingly, solitary second and third recurrences were resected with 5-year survival rates of 46 and 44 per cent, respectively. Lastly, patients with a disease-free interval (DFI) greater than 12 months tended to

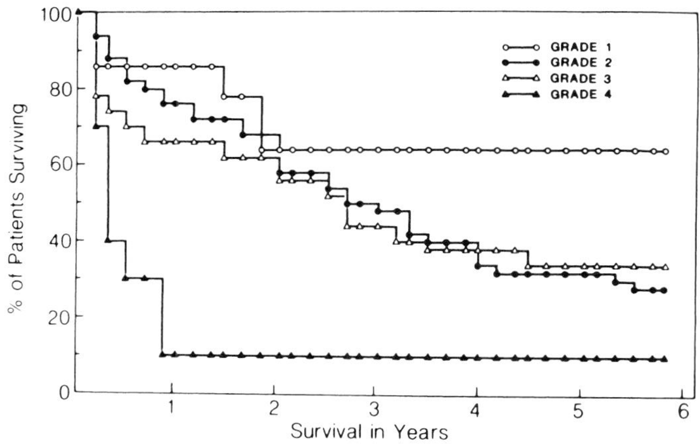

Fig. 19.2 From reference[8], page 255 (figure 6)

fare better than patients with a DFI less than 12 months: 53 versus 33 per cent 5-year survival, respectively.

In patients with metastatic disease, cytoreductive nephrectomy has been associated with spontaneous regression of metastases in up to 0.8 per cent (Onishi *et al.* 1989). In response to this many researchers have proposed that an 'immunologic mechanism' is responsible for this observation. As a result, clinical trials with different immunomodulating compounds have been devised to treat metastatic RCC. Although the response rates are still unfavorable, interleukin 2 (IL-2), the most widely studied of these agents, has been noted to produce objective responses in the range of 17–27 per cent when combined with cytoreductive surgery (Figlin 1999; Tourani *et al.* 1996; Walther *et al.* 1993). With the future elucidation of the pathogenesis of RCC, perhaps more effective therapeutic modalities will be devised for the management of this devastating malignancy. However, as it now stands there is no widely effective treatment for this disease once it escapes the confines of Gerota's fascia.

Nuclear grade

Although it has been demonstrated that stage at presentation is the most reliable prognostic indicator, because up to 30 per cent of patients with 'organ-confined' RCC experience disease progression, other prognostic indicators have been sought (Usubutun *et al.* 1998). One of these supplemental prognostic indicators is nuclear grade. A number of systems have been devised for this purpose. No one system has been demonstrated to be objectively more reliable than the others; hence different systems are utilized at different institutions. At times this makes the comparison of different patient series difficult. Most commonly, these systems use a combination of nuclear and nucleolar characteristics. Some have utilized tumor architecture and cell type as well as the aforementioned characteristics (Goldstein 1997). Most commonly, these systems contain three or four tiers. The first grading system was reported by Hand and Broders (1932); in this system it was observed that patients with high-grade tumors did worse than patients with lower-grade tumors. Since then, many others have devised systems attempting to categorize patients. Some of the

more common grading systems include ones by Fuhrman *et al.* (1982), Skinner *et al.* (1971), Thoenes *et al.* (1986), and Arner *et al.* (1965). The Fuhrman scale contains four grades. Grade 1 tumors contain cells with small, round nuclei with inconspicuous or absent nuceoli. Grade 2 tumors contain cells with slightly irregular nuclei and nucleoli. Grade 3 tumors have larger nuclei and more prominent nucleoli, and grade 4 tumors contain cells with grade 3 nuclei or bizarre multilobulated nuclei (Thrasher and Paulson 1993). Based upon survival characteristics of patients with different stages, Fuhrman and associates were able to identify groups with favorable (grade 1), intermediate (grades 2–3), and dismal prognosis (grade 4); see Fig. 19.2 (Fuhrman *et al.* 1982).

In a study of 309 patients, Skinner and associates (1971) devised a grading system (four grades) based upon nuclear morphology that allowed them to separate the patients into four groups with different survival characteristics. This correlation between grading and survival held true even for patients within similar stages.

Other series fail to demonstrate the clear distinction in survival advantage between patients with different grades. Usubutun *et al.* (1998) reported on a series of 165 patients with RCC graded according to the Thoenes, Fuhrman, Arner, and Skinner systems. They found that, only when patients were grouped into two groups, low-grade (grades 1–2) and high-grade (grades 3–4), did statistically different survival characteristics become apparent (Usubutun *et al.* 1998).

Selli *et al.* (1983) had a similar experience in that they did identify survival differences between grade 1–2 tumors compared to grade 3–4 tumors. Ultimately, they attributed at least some of these differences to the enhanced probability of undetected metastatic disease among patients with high-grade tumors.

Eventually, grade does play a role in the prognostic predictions of patients with RCC. Whether or not this prediction is independent of or dependent upon stage remains to be elucidated. Current observations suggest that patients can be viewed in at least two groups: high- and low-grade. When these grading characteristics are combined with presenting stage, more meaningful information can be gleaned.

Cell type

RCC has a number of different histologies (clear, granular, mixed, and spindle/sarcomatoid). A number of different investigators have tried to establish a link between histology and prognosis. Although no clear distinctions can be made, it appears that spindle cells have been associated with the most unfavorable prognosis (Skinner *et al.* 1971; Boxer *et al.* 1979; Bertoni *et al.* 1987; Ro *et al.* 1987; Sella *et al.* 1987; Tomera *et al.* 1983; Mani *et al.* 1995). In a series by Kanamaru *et al.* (1999) the pathologic specimens from 106 patients with RCC were reviewed. The presence of sarcomatoid histology was found to correlate with higher T category, nuclear grade, and larger tumors. Skinner *et al.* (1971) noted a correlation between spindle cell tumors and grade. In their series 25 and 75 per cent of the spindle cell lesions were grade 3 and 4 tumors, respectively. In this series pure clear cell containing tumors tended to have a better prognosis than the other histologic types (Skinner *et al.* 1971). Boxer *et al.* (1979)

observed no differences in the 5-year survival rate between patients with clear cell and granular cell tumors; however, the 10-year survival differences were 53 and 29 per cent, respectively. Upon further analysis these authors noted that, in accordance with other series, spindle cell tumors were associated with the poorest prognosis (Boxer *et al.* 1979). As histologic cell type is inextricably intertwined with presenting stage, grade, and tumor size, it is felt by many that cell type is a stage-dependent rather than an independent prognostic indicator.

Histologic pattern

The histologic pattern of RCC describes the cellular architecture of the tumor. The most common patterns are: papillary, tubular, alveolar, cystic, solid, and mixed (Golimbu *et al.* 1986). In a study by Golimbu and associates (1986), histologic patterns were noted to vary with the tumor stage. For example, as tumor stage increased from I to IV, the incidence of papillary architecture followed a stepwise decline (26, 17, 7, and 10 per cent, respectively); concomitantly the incidence of cystic tumors followed a similar decline (10, 6, 2.5, and 0 per cent, respectively) (Golimbu *et al.* 1986). It was also noted that the percentage of solid tumors increased in a stepwise incremental fashion (16, 26, 43, and 62.5 per cent, respectively) (Golimbu *et al.* 1986). With respect to survival prognosis, the patients that experienced the most favorable 5-year survival tended to have one histologic pattern as well as fewer tumors with mixed or solid architecture (Golimbu *et al.* 1986).

In a study of 121 patients with RCC, Takashi *et al.* (1993) observed that 5-year survival rates had some relation to the histologic pattern of presentation. For example, alveolar, cystic, papillary, tubular, and solid architectures have the following 5-year survival rates (68.8, 100, 40, 66.7, and 50 per cent, respectively). As no mention was made regarding the relationship of other prognostic factors to the histologic pattern, no conclusions can be made regarding the independence of the histologic pattern as a prognostic factor.

Storkel and associates(1989) reviewed 431 cases of RCC that underwent surgery noting the mortality rates for cystic, tubulo-papillary, and solid architectures to be 0, 16, and 26 per cent respectively.

Historically histologic pattern has been an unreliable prognostic indicator as there is no consensus in the literature regarding the ramifications of cellular architecture. Accordingly, histology should be evaluated in the context of the other prognostic indicators as it can support an individual clinical scenario as opposed to being a free-standing prognostic indicator.

Tumor size

In the literature tumor size has been a subject of debate with respect to its ability to provide independent prognostic information regarding survival (Targonski *et al.* 1994). Targonski *et al.* (1994) analysed a series of 93 patients with T1N0M0 and T2N0M0 tumors and concluded that size had no prognostic value in predicting survival. They did observe that, in patients with T1NallMall and T2NallMall with metastatic disease, a size cut-off of 5.0 cm did have significant prognostic value. Giuliani *et al.* (1990) evaluated a series of patients and designated three size groups: small (< 5 cm), medium (5–10 cm), and large (> 10 cm). In this series it was observed that the 5-year

survival rates were 83.5, 50, and 0 per cent, respectively. It is noteworthy that this study did not take grade or stage into account when evaluating tumor size.

Green *et al.* (1989) evaluated tumor size and took into account the influence of tumor stage and grade and determined that patients with a tumor size of < 8 cm were associated with a 95 per cent 5-year survival, whereas patients with a tumor size of > 8 cm were associated with a 65 per cent 5-year survival rate. In a series by Golimbu *et al.* (1986), a 5.0 cm tumor size cut-off value yielded interesting results. In stage I and II disease, 72 per cent of patients who died of disease had tumors greater than 5.0 cm, and in stage III disease 85 per cent of the patients who died of disease had tumors greater than 5.0 cm. Intuitively, tumor size should have some relationship to the prognosis of RCC. More series of patients will need to be evaluated with multivariate analyses of tumor size in light of other prognostic factors to further address the significance of tumor size on the prognosis of RCC.

Nuclear morphometry and DNA content

Nuclear morphometry and cellular DNA content have both been demonstrated to have predictive value in certain groups of patients. The tendency is towards a poorer prognosis for increasing nuclear area and aneuploidy (Van Brussel *et al.* 1999). Bibbo *et al.* (1987) reviewed the results of nuclear morphometry analysis in 19 patients with stage I RCC. It was observed that mean nuclear areas were 39.19 ± 17.81 μm^2 and 59.96 ± 18.17 μm^2 in patients with survival rates of greater than and less than 5 years, respectively. Additionally, patients who succumbed to metastatic disease tended to have high grade tumors as well as nuclear crowding and high mitotic densities (Bibbo *et al.* 1987).

In a series of 41 patients with stage I RCC, Tosi *et al.* (1986) observed that, when a number of morphometric characters (nuclear area, nuclear ellipsoidity, and nuclear boundary regularity) were analysed, nuclear area turned out to be the best prognostic indicator. Mean nuclear area of less than 32 μm^2 appeared to be linked to an increased 5-year survival as no patients with a mean nuclear area of less than 32 μm^2 succumbed to disease in this time period (Tosi *et al.* 1986). Although these series consist of patients with low-stage disease, other series with more extensive stage analyses yield similar results. In a study of 95 specimens, Gutierrez and associates (1992) observed that a mean nuclear area less than 35 μm^2 was associated with a 97 per cent 5-year survival rate, whereas a mean nuclear area of greater than 52 μm^2 was associated with a 17.2 per cent 5-year survival.

DNA content analysis by flow cytometry has gained popularity in the prognostic evaluation of patients with RCC since 1982 (Ljungberg *et al.* 1986). Briefly, flow cytometry allows for DNA categorization into aneuploid (an abnormal increase in cellular DNA content) and diploid (normal cellular DNA content) categories using automated cellular DNA analyses and DNA histograms (Thrasher and Paulson 1993). Different series have yielded conflicting results with respect to DNA analysis (Lanigan 1995). Some suggest a worse prognosis for aneuploid tumors (deKernion *et al.* 1989; Otto *et al.* 1984), whereas others suggest that ploidy is of no prognostic value when tumor stage and grade are factored into the analysis (Currin *et al.* 1990; Grignon *et al.*

1989). Currently, DNA ploidy analysis is both time-consuming and expensive and does not have an unequivocal role in the prognosis of RCC. As more series utilizing large numbers of patients, multivariate analyses, and inclusion of all stages (I–IV) become available, a more defined role for the utilization of DNA ploidy analysis in the evaluation of RCC will emerge.

Patient-specific factors

Age

Demographic studies focusing on age have generally demonstrated that age is not a significant factor in the prognosis of RCC (Storkel *et al.* 1989; Citterio *et al.* 1997). Many studies have focused on the pediatric patient population on the grounds that younger patients may have more aggressive tumors; however, in general the data does not support this hypothesis (Storkel *et al.* 1989; Dehner *et al.* 1970; Lack *et al.* 1985; Lieber *et al.* 1981). Similarly, age does not appear to affect the prognosis for middle-aged versus younger adults. Lieber and associates (1981) reviewed the literature and evaluated 89 patients with RCC (mean age, 37 years) and determined that middle-aged patients and younger adults had comparable survival rates. In this series the 3-, 5-, and 10-year survival rates were 60, 55, and 47 per cent, respectively.

Race and gender

Race has not been demonstrated to have any prognostic significance with respect to RCC (Thrasher and Paulson 1993). As with many of the other prognostic indicators, gender evaluation has provided equivocal results. Lieber *et al.* (1981) evaluated a series of 89 patients who were managed with nephrectomy and determined that men had a poorer prognosis than women. However, the men tended to present with higher-stage disease twice as often as the women. When stage presentation was accounted for, this difference in prognosis disappeared (Thrasher and Paulson 1993). Numerous other investigators have also demonstrated no significant gender-related differences with respect to prognosis (Selli *et al.* 1983; Nurmi 1984; Green *et al.* 1989; Ljungberg *et al.* 1988). However, there are still a minority who report a worse prognosis associated with male gender (McNichols *et al.* 1981; Lieber *et al.* 1981).

Performance status

The majority of the data regarding the relationship of performance status to the prognosis of RCC comes from patients with metastatic disease. The salient observation is that performance status has, in a number of studies, been a significant prognostic indicator with worsening performance status portending a poor prognosis (Nurmi 1984; Maldazys and deKernion 1986). Maldazys and deKernion (1986) reviewed a series of 181 cases of metastatic RCC and determined that patients with a good performance status (Karnofsky scale > 80) had a median survival of 35 months versus 7 months for patients with a poor performance status (Karnofsky

< 80) ($p < 0.0005$). Similarly, in a retrospective review of 84 patients with metastatic or recurrent RCC treated with biologic response modifiers, Mani *et al.* (1995) reported that both univariate and multivariate analyses demonstrated that poorer performance status adversely affected prognosis.

References

Arner, O., Blanck, C., and Schreeb, T. (1965). Renal adenocarcinoma; morphology—grading of malignancy—prognosis. A study of 197 cases. *Acta Chir. Scand. Suppl.* **346**, 1–51.

Barney, J. and Churchill, E. (1939). Adenocarcinoma of the kidney with metastasis to the lung: cured by nephrectomy and lobectomy. *J. Urol.* **42**, 269–76.

Bassil, B., Dosoretz, D.E., and Prout, G.R. Jr. (1985). Validation of the tumor, nodes and metastasis classification of renal cell carcinoma. *J. Urol.* **134**, 450–4.

Bertoni, F., Ferri, C., Benati, A., Bacchini, P., and Corrado, F. (1987). Sarcomatoid carcinoma of the kidney. *J. Urol.* **137**, 25–8.

Bibbo, M., Galera-Davidson, H., Dytch, H.E., Gonzalez de Chaves, J., Lopez-Garrido, J., Bartels, P.H., and Wied, G.L. (1987). Karyometry and histometry of renal-cell carcinoma. *Anal. Quant. Cytol. Histol.* **9**, 182–7.

Boxer, R.J., Waisman, J., Lieber, M.M., Mampaso, F.M., and Skinner, D.G. (1979). Renal carcinoma: computer analysis of 96 patients treated by nephrectomy. *J. Urol.* **122**, 598–601.

Citterio, G., Bertuzzi, A., Tresoldi, M., Galli, L., Di Lucca, G., Scaglietti, U., and Rugarli, C. (1997). Prognostic factors for survival in metastatic renal cell carcinoma: retrospective analysis from 109 consecutive patients. *Eur. Urol.* **31**, 286–91.

Currin, S.M., Lee, S.E., and Walther, P.J. (1990). Flow cytometric assessment of deoxyribonucleic acid content in renal adenocarcinoma: does ploidy status enhance prognostic stratification over stage alone? *J. Urol.* **143**, 458–63.

Czaplicki, M., Borkowski, A., Wesolowski, S., Kuzaka, B., Walecki, S., and Milewski, J.B. (1986). Late results of surgical treatment of renal clear-cell carcinoma. *Int. Urol. Nephrol.* **18**, 37–43.

Dehner, L.P., Leestma, J.E., and Price, E.B. Jr (1970). Renal cell carcinoma in children: a clinicopathologic study of 15 cases and review of the literature. *J. Pediatr.* **76**, 358–68.

deKernion, J.B., Mukamel, E., Ritchie, A.W., Blyth, B., Hannah, J., and Bohman, R. (1989). Prognostic significance of the DNA content of renal carcinoma. *Cancer* **64**, 1669–73.

Dinney, C.P., Awad, S.A., Gajewski, J.B., Belitsky, P., Lannon, S.G., Mack, F.G., and Millard, O.H. (1992). Analysis of imaging modalities, staging systems, and prognostic indicators for renal cell carcinoma. *Urology* **39**, 122–9.

Engelmann, U., Storkel, S., Kroehl, W., Jacobi, G., and Hohenfellner, R. (1988). Sonographische Fruherkennung asymptomatischer Nierenzellkarzinome—der Einfluss auf Uberlebensrate und prognostische Faktoren. *Urologe* **28**, 204–8.

Figlin, R.A. (1999). Renal cell carcinoma: management of advanced disease. *J. Urol.* **161**, 381–6; discussion 386–7.

Fuhrman, S.A., Lasky, L.C., and Limas, C. (1982). Prognostic significance of morphologic parameters in renal cell carcinoma. *Am. J. Surg. Pathol.* **6**, 655–63.

Giberti, C., Oneto, F., Martorana, G., Rovida, S., and Carmignani, G. (1997). Radical nephrectomy for renal cell carcinoma: long-term results and prognostic factors on a series of 328 cases. *Eur. Urol.* **31**, 40–8.

Giuliani, L., Giberti, C., Martorana, G., and Rovida, S. (1990). Radical extensive surgery for renal cell carcinoma: long-term results and prognostic factors. *J. Urol.* **143**, 468–73; discussion 473–4.

Goldstein, N.S. (1997). The current state of renal cell carcinoma grading. Union Internationale Contre le *Cancer* (UICC) and the American Joint Committee on *Cancer* (AJCC). *Cancer* **80**, 977–80.

Golimbu, M., Joshi, P., Sperber, A., Tessler, A., Al-Askari, S., and Morales, P. (1986). Renal cell carcinoma: survival and prognostic factors. *Urology* 27, 291–301.

Green, L.K., Ayala, A.G., Ro, J.Y., Swanson, D.A., Grignon, D.J., Giacco, G.G., and Guinee, V.F. (1989). Role of nuclear grading in stage I renal cell carcinoma. *Urology* 34, 310–15.

Grignon, D.J., el-Naggar, A., Green, L.K., Ayala, A.G., Ro, J.Y., Swanson, D.A., Troncoso, P., McLemore, D., Giacco, G.G., and Guinee, V.F. (1989). DNA flow cytometry as a predictor of outcome of stage I renal cell carcinoma. *Cancer* 63, 1161–5.

Guinan, P., Sobin, L.H., Algaba, F., Badellino, F., Kameyama, S., MacLennan, G., and Novick, A. (1997). TNM staging of renal cell carcinoma: Workgroup No. 3. Union International Contre le Cancer (UICC) and the American Joint Committee on Cancer (AJCC). *Cancer* 80, 992–3.

Gutierrez, J.L., Val-Bernal, J.F., Garijo, M.F., Buelta, L., and Portillo, J.A. (1992). Nuclear morphometry in prognosis of renal adenocarcinoma. *Urology* 39, 130–4.

Hand, J. and Broders, A. (1932). Carcinoma of the kidney: the degree of malignancy in relation to factors bearing on prognosis. *J. Urol.* 28, 199–216.

Hatcher, P.A., Anderson, E.E., Paulson, D.F., Carson, C.C., and Robertson, J.E. (1991). Surgical management and prognosis of renal cell carcinoma invading the vena cava. *J. Urol.* 145, 20–3; discussion 23–4.

Herrlinger, A., Schrott, K.M., Schott, G., and Sigel, A. (1991). What are the benefits of extended dissection of the regional renal lymph nodes in the therapy of renal cell carcinoma? *J. Urol.* 146, 1224–7.

Holland, J. (1973). Cancer of the kidney: natural history and staging. *Cancer* 32, 1030.

Jayson, M. and Sanders, H. (1998). Increased incidence of serendipitously discovered renal cell carcinoma. *Urology* 51, 203–5.

Kanamaru, H., Sasaki, M., Miwa, Y., Akino, H., and Okada, K. (1999). Prognostic value of sarcomatoid histology and volume-weighted mean nuclear volume in renal cell carcinoma. *BJU Int.* 83, 222–6.

Kavolius, J.P., Mastorakos, D.P., Pavlovich, C., Russo, P., Burt, M.E., and Brady, M.S. (1998). Resection of metastatic renal cell carcinoma. *J. Clin. Oncol.* 16, 2261–6.

Konnak, J.W. and Grossman, H.B. (1985). Renal cell carcinoma as an incidental finding. *J. Urol.* 134, 1094–6.

Lack, E.E., Cassady, J.R., and Sallan, S.E. (1985). Renal cell carcinoma in childhood and adolescence: a clinical and pathological study of 17 cases. *J. Urol.* 133, 822–8.

Lanigan, D. (1995). Prognostic factors in renal cell carcinoma. *Br. J. Urol.* 75, 565–71.

Libertino, J.A., Zinman, L., and Watkins, E. Jr (1987). Long-term results of resection of renal cell cancer with extension into inferior vena cava. *J. Urol.* 137, 21–4.

Lieber, M.M., Tomera, F.M., Taylor, W.F., and Farrow, G.M. (1981). Renal adenocarcinoma in young adults: survival and variables affecting prognsis. *J. Urol.* 125, 164–8.

Ljungberg, B., Stenling, R., and Roos, G. (1986). DNA content and prognosis in renal cell carcinoma. A comparison between primary tumors and metastases. *Cancer* 57, 2346–50.

Ljungberg, B., Joanssen, H., and Stenling, R. (1988). Prognostic factors in renal cell carcinoma. *Int. Urol. Nephrol.* 20, 115–21.

Ljungberg, B., Stenling, R., Osterdahl, B., Farrelly, E., Aberg, T., and Roos, G. (1995). Vein invasion in renal cell carcinoma: impact on metastatic behavior and survival. *J. Urol.* 154, 1681–4.

Maldazys, J.D. and deKernion, J.B. (1986). Prognostic factors in metastatic renal carcinoma. *J. Urol.* 136, 376–9.

Mani, S., Todd, M.B., Katz, K., and Poo, W.J. (1995). Prognostic factors for survival in patients with metastatic renal cancer treated with biological response modifiers [see comments]. *J. Urol.* 154, 35–40.

Marshall, V.F., Middleton, R.G., Holswade, G.R., and Goldsmith, E.I. (1970). Surgery for renal cell carcinoma in the vena cava. *J. Urol.* 103, 414–20.

McNichols, D.W., Segura, J.W., and DeWeerd, J.H. (1981). Renal cell carcinoma: long-term survival and late recurrence. *J. Urol.* 126, 17–23.

Medeiros, L.J., Gelb, A.B., and Weiss, L.M. (1988). Renal cell carcinoma. Prognostic significance of morphologic parameters in 121 cases. *Cancer* 61, 1639–51.

Miyao, N., Oda, T., Shigyou, M., Takeda, K., Masumori, N., Takahashi, A., Kitamura, H., and Tsukamoto, T. (1997). Pre-operatively determined prognostic factors in metastatic renal cell carcinoma. *Eur. Urol.* 31, 292–6.

Nurmi, M.J. (1984). Prognostic factors in renal carcinoma. An evaluation of operative findings. *Br. J. Urol.* 56, 270–5.

O'Donohoe, M.K., Flanagan, F., Fitzpatrick, J.M., and Smith, J.M. (1987). Surgical approach to inferior vena caval extension of renal carcinoma. *Br. J. Urol.* 60, 492–6.

Onishi, T., Machida, T., Masuda, F., Kurauchi, H., Mori, Y., Suzuki, M., Iizuka, N., Kondo, I., Furuta, N., and Shirakawa, H. (1989). Nephrectomy in renal carcinoma with distant metastasis. *Br. J. Urol.* 63, 600–4.

Otto, U., Baisch, H., Huland, H., and Kloppel, G. (1984). Tumor cell deoxyribonucleic acid content and prognosis in human renal cell carcinoma. *J. Urol.* 132, 237–9.

Parker, S.L., Tong, T., Bolden, S., and Wingo, P.A. (1997). Cancer statistics, 1997 [published erratum appears in *CA Cancer J. Clin.* 1997 Mar-Apr; 47 (2), 68]. *CA Cancer J. Clin.* 47, 5–27.

Ro, J.Y., Ayala, A.G., Sella, A., Samuels, M.L., and Swanson, D.A. (1987). Sarcomatoid renal cell carcinoma: clinicopathologic. A study of 42 cases. *Cancer* 59, 516–26.

Robson, C.J., Churchill, B.M., Anderson, W. (1969). The results of radical nephrectomy for renal cell carcinoma. *J. Urol.* 101, 297–301.

Samma, S., Yoshida, K., Ozono, S., Ohara, S., Hayashi, Y., Tabata, S., Uemura, H., Iwai, A., Hirayama, A., Hirao, Y., *et al.* (1991) Tumor thrombus and microvascular invasion as prognostic factors in renal cell carcinoma. *Jpn J. Clin. Oncol.* 21, 340–5.

Schafhauser, W., Ebert, A., Brod, J., Petsch, S., and Schrott, K.M. (1999). Lymph node involvement in renal cell carcinoma and survival chance by systematic lymphadenectomy. *AntiCancer Res.* 19, 1573–8.

Sella, A., Logothetis, C.J., Ro, J.Y., Swanson, D.A., and Samuels, M.L. (1987). Sarcomatoid renal cell carcinoma. A treatable entity. *Cancer* 60, 1313–18.

Selli, C., Hinshaw, W.M., Woodard, B.H., and Paulson, D.F. (1983). Stratification of risk factors in renal cell carcinoma. *Cancer* 52, 899–903.

Siminovitch, J.M., Montie, J.E., and Straffon, R.A. (1983). Prognostic indicators in renal adenocarcinoma. *J. Urol.* 130, 20–3.

Skinner, D.G. and Lieskovsky, G. (1988). *Diagnosis and management of genitourinary cancer.* Saunders, Philadelphia.

Skinner, D.G., Colvin, R.B., Vermillion, C.D., Pfister, R.C., and Leadbetter, W.F. (1971). Diagnosis and management of renal cell carcinoma. A clinical and pathologic study of 309 cases. *Cancer* 28, 1165–77.

Skinner, D.G., Vermillion, C.D., and Colvin, R.B. (1972). The surgical management of renal cell carcinoma. *J. Urol.* 107, 705–10.

Sosa, R.E., Muecke, E.C., Vaughan, E.D. Jr, and McCarron, J.P. Jr. (1984). Renal cell carcinoma extending into the inferior vena cava: the prognostic significance of the level of vena caval involvement. *J. Urol.* 132, 1097–100.

Storkel, S., Thoenes, W., Jacobi, G.H., and Lippold, R. (1989). Prognostic parameters in renal cell carcinoma—a new approach. *Eur. Urol.* 16, 416–22.

Takashi, M., Nakano, Y., Sakata, T., Miyake, K., and Hamajima, N. (1993). Multivariate evaluation of prognostic determinants for renal cell carcinoma. *Urol. Int.* 50, 6–12.

Targonski, P.V., Frank, W., Stuhldreher, D., and Guinan, P.D. (1994). Value of tumor size in predicting survival from renal cell carcinoma among tumors, nodes and metastases stage 1 and stage 2 patients. *J. Urol.* 152, 1389–92.

Thoenes, W., Storkel, S., and Rumpelt, H.J. (1986). Histopathology and classification of renal cell tumors (adenomas, oncocytomas and carcinomas). The basic cytological and histopathological elements and their use for diagnostics. *Pathol. Res. Pract.* 181, 125–43.

Thrasher, J.B. and Paulson, D.F. (1993). Prognostic factors in renal cancer. *Urol. Clin. N. Am.* 20, 247–62.

Tomera, K.M., Farrow, G.M., and Lieber, M.M. (1983). Sarcomatoid renal carcinoma. *J. Urol.* 130, 657–9.

Tosi, P., Luzi, P., Baak, J.P., Miracco, C., Santopietro, R., Vindigni, C., Mattei, F.M., Acconcia, A., and Massai, M.R. (1986). Nuclear morphometry as an important prognostic factor in stage I renal cell carcinoma. *Cancer* **58**, 2512–18.

Tourani, J.M., Lucas, V., Mayeur, D., Dufour, B., DiPalma, M., Boaziz, C., Grise, P., Varette, C., Pavlovitch, J.M., Pujade-Lauraine, E., Larregain, D., Ecstein, E., Untereiner, M., Vuillemin, E., Merran, S., and Andrieu, J.M. (1996). Subcutaneous recombinant interleukin-2 (rIL-2) in out-patients with metastatic renal cell carcinoma. Results of a multicenter SCAPP1 trial. *Ann. Oncol.* **7**, 525–8.

Usubutun, A., Uygur, M.C., Ayhan, A., Toklu, C., Sahin, A., Ozen, H., and Ruacan, S. (1998). Comparison of grading systems for esti-mating the prognosis of renal cell carcinoma. *Int. Urol. Nephrol.* **30**, 391–7.

Van Brussel, J.P. and Mickisch, G.H. (1999). Prognostic factors in renal cell and bladder cancer. *BJU Int.* **83**, 902–8; quiz 908–9.

Van Poppel, H., Vandendriessche, H., Boel, K., Mertens, V., Goethuys, H., Haustermans, K., Van Damme, B., and Baert, L. (1997). Microscopic vas-cular invasion is the most relevant prognosticator after radical nephrectomy for clinically nonmetastatic renal cell carcinoma. *J. Urol.* **158**, 45–9.

Walther, M.M., Alexander, R.B., Weiss, G.H., Venzon, D., Berman, A., Pass, H.I., Linehan, W.M., and Rosenberg, S.A. (1993). Cytoreductive surgery prior to interleukin-2-based therapy in patients with metastatic renal cell carcinoma. *Urology* **42**, 250–7; discussion 257–8.

20. Prognostic factors in advanced renal cell carcinoma

Paul J. Elson

Malignant tumors of the kidney account for 2.5 per cent of the cancer incidence and 2 per cent of the cancer mortality in the US. It is estimated that over 31 000 new cases will be diagnosed in 2000 and that almost 12 000 deaths will be reported (Greenlee *et al.* 2000). Renal cell carcinoma (RCC) is the most common renal malignancy reported, and recent epidemiological studies suggest that the incidence of all stages of the disease is increasing (Chow *et al.* 1999). If detected early, RCC can be cured surgically. The estimated 5-year survival for patients with disease confined to the kidney (stages T1 and T2) is approximately 90–95 per cent. However, once metastatic disease develops the prognosis for long-term survival is poor, the estimated 5-year survival being 0–20 per cent. Unfortunately, approximately one-third of patients have metastatic disease at the time of diagnosis and approximately 50 per cent of patients undergoing surgical resection for less advanced disease eventually relapse (Linehan *et al.* 1997; Figlin 1999). Effective treatment strategies for this disease are clearly needed.

The natural history of RCC is highly variable. Therefore, an important consideration in the development and evaluation of new treatments is the role of prognostic factors, which are often defined simply as pretreatment features that are predictive of outcome. Use of known prognostic factors and identification of new ones can help direct treatment strategies to the patient groups most likely to benefit from them. In addition, knowledge of prognostic factors can aid in the interpretation of clinical studies by helping to distinguish real from artifactual differences between treatments and to determine the extent to which a treatment is altering the natural history of the disease.

A number of patient- and disease-related factors are recognized as being prognostic for survival in advanced RCC. With the advent of molecular-based technologies such as reverse transcriptase polymerase chain reaction (RT-PCR) and cDNA and oligonucleotide microarrays, and the recognition that RCC is associated with immunological defects such as impaired signal transduction and apoptosis in T lymphocytes (Bukowski *et al.* 1998; Uzzo *et al.* 1999), new molecular- and genetics-based candidate prognostic factors are also being identified. Many of these candidate prognostic factors have been studied individually using univariate data analysis methods, and in groups using multivariate methods. Univariate analyses consider the prognostic importance of only the immediate factor being studied without regard to the possible impact of other factors. Multivariate methods, on the other hand, allow for the simultaneous assessment of several factors, and allow the effect of each factor to be examined while taking into account the possible impact of the others. The most commonly used statistical methods for evaluating factors associated with survival are the logrank test, for univariate analyses, and the Cox proportional hazards model for multivariate analyses. The univariate approach is a useful way to elucidate the potential value of a new prognostic factor, and individually many of the newer predictors do appear to be correlated with survival. It is important, however, that these candidate predictors also be examined within the context of recognized prognostic factors, using multivariate methods, to insure that they are providing additional independent information, and that their importance is not simply due to associations with other known factors.

The following sections summarize the factors that have been suggested to be of prognostic value in advanced RCC.

Patient- and disease-related factors

Patient and disease characteristics such as demographics, presenting symptoms, disease and treatment history, metastatic sites, grade, histology, and biochemical factors have been extensively studied as potential prognostic factors in advanced RCC. For completeness, studies that employed only univariate data analysis methods as well as those using multivariate methods are discussed below; however, emphasis is placed on the studies that employed the latter approach.

Table 20.1 summarizes the results of published studies that have examined the issue of prognostic factors in advanced RCC, and which have evaluated these 'classical' predictors using multivariate data analysis methods. For each study, Table 20.1 gives the number of patients studied, the time period during which they were treated, and the factors identified as prognostic for survival based on univariate and multivariate analysis of the data. The factors that were examined but which did not appear to be associated with survival are also given. It is important to remember when interpreting these data that all of the studies are retrospective in nature and that many combined data from different clinical trials of cytotoxic chemotherapy, hormonal therapy, and/or biologic response modifiers (BRM). However, a strength of these studies is that, although retrospective in nature, they are generally based on well-controlled prospective clinical trials. In addition sound statistical methods were used to analyse them.

Table 20.1 Multivariate analyses of patient- and disease-related factors

Reference	N	Treatment period	Factors associated with poor survival in		Factors examined but not found to influence survival
			Multivariate analysis	Univariate analysis	
Neves *et al.* 1988	158	1970–80	Recent weight loss ≥ 10%; > 1 metastatic site; high grade tumor	None	Sex and age; histology; size of the primary and side (left vs. right)
de Forges *et al.* 1988	134	1971–86	Recent weight loss > 10%*; ESR ≥ 100 vs. 50–99 vs. < 50 mm/h[2]; metastatic disease present at diagnosis; liver metastases, lung metastases > 2 cm and/or ≥ 5 per field	P.S.; prior nephrectomy; fever > 38°C	Sex; histology
Elson *et al.* 1988	610	1975–84	ECOG P.S. 3 vs. 2 vs. 1 vs. 0; recent weight loss; DTI ≤ 12 months; > 1 metastatic site[†]; prior chemotherapy	Prior nephrectomy	Sex and age; race; prior radiotherapy
Fosså *et al.* 1994	295	1975–90	ECOG P.S. 2, 3 vs. 0, 1; recent weight loss > 10%; DTI ≤ 12 months; elevated ESR[‡]	Metastatic sites; prior nephrectomy; age	Sex
Motzer *et al.* 1999	670	1975–96	ECOG P.S. > 1 vs. ≤ 1; no prior nephrectomy; hemoglobin < 13 g/dl (males), <11.5 g/dl (females); LDH > 300 U/l; corrected calcium > 10 mg/dl	Metastatic sites; DTI; prior chemotherapy[§]; prior radiotherapy[§]; serum albumin[§], and alk. phosphatase[§]	None
Landonio *et al.* 1994	156	1978–93	ECOG P.S. > 2 vs. ≤ 2; DMI < 24 months; > 2 metastatic sites; no prior nephrectomy	Sex	Age
Minasian *et al.* 1993	159	1982–86	ECOG P.S. > 1 vs. 0, 1; no prior nephrectomy	DTI	Sex and age; metastatic sites
Mani *et al.* 1995	84	1983–91	ECOG P.S. 1 vs. 0; bone metastases; sarcomatoid histology	Recent weight loss; prior nephrectomy	Sex, age, and race; DTI; prior chemotherapy; prior radiotherapy
Palmer *et al.* 1992	134	1986–90	ECOG P.S. 1 vs. 0; DTI ≤ 24 months; > 1 metastatic site[¶]	Prior nephrectomy	Sex and age; recent weight loss; prior chemotherapy; prior radiotherapy
Canobbio *et al.* 1995	73	1988–92	ECOG P.S. 1, 2 vs. 0; > 1 metastatic site	DTI	Sex and age; prior nephrectomy; prior chemotherapy
Lopez-Hänninen *et al.* 1996	215	1988–93	Extrapulmonary metastases only; bone metastases; ESR > 70 mm/h; hemoglobin < 10 g/dl; neutrophil count > 6000/ml; LDH > 280 U/l	None	P.S. and weight loss[‖]; DTI[‖]; size of the primary[‖]; prior chemotherapy[‖]; prior nephrectomy[‖]; leukocyte count[‖]; gamma GT[‖]; alk. phosphatase[‖]; CRP[‖]
Citterio *et al.* 1997	109	1988**	ECOG P.S. 2, 3 vs. 0, 1; hemoglobin ≤ 10 g/dl	Prior nephrectomy; DMI; tumor grade; metastatic sites; serum albumin, calcium, LDH, alk. phosphatase	Sex and age; serum creatinine; serum ferritin; serum triglycerides

* Authors used a combination of weight loss and sedimentation rate in multivariate analysis: no weight loss and ESR < 100 mm/h vs. weight loss and/or ESR ≥ 100mm/h.
[†] Number of metastatic sites is based on lung, hepatic, brain, and 'other'.
[‡] Authors analysed ESR as a continuous measure.
[§] Not considered in the multivariate analysis.
[¶] Number of metastatic sites is based on lung, bone, and 'other'.
[‖] Univariate analyses not performed; however, these factors were not associated with survival in the multivariate analysis.
** Date of end of study not specified.

Demographics

Most studies have found no association between survival and demographic factors such as age (Neves *et al.* 1988; Elson *et al.* 1988; Palmer *et al.* 1992; Minasian *et al.* 1993; Landonio *et al.* 1994; Canobbio *et al.* 1995; Mani *et al.* 1995; Citterio *et al.* 1997), sex (de Forges *et al.* 1988; Neves *et al.* 1988; Elson *et al.* 1988; Palmer *et al.* 1992; Minasian *et al.* 1993; Canobbio *et al.* 1995; Mani *et al.* 1995; Citterio *et al.* 1997; Fosså *et al.* 1994), and race (Elson *et al.* 1988; Mani *et al.* 1995). Exceptions to this are an early study of 101 stage IV patients by Klugo *et al.* (1977) that suggested that males have a better prognosis than females and a more recent study by Landonio *et al.* (1994) of 159 patients that, in univariate but not multivariate analyses, suggested that females have a better prognosis.

Performance status and weight loss

Performance status (P.S.) is a subjective measure of overall well-being. One of the most commonly used P.S. scales in cancer is the

Eastern Cooperative Oncology Group (ECOG) score (Oken *et al.* 1982). ECOG P.S. scores range from 0 to 5 (5 indicating death). Asymptomatic patients who have no restrictions on their activities are ECOG P.S. 0, whereas patients who are completely bedridden have an ECOG P.S. of 4. As can be seen from Table 20.1, P.S. is the most consistently reported prognostic factor for survival in advanced RCC (Elson *et al.* 1988; Palmer *et al.* 1992; Minasian *et al.* 1993; Landonio *et al.* 1994; Canobbio *et al.* 1995; Mani *et al.* 1995; Citterio *et al.* 1997; Fosså *et al.* 1994; Motzer *et al.* 1999). Patients with good P.S. (ECOG 0) are reported to have a median survival of 10–21 months (Elson *et al.* 1988; Palmer *et al.* 1992; Canobbio *et al.* 1995; Mani *et al.* 1995), whereas median survival is only 2–7 months for patients with relatively poor P.S. (ECOG > 1) (Elson *et al.* 1988; Minasian *et al.* 1993; Citterio *et al.* 1997; Motzer *et al.* 1999). The prognostic value of P.S., however, is not a universal finding. de Forges *et al.* (1988), for example, found P.S. to be of prognostic value in univariate, but not multivariate analysis of 134 patients treated with chemotherapy or hormonal therapy between 1971 and 1986. Similarly, after correcting for sites of metastatic disease pretreatment laboratory measurements (erythrocyte sedimentation rate (ESR), lactate dehydrogenase (LDH), and neutrophil count) Lopez-Hänninen *et al.* (1996) failed to find an association between P.S. and survival in 215 patients treated with interleukin 2 (IL-2)-based therapies.

Recent weight loss is a presenting symptom of many patients with advanced RCC. Like P.S. it can also be considered a measure of general health, and a number of studies have identified it as a important prognostic factor (de Forges *et al.* 1988; Neves *et al.* 1988; Elson *et al.* 1988; Fosså *et al.* 1994). Recent weight loss and P.S., however, are correlated and, therefore, when viewed independently they each may appear to be of prognostic value simply because they are both measuring aspects of the same feature, that is, general health. Studies by Elson *et al.* (1988) and Fosså *et al.* (1994), however, found weight loss to be an independent predictor of survival even after correcting for the effects of P.S.. As with P.S., the prognostic value of weight loss is not a universal finding, and several reports have found no association at all with survival (Palmer *et al.* 1992; Lopez-Hänninen *et al.* 1996) or an association in univariate but not multivariate analyses (Mani *et al.* 1995). Possible explanations for these contradictory findings are the correlation between weight loss and P.S. described above and patient selection. The reports by de Forges *et al.* (1988) and Elson *et al.* (1988), for example, included good and poor P.S. patients (ECOG P.S. 0–3) and almost half the patients in each study, 44 and 47 per cent, respectively, presented with at least some recent weight loss. In contrast, the studies by Palmer *et al.* (1992) and Mani *et al.* (1995) included only patients with good P.S. (ECOG 0, 1) and relatively few patients had a history of recent weight loss (11 and 15 per cent, respectively).

Other presenting symptoms and biochemical factors

In addition to P.S. and weight loss, investigators have also evaluated the effects on survival of inflammatory parameters such as ESR, anemia, blood counts, and laboratory measures such as serum LDH, calcium, and alkaline phosphatase.

A consistent finding in studies that have evaluated inflammatory parameters is that elevated pretreatment ESR is a poor prognostic factor for survival in advanced RCC. Ljungberg *et al.* (1995), for example, evaluated ESR and several serum markers, C-reactive protein (CRP), haptoglobin, ferritin, orosomucid, and α1-antitrypsin in a series of 170 patients with RCC. All six acute phase reactants were found to be correlated with each other and with survival in univariate analyses. However, in a multivariate analysis only ESR ($\geq$ 54 vs. < 54 mm/hour) was found to provide additional independent prognostic information after adjusting for tumor stage and grade ($p = 0.01$). Lopez-Hänninen *et al.* (1996) observed similar results in that patients with an ESR > 70 mm/hour had poorer survival than patients with an ESR $\leq$ 70 mm/hour ($p < 0.001$) and CRP was not associated with survival once ESR was accounted for in a multivariate analysis. Hoffmann *et al.* (1999), on the other hand, found both elevated ESR ($\geq$ 70 mm/hour) and elevated CRP ($\geq$ 8 mg/ml) to be independent predictors of poor survival ($p = 0.02$ in both cases). Other investigators evaluating only ESR (deForges *et al.* 1988; Fosså *et al.* 1994; Wittke *et al.* 1999), and using different cutpoints ($\geq$ 100 mm/hour, the uncoded ESR measurement, and $\geq$ 50 mm/hour, respectively) have also found it to be an independent predictor of survival.

Anemia has also consistently, though not universally, been found to negatively impact on survival in the studies in which it has been evaluated. Citterio *et al.* (1997), Lopez-Hänninen *et al.* (1996), and Wittke *et al.* (1999) all found pretreatment hemoglobin < 10 g/dl to be an independent predictor of poor survival. Correcting for other important prognostic factors, patients presenting with low hemoglobin levels had an approximately 20 per cent greater risk of death than patients with normal hemoglobins (Citterio *et al.* 1997; Wittke *et al.* 1999). Similarly, in a large series of 670 patients treated at Memorial Sloan–Kettering Cancer Center between 1975 and 1996 Motzer *et al.* (1999) found patients with pretreatment hemoglobin below the lower limit of normal (< 13 g/dl for males and < 11.5 g/dl for females) to have approximately twice the risk of death as patients with normal hemoglobin levels ($p < 0.001$) after adjusting for P.S., prior nephrectomy, elevated LDH, and corrected serum calcium levels. A study by Hoffmann *et al.* (1999), however, found no association between hemoglobin levels and survival in univariate or multivariate analyses.

Other hematological and biochemical factors that have been studied on a more limited basis include pretreatment serum LDH and calcium and pretreatment neutrophil count. Results for these factors have been mixed. In the study described above by Motzer *et al.* (1999) elevated levels of LDH (> 300 U/L) and calcium (> 10 mg/dl—corrected to represent free calcium) were identified as independent predictors of poor survival. Wittke *et al.* (1999) also identified LDH ($\geq$ 240 U/l) as an independent predictor, and Lopez-Hänninen *et al.* (1996) found LDH levels > 280 U/l and absolute neutrophil counts > 6000/μl to be prognostic. Hoffman *et al.* (1999), on the other hand, found neither serum LDH nor neutrophil count to impact on survival in multivariate analysis, although both factors were prognostic in univariate analyses. Citterio *et al.* (1997) similarly found no effect for LDH or calcium levels.

Biochemical factors that have been studied in a very limited capacity and found not to be of prognostic value include, serum levels of alkaline phosphatase (Citterio *et al.* 1997; Lopez-Hänninen *et al.* 1996; Seaman *et al.* 1996), creatinine (Citterio *et al.* 1997), albumin (Citterio *et al.* 1997), triglycerides (Citterio *et al.* 1997), gamma GT (Lopez-Hänninen *et al.* 1996), and β_2 microglobulin (Rasmuson *et al.* 1996).

Prior treatment

There is little evidence to suggest that prior radiotherapy influences survival in advanced RCC. The few studies that have examined the impact of prior radiotherapy have not found any correlation with survival (Elson *et al.* 1988; Palmer *et al.* 1992; Mani *et al.* 1995). Motzer *et al.* (1999), however, did find prior radiotherapy to be associated with poor survival in a univariate analysis. It was not, however, included as a factor in their multivariate analysis. Similarly, most studies that have evaluated prior chemotherapy have failed to find it of prognostic significance (Palmer *et al.* 1992; Canobbio *et al.* 1995; Mani *et al.* 1995; Lopez-Hänninen *et al.* 1996). However, in a review of 610 patients treated on phase II chemotherapy/hormonal therapy trials conducted by the ECOG between 1975 and 1984, Elson *et al.* (1988) found prior chemotherapy to be an independent predictor of survival after adjusting for P.S., weight loss, time from initial diagnosis to treatment for metastatic disease (DTI), and metastatic sites. Motzer *et al.* (1999) also found prior chemotherapy to be associated with poor survival in a univariate analysis. However, it was not included as a factor in their multivariate analysis, and therefore its true relation to survival is unclear. The value of prior nephrectomy as an independent prognostic factor for survival is also unclear. Several multivariate analyses (Minasian *et al.* 1993; Landonio *et al.* 1994; Motzer *et al.* 1999) have found it to be an independent predictor of improved survival. It has also been associated with improved survival in several univariate analyses (de Forges *et al.* 1988; Elson *et al.* 1988; Palmer *et al.* 1992; Mani *et al.* 1995; Citterio *et al.* 1997; Fosså *et al.* 1994). However, in these studies prior nephrectomy lost its prognostic significance once other important predictors were accounted for in multivariate analyses. Canobbio *et al.* (1995) found no association at all between prior nephrectomy and survival in a series of 73 patients treated with IL-2 and interferon α (IFNα).

Disease-related factors

Several features of RCC metastases have been extensively studied as potential prognostic factors. These include the sites of metastases, the number of involved metastatic sites, and metastasis-free interval as measured by either the time from initial diagnosis to the development of metastatic disease (DMI) or the DTI.

Common sites of metastatic spread in RCC are the lungs, liver, bone, adrenal gland, and brain (Figlin 1999). As can be seen from Table 20.1, most studies have found metastatic spread to be an important prognostic factor for survival. However, there is little consensus regarding the predictive value of individual sites. Some studies have found the presence of lung (de Forges *et al.* 1988; Elson *et al.* 1988; Palmer *et al.* 1992; Landonio *et al.* 1994), liver

(de Forges *et al.* 1988; Neves *et al.* 1988; Elson *et al.* 1988; Motzer *et al.* 1999), bone (Palmer *et al.* 1992; Landonio *et al.* 1994; Mani *et al.* 1995; Lopez-Hänninen *et al.* 1996), or brain metastases (Elson *et al.* 1988; Landonio *et al.* 1994) to be associated with poor survival while others have found no relationship between these sites and prognosis (lung (Neves *et al.* 1988; Mani *et al.* 1995; Fosså *et al.* 1994; Motzer *et al.* 1999; Lopez-Hänninen *et al.* 1996; Hoffmann *et al.* 1999; Wittke *et al.*1999), liver (Palmer *et al.* 1992; Landonio *et al.* 1994; Mani *et al.* 1995; Fosså *et al.* 1994; Motzer *et al.* 1999; Lopez-Hänninen *et al.* 1996; Hoffmann *et al.* 1999; Wittke *et al.*1999), bone (de Forges *et al.* 1988; Neves *et al.* 1988; Elson *et al.* 1988; Minasian *et al.* 1993; Motzer *et al.* 1999; Hoffmann *et al.* 1999; Wittke *et al.*1999), brain (de Forges *et al.* 1988; Hoffmann *et al.* 1999; Wittke *et al.*1999)). A more consistent finding is that the number of metastatic sites present, which can be thought of as a crude surrogate for tumor burden, is a negative predictor of survival. Correcting for other important factors, most studies have found that prognosis is inversely correlated with the number of metastatic sites present (Neves *et al.* 1988; Elson *et al.* 1988; Palmer *et al.* 1992; Landonio *et al.* 1994; Canobbio *et al.* 1995). Palmer *et al.* (1992), Landonio *et al.* (1994), and Canobbio *et al.* (1995) estimated the risk of dying to be 2–4-fold greater in patients with more than one site of metastatic disease compared to those with only a single site of involvement (> 2 sites in the study by Landonio *et al.*). Elson *et al.* (1988) estimated a 40 per cent greater risk if multiple sites were involved. This finding has not been universal, however, and studies by Minasian *et al.* (1993) and Citterio *et al.* (1997) found no association between the number of metastatic sites and survival.

Similarly to the location and number of involved metastatic sites, the evidence supporting metastasis-free interval as an independent prognostic factor has been mixed. As can be seen from Table 20.1, several studies (de Forges *et al.* 1988; Elson *et al.* 1988; Palmer *et al.* 1992; Landonio *et al.* 1994; Fosså *et al.* 1994) have found a 'short' DMI or DTI to be predictive of poor survival in multivariate analyses, while others have found it to be prognostic only in univariate analyses (Minasian *et al.* 1993; Canobbio *et al.* 1995; Citterio *et al.* 1997; Motzer *et al.* 1999), or not at all (Mani *et al.* 1995). Several different cut-points were used in these studies to define a short metastasis-free interval including metastases within 2 years of diagnosis (Palmer *et al.* 1992; Landonio *et al.* 1994; Citterio *et al.* 1997), 1 year (Elson *et al.* 1988; Minasian *et al.* 1993; Canobbio *et al.* 1995; Mani *et al.* 1995; Fosså *et al.* 1994; Motzer *et al.* 1999), and concurrent with the initial diagnosis (de Forges *et al.* 1988). Despite these differences, the studies in which metastasis-free interval was identified as an independent predictor of survival had qualitatively similar results in that patients with a short metastasis-free interval had a 50–90 per cent greater risk of dying than patients with longer intervals.

In addition to the extent of metastatic disease and metastasis-free interval, several investigators have also examined the prognostic value of tumor size, right versus left-sided primaries, histology, tumor grade, nuclear morphology, and DNA content.

Location of the primary tumor does not appear to influence survival (Neves *et al.* 1988); however, tumor size may. In a retrospective review of 2473 patients diagnosed with RCC between 1975 and 1985 Guinan *et al.* (1995) found survival to be inversely correlated with tumor size regardless of the tumor stage. Estimated 5-year survival rates for 441 stage IV patients were 28 per cent if the primary was < 5 cm, and 10–20 per cent for tumors greater than 5 cm ($p = 0.02$). In contrast, multivariate analyses by Neves *et al.* (1988) and Lopez-Hänninen *et al.* (1996) found no relationship between tumor size and survival once other important predictors were accounted for.

Several studies have examined the impact of histology on survival. Mani *et al.* (1995) reported that patients with sarcomatoid tumors had significantly worse survival than patients with other histologies. However, only five of the 84 patients studied in that series had a sarcomatoid variant. Similar findings, however, were reported in a recent study by Kanamaru *et al.* (1999) in which 34/106 patients had a sarcomatoid component present. Correcting for other important factors, such as the presence or absence of metastatic disease, Kanamaru *et al.* reported that the presence of a sarcomatoid histology was associated with an approximately threefold increase in the risk of death ($p = 0.02$). de Forges *et al.* (1988) and Neves *et al.* (1988), on the other hand, found no relationship between survival and histology. The distribution of RCC subtypes was not, however, fully described in these studies.

Tumor DNA content has been found to be of prognostic value in a number of cancers (Silvestrini 2000); however, its value in advanced RCC is unclear. Several investigators have reported the presence of aneuploid tumors to be negatively correlated with survival (Ljungberg *et al.* 1996; Ruiz-Cerda *et al.* 1999). Others, however, have found no association between prognosis and ploidy status (Nakano *et al.* 1993; Lanigan *et al.* 1993), or that aneuploidy has a positive impact on survival (Eskelinen *et al.* 1995). A possible explanation for these contradictory results is that RCC is a heterogeneous tumor and, therefore, the likelihood of defining a tumor as diploid or not is highly dependent on the number of samples taken (Ljungberg *et al.* 1996; Ruiz-Cerda *et al.* 1999).

Investigations of tumor grade have had mixed results. Neves *et al.* (1988), for example, found patients with advanced RCC and high-grade tumors to have a significantly poorer prognosis than patients with well differentiated tumors ($p < 0.001$). Citterio *et al.* (1997), however, found no association between grade and survival once the effects of P.S. and baseline hemoglobin were accounted for. Tumor grade as a potential prognostic factor has been criticized because of the subjectivity associated with its evaluation and the various systems employed (Lanigan *et al.* 1994). This has led a number of investigators to suggest assessing nuclear morphology using more quantitative measures that describe the size of the nuclei and/or their shape. The proposed size parameters include nuclear perimeter or area, length of the major and minor axes, and a measure of average nuclear volume (MNV). The shape parameters that have been studied are primarily measures of the extent to which the contours of the nuclei deviate from a perfect circle. Many of these parameters are correlated with histopathological factors such as stage and grade and, in univariate analyses, with survival (Ruiz *et al.* 1995; van der Poel *et al.* 1993; Delahunt *et al.* 1994; Artacho-Pérula *et al.* 1994; Soda *et al.* 1999). Most studies, however, have not evaluated the same set of parameters and the results of multivariate analyses have been mixed. Ruiz *et al.* (1995), for example, evaluated nuclear area, perimeter, length of the major and minor axes, and a shape factor, and found none

that were prognostic in patients with advanced disease. Similarly van der Poel *et al.* (1993) found a measure of chromatin 'texture', but no size or shape parameters to be prognostic. Delahunt *et al.* (1994), on the other hand, found departures from nuclear 'roundness' to be the only independent predictor of survival after adjusting for other important factors such as disease stage, and Artacho-Pérula *et al.* (1994) found only MNV to be important. Soda *et al.* (1999), evaluating only MNV, also found it to be of prognostic value after adjusting for disease stage and grade.

Cytogenetics

Few studies have examined the relationship between chromosomal abnormalities and survival in RCC. However, reports by Wu *et al.* (1996), Moch *et al.* (1996), and Elfving *et al.* (1997) of small series of patients suggest that indicators of genetic instability may be of prognostic value. For example, in a study of 30 nonpapillary RCC, Wu *et al.* found that loss of the long arm of chromosome 14 was associated with poor survival. Moch *et al.*, on the other hand, found loss of chromosome 9p, but not 14q to be associated with a poor outcome. Moch *et al.* also found that patients with a total of three or more chromosomal deletions had a poorer prognosis than patients with fewer than three deletions. Similarly, in a series of 50 consecutive RCC patients Elfving *et al.* (1997) reported patients with six or more chromosomal aberrations (deletions, additions, and translocations) to have shorter recurrence-free survival than patients with fewer than six aberrations.

Immunological factors

The ability to mount an effective immune response to RCC is dependent on the activation of T lymphocytes following presentation of tumor-associated antigens by antigen-presenting cells (APC) (Altman *et al.* 1990). Interleukin 10 (IL-10) is an immunosuppressive cytokine that has been shown to downregulate major histocompatibility complex (MHC) class I and II molecules on APC, thereby leading to impaired antigen presentation (Wittke *et al.* 1999). It also has a direct inhibitory effect on the growth of T lymphocytes (Taga *et al.* 1993). IL-6 is a multifunctional cytokine that has a number of immunoregulatory and proinflammatory effects including regulation of T- and B-lymphocyte differentiation and induction of acute phase protein genes, such as the CRP gene (Blay *et al.* 1992). Both IL-10 and IL-6 are secreted by RCC (Knoefel *et al.* 1997) and several investigators have evaluated the prognostic value of their levels in serum. A recent study by Wittke *et al.* (1999) found serum IL-10 levels greater than 1 pg/ml to be an independent predictor of poor survival after correcting for the effects of elevated ESR, LDH, and anemia. Similarly, studies by Blay *et al.* (1992) and Ljungberg *et al.* (1997) reported elevated serum levels of IL-6 to have a negative impact on survival. In the study by Blay *et al.*, for example, patients with detectable IL-6 levels ($n = 66$) had a median survival of 8 months compared to 16 months for patients ($n = 72$) without detectable levels ($p < 0.03$). Ljungberg *et al.* (1997), studying 66 stage IV patients and 130 patients with non-metastatic disease found serum IL-6 levels above 8.3 ng/l to be a negative predictor of survival in a univariate analysis of the stage IV patients. However, IL-6 lost its prognostic significance in a multivariate analysis, after correcting for stage, grade, and ESR. As might be expected, IL-6 levels were correlated with serum CRP levels in both studies and with ESR in the study by Ljungberg et al. (1997).

In addition to cytokine levels, several investigators have evaluated the prognostic value of monitoring peripheral blood lymphocyte subsets before and/or after treatment with interferon-based therapies. Göhring et al. (1996) found the absolute numbers of CD4$^+$ and CD8$^+$ T lymphocytes and B lymphocytes prior to the start of treatment to be positively correlated with response while no relationship was observed for pretreatment natural killer (NK) cells or the CD4$^+$/CD8$^+$ ratio. Hernberg et al. (1997), on the other hand, found an increasing CD4$^+$/CD8$^+$ ratio during treatment with vinblastine plus IFNα to be correlated with response and improved survival.

Markers of cell proliferation, apoptosis, and metastasis

Tumor growth and metastasis are dependent on numerous factors including the balance between cellular proliferation and death, the ability of tumor cells to detach from the main lesion and invade the vascular system, and the ability to stimulate the formation of new blood vessels. In recent years the prognostic value of various markers of these processes in RCC have begun to be studied.

Ki-67 and proliferative cell nuclear antigen (PCNA) are nuclear antigens expressed during the G_1, S, G_2, and M (Ki-67) phases of the cell cycle that have been studied as markers of cell proliferation. Silver-binding nucleolar organizer regions (AgNOR) are DNA loops that transcribe to ribosomal RNA, and are also thought to be indicators of proliferative activities (Tannapfel et al. 1996). Studies of Ki-67 immunostainig have consistently, but not universally, found it to be of prognostic value in RCC. Tannapfel et al. (1996) and Delahunt et al. (1995), for example, evaluated all three markers in patients with stages I–IV disease, and Aaltomaa et al. (1999) studied Ki-67 and PCNA. All three investigators found Ki-67 labeling index (LI—that is, the proportion of cells staining positively for Ki-67 antibody) to be negatively correlated with survival, even after correcting for the effects of stage. Other investigators evaluating only Ki-67 have reported similar results (Yoshino et al. 2000; Rioux-Leclercq et al. 2000). Moch et al. (1997a), on the other hand, found Ki-67 LI to be highly correlated with p53 expression ($p < 0.001$) but not with survival after adjusting for p53 overexpression. Studies of PCNA immunostaining and AgNOR counts have had mixed results. Delahunt et al. (1995) found both PCNA index and AgNOR counts to be independent predictors of survival. Lipponen et al. (1994) and Fischer et al. (1999) also found PCNA to be an important predictor, but only of disease-free survival. Tannapfel et al. (1996), however, found neither marker to be of independent prognostic value, possibly because both were highly correlated with Ki-67. Similarly, Aaltomaa et al. (1999) found no association between PCNA and survival after adjusting for the Ki-67 LI, and Yang et al. (1992) found no prognostic value for AgNOR.

Epidermal growth factor receptor (EGFR) is a transmembrane receptor for several growth factors including epidermal growth factor (EGF) and transforming growth factor alpha (TGFα) (Moch et al. 1997b; Uhlman et al. 1995). c-erb-B2 (HER-2/neu) encodes a transmembrane protein that has structural similarities to EGFR (Lipponen et al. 1994; Rasmuson et al. 1997). Overexpression of both of these proteins has been linked to increased cell proliferation; however, their prognostic value in RCC is unclear. Studies by Moch et al. (1997b), Lipponen et al. (1994), and Rasmuson et al. (1997), for example, found no association between EGFR or c-erbB-2 expression and survival, whereas Uhlman et al. (1995) found strong immunostaining for EFGR to be correlated with high-grade tumors, the presence of metastatic disease, and, in univariate analysis, survival.

Markers of cell cycle regulation and programmed cell death, or apoptosis, that have been evaluated as potential prognostic factors in RCC include immunohistochemical assessment of p53, bcl-2, c-myc, and retinoblastoma (Rb) gene products, and measurement of apoptotic bodies using the (TUNEL) assay. p53 protein is the marker that has been most extensively studied. p53 is a tumor suppressor gene that acts by arresting cell growth in the G_1 phase of mitosis in response to DNA damage (Uhlman et al. 1994; Shiina et al. 1997). In contrast to wild-type p53, p53 mutation leads to production of a protein that can be detected immunohistochemically. Though somewhat controversial, detection of the p53 protein is associated with mutated p53 and loss of its normal function, which can lead to increased cell proliferation and reduced apoptosis (Pepe et al. 2000). In RCC, assessment of p53 as a prognostic factor has had mixed results. Studies by Moch et al. (1997a) and Shiina et al. (1997), for example, found p53 expression to be correlated with tumor grade and, in multivariate analyses, was an independent predictor of poor survival. Uhlman et al. (1994) also found a positive correlation between p53 expression and grade and a negative correlation with survival. The effect on survival of p53 expression, however, was restricted to patients without metastatic disease ($n = 119$, $p < 0.01$). There was no impact on survival in patients with metastatic disease ($n = 45$, $p = 0.43$). In contrast to these studies, Lipponen et al. (1994) and Bot et al. (1994) found no association between p53 expression and survival or histopathological characteristics such as grade.

Rb is also a tumor suppressor gene and bcl-2 and c-myc are genes that play important roles in directing a cell toward either apoptosis or mitosis. Lipponen et al. (1995) evaluated expression of these genes in 26 patients with metastatic RCC and 78 patients with non-metastatic disease. None of the genes was found to be an independent predictor of survival in multivariate analysis after taking into account T-stage, nuclear grade, and mitotic index. Similarly, a recent study by Yoshino et al. (2000) of 96 RCC patients, 33 of whom had metastatic disease, failed to find an association between apoptotic index (that is, the proportion of cells staining positive by TUNEL assay) and survival after adjusting for stage, grade, Ki-67 LI, and microvessel density.

The first steps towards metastasis are the detachment of tumor cells from the primary tumor and their subsequent entrance into the circulation. These processes are mediated by several classes of cell adhesion molecules, such as the cadherins, integrins, and selectins. Several recent studies have suggested that overexpression (or loss of expression) of these molecules may be associated with a poor prognosis in RCC. Fischer *et al.* (1999), for example, evaluated two cell adhesion molecules, E-cadherin and CD44s, which have opposite effects on tissue integrity, in 137 patients with advanced ($n = 37$) or localized/locally advanced ($n = 100$) RCC. Absence or low expression of E-cadherin and high CD44s expression were found to be associated with poor disease-free survival. Katagiri *et al.* (1995) reported similar results from a study of 106 RCC patients in which absence of E-cadherin expression was correlated with advanced stage, high grade, and, in univariate analysis, poor survival. Similarly, Paradis *et al.* (1999) found positive CD44s immunostaining to be predictive of poor survival in 91 patients with localized disease. Hoffmann *et al.* (1999) evaluated serum levels of several integrins and selectins, soluble intercellular adhesion molecule-1 (sICAM-1), soluble vascular adhesion molecule-1 (sVCAM-1), and E-selectin (sELAM-1) in 99 patients with metastatic disease. Adjusting for the effects of ESR and CRP, sICAM1, but neither sVCAM-1 nor sELAM-1, was found to be an independent predictor of survival, with patients whose serum levels were below 360 ng/ml having significantly better survival than patients with higher levels ($p = 0.001$).

Integral to tumor growth and metastasis is the ability to form new blood vessels. Markers of angiogensis have not yet been extensively evaluated as potential prognostic factors; however, a recent study by Yoshino *et al.* (2000) found a significant negative correlation between microvessel density and survival, even after correcting for the effects of stage, grade, and Ki-67 LI. Jacobsen *et al.* (2000), on the other hand, evaluated vascular endothelial growth factor (VEGF) in164 patients with stage I–IV RCC and found no association between VEGF levels and survival after correcting for stage and grade.

Conclusions

Clinical factors that are easily obtained as part of the normal patient work-up have been extensively evaluated as potential prognostic factors in advanced RCC. Performance status is the most important of these identified to date. It is a subjective measure of overall functional status and clearly open to interpretation. Nevertheless, it has consistently, albeit not universally, been shown to have excellent discriminatory power in numerous studies. With the exception of P.S., most studies that have evaluated clinical factors have examined different groups of them and, therefore, it is difficult to fully assess their value as independent prognostic factors. Despite this, several clinical factors, in addition to P.S., also appear to be of prognostic value. These include weight loss, ESR levels, the presence or absence of anemia, metastasis-free interval, and tumor burden as measured by the number of involved metastatic sites. In addition to these 'classical' prognostic factors, new molecular-based technologies are helping to better define the biology of RCC and identify new prognostic factors. As discussed above, a number of immunological, genetic, and molecular factors are correlated with outcome. Their value as independent prognostic factors needs to be confirmed, however, by examining them uniformly in relatively homogeneous groups of patients and in conjunction with the classical predictors.

References

Aaltomaa, S., Lipponen, P., Ala-Opas, M., Eskelinen, M., Syrjänen, K., and Kosma, V.-M. (1999). Expresson of cyclins A and D and p21[(waf1/cip1)] proteins in renal cell carcinoma and their relation to clinicopathological variables and patient survival. *Br. J. Cancer* **80**, 2001–7.

Altman, A., Cogeshall, K., and Mustelin, T. (1990). Molecular events mediating T cell activation. *Adv. Immunol.* **48**, 227–360.

Artacho-Pérula, E., Roldán-Villalobos, R., Martínez-Cuevas, J.F., and López-Rubio, F. (1994). Nuclear quantitative grading by discriminant analysis of renal cell carcinoma samples. A patient survival evaluation. *J. Pathol.* **173**, 105–14.

Blay, J.-Y., Negrier, S., Combaret, V., Attali, S., Goillot, E., Merrouche, Y., Mercatello, A., Ravault, A., Tourani, J.M., Moskovtchenko, J.F., Philip, T., and Faurot, M. (1992). Serum level of inteleukin 6 as a prognosis factor in metastatic renal cell carcinoma. *Cancer Res.* **52**, 3317, 3322.

Bot, F.J., Godschalk, J.C.J., Krishnadath, K.K., van der Kwast, T.H.M., and Bosman, F.T. (1994). Prognostic factors in renal-cell carcinoma: immuno-histochemical detection of p53 protein versus clinico-pathological parameters. *Int. J. Cancer* **57**, 634–7.

Bukowski, R.M., Rayman, P., Uzzo, R., Bloom, T., Sandstrom, K., Peereboom, D., Olencki, T., Budd, G.T., McLain, D., Elson, P., Novick, A., and Finke, J. (1998).Signal transduction abnormalities in T lymphocytes from patients with advanced renal carcinoma: clinical relevance and effects of cytokine therapy. *Clin. Cancer Res.* **4**, 2337–47.

Canobbio, L., Rubagotti, A., Miglietta, L., Cannata, D., Curotto, A., Amoroso, D., and Boccardo, F. (1995). Prognostic factors for survival in patients with advanced renal cell carcinoma treated with interleukin-2 and interferon-α. *J. Cancer Res. Clin. Oncol.* **121**, 753–6.

Chow, W.H., Devesa, S.S., Warren, J.L., and Fraumeni, J.F. (1999). Rising incidence of renal cell cancer in the United States. *J. Am. Med. Assoc.* **281**, 1628–31.

Citterio, G., Bertuzzi, A., Tresoldi, M., Galli, L., Di Lucca, G., Scaglietti, U., and Rugarli, C. (1997). Prognostic factors for survival in metastatic renal cell carcinoma: retrospective analysis from 109 consecutive patients. *Eur. Urol.* **31**, 286–91.

de Forges, A., Rey, A., Klink, M., Ghosn, M., Kramar, A., and Droz, J.-P. (1988). Prognostic factors of adult metastatic renal carcinoma: a multivariate analysis. *Sem. Surg. Oncol.* **4**, 149–54.

Delahunt, B., Becker, R.L., Bethwaite, P.B., and Ribas, J.L. (1994). Computerized nuclear morphometry and survival in renal cell carcinoma: comparison with other prognostic indicators. *Pathology* **26**, 353–8.

Delahunt, B., Bethwaite, P.B., Thornton, A., and Ribas, J.L. (1995). Proliferation of renal cell carcinoma assessed by fixation-resistant polyclonal Ki-67 antibody labeling. *Cancer* **75**, 2714–19.

Elfving, P., Mandahl, N., Lundgren, R., Limon, J., Bak-Jensen, E., Fernö, M., Olsson, H., and Mitelman, F. (1997). Prognostic implications of cytogenetic findings in kidney cancer. *Br. J. Urol.* **80**, 698–706.

Elson, P.J., Witte, R.S., and Trump, D.L. (1988). Prognostic factors for survival in patients with recurrent or metastatic renal cell carcinoma. *Cancer Res.* **48**, 7310–13.

Eskelinen, M., Lipponen, P., and Nordling, S. (1995). Prognostic evaluation of DNA flow cytometry and histomorphological criteria in renal cell carcinoma. *Anticancer Res.* **15**, 2279–84.

Figlin, R.A. (1999). Renal cell carcinoma: management of advanced disease. *J. Urol.* **161**, 381–7.

Fischer, C., Georg, C.H., Kraus, S., Terpe, H.J., Luedecke, G., and Weidner, W. (1999). CD44s, E-cadherin and PCNA as markers of progression in renal cell carcinoma. *Anticancer Res.* **19**, 1513–18.

Fosså, S.D., Kramar, A., and Droz, J.-P. (1994). Prognostic factors and survival in patients with metastatic renal cell carcinoma treated with chemotherapy or interferon-α > *Eur. J. Cancer* **30**, 1310–14.

Göhring, B., Riemann, D., Rebmann, U., Heynemann, H., Schabel, J., and Langner, J. (1996). Prognostic value of the immunomonitoring of patients with renal cell carcinoma under therapy with IL-2/IFN-α-2 in combination with 5-FU. *Urol. Res.* **24**, 297–303.

Greenlee, R.T., Murray, T., Bolden, S., and Wingo, P.A. (2000). Cancer statistics, 2000. *CA Cancer J. Clin.* **50**, 7–33.

Guinan, P.D., Vogelzang, N.J., Fremgen, A.M., Chmiel, J.S., Sylvester, J.L., Sener, S.F., and Imperato, J.P. (1995). Renal cell carcinoma: tumor size, stage and survival. *J. Urol.* **153**, 901–3.

Hernberg, M., Muhonen, T., and Pyrhönen, S. (1997). Can the CD4+/CD8+ ratio predict the outcome of interferon-α therapy for renal cell carcinoma? *Ann. Oncol.* **8**, 71–7.

Hoffmann, R., Franzke, A., Buer, J., Sel, S., Oevermann, K., Duensing, A., Probst, M., Duensing, S., Kirchner, H., Ganser, A., and Atzpodien, J. (1999). Prognostic impact of *in vivo* soluble cell adhesion molecules in metastatic renal cell carcinoma. *Br. J. Cancer* **79**, 1742–5.

Jacobsen, J., Rasmuson, T., Grankvist, K., and Ljungberg, B. (2000). Vascular endothelial growth factor as prognostic factor in renal cell carcinoma. *J. Urol.* **163**, 343–7.

Kanamaru, H., Sasaki, M., Miwa, Y., Akino, H., and Okada, K. (1999). Prognostic value of sarcomatoid histology and volume-weighted mean nuclear volume in renal cell carcinoma. *BJU Int.* **83**, 222–6.

Katagiri, A.., Watanabe, R., and Tomita, Y. (1995). E-cadherin expression in renal cell cancer and its significance in metastasis and survival. *Br. J. Cancer* **71**, 376–9.

Klugo, R.C., Detmers, M., Stiles, R.E., Talley, R.W., and Cerny, J.C. (1977). Aggressive versus conservative management of stage IV renal cell carcinoma. *J. Urol.* **118**, 244–6.

Knoefel, B., Nuske, K., Steiner, T., Junker, K., Kosmehl, H., Rebstock, K., Reinhold, D., and Junker, U. (1997). Renal cell carcinomas produce IL-6, IL-10, IL-11, and TGF-β1 in primary cultures and modulate T-lymphocyte blast transformation. *J. Interferon Cytokine Res.* **17**, 95–102.

Landonio, G., Baiocchi, C., Cattaneo, D., Ferrari, M., Gottardi, O., Margherita, M., and Ghislandi, E. (1994). Retrospective analysis of 156 cases of metastatic renal cell carcinoma: evaluation of prognostic factors and response to different treatments. *Tumori* **80**, 468–72.

Lanigan, D., McLean, P.A., Murphy, D.M., Donovan, M.G., Curran, B., and Leader, M. (1993). Ploidy and prognosis in renal carcinoma. *Br. J. Urol.* **71**, 21–4.

Lanigan, D., Conroy, R., Barry-Walsh, C., Loftus, B., Royston, D., and Leader, M. (1994). A comparative analysis of grading systems in renal adenocarcinoma. *Histopathology* **24**, 473–6.

Linehan, M.W., Shipley, W.U., and Parkinson, D.R. (1997). Cancer of the kidney and ureter. In *Cancer: principles and practice of oncology*, 5th edn (ed. V.T. DeVita, S. Hellman, and S.A. Rosenberg). Lippincott–Raven Publishers, Philadelphia.

Lipponen, P., Eskelinen, M., Hietala, K., and Syrjännen, K. (1994). Expression of proliferating cell nuclear antigen (PC10), p53 protein and c-erbB-2 in renal adenocarcinoma. *Int. J. Cancer* **57**, 275–80.

Lipponen, P., Eskelinen, M., and Syrännen, K. (1995). Expression of tumour-suppressor gene Rb, apoptosis-suppressing protein Bcl-2, and c-Myc have no independent prognostic value in renal cell adenocarcinoma. *Br. J. Cancer* **71**, 863–7.

Ljungberg, B., Grankvist, K., and Rasmuson, T. (1995). Serum acute phase reactants and prognosis in renal cell carcinoma. *Cancer* **76**, 1435–9.

Ljungberg, B., Mehle, C., Stenling, R., and Roos, G. (1996). Heterogeneity in renal cell carcinoma and its impact on prognosis—a flow cytometric study. *Br. J. Cancer* **74**, 123–7.

Ljungberg, B., Grankvist, K., and Rasmuson, T. (1997). Serum inteleukin-6 in relation to acute-phase reactants and survival in patients with renal cell carcinoma. *Eur. J. Cancer* **33**, 1794–8.

Lopez-Hänninen, E., Kirchner, H., and Atzpodien, J. (1996). Interleukin-2 based home therapy of metastatic renal cell carcinoma: risks and benefits in 215 consecutive single institution patients. *J. Urol.* **155**, 19–25.

Mani, S., Todd, M.B., Katz, K., and Poo W.-J. (1995). Prognostic factors for survival in patients with metastatic renal cancer treated with biological response modifiers. *J. Urol.* **154**, 35–40.

Minasian, L.M., Motzer, R.J., Gluck, L., Mazumdar, M., Vlamis, V., and Krown, S.E. (1993). Interferon alfa-2a in advanced renal cell carcinoma: treatment results and survival in 159 patients with long-term follow-up. *J. Clin. Oncol.* **11**, 1368–75.

Moch, H., Presti, J.C., Sauter, G., Buchholz, N., Jordan, P., Mihatsch, M.J., and Waldman, F.M. (1996). Genetic aberrations detected by comparative genomic hybridization are associated with clinical outcome in renal cell carcinoma. *Cancer Res.* **56**, 27–30.

Moch, H., Sauter, G., Gasser, T.C., Buchholz, N., Bubendorf, L., Richter, J., Jiang, F., Dellas, A., and Mihatch, M.J. (1997*a*). p53 protein expression but not mdm-2 protein expression is associated with rapid tumor cell proliferation and prognosis in renal cell carcinoma. *Urol. Res.* **25** (suppl. 1), 25–30.

Moch, H., Sauter, G., Buchholz, N., Gasser, T.C., Bubendorf, L., Waldman, F.M., and Mihatsch, M.J. (1997*b*). Epidermal growth factor receptor expression is associated with rapid tumor cell proliferation in renal cell carcinoma. *Hum. Pathol.* **28**, 1255–9.

Motzer, R.J., Mazumdar, M., Bacik, J., Berg, W., Amsterdam, A., and Ferrara, J. (1999). Survival and prognostic stratification of 670 patients with advanced renal cell carcinoma. *J. Clin. Oncol.* **17**, 2530–40.

Nakano, E., Kondoh, M., Okatani, K., Seguchi, T., and Sugao, H. (1993). Flow cytometric analysis of nuclear DNA content in renal cell carcinoma correlated with histologic and clinical features. *Cancer* **72**, 1319–23.

Neves, R.J., Zincke, H., and Taylor, W.F. (1988). Metastatic renal cell cancer and radical nephrectomy: identification of prognostic factors and patient survival. *J. Urol.* **139**, 1173–6.

Oken, M.M., Creech, R.H., Tormey, D.C., Horton, J., Davis, T.E., McFadden, E.T., and Carbone, P.P. (1982). Toxicity and response criteria of the Eastern Cooperative Oncology Group. *Am. J. Clin. Oncol.* **5**, 649–55.

Palmer, P.A., Vinke, J., Philip, T., Negrier, S., Atzpodien, J., Kirchner, H., Oskam, R., and Franks, C.R. (1992). Prognostic factors for survival in patients with advanced renal cell carcinoma treated with recombinant interleukin-2. *Ann. Oncol.* **3**, 475–80.

Paradis, V., Ferlicot, S., Ghannam, E., Zeimoura, L., Blanchet, P., Eschwege, P., Jardin, A., Benoit, G., and Bedossa, P. (1999). CD44 is an independent prognostic factor in conventional renal cell carcinomas. *J. Urol.* **161**, 1984–7.

Pepe, S., Ruggiero, A., D'Acquisto, M., De Laurentiis, S., Sandomenico, C., Staibano, S., De Rosa, G., Lucariello, A., D'Armiento, M., and Bianco, A. (2000). Nuclear DNA content-derived parameters correlated with heterogeneous expression of p53 and bcl-2 proteins in clear cell renal carcinomas. *Cancer* **89**, 1065–75.

Rasmuson, T., Grankvist, K., and Ljungberg, B. (1996). Serum β_2-microglobulin and prognosis of patients with renal cell carcinoma. *Acta Oncol.* **35**, 479–82.

Rasmuson, T., Grankvist, K., and Ljungberg, B. (1997). Soluble ectodomain of c-*erb*B-2 oncoprotein in relation to tumour stage and grade in human renal cell carcinoma. *Br. J. Cancer* **75**, 1674–7.

Rioux-Leclercq, N., Turlin, B., Bansard, J., Patard, J., Manunta, A., Moulinoux, J., Guille, F., Ramee, M., and Lobel, B. (2000). Value of immunohistochemical Ki-67 and p53 determinations as predictive factors of outcome in renal cell carcinoma. *Urology* **55**, 501–5.

Ruiz, J.L., Hernandez, M., Martinez, J., Vera, C., and Jimenez-Cruz, J.F. (1995). Value of morphometry as an independent prognostic factor in renal cell carcinoma. *Eur. Urol.* **27**, 54–7.

Ruiz-Cerda, J.L., Hernandez, M., Sempere, A., O'Connor, J.E., Kimler, B.F., and Jimenez-Cruz, F. (1999). Intratumoral heterogeneity of DNA content in renal cell carcinoma and its prognostic significance. *Cancer* **86**, 664–71.

Seaman, E., Goluboff, E.T., Ross, S., and Sawczuk, I.S. (1996). Association of radionuclide bone scan and serum alkaline phosphatase in patients with metastatic renal cell carcinoma. *Urology* **48**, 692–5.

Shiina, H., Igawa, M., Urakami, S., Shirakawa, H., Ishibe, T., and Kawanishi, M. (1997). Clinical significance of immunohistochemically detectable p53 protein in renal cell carcinoma. *Eur. Urol.* **31**, 73–80.

Silvestrini, R. (2000). Relevance of DNA-ploidy as a prognostic instrument for solid tumors. *Ann. Oncol.* **11**, 259–61.

Soda, T., Fujikawa, K., Ito, T., Sasaki, Nishio, Y., and Miyakawa, M. (1999). Volume-weighted mean nuclear volume as a prognostic factor in renal cell carcinoma. *Lab. Invest.* **79**, 859–67.

Taga, K.H., Mostowski, H., and Tosato, G. (1993). Human interleukin-10 can directly inhibit T cell growth. *Blood* **81**, 2964–71.

Tannapfel, A., Hahn, H.A., Katalinic, A., Fietkau, R.J., Kühn, R., and Wittekind, C.W. (1996). Prognostic value of ploidy and proliferation markers in renal cell carcinoma. *Cancer* **77**, 164–71.

Uhlman, D.L., Nguyen, P.L., Manivel, J.C., Aeppli, D., Resnick, J.M., Fraley, E.E., Zhang, G., and Niehans, G.A. (1994). Association of immunohistochemical staining for p53 with metastatic progression and poor survival in patients with renal cell carcinoma. *J. Natl Cancer Inst.* **86**, 1470–75.

Uhlman, D.L., Nguyen, P., Manivel, J.C., Zhang, G., Hagen, K., Fraley, E., Aeppli, D., and Niehans, G.A. (1995). Epidermal growth factor receptor and transforming growth factor α expression in papillary and non-papillary renal cell carcinoma: correlation with metastatic behavior and prognosis. *Clin. Cancer Res.* **1**, 913–20.

Uzzo, R.G., Rayman, P., Kolenko, V., Clark, P.E., Bloom, T., Ward, A.M., Molto, L., Tannenbaum, C., Worford, L.J., Bukowski, R., Tubbs, R., His, E.D., Bander, N.H., Novick, A.C., and Finke, J.H. (1999). Mechanisms of apop-tosis in T cells from patients with renal cell carcinoma. *Clin. Cancer Res.* **5**, 1219–29.

van der Poel, H.G., Mulders, P.F.A., Oosterhof, G.O.N., Schaafsma, H.E., Hendriks, J.C.M., Schalken, J.A., and Debruyne, F.M.J. (1993). Prognostic value of karyometric and clinical characteristics in renal cell carcinoma. *Cancer* **72**, 2667–74.

Wittke, F., Hoffman, R., Buer, J., Dallmann, I., Oevermann, K., Sel, S., Wandert, T., Ganser, A., and Atzpodien, J. (1999). Interleukin 10 (IL-10): an immunosuppressive factor and independent predictor in patients with metastatic renal cell carcinoma. *Br. J. Cancer* **79**, 1182–4.

Wu, S.-Q., Hafez, G.R., Xing, W., Newton, M., Chen, X.-R., and Messing, E. (1996). The correlation between the loss of chromosome 14q with histologic tumor grade, pathologic stage, and outcome of patients with nonpapillary renal cell carcinoma. *Cancer* **77**, 1154–60.

Yang, A.H., Wang, T.Y., and Liu, H.C. (1992). Comparative study of the prognostic value of nuclear grade and silver binding nucleolar organizer region in renal cell carcinomas. *J. Pathol.* **166**, 157–61.

Yoshino, S., Kato, M., and Okada, K. (2000). Clinical significance of angio-genesis, proliferation, and apoptosis in renal cell carcinoma. *Anticancer Res.* **20**, 591–4.

Part 1, Section 3

Renal cell carcinoma: imaging and management

21. Evaluation of the renal mass and the role of renal biopsy

Ojas Shah and Samir S. Taneja

The evaluation of the renal mass has changed dramatically in recent years, largely due to the availability of imaging modalities such as ultrasound, computerized tomography (CT), and magnetic resonance imaging (MRI). In addition to enhancing our ability to evaluate known renal masses, these imaging techniques have changed the means by which most tumors are diagnosed. The number of tumors incidentally noted on radiologic examination for unrelated symptoms has increased with the increasing use of advanced radiologic imaging over the last 40 years (Rodriguez *et al.* 1995) (see Table 21.1). As such, our evaluation of the renal mass is very different from what it was 20 years ago. In this chapter, we discuss the important aspects of renal mass evaluation including a review of available diagnostic imaging modalities, differential diagnosis, and the role of invasive diagnostic techniques.

Renal mass presentation/detection

It is clear that the means by which renal masses are detected have changed dramatically in the last 20 years. In our institution, the large majority of masses are noted in asymptomatic individuals upon routine radiologic exam. This clearly has resulted in a stage migration at diagnosis as well as an impact upon the ability to treat renal tumors at the time of presentation. At our institution, 5 per cent of renal cell carcinomas (RCC) were less than 3 cm in size and 32 per cent of patients presented with metastases in the 1970s. Ten years later, when the use of newer imaging techniques increased, many RCC were detected incidentally and 25 per cent

Table 21.1 Comparison of percentage of renal masses discovered incidentally over the last 40 years*

Reference	Year ending	Total no. of cases	Incidental (%)
Riches *et al.* (1951)	1951	1746	4
Skinner *et al.* (1971)	1971	309	7
Konnack and Grossman (1985)	1973	56	13
Konnack and Grossman (1985)	1984	46	48
Lanctin and Futter (1990)	1986	202	40
Sigalow *et al.* (1991)	1987	105	47
Mevorach *et al.* (1992)	1987	235	28.5
Tsukamoto *et al.* (1991)	1988	74	40
Vallancien *et al.* (1990)	1988	126	37

* Adapted with permission from Rodriguez *et al.* (1995).

of RCCs were less than 3 cm, and the proportion of patients presenting with metastases had dropped to 17 per cent (Smith *et al.* 1989).

Tumors diagnosed in the asymptomatic individual appear to carry a better prognosis than those tumors detected upon presentation with classic symptoms. There is a stage-stratified survival advantage among individuals with incidentally noted RCC when compared to individuals with symptomatic tumors (Tsui *et al.* 2000; Sweeney *et al.* 1996). Furthermore, since the majority of incidentally noted tumors are locally confined earlier stage lesions, the routine use of radiologic studies such as CT and ultrasound has increased the role of the urologist in the management of RCC.

A number of patients with renal masses do still present symptomatically. The classic triad of flank pain, flank or abdominal mass, and gross hematuria, although only present in less than 10 per cent of patients with RCC, should prompt an evaluation of the kidneys. Often, clinical manifestations such as pain or excessive bleeding are indicative of advanced disease. Weight loss, anemia, and malaise may be signs of systemic disease, and symptoms such as fever and night sweats should suggest to the physician the possibility of large tumor volume. Overall, hematuria is the most common presenting sign, present in approximately 60 per cent of patients.

Paraneoplastic processes are common (> 10 per cent of RCC) including hypercalcemia, erythrocytosis, and pyrexia of unknown origin (Sufrin *et al.* 1989). Physical findings are limited but may include hypertension, jaundice, weight loss, cachexia, fever, or a new onset varicocele (most commonly on the left side). Laboratory studies may reveal an elevation of liver function tests (non-metastatic hepatic dysfunction called Stauffer's syndrome), anemia (hypochromic, microcytic), elevated sedimentation rate, hypercalcemia, microhematuria, or changes in the hematocrit. In individuals with a known renal mass and systemic symptoms such as paraneoplastic syndrome, the suspicion for malignancy should be high.

In a patient with symptoms such as hematuria, the intravenous urogram (IVU) remains the initial screening radiologic examination of choice because it has the sensitivity to detect a wide range of pathologic conditions. The excellent spatial resolution of this procedure provides detailed images that can detect subtleties of the collecting system that newer imaging modalities may lack, such as medullary sponge kidney, papillary necrosis, transitional cell carcinoma (TCC) of the upper tract, nephrolithiasis, and nephrocalcinosis (Demos *et al.* 1985; Kass *et al.* 1983). Ultrasound, CT, and MRI are however far superior to IVU in detecting and characterizing renal parenchymal masses because cross-sectional and multiplanar imaging can eliminate the confusion of overlapping structures and can provide excellent contrast resolution and enhancement of small lesions (Stephenson *et al.* 1984; Curry and Bissada 1997).

The relative sensitivities of IVU, ultrasound, CT scan, and MRI in the detection of parenchymal renal masses are 67, 79, 94, and 95 per cent, respectively (Warshauer *et al.* 1988; Amendola *et al.* 1988; Bartolozzi *et al.* 1991). Statistically, most renal masses are cysts, but incidental RCC can be discovered in 0.3 per cent of CT scans and, in recent series, one-third to one-half of all surgically treated RCC have been discovered incidentally (Raval and Lamki 1983; Nissenkorn and Bernheim 1995; Ozen *et al.* 1993). We recently have begun to utilize ultrasound and cytology in individuals with painless microscopic hematuria as the likelihood of a parenchymal renal mass is greater than that of collecting system abnormality. This is controversial and remains to be validated.

Upon detection of a renal mass in the symptomatic or asymptomatic individual, the approach is essentially the same. The clinician should assess the nature of the mass, the size and position, the presence of associated extrarenal lesions, and the presence of metastatic disease. The fundamental purpose of evaluation is to determine the likelihood of the lesion representing a malignancy. This can be dependent upon the appearance of the mass, its solid or cystic nature, and the clinical setting. In those cases in which a malignancy is suspected, the evaluation should also include an assessment of the stage of disease as well as its amenability to partial resection of the kidney.

Is the renal mass solid or cystic?

The first question to be answered upon identification of a symptomatic or incidental renal mass is whether it is solid or cystic. The majority of incidentally noted renal masses are benign simple cysts. Clearly, the risk of malignancy is much higher in solid masses, and the treatment approach hinges upon this observation. Several radiologic modalities are available for addressing this question, and each has its strengths and limitations. The decision of solid or cystic can generally be made from ultrasound, CT, or MRI. The inability of the IVU to distinguish solid from cystic is one of its shortcomings, and demonstrates why it is generally followed by a second study to evaluate the nature of the mass.

IVU is the initial examination in many clinical scenarios and is ideal in evaluating the collecting system in the setting of hematuria as an initial study, but it has become apparent with the availability of newer techniques that the sensitivity of IVU in detecting parenchymal masses is limited. An IVU can detect distortion in the renal shape, distortion of the collecting system, malrotation of the kidney due to mass effect, and can provide information regarding the location and function of kidneys. These findings are usually in the setting of larger renal masses, and small masses that do not distort the collecting system or periphery of the kidney will usually not be detected. Additionally, the presence of renal mass effect on IVU can accompany both solid and cystic lesions. Therefore, findings suspicious for a mass in the kidney on IVU should prompt further radiographic evaluation.

Although it does not have the specificity of CT scanning, ultrasound is very useful in differentiating solid tissue from fluid. Ultrasound is the recommended follow-up examination for a suspicious IVU because of its ability to reliably identify simple renal cysts (the majority of the masses), to further define renal masses, and to maintain cost-effectiveness in the present health care scheme (Einstein *et al.* 1995). Strict sonographic criteria exist for detection of cysts that include a smooth cyst wall, a round or oval shape without internal echoes, and good through transmission with strong acoustic shadows posteriorly (evaluation of cystic disease is discussed in detail later). Ultrasound has a sensitivity of 79 per cent for detecting solid masses, and the addition of Doppler technology has probably improved its accuracy (Kuijpers and Jaspers 1989).

Limitations of ultrasound in lesion detection stem from relatively poor spatial resolution of the modality combined with handicaps imposed by patient factors, such as obesity or bowel gas. The study can be deceptive as many necrotic or low-density solid lesions may allow partial through transmission of sound waves, making it unclear if the mass represents a solid lesion or a cystic lesion with internal debris. Additionally, many small lesions are isoechoic and cannot be distinguished from the adjacent renal tissue. As such, while ultrasound is definitive in determining the solid or cystic nature of most lesions, the CT scan remains the gold standard for determining the solid nature of a mass.

The advantages of CT scan over ultrasound are multiple, and include greater sensitivity in detecting and evaluating small renal masses, the ability to quantitate the density of the mass and its internal components including fat and fluid, detection of small amounts of vascularity through enhancement upon intravenous (IV) contrast administration, and, ultimately, more accurate staging because of improved visualization of retroperitoneal structures, vasculature, and adjacent organs. Additionally, CT scanning is less invasive and less expensive than procedures such as angiography (Jennings and Linehan 1996).

Hounsfield units (HU) are numerical representations of the relative density of the tissues imaged and reflect how they interact with the X-ray beam (see Table 21.2). The HU scale ranges from -1000 (for example, air) to $+1000$ (for example, metal). Just as in standard radiography, structures with the greatest density (bone, surgical clips) appear white, and the least dense (fat, gas) appear dark to black. The center of the scale is set at water density, which is arbitrarily assigned the number 0, with a range of $+20$ to -20 HU.

Table 21.2 Typical CT values in Hounsfield units for renal imaging*

Tissue	(–) IV contrast	(+) IV contrast
Fat	0 to –100	No change
Fluid/water	–20 to +20	No change
Fresh hematoma	30 to 70	No change
Old blood	10 to 20	No change
High attenuation cyst	50 to 90	No change
Muscle	30 to 35	40 to 45
Lymphoma	10 to 25	30 to 50
Renal parenchyma	20 to 30	200 to 300
Renal cancer	15 to 40	40 to 90

* Adapted with permission from Patel and deKernion (1997).

Simple renal cysts should fall in this range. Tissue density (unenhanced kidney, muscle, tumor) is around +20 to 30 HU, and calculi, bone, and metal occupy the high end of the scale. Fat, which attenuates the X-ray beam much less than water, looks darker and typically measures less than –50 HU. Air occupies the most negative end of the scale and appears black.

The administration of iodinated IV contrast material results in much better tissue differentiation, with the kidneys increasing attenuation in the nephrogram phase similar to an IVU due to tubular concentration of contrast material. A lesion that contains fluid and has no blood supply remains at water density after contrast administration. The typical findings of RCC on CT include a solid mass that is hypodense or isodense compared with normal renal parenchyma, with densities of +15 to 40 HU. A solid tumor is vascular and is suffused with contrast material and shows an increase in HU, although it usually appears relatively lower in density compared to the normally enhancing parenchyma. There is no universal agreement as to how much enhancement is required to establish a suspicious renal lesion; however, an increase of 10 to 20 HU over baseline should be regarded as highly indicative for a solid tumor (Curry and Bissada 1997). Secondary findings indicative of malignancy may include irregular margins, areas of necrosis, grossly enlarged lymph nodes, venous invasion, and metastases.

On noncontrast imaging, the mass may be hypodense, isodense, or hyperdense. The clinician must exercise caution in not assuming that the pre-contrast density will predict the nature of the lesion. Hyperdense cysts are defined as lesions with density of +50 to 90 HU on noncontrast imaging, but no enhancement on the post-contrast cuts (Fig. 21.1). Likewise, hypodense lesions with fluid-density on non-contrast CT may have focal or diffuse enhancement upon administration of bolus contrast (Fig. 21.2; see also Fig. 21.13). For this reason, the assumption of cystic disease cannot be made on the basis of a noncontrast scan alone.

In order to accurately define the solid or cystic nature of a mass, the study should be performed in a specific manner each time. Urologists, in addition to radiologists, should be aware of what constitutes an acceptable scan so that they can play an informed role in determining when the examination is not adequate. At our institution a high-quality CT scan dedicated to renal evaluation includes: (1) performance with modern equipment capable of thin sections (≤ 5 mm); (2) scanning before and after IV contrast; (3) an adequate amount of contrast medium (30–40 g of iodine in patients with normal renal function) injected rapidly so that a high blood concentration of contrast is present at the time of scanning; (4) accurate Hounsfield unit (HU) density measurement (Bosniak 1993). The use of measurements within multiple areas of the mass may be useful in detecting focal enhancement at the periphery of the lesion (see Figs. 21.1 and 21.2).

Helical CT scanning has the advantages of minimal motion artifact, exact duplication of cuts before and after contrast, and the ability to reconstruct images retrospectively at any level (Wolf 1998). Care must be taken to start scanning at an appropriate interval after contrast injection, ideally after a 90 to 100 second delay, because it has been shown that images obtained in the corticomedullary differentiation phase tend to make medullary lesions inconspicuous. The delay time ensures a uniform nephrogram (Yuh and Cohan 1999). Additionally, if scans are obtained too soon, there may be inadequate time for accumulation of contrast in the lesion to show enhancement (Curry and Bissada 1997). One potential limitation of early scanning is that contrast excretion has not yet occurred, and the renal pelvis cannot be fully evaluated. In selected cases, delayed images can be performed (Rodriguez *et al.* 1995). Some authors recommend that nephrogenic or excretory phase images, in addition to corticomedullary phase, should be required for optimal helical scanning for detection, characterization, and staging of renal masses (Yuh and Cohan 1999).

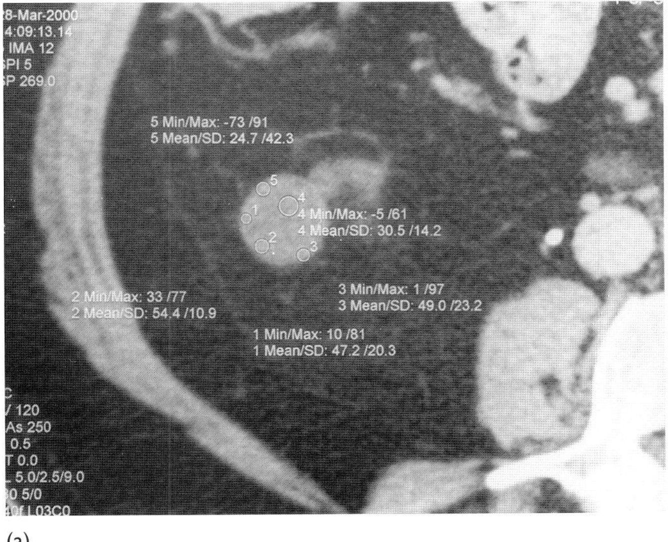

(a)

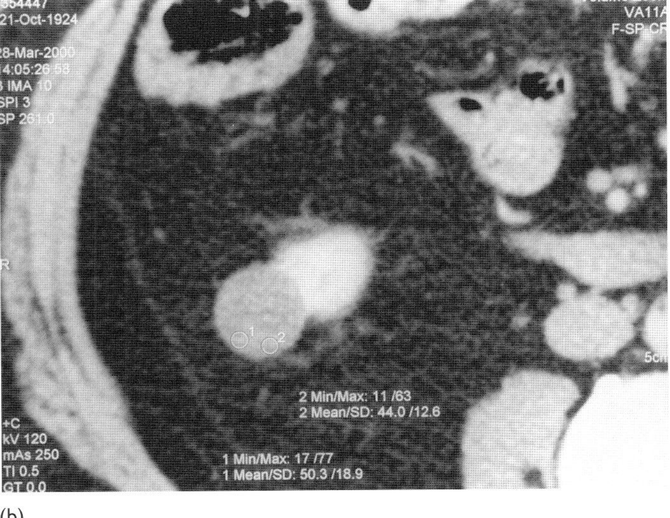

(b)

Fig. 21.1 Pre-contrast and contrast-enhanced computerized tomography (CT) images of a non-enhancing renal mass. (a) The pre-contrast image reveals a relatively high density of up to 54.4 HU. Note the heterogeneity of the lesion. (b) Upon contrast administration, no enhancement is seen despite measurement in multiple areas of the mass. The lesion was deemed a hyperdense cyst and has been clinically observed.

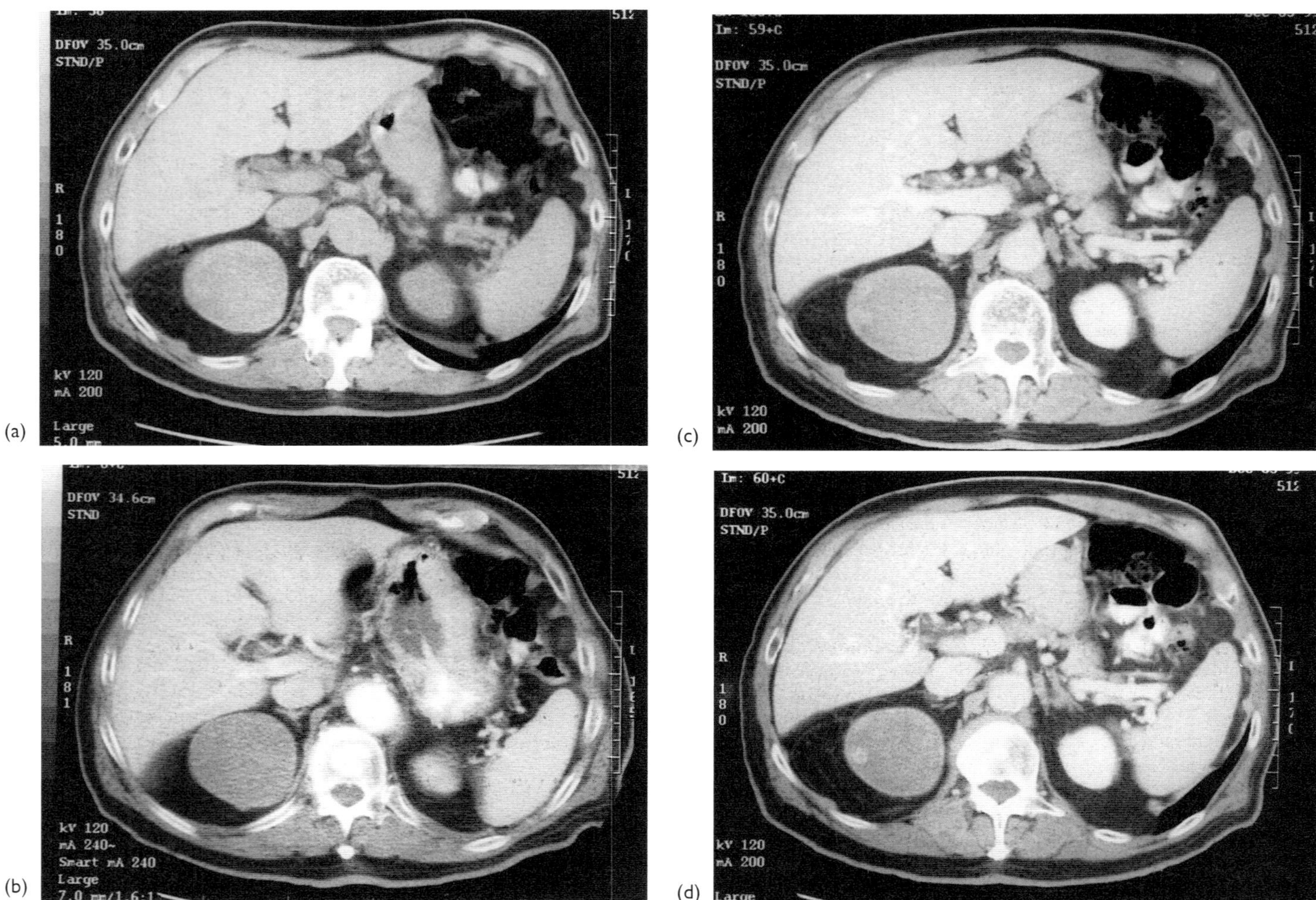

Fig. 21.2 An 82-year-old male presented with a suspicious right renal mass. (a) The pre-contrast CT images reveal a mass that is slightly hyperdense relative to the renal parenchyma. (b) The initial contrast-enhanced images do not show clear enhancement of the lesion. (c) A repeat scan performed with rapid infusion of a larger contrast bolus and early arterial phase imaging reveals peripheral enhancement within several locations in the mass. A right nephrectomy was performed revealing a centrally necrotic grade 2/4 papillary RCC.

For the routine evaluation of renal masses, MRI currently carries no significant advantage over CT (Kreft *et al.* 1997). Since the introduction of gadolinium-enhanced studies, its use has increased significantly and, in certain clinical situations, such as a patient with renal insufficiency, contrast allergy, hyperdense renal cyst, or a complicated renal cyst (discussed later), MRI is either safer or more accurate than CT. In the initial evaluation of a renal mass, MRI may be particularly useful in studying small lesions (< 2 cm) in which CT cannot identify enhancement (Fig. 21.3), lesions with minimal or equivocal enhancement (Fig. 21.4), and in assessing focal enhancement within the lesion. Additionally, when iodinated contrast cannot be given and CT scanning therefore cannot be definitive, enhancement of a renal lesion can still be determined using MRI and IV gadolinium-DTPA (diethylenetriamine pentaacetic acid).

RCC typically displays a signal intensity intermediate between normal cortex and medulla on T1-weighted images and a hyperintense signal on T2. On T1-weighted images before and after the administration of gadolinium, the presence of enhancement (vascularity) of the mass will be detected (Eilenberg *et al.* 1990) (Fig. 21.5). Gadolinium is less toxic to the kidneys at the small dose used for MRI imaging (Rofsky *et al.* 1991). Furthermore, MRI can allow for improved staging of RCC with its multiplanar imaging and improved assessment of venous involvement (discussed later). At the present time, MRI is perhaps most useful as an adjunct to CT, partly because of its greater cost, but it will undoubtedly play a larger role in the future.

Angiography has historically played a large role in the evaluation of renal masses, but, due to the advent of newer technologies such as cross-sectional imaging, it currently has an extremely limited role in the evaluative process. The typical angiographic findings with RCC include neovascularity, venous pooling, and arteriovenous fistulae. The angiographic findings of hypervascularity and hypovascularity, although suggestive of RCC and renal cyst, respectively, are not conclusive. The risks of angiography include contrast-associated renal impairment, hemorrhage, pseudoaneurysm formation, and arterial emboli. While it has been largely replaced in the evaluation of renal masses by CT or MRI,

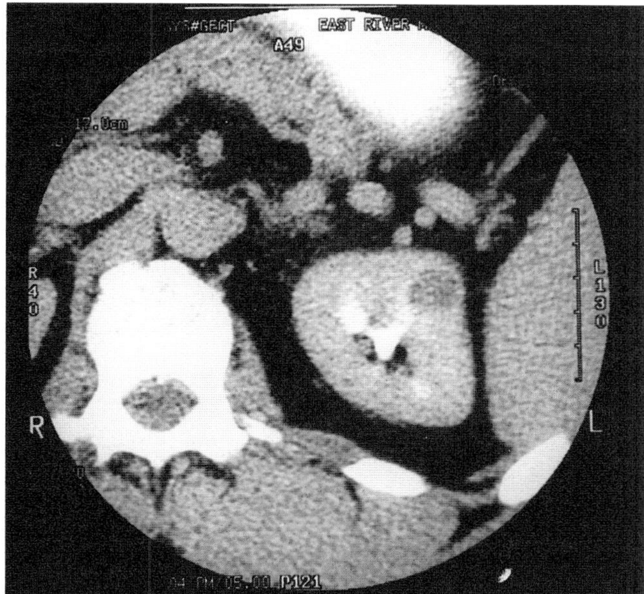

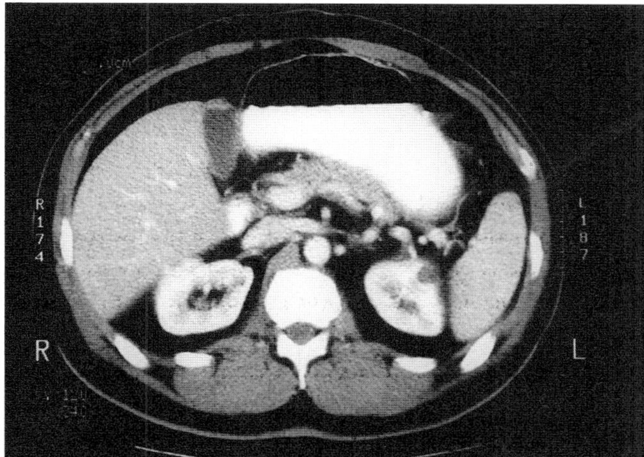

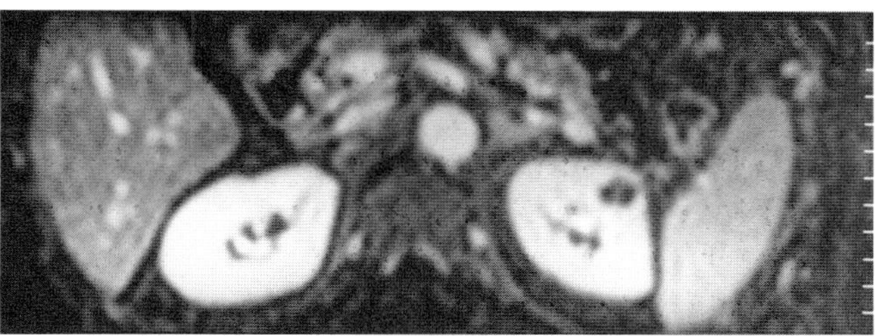

Fig. 21.3 An incidentally noted 1.2 cm renal mass. (a) Early and (b) delayed contrast-enhanced CT images reveal equivocal enhancement. (c) A gadolinium-enhanced T1-weighted MRI reveals a single septation within the lesion and no enhancement. The lesion was determined to be a minimally suspicious cyst and clinically observed.

it continues to have a role in mapping of the renal blood supply prior to therapeutic embolization of RCC or angiomyolipoma (Bosniak 1984; Oesterling *et al.* 1986; Zerhouni *et al.* 1984).

Renal nuclear medicine scans, which can differentiate parenchymal lobulations from space-occupying lesions, have essentially been replaced by CT. Their limited role can be found in the evaluation of pseudotumors, which equivocally enhance on CT (to be discussed in detail), and of differential renal function for surgical planning.

Is the renal mass benign or malignant?

Evaluation of the solid mass

Solid masses of the kidney may represent malignant or benign tumors of the kidney parenchyma, urothelial tumors, metastatic deposits, or, on rare occasions, inflammatory lesions or pseudotumors. The large majority of solid masses of the kidney represent RCC, and as such the approach is typically surgical. While histologic diagnosis is generally made upon excision, unique characteristics and clinical settings do exist for each benign and malignant tumor subtype. Recognition of these features may allow the preoperative recognition of benign tumors or inflammatory lesions such as abscess, and may save the patient unnecessary surgery. Likewise, the preoperative recognition of benign solid tumor features may prompt a less radical approach such as partial nephrectomy or embolization.

The differential diagnosis of renal masses can be divided into three categories classified by pathology: malignant, benign, and inflammatory (see Table 21.3). Malignant renal masses include RCC (85–90 per cent of all malignant renal tumors), sarcoma (2–3 per cent), urothelial tumors (6–7 per cent), lymphoma, and metastatic disease (especially lung, breast, and colon). Urothelial tumors of the renal pelvis and collecting system include 90 per cent TCC, 7–10 per cent squamous cell carcinoma, and < 1 per cent adenocarcinoma or small cell carcinoma. Benign renal masses consist of simple and acquired cysts, renal cortical adenomas, oncocytomas, angiomyolipomas, pseudotumors, and, less commonly, fibromas, leiomyomas, hemangiomas, lipomas, juxtaglomerular cell tumors/reninomas, and arteriovenous malformations. Inflammatory renal masses are renal abscesses, xanthogranulomatous pyelonephritis, and genitourinary tuberculosis.

Oncocytoma

Renal oncocytoma is a relatively common, benign solid tumor first characterized as a clinical entity by Klein and Valensi (1976); it accounts for 3 to 7 per cent of all solid renocortical tumors (Lieber 1993; Licht 1995). Most tumors are solitary; however multifocal disease has been reported (Licht *et al.* 1993; Kadesky and Fulgham 1993) and it can also be coexistent with RCC in the same (Lehmann and Blessing 1982) or opposite kidney (Kavoussi *et al.* 1985) in approximately 7 per cent of patients. The majority of these lesions are discovered incidentally, although occasionally patients present with flank or abdominal pain, hematuria, or a palpable mass.

Renal oncocytomas appear as solid, well-circumscribed masses on IVU and ultrasound with no distinctive features from RCC (Licht 1995). On CT scan, they typically appear as well-defined, relatively homogeneous, hypodense, enhancing, solid masses (Quinn *et al.* 1984; Newhouse 1993). In one study, a central

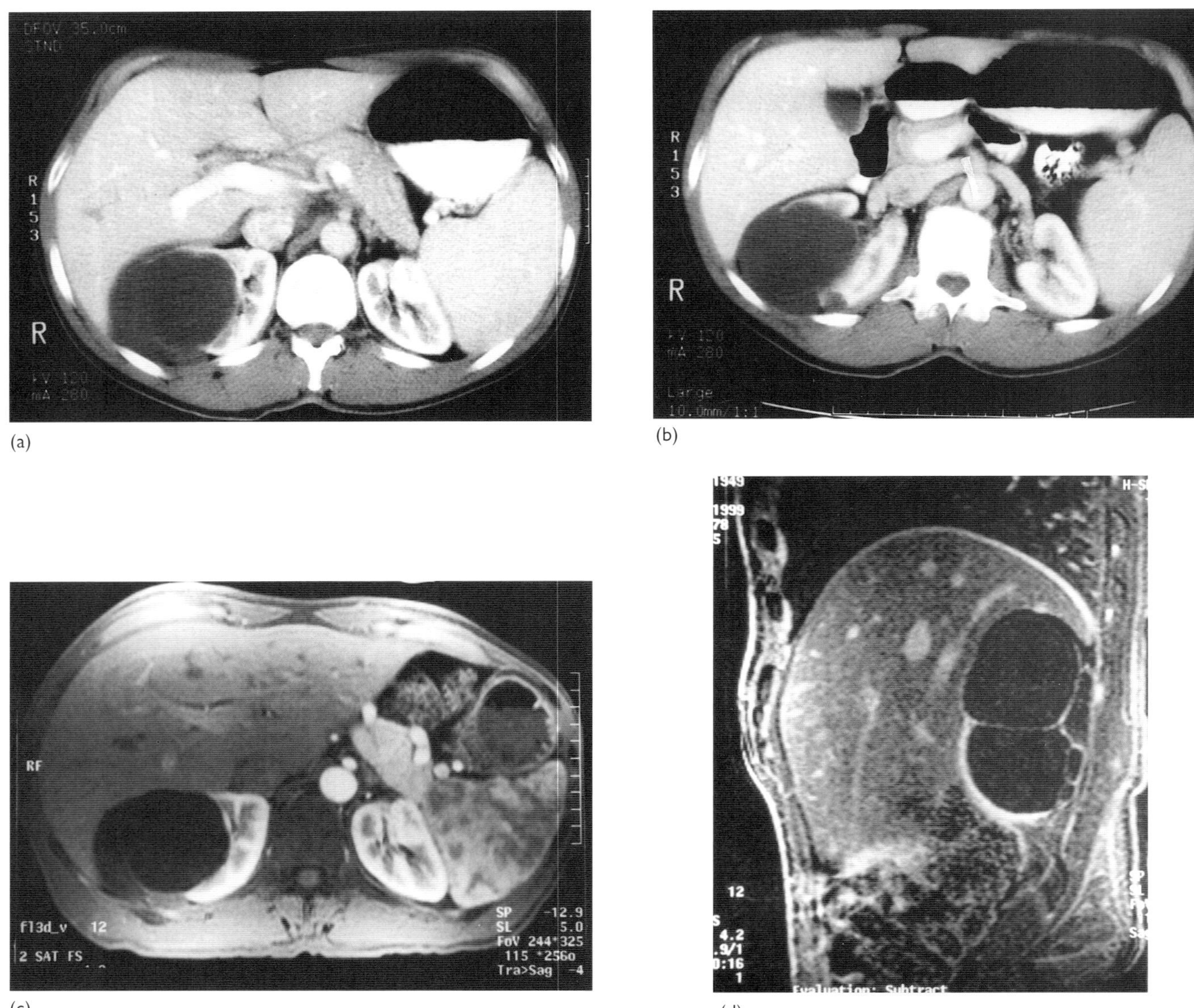

Fig. 21.4 A large complex cystic mass identified incidentally on CT. (a), (b) Contrast-enhanced CT reveals equivocal internal enhancement with internal septation. (c) T1-weighted MRI shows multiple septations with non-enhancing proteinaceous debris within the dependent compartments of the cyst. (d) Sagittal T1-weighted MR images show a cluster of multiple adjacent cysts. The mass was deemed to be a Bosniak category IIF lesion and clinically observed.

stellate scar within the lesion has been found up to 33 per cent of the time (Quinn *et al.* 1984); however, this finding is not pathognomonic (Levine and Huntrakoon 1983). Nuclear medicine scans have also been unsuccessful in differentiating these types of lesions (Lautin *et al.* 1981).

Recently, MRI has been used to attempt to differentiate oncocytoma from RCC with no specific defining characteristics being identified (Defossez *et al.* 1991). Harmon *et al.* (1996) reported that the MRI appearance of oncocytomas differs from that of RCC while evaluating 11 patients with MRI. They found that a low-intensity homogeneous mass on T1-weighted images, which appears as increased intensity on T2-weighted images; the presence of a capsule, central scar or stellate pattern; and the absence of either hemorrhage or necrosis suggest oncocytoma. These MRI findings differ somewhat from those found in RCC which typically show intermediate to high signal intensity compared to renal cortex on T1- and T2-weighted pulse sequences and usually contain evidence of either hemorrhage or necrosis.

The angiographic appearance of renal oncocytoma has classically been reported to have a distinctive spoke-wheel arterial pattern to describe the appearance of the feeding arteries in 20 to 57 per cent of cases (Ambos *et al.* 1978; Bonavita *et al.* 1980); however, this appearance has been described in RCC as well (Morra and Das 1993; Nurmi *et al.* 1984a). While a central stellate scar and a spoke-wheel pattern are suggestive of oncocytoma, the definitive diagnosis at this time with current radiologic modalities cannot be made without a pathologic diagnosis, and therefore surgical intervention is mandated.

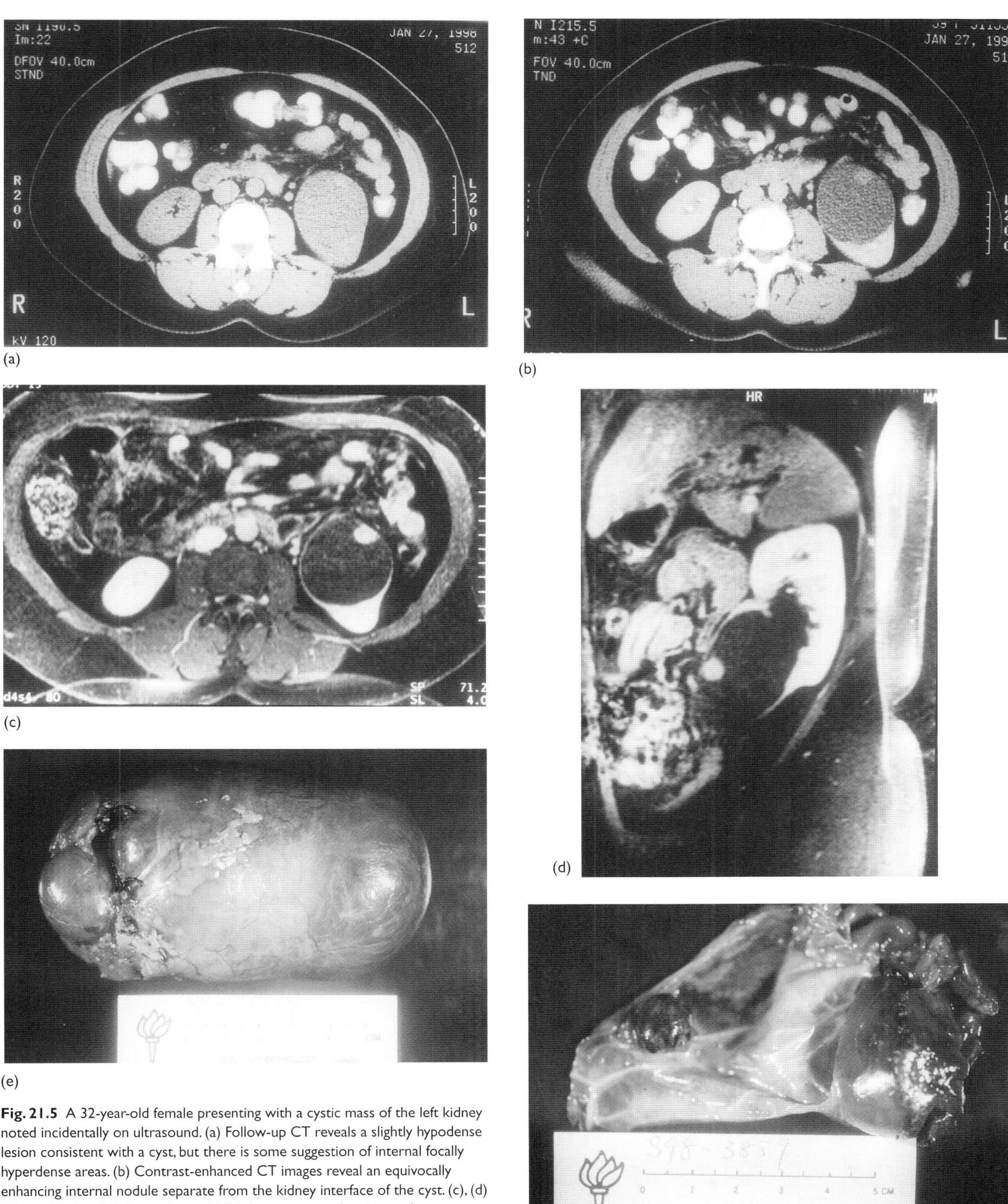

Fig. 21.5 A 32-year-old female presenting with a cystic mass of the left kidney noted incidentally on ultrasound. (a) Follow-up CT reveals a slightly hypodense lesion consistent with a cyst, but there is some suggestion of internal focally hyperdense areas. (b) Contrast-enhanced CT images reveal an equivocally enhancing internal nodule separate from the kidney interface of the cyst. (c), (d) T1-weighted gadolinium-enhanced MRI demonstrates clear internal enhancement within the cyst lumen. (e) A partial nephrectomy was performed revealing a cystic mass with (f) a single internal hemorrhagic nodule of RCC.

Table 21.3 Renal masses classified by pathology

Malignant	Benign	Inflammatory
Renal cell carcinoma	Simple cyst	Renal abscess
Urothelial carcinoma	Renal cortical adenoma	Genitourinary tuberculosis
Transitional cell carcinoma	Acquired renal cysts	Xanthogranulomatous pyelonephritis
Squamous cell carcinoma	Oncocytoma	
Adenocarcinoma	Angiomyolipoma	
Small cell carcinoma	Pseudotumor	
Sarcoma	Fibroma	
Lymphoma	Leiomyoma	
Metastasis	Hemagioma	
	Lipoma	
	Juxtaglomerular cell tumor/reninoma	

Angiomyolipoma

Angiomyolipomas are benign renal tumors that occur in a number of clinical scenarios: (1) associated with tuberous sclerosis; (2) associated with lymphangiomyomatosis; (3) discovered because of clinical symptoms resulting from bleeding of the tumor. Although as many as 80 per cent of patients with tuberous sclerosis will ultimately develop renal angiomyolipomas (Fig. 21.6), the majority of angiomyolipomas are not associated with this disease process (Jennings and Linehan 1996). The clinical presentation of this lesion is variable and is usually related to the size of

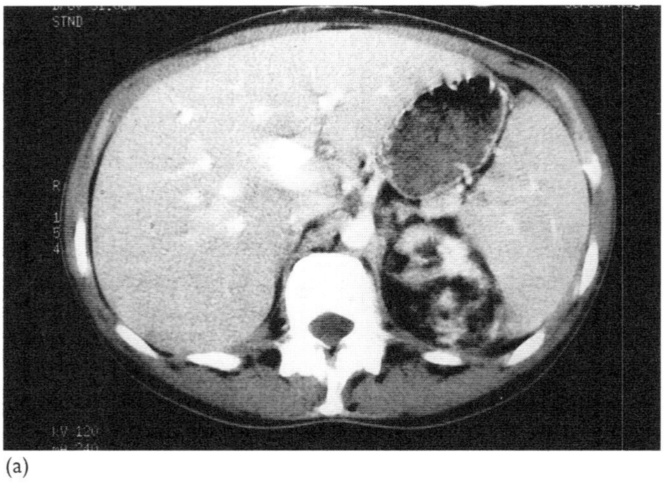

(a)

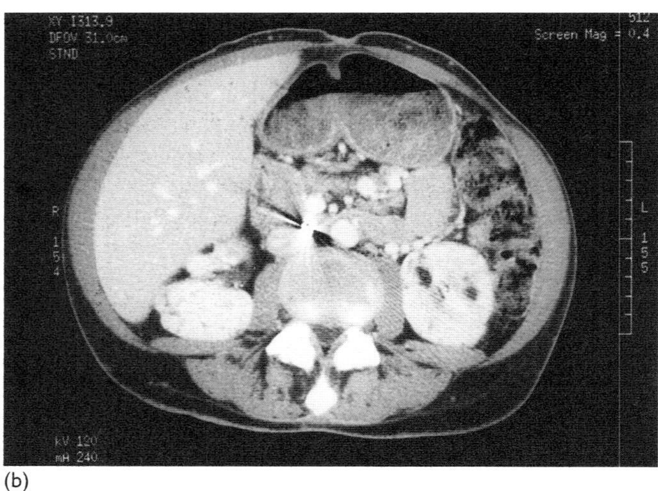

(b)

Fig. 21.6 (a), (b) Multiple bilateral angiomyolipomas in a patient with tuberous sclerosis.

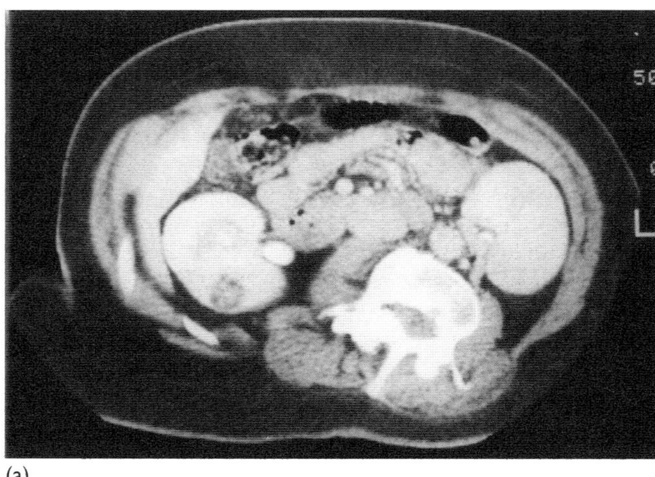

(a)

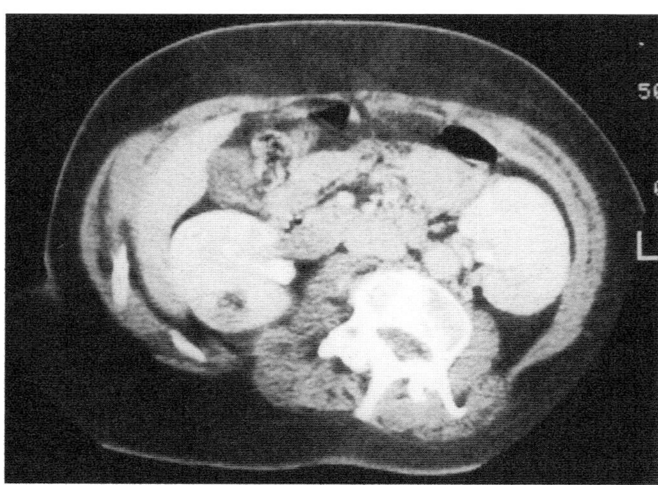

(b)

Fig. 21.7 (a), (b) Demonstration of fat density within a small renal mass pathognomonic of angiomyolipoma

the mass. Flank or abdominal pain is the most common present-ing symptom, followed by palpable mass and hematuria. Hyper-tension and anemia are also common. Patients may also present with hemorrhagic shock after the rupture of a tumor. Tumors smaller than 4 cm are typically asymptomatic (Steiner *et al.* 1993), while those larger than 4 cm are symptomatic in 46 to 82 per cent of cases (Oesterling *et al.* 1986; Steiner *et al.* 1993).

The lesion is typically solitary, asymptomatic and found inciden-tally on CT or ultrasound (Bosniak 1993). The most reliable and commonly encountered sign of angiomyolipoma is the demonstra-tion of fat within the tumor (Sherman *et al.* 1981) (Fig. 21.7). The detection of fat in the tumor enables a nonoperative histologic diag-nosis. At urography, only large tumors have sufficient fat to appear on radiographs. On ultrasound, the tumors appear with increased echogenicity secondary to the fat content. This is, however, a non-specific finding since some RCC can also be quite echogenic; there-fore the general recommendation is to obtain a CT scan to see if fat can be demonstrated.

CT is the primary modality for making the diagnosis of angiomyolipoma. The presence of fat densities (−70 to −30 HU) on CT scan is almost pathognomonic for angiomyolipoma (Fig. 21.8(a)). If a small amount of fat is suspected in a renal lesion, CT should be performed with 5 mm sections and without IV contrast to maximize the ability to identify fat. Detecting fat will establish the diagnosis and is the only radiologic finding that can differentiate angiomyolipoma from RCC (Bosniak *et al.* 1988). CT is reliable only if the fat is found within the neoplasm itself rather than at its periphery. Liposarcomas may also demonstrate fat; however these lesions are usually perirenal and generally not mistaken for angiomyolipoma (Newhouse 1993).

Angiographically, angiomyolipomas demonstrate tortuous arteries that are clearly neovascular, but do not exhibit peri-vascular cuffing or encasement seen with malignant tumors (Fig. 21.8(b)). These findings can also be found in RCC, but the

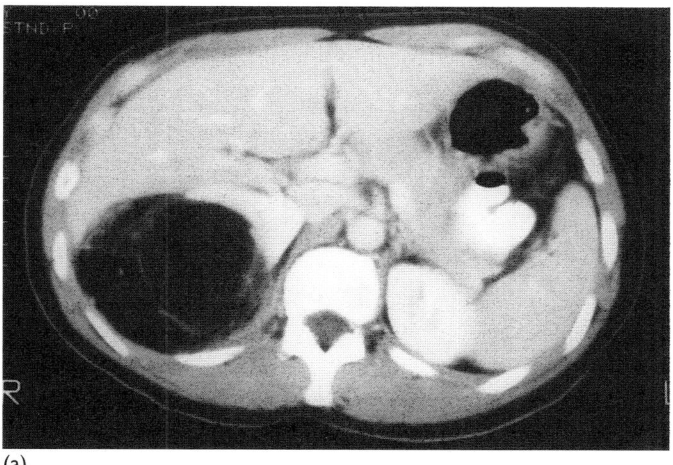

(a)

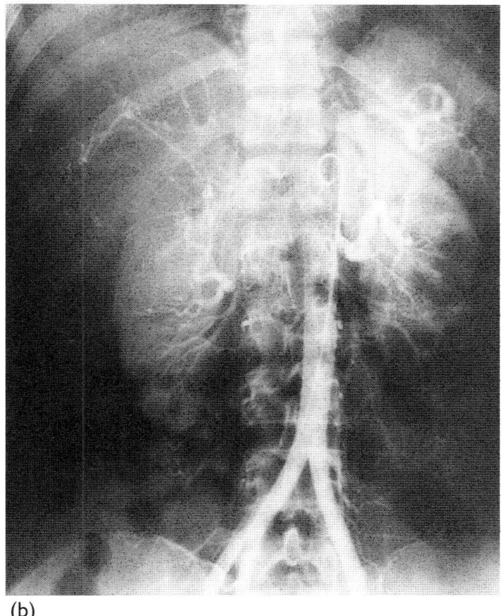

(b)

Fig. 21.8 A large right upper pole angiomyolipoma. (a) CT reveals a large mass of largely fat density. (b) Angiographic evaluation demonstrates multiple tortuous arteries representing neovascularization of the tumor.

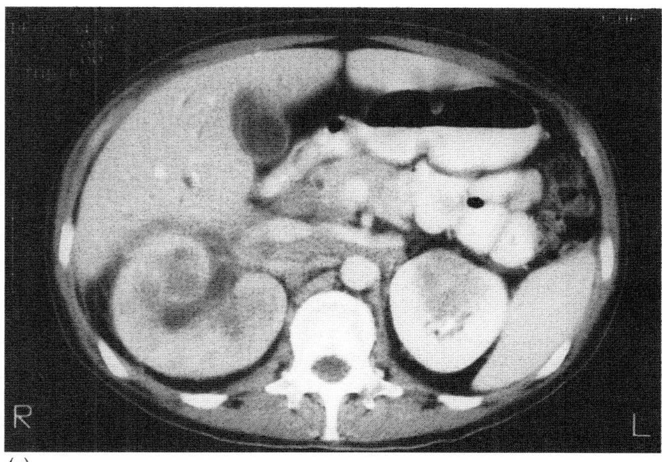

(a)

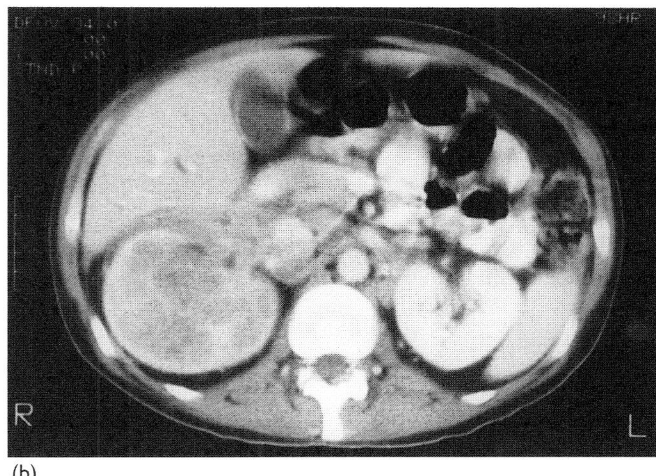

(b)

Fig. 21.9 (a), (b) A 39-year-old male with AIDS, presents with lymphoma and bilateral renal lesions. Multiple discrete masses are noted within the bilateral kidneys. Involvement of the right kidney is more extensive than the left with multiple hypodense enhancing lesions.

demonstration of arterial encasement may permit the distinction of liposarcoma from angiomyolipoma (Newhouse 1993). MRI may also occasionally be useful in the diagnosis because of the characteristic high signal intensity of fat on T1-weighted images (Jennings and Linehan 1996).

A number of reports have established that some RCC contain fat but these lesions almost always contain calcium as well (Helenon *et al.* 1993; Strotzer *et al.* 1993), and angiomyolipomas rarely contain calcification. So, if a lesion contains fat and calcification, it probably represents a carcinoma and needs removal.

Juxtaglomerular cell tumor/reninoma

Reninomas are rare but important benign tumors that present problems in diagnosis. Patients with these tumors present with severe diastolic hypertension, hypokalemia, and elevated plasma renin levels. Headache is the most common presenting symptom. The lesion is often small and may escape diagnosis with urography. On ultrasound, they are relatively echogenic and, at CT, they enhance, but less than normal parenchyma. These features are not distinguishing from RCC. The diagnosis can be suspected if the renal mass is accompanied by hypertension, hyperreninemia, and secondary hyperaldosteronism. If angiography reveals a relatively hypovascular tumor and excludes renovascular hypertension, reninoma should be strongly considered. When the tumor is small, partial nephrectomy is the appropriate treatment (Newhouse 1993).

Lymphoma

Lymphoma can frequently have renal involvement and can be ultimately demonstrated in up to one-third of patients with this disease process. Non-Hodgkin's lymphoma (NHL) is more likely than Hodgkin's disease to affect the kidneys (Newhouse 1993) and renal involvement is usually discovered during a staging CT examination. Lymphoma of the kidney most often produces multiple masses in one or both kidneys (Fig. 21.9); however it can also be present with less discrete masses or as a solitary lesion (Fig. 21.10). RCC can also occur, albeit infrequently, in patients with lymphoma. A solitary solid renal mass in a patient with an established diagnosis of lymphoma is most likely to be a lymphoma, but doubt is cast by areas of cystic degeneration and necrosis (Patel and deKernion 1997). Although Rabbani and Russo (1999) showed there is no increased risk of NHL in patients with RCC or vice versa, Anderson *et al.* (1998) and Nishikubo *et al.* (1996) have shown there is a higher than expected incidence of co-occurrence of RCC and NHL for unknown reasons.

Urography may suggest lymphoma by demonstrating a mass or masses within the renal parenchyma and by revealing ureteral displacement by retroperitoneal lymphadenopathy. Ultrasound will typically reveal one or more hypoechoic areas without evidence for a cyst wall or enhanced through transmission, providing the clue that these lesions are solid instead of cystic (Newhouse 1993).

Noncontrast CT scans will typically show multiple, homogeneous lesions that are often isodense with renal parenchyma. The lesions are usually relatively hypovascular and enhance 10 to 25 HU upon contrast administration. This enhancement is less than the normal renal parenchyma as can be seen in RCC (Horii *et al.* 1983). Extrarenal manifestations and mass effects of lymphoma are also quite common. As a rule, lymphomas show a

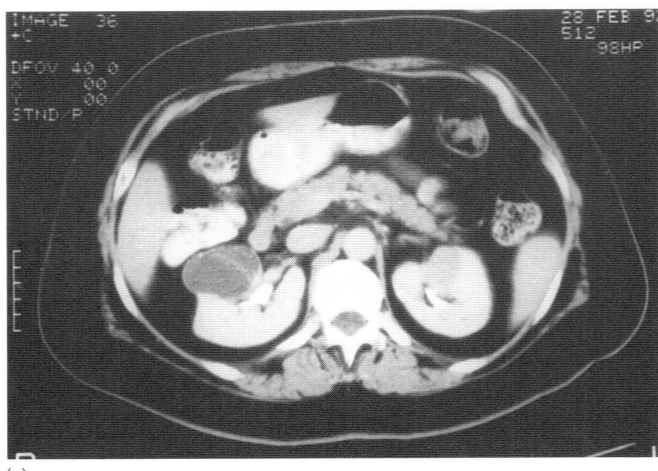

(a)

(b)

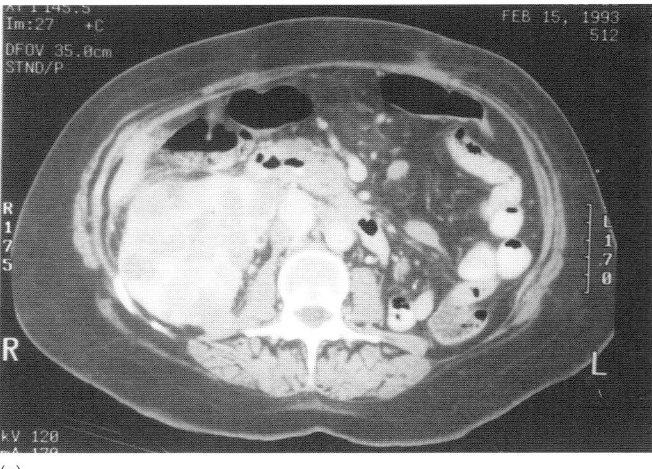

(c)

Fig. 21.10 A 56-year-old female presenting with progressive lymphoma and bilateral renal masses. (a) At initial presentation, she is noted to have a discrete solitary mass in the right kidney and an infiltrative low-attenuation lesion of the left kidney. (b) Six months later, the left disease has progressed to occupy most of the kidney. A left nephrectomy was performed. (c) Six months later, a year after the initial presentation, multiple low-attenuating lesions are noted within the residual right kidney consistent with progressive lymphoma.

slightly different angiographic pattern from the typical RCC; their neovascularity is often sparse, consists of small-diameter vessels, and reveals parallel or palisading vessels possibly caused by lymphomatous infiltration around intralobular arteries. These findings, however, can also be seen in RCC and are nondiagnostic of lymphoma (Newhouse 1993).

Therefore, in those patients in whom a renal mass is detected in the setting of known lymphoma, the diagnosis should be kept in mind, although the risk of a second malignancy is present. It is in this setting that percutaneous biopsy of the mass has an absolute indication (to be discussed later). These masses are treated nonsurgically and, if diagnosed by biopsy, treatment for lymphoma should be instituted. If the lesion persists or grows after appropriate therapy, repeat needle biopsy or resection is indicated.

Metastatic disease

Metastatic disease to the kidney is not uncommon and, although not often symptomatic, has been seen with increasing frequency because of widespread use of CT for tumor staging (Choyke *et al.* 1987; Mitnick *et al.* 1985). Renal metastases are generally small, bilateral, and multifocal. Like lymphomas, they may present as solitary or multiple lesions and can be easily missed on IVU if small (Choyke *et al.* 1987). The most common tumors that metastasize to the kidney are lung and breast cancers (see Table 21.4).

In general, there are no characteristic radiologic findings to distinguish renal metastases from primary RCC (Barbaric 1994). The sonographic appearance of metastases is typically a hypoechoic lesion, but, if small, it will be difficult to differentiate from normal parenchyma. CT is the most sensitive imaging technique. The lesions usually enhance with contrast but less than normal parenchyma.

In patients with a nonrenal primary tumor and known metastatic disease, solid renal masses are assumed to be metastases. If the lesion is truly a primary RCC, it is usually of less clinical significance in the setting of widespread disease. If a renal mass appears in a patient with a nonrenal primary without known metastases, the absence of reliable imaging necessitates percutaneous biopsy (discussed later) to differentiate the disease process. The great majority

Table 21.4 Solid tumors metastatic to the kidney

Primary site	Per cent
Lung	27
Breast	14
Stomach	12
Pancreas	7
Colon	6
Cervix	5
Esophagus	4
Prostate	4
Gall bladder	2–3
Testis	2–3
Thyroid	2–3
Bladder	2–3
Melanoma	2–3
Endometrium	1–2
Kidney	1–2
Ovary	1–2
Head and neck	1–2
Bone	1–2

of single renal masses detected in patients with a history of malignancy and with no other metastases will turn out to be primary renal malignancies (Bosniak 1993).

Renal sarcoma

Renal sarcomas have an incidence of 2 to 3 per cent of all malignant renal tumors. They have no clinical or radiologic features that distinguish them from primary RCC with any reliability (Shirkhoda and Lewis 1987). The lesions may demonstrate local advancement into surrounding organs, which is not typical of RCC. Additionally, in masses arising from the surface of the kidney or appearing to invade into the kidney from the retroperitoneum, consideration should be given to the diagnosis of sarcoma. Because there is no clear radiologic criteria for renal sarcoma, the diagnosis is usually made at resection.

Extrarenal malignancies invading the kidney

Adrenal neoplasms, retroperitoneal sarcomas, and large carcinomas arising from the stomach, pancreas, or liver may cause mass effects that can be confused with RCC or involve the kidney. Urography and occasionally CT may sometimes be unable to reveal the organ of origin. Multiplanar imaging with ultrasound or MRI may be better at differentiating the planes between the tumor and adjacent organs but this may not distinguish invasion of the kidney versus origin in the kidney. Selective angiography can occasionally demonstrate the major vessels supplying the tumor which may help elucidate the organ of origin unless the tumor has a large parasitic blood supply.

Urothelial tumors

Transitional cell carcinomas (TCC) account for 6 to 7 per cent of all malignant renal tumors and can usually be distinguished without difficulty from RCC. Urothelial tumors produce irregular mural or polypoid defects of the collecting system. Occasionally a small RCC invades the collecting system and is mistaken for a urothelial tumor; however this scenario is rare. More commonly, a centrally located, parenchymally invasive TCC may be mistaken for an RCC. The distinction can occasionally be difficult if the tumor is large or parenchymally invasive with little collecting system component, but the majority of large renal parenchymal lesions tend to be RCC. Either tumor can lead to nonfunction of the affected kidney by venous occlusion, ureteral obstruction, or parenchymal destruction, and either may cause hilar lymphadenopathy. RCC have a greater propensity to cause venous occlusion, and urothelial cancers, ureteral occlusion.

The distinction between TCC and RCC is extremely important because the surgical treatment for invasive urothelial malignancies of the renal collecting system is generally nephroureterectomy. Additionally, in the setting of metastatic disease, elective cytoreductive nephrectomy is only indicated for RCC and not TCC. The diagnosis can be made reliably with IVU, CT scan with delayed images to optimize visualization of filling defects within collecting system, and MRI. If the differentiation of the tumor is still difficult, retrograde pyelogram or ureteroscopy may be necessary. In patients with localized disease, the decision to proceed with a ureterectomy can be made upon the basis of intraoperative frozen-section pathologic diagnosis following nephrectomy. In those with known metastatic disease, percutaneous biopsy may be indicated (discussed later).

Pseudotumors

Occasionally, normal renal parenchyma or benign conditions present as a renal mass and prove difficult to distinguish from a neoplastic process. These masses, with careful attention to clinical history and imaging appearance, can be diagnosed correctly in the majority of cases. The differential diagnosis of pseudotumors includes renal anomalies, inflammatory masses (for example, chronic abscess), infarction, hematoma, localized hydronephrosis, and vascular malformations (Bosniak 1993). Renal pseudotumors caused by various anomalies such as a renal column (for example, hypertrophied column of Bertin), dysmorphism, fetal lobulation, or an unusually shaped kidney can be diagnosed correctly by showing that the lesion is identical to normal renal tissue. This can be accomplished with contrast CT scans in most cases.

In the classic literature, it is often recommended that differentiation of normal renal tissue from pathology can be made with a nuclear medicine renal scan. Only normal renal tissue concentrates any of the commonly used radioisotopes, and other masses such as cancers, cysts, angiomyolipomas, and oncocytomas typically do not, resulting in regions of diminished or absent activity (Newhouse 1993). Hypertrophied columns of Bertin are evident as areas of increased intensity. The use of nuclear renal scan has diminished in the setting of CT because CT can provide images with a spatial resolution that far exceeds that of any nuclear medicine techniques. Additionally, renal scans can have difficulty in determining normal tissue in severely scarred or deformed kidneys. A useful CT principle is that, when contrast is injected, no pathologic tissue can opacify as densely as normal renal parenchyma; therefore the differentiation of pseudotumor versus tumor can be made simply by measuring the HU of the mass.

The radiologic features of inflammation and neoplastic disease can be indistinguishable quite often and, if the clinical findings are not characteristic, these conditions can be confused. This is particularly true in the case of cystic or necrotic neoplasms versus subacute or chronic abscesses when the usual clinical findings of infection (fever, elevated white blood cell count, antibiotic treatment for a prior urinary tract infection) are not present. CT appears to be the diagnostic procedure of choice for abscesses since it provides excellent delineation of the tissue (Schaeffer 1998). CT shows renal enlargement and focal, rounded areas of decreased attenuation in the acute phase. After several days of the onset of the infection, a thick fibrotic wall begins to form around the abscess. CT of a chronic abscess shows obliteration of adjacent tissue planes, thickening of Gerota's fascia, a round or oval parenchymal mass of low attenuation, and a surrounding inflammatory wall of slightly higher attenuation that forms a ring when the scan is enhanced with contrast material. These types of lesions occasionally require percutaneous biopsy to obtain a diagnosis.

Renal infarction will appear as a sharp defect with straight margins and a rim sign on a contrast-enhanced CT. The corticomedullary phase of contrast excretion will allow the reader to determine vascular abnormalities that may present as a renal mass. Fresh blood has a characteristic appearance of high attenuation (+30 to 70 HU) on CT as well.

Evaluation of the cystic mass

The majority of incidentally noted renal masses are cystic. Approximately 70 per cent of asymptomatic renal mass lesions are simple cysts and are of no clinical significance (Lang 1973). Upon recognition of a cystic lesion, it must be determined in a rapid fashion whether any features within the cyst are suggestive of malignancy. With the advent of CT and MRI, the majority of cystic renal masses can be evaluated with high diagnostic accuracy without utilizing invasive measures. Furthermore, the role of percutaneous cyst aspiration and cystogram performance has become almost obsolete with the use of improved radiologic techniques.

Historically, cyst puncture and aspiration were performed to evaluate most cystic questionable lesions. The four major factors in helping with the diagnosis are fluid appearance, lab evaluation of the fluid, cytology, and cystogram appearance. Clear fluid that has no malignant cells, low fat and protein content, and low lactic acid dehydrogenase levels aspirated from a cyst with smooth walls is almost absolute evidence of the absence of malignancy (Lang 1977). The rate of malignancy among lesions with bloody cyst aspirates ranged from 20–70 per cent; and murky cyst aspirates, 40–50 per cent (Harris *et al.* 1975; Lang 1977; Omachi *et al.* 1992). The presence of blood in a cyst must raise the index of suspicion sufficiently to prompt further diagnostic tests. Cytology from cystic fluid has a high false-negative rate, but is extremely specific when positive and has a diagnostic rate of 20–30 per cent. Therefore, cytology and biochemical assays are frequently nondiagnostic (Bosniak 1993) except in the cases of simple cysts and thus with modern ultrasound techniques these procedures are rarely necessary. The role of percutaneous aspiration, although limited, will be discussed later.

Ultrasound's strength is the reliable identification of simple renal cysts. Increased through transmission, an anechoic internal component of the cyst, an imperceptible extrarenal wall, and a sharply demarcated intrarenal wall are hallmark features of a simple cyst. The indication for further imaging occurs when these features are not met. Since most renal lesions detected on IVU will be confirmed on ultrasound to be simple cysts, the use of ultrasound as a follow-up to IVU is a more cost-effective approach than proceeding directly to CT (Einstein *et al.* 1995).

When cysts are complicated by hemorrhage or infection, the imaging features of the cyst may be altered by internal septations, calcifications, or high attenuation. Groups of adjacent simple cysts (Fig. 21.4), multilocular cystic nephroma, cystic RCC, and tumor in the walls of a cyst can cause confusion in diagnosis (Curry and Bissada 1997). In an attempt to characterize these types of lesions and provide some logic and organization to their management, Bosniak *et al.* developed a system of categorization based on CT features discussed below (Bosniak 1986, 1991a, 1993; Bosniak and Rofsky 1996).

In 1986 Bosniak proposed a four-category classification scheme for cystic renal masses based on CT findings (see Table 21.5), which, despite its shortcomings, appears to be the best non-invasive system of classification currently available (Bosniak 1986; Goldman 1997; Wolf 1998). Category I lesions are by definition simple, benign cysts. A cyst is usually round, homogeneous, and smoothly contoured with a well-defined interface with the adjacent parenchyma. Cysts have

Table 21.5 CT criteria for Bosniak classification of cystic renal masses*

Criteria	Category			
	I	II	III[†]	IV
Wall	Thin	Thin	More than thin	Thick or nodular
Septations	None	Few, thin	More than few, moderately thickened	Numerous, thick
Calcifications	None	Few, thin	More than few, moderately thickened	Course
Enhancement	No	No	Occasionally	Yes

* Adapted with permission from Wolf (1998).
† Only 1 to 2 characteristics worse than category II but not as suspicious as category IV.

no discernible wall and have water density contents that do not enhance after administration of IV contrast. On sonography these cysts generally exhibit a sharply defined back wall, have no internal echoes, and transmit sound through them to create an acoustic shadow or posterior wall enhancement. As a result, these lesions rarely undergo CT imaging for resolution.

Category II lesions are also benign lesions that appear as minimally complicated cysts. In general, they are cysts complicated by prior hemorrhage or infection. There are three distinct features that entail placement in this category: (1) one or two delicate, nonenhancing internal septa (Reis *et al.* 1988); (2) linear, delicate calcification in the wall or septum (Waguespack and Kearse 1996); and (3) 'hyperdense' contents due to blood, protein, colloid, or iodine content (Bosniak 1993; Curry and Bissada 1997). Hyperdense cysts have higher attenuation than the surrounding kidney on noncontrast CT scans. They have a density in the range of 50 to 90 HU and remain unchanged after IV contrast infusion (Coleman *et al.* 1984; Curry *et al.* 1982; Sussman *et al.* 1984). Multiple measurements should be obtained in all portions of the lesions to rule out focal enhancement. Confirmation with ultrasound can be useful at times. To be placed in the nonsurgical category, these lesions should be less than 3 cm in size, exophytic so that the smoothness of a portion of the wall can be evaluated, round and sharply marginated, homogeneous in attenuation, and, most importantly, nonenhancing with contrast (Bosniak 1993).

Bosniak (1986) has recommended that lesions that fulfill all these criteria, on a properly performed CT scan, although not simple cysts, can be regarded as benign and do not require any further evaluation or follow-up. On CT the interior of an infected cyst or abscess often is inhomogeneous; therefore, if infection is suspected, percutaneous aspiration can be diagnostic and subsequent drainage tube placement can be therapeutic.

Bosniak (1993) amended his classification scheme to include a category IIF that incorporates any minimally complicated cyst with any degree of uncertainty (Fig. 21.4). In these lesions, a nonoperative approach is appropriate and recommended follow-up is at 3 months, 6 months, and 1 year to ensure that the lesion is not changing or growing. Examples of such lesions include hyperdense cysts (Fig. 21.1), some lesions with more calcium or thickening in the wall, or slightly more complicated septated lesions (Bosniak 1991a).

Category III lesions are moderately complicated cystic masses with features such as thick, irregular calcifications, irregular

borders, thickened or enhancing septa, uniform wall thickening, or small, nonenhancing nodules (Fig. 21.11). Multilocular cysts fall into this category. All of these lesions are considered indeter-

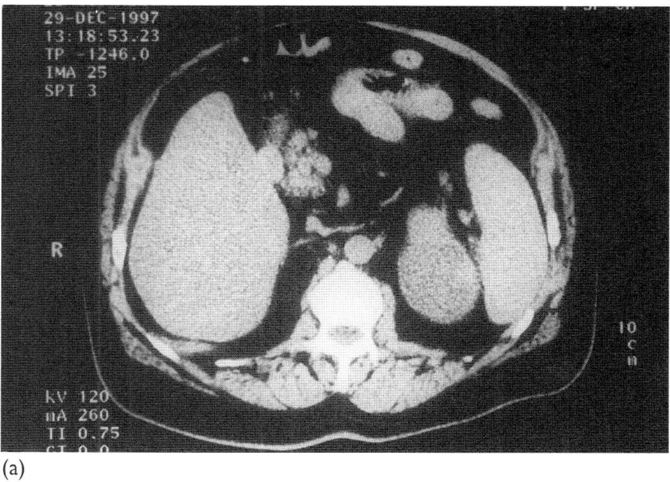

(a)

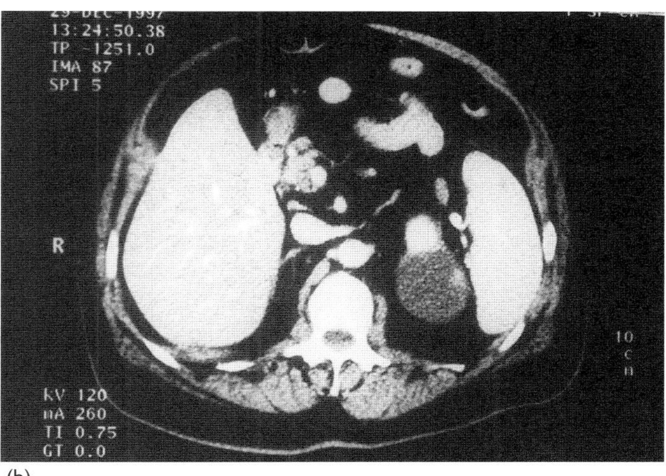

(b)

Fig. 21.11 An incidentally noted cystic mass of the left kidney in a patient with multiple right-sided solid masses (Fig. 21.14). (a) On noncontrast-enhanced CT there is a suggestion of internal high attenuation. (b) Following contrast administration, focal equivocal enhancement within an internal nodule is noted. The cyst was classified as a Bosniak category III lesion and resected by partial nephrectomy. Pathology revealed a low-grade cystic papillary RCC

Table 21.6 Evaluation of the Bosniak classification system for cystic renal masses*

Reference	No. of malignant lesions/total no. of lesions per category			
	I	II	III	IV
Aronson et al. 1991	—	0/4	4/7	5/5
Bellman et al. 1995	—	0/5	0/5	—
Wilson et al. 1996	0/7	4/5	4/4	6/6
Cloix et al. 1996	1/1	1/7	4/13	8/10
Siegel et al. 1997	0/22	1/8	5/11	26/29
Total (%)	1/30 (3)	6/29 (21)	17/40 (43)	45/50 (90)

* Adapted with permission from Wolf (1998).

minate and require pathological diagnosis; therefore resection is required for accurate diagnosis. Approximately half of these lesions will prove to be benign upon resection; however they are indistinguishable radiographically from RCC with a cystic growth pattern. Since half of these lesions are benign, it is preferable to attempt nephron-sparing surgery when technically feasible (Curry and Bissada 1997), and the size of the lesion and its position in the kidney will help determine the surgical approach.

Category IV lesions are malignant cystic masses whose appearance results from necrosis and liquefaction of a solid tumor or tumor growing within the wall of a cyst (Waguespack and Kearse 1996). Their typical appearance on CT scan is heterogeneous with a thick or nodular wall, numerous thick septations, or course calcifications. They have a density of greater than 20 HU prior to contrast injection, and they enhance with contrast. Diagnosis is usually straightforward and surgical excision is indicated.

This classification system is somewhat subjective and often relies on the quality of the CT scan and the expertise of the reader (Bosniak 1991a). However, this system is helpful in providing a framework for management of most cystic masses. Several studies have been performed to compare the radiologic evaluation of a cystic mass to the pathologic diagnosis. Five recent studies attempting to evaluate the accuracy of the Bosniak classification system are summarized in Table 21.6. The combination of these studies reveals that class I lesions have a 3 per cent chance of malignancy; class II, 21 per cent; class III, 43 per cent; and class IV, 90 per cent. The finding of one RCC in a category I lesion in the study by Cloix et al. (1996) causes concern; however in this study the CT scans were performed with 10 mm slices and the delay between contrast administration and scanning was not defined. This emphasizes the importance of a dedicated renal CT scan in order to optimize the imaging of the kidneys. This dedicated scan requires 5 mm slices at definite intervals pre- and postcontrast administration. Additionally, this study utilized the Bosniak classification system to categorize ultrasound and CT findings and obtain a total score from the findings. However, there is no defined Bosniak classification for sonographic findings and no accepted scoring system based on CT plus ultrasound discoveries. In the study by Wilson et al. (1996), the investigators discovered 80 per cent of class II lesions and 100 per cent of class III lesions were malignant . This study was based on a small series of patients in which many of the scans were not complete or dedicated CT scans and therefore not acceptable for an evaluation of the

usefulness of the Bosniak classification system. Second, only cases with pathologic proof were included in the series, eliminating hundreds of minimally complicated category II cysts that were not operated on and were left alone. Finally, this study did not fully understand the concept of enhancement. The largest and most comprehensive study of the Bosniak classification system was performed by Siegel et al. (1997). In this study, the grading of 70 cases was based on the average results of three independent readers. They found that the readers agreed on the classification in 59 per cent of the cases. This study concluded that the Bosniak classification system is useful for evaluating renal masses; however, interobserver variability in distinguishing class II and III lesions may represent difficulties in recommending surgical versus conservative management.

The role of MRI in delineating indeterminate (Bosniak category II or III) cysts is increasing with its wider availability (Hovsepian et al. 1990; Hricak et al. 1988; Marotti et al. 1987; Quint et al. 1988; Sussman et al. 1990) and is now used instead of aspiration or exploration in a number of cases in order to further evaluate these types of lesions non-invasively. A simple cyst is identifiable on MRI as having the same signal characteristics as water. It has low intensity on T1-weighted images and high signal intensity on T2-weighted images. The methemoglobin in a hemorrhagic cyst alters its appearance, so that the lesion has intermediate to high signal intensity on T1-weighted images. Signal intensity on T2-weighted images varies depending on whether red cell lysis has occurred, the amount of hemorrhage, the kinds of hemoglobin degradation, and the protein content (Hilpert et al. 1986; Roubidoux 1994). Other renal masses, such as proteinaceous cysts, RCC, and angiomyolipomas, may mimic hemorrhagic cysts in signal intensity (Fig. 21.4). Use of gadolinium is essential to show enhancement of a solid lesion (Eilenberg et al. 1990). Aside from signal characteristics, accuracy of diagnosis with MRI depends on evaluation of the same morphologic criteria used when evaluating renal lesions by CT scan (for example, wall thickening, septations, heterogeneity, enhancement). A disadvantage of MRI is its inability to detect calcifications.

We have routinely utilized MRI to characterize indeterminate or suspicious lesions on CT (Figs 21.3–21.5). Ultimately, it may have great utility in resolving issues of interobserver variability in the prediction of Bosniak category II or III cystic lesions. The increased resolution of both small and complex large lesions allows a clear distinction between proteinaceous debris and internal enhancement. While we have applied Bosniak categorization to MRI findings, this remains to be validated in a large trial. In cases of subtle abnormalities noted on CT scan, MRI can be utilized instead of aspiration or surgical excision.

The role of percutaneous biopsy

Indications

Over the last 10 years, percutaneous biopsy has replaced open surgical exploration as the procedure of choice for tissue diagnosis of the indeterminate intraabdominal mass because it is accurate, conclusive, safe, cost-effective, and can be performed in the out-patient setting. (Abe and Saitoh 1992; Richter *et al.* 2000; Wood *et al.* 1999; Smith 1991; Vassiliades and Bernardino 1991; Nadel *et al.* 1986; Charboneau *et al.* 1990; Fraser and Fairley 1995). The role of percutaneous biopsy in the evaluation of the renal mass has been a topic of great controversy. As described above, the technological progress in renal imaging has done away with most of the clinical need for renal biopsy. Renal mass biopsy can generally be performed safely with little risk of needle tract seeding, bleeding, or infection. As a result, the use of percutaneous biopsy of renal masses has increased slowly over recent decades, particularly in the US as compared with Europe (Murphy *et al.* 1985), but the indications have become well-defined and relatively narrow.

Percutaneous aspiration has been historically used to confirm the diagnosis of benign lesions such as simple cysts, complex cysts, and infections/abscesses with a high degree of accuracy (Sandler *et al.* 1986). With the advent of ultrasound, CT, and MRI, and the recognition of their ability to identify both benign and malignant processes with relatively high diagnostic accuracy, it is no longer necessary to confirm radiographically benign lesions with biopsy. In the setting of an isolated renal mass, percutaneous biopsy or aspiration should be reserved for the diagnosis of truly indeterminate lesions.

Solid or complex cystic renal masses (as discussed in the prior sections) are often found incidentally or discovered during the search for metastatic disease from a nonrenal primary malignancy. The patient's clinical history can occasionally give some indication as to the differential diagnosis; however it is often insufficient to establish a precise diagnosis. Biopsy or fine needle aspiration is often indicated in this setting for differentiating metastatic disease, lymphoma, or renal abscess from primary RCC because the treatments are different for each clinical scenario (Herts and Baker 1995; Vassiliades and Bernadino 1991; Nadel *et al.* 1986; Curry, 1995; Bosniak 1991; Nicefero and Coughlin 1993; Cristallini *et al.* 1991, Wood *et al.* 1999; Wolf 1998).

Patients with a history of nonrenal, nonlymphomatous primary malignancy and a solitary renal mass are much more likely to have a metastatic lesion than RCC (Wood *et al.* 1999; Patel and deKernion 1997) One study has shown that 85 per cent of patients with a renal mass and a nonrenal, nonlymphomatous primary malignancy had metastatic disease, and only 15 per cent had RCC as a second primary malignancy (Cristallini *et al.* 1991). Metastatic lesions in the kidney are particularly common with

Table 21.7 Indications for percutaneous biopsy of indeterminate renal masses

1	Clinical or radiographic evidence to suggest a diagnosis other than primary RCC (e.g. metastatic disease, lymphoma, or renal abscess)
2	Diagnosis of renal mass in patients with disseminated metastasis of unknown primary
3	When a renal lesion persists after the remainder of lymphomatous disease bulk regresses with systemic chemotherapy
4	When a discernible solid parenchymal abnormality persists after appropriate antibiotic therapy of a renal abscess
5	Patients with relative contraindications to surgery or significant co-morbidities (relative indication)
6	Suspicion of benign renal tumor or indeterminate lesion by diagnostic imaging (relative indication)

lung and breast carcinomas. A history of lymphoma, or secondary evidence of lymphoma such as splenomegaly or lymphadenopathy, should suggest the possibility that a small solitary renal mass may be lymphoma. These observations have important clinical implications, since many of these processes have nonsurgical treatment options (for example, abscess, hemorrhagic cyst, hematoma, infarct, inflammatory pseudotumor, metastasis, lymphoma, and other neoplasms). Therefore fine needle aspiration or biopsy is strongly indicated in these cases (see Table 21.7).

Other indications for biopsy include patients with disseminated metastatic disease, unresectable tumors, or other contraindications to surgical intervention (Nicefero and Coughlin 1993). In patients with an unknown primary malignancy and disseminated metastases or unresectable renal masses, percutaneous biopsy can be used to confirm a renal primary malignancy. This may be particularly useful in individuals under consideration for cytoreductive nephrectomy prior to immunotherapy protocol. Authors have previously reported identification of nonrenal malignancies in individuals undergoing cytoreductive nephrectomy for immunotherapeutic protocol.

In patients with medical contraindications for surgical intervention, documentation of benign disease would obviate surgery, and confirmation of malignancy might influence treatment plans regarding treatment of co-morbidities and management of the renal mass. The widespread use of radiologic imaging (particularly CT) has led to an enormous increase in the detection of incidental, small indeterminate renal masses (Curry 1995; Smith *et al.* 1989). Conservative management would be more appealing for lesions with low malignant potential, particularly in the setting of advanced age or significant co-morbid disease. Fine needle aspiration can also provide the diagnosis of low-grade RCC which could be followed non-invasively. Recent data suggests that small, solid, asymptomatic renal masses grow slowly (less than 1 cm/year) and that their risk for metastasis is low (Bosniak 1995; Birnbaum *et al.* 1990).

Percutaneous biopsy is not necessary in a solitary renal mass without a history of another primary malignancy and which radiographically appears as a typical RCC (Bosniak type IV lesion). This is especially true for patients in whom conservative surgery is not an option (large, centrally located masses) (Novick *et al.* 1989; Provet *et al.* 1991; Thrasher *et al.* 1994). There is little to be gained by biopsy in these situations unless the patient is not a surgical candidate. Biopsy is also probably not indicated in suspected cases of TCC. Radical nephroureterectomy with resection of a cuff of urinary bladder remains the recommended surgical treatment because of the high incidence of multiplicity and tumor seeding. The tumor seeding also makes percutaneous biopsy of this particular type of lesion a relative contraindication. Other contraindications to biopsy include uncorrectable bleeding disorders and lack of safe access.

Techniques

The need for a good screening history for bleeding disorders is an essential part of the evaluation prior to a renal biopsy. The history should include questions regarding bleeding problems following surgical or dental procedures, family history of bleeding disorders or hypercoagulable states, and medications (such as aspirin, nonsteroidal anti-inflammatory drugs, heparin, warfarin). It should also include history of bruising, petechiae, or purpura.

Initial bloodwork evaluation in patients with a normal bleeding history includes testing for platelets, prothrombin time (PT), and partial thromboplastin time (PTT) prior to any invasive procedure. The PT and PTT test for secondary hemostasis via the coagulation factors/cascade. The ratio of PT to a control, the international normalized ratio (INR), is used at our institution to determine coagulation factors instead of PT alone. An INR of less than 1.4 and platelet counts greater than 50 000/mm^3 are considered adequate for normal hemostasis. Based on the combination of history and laboratory evaluation, further hematologic consultation and testing should be performed in the appropriate clinical situations.

Aspirin should be stopped 7 days prior to biopsy. Warfarin and heparin also need to be stopped prior to the biopsy. If the indications for warfarin are absolute (such as mechanical valve, paroxysmal atrial fibrillation, deep venous thrombosis/pulmonary embolism, or stroke), it is common practice to convert the patients on warfarin to heparin prior to the procedure. Heparin should be discontinued approximately 4 to 6 hours before the biopsy.

Percutaneous renal biopsies can be performed using CT, ultrasound, or fluoroscopy. In Europe and Japan, biopsies are more often performed using ultrasound guidance (Leiman 1990; Helm et al. 1983; Orell et al. 1985; Juul et al. 1985; Torp-Pedersen et al. 1991; Abe and Saitoh 1992), while in the US biopsy tends to more commonly performed under CT guidance (Nadel et al. 1986; Nicefero and Coughlin 1993). This is probably due to the availability of equipment in these different regions (Herts and Baker 1995). In the US access to equipment is not generally a factor and the decision to use CT or ultrasound should be based on lesion size, its accessibility and visualization on each radiologic tool, and the radiologist's familiarity and preference.

The general procedures of CT- and ultrasound-guided biopsies are similar, but there are relative advantages and disadvantages for each. CT-guided procedures may be more expensive and time-consuming as compared to ultrasound (Gazelle and Haaga 1989). IV contrast material may also be necessary for CT-guided biopsies to help identify the lesion, because masses are often isodense or unenhanced on CT. Ultrasound has the advantage of real-time imaging and allows the radiologist to compensate for patients who have difficulty controlling their respirations. The major limitation to ultrasound is that small or isoechoic lesions can be difficult to evaluate sonographically. Another limitation is ultrasound's inability to visualize the route of access to ensure that bowel is not present in the needle track.

The preferred access to a renal mass is via the shortest route and does not traverse bowel or solid organs. However, some masses can only be reached via a transhepatic or transplenic approach (especially masses in the upper pole). These masses can be biopsied with small needles with relative safety. The only organ that should be avoided is the pancreas. For CT-guided procedures it is best to use an axial plane; for ultrasound-guided, an oblique approach. Once the approach has been determined, the patient should be prepped and draped in standard fashion, and local anesthesia can be obtained with lidocaine.

CT-guided biopsies are performed without the use of a needle guide. Patients are placed in a supine, prone, or decubitus position to provide the optimal access to the mass. CT is used to image the location of the needle during its placement. The patients are carefully coached by the radiologist as to when to stop and resume breathing. The patient's breath should always be held during needle advancement. Patients who are not able to cooperate appropriately are not ideal for CT-directed biopsy and may be better suited for ultrasound guidance.

Ultrasound-guided biopsy can be performed freehand or with a needle guide attached to the transducer. The freehand method allows independent movement of both the sampling needle and transducer which allows the experienced operator more flexibility. The needle guide identifies a path for the needle at fixed angles, which allows for direct placement and visualization of the sampling needle along a specific route.

Many different sizes and types of needles can be used for the biopsy or aspiration. In general, smaller needle sizes are used for renal biopsies compared to other organs because the risk of bleeding is less (Gazelle et al. 1992). Although fine needles (17 to 22 gauge) have a lower complication rate than larger needles (14 and 15 gauge) (Meola et al. 1994; Cozens et al. 1992; Tung et al. 1992), the difference between 22- and 18-gauge needles is not as well-established in the kidney as in the liver (Wood et al. 1999). Therefore, the size and type of needle used is probably less important than proper use of the needle and operator experience.

Complications

The major complications of percutaneous renal biopsy are bleeding, pneumothorax, and tumor seeding along the needle tract. Bleeding has been cited as the most frequent complication (Vassiliades and Bernardino 1991). In the study by Nadel et al. (1986), the rate of significant complications was 6 per cent, and only one of 51 biopsies in their series required transfusion. CT evidence of perirenal hemorrhage has been reported to be as high as 91 per cent in a series of 200 biopsies (Ralls et al. 1987). This same series showed that CT was more sensitive and accurate than ultrasound in detecting postbiopsy hemorrhage, with a sensitivity of at least 91 per cent compared to 70 per cent for ultrasound (Ralls *et al.* 1987). Gross hematuria will occur in 5 to 7 per cent of patients but is usually self-limited and resolves in approximately 3 days (Vassiliades and Bernardino 1991). Persistent gross hematuria can be caused by the formation of an arteriovenous fistula or laceration of a large vessel.

Pneumothorax can occur when the approach for upper pole lesions traverses the pleural space, typically in a posterior intercostal approach. There are also higher risks of puncturing the spleen or liver while using the posterior approach. When patients lie prone during renal biopsies, the posterior segments of the lower lobes of both lungs often extend quite inferiorly. This can be seen in 14 to 29 per cent of patients (Hopper and Yakes 1990). Angling the approach, placing the patient in an oblique or decubitus position, or performing the biopsy during the expiration phase will minimize the risk of puncturing other organs.

A significant concern of percutaneous biopsy is the risk of tumor seeding along the needle tract. Large series of percutaneous biopsies of abdominal masses in general and a review of the medical literature revealed that tumor seeding occurred in less than 0.01 per cent of cases (Herts and Baker 1995; Smith 1984, 1991), although it is likely that the true incidence is underestimated. In Smith's (1991) review, most cases of tumor seeding occurred within 2 to 6 months from time of biopsy. Percutaneous biopsy of TCC appears to carry a higher risk of tract seeding in some authors' experience (Herts and Baker 1995). Our literature search has identified seven reported cases of needle tract seeding from percutaneous biopsies of renal masses (see Table 21.8). The risk of seeding tumor cells is not appreciably greater for the kidneys than for other organs (Auvert *et al.* 1982; Juul *et al.* 1985; Abe and Saitoh 1992). The tract seeding consisted of RCC (four cases), oncocytoma (one case), TCC (one case), and angiomyoliposarcoma (one case).

Because of the small risk of needle tract seeding, it is favorable to choose a direct tract route that avoids puncture of other organs. If a recurrent tumor is detected at the needle tract site, it should be resected. Leal (1992) reported biopsy results obtained via a transureteral aspiration catheter, and transvenous biopsies of renal masses invading the renal vein or inferior vena cava have also been performed (Coel and Chalmers 1975; Wendth *et al.* 1976), thereby avoiding tract seeding with contiguous organs or skin.

Death from percutaneous biopsy is rare but is a potential complication. In Smith's review (1991) of the literature, the death rate from four large studies was less than 0.1 per cent. He also analysed data from questionnaires of complications from more than 16 000 percutaneous biopsies, which revealed a death rate of 0.031 per cent. The majority of these deaths occurred secondary to bleeding complications. To date, none have been reported to have occurred due to renal mass biopsy.

Results of percutaneous biopsy

There have been several studies that have evaluated the sensitivity, specificity, positive and negative predictive value, accuracy, and retrieval rates of both cytological and histological renal biopsy samples (Nadel *et al.* 1986; Murphy *et al.* 1985; Nicefero and Coughlin 1993; Cristallani *et al.* 1991; Leiman 1990; Helm *et al.* 1983; Orell *et al.* 1985; Juul *et al.* 1985; Torp-Pedersen *et al.* 1991; Abe and Saitoh, 1992; Wolf 1998) using a variety of biopsy techniques, needle sizes and types, and forms of radiologic guidance. These reports show the sensitivity of biopsy to be 80 to 92 per cent for cytology and 70 to 92 per cent for histology. The specificity is reported to be approximately 83 to 100 per cent for cytology and as high as 100 per cent for histology. Positive and negative predictive values ranged from 90 to 95 per cent, and accuracy is between 87 to 93 per cent for both cytology and histology (Nicefero and Coughlin 1993; Cristallani *et al.* 1991; Helm *et al.* 1983; Juul *et al.* 1985). The retrieval rate, the rate of obtaining adequate cytological and histological specimens, varied from 70 to 98 per cent (Herts and Baker 1995). These studies incorporated a number of individuals with large locally advanced lesions, metastatic disease, and multiple biopsy attempts. Therefore inclusion of larger, more advanced lesions and a more aggressive biopsy technique may be likely to contribute to the high sensitivity, specificity, and predictive values reported in some series.

Dechet *et al.* (1999) studied intraoperative frozen needle biopsies of solid renal masses and found greater than 75 per cent accuracy with 94 per cent positive predictive value for carcinoma. Unfortunately, they found a large degree of inaccuracy for benign lesions and discouraged the routine use of intraoperative frozen needle biopsy to guide surgical decision-making In our review of the literature, the overall sensitivity, specificity, positive predictive value, and negative predictive value for the detection of malig-

Table 21.8 Tumor seeding of needle tract after biopsy of a renal mass*

Reference	Needle (gauge)	Time to presentation	Pathology
Gibbons *et al.* 1977	18	20 months	RCC
Auvert *et al.* 1982	Not noted	84 months	Oncocytoma
Kiser *et al.* 1986	14	3 weeks	RCC
Wehle and Grabstald 1986	20	48 months	RCC
Shenoy *et al.* 1991	23	12 months	RCC
Abe and Saitoh 1992	14–18	30 months	Angiomyoliposarcoma[†]
Slywotzsky and Maya 1994	22	8 months	TCC

* Adapted with permission from Wolf (1998).
[†] The biopsy diagnosed medullary fibroma, the surgical specimen revealed angiomyolipoma, and the recurrent tumor histology was liposarcoma.

Table 21.9 Fine needle aspiration or biopsy of renal masses*

| Reference | No. of definitive samples | Sample type[†] | Number of samples with | | True-[‡] | | False-[‡] | |
			Metastases	Pathology confirmed	Positive	Negative	Positive	Negative
Juul *et al.* 1985	285	Aspiration			185	61	14	25
Orell *et al.* 1985	80	Aspiration		58	62	12	1	5
Nadel *et al.* 1986	30	Aspiration			14	15	0	1
Holmberg *et al.* 1988	60	Aspiration			20	36	1	3
Pilotti *et al.* 1988	124	Aspiration		32	60	63	1	0
Leiman 1990	113	Aspiration	31	63	76	27	2	8
Haubek *et al.* 1991	161	Aspiration			112	28	4	17
Torp-Pederson *et al.* 1991	131	Aspiration		61	76	41	7	7
Torp-Pederson *et al.* 1991	106	Biopsy		61	60	38	0	8
Cristallini *et al.* 1991	72	Aspiration		27	33	34	1	4
Abe and Saitoh 1992	35	Biopsy	1	21	23	9	0	3
Mondal and Ghosh 1992	92	Aspiration	0	92	80	6	2	4
Nicefero and Coughlin 1993	10	Aspiration	10	0	9	0	0	1
Nicefero and Coughlin 1993	13	Aspiration	0	6	3	8	0	2
Campbell *et al.* 1997	16	Aspiration	0	16	10	0	0	6
Wood *et al.* 1999	79	Aspiration	6	74	49	25	0	5
Totals	1407			872[§]	403[§]	33[§]	99[§]	

* Adapted with permission from Wolf (1998).
[†] Aspiration samples that were insufficient have been deleted from the tabulated data when possible. From those studies, approximately 5% of the samples obtained from the fine needle aspiration were insufficient.
[‡] Determination of positive or negative cancer specimens was as defined by the individual authors. In some cases angiomyolipomas were considered malignant.
[§] Sensitivity 90%; specificity 92%; positive predictive value 96%; negative predictive value 80%.

nancy versus benign disease by fine needle aspiration or biopsy in 1407 cases were 90, 92, 96, and 80 per cent, respectively (summarized in Table 21.9). In these series, 69 per cent of the lesions were ultimately deemed malignant.

Tumor-grading reliability from the specimens has also been reported (Nurmi *et al.* 1984*b*; Cajulis *et al.* 1993, Campbell *et al.* 1997). Concordance of the final nuclear grade varied in the studies from 32 to 76 per cent. In the series by Nurmi *et al.* (1984*b*) on *ex vivo* specimens, differing grades were seen in the same specimen in 25 per cent of the cases.

Staging of the renal mass

Once sufficient suspicion of malignancy within a renal mass has been achieved, the evaluation should proceed to staging of the lesion. Such staging should include assessment of the local advancement of the mass with particular attention to invasion of local organs, vasculature, and collecting system; presence of lymphadenopathy; and the presence of multifocality within the ipsilateral or contralateral kidney. The stage at the time of treatment has direct correlation with prognosis; therefore thorough staging is of the utmost importance prior to beginning treatment. The stage of the tumor will also have an impact upon determining the surgical approach to the patient, the feasibility of partial resection of the kidney, and the necessity for additional testing such as chest CT and bone scan.

The history of staging RCC has evolved dramatically with the introduction of newer imaging modalities. Currently, the choice of imaging method to determine the tumor stage depends on numerous factors. It depends on the preference of the surgeon and the radiologic expertise and equipment of a given medical center. In the current emphasis on cost containment, some attention should be given to methods that reduce the overall expense by eliminating redundant evaluation. Therefore a well thought out and rational imaging approach is essential to the work-up of renal masses and their staging.

In the majority of cases, CT scan is all that is necessary to properly stage the renal mass after history, physical examination, and laboratory testing. We are generally unwilling to operate upon a solid mass diagnosed upon ultrasound alone because of the absence of anatomic information. Dynamic contrast-enhanced CT scanning is now accepted as the most effective method available for staging the majority of patients with renal masses (McClennan and Deyoe 1994; Newhouse 1993), and this is generally our test of choice. Cross-sectional imaging allows survey of the adjacent organs, lymph nodes, bones, and retroperitoneum in a single test. If CT scan evaluation reveals adjacent organ infiltration or distant metastases, evaluation may stop, except for obtaining a tissue diagnosis of the lesions (Levine 1987). Overall CT scan accuracy rates for staging RCC range from 61 to 91 per cent but, if errors due to perinephric invasion in stage I and II are excluded since these are generally treated in the same manner, the accuracy rate can be as high as 96 per cent (Johnson *et al.* 1987; London *et al.* 1989; Richie *et al.* 1983; Zeman *et al.* 1988). Furthermore, many of the studies on CT scanning were performed before the introduction of helical scanning, which probably limits the accuracy of these studies. The overall accuracy in staging RCC with

MRI has been reported to be between 82 and 96 per cent (Hricak *et al.* 1985, 1988; Choyke *et al.* 1984). If CT scan fails to completely stage the tumor extension for any number of reasons to be discussed, it is then appropriate to move to other imaging modalities such as MRI, ultrasound, or, rarely, angiography.

Many authors have recently suggested that MRI is comparable or even better than CT for the staging of renal masses (Hricak *et al.* 1985, 1988; Karstaedt *et al.* 1986; Fein *et al.* 1987; Amendola 1989; Semelka *et al.* 1992). MRI may be performed in sagittal, coronal, or oblique views, unlike CT scan, which primarily performs imaging in a transaxial plane. With the advent of helical CT scanning and volume-rendered CT and MRI, the imaging data can be created into multiplanar or three-dimensional reconstructions. The ability of MRI to perform direct orthogonal scanning planes can be very helpful, particularly in studying the vasculature. The intrinsic soft-tissue contrast of MRI exceeds that of CT scan and permits the distinction of tissues of similar consistency and density on CT. Compared to CT scan, the primary advantages of MRI include the ability to determine tumor extension, vascular patency, distinction of collateral vessels from lymph-node metastases, and delineation of soft-tissue planes (Amendola 1989; Benson *et al.* 1989; Fritzsche 1989).

Tumor stage

Local invasion

Stage I tumors are confined to the renal capsule while stage II tumors extend into the perinephric fat. Although stage II tumors have a worse prognosis than stage I, the inability to accurately distinguish these two stages radiographically has little impact on treatment in the majority of cases since the surgical option between radical and partial nephrectomy is the same. CT scan findings in stage II tumors are tumor extension into the perinephric fat, thickening of the renal fascia, obliteration or blurring of the perinephric fat, adrenal gland involvement, or visible collateral vessels (Bechtold and Zagoria 1997).

Centrally located tumors are easily identified as stage I on CT; however, if a tumor is exophytic, the differentiation between stage I and II cannot be made on CT scan reliably (Zagoria *et al.* 1995). Compared to MRI, CT scan is less sensitive in detecting tumor extension in lymphatics versus small collateral blood vessels. It is also unable to detect microscopic invasion of perinephric fat or distinguish inflammatory changes from tumor infiltration (Bechtold and Zagoria 1997). Perinephric stranding or interstitial infiltration is often seen with stage I and II tumors, however such stranding can also be confused with stranding often seen in resolving hematoma, fat necrosis, dilated collateral vessels, or edema of the perinephric connective tissue septa (Weyman *et al.* 1980; Zagoria *et al.* 1995). Perinephric invasion accounts for more than half of the staging errors on CT scan; therefore some experts recommend that stage II tumors cannot be diagnosed reliably on CT scan unless a soft-tissue mass of at least 1 cm is present in the perinephric space (Johnson *et al.* 1987). Thus, perinephric infiltration on CT scan can be diagnosed with only a sensitivity of 46 per cent and a specificity of 98 per cent (Johnson *et al.* 1987).

Tumors with direct extension into adjacent organs can be difficult to identify on CT alone. Adjacent organ invasion identification with CT scan has an accuracy of approximately 60 per cent with a sensitivity and specificity of approximately 60 and 100 per cent, respectively (Johnson *et al.* 1987). Direct invasion can only be diagnosed confidently when there is enlargement or a density difference in the adjacent organ, and not just by finding an absent soft-tissue plane between tumor and adjacent structure (Johnson *et al.* 1987). Direct extension of renal masses can occur into the adrenal, liver, colon, spleen, or iliopsoas musculature. Of these cases, hepatic extension is probably the most critical to identify preoperatively. Additionally, if a suspicion of colonic invasion exists, then preoperative bowel prep should be performed with a plan for possible resection. If suspected on CT, follow-up MRI may be advisable prior to undertaking resection.

As in the case of CT scan, MRI is not reliable in differentiating stage I and stage II lesions; however, as stated previously, this distinction has little impact on therapy (Bechtold and Zagoria 1997). Multiplanar imaging enables MRI to more accurately determine if an extrinsic mass is infiltrating the kidney or if the mass is originating from the kidney (Hricak *et al.* 1988). In particular, MRI is useful in distinguishing tumors arising from the kidney as opposed to the adrenal gland (Hricak *et al.* 1988). On spin echo imaging, adjacent organ invasion is seen as irregular and inhomogeneous changes in the signal intensity and obliteration of the soft-tissue plane between the organs. MRI is also useful in detecting liver metastases from RCC, but is not reliable in diagnosing lung metastases (Amendola 1989, Bechtold and Zagoria 1997). The positive and negative predictive value of MRI for direct invasion of liver, spleen, and psoas muscle is 74 per cent and 98 to 100 per cent, respectively (Hricak *et al.* 1988).

Venous invasion

Stage IIIA tumors invade venous structures including the renal vein or vena cava. In historical series, up to 20 per cent of RCC extend into the renal vein, and 10 per cent progress into the inferior vena cava (IVC) (Hatcher *et al.* 1992; Kearney *et al.* 1981; Skinner *et al.* 1972). Ultrasound can be very helpful in evaluating the intrahepatic IVC, proximal IVC, and right atrium for tumor thrombus (Levine 1987; McClennan and Deyoe 1994). Tumor thrombus appears as a solid, hyperechoic, or hypoechoic mass. If it is non-occlusive, it often moves within the flowing blood beside it. Lymph nodes when visible appear as soft-tissue masses and are characteristically anechoic without posterior acoustic enhancement (Bechtold and Zagoria 1997). Ultrasound's sensitivity is approximately 54 per cent in detecting thrombus in the distal renal vein or IVC and approximately 100 per cent in the intrahepatic IVC (Kallman *et al.* 1992; Didier *et al.* 1987; Schwerk *et al.* 1985).

CT scan is approximately 78 and 96 per cent accurate in the detection of tumor extension into the renal vein and IVC, respectively. CT scan findings in stage IIIA disease include venous enlargement, which occurs in the renal vein and IVC in 24 and 15 per cent of cases, respectively; abrupt changes in the caliber of the vein, which occur in the renal vein and IVC in 3 and 10 per cent, respectively; or intraluminal areas of decreased density (Zagoria *et al.* 1990; Amendola 1989; Levine 1987). A persistent filling defect in the venous system is associated with a 0 per cent false-positive rate (Johnson *et al.* 1987; Zeman *et al.* 1988).

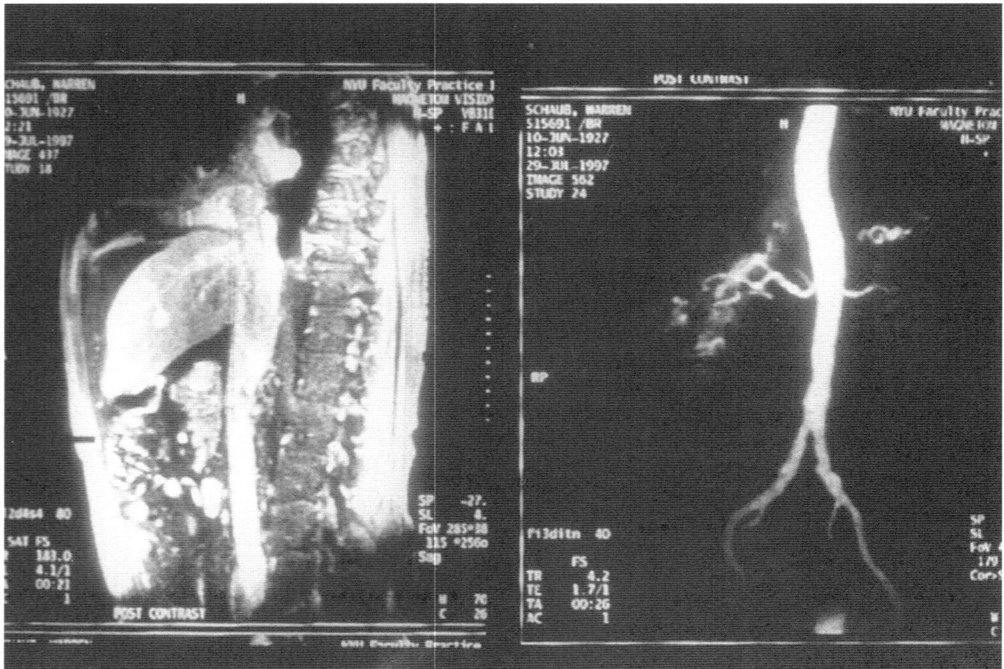

Fig. 21.12 Demonstration of a caval tumor thrombus extending to the right atrium in a patient with a large right renal tumor. The arrow indicates the atrial extension of the caval thrombus (left). MR angiogram reveals arterial vascularity within the tumor thrombus.

The diagnosis of venous invasion is strengthened by the presence of clot within collateral vessels (Zagoria *et al.* 1995). Thrombus may be bland (simple blood clot) or tumoral, which can be distinguished on CT scan by identifying a solid mass directly extending into the venous system (Zagoria *et al.* 1995). The most helpful finding to differentiate a tumor thrombus from a bland one is the presence of tumor enhancement within the vein secondary to neovascularity (Handel *et al.* 1983). However this finding only appears in 2 per cent of cases of tumor thrombus (Zagoria *et al.* 1990). The hypervascularity of RCC also can create many false-positive and false-negative results in stage IIIA tumors (Zeman *et al.* 1988). It can be difficult to distinguish between intraluminal tumor thrombus and extrinsic caval compression caused by a large primary tumor or enlarged lymph nodes, particularly on right-sided tumors (Levine 1987).

For these reasons, when a suspicion of venous thrombus exists, MRI is generally the preferred evaluative study (Fig. 21.12). Spin echo sequences are used to assess thrombus by depicting it as an area of increased signal intensity compared to blood, which typically has a low signal intensity. Gradient echo sequences are also used to assess thrombus by depicting flowing blood as a bright signal as opposed to thrombus which has a low signal intensity. These gradient images can be useful in cases with marked caval compression by bulky tumor mass (Roubidoux *et al.* 1992). MRI can also be of help in distinguishing bland from tumor thrombus and detecting vein wall invasion (Ford *et al.* 1985). The tumor thrombus exhibits intensity changes on MRI similar to those of the main tumor mass (Hricak *et al.* 1985), and may enhance with gadolinium allowing differentiation from bland thrombus

(Eilenberg et al. 1990). The spin echo imaging has a sensitivity and specificity of 82 and 97 per cent, respectively, in identifying caval thrombus; 65 and 81 per cent, respectively, in identifying renal vein tumor (Horan *et al.* 1989; Roubidoux *et al.* 1992). Overall accuracy in detecting invasion of the caval wall by MRI has been reported to be 63 per cent (Myneni *et al.* 1991).

As with CT and MRI, angiography has limitations when evaluating the patient with a bulky tumor that compresses or deviates the blood vessels (Horan *et al.* 1989). These masses can distort the vessels enough to create false-positive readings. Also false-positive findings may occur when normal, unopacified blood enters the vena cava from the renal vein giving the appearance of a filling defect (Zagoria *et al.* 1995). However this pitfall can be reduced by supplementing venacavography with selective renal venography (Bechtold and Zagoria 1997). Venography should be reserved for cases where CT or MRI is inconclusive or indeterminate, such as when a bulky tumor is adjacent to the IVC. In these cases, venography is complementary to MRI/MRA (magnetic resonance angiography), and, when combined, these have an accuracy near 100 per cent (Benson *et al.* 1989; Horan *et al.* 1989).

Lymphatic invasion

Stage IIIB tumors are associated with lymph node involvement. Patients with lymph node metastases and venous extension have a poor prognosis and treatment options are typically nonsurgical (London *et al.* 1989). CT scan has a sensitivity and specificity of approximately 83 and 88 per cent, respectively, in detecting lymphadenopathy related to RCC (Johnson *et al.* 1987). The detection of abnormal lymph nodes can be difficult; however, the involvement is inferred when a node exceeds a size criterion or when several nodes are clustered (Bechtold and Zagoria 1997). Lymph nodes greater than 2 cm have an extremely high correlation with metastatic disease (Levine 1987). This is pertinent since this size lymph node is found in up to 32 per cent of tumors (Zagoria *et al.* 1990). Some authorities, however, have advocated labeling lymph

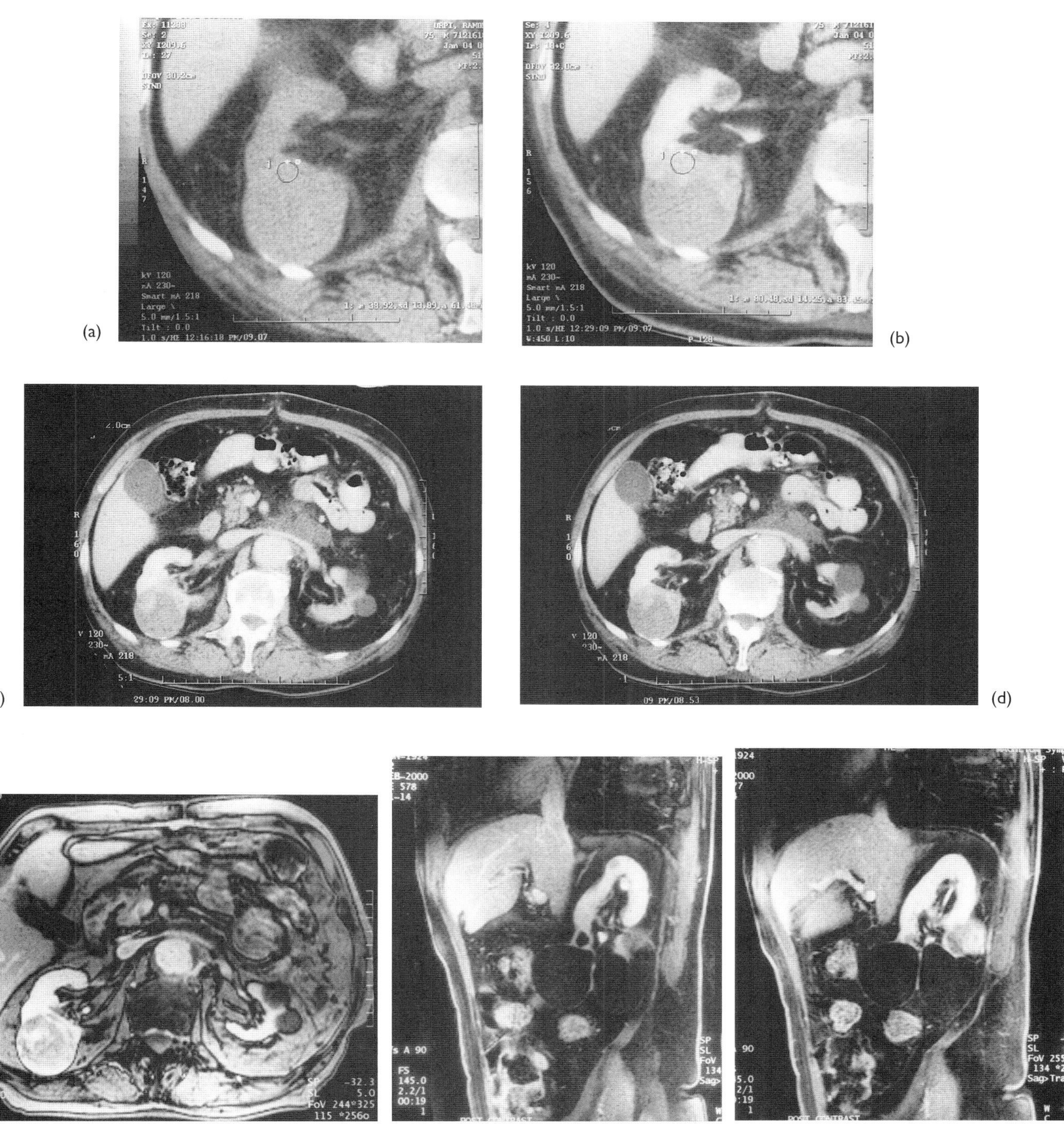

Fig. 21.13 An incidentally noted low-attenuating lesion of the right kidney at the time of abdominal aortic aneurysm repair. (a) On noncontrast CT the lesion is noted to be isodense with the kidney measuring 38.92 HU. (b) Upon contrast administration, internal focal enhancement is noted to a density of 80.48 HU. (c), (d) CT reveals the location of the tumor to be quite central in the kidney with a contralateral atrophic kidney. (e) Preoperative planning three-dimensional T2-weighted MRI demonstrates direct juxtaposition of the lower pole collecting system to the tumor predicting necessity for collecting system injury at the time of partial nephrectomy. (f) Sagittal T1-weighted gadolinium-enhanced images demonstrate a single segmental artery entering the tumor bed and (g) map access to the hilar tumor bed through two large lower pole simple cysts.

nodes as abnormal when greater than 1 cm to improve detection sensitivity (Fritzsche 1989), but others state this size should still be considered indeterminate secondary to the high false-positive rate (Johnson *et al.* 1987). When using the size criteria of 1 cm or greater, the false-positive rate of lymph node involvement is between 3 and 43 per cent (Fein *et al.* 1987; Johnson *et al.* 1987; Hatcher *et al.* 1992). There is also at least a 4 per cent false-negative rate in detection of microscopic tumor invasion of normal-sized lymph nodes (Studer *et al.* 1990). Lymph node enlargement can also be secondary to inflammatory changes, particularly in the presence of tumor necrosis or tumor thrombus (Studer *et al.* 1990).

Preoperative planning

With the emergence of partial nephrectomy as an effective and indicated treatment for small peripherally located renal tumors, the role of preoperative imaging has extended to intrarenal evaluation with the intent of determining the feasibility of partial resection. In general, lesions that are < 4 cm, peripherally located, and solitary are ideal for partial nephrectomy. Bilateral tumors are present in approximately 4 per cent of cases (Russo 2000) and 7–25 per cent of cases are multifocal (Mukamel *et al.* 1988; Cheng *et al.* 1991; Nissenkorn and Bernheim 1995; Whang *et al.* 1995; Kletscher *et al.* 1995; Wunderlich *et al.* 2000; Campbell *et al.* 1996; Schlichter *et al.* 2000) With improved imaging techniques, surgeons have now begun to consider larger lesions for elective partial nephrectomy, provided the lesion is not invading into the centrally located vascular structures of the kidney.

As such, the ability of individual imaging modalities to predict vascular invasion, collecting system invasion, and multifocality has become of paramount importance. Standard CT and MRI techniques allow excellent delineation of the size and position of an individual tumor. As described above, MRI may be more accurate in the evaluation of small renal vein tumor invasion. CT has the limitation of poor delineation of subcentimeter renal lesions which may represent multifocal disease. In this regard, MRI once again provides a greater ability to detect small lesions because of its three-dimensional imaging capability.

Angiography may provide a comprehensive map of the renal vasculature to aid the surgeon and directly visualize the IVC lumen. However, newer imaging modalities such as CT or MRA can also visualize the vasculature non-invasively. Gadolinium-enhanced MRA has been found to be 90–100 per cent accurate; and its reliability is comparable to conventional angiography in determining renal vascular anatomy in living kidney donors without any of the associated potential angiographic complications (Buzzas *et al.* 1997; Gourlay *et al.* 1995; Nelson *et al.* 1999; Choyke *et al.* 1997).

The latest development in three-dimensional imaging is volume-rendering, which allows real-time interactive stereoscopic viewing without preliminary editing, and presents complex renal parenchymal and vascular anatomy in a format familiar to the surgeon and consistent with intraoperative findings. Three-dimensional volume-rendered CT was prospec-

tively evaluated in 60 patients undergoing nephron-sparing surgery for RCC at the Cleveland Clinic Foundation. The number and location of lesions had an accuracy of 100 per cent and enhancement and diagnostic characteristics were consistent with pathological findings in 98 per cent of cases. Ninety-six percent of renal arteries and 93 per cent of renal veins were detected with this technique (Coll *et al.* 1999).

We have recently utilized three-dimensional volume-rendered MRI for preoperative planning of partial nephrectomy (Fig. 21.13). In the technique, the position of the tumor along with its relationship to centrally located intrarenal structures is evaluated in volume-rendered three-dimensional images that allow sectioning of kidney in any plane using computer reconstruction. Images are obtained during an arteriographic phase for evaluation of tumor vessels, nephrographic phase for evaluation of tumor interfaces, and delayed lasix–urogram phase for evaluation of the relationship to the collecting system. We have used the technique to determine the feasibility of partial resection as well as the intraoperative plan.

In a preliminary evaluation of 27 consecutive renal tumors, 14 tumors were selected for partial nephrectomy, and 13 for radical nephrectomy (unpublished data). Preoperative images were compared with intraoperative ultrasound and pathologic findings. Multifocality was identified down to a size cut-off of 5 mm in 100 per cent of cases (Fig. 21.14). Nodal metastases were identified with a sensitivity of 80 per cent and specificity of 91 per

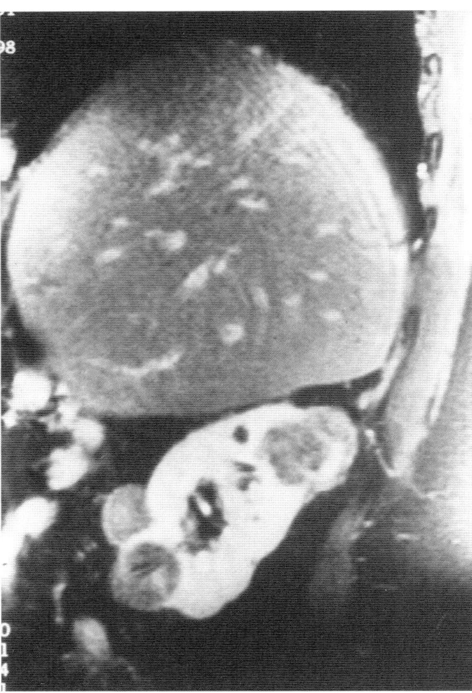

Fig. 21.14 Multifocal renal tumors in an individual with bilateral RCC (see Fig. 21.11). Sagittal section T1-weighted gadolinium-enhanced MRI reveals multiple solid enhancing masses within the kidney. Upper and lower pole partial nephrectomy was performed revealing four moderately differentiated papillary renal RCC, the smallest measuring 6 mm. All were identified on the preoperative planning MRI.

cent. Involvement of the collecting system was noted with a sensitivity of 89 per cent and specificity of 83 per cent, while injury to the collecting system was predicted with 100 per cent accuracy. Preoperative prediction of tumor stage was performed with 88 per cent accuracy. The effects on surgical outcome remain to be identified.

The evaluation of a patient with a renal mass has undergone dramatic changes in recent years with the technologic advances in the fields of radiologic imaging, including ultrasound, CT, and MRI. These new imaging techniques have also led to a dramatic increase in the identification of incidental renal masses. In approaching a patient with a renal mass, the physician must first understand the differential diagnosis of renal lesions, the characteristic features of each type, the available diagnostic imaging modalities, the role of invasive diagnostic techniques, and the staging of malignant disease. The ultimate goal is to provide information useful in understanding the different radiologic modalities and creating a framework for the successful identification of a renal lesion. From this framework, indeterminate lesions will also be identifiable and options for their further evaluation have also been presented. Obtaining a diagnosis will allow the physician to determine the appropriate management options and the role of surgical intervention.

Acknowledgement
We would like to thank Dr Morton A. Bosniak, Professor of Radiology and Urology, New York University School of Medicine, for his support, advice, and assistance in preparing this manuscript.

References

Abe, M. and Saitoh, M. (1992). Selective renal tumour biopsy under ultrasonic guidance. *Br. J. Urol.* **70**, 7–11.

Ambos, M.A., Bosniak, M.A., Valensi, Q.J., Madayag, M.A., and Lefleur, R.S. (1978). Angiographic patterns in renal oncocytomas. *Radiology* **129**, 615–22.

Amendola, M.A. (1989). Comparison of MR imaging and CT in the evaluation of renal masses. *Crit. Rev. Diagn. Imaging* **29**, 117–50.

Amendola, M.A., Bree, R.L., Pollack, H.M., Francis, I.R., Glazer, G.M., Jafri, S.Z., and Tomaszewski, J.E. (1988). Small renal cell carcinomas: resolving a diagnostic dilemma. *Radiology* **166**, 637–41.

Anderson, C.M., Pusztai, L., Palmer, J.L., Cabanillas, F., and Ellerhorst, J.A. (1998). Coincident renal cell carcinoma and nonHodgkin's lymphoma: the M.D. Anderson experience and review of the literature. *J. Urol.* **159**, 714–17.

Aronson, S., Frazier, H.A., Baluch, J.D., Hartman, D.S., and Christenson, P.J. (1991). Cystic renal masses: usefulness of the Bosniak classification [see comments]. *Urol. Radiol.* **13**, 83–90.

Auvert, J., Abbou, C.C., and Lavarenne, V. (1982). Needle tract seeding following puncture of renal oncocytoma. *Prog. Clin. Biol. Res.* **100**, 597–8.

Barbaric, Z.L. (1994). *Principles of genitourinary radiology*. Thieme Medical Publishers, New York.

Bartolozzi, C., Caramella, D., and Zampa, V. (1991). [Problems and errors of magnetic resonance in the diagnosis of renal masses]. *Radiol. Med.* (*Torino*) **82**, 253–9.

Bechtold, R. E. and Zagoria, R. J. (1997). Imaging approach to staging of renal cell carcinoma. *Urol. Clin. N. Am.* **24**, 507–22.

Bellman, G.C., Yamaguchi, R., and Kaswick, J. (1995). Laparoscopic evaluation of indeterminate renal cysts. *Urology* **45**, 1066–70.

Benson, M.A., Haaga, J.R., and Resnick, M.I. (1989). Staging renal carcinoma. What is sufficient? *Arch. Surg.* **124**, 71–3.

Birnbaum, B.A., Bosniak, M.A., Megibow, A.J., Lubat, E., and Gordon, R.B. (1990). Observations on the growth of renal neoplasms. *Radiology* **176**, 695–701.

Bonavita, J.A., Pollack, H.M., and Banner, M.P. (1980). Renal oncocytoma: further observations and literature review. *Urol. Radiol.* **2**, 229–34.

Bosniak, M.A. (1984). The changing approach to the management of renal angiomyolipomas. *Urol. Radiol.* **6**, 194–5.

Bosniak, M.A. (1986). The current radiological approach to renal cysts. *Radiology* **158**, 1–10.

Bosniak, M.A. (1991*a*). Difficulties in classifying cystic lesions of the kidney [comment]. *Urol. Radiol.* **13**, 91–3.

Bosniak, M.A. (1991*b*). The small (less than or equal to 3.0 cm) renal parenchymal tumor: detection, diagnosis, and controversies [published erratum appears in *Radiology* 1991 Oct. 181(1):289]. *Radiology* **179**, 307–17.

Bosniak, M.A. (1993). Problems in the radiologic diagnosis of renal parenchymal tumors. *Urol. Clin. N. Am.* **20**, 217–30.

Bosniak, M.A. (1995). Observation of small incidentally detected renal masses. *Sem. Urol. Oncol.* **13**, 267–72.

Bosniak, M.A. and Rofsky, N.M. (1996). Problems in the detection and characterization of small renal masses [letter; comment]. *Radiology* **200**, 286–7.

Bosniak, M.A., Megibow, A.J., Hulnick, D.H., Horii, S., and Raghavendra, B.N. (1988). CT diagnosis of renal angiomyolipoma: the importance of detecting small amounts of fat. *Am. J. Roentgenol.* **151**, 497–501.

Bosniak, M.A., Birnbaum, B.A., Krinsky, G.A., and Waisman, J. (1995). Small renal parenchymal neoplasms: further observations on growth [see comments]. *Radiology* **197**, 589–97.

Buzzas, G.R., Shield, C.F., III, Pay, N.T., Neuman, M.J., and Smith, J.L. (1997). Use of gadolinium-enhanced, ultrafast, three-dimensional, spoiled gradient-echo magnetic resonance angiography in the preoperative evaluation of living renal allograft donors. *Transplantation* **64**, 1734–7.

Cajulis, R.S., Katz, R.L., Dekmezian, R., el-Naggar, A., and Ro, J.Y. (1993). Fine needle aspiration biopsy of renal cell carcinoma. Cytologic parameters and their concordance with histology and flow cytometric data. *Acta Cytol.* **37**, 367–72.

Campbell, S.C., Fichtner, J., Novick, A.C., Steinbach, F., Stockle, M., Klein, E.A., Filipas, D., Levin, H.S., Storkel, S., Schweden, F., Obuchowski, N.A., and Hale, J. (1996). Intraoperative evaluation of renal cell carcinoma: a prospective study of the role of ultrasonography and histopathological frozen sections. *J. Urol.* **155**, 1191–5.

Campbell, S.C., Novick, A.C., Herts, B., Fischler, D.F., Meyer, J., Levin, H.S., and Chen, R.N. (1997). Prospective evaluation of fine needle aspiration of small, solid renal masses: accuracy and morbidity. *Urology* **50**, 25–9.

Charboneau, J.W., Reading, C.C., and Welch, T.J. (1990). CT and sonographically guided needle biopsy: current techniques and new innovations [see comments]. *Am. J. Roentgenol.* **154**, 1–10.

Cheng, W.S., Farrow, G.M., and Zincke, H. (1991). The incidence of multicentricity in renal cell carcinoma [see comments]. *J. Urol.* **146**, 1221–3.

Choyke, P.L., Kressel, H.Y., Pollack, H.M., Arger, P.M., Axel, L., and Mamourian, A.C. (1984). Focal renal masses: magnetic resonance imaging. *Radiology* **152**, 471–7.

Choyke, P.L., White, E.M., Zeman, R.K., Jaffe, M.H., and Clark, L.R. (1987). Renal metastases: clinicopathologic and radiologic correlation. *Radiology* **162**, 359–63.

Choyke, P.L., Walther, M.M., Wagner, J.R., Rayford, W., Lyne, J.C., and Linehan, W.M. (1997). Renal cancer: preoperative evaluation with dual-phase three-dimensional MR angiography. *Radiology* **205**, 767–71.

Cloix, P., Martin, X., Pangaud, C., Marechal, J.M., Bouvier, R., Barat, D., and Dubernard, J.M. (1996). Surgical management of complex renal cysts: a series of 32 cases [see comments]. *J. Urol.* **156**, 28–30.

Coel, M.N. and Chalmers, J. (1975). Percutaneous catheter transcaval tumor biopsy. *Radiology* **116**, 222.

Coleman, B.G., Arger, P.H., Mintz, M.C., Pollack, H.M., and Banner, M.P. (1984). Hyperdense renal masses: a computed tomographic dilemma. *Am. J. Roentgenol.* **143**, 291–4.

Coll, D.M., Uzzo, R.G., Herts, B.R., Davros, W.J., Wirth, S.L., and Novick, A.C. (1999). 3-dimensional volume rendered computerized tomography for preoperative evaluation and intraoperative treatment of patients undergoing nephron sparing surgery. *J. Urol.* **161**, 1097–102.

Cozens, N.J., Murchison, J.T., Allan, P.L., and Winney, R.J. (1992).Conventional 15 G needle technique for renal biopsy compared with ultrasound-guided spring-loaded 18 G needle biopsy. *Br. J. Radiol.* **65**, 594–7.

Cristallini, E.G., Paganelli, C., and Bolis, G.B. (1991). Role of fine-needle aspiration biopsy in the assessment of renal masses. *Diagn. Cytopathol.* **7**, 32–5.

Curry, N.S. (1995). Small renal masses (lesions smaller than 3 cm): imaging evaluation and management. *Am. J. Roentgenol.* **164**, 355–62.

Curry, N.S. and Bissada, N.K. (1997). Radiologic evaluation of small and indeterminant renal masses. *Urol. Clin. N. Am.* **24**, 493–505.

Curry, N.S., Brock, G., Metcalf, J.S., and Sens, M.A. (1982). Hyperdense renal mass: unusual CT appearance of a benign renal cyst. *Urol. Radiol.* **4**, 33–5.

Dechet, C.B., Sebo, T., Farrow, G., Blute, M.L., Engen, D.E., and Zincke, H. (1999). Prospective analysis of intraoperative frozen needle biopsy of solid renal masses in adults. *J. Urol.* **162**, 1282–4; discussion 1284–5.

Defossez, S.M., Yoder, I.C., Papanicolaou, N., Rosen, B.R., and McGovern, F. (1991). Nonspecific magnetic resonance appearance of renal onco-cytomas: report of 3 cases and review of the literature. *J. Urol.* **145**, 552–4.

Demos, T.C., Schiffer, M., Love, L., Waters, W.B., and Moncada, R. (1985). Normal excretory urography in patients with primary kidney neoplasms. *Urol. Radiol.* **7**, 75–9.

Didier, D., Racle, A., Etievent, J.P., and Weill, F. (1987). Tumor thrombus of the inferior vena cava secondary to malignant abdominal neoplasms: US and CT evaluation. *Radiology* **162**, 83–9.

Eilenberg, S.S., Lee, J.K., Brown, J., Mirowitz, S.A., and Tartar, V.M. (1990). Renal masses: evaluation with gradient-echo Gd-DTPA-enhanced dynamic MR imaging. *Radiology* **176**, 333–8.

Einstein, D.M., Herts, B.R., Weaver, R., Obuchowski, N., Zepp, R., and Singer, A. (1995). Evaluation of renal masses detected by excretory urography: cost-effectiveness of sonography versus CT. *Am. J. Roentgenol.* **164**, 371–5.

Fein, A.B., Lee, J.K., Balfe, D.M., Heiken, J.P., Ling, D., Glazer, H.S., and McClennan, B.L. (1987). Diagnosis and staging of renal cell carcinoma: a comparison of MR imaging and CT. *Am. J. Roentgenol.* **148**, 749–53.

Ford, K.K., Braun, S.D., Miller, G.A., Jr, Newman, G.E., and Dunnick, N.R. (1985). Intravenous digital subtraction angiography in the preoperative evaluation of renal masses. *Am. J. Roentgenol.* **145**, 323–6.

Fraser, I.R. and Fairley, K.F. (1995). Renal biopsy as an outpatient procedure. *Am. J. Kidney Dis.* **25**, 876–8.

Fritzsche, P.J. (1989). Current state of MRI in renal mass diagnosis and staging of RCC. *Urol. Radiol.* **11**, 210–14.

Gazelle, G.S. and Haaga, J.R. (1989). Guided percutaneous biopsy of intra-abdominal lesions. *Am. J. Roentgenol.* **153**, 929–35.

Gazelle, G.S., Haaga, J.R., and Rowland, D.Y. (1992). Effect of needle gauge, level of anticoagulation, and target organ on bleeding associated with aspiration biopsy. Work in progress. *Radiology* **183**, 509–13.

Gibbons, R.P., Bush, W.H., Jr, and Burnett, L.L. (1977). Needle tract seeding following aspiration of renal cell carcinoma. *J. Urol.* **118**, 865–7.

Goldman, S.M. (1997). Editorial comment. *J. Urol.* **157**, 1524.

Gourlay, W.A., Yucel, E.K., Hakaim, A.G., O'Meara, Y.M., Mesler, D.E., Kerr, K., and Cho, S.I. (1995). Magnetic resonance angiography in the evaluation of living-related renal donors. *Transplantation* **60**, 1363–6.

Handel, D.B., Heaston, D.K., Korobkin, M., Silverman, P.M., and Dunnick, N.R. (1983). Circumaortic left renal vein with tumor thrombus: CT diagnosis with angiographic and pathologic correlation. *Am. J. Roentgenol.* **141**, 97–8.

Harmon, W.J., King, B.F., and Lieber, M.M. (1996). Renal oncocytoma: magnetic resonance imaging characteristics. *J. Urol.* **155**, 863–7.

Harris, R.D., Goergen, T.G., and Talner, L.B. (1975). The bloody renal cyst aspirate: a diagnostic dilemma. *J. Urol.* **114**, 832–5.

Hatcher, P.A., Paulson, D.F., and Anderson, E.E. (1992). Accuracy in staging of renal cell carcinoma involving vena cava. *Urology* **39**, 27–30.

Haubek, A., Lundorf, E., and Lauridsen, K.N. (1991). Diagnostic strategy in renal mass lesions. *Scand. J. Urol. Nephrol. Suppl.* **137**, 35–9.

Helenon, O., Chretien, Y., Paraf, F., Melki, P., Denys, A., and Moreau, J.F. (1993). Renal cell carcinoma containing fat: demonstration with CT [see comment]. *Radiology* **188**, 429–30.

Helm, C.W., Burwood, R.J., Harrison, N.W., and Melcher, D.H. (1983). Aspiration cytology of solid renal tumours. *Br. J. Urol.* **55**, 249–53.

Herts, B.R. and Baker, M.E. (1995). The current role of percutaneous biopsy in the evaluation of renal masses. *Sem. Urol. Oncol.* **13**, 254–61.

Hilpert, P.L., Friedman, A.C., Radecki, P.D., Caroline, D.F., Fishman, E.K., Meziane, M.A., Mitchell, D.G., and Kressel, H.Y. (1986). MRI of hemor-rhagic renal cysts in polycystic kidney disease. *Am. J. Roentgenol.* **146**, 1167–72.

Holmberg, G., Hietala, S.O., and Ljungberg, B. (1988). A comparison of radio-logic methods in the diagnosis of renal mass lesions. *Scand. J. Urol. Nephrol.* **22**, 187–96.

Hopper, K.D. and Yakes, W.F. (1990). The posterior intercostal approach for percutaneous renal procedures: risk of puncturing the lung, spleen, and liver as determined by CT. *Am. J. Roentgenol.* **154**, 115–17.

Horan, J.J., Robertson, C.N., Choyke, P.L., Frank, J.A., Miller, D.L., Pass, H.I., and Linehan, W.M. (1989). The detection of renal carcinoma extension into the renal vein and inferior vena cava: a prospective comparison of venacavography and magnetic resonance imaging. *J. Urol.* **142**, 943–7; discussion 947–8.

Horii, S.C., Bosniak, M.A., Megibow, A.J., Raghavendra, B.N., Subramanyam, B.R., and Rothberg, M. (1983). Correlation of CT and ultrasound in the evaluation of renal lymphoma. *Urol. Radiol.* **5**, 69–76.

Hovsepian, D.M., Levy, H., Amis, E.S., Jr, and Newhouse, J.H. (1990). MR eval-uation of renal space-occupying lesions: diagnostic criteria. *Urol. Radiol.* **12**, 74–9.

Hricak, H., Amparo, E., Fisher, M.R., Crooks, L., and Higgins, C.B. (1985). Abdominal venous system: assessment using MR. *Radiology* **156**, 415–22.

Hricak, H., Thoeni, R.F., Carroll, P.R., Demas, B.E., Marotti, M., and Tanagho, E.A. (1988). Detection and staging of renal neoplasms: a reassessment of MR imaging. *Radiology* **166**, 643–9.

Jennings, S.B. and Linehan, W.M. (1996). Renal, perirenal, and ureteral neoplasms. In *Adult and pediatric urology* (ed. J.Y. Gillenwater, J.T. Grayhack, S.S. Howards, and J.W. Duckett), pp. 643–94. Mosby, St Louis.

Johnson, C.D., Dunnick, N.R., Cohan, R.H., and Illescas, F.F. (1987). Renal adenocarcinoma: CT staging of 100 tumors. *Am. J. Roentgenol.* **148**, 59–63.

Juul, N., Torp-Pedersen, S., Gronvall, S., Holm, H.H., Koch, F., and Larsen, S. (1985). Ultrasonically guided fine needle aspiration biopsy of renal masses. *J. Urol.* **133**, 579–81.

Kadesky, K.T. and Fulgham, P.F. (1993). Bilateral multifocal renal oncocytoma: case report and review of the literature. *J. Urol.* **150**, 1227–8.

Kallman, D.A., King, B.F., Hattery, R.R., Charboneau, J.W., Ehman, R.L., Guthman, D.A., and Blute, M.L. (1992). Renal vein and inferior vena cava tumor thrombus in renal cell carcinoma: CT, US, MRI and venacavography. *J. Comput. Assist. Tomogr.* **16**, 240–7.

Karstaedt, N., McCullough, D.L., Wolfman, N.T., and Dyer, R.B. (1986). Magnetic resonance imaging of the renal mass. *J. Urol.* **136**, 566–70.

Kass, D.A., Hricak, H., and Davidson, A.J. (1983). Renal malignancies with normal excretory urograms. *Am. J. Roentgenol.* **141**, 731–4.

Kavoussi, L.R., Torrence, R.J., and Catalona, W.J. (1985). Renal oncocytoma with synchronous contralateral renal cell carcinoma. *J. Urol.* **134**, 1193–6.

Kearney, G.P., Waters, W.B., Klein, L.A., Richie, J.P., and Gittes, R.F. (1981). Results of inferior vena cava resection for renal cell carcinoma. *J. Urol.* **125**, 769–73.

Kiser, G.C., Totonchy, M., and Barry, J.M. (1986). Needle tract seeding after percutaneous renal adenocarcinoma aspiration. *J. Urol.* **136**, 1292–3.

Klein, M.J. and Valensi, Q.J. (1976). Proximal tubular adenomas of kidney with so-called oncocytic features. A clinicopathologic study of 13 cases of a rarely reported neoplasm. *Cancer* **38**, 906–14.

Kletscher, B.A., Qian, J., Bostwick, D.G., Andrews, P.E., and Zincke, H. (1995). Prospective analysis of multifocality in renal cell carcinoma: influence of histological pattern, grade, number, size, volume and deoxyribonucleic acid ploidy. *J. Urol.* **153**, 904–6.

Konnak, J.W. and Grossman, H.B. (1985). Renal cell carcinoma as an incidental finding. *J. Urol.* **134**, 1094–6.

Kreft, B.P., Muller-Miny, H., Sommer, T., Steudel, A., Vahlensieck, M., Novak, D., Muller, B.G., and Schild, H.H. (1997). Diagnostic value of MR imaging in comparison to CT in the detection and differential diagnosis of renal masses: ROC analysis. *Eur. Radiol.* **7**, 542–7.

Kuijpers, D. and Jaspers, R. (1989). Renal masses: differential diagnosis with pulsed Doppler US. *Radiology* **170**, 59–60.

Lanctin, H.P. and Futter, N.G. (1990). Renal cell carcinoma: incidental detection. *Can. J. Surg.* **33**, 488–90.

Lang, E.K. (1973). Roentgenographic assessment of asymptomatic renal lesions. An analysis of the confidence level of diagnoses established by sequential roentgenographic investigation. *Radiology* **109**, 257–69.

Lang, E.K. (1977). Renal cyst puncture and aspiration: a survey of complications. *Am. J. Roentgenol.* **128**, 723–7.

Lautin, E.M., Gordon, P.M., Friedman, A.C., McCormick, J.F., Fromowitz, F.B., Goldman, M.J., and Sugarman, L.A. (1981). Radionuclide imaging and computed tomography in renal oncocytoma. *Radiology* **138**, 185–90.

Leal, J.J. (1992). A new procedure for biopsy of a solid renal mass: transurethral approach under fluoroscopic control. *J. Urol.* **148**, 98–100.

Lehmann, H.D. and Blessing, M.H. (1982). Renal oncocytoma (pathology, preoperative diagnosis, therapy). *Prog. Clin. Biol. Res.* **100**, 589–96.

Leiman, G. (1990). Audit of fine needle aspiration cytology of 120 renal lesions. *Cytopathology* **1**, 65–72.

Levine, E. (1987). Renal cell carcinoma: radiological diagnosis and staging. *Sem. Roentgenol.* **22**, 248–59.

Levine, E. and Huntrakoon, M. (1983). Computed tomography of renal oncocytoma. *Am. J. Roentgenol.* **141**, 741–6.

Licht, M.R. (1995). Renal adenoma and oncocytoma. *Sem. Urol. Oncol.* **13**, 262–6.

Licht, M.R., Novick, A.C., Tubbs, R.R., Klein, E.A., Levin, H.S., and Streem, S.B. (1993). Renal oncocytoma: clinical and biological correlates. *J. Urol.* **150**, 1380–3.

Lieber, M.M. (1993). Renal oncocytoma. *Urol. Clin. N. Am.* **20**, 355–9.

London, N.J., Messios, N., Kinder, R.B., Smart, J.G., Osborn, D.E., Watkin, E.M., and Flynn, J.T. (1989). A prospective study of the value of conventional CT, dynamic CT, ultrasonography and arteriography for staging renal carcinoma. *Br. J. Urol.* **64**, 209–17.

Marotti, M., Hricak, H., Fritzsche, P., Crooks, L.E., Hedgcock, M.W., and Tanagho, E.A. (1987). Complex and simple renal cysts: comparative evaluation with MR imaging. *Radiology* **162**, 679–84.

McClennan, B.L. and Deyoe, L.A. (1994). The imaging evaluation of renal cell carcinoma: diagnosis and staging. *Radiol. Clin. N. Am.* **32**, 55–69.

Meola, M., Barsotti, G., Cupisti, A., Buoncristiani, E., and Giovannetti, S. (1994). Free-hand ultrasound-guided renal biopsy: report of 650 consecutive cases [see comments]. *Nephron* **67**, 425–30.

Mevorach, R.A., Segal, A.J., Tersegno, M.E., and Frank, I.N. (1992). Renal cell carcinoma: incidental diagnosis and natural history: review of 235 cases. *Urology* **39**, 519–22.

Mitnick, J.S., Bosniak, M.A., Rothberg, M., Megibow, A.J., Raghavendra, B.N., and Subramanyam, B.R. (1985). Metastatic neoplasm to the kidney studied by computed tomography and sonography. *J. Comput. Assist. Tomogr.* **9**, 43–9.

Mondal, A. and Ghosh, E. (1992). Fine needle aspiration cytology (FNAC) in the diagnosis of solid renal masses—a study of 92 cases. *Ind. J. Pathol. Microbiol.* **35**, 333–9.

Morra, M.N. and Das, S. (1993). Renal oncocytoma: a review of histogenesis, histopathology, diagnosis and treatment. *J. Urol.* **150**, 295–302.

Mukamel, E., Konichezky, M., Engelstein, D., and Servadio, C. (1988). Incidental small renal tumors accompanying clinically overt renal cell carcinoma. *J. Urol.* **140**, 22–4.

Murphy, W.M., Zambroni, B.R., Emerson, L.D., Moinuddin, S., and Lee, L.H. (1985). Aspiration biopsy of the kidney. Simultaneous collection of cytologic and histologic specimens. *Cancer* **56**, 200–5.

Myneni, L., Hricak, H., and Carroll, P.R. (1991). Magnetic resonance imaging of renal carcinoma with extension into the vena cava: staging accuracy and recent advances. *Br. J. Urol.* **68**, 571–8.

Nadel, L., Baumgartner, B.R., and Bernardino, M.E. (1986). Percutaneous renal biopsies: accuracy, safety, and indications. *Urol. Radiol.* **8**, 67–71.

Nelson, H.A., Gilfeather, M., Holman, J.M., Nelson, E.W., and Yoon, H.C. (1999). Gadolinium-enhanced breathhold three-dimensional time-of-flight renal MR angiography in the evaluation of potential renal donors. *J. Vasc. Interv. Radiol.* **10**, 175–81.

Newhouse, J.H. (1993). The radiologic evaluation of the patient with renal cancer. *Urol. Clin. N. Am.* **20**, 231–46.

Niceforo, J. and Coughlin, B.F. (1993). Diagnosis of renal cell carcinoma: value of fine-needle aspiration cytology in patients with metastases or contraindications to nephrectomy. *Am. J. Roentgenol.* **161**, 1303–5.

Nishikubo, C.Y., Kunkel, L.A., Figlin, R., Belldegrun, A., Rosen, P., Elashoff, R., Wang, H., and Territo, M.C. (1996). An association between renal cell carcinoma and lymphoid malignancies. A case series of eight patients [see comments]. *Cancer* **78**, 2421–6.

Nissenkorn, I. and Bernheim, J. (1995). Multicentricity in renal cell carcinoma. *J. Urol.* **153**, 620–2.

Novick, A.C., Streem, S., Montie, J.E., Pontes, J. E., Siegel, S., Montague, D.K., and Goormastic, M. (1989). Conservative surgery for renal cell carcinoma: a single-center experience with 100 patients. *J. Urol.* **141**, 835–9.

Nurmi, M., Satokari, K., and Alanen, K. (1984*a*). Angiography in renal oncocytoma: a report on 13 cases. *Eur. Urol.* **10**, 303–5.

Nurmi, M., Tyrkko, J., Puntala, P., Sotarauta, M., and Antila, L. (1984*b*). Reliability of aspiration biopsy cytology in the grading of renal adenocarcinoma. *Scand. J. Urol. Nephrol.* **18**, 151–6.

Oesterling, J.E., Fishman, E.K., Goldman, S.M., and Marshall, F.F. (1986). The management of renal angiomyolipoma. *J. Urol.* **135**, 1121–4.

Omachi, T., Sakamoto, W., Kishimoto, T., Kawano, M., Oyama, A., Kamizuru, M., Maekawa, M., Hagihara, S., and Nakamura, K. (1992). [A case of renal cyst associated with renal cell carcinoma– characteristics of intracystic fluid associated with renal cell carcinoma from Japanese reports]. *Hinyokika Kiyo* **38**, 323–6.

Orell, S.R., Langlois, S.L., and Marshall, V.R. (1985). Fine needle aspiration cytology in the diagnosis of solid renal and adrenal masses. *Scand. J. Urol. Nephrol.* **19**, 211–16.

Ozen, H., Colowick, A., and Freiha, F.S. (1993). Incidentally discovered solid renal masses: what are they? *Br. J. Urol.* **72**, 274–6.

Patel, A. and DeKernion, J.B. (1997). Diagnosis and staging of renal cell cancer. In *Urologic oncology* (ed. J.E. Oesterling and J.P. Richie), pp. 147–73. W.B. Saunders, Philadelphia.

Pilotti, S., Rilke, F., Alasio, L., and Garbagnati, F. (1988). The role of fine needle aspiration in the assessment of renal masses. *Acta Cytol.* **32**, 1–10.

Provet, J., Tessler, A., Brown, J., Golimbu, M., Bosniak, M., and Morales, P. (1991). Partial nephrectomy for renal cell carcinoma: indications, results and implications. *J. Urol.* **145**, 472–6.

Quinn, M.J., Hartman, D.S., Friedman, A.C., Sherman, J.L., Lautin, E.M., Pyatt, R.S., Ho, C.K., Csere, R., and Fromowitz, F.B. (1984). Renal oncocytoma: new observations. *Radiology* **153**, 49–53.

Quint, L.E., Glazer, G.M., Chenevert, T.L., Fechner, K.P., Gikas, P.W., Shireman, P.K., Grossman, H.B., and Li, K.C. (1988). *In vivo* and *in vitro* MR imaging of renal tumors: histopathologic correlation and pulse sequence optimization. *Radiology* **169**, 359–62.

Rabbani, F. and Russo, P. (1999). Lack of association between renal cell carcinoma and non-Hodgkin's lymphoma. *Urology* **54**, 28–33.

Ralls, P.W., Barakos, J.A., Kaptein, E.M., Friedman, P.E., Fouladian, G., Boswell, W.D., Halls, J., and Massry, S.G. (1987). Renal biopsy-related hemorrhage: frequency and comparison of CT and sonography. *J. Comput. Assist. Tomogr.* **11**, 1031–4.

Raval, B. and Lamki, N. (1983). Computed tomography in detection of occult hypernephroma. *J. Comput. Tomogr.* **7**, 199–207.

Reis, M., Faria, V., Lindoro, J., and Adolfo, A. (1988). The small cystic and noncystic noninflammatory renal nodules: a postmortem study. *J. Urol.* **140**, 721–4.

Riches, E.W., Griffiths, I.H., and Thackray, A.C. (1951). New growths of the kidney and ureter. *Br. J. Urol.* **23**, 297.

Richie, J.P., Garnick, M.B., Seltzer, S., and Bettmann, M.A. (1983). Computerized tomography scan for diagnosis and staging of renal cell carcinoma. *J. Urol.* **129**, 1114–16.

Richter, F., Kasabian, N.G., Irwin, R.J., Jr, Watson, R.A., and Lang, E.K. (2000). Accuracy of diagnosis by guided biopsy of renal mass lesions classified indeterminate by imaging studies. *Urology* **55**, 348–52.

Rodriguez, R., Fishman, E.K., and Marshall, F.F. (1995). Differential diagnosis and evaluation of the incidentally discovered renal mass. *Sem. Urol. Oncol.* **13**, 246–53.

Rofsky, N.M., Weinreb, J.C., Bosniak, M.A., Libes, R.B., and Birnbaum, B.A. (1991). Renal lesion characterization with gadolinium-enhanced MR imaging: efficacy and safety in patients with renal insufficiency [see comments]. *Radiology* **180**, 85–9.

Roubidoux, M.A. (1994). MR imaging of hemorrhage and iron deposition in the kidney. *Radiographics* **14**, 1033–44.

Roubidoux, M.A., Dunnick, N.R., Sostman, H.D., and Leder, R.A. (1992). Renal carcinoma: detection of venous extension with gradient-echo MR imaging. *Radiology* **182**, 269–72.

Russo, P. (2000). Renal cell carcinoma: presentation, staging, and surgical treatment. *Sem. Oncol.* **27**, 160–76.

Sandler, C.M., Houston, G.K., Hall, J.T., and Morettin, L.B. (1986). Guided cyst puncture and aspiration. *Radiol. Clin. N. Am.* **24**, 527–37.

Schaeffer, A.J. (1998). Infections of the urinary tract. In *Campbell's urology*, 7th edn (ed. P.C. Walsh, A.B. Retik, E.D. Vaughan, and A.J. Wein), pp. 533–614. W.B. Saunders, Philadelphia.

Schlichter, A., Wunderlich, H., Junker, K., Kosmehl, H., Zermann, D.H., and Schubert, J. (2000). Where are the limits of elective nephron-sparing surgery in renal cell carcinoma? *Eur. Urol.* **37**, 517–20.

Schwerk, W.B., Schwerk, W.N., and Rodeck, G. (1985). Venous renal tumor extension: a prospective US evaluation. *Radiology* **156**, 491–5.

Semelka, R.C., Shoenut, J.P., Kroeker, M.A., MacMahon, R.G., and Greenberg, H.M. (1992). Renal lesions: controlled comparison between CT and 1.5-T MR imaging with nonenhanced and gadolinium-enhanced fat-suppressed spin-echo and breath-hold FLASH techniques [see comments]. *Radiology* **182**, 425–30.

Shenoy, P.D., Lakhkar, B.N., Ghosh, M.K., and Patil, U.D. (1991). Cutaneous seeding of renal carcinoma by Chiba needle aspiration biopsy. Case report. *Acta Radiol.* **32**, 50–2.

Sherman, J.L., Hartman, D.S., Friedman, A.C., Madewell, J.E., Davis, C.J. and Goldman, S.M. (1981). Angiomyolipoma: computed tomographic–pathologic correlation of 17 cases. *Am. J. Roentgenol.* **137**, 1221–6.

Shirkhoda, A. and Lewis, E. (1987). Renal sarcoma and sarcomatoid renal cell carcinoma: CT and angiographic features. *Radiology* **162**, 353–7.

Siegel, C.L., McFarland, E.G., Brink, J.A., Fisher, A.J., Humphrey, P., and Heiken, J.P. (1997). CT of cystic renal masses: analysis of diagnostic performance and interobserver variation [see comments]. *Am. J. Roentgenol.* **169**, 813–18.

Sigalow, D.A., Waldbaum, R.S., and Lowe, F.C. (1991). Identification of asymptomatic renal cell carcinomas utilizing modern radiographic techniques [see comments]. *NY State J. Med.* **91**, 200–2.

Skinner, D.G., Colvin, R.B., Vermillion, C.D., Pfister, R.C., and Leadbetter, W.F. (1971). Diagnosis and management of renal cell carcinoma. A clinical and pathologic study of 309 cases. *Cancer* **28**, 1165–77.

Skinner, D.G., Pfister, R.F., and Colvin, R. (1972). Extension of renal cell carcinoma into the vena cava: the rationale for aggressive surgical management. *J. Urol.* **107**, 711–16.

Slywotzky, C. and Maya, M. (1994). Needle tract seeding of transitional cell carcinoma following fine-needle aspiration of a renal mass. *Abdom. Imaging* **19**, 174–6.

Smith, E.H. (1984). The hazards of fine-needle aspiration biopsy. *Ultrasound Med. Biol.* **10**, 629–34.

Smith, E.H. (1991). Complications of percutaneous abdominal fine-needle biopsy. Review. *Radiology* **178**, 253–8.

Smith, S.J., Bosniak, M.A., Megibow, A.J., Hulnick, D.H., Horii, S.C., and Raghavendra, B.N. (1989). Renal cell carcinoma: earlier discovery and increased detection [see comments]. *Radiology* **170**, 699–703.

Steiner, M.S., Goldman, S.M., Fishman, E.K., and Marshall, F.F. (1993). The natural history of renal angiomyolipoma. *J. Urol.* **150**, 1782–6.

Stephenson, T.F., Iyengar, S., and Rashid, H.A. (1984). Comparison of computerized tomography and excretory urography in detection and evaluation of renal masses. *J. Urol.* **131**, 11–13.

Strotzer, M., Lehner, K.B., and Becker, K. (1993). Detection of fat in a renal cell carcinoma mimicking angiomyolipoma [see comments]. *Radiology* **188**, 427–8.

Studer, U.E., Scherz, S., Scheidegger, J., Kraft, R., Sonntag, R., Ackermann, D., and Zingg, E.J. (1990). Enlargement of regional lymph nodes in renal cell carcinoma is often not due to metastases. *J. Urol.* **144**, 243–5.

Sufrin, G., Chasan, S., Golio, A., and Murphy, G.P. (1989). Paraneoplastic and serologic syndromes of renal adenocarcinoma. *Sem. Urol.* **7**, 158–71.

Sussman, S., Cochran, S.T., Pagani, J.J., McArdle, C., Wong, W., Austin, R., Curry, N., and Kelly, K.M. (1984). Hyperdense renal masses: a CT manifestation of hemorrhagic renal cysts. *Radiology* **150**, 207–11.

Sussman, S.K., Glickstein, M.F., and Krzymowski, G.A. (1990). Hypointense renal cell carcinoma: MR imaging with pathologic correlation. *Radiology* **177**, 495–7.

Sweeney, J.P., Thornhill, J.A., Graiger, R., McDermott, T.E., and Butler, M.R. (1996). Incidentally detected renal cell carcinoma: pathological features, survival trends and implications for treatment [see comments]. *Br. J. Urol.* **78**, 351–3.

Thrasher, J.B., Robertson, J.E., and Paulson, D.F. (1994). Expanding indications for conservative renal surgery in renal cell carcinoma. *Urology* **43**, 160–8.

Torp-Pedersen, S., Juul, N., Larsen, T., Karstrup, S., Sehested, M., and Glenthoj, A. (1991). US-guided fine needle biopsy of solid renal masses—comparison of histology and cytology. *Scand. J. Urol. Nephrol. Suppl.* **137**, 41–3.

Tsui, K.H., Shvarts, O., Smith, R.B., Figlin, R., de Kernion, J.B., and Belldegrun, A. (2000). Renal cell carcinoma: prognostic significance of incidentally detected tumors. *J. Urol.* **163**, 426–30.

Tsukanoto, T., Kumanoto, Y., Yamazaki, K., Miyao, N., Takahashi, A., Masumori, N., and Satoh, M. (1991). Clinical analysis of incidentally found renal cell carcinoma. *Eur. Urol.* **19**, 109–113.

Tung, K.T., Downes, M.O., and O'Donnell, P.J. (1992). Renal biopsy in diffuse renal disease—experience with a 14-gauge automated biopsy gun. *Clin. Radiol.* **46**, 111–13.

Vallancien, G., Torres, L.O., Gurfinkel, E., Veillon, B., and Brisset, J.M. (1990). Incidental detection of renal tumours by abdominal ultrasonography. *Eur. Urol.* **18**, 94–6.

Vassiliades, V.G. and Bernardino, M.E. (1991). Percutaneous renal and adrenal biopsies. *Cardiovasc. Intervent. Radiol.* **14**, 50–4.

Waguespack, R. L. and Kearse, W. S., Jr (1996). Renal cell carcinoma arising from the free wall of a renal cyst. *Abdom. Imaging* **21**, 71–2.

Warshauer, D.M., McCarthy, S.M., Street, L., Bookbinder, M.J., Glickman, M.G., Richter, J., Hammers, L., Taylor, C., and Rosenfield, A.T. (1988). Detection of renal masses: sensitivities and specificities of excretory urography/linear tomography, US, and CT. *Radiology* **169**, 363–5.

Wehle, M. J. and Grabstald, H. (1986). Contraindications to needle aspiration of a solid renal mass: tumor dissemination by renal needle aspiration. *J. Urol.* **136**, 446–8.

Wendth, A.J., Jr, Garlick, W.B., Pantoja, G.E., and Shamoun, J. (1976). Transcatheter biopsy of renal carcinoma invading the inferior vena cava. *J. Urol.* **115**, 331–2.

Weyman, P.J., McClennan, B.L., Stanley, R.J., Levitt, R.G., and Sagel, S.S. (1980). Comparison of computed tomography and angiography in the evaluation of renal cell carcinoma. *Radiology* **137**, 417–24.

Whang, M., O'Toole, K., Bixon, R., Brunetti, J., Ikeguchi, E., Olsson, C.A., Sawczuk, T.S., and Benson, M.C. (1995). The incidence of multifocal renal cell carcinoma in patients who are candidates for partial nephrectomy. *J. Urol.* **154**, 968–70; discussion 970–1.

Wilson, T.E., Doelle, E.A., Cohan, R.H., Wojno, K., and Korobkin, M. (1996). Cystic renal masses: a reevaluation of the usefulness of the Bosniak classification system. *Acad. Radiol.* **3**, 564–70.

Wolf, J.S., Jr (1998). Evaluation and management of solid and cystic renal masses. *J. Urol.* **159**, 1120–33.

Wood, B.J., Khan, M.A., McGovern, F., Harisinghani, M., Hahn, P.F., and Mueller, P.R. (1999). Imaging guided biopsy of renal masses: indications, accuracy and impact on clinical management [see comments]. *J. Urol.* **161**, 1470–4.

Wunderlich, H., Schlichter, A., Zermann, D., Reichelt, O., Kosmehl, H., and Schubert, J. (2000). Multifocality in renal cell carcinoma: a bilateral event? *Urol. Int.* **63**, 160–3.

Yuh, B.I. and Cohan, R.H. (1999). Different phases of renal enhancement: role in detecting and characterizing renal masses during helical CT. *Am. J. Roentgenol.* **173**, 747–55.

Zagoria, R.J., Wolfman, N.T., Karstaedt, N., Hinn, G.C., Dyer, R.B., and Chen, Y.M. (1990). CT features of renal cell carcinoma with emphasis on relation to tumor size. *Invest. Radiol.* **25**, 261–6.

Zagoria, R.J., Bechtold, R.E., and Dyer, R.B. (1995). Staging of renal adenocarcinoma: role of various imaging procedures. *Am. J. Roentgenol.* **164**, 363–70.

Zeman, R.K., Cronan, J.J., Rosenfield, A.T., Lynch, J.H., Jaffe, M.H., and Clark, L.R. (1988). Renal cell carcinoma: dynamic thin-section CT assessment of vascular invasion and tumor vascularity. *Radiology* **167**, 393–6.

Zerhouni, E.A., Schellhammer, P., Schaefer, J.C., Drucker, J.R., Jaffe, A.H., Gonzales, J.E., Edwards, O.E., and Lampton, L.D. (1984). Management of bleeding renal angiomyolipomas by transcatheter embolization following CT diagnosis. *Urol. Radiol.* **6**, 205–9.

22. Role of the excretory urogram in contemporary uroradiologic practice

Steven S. Raman, Sherelle Laifer-Narin, and Sachiko T. Cochran

Indications and contraindications for the excretory urogram

The indications for the intravenous urogram (excretory urogram, IVU, IVP) have changed significantly in the last 20 years with the advent of sophisticated cross-sectional imaging. The IVU remains the initial test of choice in adults to survey the urothelium and pyelocaliceal systems and is an essential diagnostic study for the patient with hematuia. The role of the IVU in the detection of renal and adrenal parenchymal masses is now secondary to helical computerized tomography (CT) and ultrasound (US). In a classic study, Warshauer *et al.* (1988) reported that the IVU was 67 per cent sensitive for the detection for renal masses versus 79 per cent for conventional sonography and 94 per cent for conventional CT. As Dunnick (1992) has stated, 'We cannot rely on a negative excretory urogram to exclude a renal tumor in a patient with unexpected persistent hematuria or other signs strongly suggestive of a renal tumor.' US, conventional CT, and magnetic resonance imaging (MRI) are more sensitive and specific for smaller tumors (< 3 cm) and have the advantage of accurately characterizing and staging solid renal masses (Bosniak 1991*a*; Smelka *et al.* 1991). However, utilizing one imaging modality over another is often dictated by local expertise and availability of competing technologies such as spiral or multidetector-row CT, CT urography, high-field strength MRI–urography, and latest-generation sonography.

Performance of the IVU is somewhat contingent on the overall medical condition of the patient. The IVU should not be performed in diabetics with marginal or poor renal function (rising creatinine or creatinine > 2 mg/dl) since the contrast load may precipitate acute renal failure. In this population of patients, the information derived from the IVU will be marginal due to poor concentration ability. Competing imaging modalities usually provide adequate information, especially with regards to renal parenchyma.

Technique

The technical performance of the excretory urogram is varied, but a high-quality technique is critical to demonstrate normal renal anatomy and a wide range of abnormalities (Hattery *et al.* 1988). Ideally, the colon should be prepared free of stool to improve renal conspicuity. Tomography is helpful to blur bowel gas while keeping the kidneys in focus. This is especially helpful in the middle-aged and elderly patient, since advanced age is a risk factor for the development of parenchymal masses. A plain radiograph (scout film) is performed for screening large renal masses or calculi and to gauge skeletal abnormalities. Depending on the patient's age, weight, and renal status, an appropriate contrast material is chosen and a dose typically between 15 and 30 g of iodine is rapidly injected within 1 to 2 minutes. Rapid injection leads to a more robust and dense nephrogram. The chief drawback to rapid injection is a slightly increased incidence of minor reactions such as flushing, nausea, and vomiting (Hattery *et al.* 1988). Drip infusion techniques generally deliver 25–50 g of iodine over a longer time and result in a prolonged combined nephrogram and pyelogram phase, but are not considered optimal.

Although an adequate discussion is beyond the scope of this chapter, as with any radiographic technique, proper exposure factors are essential. A three-phase 500 mA generator, Bucky diaphragm, and low kilovoltage technique (65–75 kV) are needed for detail to resolve small abnormalities such as calcifications (Hattery *et al.* 1988).

The nephrographic enhancement phase relies on a combination of vascular and tubular opacification with early films (20–60 s) imaging chiefly the vascular phase and later films (60–120 s) imaging the total renal parenchyma. The pyelogram phase follows the initial nephrogram. Tomograms are performed early (1 minute) for best evaluation of renal parenchyma. This is followed by a coned (collimated) view of the kidneys at 5 minutes. If function is not delayed and the patient has no contraindications (renal stone, aortic aneurysm, etc.), then compression balloons may be applied over the sacral promontory to better distend and define the pelvocaliceal system. Coned anteroposterior (AP) and bilateral obliques are acquired. Compression is then released and a 14 × 17 compression release film is obtained to examine the ureters. Prone and upright views are obtained as indicated to fill the ureters. A post-void AP view is taken coned to the bladder.

Intravenous contrast materials

A wide choice of intravenous (IV) contrast materials are available for urography. The choice must be based on experience, patient population, and cost. Urographic contrast agents date back to pioneering work undertaken between 1895 and 1923, primarily in Germany and the US. Osborne, Sutherland, Scholl, and Rowntree (1923) published the first report describing IVU. All currently available agents are based on a tri-iodinated benzene ring and are classified as ionic or non-ionic monomers or dimers. The 'ionic agents', such as iothalamic acid (Conray®) and diatrizoic acid (Hypaque®), are salts of sodium or meglumine and dissociate in solution into ions, yielding osmolar loads 5–7 times that of serum. Consequently, these agents are known as high-osmolality contrast agents (HOCM). The 'non-ionic agents' are water-soluble but do not dissociate and are classified as low-osmolality contrast agents (LOCM). The newer LOCM agents, ioxaglate (Hexabrix®), iohexol (Omnipaque®), iopamidol (Isovue®), and ioversol (Optiray®), have osmolalities approximately 2 to 3 times that of serum. A newer class of isoosmotic agents has been under development for the past decade (McClennan 1990; Morris 1993; Ellis *et al.* 1996; Byrd and Sherman 1979). Improved quality of nephrographic opacification with the LOCM agents when compared to more traditional agents has been demonstrated (Sparato *et al.* 1987).

Adverse reactions to contrast agents

Adverse reactions to contrast agents may result in dose-dependent and non-dose-dependent reactions. Dose-dependent nephrotoxicity resulting from contrast media has been variably reported. Most studies have examined the older ionic agents. A study by Levy *et al.* (1996) reported a 1 per cent incidence of nephrotoxicity (25 per cent rise in creatinine within 2 days postcontrast) in 16 248 hospitalized patients. Other studies have reported up to 30 per cent of the hospitalized population in some studies and may range in severity from transient renal dysfunction to severe oliguric failure requiring dialysis (McClennan 1990; Morris 1993; Ellis *et al.* 1996; Byrd and Sherman 1979). In most patients, acute tubular necrosis is usually self-limited with return to baseline within 2 weeks (peak at 5 days). Patients at notably high risk (Table 22.1) include diabetics with creatinine level over 3 mg/dl. Other common risk factors include congestive heart failure (CHF), hepatic failure, multiple myeloma, dehydration, hypertension, and proteinuira. LOCM agents are preferred for high-risk patients due to their decreased risk of nephrotoxicity. In patients without known risk factors, no significant reduced nephrotoxicity risk has been demonstrated (Berns and Rudnick 1992; Katholi *et al.* 1993).

Nonrenal adverse reactions may be classified as allergic (idiosyncratic) or dose-dependent (chemotoxic). Idiosyncratic reactions, which may be mediated by a complex pathway involving IgE, complement, and other mediators, may be classified as mild (single episode of nausea, emesis, vertigo fever, chills,

Table 22.1 Risk factors for acute renal failure precipitated by contrast media (Ellis *et al.* 1996)

Diabetes-related renal insufficiency (creatinine > 1.5 mg/dl)
Renal insufficiency
Dehydration
Cardiac and vascular disorders with diuretic use
Age > 75 years
Multiple myeloma with dehydration
Hypertension
Uricosuria

urticaria), moderate (widespread urticaria, severe skin swelling, mild largyngospasm or bronchospasm), or severe (severe bronchospasm, severe laryngoedema, hypotension, or arrythmia). Mild reactions require a short period of observation and are generally not treated. Moderate reactions require medical treatment (benedryl for skin reactions, subcutaneous epinephrine (adrenaline) for bronchospasm or laryngospasm). Severe reactions can be life-threatening and may require IV epinephrine, airway protection, and blood pressure support. All three categories of reactions are much less common with the LOCM agents; moderate reactions are reported to be one-fifth as common as with HOCM agents (Siegle *et al.* 1991; Lasser *et al.* 1987). The non-ionic agents are generally in widespread use in developed countries and should be used for any patients with prior allergic reactions. Patients with allergic reactions to the non-ionic agents have a 5 per cent risk of recurrent allergic reactions when re-exposed to non-ionic agents.

If ionic agents must be used, patients must be judiciously questioned about all prior allergies since those allergic to seafood (especially shellfish) or drugs or those with asthma have a twofold increased risk of a contrast allergy. Those with previous contrast allergy have a threefold increased risk. For all patients except those with prior life-threatening contrast allergy (laryngospasm, anaphylaxis), premedication with a regimen of corticosteroids and antihistamines should be used to significantly decrease the chances of both minor and life-threatening reactions (Siegle *et al.* 1991).

The normal excretory urogram

The kidneys and adrenals lie in the perinephric space of the retroperitoneum along with blood vessels, fat, and lymphatics. The kidneys and adrenals lie obliquely, paralleling the psoas muscles. The upper poles are slightly posterior and the lower poles are slightly anterior in orientation. Normal renal size is related to body surface area. Each kidney measures approximately 11–13 cm in the adult with variations based on size and sex. There are significant congenital variations in the position and orientation of both kidneys encountered in routine practice.

Analysis of the IVU in the nephrographic phase is generally best for parenchymally based primary or metastatic space-occupying lesions. For lesion characterization, cross-sectional imaging techniques are necessary. The urographic or pyelographic phase is best for detecting transitional cell carcinomas (TCC) and other tumors of the urothelium. A systematic analysis must be performed on each nephrogram accounting for bilateral symmetry with respect to size, shape, axis, and enhancement. Renal parenchymal enhancement and enhancement of the collecting system should be symmetric. Renal contours should be smooth or lobular. Focal bulges in contour must be explained since tumors of renal parenchyma or renal capsule may produce this finding. On the pyelogram, the calyces must be evaluated with regard to symmetry and their relationship to the outer renal contour. Any caliceal and infundibular splaying, stretching, irregularity or filling defects must be explained (Newhouse and Pfister 1979).

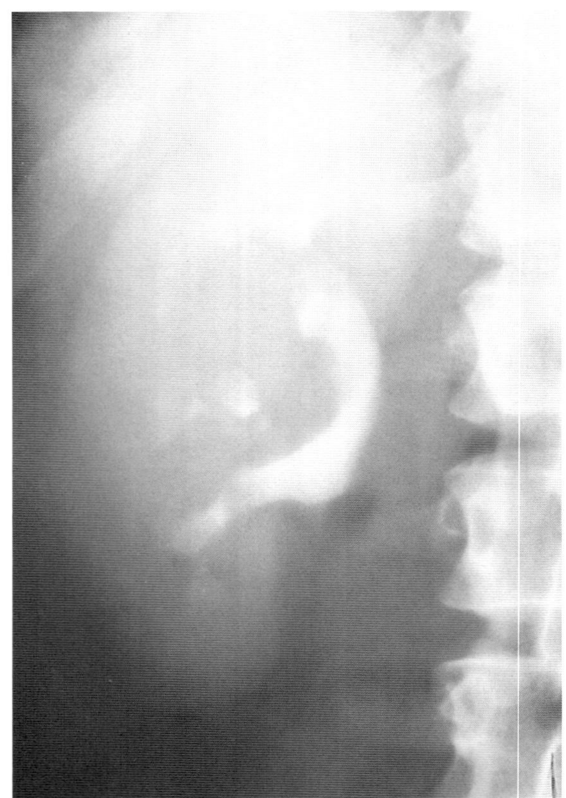
(a)

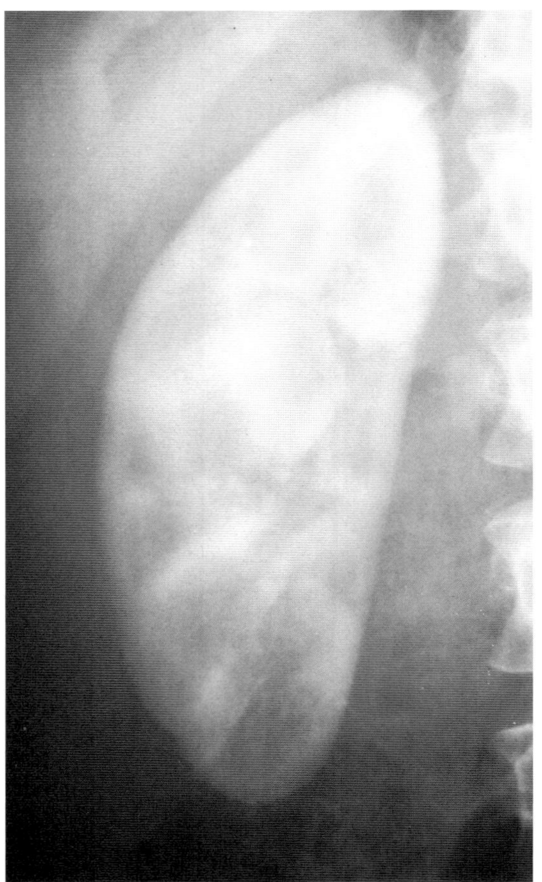
(b)

Fig. 22.1 (a) On IVU, the right upper pole infundibula are splayed and the posterior upper pole calyx is diminutive (confirmed on oblique views). (b) Corresponding arteriogram in the corticomedullary phase shows normal enhancement of cortex in the region corresponding to cortical rest.

Tumors of parenchymal origin

The pseudotumor

Normal renal tissue may be lobular in contour and sometimes be confused for a mass. These variants may be congenital or acquired. The most common congenital entity includes a thick column of Bertin (Figs 22.1 and 22.2), which typically occurs at the junction of the upper one-third and lower two-thirds of the kidney, splaying the collecting system or resulting in a bifid system. Typically, no outer contour defect is present on the IVU (Feldman *et al.* 1978). Other congenital variants producing pseudotumors on IVU include juxtahilar bulges which are more common in the infrahilar region, cortical bulges (dysmorphisms), asymmetric fetal lobulations, and dromedary humps (Figs 22.3 and 22.4). These findings can usually be confirmed as normal by cross-sectional techniques or less frequently with technetium 99m–dimercaptosuccinic acid (DMSA) scans.

Acquired pseudotumors are related to normal or hypertrophied normal parenchyma adjacent to regions of scarring typically related to insults from pyelonephritis or reflux nephropathy. Again, correlation with clinical history and cross-sectional techniques is essential.

Renal lesions

Discrete space occupying renal lesions arising in the cortex or corticomedullary junction may deform the bean-shaped contour of the kidney at excretory urography or may cause caliceal distortion. All lesions must be evaluated for uniformity of contour, calcifications, and contrast enhancement.

Cystic lesions

Although renal cysts and cystic lesions account for 95 per cent of space-occupying renal lesions, they are difficult to differentiate from other renal lesions at excretory urography. Size and location are key for initial detection. Large cysts (> 3 cm) may splay, compress, displace, or distort calyces and/or deform the renal contour (Figs 22.5–22.7). Nephrotomograms are required for diagnostic confidence but all methods are inferior to CT, US, or MRI. The urographic criteria to diagnose a simple cyst include (Bosniak 1986*a*):

(1) internal fluid density without enhancement;
(2) pencil-thin nearly imperceptible wall;
(3) no mural nodularity;
(4) extension of at least 50 per cent of mass beyond the renal contour.

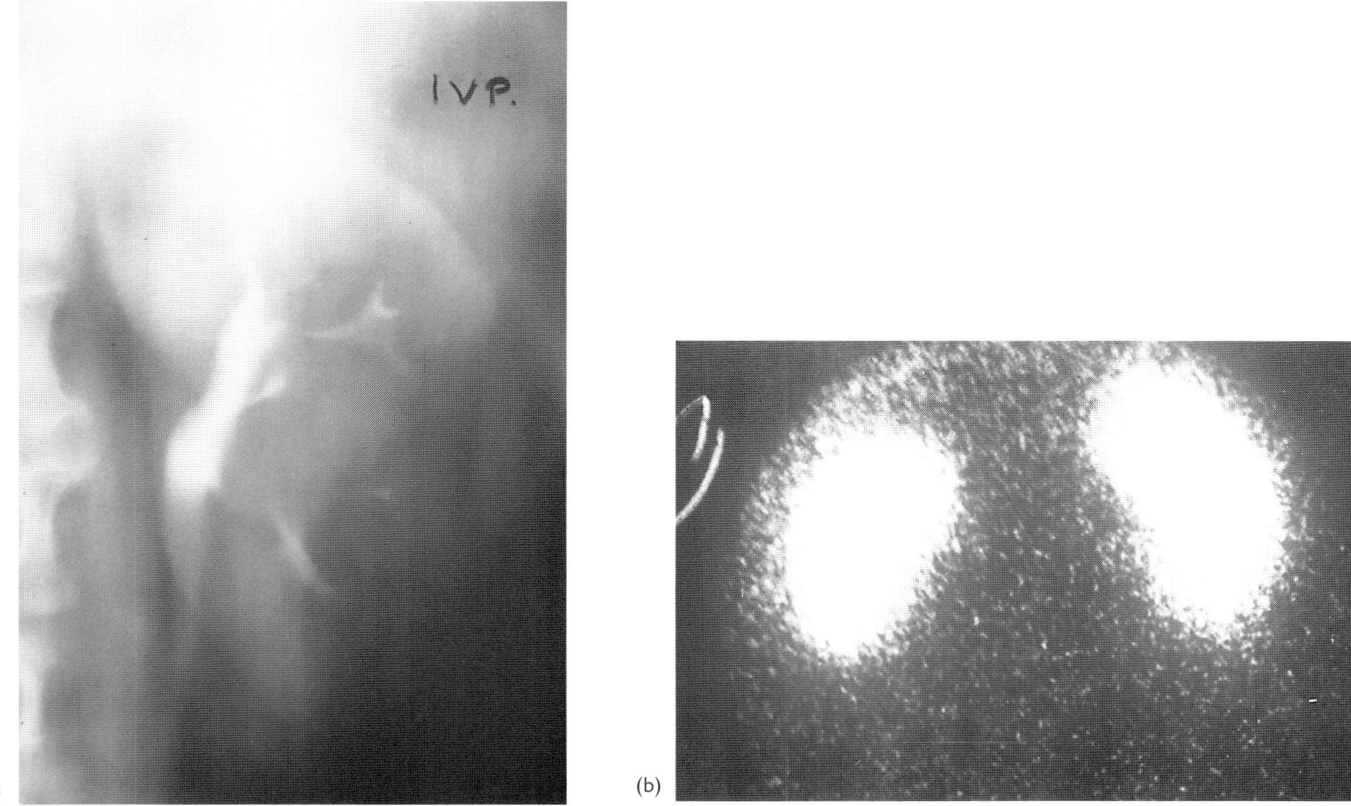

Fig. 22.2 (a) There is splaying of the interpolar and lower pole calyces. (b) Corresponding Tc99m–DMSA scan shows normal renal tissue confirming a cortical rest or column of Bertin.

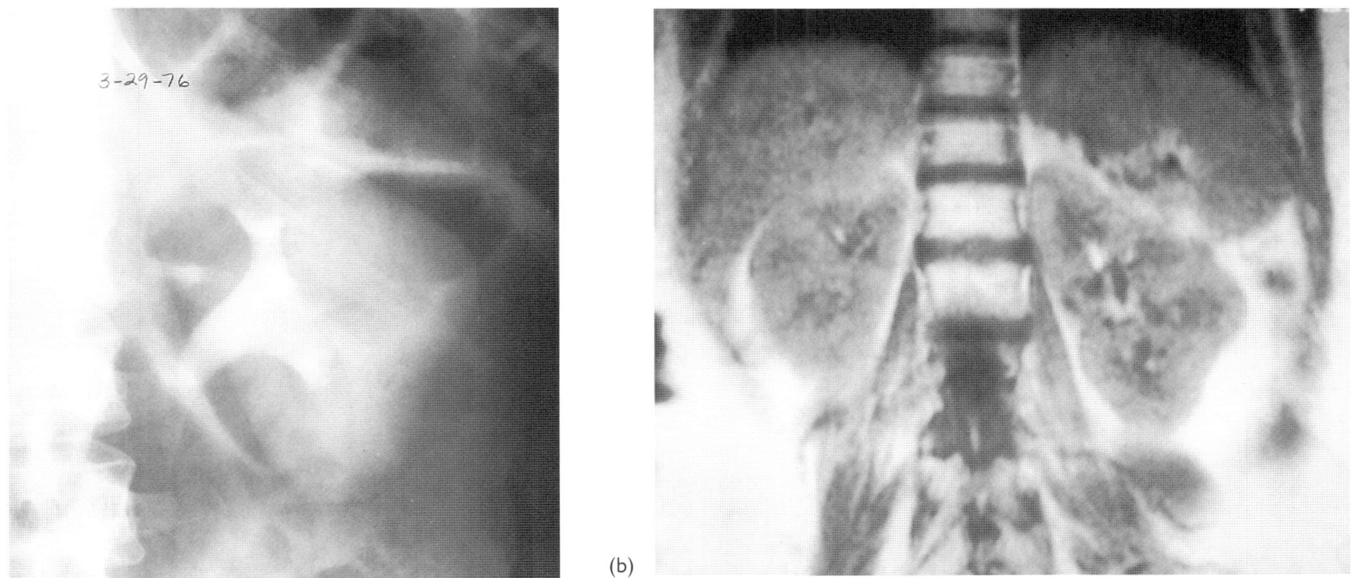

Fig. 22.3 (a) IVU demonstrates a focal cortical bulge at the interpolar region associated with an accompanying calyx. (b) Corresponding angiogram shows no evidence of neovascularity or displacement in the region to suggest tumor

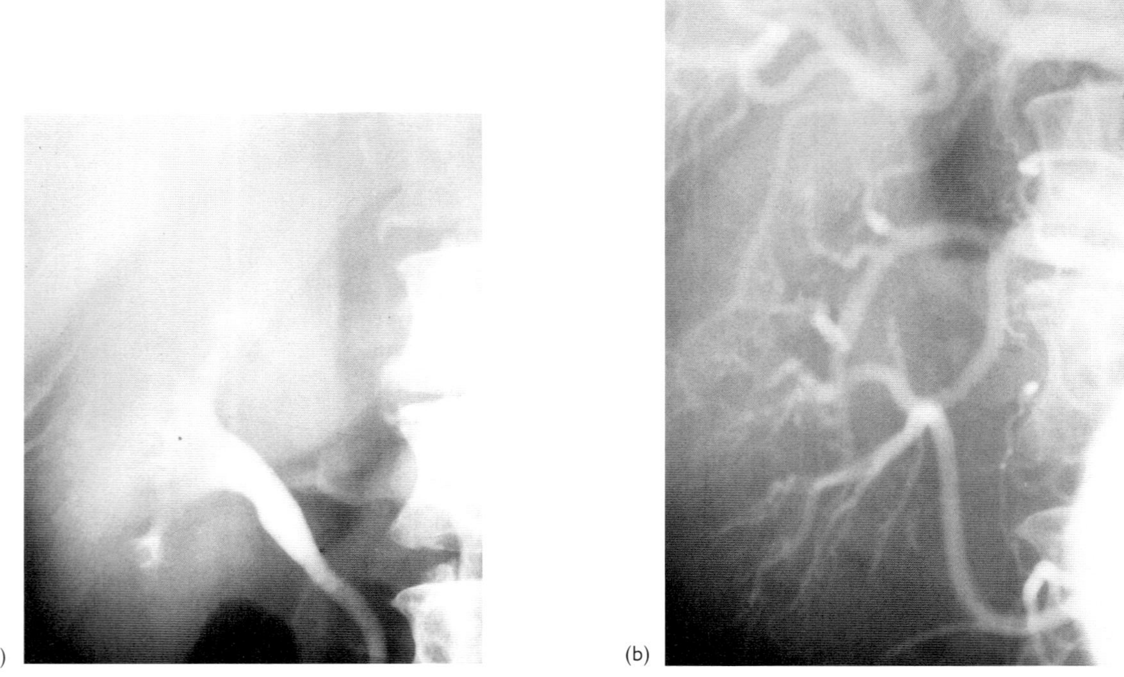

Fig. 22.4 (a) Excretory phase of IVU shows excess renal tissue at the superomedial border of the right kidney. (b) Corresponding angiogram shows no evidence of neovascularity or displacement in the region to suggest tumor.

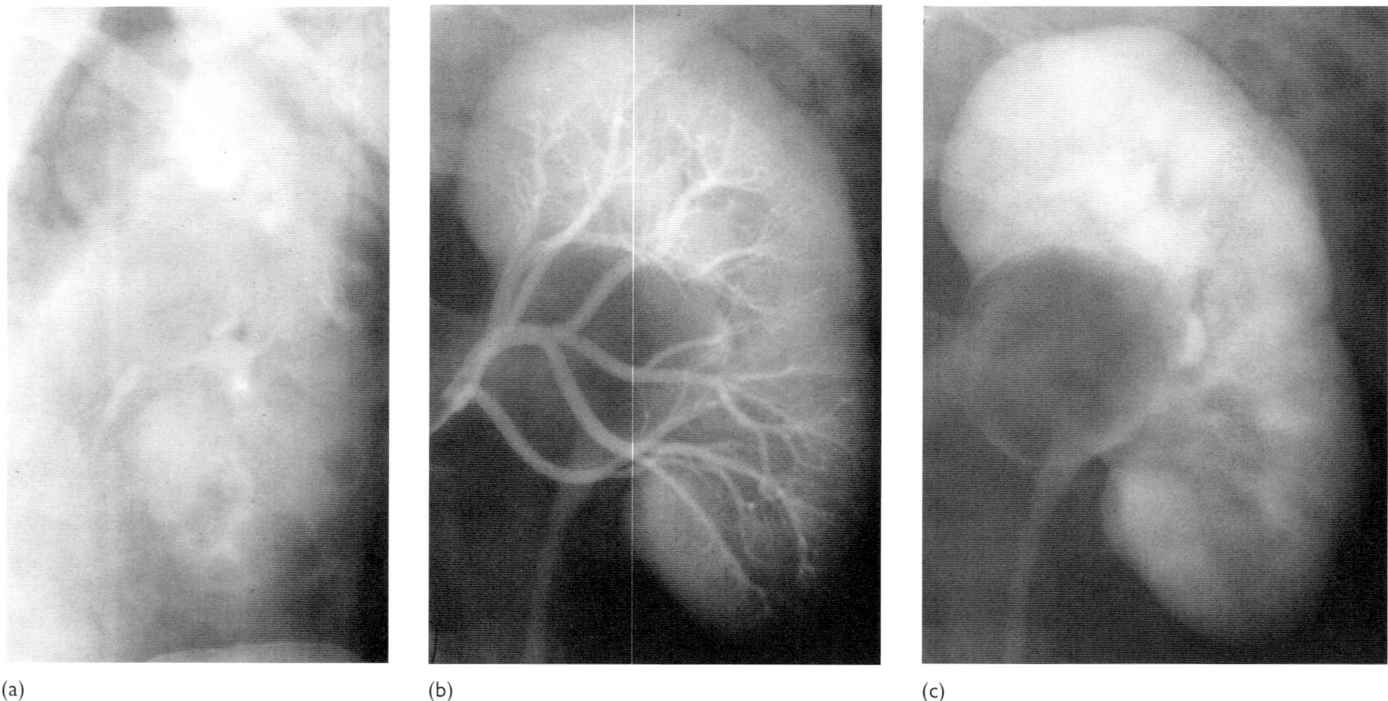

Fig. 22.5 (a) Excretory phase of IVU demonstrates a large contour defect in the left renal pelvis with splaying of the calyces. (b) Arterial phase and (c) nephrogram phase from a selective renal angiogram demonstrate a well defined, non-enhancing low-density lesion with thin walls most compatible with a renal sinus cyst. A simple cyst was confirmed by cyst puncture (not shown).

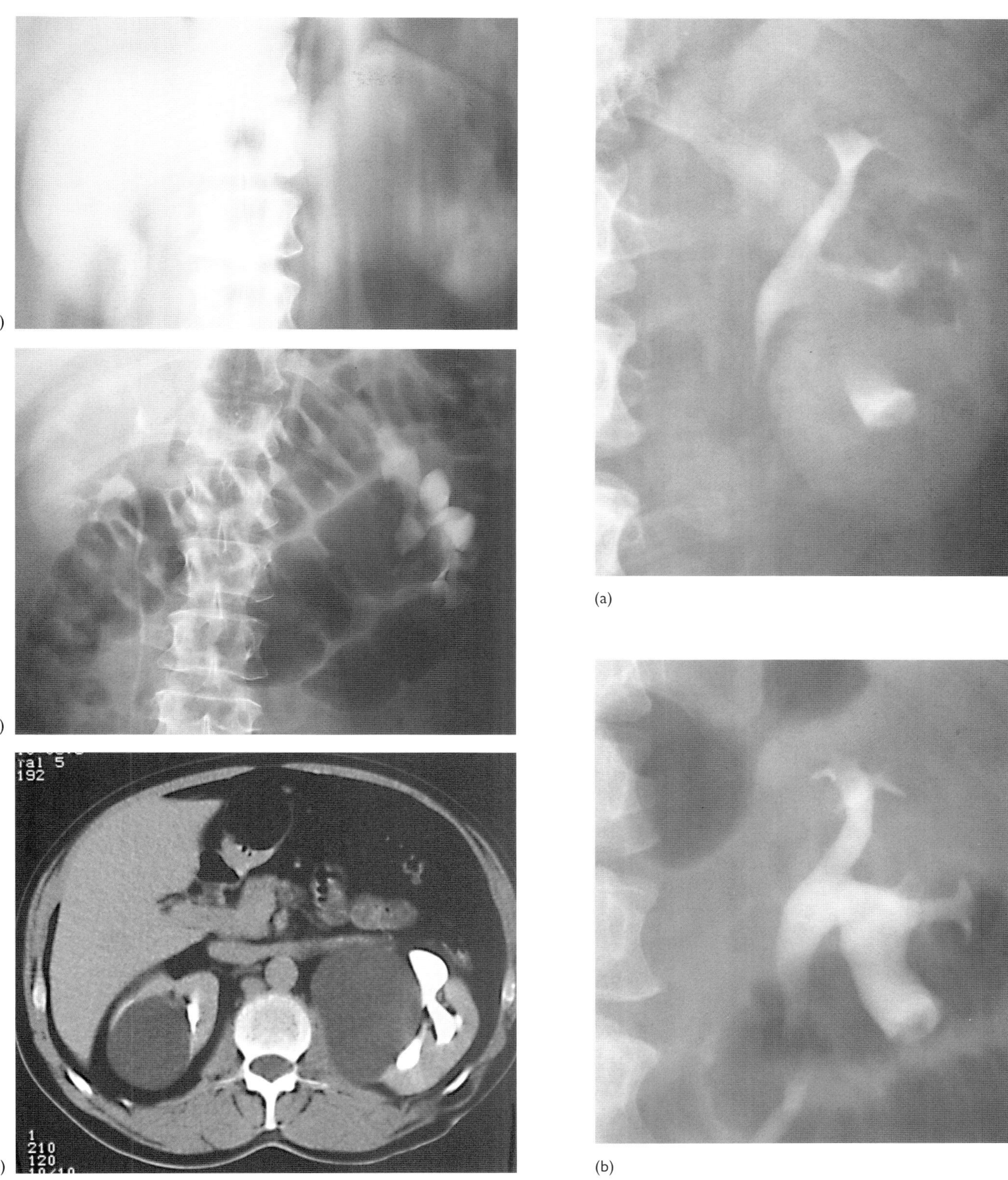

Fig. 22.6 (a) Nephrotomogram from IVU demonstrates left central low-density lesion (arrows) with a more subtle right upper pole lesion (arrowheads). (b) Excretory phase of IVU demonstrates splaying of right upper pole calyces and marked lateral splaying of left-sided calyces. (c) Contrast-enhanced CT scan confirms bilateral parapelvic cysts.

Fig. 22.7 (a) Excretory phase of IVU shows effacement of the central calyces on the left side. (b) No intrinsic collecting system abnormality was noted on the corresponding retrograde pyelogram. A simple parapelvic cyst was later confirmed on sonography (not shown).

The 'claw sign' or 'beak sign' of normal renal tissue at the margin of a cyst is a suggestive but nonspecific sign of a cyst. Characteristic features of cystic lesions have been classified by Bosniak to risk-stratify the work-up of simple cysts. The classification relies on cross-sectional imaging and cannot be applied to IVU alone. Lesions adhering to the features mentioned above are graded as class I, which requires no follow-up or intervention. Cystic renal lesions complicated by hemorrhage, infection, linear mural calcifications, or less than three thin, smooth septations are classified as class II. Although both class I and II require no surgical intervention, class II lesions need follow-up at 3 month intervals for 2 years to assure stability. Class III and IV lesions are more complex with indeterminate features on cross-sectional imaging. These lesions usually require surgical intervention (Bosniak 1986b). Hemorrhagic cysts are usually non-enhancing but high in density. A small fraction of hemorrhagic lesions may be caused by an underlying bleeding neoplasm. Infected cystic lesions may have thick, irregular walls and possibly internal gas with abscess formation. Renal cell carcinoma (RCC) may arise in cyst walls and present as a mural nodule, which is difficult to both detect and exclude by excretory urography alone (Fig. 22.8). Calcifications within cysts must be carefully evaluated since irregular clusters and clumps may indicate a cystic renal cell tumor (Fig. 22.9) (Bosniak 1991b; Daniel et al. 1972).

Multilocular cystic tumors are known by a variety of names with the preferred terminology being multilocular cystic nephroma or cystic partially differentiated nephroblastoma. They have a bimodal distribution typically seen in young boys (< 2 years old) and middle-aged women. Nephrotomograpy during excretory urography may demonstrate a septated low-density mass sometimes 'protruding' into the renal pelvis (Agrons et al. 1995) (Figs 22.10 and 22.11).

Solid renal lesions

Although many solid and cystic lesions may present with identical imaging findings, RCC must be excluded by alternative imaging modalities in nearly all lesions not displaying the specific features of a simple cyst.

Findings that increase the radiological suspicion for a renal neoplasm include irregular or coarse calcifications, contour deformities, malalignment of axis, and distortion of infundibula, calyces, and renal pelvis (Bosniak 1986b). Filling defects are occasionally caused by bleeding related to RCC but much more commonly by urothelial tumors.

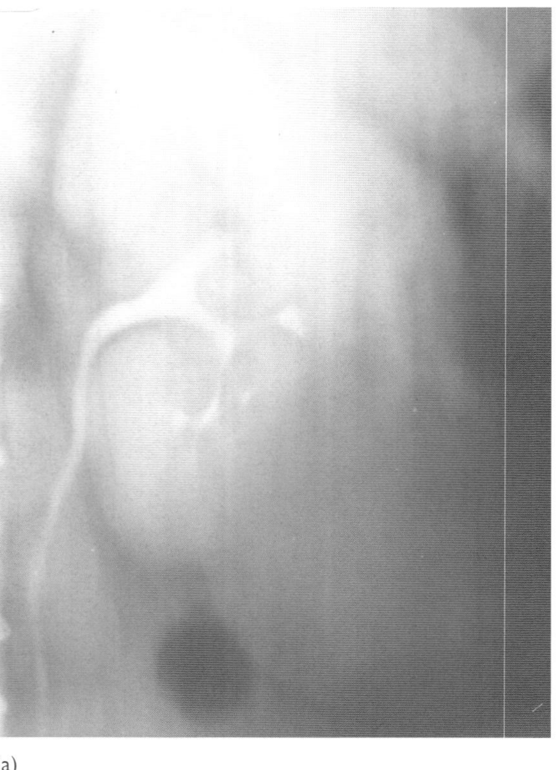

(a)

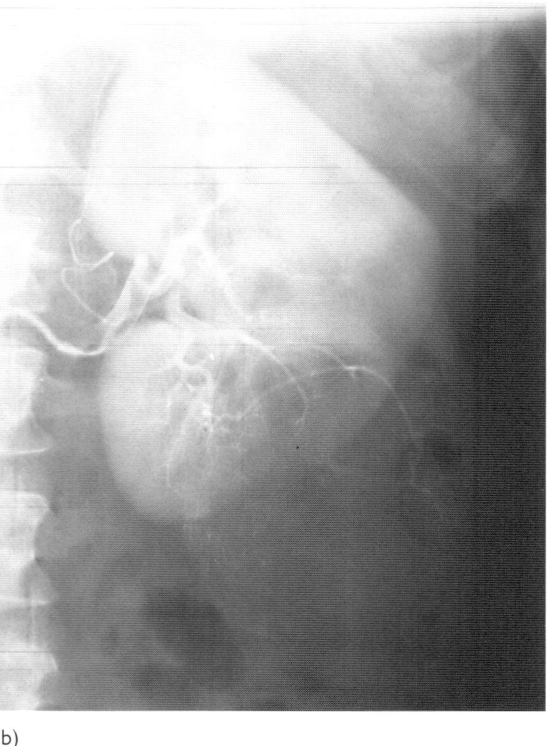

(b)

Fig. 22.8 (a) Nephrotomogram from an excretory phase of IVU demonstrates an exophytic left lower pole low-density lesion. No discrete 'claw sign' of surrounding normal kidney is demonstrated. The walls are imperceptible. (b) On the subsequent angiogram, distinct neovascularity was demonstrated and a cystic RCC was confirmed at nephrectomy. All cystic renal lesions must be carefully scrutinized with cross-sectional imaging to avoid missing the occasional cystic RCC

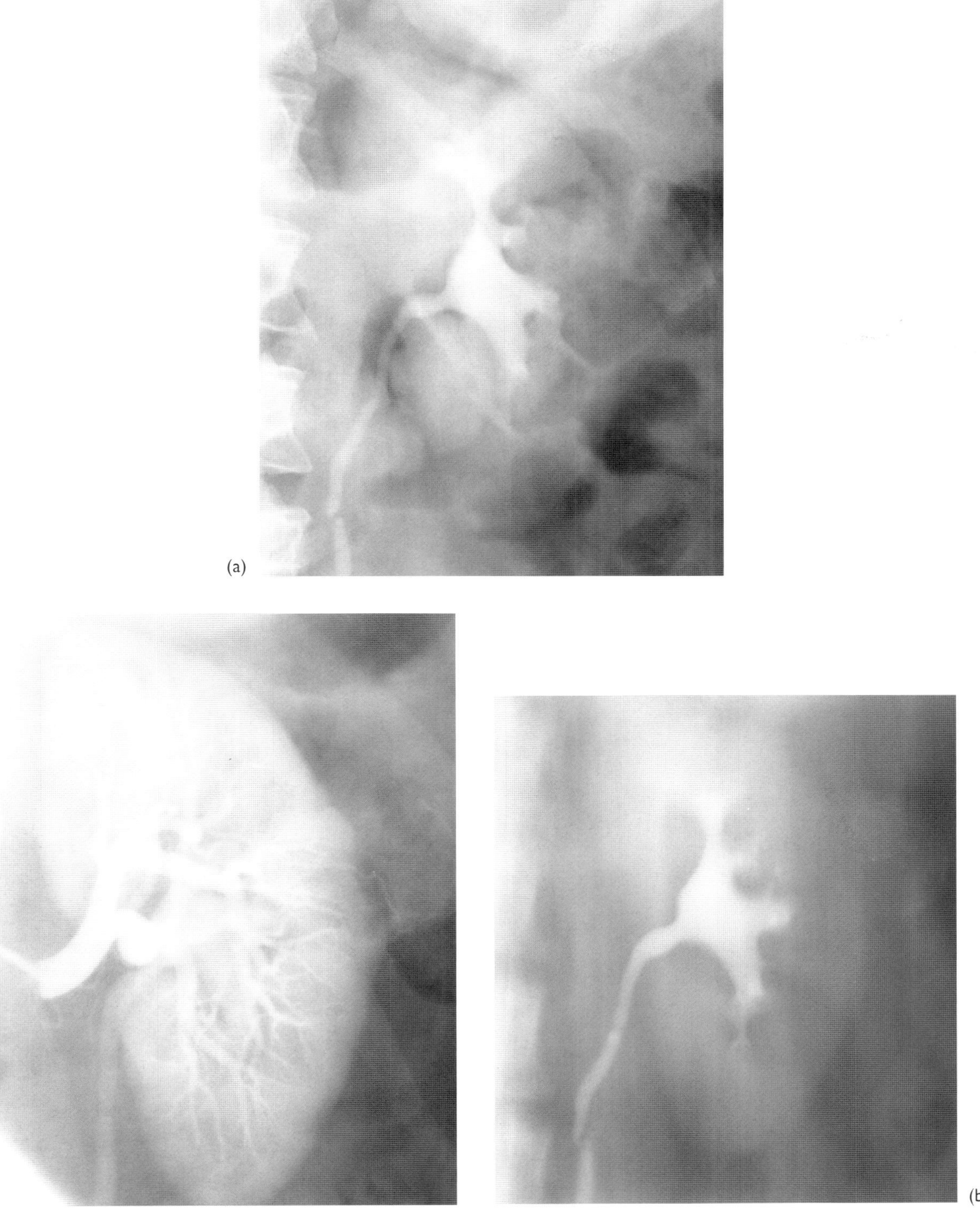

Fig. 22.9 A 50-year-old man with left flank pain. (a) 10 minute post-injection film from IVU demonstrates an exophytic left midpole calcified 3 cm mass. (b) 12 cm nephrotomogram 15 minutes post-injection highlights the rim calcifications. (c) Angiogram demonstrates the peripheral neovascularity.

Calcifications may be found in up to 10 per cent of RCC and 1 per cent of cysts on excretory urography. The pattern of calcifications is relatively nonspecific but location is important. Although peripheral rim-like calcifications are nonspecific, central calcifications are more specific for neoplasms. Renal tumors may rarely ossify. All calcified masses should be followed up with contrast-enhanced CT for characterization (Daniel *et al.* 1972) (Figs 22.12–22.14).

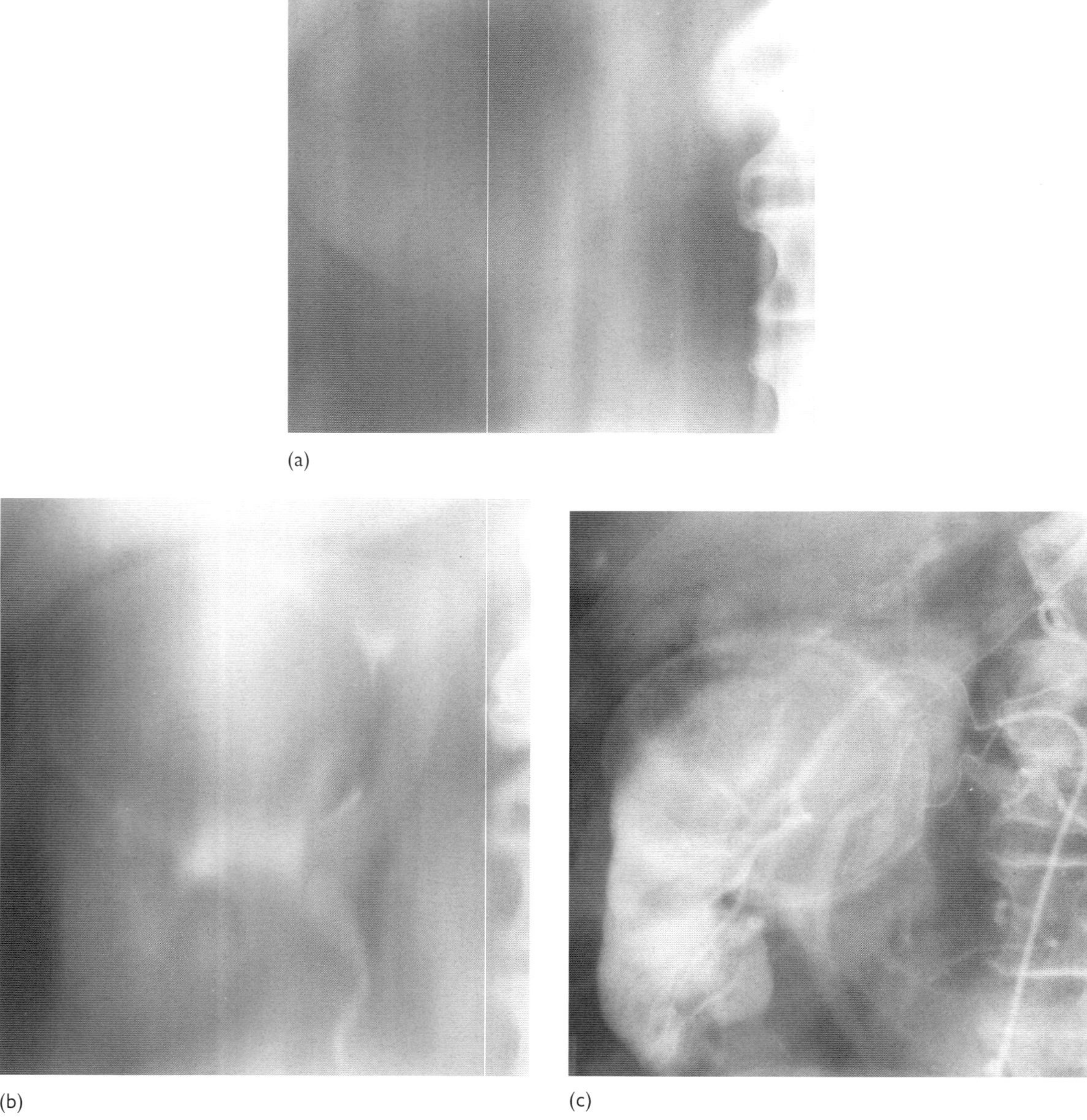

(a)

(b)   (c)

Fig. 22.10 (a) Scout tomogram detected a mass. (b) On the 10 min right posterior oblique tomogram, the lesion is thick-walled and effaces the right upper pole calyces. (c) Corresponding angiogram in corticomedullary phase demonstrates mural enhancement. The lesion was subsequently proven to be a multilocular cystic nephroma.

On excretory urography, masses that distort the outer renal contour are best detected on the medial, lateral, or oblique margins of the kidney (Figs 22.15 and 22.16). Lesions on the anterior or posterior surfaces are relatively poorly detected. Large lesions at the upper and lower poles may deviate the renal axis. Upper pole lesions may cause straightening of the kidney along a vertical axis, whereas lower pole lesions may cause horizontal deviation.

RCC and other masses may protrude into the renal pelvis if central in location. Other findings include caliceal or infundibular displacement, distortion, or invasion. RCC may rarely mimic transitional cell carcinoma (TCC), causing a focal hydrocalyx, amputated calyx, or hydronephrosis due to obstruction at the renal pelvis or in the proximal ureter (Newhouse and Pfister 1979) (Figs 22.17–22.21).

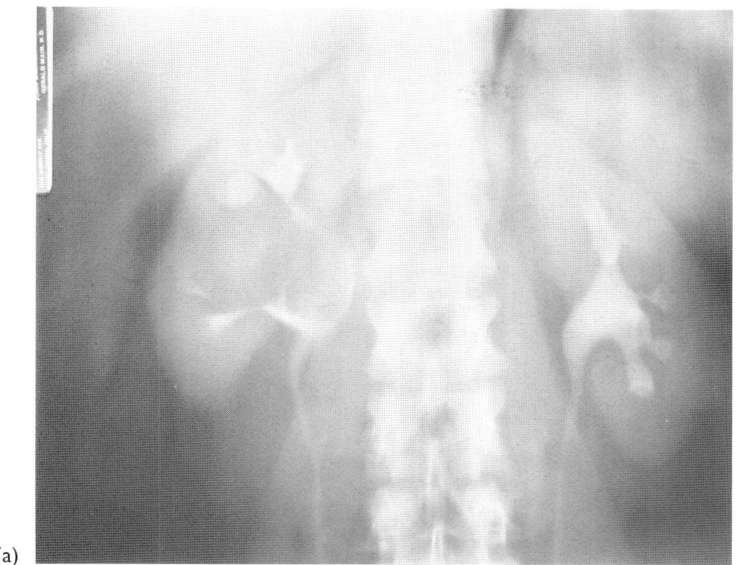

(a)

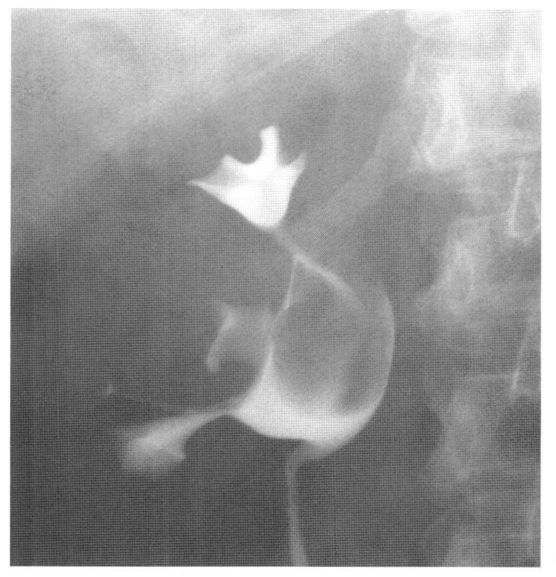

(b)

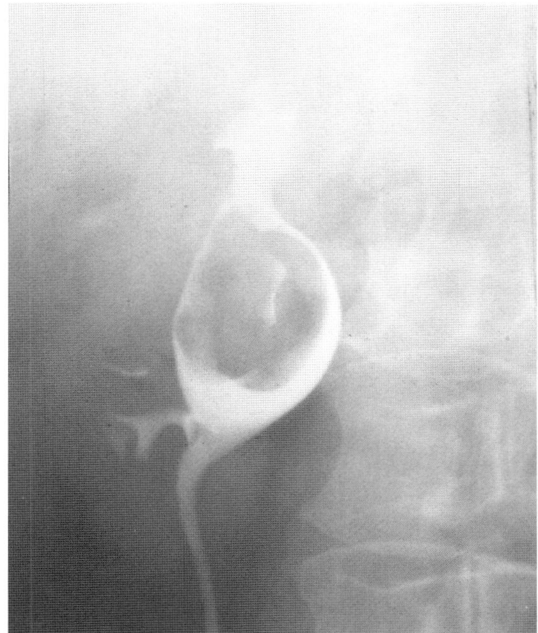

(c)

Fig. 22.11 (a) Excretory phase of IVU demonstrates mass effect in the renal parenchyma with caliceal effacement. The lesion also bulges into the renal pelvis. (b), (c) On AP and RPO retrograde pyelogram, the lobulated lesion appears as a filling defect within the renal pelvis.

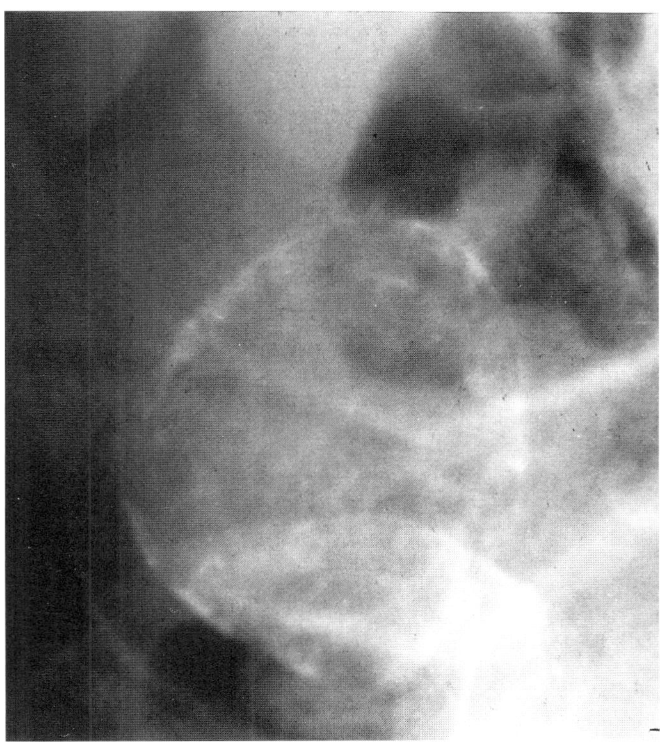

Fig. 22.12 A 51-year-old man with right flank pain. A 10 minute post-injection excretory phase IVU image demonstrates extensive dystrophic calcifications within a right inferior pole renal mass.

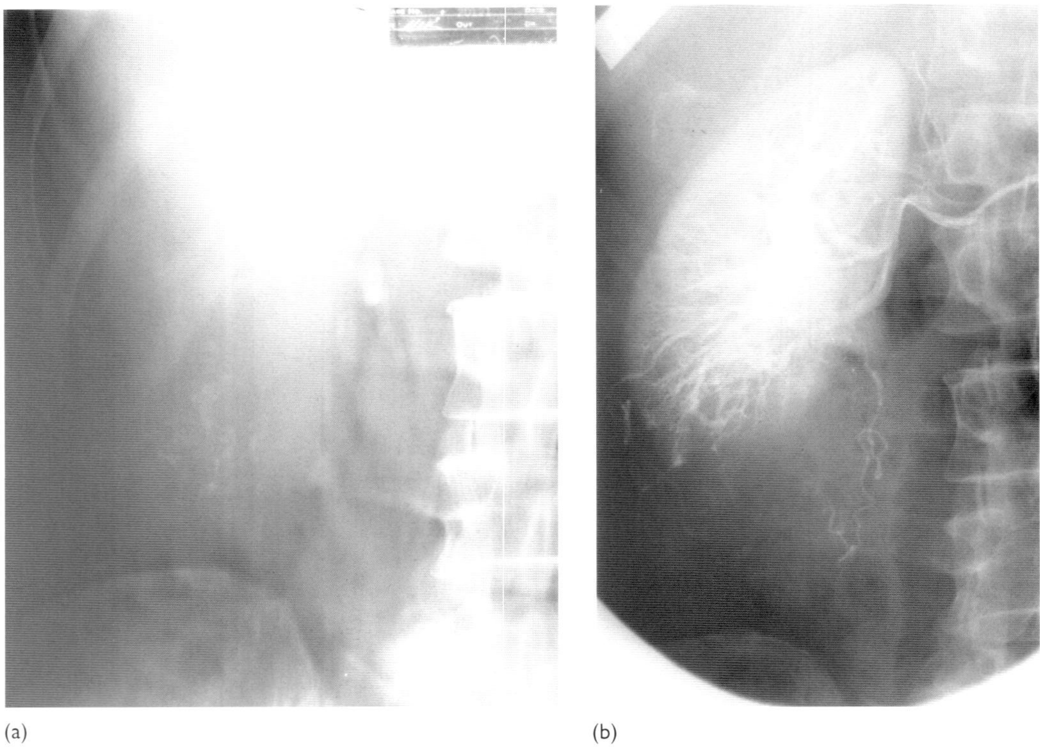

(a)   (b)

Fig. 22.13 A 57-year-old man with hematuria. (a) Excretory phase of IVU demonstrates dystropic calcifications in exophytic right lower pole renal mass. (b) A follow-up angiogram done 10 days later demonstrates the tumor neovascularity in this RCC.

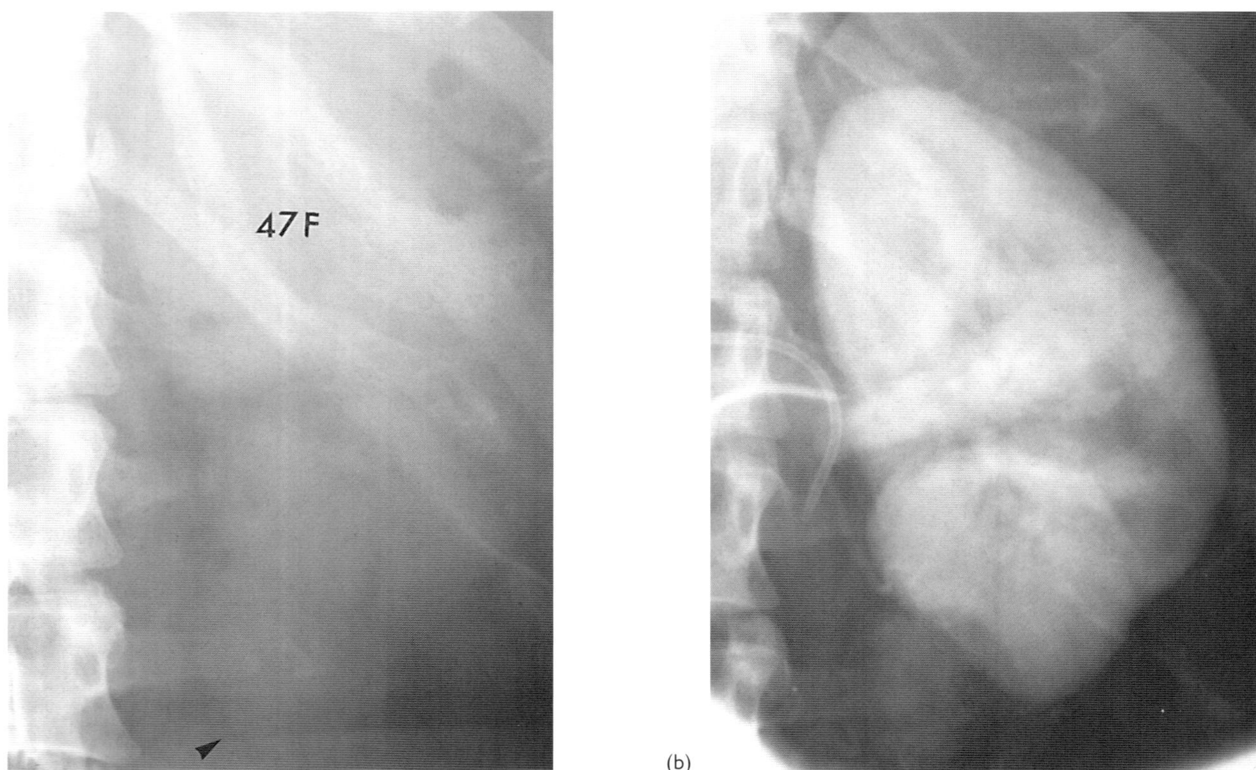

(a)   (b)

Fig. 22.14 A 47-year-old woman with hematuria. (a) On the 5 minute post-injection view, a lobular exophytic renal mass is present with coarse dystrophic calcifications adjacent to the lumbar transverse process (arrowhead). (b) Follow-up nephrogram from an angiogram demonstrates neovascularity.

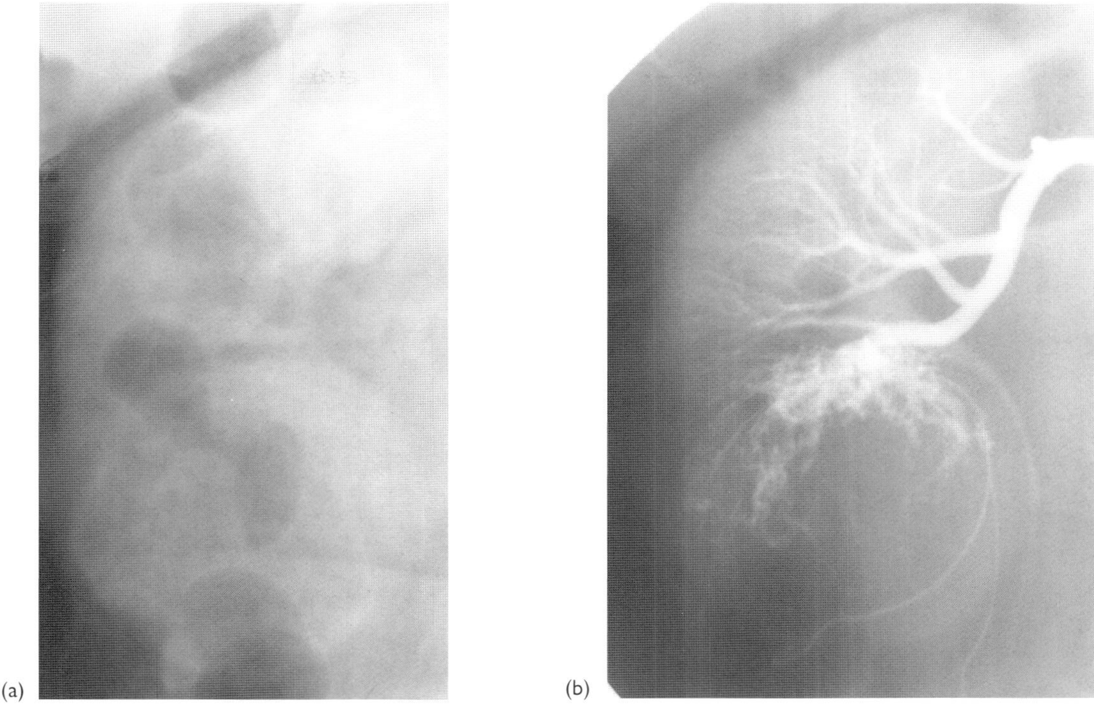

Fig. 22.15 A 77-year-old man with hematuria. (a) One minute post-contrast film demonstrates a hypervascular mass deforming the right lower pole. `(b) A right renal angiogram performed 3 months later demonstrates peripheral neovascularity.

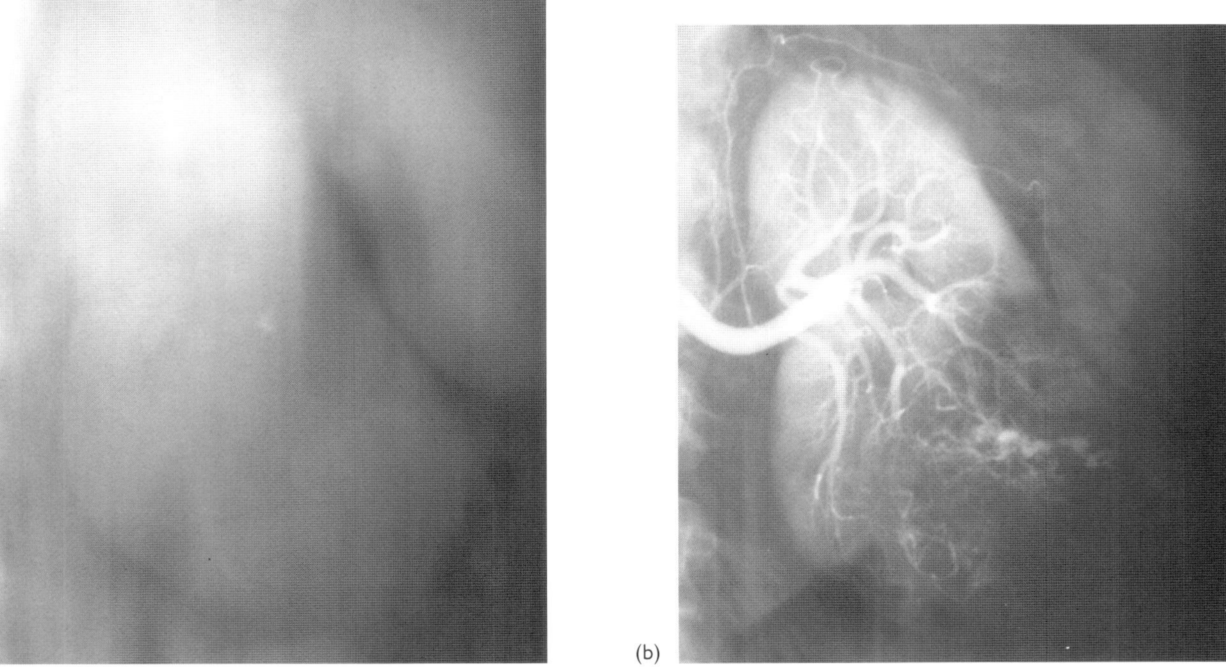

Fig. 22.16 A 73-year-old woman with left flank pain. (a) Two minute left nephrotomogram demonstrates a lower pole contour-deforming renal mass with focal associated calcifications. (b) The associated neovascularity is confirmed on an angiogram 10 days later.

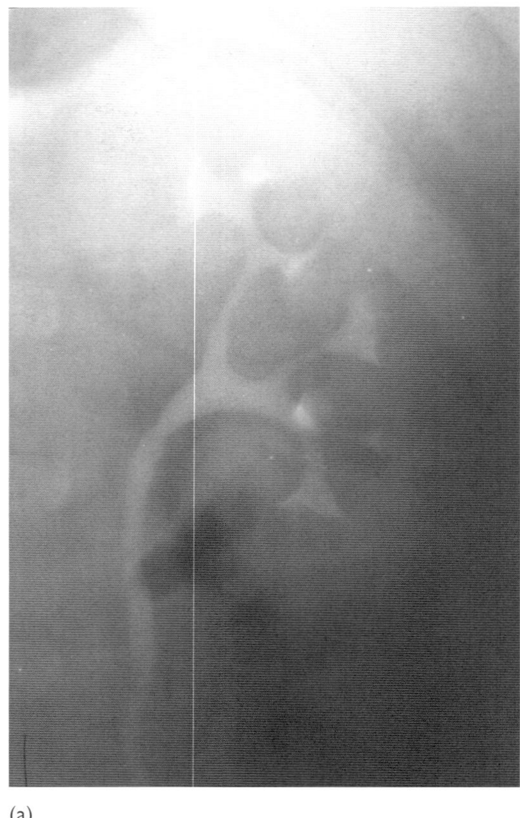

(a)

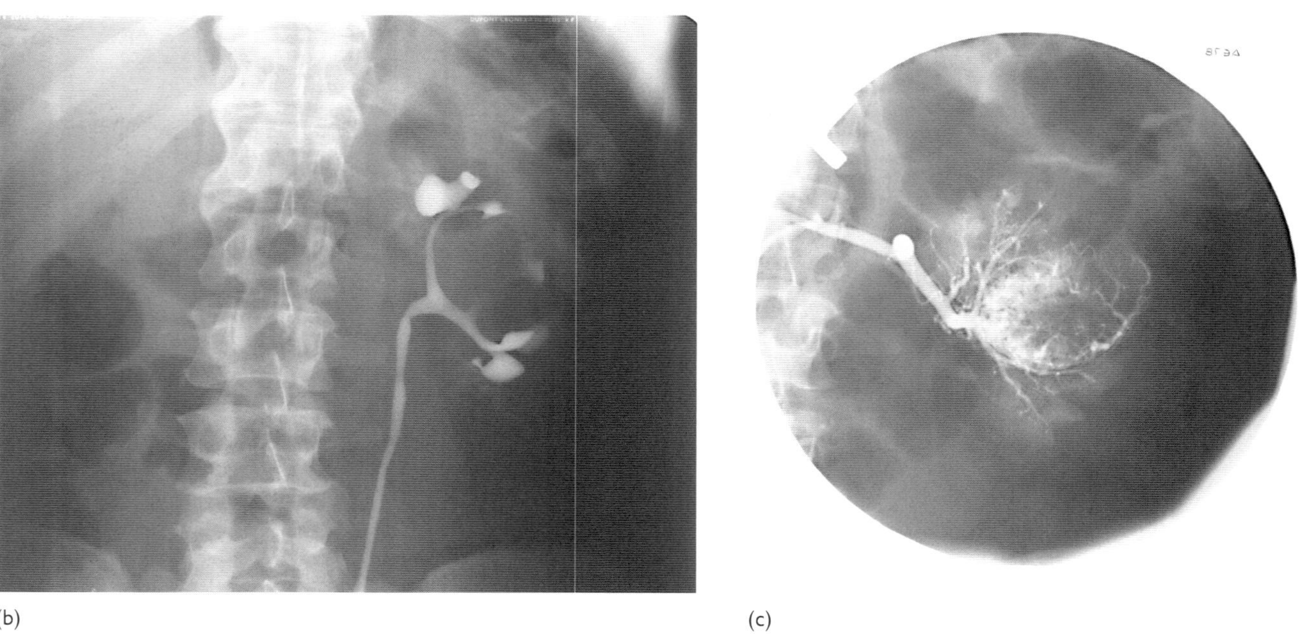

(b)   (c)

Fig. 22.17 A 50-year-old man with persistent microscopic hematuria. (a) IVU in 1968 shows a normal left nephrotomogram. (b) Retrograde pyelogram 7 years later shows splaying of the central calyces. (c) A hypervascular mass is confirmed on a left renal angiogram.

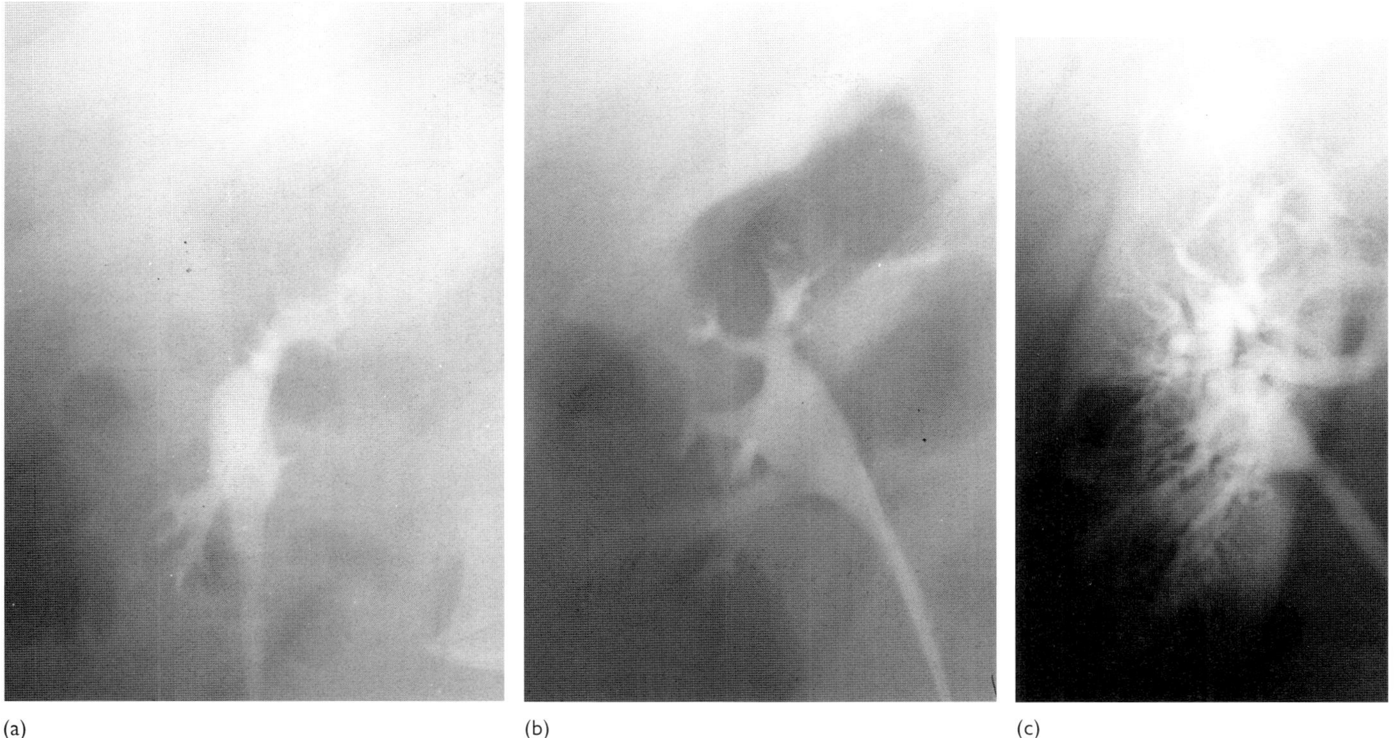

Fig. 22.18 A 42-year-old man with gross hematuria. Outside IVU was interpreted as normal. (a) Right posterior oblique excretory phase IVU shows both upper pole caliceal irregularity and a contour-deforming right upper pole mass. (b) Subsequent retrograde pyelogram better demonstrates the irregular right upper pole calyx. (c) Neovascularity characteristic of RCC is confirmed on renal arteriogram

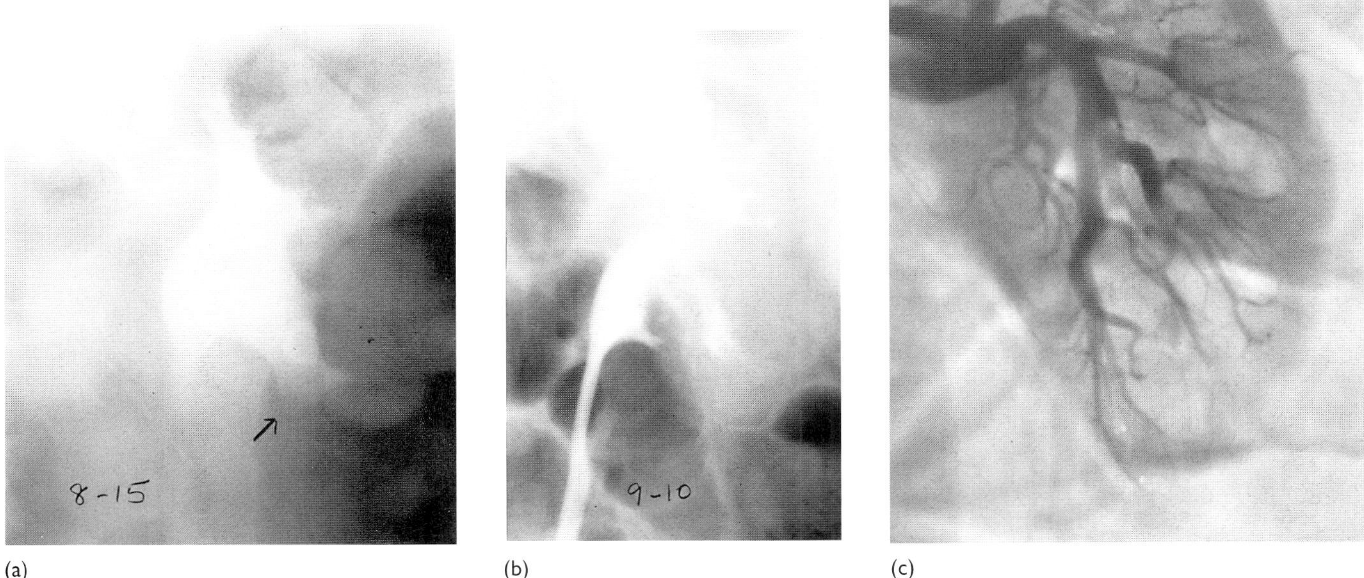

Fig. 22.19 (a) Excretory phase of IVU demonstrates a subtle attenuation of the left inferior pole calyx. (b) The calyx is irregular on retrograde pyelography. Differential favored a TCC. (c) Subtle neovascularity was present on a selective left renal angiogram. A small RCC was confirmed at surgery. Prognosis of RCC with pelvocaliceal invasion is poor.

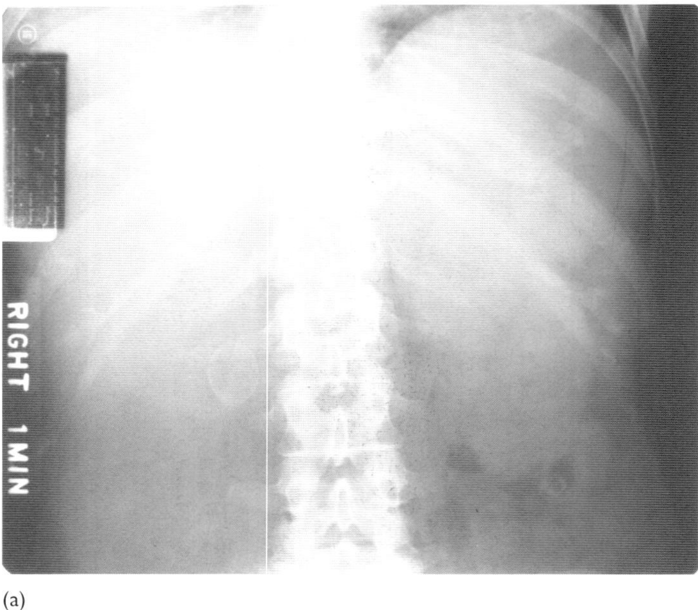

(a)

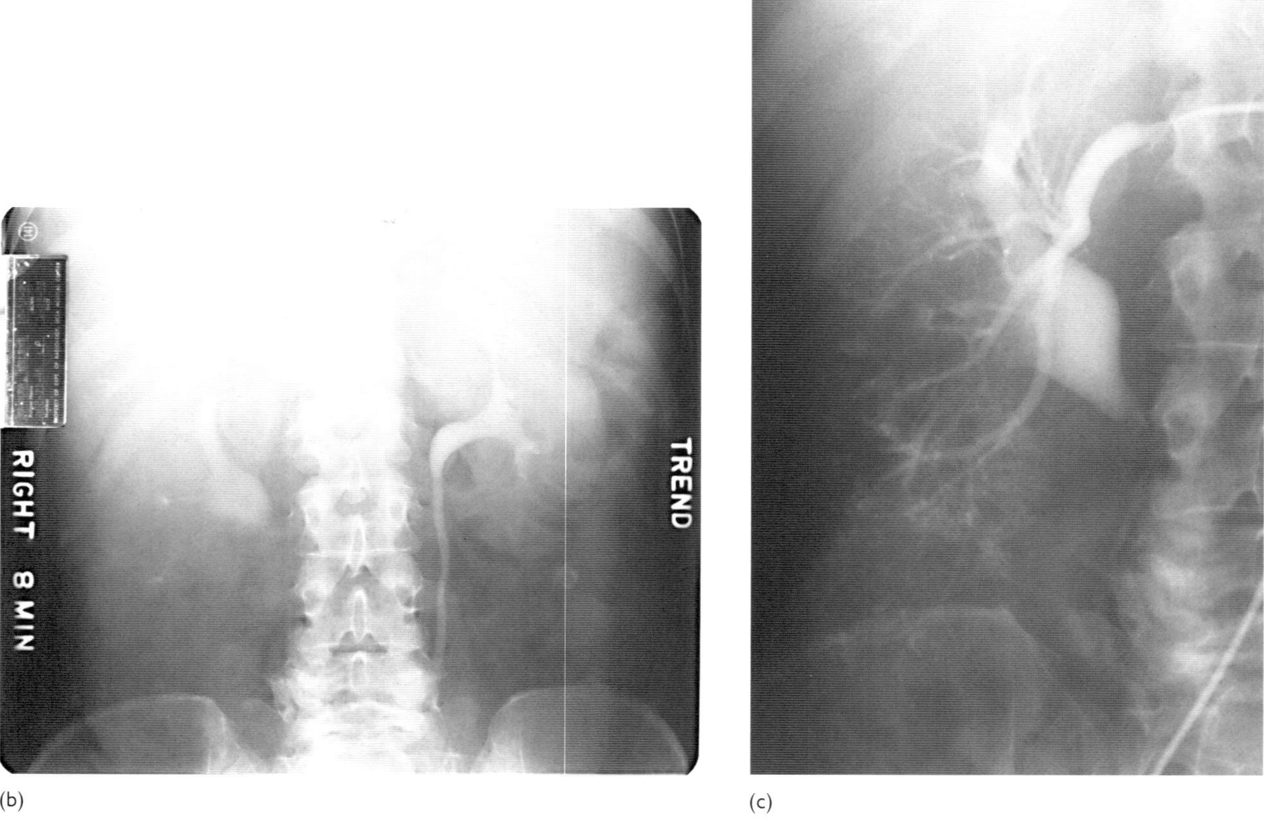

(b)   (c)

Fig. 22.20 (a) One minute film from an IVU demonstrates an abnormally enlarged contour to the right lower pole. (b) On the pyelogram phase, the mass deforms the right lower pole calyces and invades the middle and lower pole calyces and the right renal pelvis. (c) Tumor neovascularity in the right lower pole is demonstrated on a selective right renal angiogram.

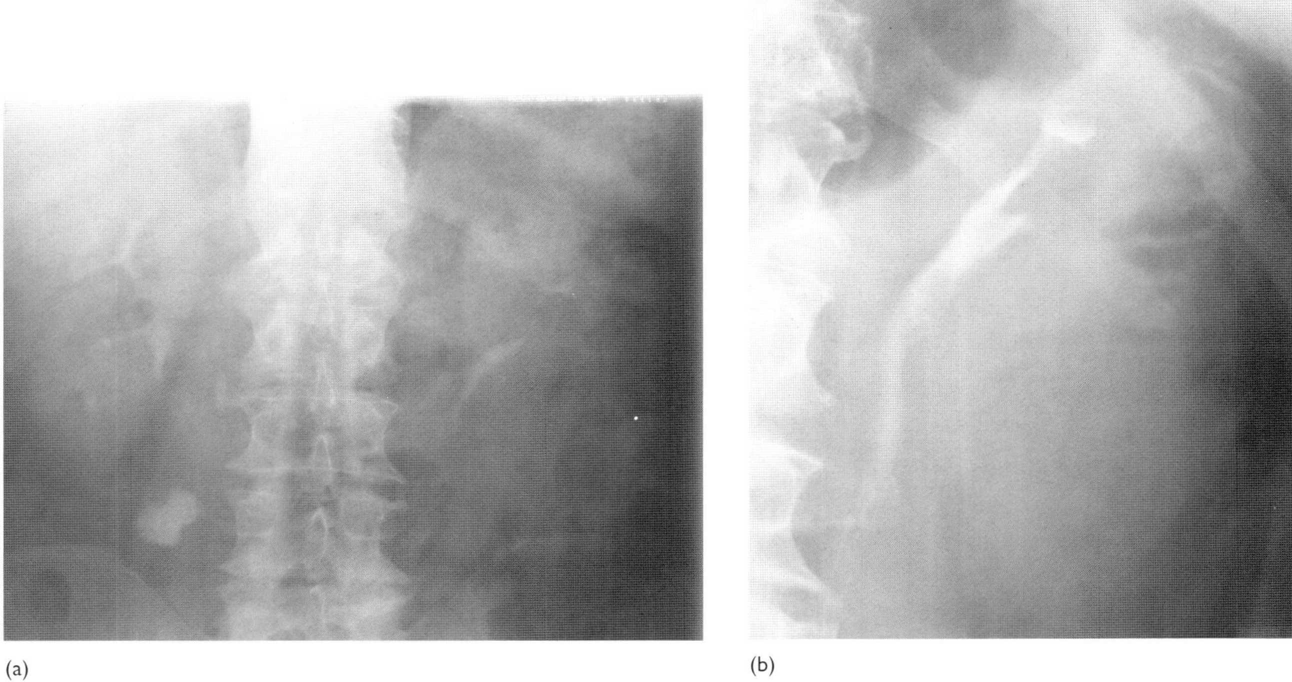

Fig. 22.21 (a) Contour-deforming left lower pole renal mass is demonstrated on excretory phase of IVU. The pelvis is deformed with irregular contour. (b) The retrograde pyelogram demonstrates filling defects in the ureter with irregular invasion centrally from a RCC.

Renal malignancies may also be detected as they usually differ in density when compared to the surrounding parenchyma on excretory urography. Large RCC may cause an absent or delayed nephrogram unilaterally due to tumor thrombus in the renal vein or inferior vena cava (IVC) (Newhouse and Pfister 1979).

Although most solid renal masses will be RCC, the differential diagnosis includes pseudotumors, primary and metastatic neoplasms, and lymphoma. Pseudotumors may be caused by a variety of conditions, including a prominent column of Bertin, fetal renal lobulations, and reflux-nephropathy-induced scarring with compensatory hypertrophy. Pseudotumors may be differentiated from true lesions by CT, MRI, US, or nuclear medicine scans.

Primary renal lesions mimicking RCC include renal adenoma and oncocytoma. Although some specific imaging features have been described, especially for oncocytoma, the lesion cannot be diagnosed by imaging alone and usually must be surgically resected (Quinn *et al.* 1984). Renal angiomyolipomas are heterogeneous in size and appearance. They are rarely diagnosed on IVU unless they predominantly contain fat. The diagnosis can usually be confirmed with CT or MRI (Bosniak 1981). TCC may invade renal parenchyma from the urothelium. They are usually infiltrative in nature, but may be expansile, and mimic a central RCC. Whereas RCC is usually a vascular tumor that enhances avidly, TCC is hypovascular and enhances poorly. Renal sarcomas may present as a solitary renal mass. A single renal mass may be due to lymphoma, although mutifocal or diffuse lesions are more common. Most lymphomas are hypovascular and will enhance poorly after contrast administration.

Hematogenous metastases to the kidney may arise from lung, breast, colon, melanoma, and contralateral kidney (Fig. 22.22). Due to their small size and cortical location, smaller metastases are not usually not detected on excretory urography. When metastases enlarge, radiographic or excretory urography mimic RCC.

Tumors of the urothelium

In current state of the art radiological practice, the IVU is best suited for evaluation of the upper urothelial tract, including the calyces, infundibula, renal pelvis, and the ureter. Transitional cell carcinoma (TCC) remains the most common primary urothelial malignancy in the developed world. With adherence to optimal IVU technique, including bowel preparation, tomography, and compression views, the renal collecting system can be well evaluated.

Although TCC occurs much more commonly in the lower ureter and bladder, the risk of upper tract disease significantly increases in certain high-risk groups such as smokers and factory workers exposed to plastics and aniline dyes. Patients with prior bladder cancer also have a 2–4 per cent risk of metachronous disease in the upper tracts.

The basic radiological findings of a TCC on excretory urography would be a filling defect in the renal calyces, infundibula, or collecting system. The filling defects may be solitary or multiple with smooth, irregular, or cauliflower-like papillary contour

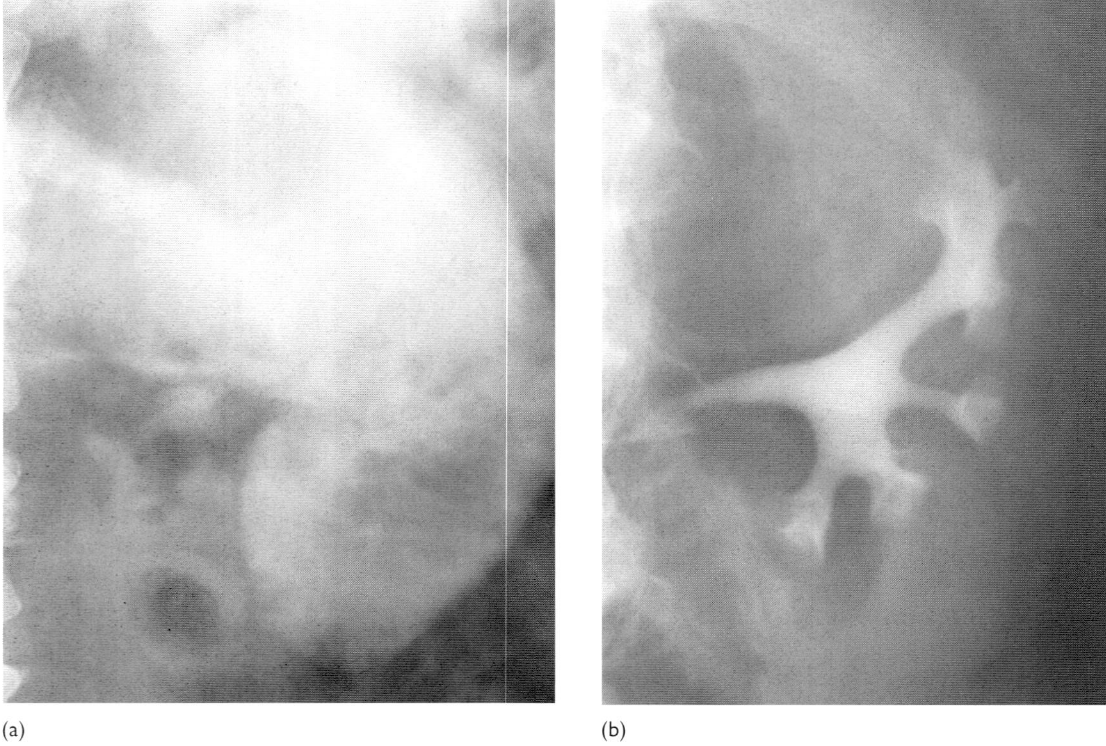

(a)   (b)

Fig. 22.22 (a) On the parenchymal phase of the IVU, an abnormally large contour is present in the left upper pole suggesting a large mass. (b) This lesion splays the upper pole calyces laterally on the excretory phase. Metastasis from malignant melanoma was confirmed at surgery.

(Leder and Dunnick 1990) (Figs 22.23–22.25). However, the tumor can produce a number of characteristic patterns due to its pattern of spread. Five of the most common IVU presentations as described by Lowe *et al.* (1976) are: (1) single or multiple discrete filling defects (35 per cent); (2) filling defects within distended calyces (26 per cent); (3) caliceal obliteration (amputation) (19 per cent); (4) ureteropelvic junction (UPJ) obstruction by tumor causing hydronephrosis; (5) decreased concentration due to longstanding UPJ obstruction without hydronephrosis (Fig. 22.26). Large TCC may diffusely enlarge the kidney as they invade renal parenchyma. Filling defects of the renal collecting systems must be followed up with further imaging including retrograde pyelograms and additional tests such as ureteroscopy and selective brushings for cytology (Figs 22.27 and 22.28).

The adrenal gland

Space-occupying masses of the adrenal glands are best detected and characterized by cross-sectional techniques, especially CT and MRI, which in most cases can provide a specific diagnosis or a narrow differential. On excretory urography, meticulous technique and nephrotomography is essential for detection. For adrenocortical tumors and pheochromocytoma, a detection rate of 80 per cent was reported for nephrotomography in the era prior to cross-sectional imaging (Hamberger *et al.* 1982). Indeed, Hamberger *et al.* (1982) noted that the accuracy of preoperative

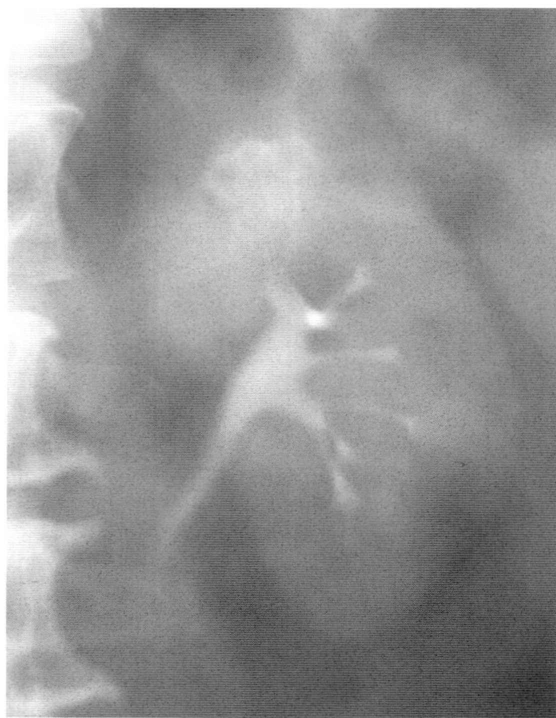

Fig. 22.23 Excretory phase of a left nephrotomogram demonstrates an irregular filling defect within the left upper pole calyx that proved to be TCC.

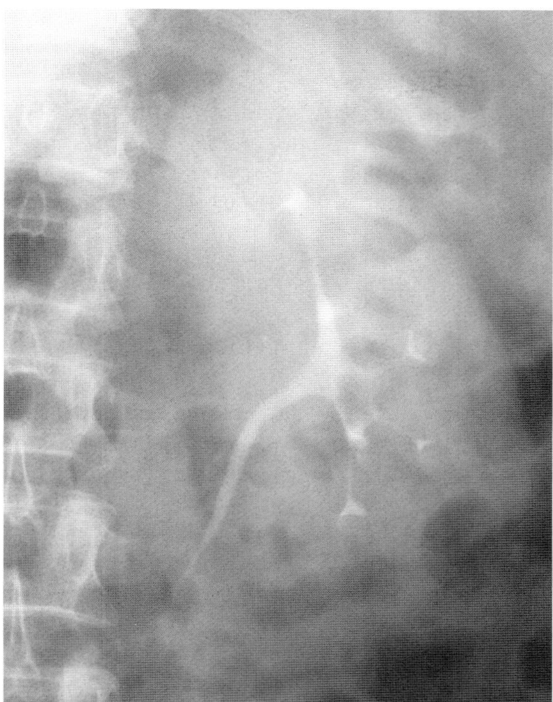

Fig. 22.24 Excretory phase of an IVU demonstrates a central filling pelvic defect just above the inferior pole that was confirmed to be TCC at surgery.

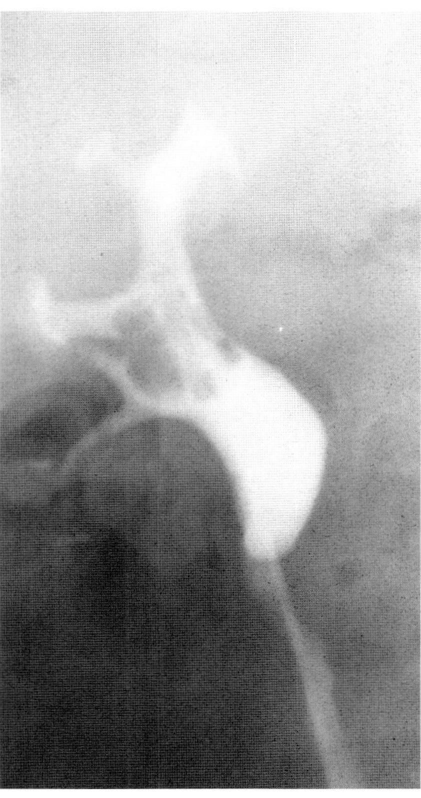

Fig. 22.25 Retrograde pyelogram demonstates a large right central filling defect. TCC can sometimes grow large with mass effect. However they usually enchance poorly relative to RCC.

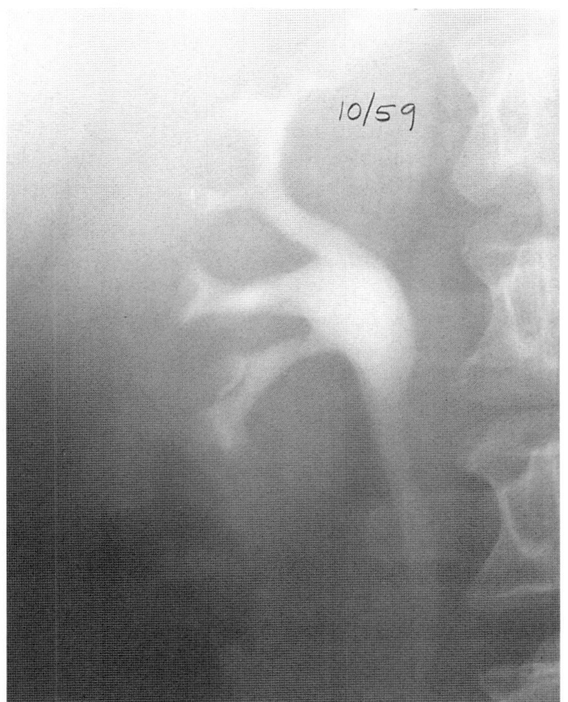

(a)

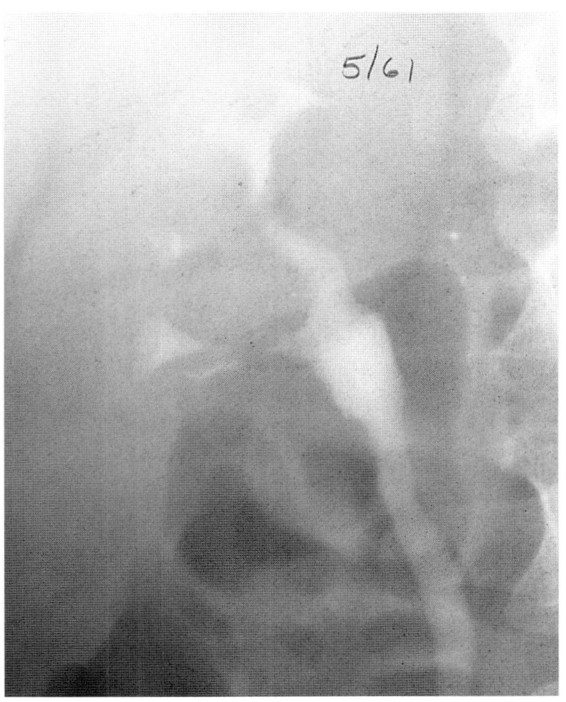

(b)

Fig. 22.26 (a) The excretory phase of an IVU was unremarkable. (b) Two years later, the right lower pole calyces have become attenuated with surrounding infundibular stenosis.

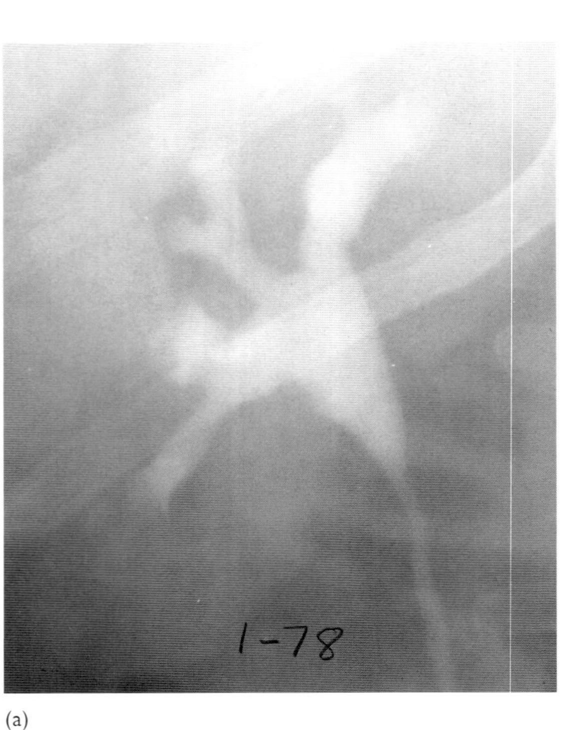

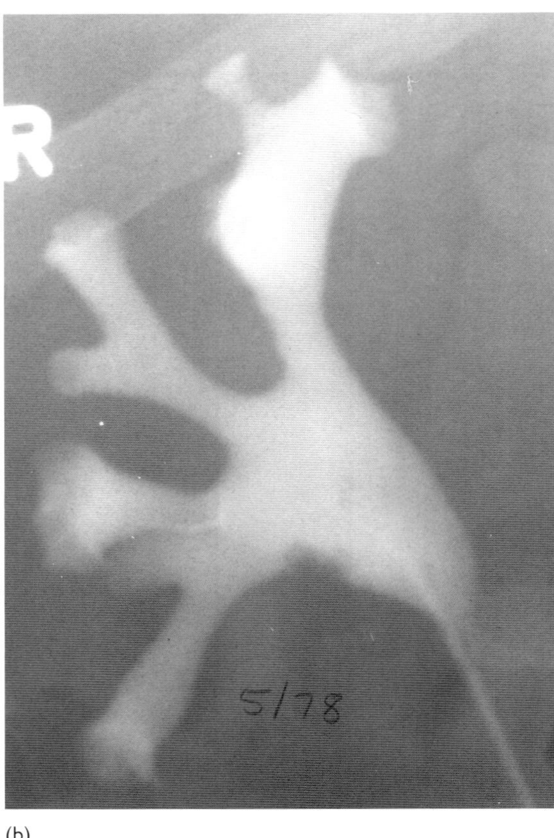

(a)   (b)

Fig. 22.27 (a) The excretory phase of IVU demonstrates a focal irregularity at the inferior margin of the pelvis. (b) This was confirmed on a retrograde pyelogram and proved to be TCC on cytology.

localization of adrenal tumors increased rapidly from 50 to 98 per cent during the 1970s as nephrotomography and then CT scans became widespread. Although the differential diagnosis for an adrenal mass is broad (Table 22.3), 90 per cent of lesions are either adenomas or metastasis. The value of excretory urography lies in detecting larger (3–5 cm) masses, both benign and neoplastic disease, and imaging associated features such as skeletal changes (osteoporosis and/or metastasis), pattern of calcifications (common in neonatal adrenal hemorrhage and neuroblastoma), and associated nephrolithiasis.

Preparation of patients with adrenal lesions may become an issue if there is clinical evidence for an endocrine dysfunction especially with Conn's syndrome or congenital adrenal hyperplasia (in pediatric populations). Patients with known medullary tumors such as pheochromocytoma will need alpha blockade to avoid the uncommon but potentially serious consequences of pressor effects and 'pheo crisis' (Pikering *et al.* 1975).

On excretory urography, right-sided adrenal masses will flatten or depresses the right upper renal pole with inferior and sometimes lateral renal displacement. Adrenal and other extrarenal lesions usually do not distort calyces. A large lesion may also displace or compress liver (Fig. 22.29). These lesions must be differentiated from exophytic liver and renal masses. When detected, patients proceed to CT or MRI to characterize and stage

Table 22.3 Differential diagnosis for lesions of the adrenal gland

Benign lesions	Infections and inflammatory conditions	Malignant lesions
Primary tumors	Granulomatous	Adrenal cortical carcinoma
Adenoma	Tuberculosis, fungus	Malignant pheochromocytoma
Nonfunctioning	Sarcoid	Neuroblastoma
Functioning		Metastasis
Cushing syndrome		
Conn's producing		
Pheochromocytoma		
Myelolipoma		
Cysts		
Hemorrhage		

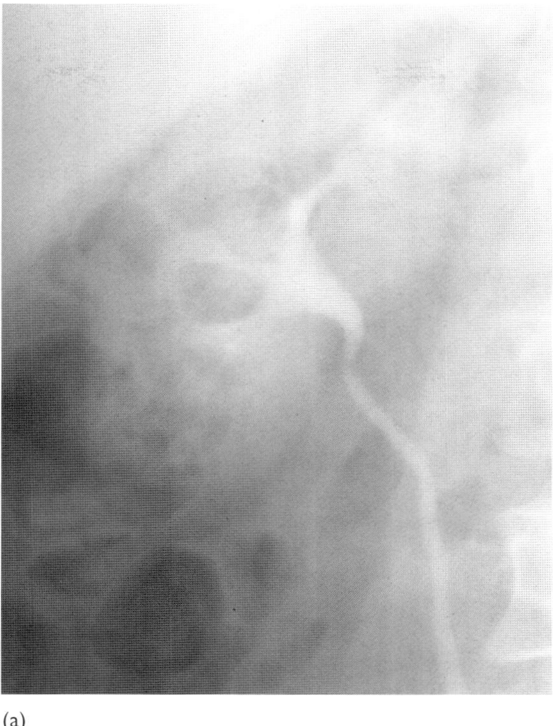

(a)

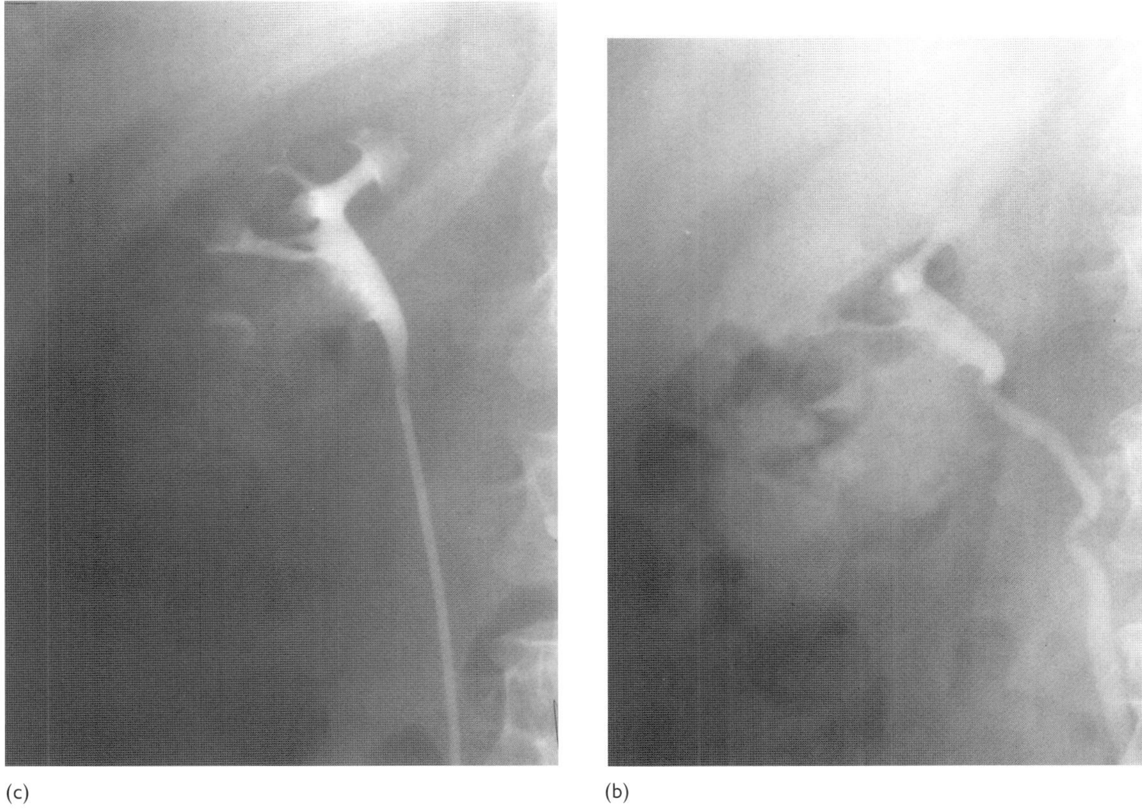

(c)

(b)

Fig. 22.28 (a) The excretory phase of an IVU demonstrates mild irregularity and attenuation of the right lower pole calyces. No definite malignancy could be detected on subsequent retrograde study (not shown). (b) Follow-up excretory urogram 1 year later shows truncation of the right lower pole calyces and (c) retrograde pyelogram confirms a mass that proved to be TCC.

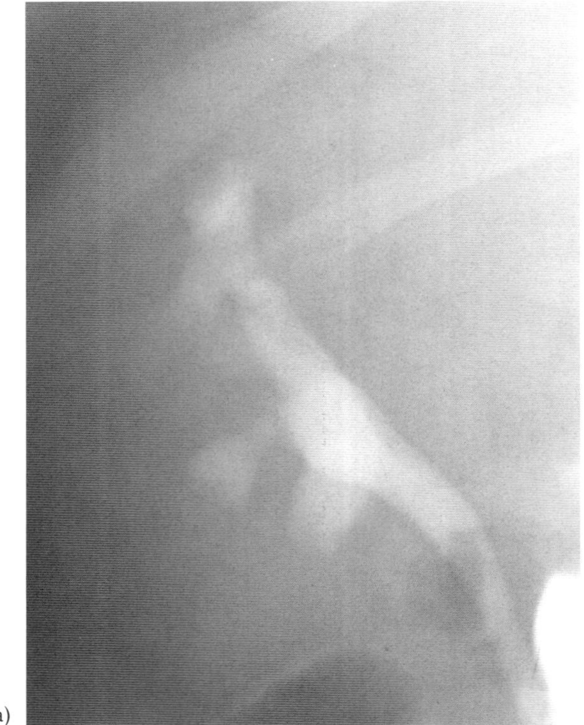

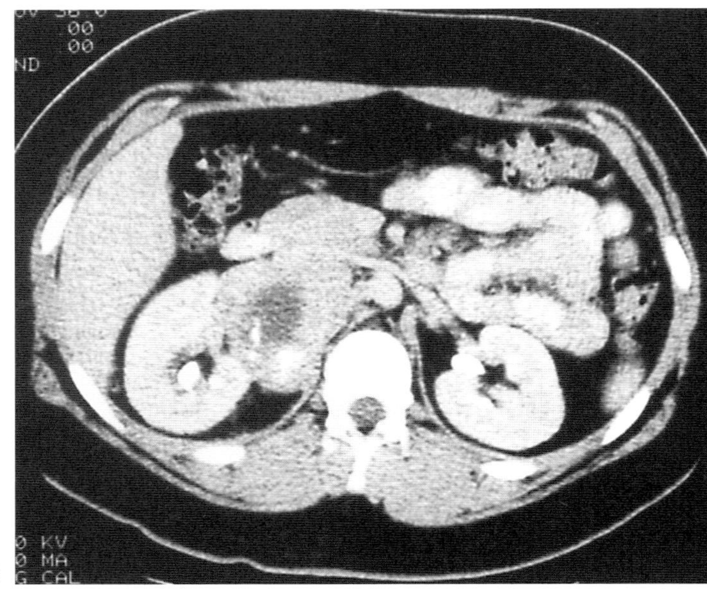

(a)

(b)

Fig. 22.29 (a) The excretory phase of an IVU demonstrates upper pole deviation of the axis of the right kidney. There is no caliceal distortion, suggesting that the lesion may be extrarenal in origin. (b) CT confirms the right adrenal mass with invasion of the IVC.

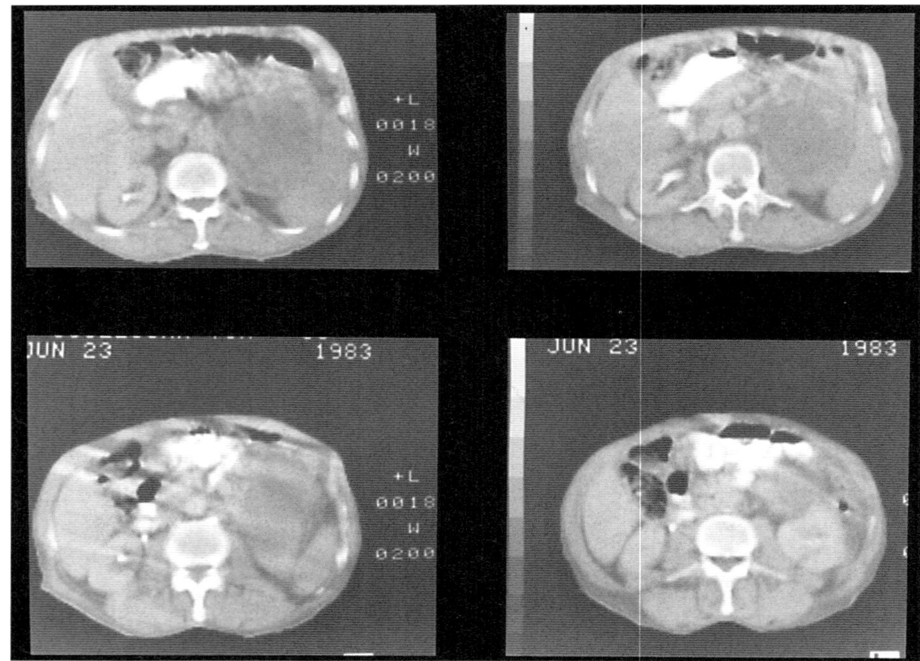

Fig. 22.30 Corresponding delayed phase of contrast-enhanced CT shows large left adrenal mass that was adrenocortical carcinoma.

the lesion, with respect to invasion locally, portal venous invasion, and metastasis. Angiography may be useful to map feeding arteries.

On the left side, adrenal tumors tend to displace the kidney inferolaterally, and deform the left upper renal pole (Fig. 22.30). Sometimes, these lesions will invade the kidney, making accurate localization more challenging. Benign lesions mimicking adrenal tumors include the gastric fundus which disappears in the prone position, and accessory spleen, which may be distinguished on CT or sulfur colloid nuclear medicine scan.

Calcifications, typically found in neuroblastomas, are generally nonspecific within adult tumors since approximately 10 per cent of adrenal cortical carcinomas calcify. Twenty per cent of adrenal cysts may calcify, typically in an 'eggshell' or peripheral pattern. Some metastasis, granulomatous disease of the adrenals, and myelolipoma may all contain calcifications. CT is the modality of choice for sorting out these entities and guiding biopsy as necessary.

Summary

The IVU continues to be widely employed despite rapid advances in cross-sectional imaging. The IVU is the procedure of choice for evaluation of the upper tract urothelium. When performed optimally, it remains useful for a variety of non-neoplastic renal problems. Although larger renal and adrenal masses may be detected on the IVU, it cannot be relied upon to exclude them. Therefore negative IVUs and those demonstrating a space-occupying lesion in the kidneys and adrenals will need further characterization and potential staging with sonography, CT, or MRI. Filling defects detected in the collecting systems and renal pelvis will need a retrograde examination.

References

Agrons, G., Wagner, B., Davidson, A., *et al.* (1995). Multilocular cystic renal tumor in children: Radiologic–pathologic correlation. *Radiographics* **15**, 653–.

Berns, J.S. and Rudnick, M.R. (1992). Radiocontrast media associated nephro-toxicity. *Kidney* **24**, 1–5.

Bosniak, M. (1981). Angiomyolipoma (hamartoma) of the kidney. A preoperative diagnosis is possible in virtually every case. *Urol. Radiol.* **135**, 3.

Bosniak, M. (1986*a*). The current radiological approach to renal cysts. *Radiology* **158**, 1.

Bosniak, M. (1986*b*). Difficulties in classifying cystic lesions of the kidney. *Radiology* **158**, 1–5.

Bosniak, M.A. (1991*a*). The small (≤ 3.0 cm) renal parenchymal tumor: detection, diagnosis and controversies. *Radiology* **179**, 307–17.

Bosniak, M. (1991*b*). Difficulties in classifying cystic lesions of the kidney. *Urol. Radiol.* **13**, 91.

Byrd, L. and Sherman, R. (1979). Radiocontrast-induced acute renal failure: a clinical and pathophysiologic review. *Medicine* **58**, 270–9.

Daniel, W., Hartman, G., Witten, D., *et al.* (1972). Calcified renal masses: a review of ten years' experience at the Mayo Clinic. *Radiology* **103**, 503.

Disler, D. and Chew, F. (1992). Adrenal pheochromocytoma. *Am. J. Roentgenol.* **158**, 1056.

Dunnick, N.R. (1992). Renal lesions: great strides imaging. *Radiology* **182**, 305–6.

Ellis, J., Cohan, R., Sonnad, S., and Cohan, N. (1996). Selective use of radio-graphic low-osmolality contrast media in the 1990's. *Radiology* **200**, 297.

Feldman, A.E., Pollack, H.M., Perri, A.J. Jr, *et al.* (1978). Renal pesudotumors: an anatomic–radiologic classification. *J. Urol.* **120**, 133.

Hamberger, B. *et al.* (1982). Adrenal surgery: trends during the seventies. *Am. J. Surg.* **144**, 523–6.

Hattery, R.R., Williamson, B., Hartman, G.W., LeRoy, A.J., and Witten, D.M. (1988). Intravenous urographic technique. *Radiology* **167**, 593–9.

Katholi, R., Taylor, G., Woods, W., *et al.* (1993). Nephrotoxicity of nonionic low osmolality contrast media: a prospective double-blind randomized comparison in human beings. *Radiology* **186**, 183–7.

Katzberg, R.W. (1997). Urography into the 21st century. *Radiology* **204**, 297–312.

Lasser, E., Berry, C., Talner, L., *et al.* (1987). Pretreatment with corticosteroids to alleviate reactions to intravenous contrast material. *New Engl. J. Med.* **317**, 845–9.

Leder, R. and Dunnick, N. (1990). Transitional cell carcinomal of the pelvica-lyces and ureter. *Am. J. Roentgenol.* **155**, 713.

Lee, M., Hahn, P., Papanicolau, N., *et al.* (1991). Benign and malignant adrenal masses: CT distinctions with attenuation coefficients, size and observer analysis. *Radiology* **179**, 425–8.

Levy, E.M., Viscoli, C., and Horwitz, R. (1996). The effect of acute renal failure on mortality: a cohort analysis. *J. Am. Med. Assoc.* **275**, 1489–94.

Lowe, P. and Roylance, J. (1976). Transitional cell carcinoma of the kidney. *Clin. Radiol.* **27**, 503.

McClennan, B. (1990). Ionic and nonionic iodinated contrast media: evolution and strategies for use. *Am. J. Roentgenol.* **155**, 225–33.

Morris, T.W. (1993). X-ray contrast media: where are we now and where are we going? *Radiology* **188**, 11–16.

Newhouse, J. and Pfister, R. (1979). The nephrogram. *Rad. Clin. N. Am.* **17**, 213–26.

Osborne, E., Sutherland, C., Scholl, A., and Rowntree, L. (1923). Roentgenography of urinary tract during excretion of sodium iodide. *J. Am. Med. Assoc.* **80**, 368–73.

Pikering, R., Hartman, G., Weeks, R., *et al.* (1975). Excretory urographic local-ization of adrenal cortical tumors and pheochromocytomas. *Radiology* **114**, 345.

Quinn, M., Hartman, D., Friedman, A., *et al.* (1984). Renal oncocytoma: new observations. *Radiology* **153**, 49.

Siegle, R.L., Halvorsen, R.A., Dillon, J., and Gavant, M.L. (1991). The use of iohexol in patients with prior reactions to ionic contrast material. A multi-center clinical trial. *Invest. Radiol.* **26**, 411–16.

Smelka, R.C., Shoenut, J.P., Kroeker, M.A., MacMahon, R., and Greenberg, H.M. (1992). Renal lesions: controlled comparison between CT and 1.5 T MR imaging with nonenhanced and gadolinium-enhanced fat-suppressed spin-echo and breath-hold FLASH technique. *Radiology* **182**, 425–30.

Sparato, R., Katzberg, R., Fischer, H., and McMannis, M. (1987). High dose clinical urography with the low-osmolality contrast agent. *Radiology* **162**, 9–14.

Warshauer, D.M., McCarthy, S.M., Street, L., *et al.* (1988). Detection of renal masses: sensitivities and specificities of excretory urography/linear tomography, US and CT. *Radiology* **169**, 363–5.

Wolf, G., Arenson, R., and Cross, A. (1989). A prospective trial of ionic vs nonionic contrast agents in routine clinical practice. *Am. J. Roentgenol.* **152**, 939–44.

23. Radiologic imaging: computerized tomography and magnetic resonance imaging

Zoran L. Barbaric

Terminology

Before attempting to describe how computerized tomography (CT) and magnetic resonance imaging (MRI) contribute to diagnosis, staging, and follow- up of renal and adrenal carcinoma, a few words about the terminology a radiologist uses will hopefully make this chapter more understandable to the practising clinician.

Both CT and MRI studies can be obtained with or without contrast material. Sometimes both studies are required. CT contrast is iodine-based and injected intravenously with a power injector at a rate of 1–5 cm^3/s for a total of 100–150 cm^3. Intravenous (IV) CT contrast is contraindicated in patients with impaired renal function (creatinine < 1.5 mg/dl) and a history of prior severe allergic reaction. MRI contrast is gadolinium-based and is also power injected at a rate of 1–5 cm^3/s for a total dose of 10–20 cm^3. It can be used safely in patients with moderate renal impairment and those with known allergy to CT contrast or iodine.

CT cuts may be acquired one at a time, usually one per second. The patient may be asked to suspend respiration for each cut. The cuts may be of different thickness such as 10, 7, 5, or 3 mm. Fewer thick cuts will be needed to cover the entire abdomen. Spiral or helical CT refers to continuous acquisition of images while the patient is moved through the gantry on a motorized tabletop. Continuous acquisition requires the patient to suspend respiration for 10 to 20 seconds. Spiral CT imaging allows for some significant advantages over single-slice image acquisition. These include vascular imaging, retrospective reconstruction at spacing smaller than collimation, reduction of partial volume-averaging (see below), and, in some instances, decreased radiation exposure compared to that of conventional CT (Silverman *et al.* 1994). Using a simple mouse-guided cursor, X-ray attenuation over any part of an acquired image can be obtained and expressed in Hounsfield units (HU), so-named in honor of the inventor of CT.

Each set of MR image acquisitions is called a sequence. Most studies consist of at least two sequences. MR images are usually acquired simultaneously for a period that may last 2–5 minutes. Such prolonged imaging inevitably invites some artifacts induced by respiration, peristalsis, cardiac contractions, and blood flow. Newer sequences are now available whereby the entire set of images may be obtained in 20 seconds, that is, during one breath-hold (Semelka *et al.* 1992). This is especially useful when IV MR contrast is used, because the imaging is done at the time of maximum contrast concentration in the area of interest. Lastly, there are now 'single shot' sequences that acquire images one by one, needing only one second per image.

Two other MR terms are of importance to fully understand this chapter. The first is 'fat suppression'. Unlike CT where one measures X-ray attenuation, MR directs a radio signal into the body and listens for resonance. The resonance is the MR signal returning from the tissues. Fat is one of the tissues with very high signal strength, which is portrayed as white on printed MR images. Special sequences are used to suppress the signal specifically coming from the fat and portray it as dark on printed images. Thus it is possible to diagnose the presence or absence of fat by comparing two MR sequences.

The second term—'in- and out-of-phase' or 'opposing phase' gradient echo sequences—applies to situations where some lipid-laden and normal cells are intermixed within a tumor. Tumors containing such a mixture of cells will have a normal signal on 'in-phase' sequence, but their signal will dramatically decrease on 'out-of-phase' or 'opposing phase' sequence and they will appear dark. Such a 'drop in signal' is useful in differentiating benign adrenal adenoma from metastasis.

Renal carcinoma

Enhancement

Enhancement is the change in X-ray beam attenuation (CT) or change in signal intensity (MRI) on images obtained after IV injection of contrast material, compared to images obtained prior to the injection. Most solid renal tumors enhance following IV injection of radiographic or MR contrast material. The change in attenuation or signal intensity happens as contrast transverses the tumor capillary bed and migrates into extracellular spaces. The degree of enhancement is to a large degree proportional to the abundance of neovascularity within the tumor (Figs 23.1 and 23.2). Consequently, enhancement will be greatest shortly after arrival of the contrast bolus to the organ, usually 2–3 minutes after IV injection. Change in attenuation of at least 15–20 HU from the baseline pre-contrast scan to the post-contrast scan is diagnostic of a solid neoplasm. The degree of attenuation is usually higher (40–80 HU).

In MR imaging there are no Hounsfield units. The degree of enhancement is expressed in relative value units (RVU) that portray

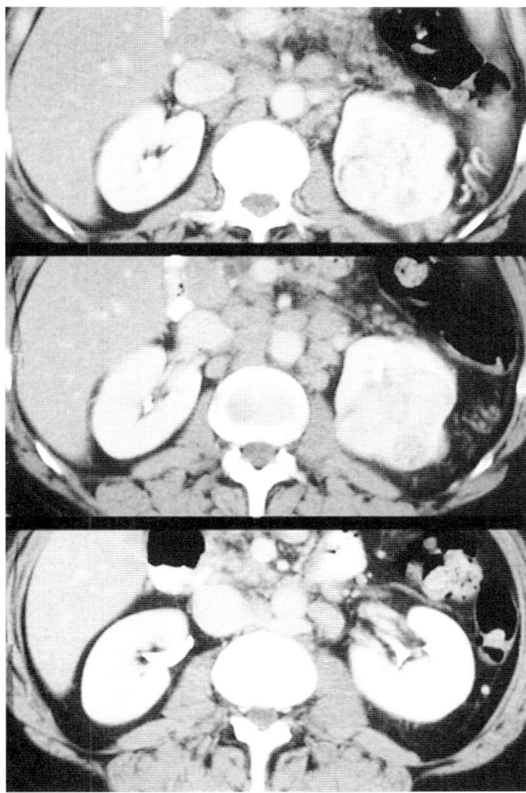

Fig. 23.1 A composite of three CT cuts shows an enhancing heterogeneous mass in the left kidney that proved to be a renal carcinoma. There are also multiple enlarged periaortic and aortocaval lymph nodes. Notice tumor-free retroaortic left renal vein on the bottom image.

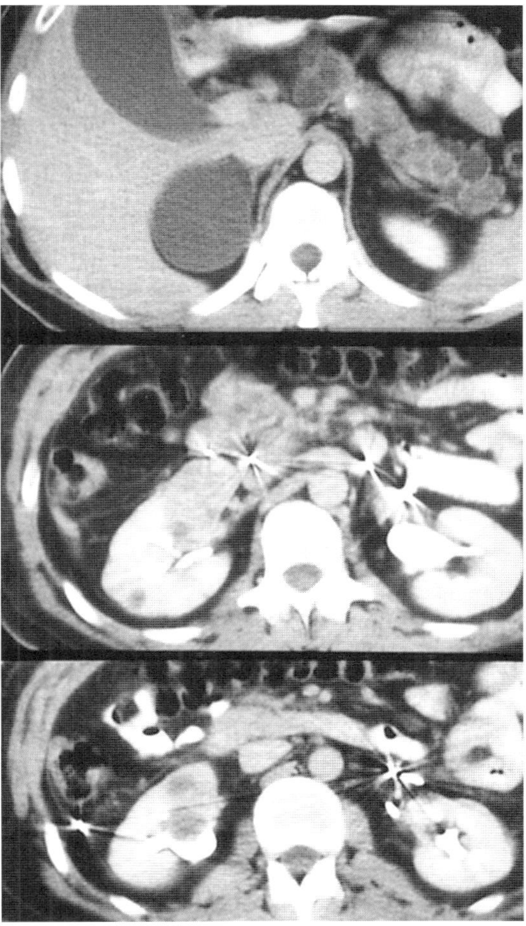

Fig. 23.2 Excellent example of tumor enhancement. In this patient with von Hippel–Lindau disease there is an enhancing right renal tumor (middle and lower images). Right upper pole renal cyst, gall bladder, and several small pancreatic cysts do not enhance as there is no vasculature within their lumens.

relative MR signal strength. Absolute values are not possible due to the variety of different machines and imaging sequences. The best MR sequences for evaluation of renal carcinoma seem to be breath-hold, gadolinium-enhanced, fat-saturated sequences (Fig. 23.3) (Eilenberg *et al.* 1990).

Enhancement alone is not diagnostic of a renal carcinoma but of a solid neoplasm. There are some 40–50 malignant, benign, and inflammatory renal tumors and several pseudotumors, so that a definitive histologic diagnosis by any imaging modality is seldom possible. Statistically, however, a newly discovered enhancing tumor is likely to be a renal carcinoma in 80–85 per cent of cases. Differentiation from two more common benign renal tumors, angiomyolipoma and oncocytoma, is possible to some extent.

Texture

As far as angiomyolipoma is concerned, diagnosis is readily made on both CT and MR imaging. This is because this tumor, in addition to vascular and muscular elements, also contains a moderate amount of fatty tissue, and fat is easily diagnosed by both modalities. Fat has a low attenuation value and will measure around – 50 HU on pre-contrast CT scan. Therefore, even a small amount of fatty tissue within a solid enhancing tumor should be diagnostic of angiomyolipoma (Fig. 23.4) (Bosniak *et al.* 1988). There are exceptions to this rule, such as when there is abundant dystrophic

calcification within the tumor. In this circumstance a renal carcinoma must be considered (Strotzer *et al.* 1993; Helemon *et al.* 1993). Or, a large renal carcinoma may engulf renal sinus fat in such a way as to mimic fat in an angiomyolipoma. Also, intratumoral fat has been described in one case of renal oncocytoma (Prando 1991) and several cases of renal liposarcoma and Wilms' tumor (Williams *et al.* 1994). In general, diagnosis of an angiomyolipoma is usually very simple and pre-contrast CT alone is sufficient.

MRI is also excellent for detecting and confirming presence of fat within the tumor. On most MRI sequences used to image the kidneys, fat exhibits a strong MR signal and generally appears bright on printed images. With a simple push of the button, a set of images can be obtained where the fat is suppressed; that is, all fat, whether subcutaneous, retroperitoneal, or within the tumor, will send no signal to the receiving coil and the resulting image will show all fat as dark tissue. Being able to discriminate between certain tissue types is one of many powerful attributes of MRI.

Oncocytoma is more of a problem. Some findings are suggestive, but not diagnostic of this tumor, as most are also seen in

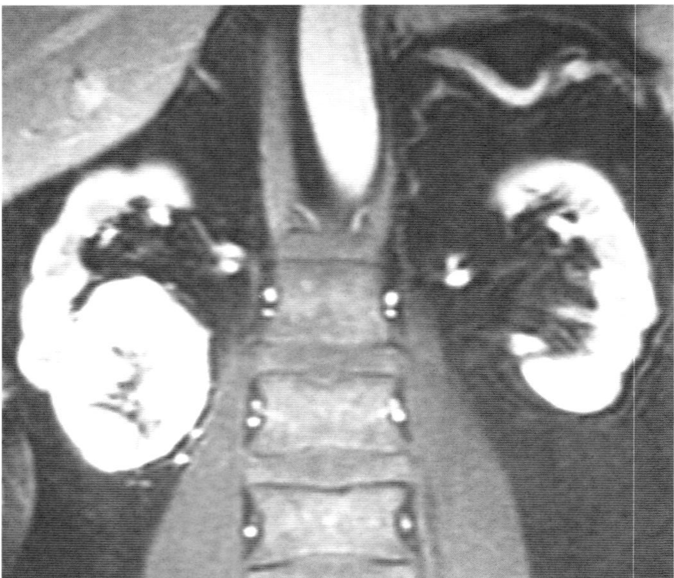

Fig. 23.3 Unlike CT, image acquisition on MRI can be in any plane. Here, in the coronal plane, there is post-contrast enhancement of right lower pole neoplasm, renal parenchyma, and aorta. Perinephric fat appears dark because a fat suppression sequence was used. Otherwise, the fat would appear bright

renal carcinoma (Davidson *et al.* 1992; Endress and Chita 1992; Tikkakoski *et al.* 1991; Selzman *et al.* 1994). On CT, homogeneous enhancement and a central scar, sometimes stellate in appearance, should at least suggest the presence of this tumor, especially if a homogeneous pattern is found on ultrasound (Quinn *et al.* 1984; Neisius *et al.* 1988). On MRI a mass with lower intensity than that of the cortex, a central scar or stellate pattern, a well-defined capsule, and absence of hemorrhage and necrosis are suggestive of

this tumor (Harmon *et al.* 1996; Defosses *et al.* 1991). Notice, however, that both angiomyolipomas and oncocytomas do enhance.

Lack of enhancement

If after IV injection of contrast material a renal mass does not enhance, it could be a simple cyst, cystic carcinoma, papillary carcinoma, infarct, or inflammation. This is where the morphological attributes of these lesions as seen on CT and MRI become extremely important.

The term 'complex cyst' was introduced to try to simplify differentiation between some of these entities.. A somewhat complex cyst (Bosniak class II) has a few septa or some thin curvilinear wall calcification. A more complex cyst (Bosniak class III) either has a thick wall (Figs 23.5 and 23.6(a),(b)), more than a few septations, thick wall calcification (Fig. 23.7), and a thick septum that may enhance or a nodular cyst base (Fig. 23.8) (Bosniak 1986; Aronson *et al.* 1991). In the first instance, the renal mass is re-evaluated with CT or ultrasound in 6 months; in the second instance, it is considered a neoplasm and treated accordingly. Simple cysts do not enhance; they have a thin wall and an attenuation value close to 0 HU (Bosniak class I). A mostly necrotic tumor (Bosniak class IV) is usually not a diagnostic problem (Figs 23.9 and 23.10).

Some cysts on CT are of a very high density, up to 80 HU. These are either hemorrhagic cysts or cysts with a high protein content (Sussman *et al.* 1984; Fishman *et al.* 1983). They are considered benign if they do not enhance and if there is no evidence of other 'complex cyst' attributes (Fig. 23.11 (a), (b)).

If infarct or focal pyelonephritis is suspected, repeat of imaging at an interval of several weeks is almost always sufficient to exclude neoplasm. Mass effects associated with these entities disappear over time and in many instances a parenchymal scar develops.

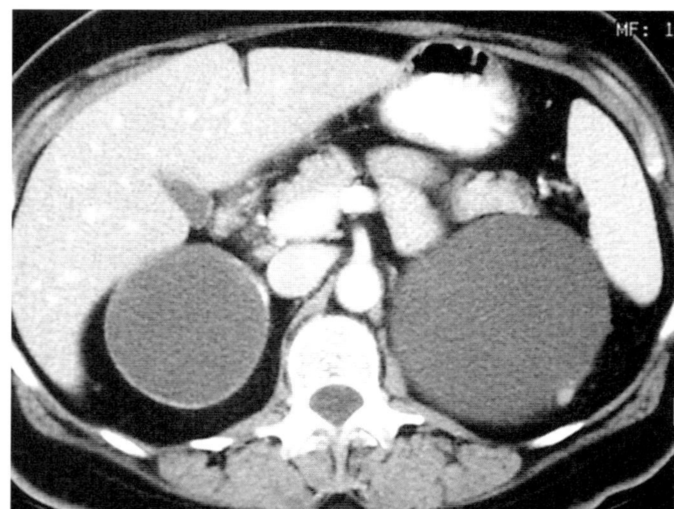

Fig. 23.4 Bleeding left renal angiomyolipoma. Fatty tumor in the lower pole of the left kidney has similar attenuation to that of retroperitoneal and subcutaneous fat and, by placing a cursor in the middle of the mass, −50 HU was measured. Crescent of dense material at the left periphery of the mass is a fresh blood clot. Large angiomyolipomas tend to bleed.

Fig. 23.5 Excellent example of Bosniak class III lesion in the right upper pole. The best way to appreciate the increased wall thickness is to compare with simple left upper pole renal cyst where the wall thickness is imperceptible.

(a)

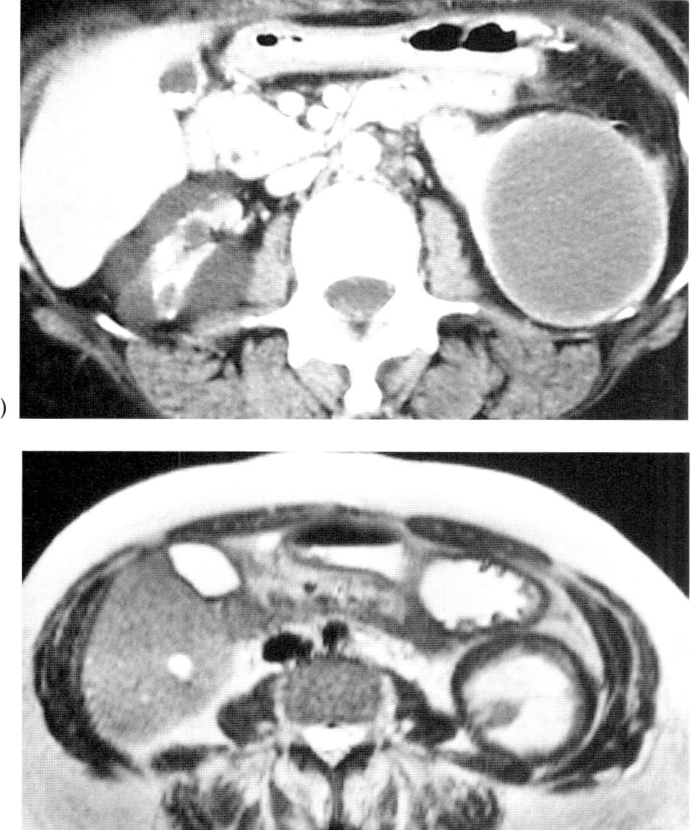

(b)

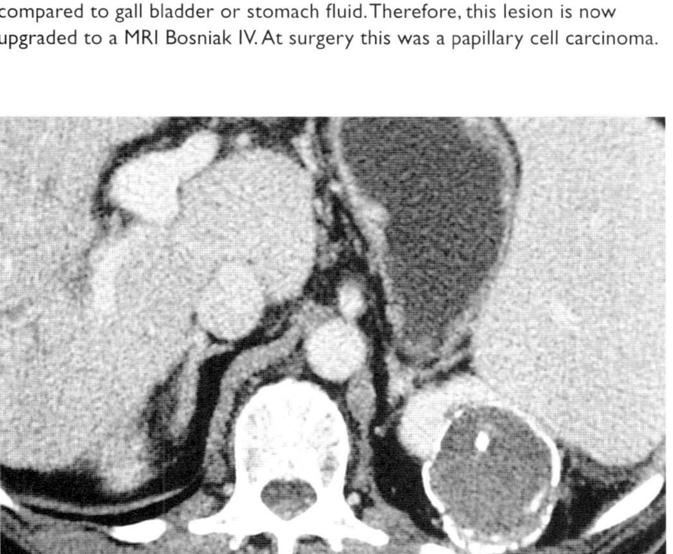

Fig. 23.6 (a) CT in a patient with end-stage renal disease and acquired cystic renal disease shows multiple right renal cysts and a thick-walled left lower pole renal cyst. Therefore, this is a Bosniak class III lesion. (b) MRI without IV contrast on the same patient shows to much better advantage the markedly thickened wall and a dark internal nodule. In addition, the high signal within the lesion is somewhat heterogeneous and not as strong as compared to gall bladder or stomach fluid. Therefore, this lesion is now upgraded to a MRI Bosniak IV. At surgery this was a papillary cell carcinoma.

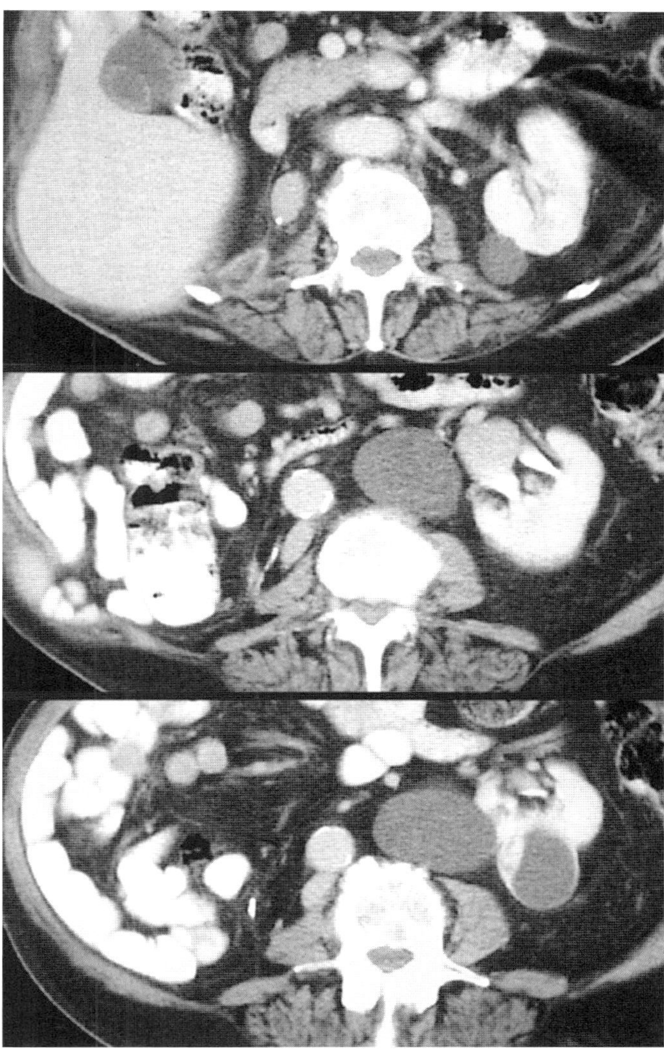

Fig. 23.8 A composite of three CT cuts in a patient with a solitary left kidney. There are three left renal cysts. The small upper pole and large middle cyst have thin walls and smooth base. The posterior, left lower pole cyst has thick wall and a nodule at its medial base. Note also a gallstone.

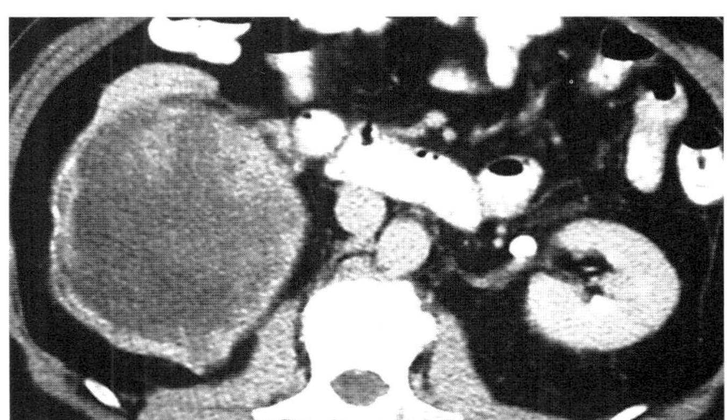

Fig. 23.7 Example of thick wall calcification and a suggestion of a septal calcification.

Fig. 23.9 Contrast-enhanced CT shows a necrotic right renal carcinoma. Bosniak class IV.

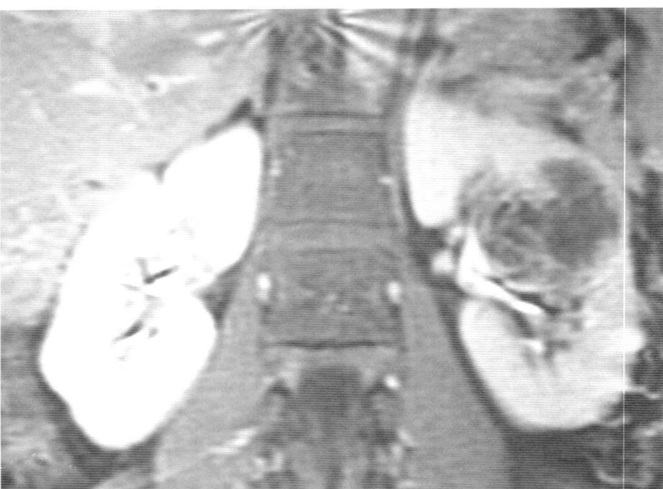

Fig. 23.10 Enhanced MRI of a partially cystic-necrotic renal carcinoma with enhancing solid elements. Bosniak class IV.

Low-density renal lesions (LDRL) too small to characterize

When the diameter of a renal lesion is less than the slice thickness it is not possible to measure true attenuation values because of contamination from adjacent normal parenchyma. This, in radiologic terms, is referred to as 'partial volume-averaging'. Thus a simple 5–10 mm renal cyst may have higher apparent measured HU values such that a small solid neoplasm cannot be excluded. Because statistically these LDRL lesions are probably simple cysts, any further work-up is likely to be expensive. By having the qualifier 'too small to characterize' appear on the report, the radiologist has in effect placed the responsibility of deciding upon any further work-up squarely on the shoulders of the referring physician. This is mainly because the radiologist is unfamiliar with the overall clinical situation. Possible courses of action depending on the clinical situation are: (1) directed renal CT using 3 mm thin cuts, with and without contrast, within the next 6–9 months; (2) directed MRI using the single-shot fast spin echo (SSFSE) slab technique to show even the smallest of cysts; (3) renal ultrasound (Davidson *et al.* 1997).

Imaging of local tumor extension

Renal carcinoma may involve regional lymph nodes, propagate along the venous channels into renal vein, inferior vena cava, and right heart, and, by direct extension, into the ipsilateral adrenal gland, renal fascia and psoas muscle.

On either CT or MRI the only manifestation of lymph node metastasis is globular enlargement of the affected node (see Fig. 23.1). Retroperitoneal nodes larger than 1 cm in short axis are abnormal. When there is regional lymph node enlargement in the presence of renal carcinoma, 50 per cent of the lymph nodes are hyperplastic, and therefore indistinguishable from nodes harboring metastases (Studer *et al.* 1990). At the present time there is no reliable way to differentiate between metastatic and hyperplastic nodes. There are studies in Europe addressing this problem with

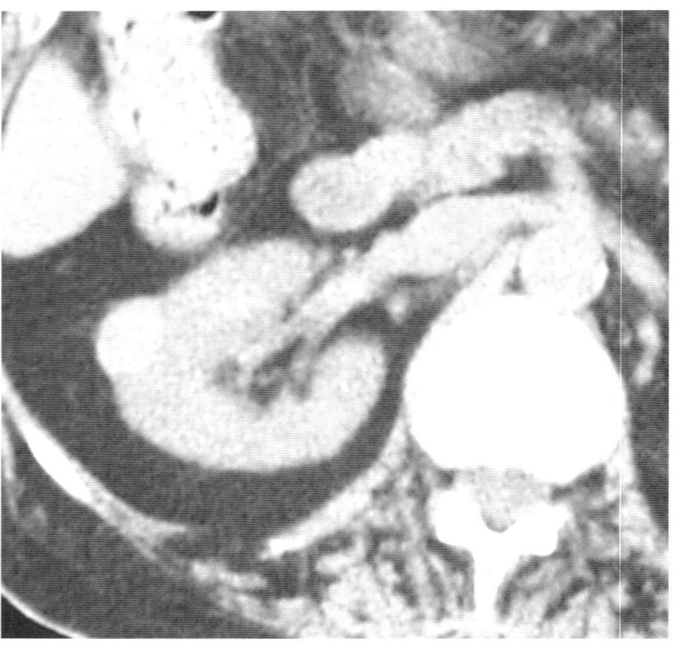

(a)

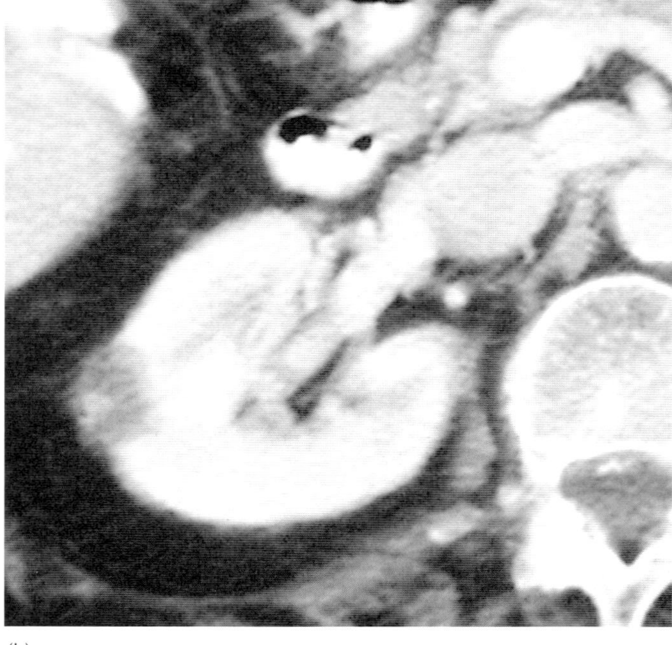

(b)

Fig. 23.11 (a) Pre-contrast CT. A small hyperdense right renal cyst is present. These hemorrhagic cysts are usually benign provided they do not enhance after IV contrast and show no other attributes of a complex cyst. (b) Post-contrast CT in the same patient. The cyst appears of relatively low density compared with the enhancing renal parenchyma around it. Most of the cyst did not measurably enhance apart from a small peripheral nodule, which proved to be a small carcinoma within a hemorrhagic cyst

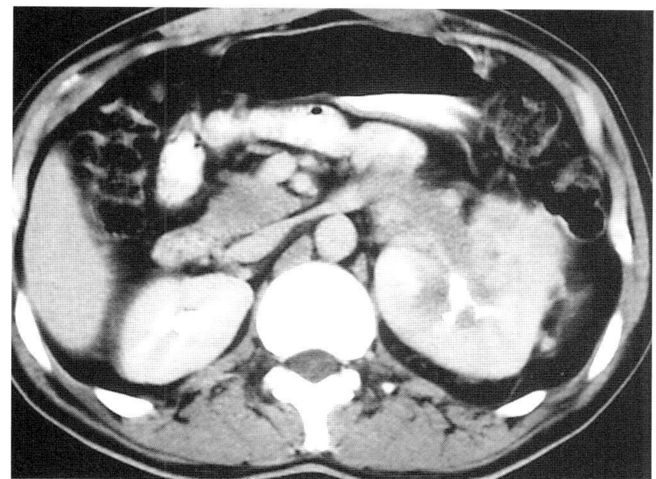

Fig. 23.12 Post-contrast CT shows renal carcinoma extending into proximal left renal vein. More distal left renal vein (anterior to the aorta) is tumor-free which would permit renal vein ligation at the cava.

nodal enlargement associated with prostate and bladder carcinomas. They involve IV administration of a colloidal suspension of minute ferric particles. Phagocytized by the lymph node's reticuloendothelial system, the ferric particles will change the MR signal in normal lymph nodes. In a node harboring metastasis, the reticuloendothelial system is replaced with tumor and no change in signal is expected. Fibro-fatty changes are diagnosed with fat suppression sequences (Barentsz *et al.* 1997). This very fine colloidal suspension is awaiting approval in the US and has yet to be tested in renal carcinomas.

One of the common features of renal carcinoma is its growth into the renal vein (Fig. 23.12), inferior vena cava (IVC), and even the right heart. At times the tumor may extend as far as the pulmonary artery and it can also grow against the blood flow into infrarenal IVC, contralateral renal vein, and ipsilateral gonadal vein. The exact delineation of tumor thrombus and its extent will determine operative approach, patient positioning, need for cardiac pump and thoracic surgery involvement, etc. (Stief *et al.* 1995). Both CT and MRI can be used in diagnosis of venous propagation, with MRI having somewhat better sensitivity (Semelka *et al.* 1993).

CT is the most common means to diagnose renal carcinoma. This is probably because, along with IV pyelography (IVP), it is the imaging study of choice for evaluating hematuria. The trend in the last several years has been to combine these two studies into one (CTU or CT–IVP). Such combination allows for detailed evaluation of renal calculi (something MRI is not especially good at) as well as renal neoplasms, including carcinoma. Also, at the present time, CT is somewhat cheaper than MRI. Therefore, whenever a neoplasm is detected on CT or CTU, attention should be paid to a possible tumor thrombus.

On CT a tumor thrombus is identified as a 'filling defect' within the vein (Fig. 23.13 (a), (b)). After a compact bolus injection contrast will appear quickly in the renal vein and show it to be free of filling defects. It is somewhat more difficult to diagnose an IVC tumor because of the dilutional effect of non-opacified blood from the lower limbs admixing with fully opacified renal vein blood.

It is obvious that faster acquisition and thinner CT cuts will help better delineate venous tumor thrombus. Breath-hold helical (spiral) CT allows for increased sensitivity and also allows computer-generated reconstruction in different planes or the use of one of several three-dimensional reconstruction techniques, such as maximum intensity projection (MIP). Attention should be paid to congenital anomalies, such as retroaortic or circumaortic left renal vein and left IVC. A tumor within these vessels may be misdiagnosed as nodal metastasis.

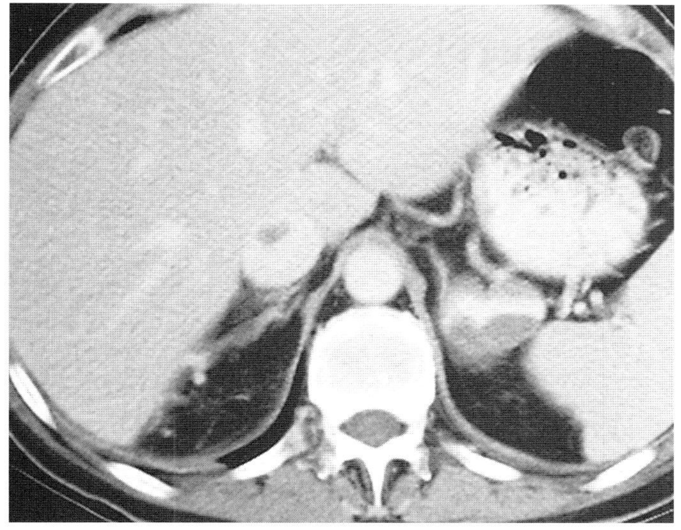

(a)

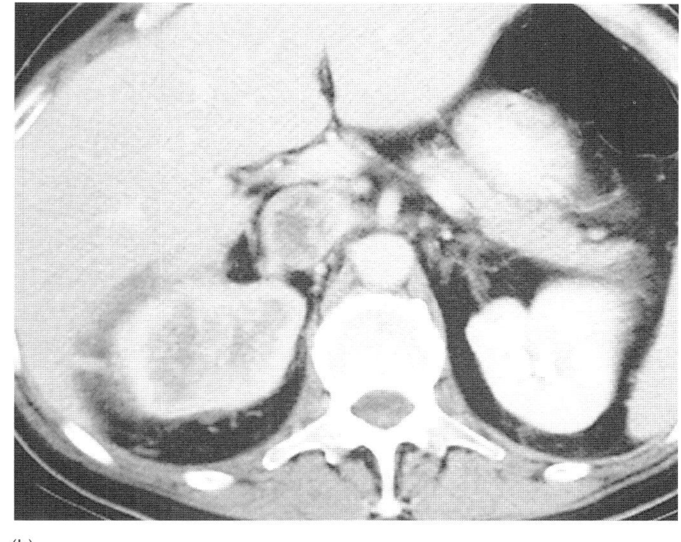

(b)

Fig. 23.13 (a) Contrast-enhanced CT shows the most cephalad extension of a tumor thrombus that appears as a 'filling defect' within contrast-enhanced IVC and is well below the hepatic veins' confluence. (b) In the same patient, several cuts below, a right upper pole renal carcinoma and a tumor thrombus in the infrahepatic IVC are clearly identified.

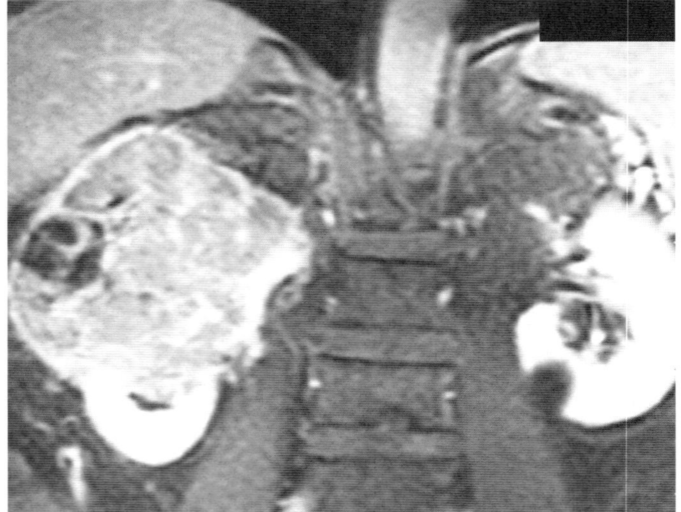

(a)

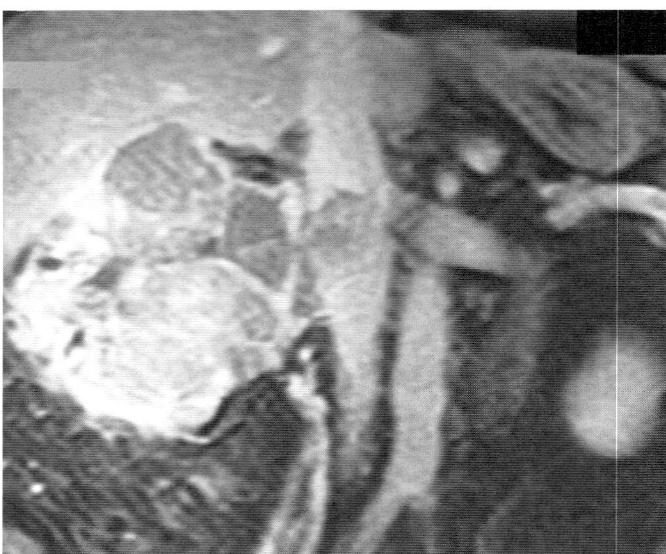

(b)

Fig. 23.14 (a) Contrast-enhanced, fat-suppressed sequence in coronal plane shows a large right renal carcinoma and a small left lower pole renal cyst. (b) On a more anterior cut vena cava and left renal vein are clearly seen. A filling defect in the inferior vena cava is the tumor thrombus.

MRI seems to be moderately better than CT in detection and evaluation of the extent of a tumor thrombus (Helenon *et al.* 1992). This is because MRI signal discrimination between blood and tumor is extraordinary. This visible difference between blood and tumor may be further amplified by using one of several sequences that optimize vascular conspicuity (Fig. 23.14 (a), (b)).

If at all uncertain of CT findings one should resort to other imaging modalities. Ultrasound and color Doppler imaging can be tried, except in bulky tumors where they have a limited ability to predict venous tumor extension (McGahan *et al.* 1993). Transesophageal echocardiography can be used to evaluate atrial tumor thrombus (Treiger *et al.* 1991). Intraoperative sonography has also been recommended (Harris *et al.* 1994).

Ipsilateral adrenal gland

If the ipsilateral adrenal gland appears normal on a well executed CT study it is likely to be tumor-free. Nephrectomy with sparing of the ipsilateral adrenal gland may be contemplated. This is especially true if the primary renal tumor is in the lower pole. However, upper pole renal carcinoma and venous involvement have a high probability of local extension into the adrenal gland. Needless to say, the opposite gland should be scrutinized for telltale signs of hematogenous metastases.

CT and MRI after radical nephrectomy and nephron-sparing surgery

A chest radiograph is suggested every 6 months for early detection of pulmonary metastases (Sandock *et al.* 1995). In many institutions follow-up by abdominal CT at yearly intervals is almost routine because early detection of local recurrence allows for early administration of alternative therapies.

Imaging of distant metastases

CT has a definite edge over MRI in pulmonary metastases primarily because of respiratory and cardiac motion artifacts associated with the latter. Helical (spiral) CT does even better since the acquisition is obtained quickly in a single breath-hold. Also, the chance of missing a small metastasis due to different inspiratory efforts between slices is eliminated (Paranjpe and Bergin 1994; Kauczor *et al.* 1994).

The most common metastases are to the lungs. CT is much more sensitive than a simple chest X-ray in detecting these round, nodular lesions in their early stages. Metastases to bones are osteolytic and may be solitary and large. At times there is a large soft-tissue component associated with the destructive change in the bone (Fig 23.15). Metastases to the vertebra may produce cord compression. For evaluation of these and brain metastases, MRI is the method of choice.

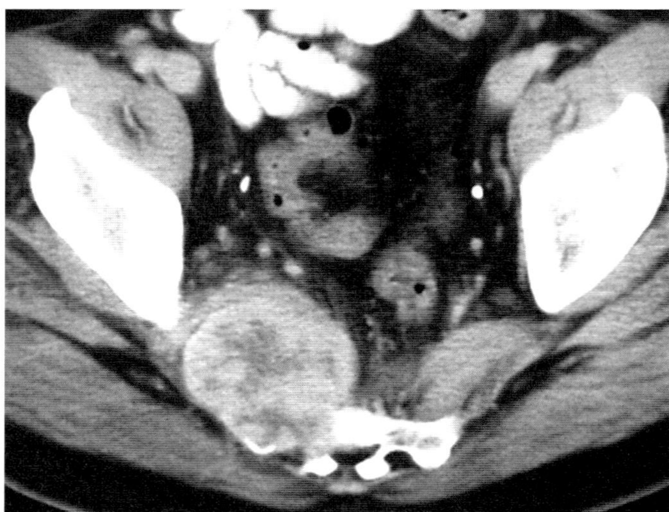

Fig. 23.15 Enhancing osteolytic metastasis to the right sacrum with a large soft-tissue component involving right pyryformis muscle.

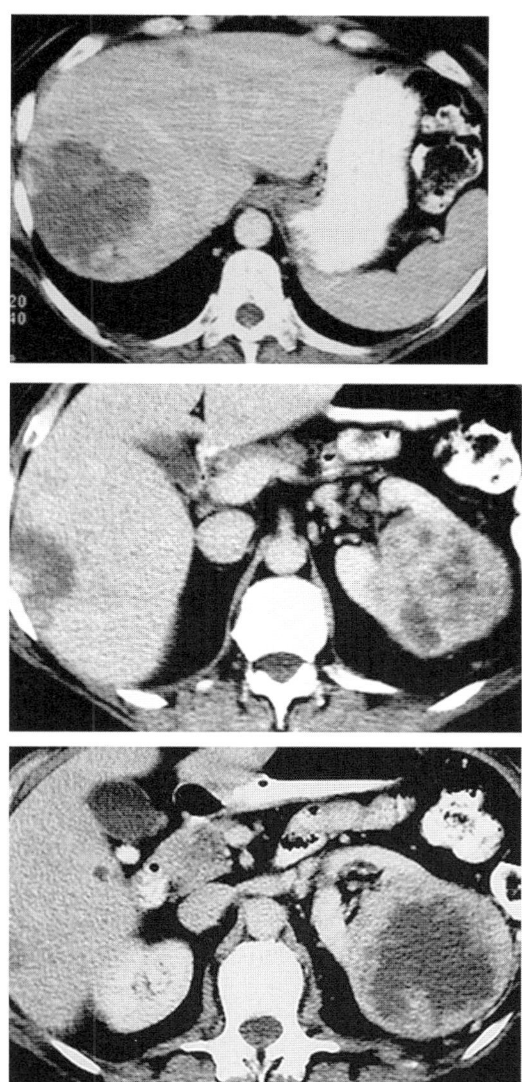

Fig. 23.16 Post-contrast CT. A composite of three cuts shows a necrotic left renal carcinoma. In the right liver lobe there is a low-density mass that resembles in appearance the left renal neoplasm. Peripheral enhancement and nodularity at the base are the telltale signs of a liver hemangioma. A 5–10 minute delayed scan would confirm the diagnosis if the liver mass became uniformly dense.

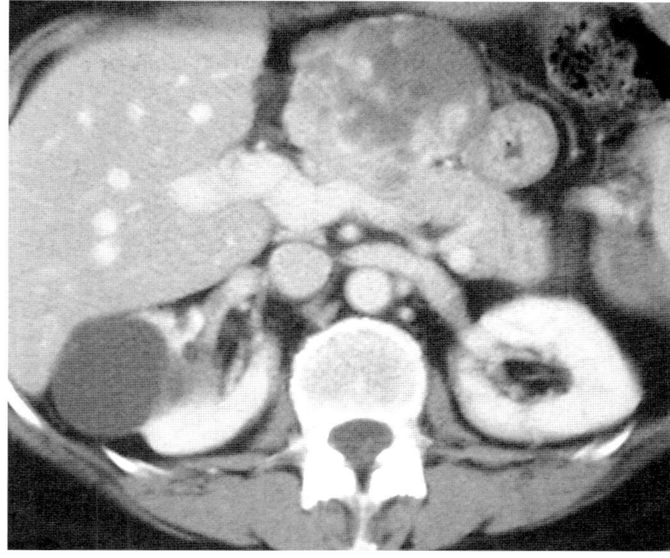

(a)

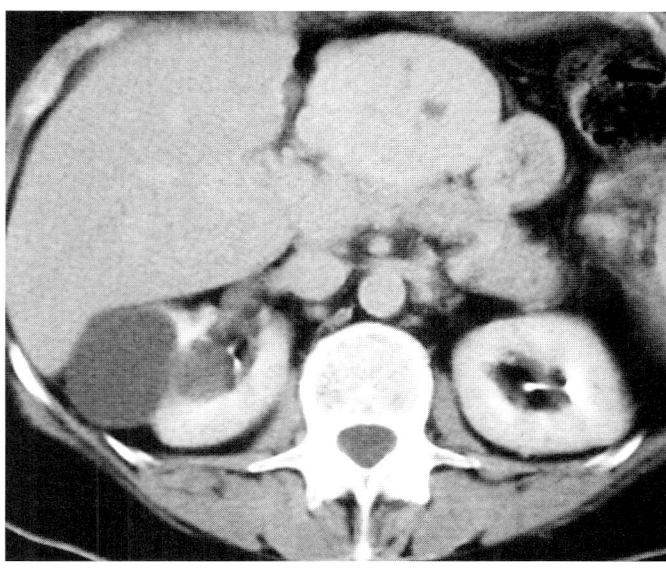

(b)

Fig. 23.17 (a) Contrast-enhanced CT. There is a large mass in the left lobe of the liver that shows peripheral nodular enhancement. (b) On 10 minute delayed scan the mass is now uniformly opacified with the exception of the very center. This central scar is also typical of hemangioma.

Liver metastases are also common. They are usually hypervascular and enhance on post-contrast scans. Two very common benign liver lesions, liver cyst and liver hemangioma, are always distinguished in differential diagnosis. Cyst does not enhance. Hemangioma has a very distinctive pattern on CT. On pre-contrast scan this is usually a low-density lesion. On post-contrast scan enhancement is gradual and begins at the periphery as nodular protuberances (Fig. 23.16). When this is detected, 5–10 minute delayed cuts are obtained. On these the hemangioma becomes of uniform density, sometimes with a central lucency that represents a scar (Fig. 23.17 (a), (b)). This pattern is diagnostic of hemangioma. Liver metastases may also have a lucent center but will not fill on delayed cuts (Fig. 23.18). On MRI

hemangioma also has a very distinct appearance on special sequences that use very heavy T2 weighting. Hemangioma exhibits a very strong signal and appears very bright.

Other less common metastases are to subcutaneous tissues, spleen, psoas, epididymis, and pancreas. Pancreatic metastases are usually difficult to diagnose in early stages (Fig. 23.19). Later, as they grow and depending on their location, they can cause common bile duct obstruction, invade the splenic vein, and propagate along the portal vein. Local recurrence in the ipsilateral renal bed is common after radical nephrectomy.

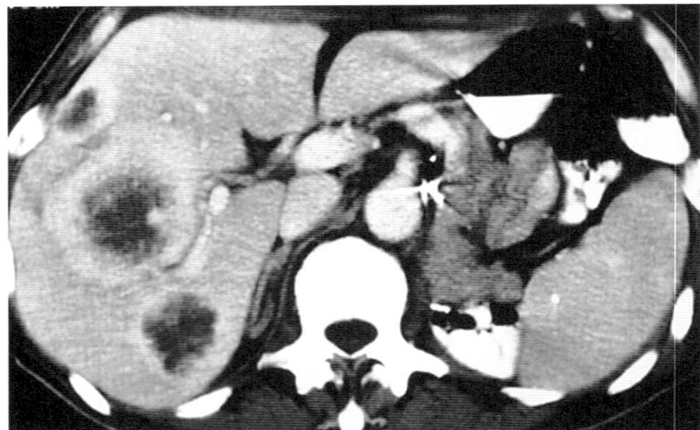

Fig. 23.18 Contrast-enhanced CT showing liver metastases from renal carcinoma after left radical nephrectomy. Although these metastases may look like hemangiomas, there is no uniform fill-in with contrast on delayed cuts.

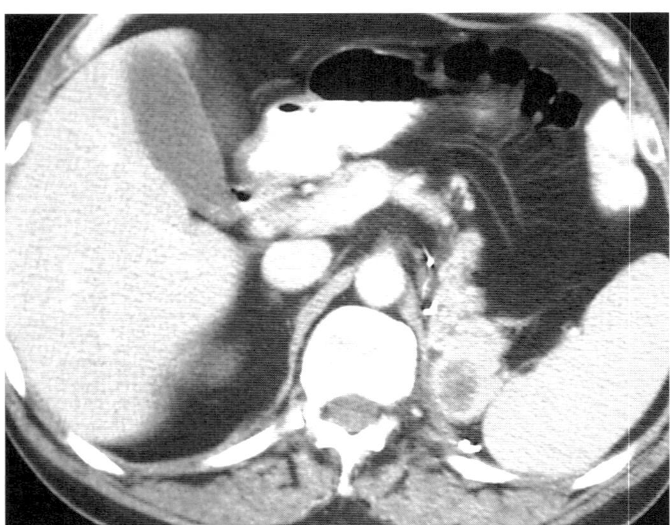

Fig. 23.19 Metastasis in the tail of the pancreas after left radical nephrectomy.

Hematogenous metastases to adrenal gland

Metastases to the adrenal gland need to be differentiated from all too common benign adrenal adenomas. Fortunately, this is possible because adenomas contain a mixture of clear and compact cells. Clear cells contain cytoplasmatic lipids and, since there is a preponderance of clear cells within the tumor, the attenuation values on CT should be low. Indeed, an adrenal nodule of 10 HU or less is almost always an adenoma or an adrenal cyst, while from 10 to 18 HU the probability of an adenoma is 98 per cent (Korobkin *et al.* 1996). Since most adrenal adenomas are small, one should use thin, 3 mm cuts without contrast to eliminate partial volume-averaging.

Adenomas and metastases will enhance following IV CT contrast injection. The degree of maximum enhancement is not helpful in differentiation because all enhance about the same. The differentiating feature is that adenomas 'disenhance' at a much faster rate compared to that of other solid tumors (Boland *et al.* 1997; Szolar and Kammerhuber 1997). On delayed cuts adenomas will have attenuation values less than 37 HU. If repeated cuts are obtained 15 minutes after the first set of post-contrast cuts, the adenomas will 'disenhance' 50 per cent or more compared to maximum enhancement (Fig. 23.20 (a)–(c)). A nodule with maximum enhancement of up to 80 HU, which at 15 minutes measures 30 HU, is certainly an adenoma.

Differentiation of adenomas from metastases by MRI is possible using in-phase and out-of-phase (opposing phase) gradient echo sequences. Because an adenoma contains clear cells with abundant cytoplasmatic lipids, on the out-of-phase sequence the signal will 'drop' and the adenoma will appear dark (Fig. 23.21 (a), (b)) (Korobkin *et al.* 1995; Mayo-Smith *et al.* 1995). Metastases

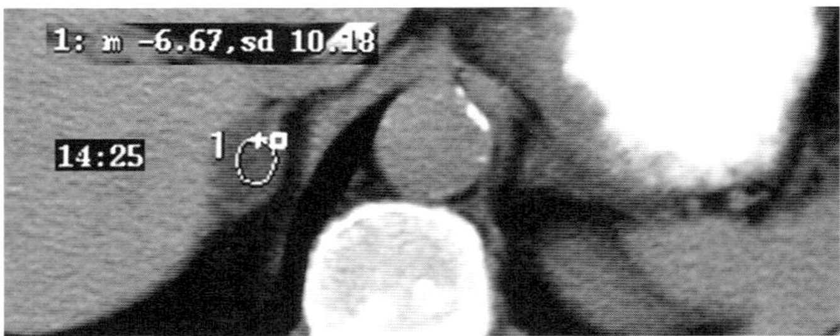

(a)

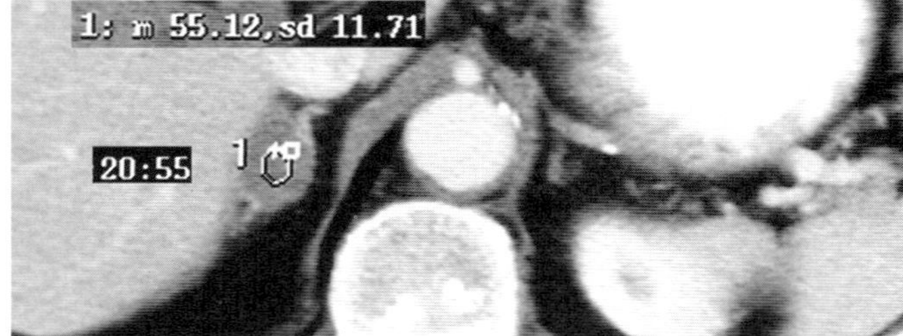

(b)

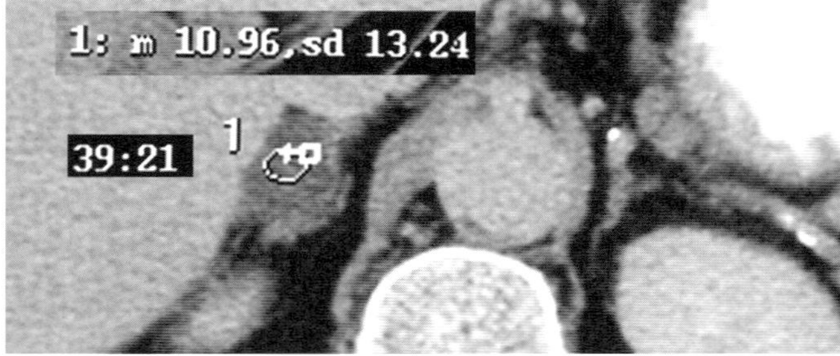

(c)

Fig. 23.20 CT findings in adrenal adenoma. (a) A rounded cursor is placed over the right adrenal nodule. Time is displayed to the right of the nodule and HU on the top. Attenuation value is −6 HU, which is diagnostic of an adenoma. (b) Following IV injection of contrast material the nodule enhances to 55 HU confirming that this as a solid tumor. Compare also aorta on pre- and post-contrast scan to verify presence of contrast. (c) Some 19 minutes after the post -contrast scan a repeat set of images was obtained to check for disenhancement. Attenuation value at this time is 11 HU, confirming again that this is a benign adrenal adenoma.

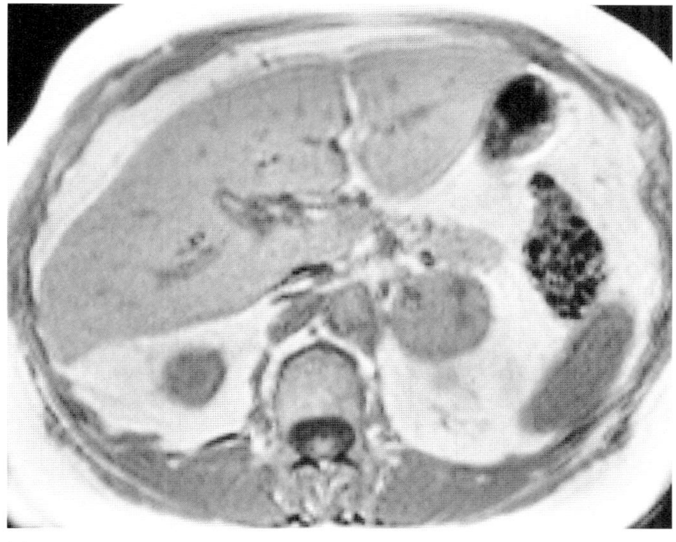

(a)

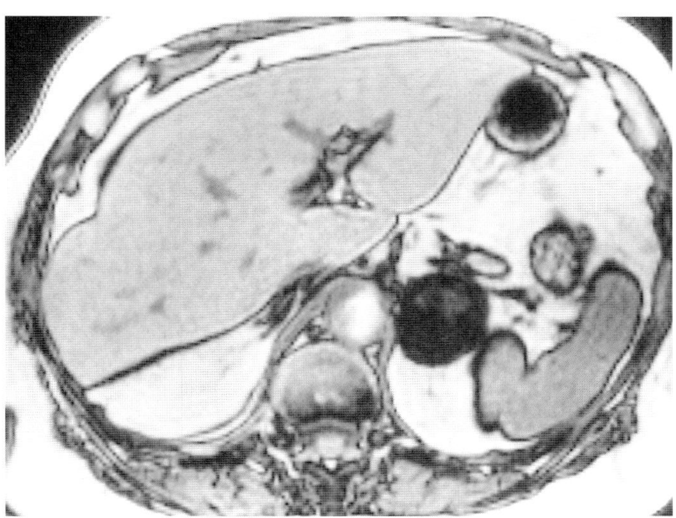

(b)

Fig. 23.21 (a) In-phase sequence shows large left adrenal nodule that has similar signal intensity to that of spleen and liver. (b) Out-of-phase (opposing phase) sequence shows marked 'drop in signal' from the nodule, which appears dark compared to the spleen and liver. This is very typical of adrenal adenomas.

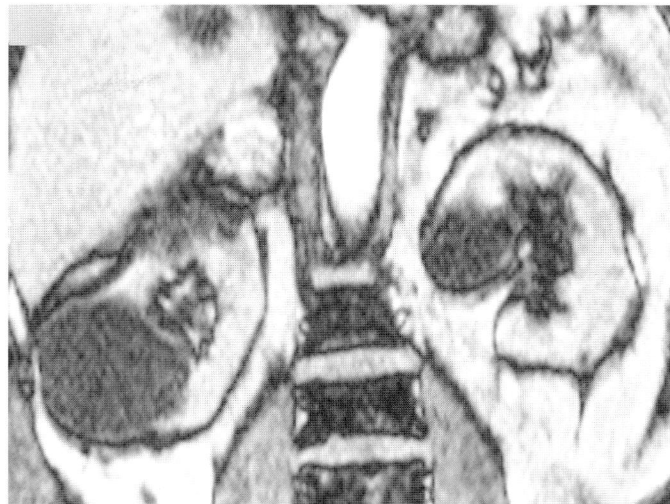

Fig. 23.22 Out-of-phase sequence that shows several low-signal bilateral renal cysts (dark), and a right adrenal tumor that did not 'drop' the signal. Biopsy showed metastasis from renal cell carcinoma.

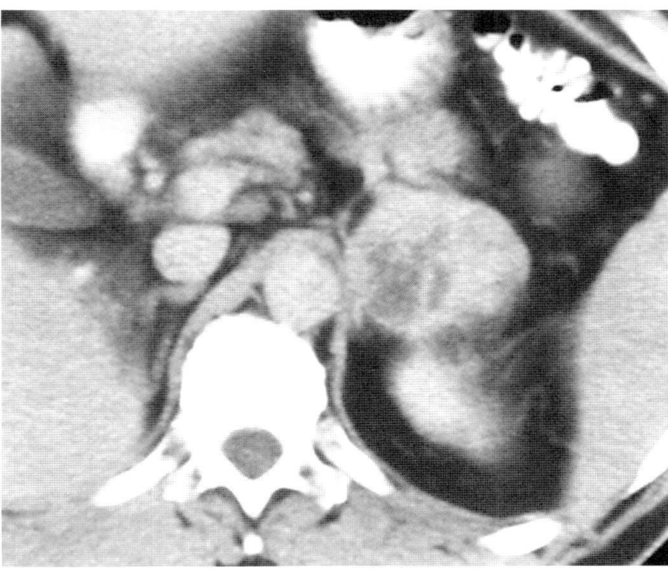

Fig. 23.23 Newly discovered small adrenal carcinoma is less than 5 cm in diameter and there is no evidence of local infiltration or lymphadenopathy.

will not drop in signal and there will be no difference in signal intensity on two sequences. These sequences are very fast and can be acquired in two breath-holds.

CT or ultrasound-guided adrenal biopsy can be employed in cases that are unresolved by above methods. Positive predictive value is high and complication rate is less than 3 per cent (Welch *et al.* 1994).

Adrenal cortical carcinoma

At discovery, adrenal carcinomas are usually large. This is especially true if the tumor is endocrinologically inactive and produces few or no hormones. 'Functioning' adrenal carcinomas may produce varying degrees of virilization, feminization, precocious puberty, Cushing's syndrome, or hyperaldosteronism and are thus more likely to be diagnosed earlier (Fig. 23.23).

Compared with highly vascular renal carcinoma, adrenal cortical tumors are usually somewhat hypovascular. As seen on CT, the degree of enhancement is comparatively less. As the tumor overgrows its vascular supply, areas of necrosis and dystrophic calcification commonly develop (Fig. 23.24(a)). Heterogeneous enhancement is seen on CT and MRI. Areas of intratumoral hemorrhage are seen as high-attenuation geographic areas on pre-contrast CT scan. High signal is seen on T1- and T2-weighted sequences, which is typical for old hemorrhages.

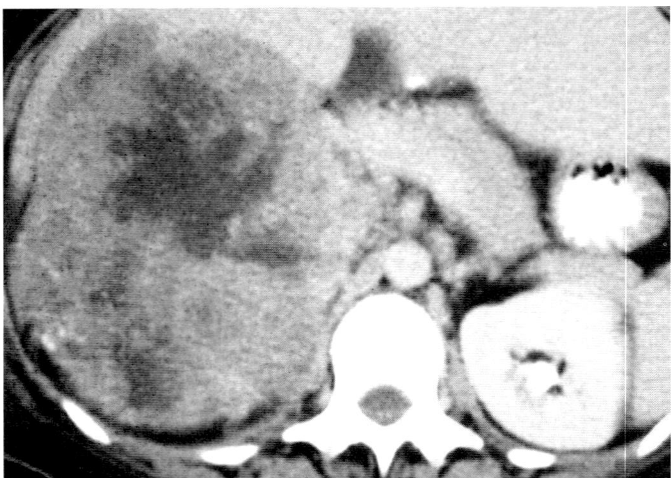

(a)

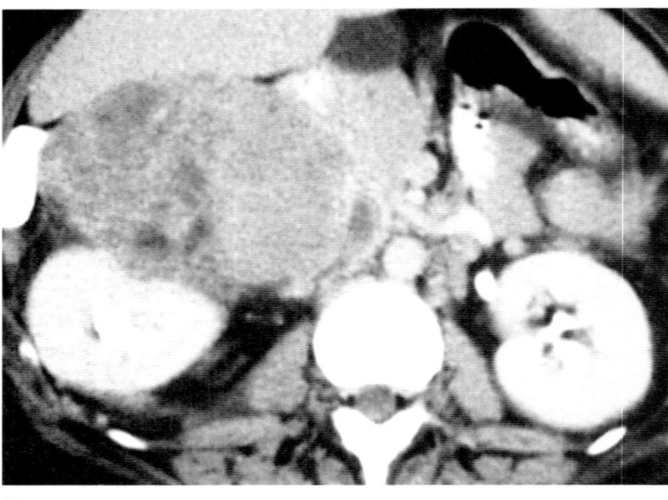

(b)

Fig. 23.24 (a) Large heterogeneous right adrenal carcinoma. (b) IVC invasion is seen to the right of the aorta.

Many adrenal cortical carcinomas contain cells with high cytoplasmatic lipids. For this reason many exhibit low attenuation on CT and also tend to drop in signal on in-phase–out-of-phase gradient echo MR sequences (Schlund *et al.* 1995). To some extent this interferes in differentiating benign adenomas from adrenal carcinomas and it is for this reason that we come back to the large size, tumor necrosis, and intratumoral hemorrhage as the most important indicators of malignancy. Interestingly, some 70 per cent of renal carcinomas contain clear cells, which are also rich in glycogen and lipids. However, their signal does not drop sufficiently on 'out-of-phase' sequence to allow reliable histologic diagnosis or differentiation from oncocytoma.

Because of their large size it is often difficult on CT to decide if the tumor is renal or adrenal in origin. Reformatting images in different planes, especially the parasaggital plane, over the kidney and adrenal gland provides tremendous help in resolving this

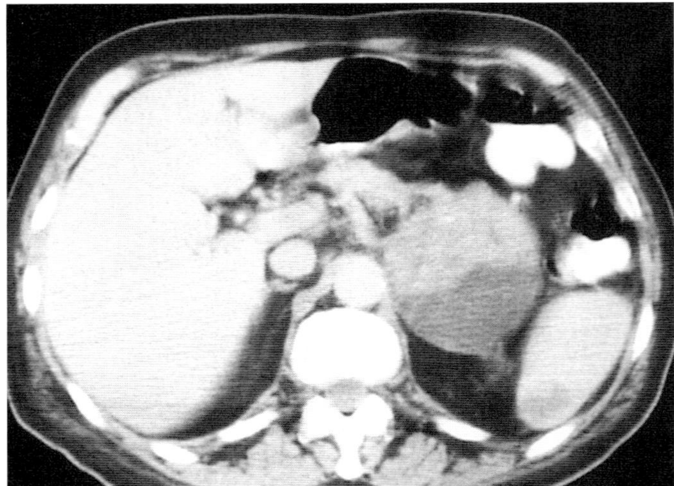

Fig. 23.25 Left adrenal carcinoma and metastasis to the spleen.

problem. Low attenuation on CT and drop in signal on MRI favors adrenal carcinoma.

Similarly to renal carcinoma, adrenal cortical carcinoma often propagates inside the veins; on the left via left renal vein, and on the right into the IVC (Fig. 23.24 (b)), via the rather short right adrenal vein. Venous tumor thrombus is best seen on MRI (Lee *et al.* 1994).

Staging of adrenal carcinoma depends on its size and local extension:

stage I   the tumor is less than 5 cm, without nodal or local invasion;
stage II   the tumor is larger than 5 cm, without nodal or local invasion;
stage III positive nodes *or* local invasion;
stage IV   positive nodes *and* local invasion, or distant metastases.

Metastases are to lungs, bones, liver, and spleen (Fig. 23.25). Lung metastases are round, 'cannon ball' nodules. Bone metastases are osteolytic.

References

Aronson, S., Frazier, H.A., Baluch, J.D., *et al.* (1991). Cystic renal masses: usefulness of the Bosniak classification. *Urol. Radiol.* **13**, 83.

Barentsz, J.O., Mitjes, J.A., and Ruijs, J.H.J. (1997). What's new in bladder imaging? *Urol. Clin. N. Am.* **24**, 583.

Boland, G.W., Hahn, P.F., Pena, C., *et al.* (1997). Adrenal masses: characterization with delayed contrast-enhanced CT. *Radiology* **202**, 693–8.

Bosniak, M.A. (1986). The current radiological approach to renal cysts. *Radiology* **158**, 1–10.

Bosniak, M.A., Megibow, A.J., Hulnick, D.H., *et al.* (1988). CT diagnosis of renal angiomyolipoma: the importance of detecting small amounts of fat. *Am. J. Roentgenol.* **151**, 497–500.

Davidson, A.J., Hayes, W.S., Hartman, D.S., *et al.* (1993). Renal oncocytoma and carcinoma: failure of differentiation with CT. *Radiology* **186**, 693–6.

Davidson, A.J., Hartman, D.S., Choyke, P., *et al.* (1997). Radiologic assessment of renal masses: implication for patient care. *Radiology* **202**, 297–302.

Defosses, A.M., Yoder, I.C., Papanicolaou, N., *et al.* (1991). Nonspecific magnetic resonance appearance of renal oncocytomas: report of 3 cases and review of the literature. *J. Urol.* **145**, 552–4.

Eilenberg, S.S., Lee, J.K., Brown, J., *et al.* (1990). Renal masses: evaluation with gradient-echo GD–DTPA-enhanced dynamic MR imaging. *Radiology* **176**, 333–8.

Endress, C. and Chita, M.A. (1992). Renal cell carcinoma simulating oncocytom [letter]. *Am. J. Roentgenol.* **158**, 920.

Fishman, M.C., Pollack, H.M., Arger, P.H., and Banner, M.P. (1983). High protein content: another cause of CT hyperdense renal cyst. *J. Comput. Assist. Tomogr.* **7**, 1103–6.

Harmon, W.J., King, B.F., and Lieber, M.M. (1996). Renal oncocytoma: magnetic resonance imaging characteristics. *J. Urol.* **155**, 863–7.

Harris, D.D., Ruckle, H.C., Gaskill, D.M., *et al.* (1994). Intraoperative ultrasound: determination of the presence and extent of vena caval tumor thrombus. *Urology* **44**, 189–93.

Helenon, O., Denys, A., Chretien, Y., *et al.* (1992). Role of MRI in the diagnosis of cancer of the kidney. *J. d'Urologie* **98**, 3–13.

Helemon, O., Chretien, Y., Paret, F., *et al.* (1993). Renal cell carcinoma containing fat: demonstration with CT. *Radiology* **188**, 420–6.

Kauczor, H.U., Hansen, M., and Schweden, F., *et al.* (1994). Computerized tomography in diagnosis of lung metastases: improvement with the spiral technique. *Radiology* **34**, 569–75.

Korobkin, M., Lombardi, T.J., Aisen, A.M., *et al.* (1995). Characterization of adrenal masses with chemical shift and gadolinium-enhanced MR imaging. *Radiology* **197**, 411–15.

Korobkin, M., Brodeur, F.J., Yutzy, G.G., *et al.* (1996). Differentiation of adrenal adenomas from nonadenomas using CT attenuation values. *Am. J. Roentgenol.* **166**, 531–6.

Lee, M.J., Mayo-Smith, W.W., Hahn, P.F., *et al.* (1994). State of the art MR imaging of the adrenal gland. *Radiographics* **14**, 1015.

Mayo-Smith, W.W., Lee, M.J., McNicholas, M.M.J., *et al.* (1995). Chararcterization of adrenal masses (< 5 cm) by use of chemical shift MR imaging: observer performance versus quantitative measures. *Am. J. Roentgenol.* **165**, 91–4.

McGahan, J.P., Blake, L.C., deVere White, R., *et al.* (1993). Color flow sonographic mapping of intravascular extension of malignant renal tumors. *J. Ultrasound Med.* **12**, 403–9.

Neisius, D., Braedel, H.U., Schindler, E., *et al.* (1988). Computed tomographic and angiographic findings in renal oncocytoma. *Br. J. Radiol.* **61**, 1019–25.

Paranjpe, D.V. and Bergin, C.J. (1994). Spiral CT of the lungs: optimal technique and resolution compared with conventional CT. *Am. J. Roentgenol.* **162**, 561–7.

Prando, A. (1991). Intratumoral fat in a renal cell carcinoma [letter]. *Am. J. Roentgenol.* **156**, 871.

Quinn, M.J., Hartman, D.S., Friedman, A.C., *et al.* (1984). Renal oncocytoma: new observations. *Radiology* **153**, 49–53.

Sandock, D.S., Seftel, A.D., and Resnick, M.I. (1995). A new protocol for the follow up of renal cell carcinoma based on pathological stage. *J. Urol.* **154**, 28.

Schlund, J.F., Kenney, P.J., Brown, E.D., *et al.* (1995). Adrenocortical carcinoma: MR imaging appearance with current techniques. *J. Mag. Reson. Imaging* **5**, 171–3.

Selzman, A.A., Hampel, N., and Hassan, M.O. (1994). Renal oncocytoma arising from a renal cyst: a case report and review of the literature. *J. Urol.* **151**, 1610–11.

Semelka, R.C., Shoenut, J.P., Kroeker, M.A., *et al.* (1992). Renal lesions: controled comparisson between CT and 1.5 T MR imaging with non-enhanced and gadolinium-enhanced fat-suppressed spin-echo and breath-hold FLASH techniques. *Radiology* **182**, 425–500.

Semelka, R.C., Shoenut, J.P., Magro, C.M., *et al.* (1993). Renal cancer staging: comparison of contrast-enhanced CT and gadolinium-enhanced fat-suppressed spin-echo and gradient-echo MR imaging. *J. Mag. Reson. Imaging* **3**, 597–602.

Silverman, S.G., Lee, B.Y., Seltzer, S.E., *et al.* (1994). Small hyperechoic renal masses: correlation of spiral CT features and pathologic findings. *Am. J. Roentgenol.* **163**, 597–601.

Stief, C.G., Schafers, H.J., Kuczyk, M., *et al.* (1995). Renal-cell carcinoma with intracaval neoplastic extension: stratification and surgical technique. *World J. Urol.* **13**, 166–70.

Strotzer, M., Lehner, K.B., and Becker, K. (1993). Detection of fat in a renal cell carcinoma mimicking angiomyolipoma. *Radiology* **188**, 427–8.

Studer, U.E., Scherz, S., Scheidegger, J., *et al.* (1990). Enlargement of regional lymph nodes in renal cell carcinoma is often not due to metastases. *J. Urol.* **144**, 243–5.

Sussman, S., Cochran, S.T., Pagani, J.J., *et al.* (1984). Hyperdense renal masses: a CT manifestation of hemorrhagic renal cyst. *Radiology* **150**, 207–11.

Szolar, D.H. and Kammerhuber, F. (1997). Quantitative CT evaluation of adrenal gland masses: a step forward in the differentiation between adenomas and nonadenomas? *Radiology* **202**, 517–601.

Tikkakoski, T., Paivansalo, M., Alanen, A., *et al.* (1991). Radiologic findings in renal oncocytoma. *Acta Radiol.* **32**, 363–7.

Treiger, B.F.G., Humphrey, L.S., Peterson, C.V. Jr, *et al.* (1991). Transesophageal echocardiography in renal cell carcinoma: an accurate diagnostic technique for intracaval neoplastic extension. *J. Urol.* **145**, 1138–40.

Welch, T.J., Sheedy, P.F., Stephens, D.H., *et al.* (1994). Percutaneous adrenal biopsy: review of a 10-year experience. *Radiology* **193**, 341–5.

Williams, M.A., Schropp, K.P., and Noe, H.N. (1994). Fat containing renal mass in childhood: a case report of teratoid Wilms tumor. *J. Urol.* **151**, 1662–3.

24. Ultrasound imaging

Sherelle Laifer-Narin

Ultrasound is the modality of choice for the initial evaluation of the kidneys in many clinical situations. According to the American College of Radiology appropriateness criteria, patients presenting with acute flank pain, hematuria, voiding obstruction secondary to prostate disease and an indeterminate renal mass should be referred to ultrasound (Caskey 2000).

A methodical approach to the evaluation of a renal mass includes determination of the location of a mass, the number of masses present, the echogenicity of a mass, and the contour and edge definition of a mass. Multiple longitudinal and transverse gray-scale images of the kidneys are obtained. Color, power, and spectral Doppler imaging are performed as necessary for evaluation of renal vessels, renal perfusion, and renal masses.

Ultrasound has become the primary examination for the differentiation between cystic and solid renal masses (Baltarowich and Kurtz 1987). This determination is significant for categorizing lesions that will require no further imaging, lesions that require follow-up, and lesions that must be treated surgically (Curry 1995). As ultrasound is relatively cheap, fast, and non-invasive, it is an excellent modality in the initial assessment of a renal mass (Baltarowich and Kurtz 1987).

Cystic renal masses

A renal mass that meets the criteria of a simple renal cyst requires no further evaluation. Simple cysts, by definition, have a well-defined, imperceptible far wall, absent internal echoes, smooth contours, and demonstrate distal through-transmission (Thurston and Wilson 1998; Coleman 1985) (Fig. 24.1). A complex renal cyst does not meet the strict criteria of a simple cyst and may contain internal echoes, septations, calcifications, and mural nodularity or a perceptible wall (Fig. 24.2). Complex cysts with benign type features may be serially followed, whereas those with malignant type features require surgical removal to exclude malignancy. Computerized tomography (CT) scan may be performed to evaluate for enhancement following contrast material, including surgical treatment (Curry 1995).

A cyst classification system has been developed by Bosniak to categorize renal cystic masses. Category I lesions are simple cysts. There is no definable wall, they are smoothly marginated are anechoic, and demonstrate through-transmission of the sound wave. Category II lesions are benign lesions requiring no further follow-up. They may contain one or two thin, internal septa, may have a calcific focus in the wall or septa, or demonstrate high

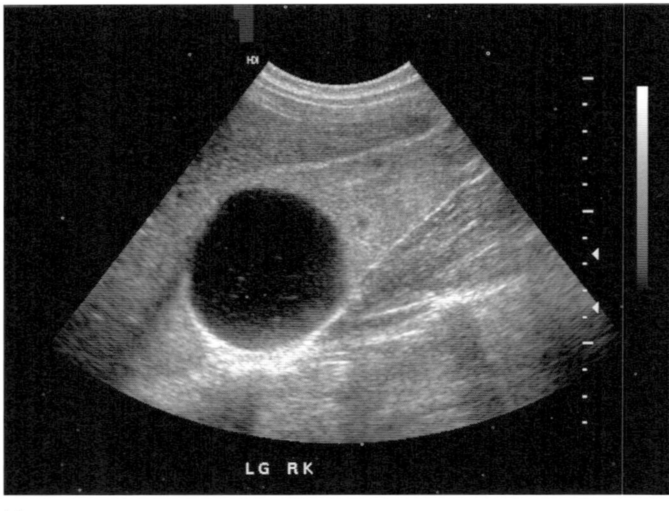

(a)

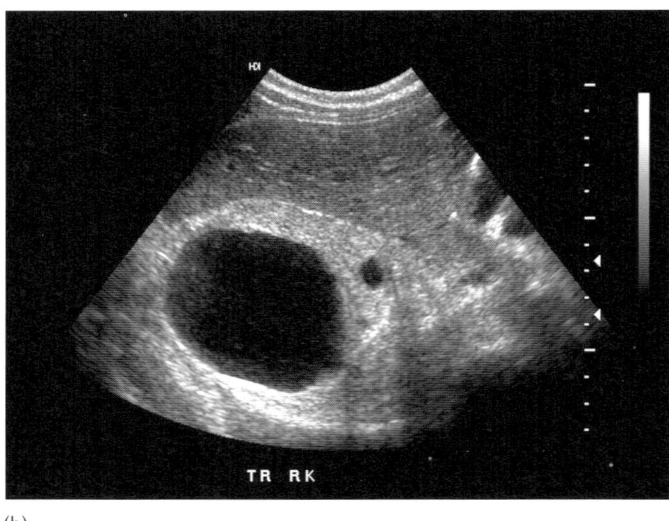

(b)

Fig. 24.1 (a) Longitudinal and transverse images of the right kidney demonstrate a simple cyst of the right upper pole. (b) It is round, anechoic, smoothly marginated, with a sharp back wall, and demonstrates excellent through transmission.

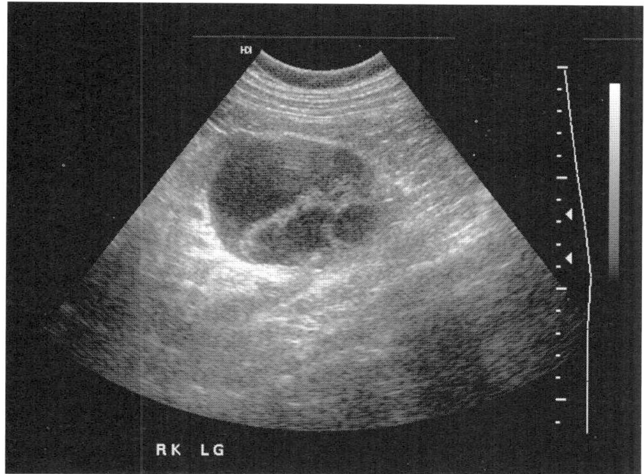

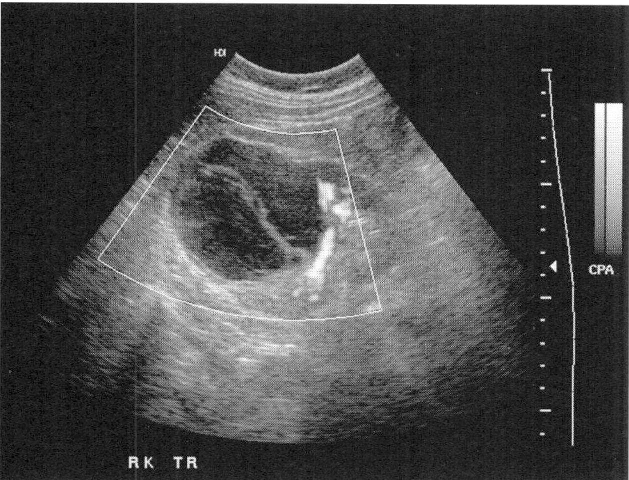

Fig. 24.2 Complex (hemorrhagic) renal cyst. 52-year-old male, pedestrian involved in a motor vehicle accident. A right renal cyst containing thick, irregular separations is present. Power Doppler imaging does not demonstrate internal vascularity. This was thought to be a traumatic, hemorrhagic cyst. Repeat imaging 9 months later demonstrated resolution of this complex cyst.

attenuation secondary to high content of protein, heme, or iodine. Category IIF lesions are minimally complex cysts requiring follow-up to ensure stability in size and appearance. These are benign type lesions that exhibit some 'suspicious' features. Category III lesions are those with malignant characteristics, exhibiting thick septations, chunky calcifications, irregular margins, wall thickening, multilocular mass, or soft-tissue nodularity. Category IV lesions are neoplasms with cystic necrosis, or solid tumors occurring within the wall of a cyst. Category III and IV lesions must be treated surgically (Curry 1995).

The majority of isolated simple cystic renal masses are benign, simple, renal cortical cysts. Other purely cystic renal masses include solitary parapelvic cysts, an extrarenal pelvis, a pyelogenic cyst, and a focal region of caliectasis. Less commonly, a hematoma may be purely cystic. Vascular abnormalities such as arteriovenous malformation or fistula, aneurysm, and pseudoaneurysm may also

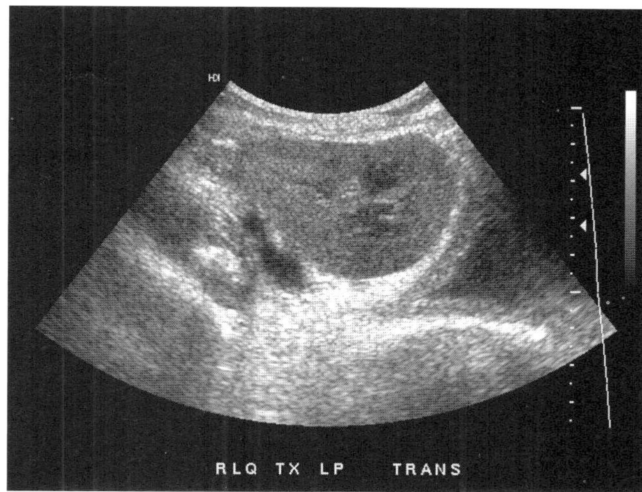

(a)

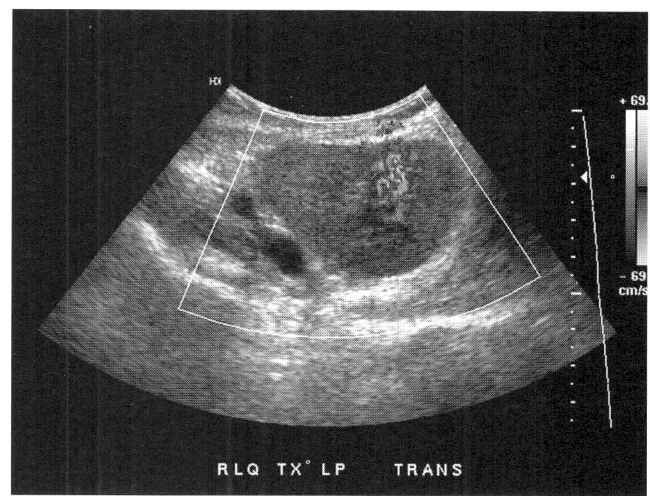

(b)

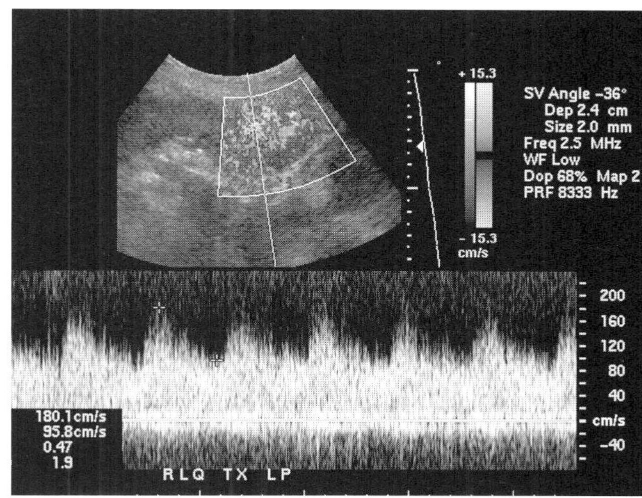

(c)

Fig. 24.3 Intrarenal arteriovenous fistula. (a) A small anechoic mass is present in the kidney. (b) Color and (c) spectral Doppler examination demonstrates low resistance, turbulent, arterial flow consistent with an arteriovenous fustula.

be purely cystic; however, these can be differentiated with the use of color and spectral Doppler ultrasound (Baltarowich and Kurtz 1987) (Fig. 24.3).

Simple renal cysts may be multiple and bilateral. After age 30, an increasing number of patients develop renal cysts, and there are a greater number of cysts per patient. Autopsy results demonstrate that 50 per cent of patients older than 50 years of age have one or more detectable cysts upon visual inspection (Thurston and Wilson 1998; Baltarowich and Kurtz 1987).

Autosomal dominant adult polycystic kidney disease is a hereditary renal disorder manifested by a large number of bilateral cortical and medullary cysts. The cysts are asymmetric, of varying size, and may be complicated by hemorrhage, infection, stone formation, cyst rupture, and obstruction (Thurston and Wilson 1998). Manifestations of the disease do not present until adulthood, usually the fourth or fifth decade. Eventually, renal failure will develop in 50 per cent of patients. There is no increased predilection for renal cell carcinoma in patients who are not on dialysis (Figs 24.4–24.6).

Acquired renal cystic disease may occur in patients with end-stage renal disease and in those on chromic dialysis (Baltarowich and Kurtz 1987). The pathogenesis is unclear, but may be secondary to induction of epithelial hyperplasia and tubular obstruction by toxic substances. Multiple cortical and medullary cysts develop that are small and bilateral (Thurston and Wilson 1998) (Fig. 24.7).

Multicystic dysplastic kidney is a developmental anomaly associated with genitourinary tract obstruction during embryogenesis, manifested on sonography as multiple noncommunicating cysts with limited or no normal renal parenchyma. Multicystic dysplastic kidney is usually unilateral and detected in the fetus or newborn. There is poor, if any renal function. If bilateral, it is incompatible with life.

Multilocular cystic nephroma is a benign, encapsulated renal mass composed of multiple, noncommunicating cysts. There is a bimodal age and sex distribution, with masses found in pediatric males, and females between 40 and 60 years of age.

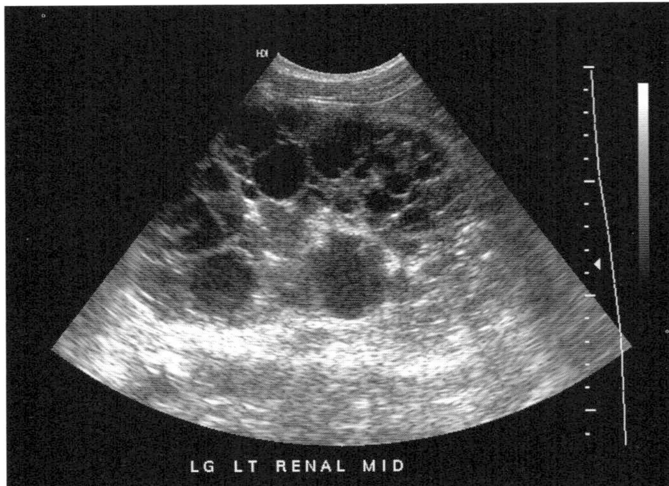

Fig. 24.5 A 55-year-old male with adult polycystic kidney disease. Longitudinal image of the left kidney demonstrates innumerable cysts.

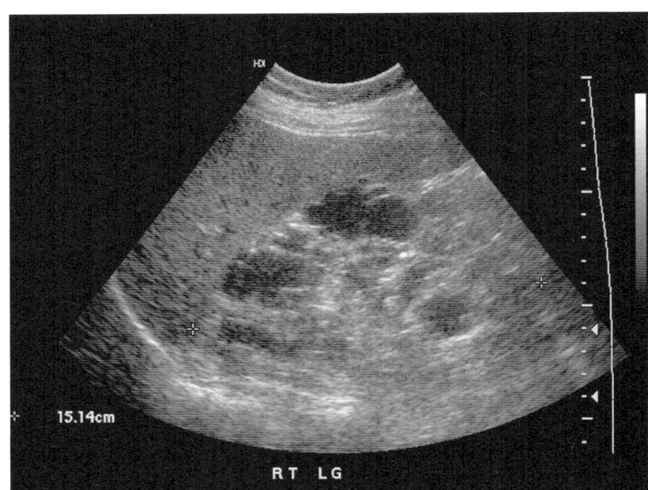

(a)

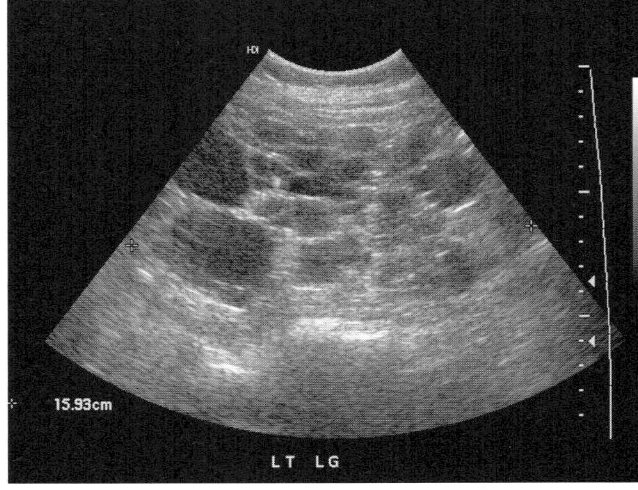

(b)

Fig. 24.6 A 55-year-old female with adult polycystic kidney disease. (a), (b) Longitudinal images of the kidneys demonstrate bilaterally enlarged kidneys containing multiple cysts.

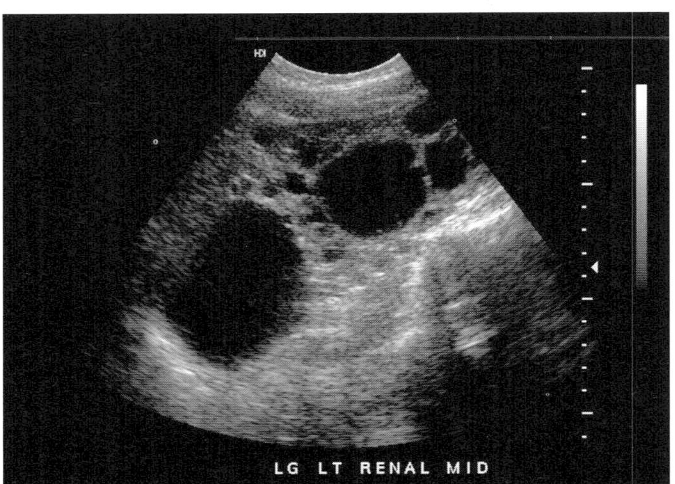

Fig. 24.4 A 32-year-old female with adult polycystic kidney disease. Longitudinal image of the right kidney demonstrates multiple cysts of varying sizes.

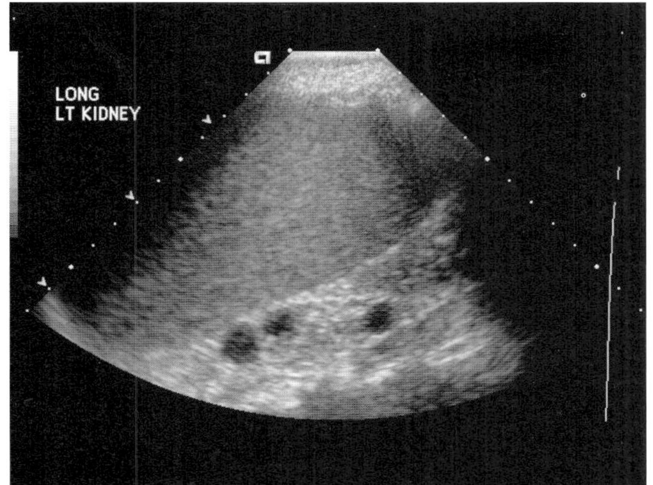

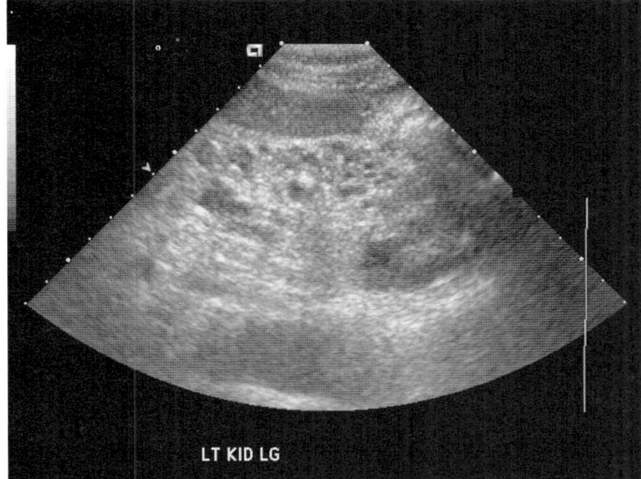

(a)

(b)

Fig. 24.7 Acquired cystic disease. (a), (b) Two different patients with history of end-stage renal disease and chronic dialysis. The kidneys are markedly echogenic and shrunken, containing small cysts.

Solid renal masses

Solid renal masses may be peripheral or central in location, and may be hypoechoic, isoechoic, or hyperechoic compared to normal renal cortex (Baltarowich and Kurtz 1987). Solid renal masses that can be detected with ultrasound include renal cell carcinoma, transitional cell carcinoma, squamous cell carcinoma, adenocarcinoma, oncocytoma, angiomyolipoma, lymphoma, leukemia, and metastases.

Renal cell carcinoma (RCC) is the most common primary malignant tumor of the kidney, comprising more than 80 per cent of primary malignant renal tumors. The majority of RCC occur sporadically; however, there is a familial association, and an association with von Hippel–Lindau disease, tuberous sclerosis, and acquired cystic kidney disease (Thurston and Wilson 1998; Caskey 2000).

On ultrasound, tumors are solid and of variable echogenicity. Charboneau *et al.* (1983) have demonstrated that 86 per cent of RCC are isoechoic, while others have demonstrated that small RCC (< 3 cm) are hyperechoic compared to normal renal parenchyma. RCC may also appear heterogeneous with intratumoral cystic spaces, may demonstrate a hypoechoic rim consistent with a pseudocapsule on histology, and may contain calcifications. These calcifications may be punctate, curvilinear, diffuse, central, or peripheral. RCC usually demonstrate an irregular contour, with poorly defined margins. Doppler ultrasound is useful in demonstrating tumor neovascularity, and the combination of both grayscale and color/Doppler imaging is advantageous in detecting tumor thrombus within the renal vein and inferior vena cava (Caskey 2000) (Figs 24.8 and 24.9).

Transitional cell carcinoma (TCC) may affect the renal pelvis, ureter, or urinary bladder. TCC of the renal pelvis accounts for 7 per cent of all primary renal tumors, is more common in men than women (4:1), and the majority of patients will present with gross or microscopic hematuria. The sonographic appearance of TCC is variable, and imaging the renal sinus can be challenging, with renal sinus fat simulating a mass. The papillary form of TCC

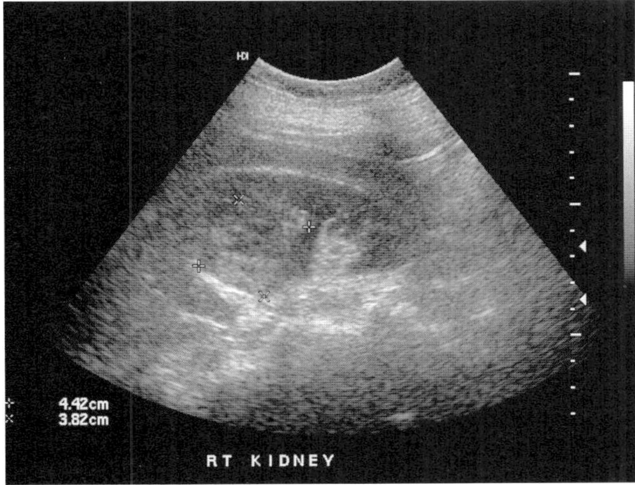

(a)

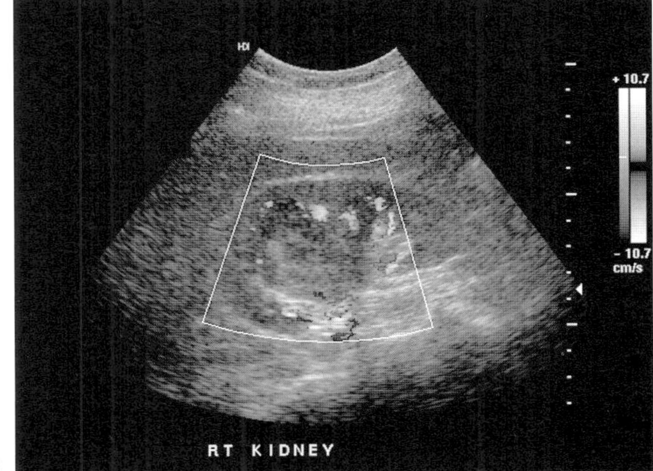

(b)

Fig. 24.8 Renal cell carcinoma. (a) Longitudinal image of the right kidney demonstrates a renal mass, that is relatively isoechoic to normal renal parenchyma. (b) Color Doppler imaging demonstrates vessels splayed around the mass.

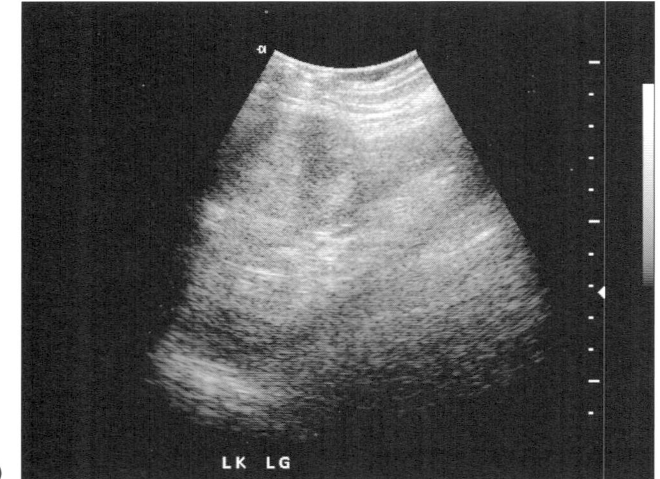
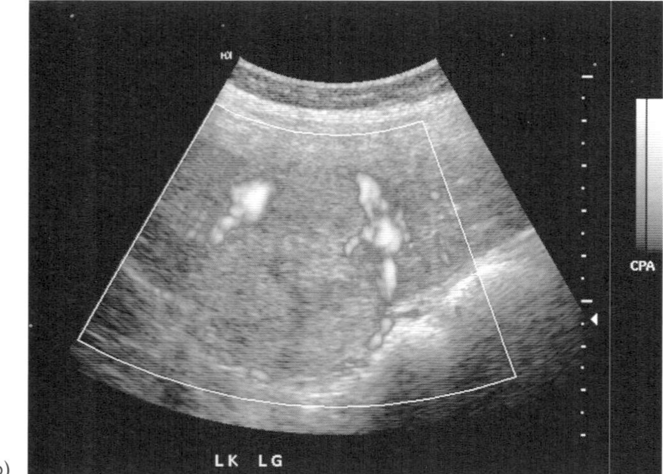
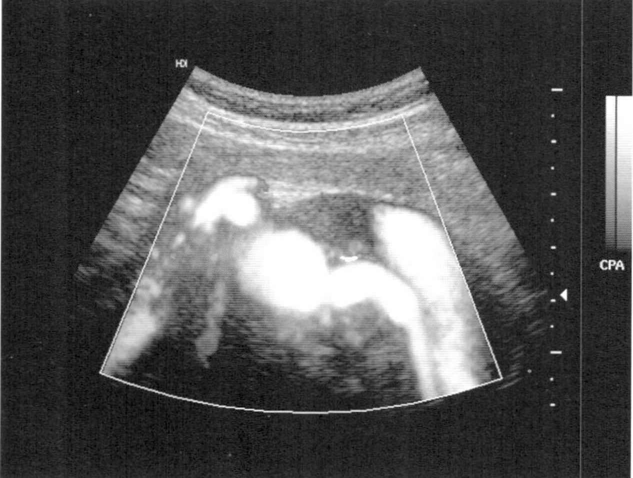

will present as a discrete, solid, central mass of decreased echogenicity, with or without associated hydronephrosis. The kidney is distorted and enlarged but there is maintenance of the reniform shape. The nonpapillary TCC is a nodular or flat tumor and is difficult to see. It demonstrates mucosal thickening, and is often high-grade and infiltrating (Thurston and Wilson 1998).

TCC of the urinary bladder is a common malignant tumor, with a male:female predominance of 3:1, and peak incidence in patients aged 50–70. The sonographic appearance is that of a focal mass within the urinary bladder or of diffuse wall thickening.

Squamous cell carcinoma is a rare malignant tumor arising from the urothelium and represents up to 15 per cent of renal pelvic tumors. Squamous cell carcinomas tend to be solid, flat, and infiltrative, and are seen on ultrasound as a diffuse renal enlargement with maintenance of the reniform shape. Associated renal stones may be present in 50 per cent of cases.

Adenocarcinomas of the genitourinary system are rare. The majority of patients will present with urinary tract infections and hematuria, and many will have staghorn calculi.

Oncocytomas are usually benign renal masses, which are indistinguishable sonographically from the RCC. These tumors are composed of epithelial cells containing granular eosinophilic cytoplasm and present as a solid renal mass, variable in appearance and echogenicity. Oncocytomas represent between 3–7 per cent of all renal tumors, and comprise approximately 5 per cent of tumors thought to be RCC on imaging. They are of variable echogenicity on ultrasound, and may be homogeneous or heterogeneous in appearance. A central scar, necrosis, or calcifications may be present (Thurston and Wilson 1998; Goiney *et al.* 1984) (Figs 24.10 and 24.11).

Renal adenomas are solid, epithelial masses that are often detected incidentally on imaging studies performed for reasons other than genitourinary symptoms, or discovered during autopsies. As they are indistinguishable from RCC both radiologically and histologically, definitive diagnosis and treatment can only be accomplished following surgical excision (Licht 1995; Diaz *et al.* 1999) (Fig. 24.12).

Fig. 24.9 RCC with renal vein invasion. (a) Sonography of the left kidney demonstrates a well demarcated, partially exophytic renal mass. (b) Power Doppler examination demonstrates blood flow encompassing the mass. (c) Power Doppler of the midabdomen in the region of the aorta and inferior vena cava demonstrates a flow void within the left renal vein as it courses toward the inferior vena cava consistent with tumor thrombus.

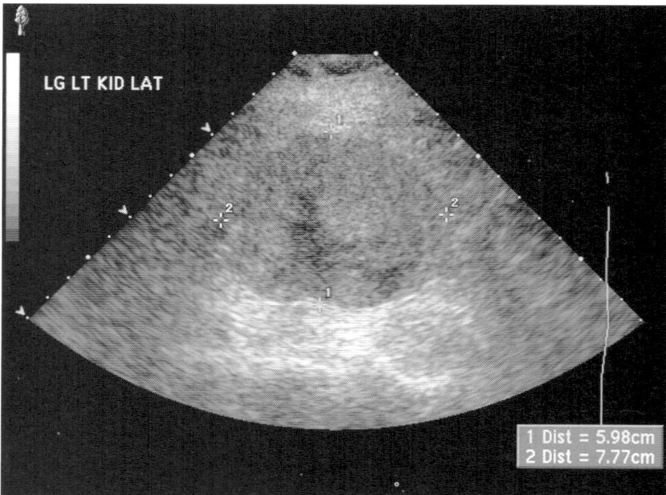

Fig. 24.10 An exophytic, solid mass is projecting off the left kidney, suspicious for malignancy. The patient underwent radical nephrectomy. Pathology revealed this mass to be a benign oncocytoma.

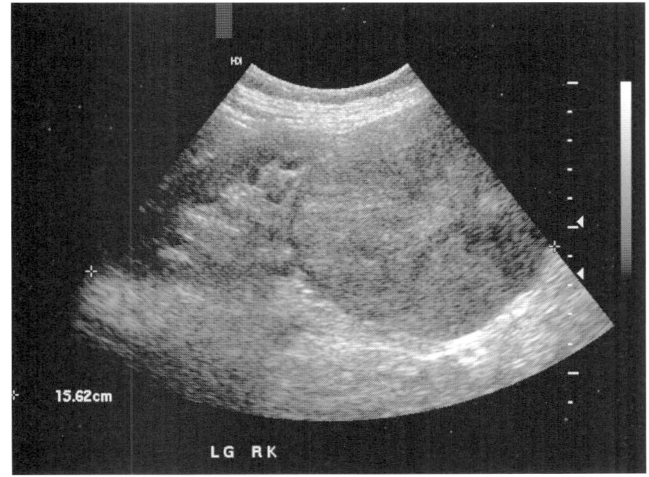

(a)

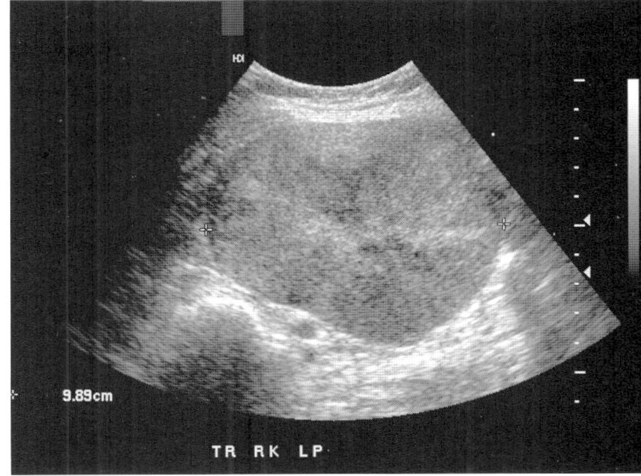

(b)

Fig. 24.11 (a) Longitudinal image of the right kidney demonstrates a large, exophytic solid mass projecting off the lower pole. (b) On a transverse image there is the appearance of a central scar radiating to the periphery. This proved to be an oncocytoma.

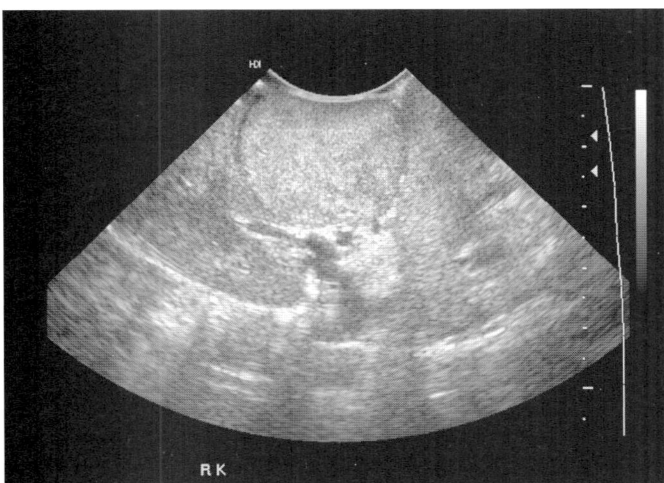

Fig. 24.12 Intraoperative ultrasound of the right kidney demonstrates an isoechoic solid renal mass, suspicious for RCC. This proved to be a renal cell adenoma.

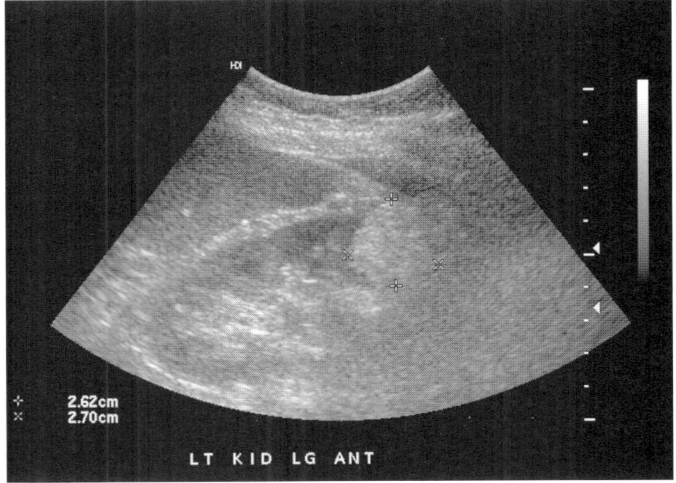

Fig. 24.13 A solid, echogenic mass is seen in the lower pole of the kidney, consistent with an angiomyolipoma.

Angiomyolipomas are benign renal tumors containing variable amounts of adipose tissue, smooth muscle, and blood vessels. Tumors may occur sporadically, or may be present in patients with tuberous sclerosis. Sporadic tumors are most prevalent unilaterally and predominate in middle aged women. Small tumors are usually asymptomatic. However, with tumor growth, there may be hemorrhage, and patients may present with flank pain, hematuria, and/or palpable mass.

As many as 80 per cent of patients with tuberous sclerosis will have at least one or more angiomyolipomas, and as many as 50 per cent of patients with angiomyolipoma will demonstrate characteristics of tuberous sclerosis (mental retardation, epilepsy, and facial sebaceous adenomas). In patients with tuberous sclerosis, tumors are often multiple and bilateral.

The sonographic appearance of angiomyolipomas depends on the proportion of fatty elements, smooth muscle and vascular elements, and hemorrhage. Tumors containing a large amount of fatty element will appear brightly echogenic, with attenuation of the sound beam posteriorly. Tumors predominating in muscle or vascular elements may appear hypoechoic. Tumors that have hemorrhaged may appear heterogeneous and variable in appearance (Caskey 2000; Thurston and Wilson 1998) (Figs 24.13 and 24.14).

As the sonographic appearance of an echogenic renal mass is suggestive but not specific for angiomyolipoma, a CT scan must be performed to confirm that fatty nature of the tumor. Small, asymptomatic angiomyolipomas may be followed with serial diagnostic examinations to assess for stability in size versus growth; however, surgery is often performed if tumors are large, symptomatic, or have hemorrhaged. Patients with actively bleeding angiomyolipomas may be treated with embolization.

The kidney is devoid of lymphoid tissue. However, lymphoma may involve the kidney by hematogenous dissemination or con-

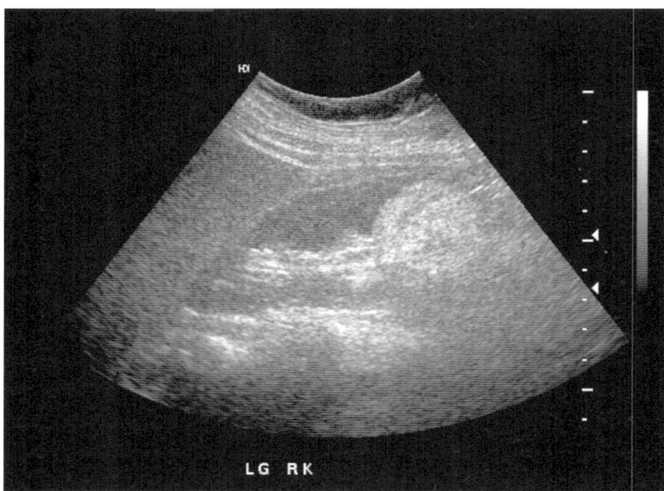

Fig. 24.14 A second patient with a solid, echogenic mass in the lower right pole of the kidney, consistent with an angiomyolipoma.

tiguous extension of retroperitoneal disease. Non-Hodgkin's lymphoma more commonly involves the kidney than Hodgkin's lymphoma. The sonographic appearance of renal lymphoma is dependent on four different patterns of involvement: focal parenchymal involvement; diffuse infiltration; invasion from a retroperitoneal mass; and perirenal involvement (Thurston and Wilson 1998) (Fig. 24.15).

Leukemia may involve the kidney in a focal or diffuse manner. Focal lesions may occur, and may be single or multiple. Diffuse involvement may manifest as diffuse renal enlargement, coarsened echo texture with distortion of the central renal sinus fat, or diffusely decreased echogenicity.

Metastatic disease to the kidneys usually occurs via hematogenous spread and may result from lung, breast, contralateral RCC, colon, stomach, cervical, ovarian, pancreatic, or prostatic primaries. Three patterns of involvement include a solitary mass, multiple masses, or a diffusely infiltrative mass. Choyke *et al.* (1987) discovered that a new renal mass in a patient with advanced cancer is more likely to be a metastatic lesion than a primary tumor. In a patient with a known primary tumor or one in remission and no evidence of metastatic disease, a biopsy must be performed to determine if a newly discovered renal lesion is a primary RCC rather than a metastatic lesion (Fig. 24.16).

Amyloidosis is a systemic disease that may involve the kidney and may be primary or secondary. Secondary amyloidosis may occur in patients with multiple myeloma, rheumatoid arthritis, tuberculosis, familial Mediterranean fever, RCC, and Hodgkin's disease. Diffuse disease is manifested as symmetrical enlargement of the kidneys. As the disease progresses, there is renal cortical atrophy and increased cortical echogenicity. Focal disease may be manifest as discrete renal masses, calcifications, focal hemorrhage, or amyloid deposits, and perirenal masses (Urban *et al.* 1993) (Fig. 24.17).

A normal variant that may present as a renal pseudomass is the hypertrophied column of Bertin. This appearance is caused by incomplete fusion of two embryological subkidneys. A renal pseudomass often occurs at the junction of the upper and middle third of the kidney, contains renal cortex continuous with adjacent renal cortex, appears as a projection of cortex into the renal sinus, and is isoechoic to adjacent renal cortex (Yeh *et al.* 1992; Lafortune *et al.* 1986). Demonstration of arcuate arteries by color Doppler within the hypertrophied column of Bertin indicates that this is not a renal tumor (Thurston and Wilson 1998). However, tumor must be considered if vessels are seen to be splayed around an indeterminate mass, and further imaging studies will be required to differentiate a true tumor from renal pseudomass (Fig. 24.18).

Renal sinus lipomatosis may simulate TCC of the collecting system. Renal sinus lipomatosis is manifested by renal parenchymal atrophy with massive fat deposition in the renal sinus. It is often associated with long-standing inflammation and calculous disease. The increased renal sinus fat may be echogenic in appear-

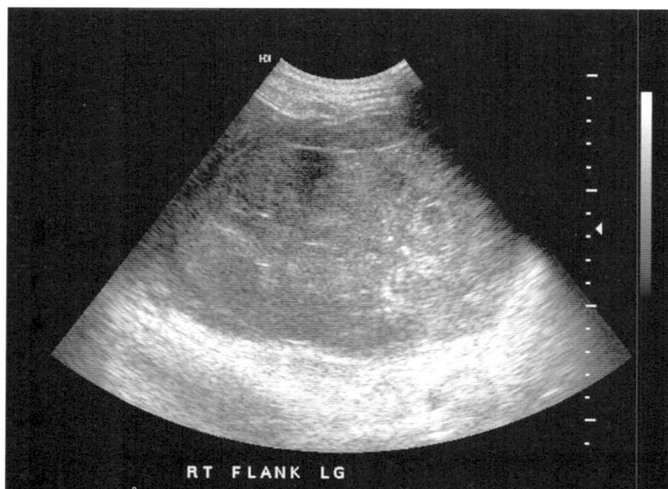

Fig. 24.15 Lymphoma. A large heterogeneous retroperitoneal mass is seen to be encompassing the region of the right kidney and invading the right kidney.

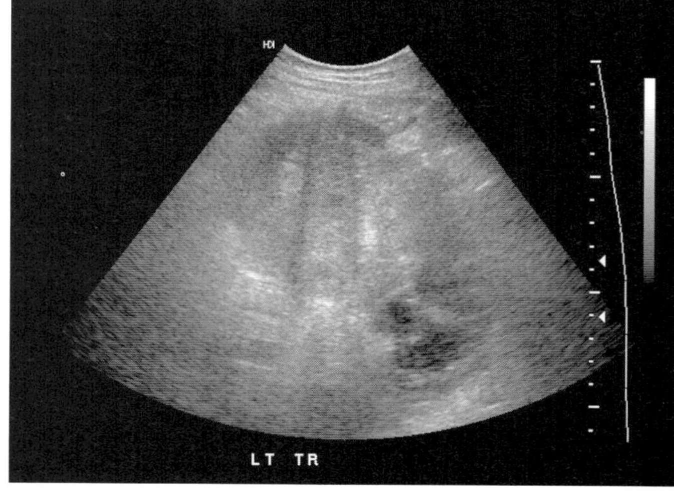

Fig. 24.16 A solid mass is identified in the upper pole of the left kidney, which proved to be a solitary lung metastasis.

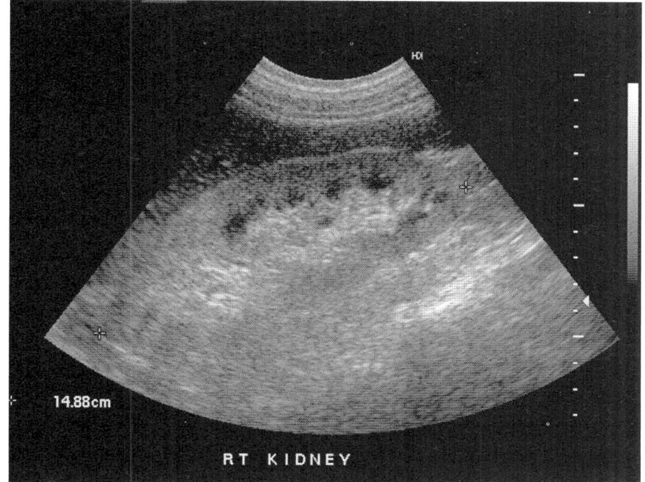
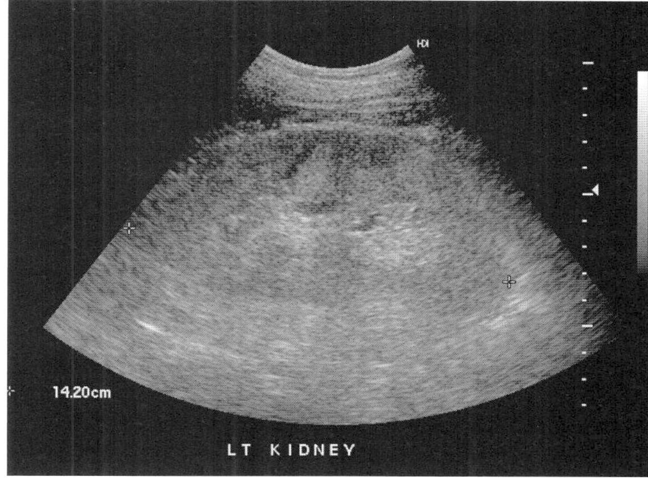

Fig. 24.17 A 52-year-old male with a history of multiple myeloma. (a), (b) The kidneys are enlarged and increased in echogenicity bilaterally, consistent with secondary amyloidosis.

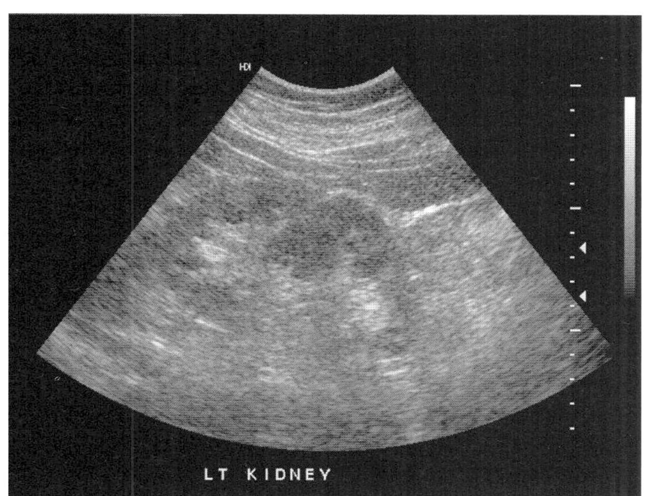
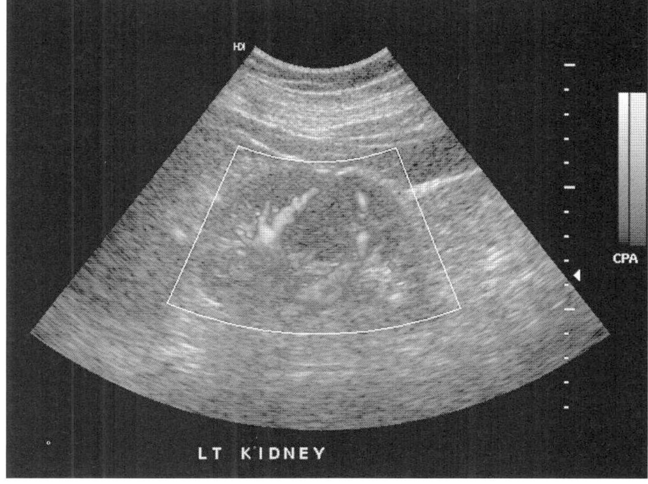

Fig. 24.18 (a) An isoechoic solid renal mass is present in the left kidney. (b) Power Doppler examination of this indeterminate mass demonstrates splaying of renal vessels, causing suspicion for a renal neoplasm. On CT this proved to be normal renal tissue, consistent with a hypertrophied column of Bertin.

ance (Subramanyam *et al.* 1983), or may be relatively echo-free (Yeh *et al.* 1977) (Fig. 24.19).

Recently developed ultrasound techniques

Recently developed ultrasound techniques that aid in the assessment of a renal mass include power Doppler ultrasound, intraoperative ultrasound, native tissue harmonic imaging, ultrasound contrast agents, and three-dimensional ultrasound.

Power Doppler ultrasound is a technique useful in evaluating the renal vasculature. Power Doppler evaluates the Doppler shift amplitude, as opposed to the mean frequency shift utilized in conventional color Doppler imaging. The sensitivity of imaging small vessels is greatly increased (3–5× that of conventional color Doppler), and intrarenal and cortical vessels are well depicted. If gray-scale images are equivocal for the presence or absence of a renal mass, power Doppler may demonstrate normal parenchymal flow, or may demonstrate splaying of vessels around a true, solid mass.

Intraoperative ultrasound is playing an important role in determination of whether a patient may undergo a partial versus radical nephrectomy. In patients undergoing partial nephrectomy, ultrasound can delineate a tumor relative to the renal hilum, and can demarcate the surgical margin boundary. This permits preservation of the maximum amount of uninvolved parenchyma, while still obtaining negative surgical margins. Color and power Doppler ultrasound identify arteries, veins, and the renal collecting system near the potential resection site, and renal parenchymal thickness between vessel and tumor may be calculated. Vessels encompassing a mass are depicted, facilitating dissection and tumor excision (Fig. 24.20).

In addition to the determination of the feasibility of partial versus radical nephectomy, intraoperative ultrasound is useful in

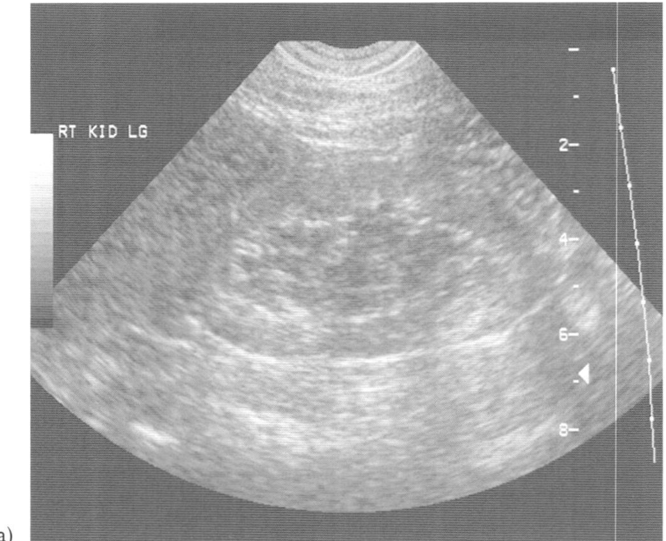

(a)

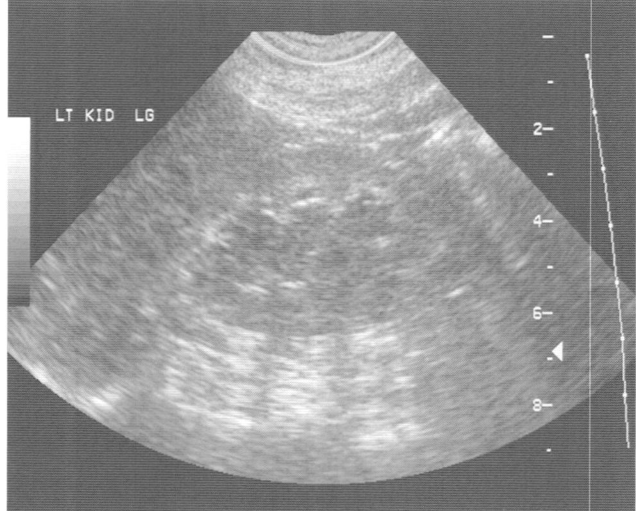

(b)

Fig. 24.19 Renal sinus lipomatosis. (a), (b) Examination of the kidneys demonstrates proliferation of the renal sinus fat, which is decreased in echogenicity relative to the renal cortex.

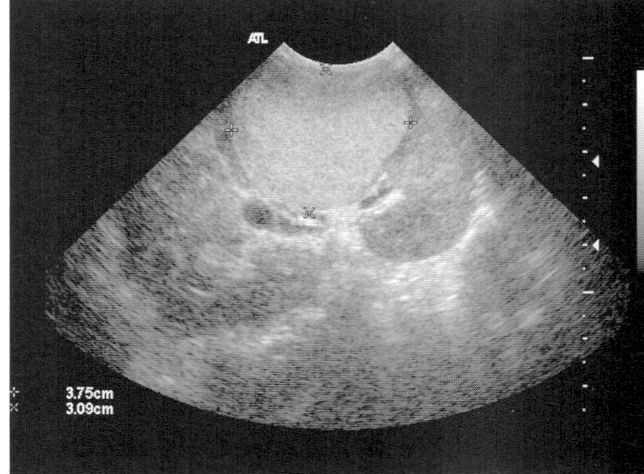

(a)

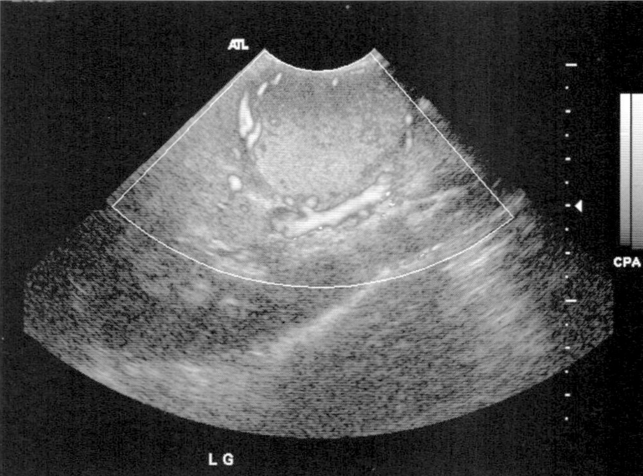

(b)

Fig. 24.20 Renal cell carcinoma. (a) Intraoperative ultrasound demonstrates an echogenic, solid renal mass impinging upon the right renal collecting system. (b) Power Doppler ultrasound demonstrates vessels encompassing the mass, in close proximity to the collecting system.

the evaluation of preoperative indeterminate lesions. Advantages of intraoperative ultrasound include closer proximity to a tumor without interference from intervening organs, bowel, and soft tissue, and the use of higher frequency transducers leading to greater resolution. Indeterminate lesions are accurately characterized, and the location and extent of tumor are better defined.

Native tissue harmonic imaging permits improvement in contrast resolution and signal–noise ratio. This enhancement in gray-scale imaging utilizes returning vibrations at a multiple of the fundamental frequency (first harmonic) from that used in conventional scanning. Reverberations and artifacts are greatly reduced, and there is improvement in the capability of distinguishing subtle, solid masses from normal parenchyma, and differentiating between simple cysts and hypoechoic masses

(Caskey 2000). Pulse inversion technology is an adaptation of harmonic imaging, allowing only signals from the contrast to be displayed (van Ophoven *et al.* 1999).

Ultrasound contrast agents utilize microbubbles that are injected intravenously into a patient. These agents undergo a phase change when injected into the bloodstream, converting from a liquid at room temperature to a gas at body temperature. Microbubbles are produced, and it is the aim that these microbubbles will increase the signal that returned to the ultrasound transducer. Using harmonic imaging and pulse inversion technology, there is a dramatic enhancement of contrast signal, improving the capability of differentiating tumoral blood flow from normal tissue vascularity (van Ophoven *et al.* 1999) (Fig. 24.21).

Conclusions

Ultrasound is an excellent, primary modality for renal imaging. Information is obtained regarding the presence or absence of a

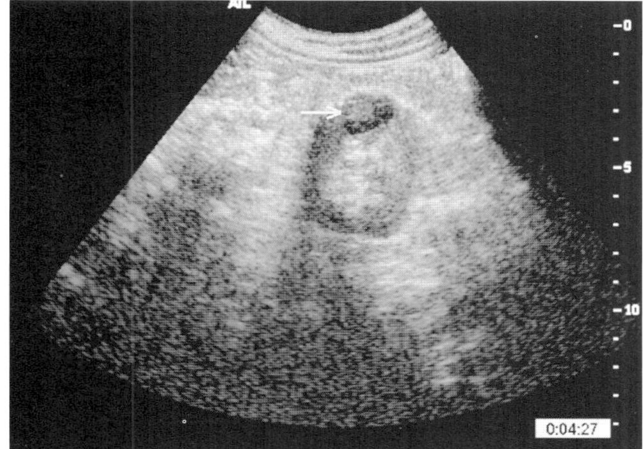

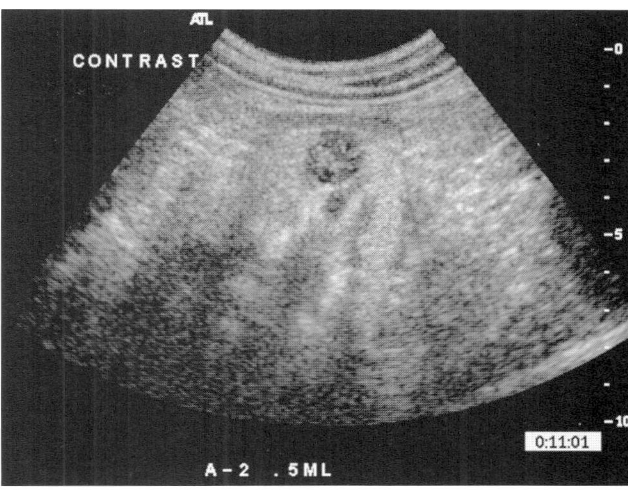

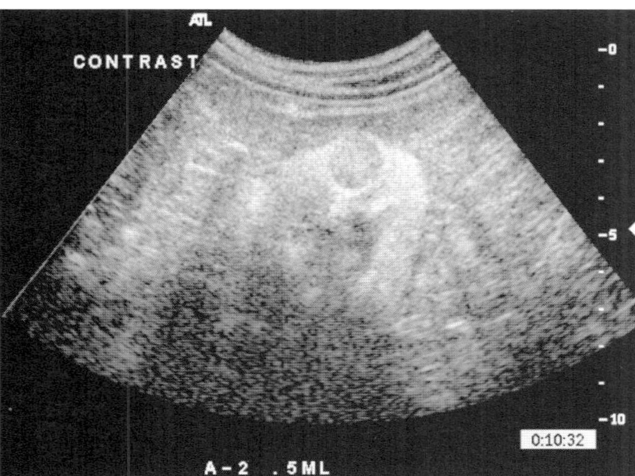

Fig. 24.21 Cystic renal cell carcinoma. (a) Conventional gray-scale images demonstrate a complex cystic renal mass. (b) Following injection of contrast, the arterial phase demonstrates gray-scale enhancement and internal vascularity in the complex cystic mass. (c) Images performed with pulse inversion demonstrate intense enhancement of normal renal parenchyma and of the complex cystic mass, indicating this to be a solid neoplasm, and not a cystic mass with debris or hemorrhage.

renal mass, and the nature of a mass, be it cystic, solid, or complex in appearance. With the advent of color, power, and spectral Doppler imaging, information is obtained regarding the renal vasculature, presence or absence of flow within a mass, and proximity of a mass to renal hilar vessels. Partial nephrectomy is now a viable option for many patients undergoing surgical excision of a renal mass. New techniques including tissue harmonic imaging and ultrasound contrast agents promise greater capability in detection and diagnosis of renal masses.

References

Baltarowich, O.H. and Kurtz, A.B. (1987). Sonographic evaluation of renal masses. *Urol. Radiol.* **9**, 79–87.

Caskey, C.I. (2000). Ultrasound techniques for evaluating renal masses, renal obstruction, and other upper tract pathology. *Ultrasound Quart.* **16**, 23–39.

Charboneau, J.W., Hattery, R.R., Ernst, E.C. III, *et al.* (1983). Spectrum of sonographic findings in 25 renal masses other than benign simple cyst. *Am. J. Roentgenol.* **140**, 87–94.

Choyke, P.L., White, E.M., Zeman, R.K., *et al.* (1987). Renal metastases: clinicopathologic and radiologic correlation. *Radiology* **162**, 359–63.

Coleman, B.G. (1985). Ultrasound of the upper genitourinary tract. *Urol. Clin. N. Am.* **12**, 633–44.

Curry, N.S. (1995). Small renal masses (lesions smaller than 3 cm): imaging evaluation and management. *Am. J. Roentgenol.* **164**, 355–62.

Diaz, J.I., Ora, L.B., and Hakam, A. (1999). The Mainz classification of renal cell tumors. *Cancer Control* **6**, 571–9.

Goiney, R.C., Goldenberg, L., Cooperberg, P.L., *et al.* (1984). Renal oncocytoma: sonographic analysis of 14 cases. *Am. J. Roentgenol.* **143**, 1001–4.

Lafortune, M., Constantin, A., Breton, G., *et al.* (1986). Sonography of the hypertrophied column of Bertin. *Am. J. Roentgenol.* **146**, 53–6.

Licht, M.R. (1995). Renal adenoma and oncocytoma. *Sem. Urol. Oncol.* **13**, 262–6.

Subramanyam, B.R., Bosniak, M.A., Horii, S.C., *et al.* (1983). Replacement lipomatosis of the kidney: diagnosis by computed tomography and sonography. *Radiology* **148**, 791–2.

Thurston, W. and Wilson, S.R. (1998). The urinary tract. In *Diagnostic ultrasound*, 2nd edn, pp. 329–99. Mosby, St. Louis.

Urban, B.A., Fishman, E.K., Goldman, S.M., *et al.* (1993). CT evaluation of amyloidosis: spectrum of disease. *Radiographics* **13**, 1295–308.

van Ophoven, A., Tsui, K.H., Shvarts, O., Laifer-Narin, S., *et al.* (1999). Current status of partial nephrectomy in the management of kidney cancer. *Cancer Control* **6**, 560–70.

Yeh, H.C., Mitty, H.A., and Wolf, B.S. (1977). Ultrasonography of renal sinus lipomatosis. *Radiology* **124**, 799–801.

Yeh, H.C., Halton, K.P., Shapiro, R.S., *et al.* (1992). Junctional parenchyma: revised definition of hypertrophic column of Bertin. *Radiology* **185**, 725–32.

25. PET imaging in renal cancer

Marc Seltzer and Jean Emmanuel Filmont

Background

Positron emission tomography (PET) is a biological whole-body imaging modality that allows clinicians and research scientists to non-invasively image biochemical processes such as the glucose utilization of tumors. Over the past several years, PET has emerged as an important clinical tool for diagnosing, staging, and monitoring therapy in patients with cancer. Unlike computed tomography (CT) or magnetic resonance imaging (MRI), which primarily examine anatomy, PET provides a functional assessment of tumor biology.

PET imaging requires access to a medical cyclotron that produces positron-emitting radioisotopes such as fluorine-18, nitrogen-13, and carbon-11. These radioisotopes can be incorporated into endogenous biochemicals such as glucose to make a positron-emitting radiopharmaceutical. The intravenously injected radiotracer accumulates in organ tissues and tumors according to their biochemical function. For example, tumors that have a high glucose metabolic rate will incorporate large amounts of the radioactive glucose analog 18-Fluoro-2-deoxy-D-glucose.

The principle of PET detection is shown in Fig. 25.1. The radioisotope portion of the radiopharmaceutical emits a positron (positively charged electron), which travels several millimeters in tissue before colliding with a negatively charged electron in the tissue. The annihilation event results in the production of two 511 keV photons (gamma rays) that are emitted from the body 180 degrees apart. The two photons are detected by two oppositely positioned detectors that define a line of coincidence along which the annihilation event occurred. A ring of multiple detectors is used to simultaneously define multiple lines of coincidence across the body that can subsequently be mathematically reconstructed to create a three-dimensional image of positron annihilation events in the body. The half-life of the most commonly used PET radiopharmaceuticals is less than 2 hours and the injected doses are comparable to those used in standard nuclear medicine procedures such as bone scintigraphy. The amount of whole-body radiation exposure the patient receives is approximately the same as that from a regional CT scan (Jones *et al.* 1982).

The radiopharmaceutical that is currently used clinically for tumor imaging with PET is the glucose analog, 18-Fluoro-2-deoxy-D-glucose (FDG). The utility of FDG–PET in oncologic imaging is based on the observation that may types of cancers have an accelerated rate of glycolysis (Warburg 1931; 1956).

This amplification is necessary because oxidative metabolism is markedly reduced in tumor cells, which rely on ATP generated from anaerobic glycolysis. Glucose metabolism needs to be amplified to meet the energy requirements of rapidly growing cancer cells. After intravenous bolus injection, FDG enters the tissue and is phosphorylated into $FDG\text{-}6\text{-}PO_4$ by the action of hexokinase. Unlike $glucose\text{-}6\text{-}PO_4$, $FDG\text{-}6\text{-}PO_4$ is not metabolized further in the glycolytic pathway and remains intracellularly trapped. The distribution of $FDG\text{-}6\text{-}PO_4$ in normal and abnormal tissue can therefore be imaged with PET. The intracellular concentration of $FDG\text{-}6\text{-}PO_4$ is roughly proportional to the rate of glucose utilization of the tissue. High uptake of FDG is common in many types of malignancies (Warburg 1931; 1956; Phelps *et al.* 1979; Di Chiro *et al.* 1982). High uptake of FDG is also seen in normal brain tissue (due to the high glucose metabolism in the brain), normal myocardial tissue (due to high myocardial glucose demand in the postprandial state), and in the kidneys and bladder (due to renal excretion of FDG). In addition, a low level of FDG activity is present in other tissues such as liver, muscle, and bowel.

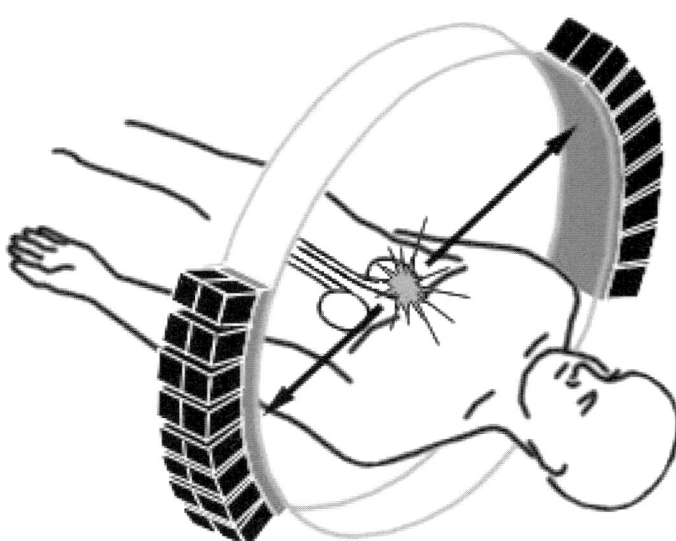

Fig. 25.1 Schematic representation of a position annhilation event in a renal tumor. The resulting 511 keV photons travel along a line of coincidence (arrows) and are detected by a full ring of crystal detectors that surrounds the body.

FDG–PET has been demonstrated in numerous studies to be an accurate modality for staging a variety of cancer types including lung (Nolop *et al.* 1987); Kubota *et al.* 1990, 1997; Gupta *et al.* 1992; Patz *et al.* 1993; Slosman *et al.* 1993; Dwamena *et al.* 1999; Coleman 1999), breast (Wahl *et al.* 1991*a, b*; Tse *et al.* 1992; Adler *et al.* 1993; Nieweg *et al.* 1993; Hoh and Schiepers 1999; Schelling *et al.* 2000), head and neck (Haberkorn *et al.* 1991; Bailet *et al.* 1992; Rege *et al.* 1994; Lowe *et al.* 2000; McGuirt *et al. 1998), colorectal (*Yonekura *et al.* 1982; Strauss *et al.* 1989; Gupta *et al.* 1993; Goldberg *et al.* 1993; Schiepers *et al.* 1995; Valk *et al.* 1999), lymphoma (Paul 1987; Okade *et al.* 1991, 1992; Leskinen-Kallio *et al.* 1991; Stumpe *et al.* 1998; Mikhaeel *et al.* 2000; Delbeke 1999), esophagus (Hoegerle *et al.* 2000; Flanagan *et al.* 1997), thyroid (Adler and Bloom 1993; Bloom *et al.* 1993; Bi and Lu 2000), ovarian (Casey *et al.* 1994; Karlan *et al.* 1993; Yuan *et al.* 1999), musculoskeletal (Adler *et al.* 1991; Kern *et al. 1988), and melanoma (Hoh et al. 1993*; Paquet *et al.* 1998; Eigtved *et al.* 2000; Dietlein *et al.* 1999). In the US the following indications for PET scanning are approved for reimbursement by the Health Care Finance Administration (HCFA): characterization of solitary pulmonary nodules, staging and restaging of non-small cell lung cancer, lymphoma, melanoma, colorectal, head and neck, and breast cancer.

A limited number of studies have been performed to determine the role of FDG–PET in renal cell carcinoma (RCC). The indications that have been investigated are characterization of indeterminate renal masses, primary staging, re-staging after primary local or systemic treatment, and monitoring the effects of systemic therapy.

Characterization of solid renal masses

Three investigations used FDG–PET for assessing the malignant nature of a solid renal mass (see Table 25.1).

Bachor *et al.* (1996) studied 29 patients with solid renal masses, all of whom underwent FDG–PET before surgery. PET results were compared to surgical pathologic findings. Twenty-six patients had a histologic diagnosis of RCC. PET was true positive for malignancy in 20 patients but was falsely negative in 6 patients. Three patients with benign pathology (angiomyolipoma, pericytoma, and pheochromocytoma) were falsely positive by PET, indicating that some benign lesions have increased glucose metabolic activity.

Goldberg *et al.* (1997) performed 26 PET studies in 21 patients. They evaluated the ability of FDG–PET to characterize solid renal masses ($n = 10$ patients) and Bosniak type III indeterminate renal cysts ($n = 11$ patients) as malignant or benign. PET correctly classified solid lesions as malignant in 9 of 10 patients subsequently confirmed histologically by surgery or biopsy (6 RCC, 3 lymphoma). One patient with bilateral RCC was falsely negative by PET. PET correctly classified indeterminate renal cysts as benign in 7 of 8 patients confirmed by surgery or needle aspiration. PET was falsely negative in one patient with a 4 mm papillary neoplasm. The authors suggested that a positive FDG–PET scan in the appropriate clinical setting may obviate the need for cyst aspiration in indeterminate renal masses.

More recently, Montravers *et al.* (2000) performed FDG–PET scans in 13 patients with renal masses who subsequently had nephrectomy or surgical resection. Nine tumors were proven malignant and 4 benign. All malignant tumors were correctly characterized by PET (7 RCC, 2 carcinosarcomas). PET was false-positive in one patient with renal tuberculosis. PET was true-negative in 3 patients with benign masses (1 angiomyolipoma, 2 complex benign renal cysts), and false-negative in 1 patient with a 3 cm RCC.

In order to investigate why some renal malignancies are negative on FDG–PET, Miyauchi *et al.* (1996), compared several biological characteristics of renal tumors with the degree of FDG uptake and lesion detection by FDG–PET. They studied 11 patients with newly diagnosed RCC and compared the results of FDG–PET with the expression of glucose transporters (Glut-1, 2, 4, 5), tumor size, and tumor grade. They concluded that renal cancers well visualized by FDG–PET have higher grade, higher Glut-1 expression, and tend to be larger than poorly imaged tumors.

In addition to the biological characteristics of renal malignancies, the normal renal excretion of FDG may result in residual parenchymal activity as well as pooling of excreted tracer in the pelvicaliceal system, which may limit the ability to visualize renal malignancies. Furthermore, lesions less than 1 cm in size or cystic lesions with mural malignancy may be below the spatial resolution of existing PET scanners (currently approximately 7 mm).

While further studies examining larger numbers of patients are required, the current literature suggests that PET has a limited role for characterizing renal masses. In masses that are classified indeterminate by conventional imaging (CT, MRI), the high positive predictive value of PET indicates that PET may be useful for further non-invasive characterization particularly in those patients in whom surgical resection or biopsy is not feasible. A negative PET scan, however, does not exclude malignancy.

Table 25.1 Results from using FDG–PET to assess the malignant nature of a solid renal mass

Reference	N	Sensitivity (%)	Specificity (%)	Accuracy (%)	PPV* (%)	NPV* (%)
Bachor *et al.* 1996	29	20/26 (76)	0/3	20/29 (69)	20/23 (87)*	0/6
Goldberg *et al.* 1997	21	9/11 (82)	9/9 (100)	18/21 (85)	9/9 (100)	9/11 (82)
Montravers *et al.* 2000	13	8/9 (88)	3/4 (75)	11/13 (85)	8/9 (88)	3/4 (75)

* PPV, positive predictive value; NPV, negative predictive value.

Primary staging

Kocher *et al.* (1994) performed presurgical staging with PET in 10 patients with renal cancer and found that PET predicted the presence or absence of lymph node metastases in all cases (3 positive, 7 negative). Bachor *et al.* (1996) reported that FDG–PET correctly identified regional lymph node metastases in 3 of 26 patients. Finally, Montravers *et al.* (2000) found that PET correctly staged 11 of 12 patients (4 true positive, 7 true negative). The sites of positive PET findings were in the bone ($n = 3$), lung ($n = 1$).

While the existing data indicate that staging of regional and distant sites of metastases is possible using FDG–PET, further studies in larger numbers of patients are needed to define the accuracy of PET for primary staging as well as the ability of PET to provide information additional to that supplied by conventional imaging modalities such as CT and MRI.

Re-staging

The most promising role of PET is for the detection of recurrent disease following local and/or systemic therapy. Anatomic imaging modalities (for example, CT, MRI) are limited in their ability to differentiate local tumor recurrence from scarring secondary to surgery or chemotherapy. As a whole-body metabolic imaging modality, FDG–PET has the potential to be a valuable adjunct to anatomic imaging for determining the presence of active tumor involvement in the postsurgical resection bed and for identifying occult metastases at distant sites in the body (Fig. 25.2).

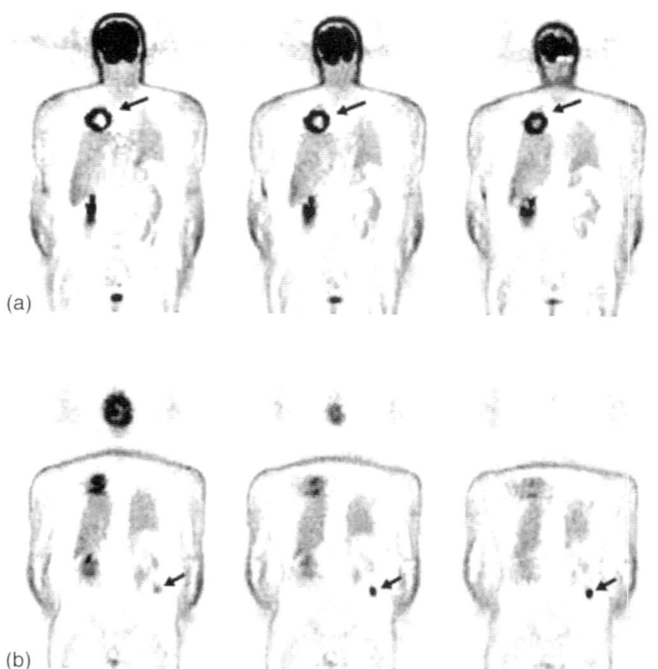

Fig. 25.2 Coronal whole-body FDG–PET images of a patient with recurrent RCC. The PET study demonstrates evidence for metastases in (a) the right upper lung (arrow) and (b) in the soft tissue of the left flank (arrow). Both lung and flank lesions were subsequently proven by biopsy to be metastases.

Montravers *et al.* (2000) performed FDG–PET in 7 patients with suspected recurrent disease after nephrectomy. PET visualized metastatic foci in 4 patients, all of which were histologically confirmed by biopsy or surgery. The other 3 patients were negative on FDG–PET and were classified as probable true-negatives based on clinical follow-up data. In 2 patients, PET correctly determined the presence of local tumor involvement in the renal bed.

Safaei *et al.* (2000) assessed the utility of FDG–PET for re-staging 36 patients with advanced RCC. In this retrospective study, the authors evaluated the value of whole-body PET used in addition to conventional imaging (including CT, MRI, ultrasound, plain radiography, and bone scintigraphy). In a patient-based analysis, PET correctly classified the clinical stage in 32 of 36 (89 per cent) and was incorrect in 4 patients (11 per cent). In a lesion-based analysis, PET correctly classified 21 of 25 (81 per cent) lesions that were subsequently biopsy proven. PET was true-positive in 14, true-negative in 7, false-positive in 1, and false-negative in 3 lesions resulting in a sensitivity of 82 per cent, specificity of 88 per cent, and diagnostic accuracy of 81 per cent.

While more studies are required that compare conventional imaging to PET, the current data suggests that PET has the ability to identify local and distant sites of recurrent disease and that PET adds additional staging information to conventional imaging modalities.

Monitoring therapy

Currently, monitoring therapy of RCC is based on conventional imaging during and after therapy, including CT or MRI of the chest, abdomen, pelvis, and bone scintigraphy.

Hoh *et al.* (1996) used whole-body FDG–PET to stage 22 patients who were receiving interleukin-2 based therapy. All patients were staged with conventional imaging every 3 to 6 months. PET images were scored as positive or negative for lesions and were compared to changes in anatomical lesion size based on conventional studies, which included CT of the chest, abdomen, and pelvis, MRI, and bone scintigraphy. In 10 patients who were proven to have active progressive disease, PET revealed active foci in all 10 patients while only 7 of 10 had progression of lesion size by CT. In one patient with stable disease, PET was positive and CT showed no change in lesion size. In 5 patients with partial response, PET and conventional imaging results were mixed. PET scans were negative in all 5 patients with complete remission. This data suggests that whole-body PET may be useful for monitoring the effect of systemic therapy in RCC and that whole-body PET may provide additional prognostic value above that of conventional imaging.

Hoh *et al.* (1997) further evaluated the prognostic value of metabolic imaging using FDG–PET in patients receiving biological therapy for metastatic RCC. This study included 25 patients, all of whom were re-staged with conventional imaging and FDG–PET at the end of treatment. In 9 of 25 patients, conventional imaging demonstrated an increase in lesion size and all lesions were positive by PET. Of the remaining 16 patients, conventional imaging showed stable, decreasing, or complete regression of metastatic disease. In 6 of 16 whole-body PET was completely negative, but in 10 patients, PET was positive in one or more metastatic sites. The authors followed all patients for an average of 20 months and correlated mortality with the results of conventional and PET imaging. When conventional imaging and PET were concordantly negative, the mortality was 0 per cent. When conventional imaging was negative and PET was positive, mortality was 20 per cent and when both imaging modalities were positive, mortality was 44 per cent. This data suggests that FDG–PET adds additional prognostic information, particularly in patients with stable or resolving metastatic lesions on conventional imaging.

Conclusion

For characterizing solid renal masses, PET has a high positive predictive value and therefore may be a useful modality for evaluating lesions that have indeterminate characteristics by conventional imaging. A negative PET scan, however, cannot exclude the presence of malignancy for several reasons including low tumor grade, decreased expression of glucose transporters, and the presence of normal renal excretion of tracer, which may mask a small parenchymal tumor. For primary staging, whole-body FDG–PET can be used to survey the body for regional and distant sites of disease but the accuracy of PET has not been determined in large number of patients nor has it been rigorously compared to conventional imaging modalities. For re-staging, PET appears to provide additional information over anatomic imaging due to its ability to distinguish scar from viable tumor involvement in the local resection bed and at distant sites in the body. Finally, PET holds promise for providing additional prognostic information to conventional imaging and may prove useful for monitoring response to therapy in patients with advanced disease. Additional studies are ongoing to further define the role of PET in the management of metastatic renal cancer.

References

Adler, L.P. and Bloom, A.D. (1993). Positron emission tomography of thyroid masses. *Thyroid* **3** (3), 195–200.

Adler, L.P., Blair, H.F., Makley, J.T., Williams, R.P., Joyce, M.J., Leisure, G., *et al.* (1991). Noninvasive grading of musculoskeletal tumors using PET. *J. Nucl. Med.* **32** (8), 1508–12.

Adler, L.P., Crowe, J.P., al-Kaisi, N.K., and Sunshine, J.L. (1993). Evaluation of breast masses and axillary lymph nodes with [F-18]2-deoxy-2-fluoro-D-glucose PET. *Radiology* **187** (3), 743–50.

Bachor, R., Kocher, F., Gropengiesser, F., Reske, S.N., and Hautmann, R.E. (1995). Positron emission tomography: introduction of a new imaging technique for urological tumors and initial clinical resuts. *Urologe Ausgabe A* **34** (2), 138–42.

Bailet, J.W., Abemayor, E., Jabour, B.A., Hawkins, R.A., Ho, C., and Ward, P.H. (1992). Positron emission tomography: a new, precise imaging modality for detection of primary head and neck tumors and assessment of cervical adenopathy. *Laryngoscope* **102** (3), 281–8.

Bi, J. and Lu, B. (2000). Advances in the diagnosis and management of thyroid neoplasms. *Curr. Opin. Oncol.* **12** (1), 54–9.

Bloom, A.D., Adler, L.P., and Shuck, J.M. (1993). Determination of malignancy of thyroid nodules with positron emission tomography. *Surgery* **114** (4), 728–34; discussion 734–5.

Casey, M.J., Gupta, N.C., and Muths, C.K. (1994). Experience with positron emission tomography (PET) scans in patients with ovarian cancer. *Gynecol. Oncol.* **53** (3), 331–8.

Coleman, R.E. (1999). PET in lung cancer. *J. Nucl. Med.* **40** (5), 814–20.

Delbeke, D. (1999). Oncological applications of FDG PET imaging: brain tumors, colorectal cancer, lymphoma and melanoma. *J. Nucl. Med.* **40** (4), 591–603.

Di Chiro, G., De La Paz, R.L., Brooks, R.A., Sokoloff, L., Kornblith, P.L., Smith, B.H., *et al.* (1982). Glucose utilization of cerebral gliomas measured by [18F]fluorodeoxyglucose and positron emission tomography. *Neurology* **32** (12), 1323–9.

Dietlein, M., Krug, B., Groth, W., Smolarz, K., Scheidhauer, K., Psaras, T., *et al.* (1999). Positron emission tomography using 18F-fluorodeoxyglucose in advanced stages of malignant melanoma: a comparison of ultrasonographic and radiological methods of diagnosis. *Nucl. Med. Commun.* **20** (3), 255–61.

Dwamena, B.A., Sonnad, S.S., Angobaldo, J.O., and Wahl, R.L. (1999). Metastases from non-small cell lung cancer: mediastinal staging in the 1990s—meta-analytic comparison of PET and CT. *Radiology* **213** (2), 530–6.

Eigtved, A., Andersson, A.P., Dahlstrom, K., Rabol, A., Jensen, M., Holm, S., *et al.* (2000). Use of fluorine-18 fluorodeoxyglucose positron emission tomography in the detection of silent metastases from malignant melanoma. *Eur. J. Nucl. Med.* **27** (1), 70–5.

Flanagan, F.L., Dehdashti, F., Siegel, B.A., Trask, D.D., Sundaresan, S.R., Patterson, G.A., *et al.* (1997). Staging of esophageal cancer with 18F-fluorodeoxyglucose positron emission tomography. *Am. J. Roentgenol.* **168** (2), 417–24.

Goldberg, M.A., Lee, M.J., Fischman, A.J., Mueller, P.R., Alpert, N.M., and Thrall, J.H. (1993). Fluorodeoxyglucose PET of abdominal and pelvic neoplasms: potential role in oncologic imaging. *Radiographics* **13** (5), 1047–62.

Goldberg, M.A., Mayo-Smith, W.W., Papanicolaou, N., Fischmann, A.J., and Lee, M.J. (1997). FDG PET characterization of renal masses: preliminary experience. *Clin. Radiol.* **52** (7), 510–15.

Gupta, N.C., Frank, A.R., Dewan, N.A., Redepenning, L.S., Rothberg, M.L., Mailliard, J.A., *et al.* (1992). Solitary pulmonary nodules: detection of malignancy with PET with 1-[F-18]-fluoro-2-deoxy-D-glucose. *Radiology* **184** (2), 441–4.

Gupta, N.C., Falk, P.M., Frank, A.L., Thorson, A.M., Frick, M.P., and Bowman, B. (1993). Pre-operative staging of colorectal carcinoma using positron emission tomography. *Nebr. Med. J.* **78** (2), 30–5.

Haberkorn, U., Strauss, L.G., Reisser, C., Haag, D., Dimitrakopoulou, A., Ziegler, S., *et al.* (1991). Glucose uptake, perfusion, and cell proliferation in head and neck tumors: relation of positron emission tomography to flow cytometry [see comments]. *J. Nucl. Med.* **32** (8), 1548–55.

Hoegerle, S., Altehoefer, C., and Nitzsche, E.U. (2000). Staging an esophageal carcinoma by F-18 fluorodeoxyglucose whole-body positron emission tomography. *Clin. Nucl. Med.* **25** (3), 219–20.

Hoh, C.K. and Schiepers, C. (1999). 18-FDG imaging in breast cancer. *Sem. Nucl. Med.* **29** (1), 49–56.

Hoh, C.K., Hawkins, R.A., Glaspy, J.A., Dahlbom, M., Tse, N.Y., Hoffman, E.J., *et al.* (1993). Cancer detection with whole-body PET using 2-[18F]fluoro-2-deoxy-D-glucose. *J. Comput. Assist. Tomogr.* **17** (4), 582–9.

Hoh, C.K., Figlin, R.A., Belldegrun, A., Moon, D.H., Franklin, J., Phelps, M.E., *et al.* (1996). Evaluation of renal cell carcinoma with whole body FDG PET. *J. Nucl. Med.* **37** (5 suppl.), 141P.

Hoh, C.K., Figlin, R.A., Seltzer, M.A., Belldegrun, A., Franklin, J., Gitliz, B., *et al.* (1997). Prognostic value of a whole body FDG PET vs. conventional imaging for the evaluation of biologic therapy in renal cell carcinoma. *J. Nucl. Med.* **38** (5 suppl.), 145P

Jones, S.C., Alavi, A., Christman, D., Montanez, I., Wolf, A.P., and Reivich, M. (1982). The radiation dosimetry of 2[F-18]fluoro-2-deoxy-D-glucose in man. *J. Nucl. Med.* **23** (7), 613–17.

Karlan, B.Y., Hawkins, R., Hoh, C., Lee, M., Tse, N., Cane, P., *et al.* (1993). Whole-body positron emission tomography with 2-[18F]-fluoro-2-deoxy-D-glucose can detect recurrent ovarian carcinoma. *Gynecol. Oncol.* **51** (2), 175–81.

Kern, K.A., Brunetti, A., Norton, J.A., Chang, A.E., Malawer, M., Lack, E., *et al.* (1988). Metabolic imaging of human extremity musculoskeletal tumors by PET. *J. Nucl. Med.* **29** (2), 181–6.

Kocher, F., Grimmel, S., Hautmann, R.E., and Reske, S.N. (1994). Positron emission tomography. Introduction of a new procedure in diagnosis of urologic tumors and initial clinical results. *J. Nucl. Med.* **35** (5), 223P.

Kubota, K. Matsuzawa, T., Fujiwara, T., Ito, M., Hatazawa, J., Ishiwata, K., *et al.* (1990). Differential diagnosis of lung tumor with positron emission tomography: a prospective study. *J. Nucl. Med.* **31** (12), 1927–32.

Kubota, K., Yamada, S., Fukuda, H., Tanida, T., Saitou, Y., Takahashi, J., *et al.* (1997). Cost effectiveness analysis of FDG–PET in the differential diagnosis and staging of lung cancer in Japan. *Kaku Igaku* **34** (5), 329–36.

Leskinen-Kallio, S., Ruotsalainen, U., Nagren, K., Teras, M., and Joensuu, H. (1991). Uptake of carbon-11-methionine and fluorodeoxyglucose in non-Hodgkin's lymphoma: a PET study. *J. Nucl. Med.* **32** (6), 1211–18.

Lowe, V.J., Boyd, J.H., Dunphy, F.R., Kim, H., Dunleavy, T., Collins, B.T., *et al.* (2000). Surveillance for recurrent head and neck cancer using positron emission tomography. *J. Clin. Oncol.* **18** (3), 651–8.

McGuirt, W.F., Greven, K., Williams, D. III, Keyes, J.W. Jr, Watson, N., Cappellari, J.O., *et al.* (1998). PET scanning in head and neck oncology: a review. *Head Neck* **20** (3), 208–15.

Mikhaeel, N.G., Timothy, A.R., Hain, S.F., and O'Doherty, M.J. (2000). 18-FDG–PET for the assessment of residual masses on CT following treatment of lymphomas. *Ann. Oncol.* **11** (suppl. 1), 147–50.

Miyauchi, T., Brown, R.A., Grossman, H.B., Wojno, K., and Wahl, R.L. (1996). Correlation between visualization of primary renal camera by FDG–PET. *J. Nucl. Med.* **37** (5 suppl.), 64P.

Montravers, F., Grahek, D., Kerrou, K., Younsi, N., Doublet, J.D., Gattegno, B., *et al.* (2000). Evaluation of FDG uptake by renal malignancies (primary tumor or metastases) using a coincidence detection gamma camera. *J. Nucl. Med.* **41** (1), 78–84.

Nieweg, O.E., Kim, E.E., Wong, W.H., Broussard, W.F., Singletary, S.E., Hortobagyi, G.N., *et al.* (1993). Positron emission tomography with fluorine-18-deoxyglucose in the detection and staging of breast cancer. *Cancer* **71** (12), 3920–5.

Nolop, K.B., Rhodes, C.G., Brudin, L.H., Beaney, R.P., Krausz, T., Jones, T., *et al.* (1987). Glucose utilization *in vivo* by human pulmonary neoplasms. *Cancer* **60** (11), 2682–9.

Okada, J., Yoshikawa, K., Imaseki, K., Minoshima, S., Uno, K., Itami, J., *et al.* (1991). The use of FDG–PET in the detection and management of malignant lymphoma: correlation of uptake with prognosis. *J. Nucl. Med.* **32** (4), 686–91.

Okada, J., Yoshikawa, K., Itami, M., Imaseki, K., Uno, K., Itami, J., *et al.* (1992). Positron emission tomography using fluorine-18-fluorodeoxyglucose in malignant lymphoma: a comparison with proliferative activity. *J. Nucl. Med.* **33** (3), 325–9.

Paquet, P., Hustinx, R., Rigo, P., and Pierard, G.E. (1998). Malignant melanoma staging using whole-body positron emission tomography. *Melanoma Res.* **8** (1), 59–62.

Patz, E.F. Jr, Lowe, V.J., Hoffman, J.M., Paine, S.S., Burrowes, P., Coleman, R.E., *et al.* (1993). Focal pulmonary abnormalities: evaluation with F-18 fluorodeoxyglucose PET scanning. *Radiology* **188** (2), 487–90.

Paul, R. (1987). Comparison of fluorine-18-2-fluorodeoxyglucose and gallium-67 citrate imaging for detection of lymphoma. *J. Nucl. Med.* **28** (3), 288–92.

Phelps, M.E., Huang, S.C., Hoffman, E.J., Selin, C., Sokoloff, L., and Kuhl, D.E. (1979). Tomographic measurement of local cerebral glucose metabolic rate in humans with (F-18)2-fluoro-2-deoxy-D-glucose: validation of method. *Ann. Neurol.* **6** (5), 371–88.

Rege, S., Maass, A., Chaiken, L., Hoh, C.K., Choi, Y., Lufkin, R., *et al.* (1994). Use of positron emission tomography with fluorodeoxyglucose in patients with extracranial head and neck cancers. *Cancer* **73** (12), 3047–58.

Safaei, A., Figlin, R., Hoh, C.K., Silverman, D.H., Seltzer, M.A., Phelps, M.E., *et al.* (2000). The usefulness of F18 deoxy-glucose whole body positron emission tomography (PET) for re-staging of renal cell cancer. *Clinical Nephrology*, vol. 57, No 1/2002, 56–62.

Schelling, M., Avril, N., Nahrig, J., Kuhn, W., Romer, W., Sattler, D., *et al.* (2000). Positron emission tomography using [(18)F] fluorodeoxyglucose for monitoring primary chemotherapy in breast cancer. *J. Clin. Oncol.* **18** (8), 1689–95.

Schiepers, C., Penninckx, F., De Vadder, N., Merckx, E., Mortelmans, L., Bormans, G., *et al.* (1995). Contribution of PET in the diagnosis of recurrent colorectal cancer: comparison with conventional imaging. *Eur. J. Surg. Oncol.* **21** (5), 517–22.

Slosman, D.O., Spiliopoulos, A., Couson, F., Nicod, L., Louis, O., Lemoine, R., *et al.* (1993). Satellite PET and lung cancer: a prospective study in surgical patients. *Nucl. Med. Commun.* **14** (11), 955–61.

Strauss, L.G., Clorius, J.H., Schlag, P., Lehner, B., Kimmig, B., Engenhart, R., *et al.* (1989). Recurrence of colorectal tumors: PET evaluation. *Radiology* **170** (2), 329–32.

Stumpe, K.D., Urbinelli, M., Steinert, H.C., Glanzmann, C., Buck, A., and von Schulthess, G.K. (1998). Whole-body positron emission tomography using fluorodeoxyglucose for staging of lymphoma: effectiveness and comparison with computed tomography. *Eur. J. Nucl. Med.* **25** (7), 721–8.

Tse, N.Y., Hoh, C.K., Hawkins, R.A., Zinner, M.J., Dahlbom, M., Choi, Y., *et al.* (1992). The application of positron emission tomographic imaging with fluorodeoxyglucose to the evaluation of breast disease. *Ann. Surg.* **216** (1), 27–34.

Valk, P.E., Abella-Columna, E., Haseman, M.K., Pounds, T.R., Tesar, R.D., Myers, R.W., *et al.* (1999). Whole-body PET imaging with [18F]fluoro-deoxyglucose in management of recurrent colorectal cancer. *Arch. Surg.* **134** (5), 503–11; discussion 511–13.

Wahl, R.L., Cody, R.L., Hutchins, G., and Mudgett, E. (1991*a*). Positron-emission tomographic scanning of primary and metastatic breast carcinoma with the radiolabeled glucose analogue 2-deoxy-2-[18F]fluoro-D-glucose [letter]. *New Engl. J. Med.* **324** (3), 200.

Wahl, R.L., Cody, R.L., Hutchins, G., and Mudgett, E. (1991*b*). Primary and metastatic breast carcinoma: initial clinical evaluation with PET with the radiolabeled glucose analogue 2-[F-18]-fluoro-2-deoxy-D-glucose. *Radiology* **179** (3), 765–70.

Warburg, O.H., Wind, F., and Neglers, E. (1930). On the metabolism of tumors in the body. In: Warburg, O.H. (ed) *Metabolism of Tumors*. London: Constable, 254–70.

Warburg, O.H. (1956). On the origins of cancer cells. *Science* **123**, 309–14.

Yonekura, Y., Benua, R.S., Brill, A.B., Som, P., Yeh, S.D., Kemeny, N.E., *et al.* (1982). Increased accumulation of 2-deoxy-2-[18F]fluoro-D-glucose in liver metastases from colon carcinoma. *J. Nucl. Med.* **23** (12), 1133–7.

Yuan, C.C., Liu, R.W., Wang, P.H., Ng, H.T., and Yeh, S.H. (1999). Whole-body PET with (fluorine-18)-2-deoxyglucose for detecting recurrent ovarian carcinoma. Initial report. *J. Reprod. Med.* **44** (9), 775–8.

26. Therapeutic options for localized disease

James E. Montie and Ricardo Beduschi

Renal cell carcinoma (RCC) is the most common malignancy of the kidney and constitutes approximately 85 per cent of all primary renal cancers and roughly 3 per cent of all adult malignancies. Radical nephrectomy, as described by Robson *et al.* (1969), has been the standard treatment for clinically localized RCC for the past 30 years. Nevertheless, management of clinically localized RCC has evolved considerably in the last few years. Radical nephrectomy is no longer regarded as the only curative therapy available, and surgical removal of the entire organ is no longer required in all cases of RCC. The widespread use of ultrasound, computerized tomography (CT), and magnetic resonance imaging (MRI) as diagnostic tools in patients with symptoms unrelated to the urinary tract has permitted detection of solid renal tumors, many of which ultimately prove to be renal cancers. Nevertheless, the untreated natural history of these tumors is uncertain. Several reports have suggested that small, incidentally detected reduced RCC tend to behave less aggressively than symptomatic RCC and, therefore, a more conservative approach would be reasonable. The management of these small tumors has stimulated the investigation of alternative methods for treating localized renal cancer.

One alternative, nephron-sparing surgery, has evolved as a safe, reliable way of removing small tumors, apparently without compromising survival. The advent of laparoscopy adds another variable to this controversial issue and emerges as an attractive option for either a total or a partial nephrectomy in selected cases. Lastly, several procedures to ablate a benign or malignant lesion of the kidney are currently under investigation in several centers worldwide.

The aim of this chapter is to review the therapeutic options currently available for the management of clinically localized RCC of the kidney, an exciting and expansive area in modern urology.

Rationale for treatment decisions

Treatment for RCC is strongly influenced by clinical staging at presentation. The stage of a disease is an important predictor of outcome, and 5-year survival is significantly better in earlier stages (T1/T2/T3) than in the more advanced stage (T4). In earlier series, approximately 30 per cent of the patients had metastatic disease at presentation, and long-term survival was no better than 15 per cent even after radical nephrectomy. Recently, there has been an increase in incidentally detected masses, and cure may be achieved using a simple or partial nephrectomy. Because today more tumors are diagnosed earlier at less advanced stages, therapeutic options may vary from observation to open radical nephrectomy depending on the patient's age and preference for treatment, medical condition, and the malignant potential of the tumor.

Conservative management

The clinical significance of incidentally detected solid renal masses has not been completely defined, and management of these tumors remains controversial. Several reports have suggested that small, incidentally detected tumors are of lower pathologic tumor stage than symptomatic RCC and, consequently, tend to have a better prognosis. To evaluate the growth and behavior of such lesions, Bosniak *et al.* (1996) followed 72 small renal tumors (from 0.2 to 3.5 cm) in a series of patients who refused surgery or were poor surgical candidates with serial CT and ultrasound over a period ranging from 1.75 to 10.3 years. They reported that this type of tumor tends to grow slowly, at 0.35 cm/year or less, and, moreover, that none of the patients developed metastatic disease during the follow-up period. They concluded that a close follow-up with serial imaging studies is a reasonable option for elderly or high surgical risk patients with tumors measuring less than 3 cm in diameter. One possible trade-off is that the true malignant potential of these lesions cannot be reliably assessed with this approach and, although small, there is always a risk for progression of the disease and development of metastasis. Attempts to assess the malignant potential of small solid renal masses with CT-guided fine-needle aspiration failed to provide clear benefits that would justify the risks of the procedure (Campbell *et al.* 1997).

Although the basis for cancer cure is early diagnosis and removal of the cancer before metastasis, some of these incidentally detected small kidney tumors may, in fact, grow slowly and, just as in other kinds of cancers, for example, prostate cancer, surgical removal may not always be necessary. Watchful waiting might be a reasonable option for senior citizens in poor health who are known to have tumors less than 3 cm in diameter. If selected as the treatment of choice, close follow-up should include periodic CT scans or MRI. Surgery should be considered if the tumor changes in size substantially.

Surgical management

Radical nephrectomy has been the standard treatment for localized RCC for the past 30 years, since its description in the early 1960s. The rationale for using radical nephrectomy rather than simple nephrectomy relies on the fact that renal capsular penetration and extension into perinephric fat can occur even with small tumors and, consequently, removal of the adjacent fat would increase the chance of a cure. Although both techniques have never been compared in a prospective randomized fashion, several series have shown an improved survival rate in patients treated with radical nephrectomy.

In recent years, nephron-sparing surgery (NSS; partial nephrectomy) has also emerged as an effective form of treatment for localized RCC, mainly for patients with low-stage tumors. In these patients, long-term survival free of cancer is comparable with that obtained after radical nephrectomy. This form of treatment is especially attractive for patients with some degree of renal insufficiency, bilateral cancer, or a solitary kidney. Surgical resection is clearly the most effective way to control renal cancer, and excellent results can be expected with both radical and partial nephrectomy.

Radical nephrectomy

Widely adopted in the early 1960s (Robson *et al.* 1969), radical nephrectomy is classically defined as removal of the kidney, perinephric fat and lymphatics, and ipsilateral adrenal gland within Gerota's fascia. Several aspects of radical nephrectomy are currently under re-evaluation, and most investigators believe that such a wide dissection may not be necessary. The role of ipsilateral adrenalectomy is under reassessment. Metastasis to the adrenal gland is relatively uncommon after radical nephrectomy, occurring in less than 5 per cent of the surgical specimens, and when they occur there is a frequent association with advanced local-regional disease or distant metastasis, when ipsilateral adrenalectomy is unlikely to promote cure or improve survival (Sagalowsky *et al.* 1994; Shalev *et al.* 1995; Gill *et al.* 1994). Today, the consensus is that adrenalectomy should be performed only for large tumors involving the upper pole of the kidney, when direct extension of the tumor into the adrenal gland is more likely to occur, a mass is present in the adrenal on preoperative imaging, and sparing the adrenal gland is not only technically difficult but may also compromise surgical margins. The benefit of extensive lymphadenectomy remains controversial as well and, in most cases, the value of node dissection is limited to the prognostic factor it provides. Lymph node involvement is an important prognostic factor and, as verified in several series, survival in patients with extensive node involvement is usually poor, with less than 5 per cent of the patients surviving more than 10 years. Nodal involvement is found in approximately 10 to 20 per cent of the patients undergoing surgery without evidence of distant metastasis. Eventually, distant metastasis becomes evident in almost all of these patients, and long-term survival is poor despite extensive node dissection (Giuliani *et al.* 1990; Philips and Messing 1993; Herrlinger *et al.* 1991).

Multiple studies have reported the outcome of patients treated with radical nephrectomy (Thrasher and Paulson 1993; Skinner *et al.* 1971; Middleton and Presto 1973; Selli *et al.* 1983). Survival appears to be influenced primarily by the anatomical extension of the primary tumor. Patients with early-stage disease (pathologic stage T1/T2) tend to have better outcomes if the tumor is excised completely, as opposed to pathologic stages T3/T4, which present a higher recurrence rate even after complete removal of the tumor. Five-year survival after radical nephrectomy ranges from 60 to 85 per cent for patients with T1 disease, from 45 to 80 per cent for those with T2 disease, 15 to 35 per cent for patients with T3 disease, and 0 to 10 per cent for those with T4 disease. Overall, the survival rate after radical nephrectomy is close to 80 per cent (Couillard and deVere White 1993; Rabinovitch *et al.* 1994; Skinner *et al.* 1972; McNichols *et al.* 1981). Between 25 and 30 per cent of the patients with localized disease relapse after radical nephrectomy; the majority present with metastasis to distant organs. The lungs, liver, and bone are the most common sites for distant metastasis. Local recurrence following radical surgery is a relatively rare event, occurring in less than 5 per cent of the cases, and does not always predispose to development of metastatic disease (Couillard and deVere White 1993). The median time for relapse varies according to the initial pathologic stage. Typically, 85 per cent of the relapses occur within 3 years after surgery, and the median time for recurrence after radical nephrectomy is 15 to 18 months (Couillard and deVere White 1993). Extension of the tumor into the renal vein or the inferior vena cava does not appear to compromise outcome. When the thrombus is completely resected, a 5-year survival of approximately 50 per cent can be achieved (American Cancer Society 1989). In contrast, regional lymph node involvement can be considered an independent predictor of treatment failure. Five-year survival is less than 30 per cent in patients with positive lymph nodes, and it is less than 5 per cent at 10 years (Couillard and deVere White 1993).

In summary, the data currently available support radical nephrectomy as the most reliable treatment for local control of RCC. Local recurrence after surgery is uncommon. Undetected metastatic disease, occult at the time of the initial diagnosis, is likely to be the main determinant of treatment failure and will ultimately be responsible for the patient's death.

Nephron-sparing surgery (partial nephrectomy)

In the past few years, NSS has established itself as an efficient alternative for treatment of localized RCC. Local control of the cancer can be safely achieved with NSS when tumors are small and favorably located within the organ. NSS was initially used in situations requiring preservation of functioning renal parenchyma, such as in patients with a solitary kidney, bilateral cancers, or chronic renal failure. Excellent success rates in terms of local control of the disease and long-term survival free of cancer stimulated investigators to apply this concept in patients with a normal contralateral kidney. Today, it is apparent that NSS may be as effective as radical nephrectomy in the treatment of localized RCC in patients with a normal contralateral organ, particularly for low-stage RCC (Morgan and Zincke 1990; Steinbach *et al.* 1992; Licht *et al.* 1994).

The rate of local recurrence in the partially resected kidney was initially reported as ranging from 4 to 10 per cent (Moll *et al.* 19??; Thrasher *et al.* 1994; Novick *et al.* 1989), which is slightly higher than that seen after radical nephrectomy. This is likely to represent progression of microscopic tumor that was not removed after partial nephrectomy. Nevertheless, local recurrence did not appear to compromise outcome and, according to most series, the overall survival was comparable to that seen after radical nephrectomy for tumors of similar pathologic stage (Marberger *et al.* 1981; Steinbach *et al.* 1995; Provet *et al.* 1991). In one of the largest series assessing the efficacy of NSS as a treatment for localized RCC, an overall 5-year survival rate of 81 per cent and a cancer-specific 5-year survival rate of 93 per cent were reported (Novick 1998). Local recurrence in the remnant kidney was observed in only 2.7 per cent of the patients, and distant metastasis occurred in 5.5 per cent of the cases. Ninety-eight per cent of the patients maintained some function in the partially resected unit, and the mean postoperative serum creatinine level in this set of patients was 1.8 mg/ml, proving the efficacy of the surgical technique to preserve functioning renal parenchyma. Evaluating patterns of recurrence after NSS, investigators from the same institution reported the outcome of 327 patients who underwent NSS for sporadic localized RCC (Hafez *et al.* 1997). Local recurrence occurred in 38 patients (11.6 per cent), and was more frequent in tumors with more advanced pathological stages (0, 2.0, 8.2, and 10.6 per cent for stages T1, T2, T3a, and T3b, respectively). Thirteen patients (4 per cent) had local recurrence, six with isolated lesion in the partially resected kidney, and seven with concurrent metastasis. All of these patients underwent further treatment, either with radical nephrectomy (four patients) or a second partial nephrectomy (two patients). Of those, one died of metastatic disease, three are free of disease, and two died of unrelated causes after a mean survival of 52.4 months. A total of 25 patients (7.6 per cent) had metastatic disease without local recurrence, which occurred more frequently in pathologic stage T3 than in stages T1/T2. A 5-year overall survival of 92 per cent and cancer-specific survival rates of 95 per cent for pathological tumor stage T1, 85 per cent for stage T2, and 82 per cent for stage T3 were reported (Novick 1998). This study not only confirms the efficiency of NSS for incidental RCC, but also provides important information for the surveillance of patients undergoing this form of treatment. Since the risk of local recurrence or metastatic disease is directly related to the initial pathologic tumor, patients with more advanced tumor stages (T3, etc.) require closer surveillance than those with earlier pathologic tumor stages (T1/T2).

The role of NSS in patients with RCC and a normal contralateral kidney has also been investigated (Licht and Novick 1993; Butler *et al.* 1995; Lemer *et al.* 1996). Most studies showed that patients with a single, localized tumor, measuring less than 4 cm in diameter, who were treated with NSS had the same overall survival and cancer-specific survival as those treated with radical surgery. Thus, patients with low pathologic stage RCC can be effectively and safely managed with NSS. NSS should be considered even if the contralateral kidney is normal.

Tumor location also does not appear to influence treatment outcome in patients undergoing NSS for small sporadic RCC (Hafez *et al.* 1998). Radical surgery and NSS are equally effective in treating both centrally and peripherally located small incidental tumors. However, locating small central tumors during surgery can be challenging depending on the size of the tumor. Intra-operative Doppler ultrasound is a valuable tool used in surgery that can identify even small tumors with precision, making tumor removal with an adequate surgical margin easier.

In summary, NSS is clearly indicated for patients with localized RCC with a concurrent deficit of renal function. It can be safely performed even in patients with a normal contralateral kidney with a solitary, less than 4 cm renal mass. The long-term impact of this remnant kidney in the renal function of patients with a normal opposite kidney has not been well investigated, but it may be a beneficial technique to use for an asynchronous tumor.

Laparoscopic radical nephrectomy

The first laparoscopic total nephrectomy for renal cancer was performed in 1990, and since then this surgical technique has been intensively investigated worldwide. Several series have reported the efficacy of laparoscopic radical nephrectomy for the management of patients with RCC (Kavoussi *et al.* 1993; Suzuki *et al.* 1995; Nishiyama and Terunuma 1995; McDougall *et al.* 1996; Himpens *et al.* 1994). The laparoscopic approach offers some clear advantages and disadvantages when compared to open surgery.

Most urologists prefer the transperitoneal approach, mainly because the anatomic landmarks are better defined and it provides a larger working space. The surgical steps are exactly the same for an open procedure, with dissection of the kidney within an intact Gerota's fascia, individual dissection of the renal vessels, and ligature of the renal artery before securing the renal vein. Removal of the specimen after laparoscopic surgery is achieved either by morcellating the specimen or by extending the incision of one of the portal sites and removing the intact organ within an entrapment sack. Although there have been no reports of peritoneal or portal site tumor seeding, morcellation still represents a disadvantage, since it disrupts the structure of the specimen, preventing pathologic staging of the tumor. Ideal candidates for laparoscopic radical nephrectomy are patients with localized tumors less than 7 cm in diameter with no renal vein or inferior vena cava involvement or perirenal extension (T1- and T2-stage disease). In this setting of patients, the operative time following laparoscopic radical nephrectomy is reported to range from 2.5 to 5.5 hours. The short-term cancer-free survival rate following laparoscopic radical nephrectomy is comparable to those seen after open radical nephrectomy, with most series reporting that 97 per cent of the patients are free of recurrence after 1.5 years of follow-up. Longer follow-up data is not available in the literature. Patients report less postoperative pain, have a shorter hospital stay, and shorter convalescence following laparoscopic radical nephrectomy. The main advantage appears to be that most patients are able to return to normal activity more quickly after laparoscopic surgery. Nevertheless, laparoscopic surgeries are lengthy, technically more complex procedures that require highly trained surgeons, and in general end up being more expensive than open surgeries. Series comparing the results of open versus laparoscopic radical nephrectomy show that the laparoscopic approach averages 2.5 hours longer than the open procedure, but the need for postoperative analgesic, hospital stay, and convalescence are reduced by 80, 43, and 63 per cent, respectively (Parra *et al.* 1995; Guillonneau *et al.* 1996; Kerbl *et al.* 1994). Major complications with the laparoscopic approach are not frequently seen, and the mortality rate is also very low (Gill *et al.* 1995).

The initial success with the transperitoneal approach stimulated investigators to perform laparoscopic nephrectomy by the retroperitoneal approach. It seemed logical and appealing since the kidney is an extraperitoneal organ. This approach proved to be challenging and technically more difficult than the transperitoneal approach. The smaller retroperitoneal space provides a suboptimal pneumoperitoneum for retroperitoneoscopic nephrectomy. A breakthrough for this approach came with the development of a balloon that allows atraumatic dilatation of the retroperitoneum space providing adequate working space for laparoscopic surgery in the retroperitoneum. Clinical indications for this approach are in general the same as for the transperitoneal approach. Morbid obesity and retroperitoneal scarring may render the procedure technically more difficult because of retroperitoneal fat and altered anatomical landmarks. This approach has not reached the widespread clinical acceptance that the transperitoneal approach has, primarily because of concerns about technical difficulty. Currently, only a few centers are offering this kind of treatment and very few reports have documented its success rate. Initial results with this technique for RCC less than 8 cm in diameter are comparable with those of the transperitoneal approach in terms of average operating time and hospitalization stay. However, wider use of the procedure is required before retroperitoneal laparoscopic radical nephrectomy is widely recognized as an accepted treatment modality for localized RCC.

One limitation to laparoscopic surgery, either transperitoneal or retroperitoneal, is the size of the tumor and/or the tumor thrombus. Tumors larger than 8 cm or involvement of the renal vein or the inferior vena cava by tumor thrombus have been regarded as absolute contraindications of the laparoscopic approach. Trying to improve the clinical spectrum of laparoscopy, investigators have developed a device that allows surgeons to introduce one hand into the abdominal cavity through a small midline incision while operating a laparoscopic camera and instruments with the other hand. Hand-assisted laparoscopy allows the removal of larger tumors while preserving the benefits of a minimally invasive procedure. Compared to standard laparoscopy, hand assistance decreases operative time and allows the intact removal of even large tumors without significant changes in postoperative pain, postoperative ileus, return of bowel function, or postoperative convalescence (Wolf *et al.* 1998; Nakada *et al.* 1997; Nishiyama and Terunuma 1995). Preliminary reports reveal that the average operative time for hand-assisted laparoscopic nephrectomy is approximately 75 per cent of the average time for standard laparoscopy, with similar findings in terms of hospital stay, return to normal activity, and pain control (Wolf *et al.* 1998). Visual orientation is much improved with manual palpation of the kidney, making laparoscopic surgery attractive even for the surgeon who is not familiar or trained in laparoscopic techniques. Situations that require intact specimen removal (for example, RCC that are considered too big for standard laparoscopy but not large enough to require open surgery and nephroureterectomy) are the ideal circumstances for

the use of this technical innovation. Hand-assisted laparoscopic partial nephrectomy for small RCC is currently under investigation at the University of Michigan. The preliminary results are promising. Manual compression of the kidney during resection of the renal parenchyma allows a much better control of bleeding, making laparoscopic partial resection another viable alternative for removing small RCC.

Surgical ablation of renal neoplasms

Numerous ablative procedures are routinely performed by most urologists to treat benign and malignant conditions of the upper tracts, prostate, bladder, and urethra, and it may not be long before they start playing a significant role in the treatment of small, incidental RCC. Evolving technology has allowed scientists to deliver energy more accurately to certain areas of the kidney, targeting specifically the cancerous tissue, making these treatments safer and more cost-effective.

Several ablative techniques are currently under investigation, in both clinical and experimental settings, and it would not be surprising to see these (for example, laser, cryotherapy, or thermotherapy) being used in clinical urologic practice in the near future. The trend toward minimally invasive treatment for RCC remains investigational and should not be recommended as the primary treatment for renal cancer. The initial results from several forms of ablative treatments are just becoming available. These results should be viewed with caution until more definitive data are available that establish their treatment efficiency.

Cryotherapy is the most studied form of ablative technique for RCC, probably because most urologists feel comfortable with this method from previous experience with prostate cancer. The objective of cryosurgery is to ablate the cancerous tissue that would be removed with conventional surgical excision. The tumor tissue, with a surrounding margin of healthy renal parenchyma, is quickly frozen. The devitalized tissue is slowly replaced by granulation and fibrous tissue. Examination of the renal cryolesion in the early postoperative period shows a large area of coagulative necrosis that contracts in size over time. Approximately 1 month after cryosurgery, histological analysis of the frozen area reveals replacement of the normal renal parenchyma by chronic inflammation, fibrotic glomeruli, hemosiderin deposits, and necrotic tissue, with no signs of viable nephrons (Breining *et al.* 1974). By 3 months, the area of necrosis is totally reabsorbed and replaced by fibrosis. The functional impact of cryoablation is determined by the nadir temperature achieved at the cryoprobe and by the amount of renal parenchyma destroyed by the ice ball. Complete renal tissue ablation occurs at temperatures of −20°C or lower.

Cryoablation has been tested in clinical settings with open, percutaneous, and laparoscopic approaches (Uchida *et al.* 1995; Delworth *et al.* 1996; Gill *et al.* 1998). Gill *et al.* (1998) reported the results of laparoscopic cryotherapy in a series of patients with small (less than 4 cm), peripherally, exophytic localized renal tumors distantly located from the renal collecting system. The total surgical time of the procedure was 2.4 hours, and the cryoablation time was 12.9 minutes. No major complications were observed in the study, hospital stay was less than 23 hours, and renal function was preserved in all cases. CT-guided biopsy of the cryoablated area was negative for tumors in the first 12 patients who completed 6 months of follow-up, but even the authors agree that a negative biopsy does not guarantee complete destruction of the cancer. Long-term follow-up to determine local recurrence and cancer-free survival rates and also the chronic impact of cryoablation in the renal calyces and pelvis is critical before accepting cryotherapy as a valuable tool for treatment of RCC.

Radiofrequency interstitial tumor ablation (RITA) is another form of tissue ablation that has been investigated *in vivo* and *in vitro* as a treatment for small renal tumors. Zlotta *et al.* (19??) treated renal lesions with RITA before and after radical nephrectomy in a selected group of patients with tumors less than 3 cm in diameter. The procedure was performed under local anesthetic and was well tolerated. Reduction in the tumor lesions was seen in the immediate postoperative period, but no long-term follow-up has been reported. In animal models, RITA-induced histologic changes are similar to those seen after cryoablation, with normal renal tissue being replaced by necrotic tissue (Leveillee *et al.* 1996).

Microwave thermotherapy is another ablative tool that is currently being investigated in experimental models. The transmission of microwaves through tissue generates an electromagnetic field that causes ionic or polarized molecules to vibrate, converting radiant energy into heat inside the tissue causing cell death. Thermotherapy has been tested as an ablative technique in an experimental laparoscopic model (Kigure *et al.* 1996). Rabbits with VX-2 tumors treated with microwave thermotherapy had significantly longer survival rates than untreated rabbits. To our knowledge, microwave thermotherapy has not yet been investigated as an alternative treatment for RCC in humans.

Conclusion

Treatment for localized RCC has changed considerably in the last decade. Radical nephrectomy is no longer accepted as the 'only hope for cure for renal cell carcinoma' as described by Robson *et al.* (1969). The widespread use of imaging studies in patients with nonspecific symptoms has increased the number of solid renal masses incidentally detected in patients with no urologic symptoms, and many of these incidental masses ultimately prove to be RCC. The clinical significance of these tumors has not been established, and there is evidence suggesting that they tend to be smaller and of a lower pathologic stage than symptomatic or suspected RCC. This makes the management of these lesions extremely controversial. Radical nephrectomy has been the standard treatment for localized RCC for the past 30 years, and it does provide excellent results in terms of overall survival and cancer-specific survival. Nevertheless, recent studies have demonstrated that NSS is just as effective in treating localized RCC and should be considered even in patients with a normal contralateral kidney. The technical success rate with NSS is excellent and long-term patient survival free of cancer is comparable to that obtained after radical nephrectomy, especially for small RCC (less than 4 cm). The benefits of renal function preservation are counterbalanced by a higher risk of postoperative local recurrence, which occurs in 4 to 10 per cent of the cases that are likely to present undetected tumors in the partially resected kidney.

With a better understanding of tumor biology and recent trends in tumor presentation, the importance of ipsilateral adrenalectomy and extensive lymph node dissection is also being reassessed. The value of lymphadenectomy is limited to the prognostic information it provides, since nodal involvement is strongly associated with a poor prognosis. Removal of the adrenal gland is also unlikely to improve survival and should be reserved for situations when large upper pole masses are being removed, when sparing the adrenal gland is technically difficult and may compromise surgical margins.

Laparoscopic radical nephrectomy has also emerged as a safe and efficient treatment for renal malignancy. When compared to radical nephrectomy, it offers all the benefits of a minimally invasive procedure: less postoperative pain, shorter hospital stay, less convalescence, quick return to normal activities, and cosmetic benefits. Nonetheless, the hospital costs for radical or laparoscopic radical nephrectomy are approximately 11 per cent higher than those for open radical nephrectomy, mainly due to increased operative time. Ideal candidates for a laparoscopic approach are patients with tumors less than 8 cm in diameter, without thrombus in the renal vein or inferior vena cava. A viable alternative to traditional laparoscopy is hand-assisted laparoscopy. Manual palpation of the kidney improves the visual orientation and allows surgical removal of tumors that cannot be removed by standard laparoscopy—with the same efficacy and morbidity. The advantages of retroperitoneal laparoscopy over more traditional transperitoneal laparoscopy will remain unsettled until the techniques become available in more centers and a randomized study is designed to compare both approaches.

As for minimally invasive ablative techniques, it may not be much longer before they become part of the armamentarium used to treat RCC. Several ablative procedures are currently under investigation at multiple centers. However, cryotherapy is the only form of ablative treatment that has been seriously investigated in humans, and the results should be interpreted with caution until long-term follow-up is available. Although promising, tissue ablation should not be recommended for the treatment of localized RCC.

Summary

New trends in the diagnosis of RCC have changed significantly the way its treatment is managed. Evidence suggests that small, incidental renal masses have a lower malignant potential than symptomatic lesions and, consequently, can be managed more conservatively. Watchful waiting with serial follow-up examinations and imaging studies are reasonable options in elderly or poor surgical risk patients with incidentally detected, well marginated tumors measuring less than 3 cm in diameter that remain stable over time.

Open radical nephrectomy remains the standard treatment for patients with large tumors, thrombus in the renal vein and inferior vena cava, with perinephric extension.

NSS is particularly suitable for low-stage RCC when there is a need to preserve renal function, such as in patients with bilateral tumors, tumors affecting a solitary kidney, or chronic renal failure. In this setting of patients, the success rate in terms of overall survival and cancer-specific survival is comparable to that obtained after radical nephrectomy.

Management of the incidentally discovered small RCC (less than 4 cm) in patients with a normal contralateral kidney remains controversial. Nevertheless, we believe that NSS could be the treatment of choice for these patients. The data suggests that this approach is as effective as radical nephrectomy in providing effective curative treatment. Although the long-term advantage of NSS with a normal contralateral kidney remains to be proven, the low morbidity and the efficacy of this procedure justifies the approach.

Laparoscopic hand-assisted or traditional radical nephrectomy is an emerging concept that is efficacious and safe in selected patients and, in our opinion, should be the treatment of choice when radical nephrectomy is indicated and there is no venous involvement by tumor. It provides the same efficacy in terms of cancer control with all the benefits of a minimally invasive therapy, and patients require less analgesic postoperatively, have a faster recovery, and a shorter hospital stay. Laparoscopic procedures are longer and technically more complex and the learning curve slow, but we believe it is beneficial in particular patients.

Surgical ablation of renal neoplasms is still in its infancy. Initial reports with cryotherapy have just been released, but long-term follow-up and further studies are required before considering cryoablation as a viable treatment for RCC.

References

American Cancer Society (1989). *Kidney cancer: a report by Illinois hospitals on cases diagnosed in 1975–1985*, Report no. 12 of results in treating cancer. American Cancer Society, Chicago.

Bosniak, M.A., Krinsky, G.A., and Waisman, J. (1996). Management of small incidental renal parenchymal tumors by watchful waiting in selected patients based on observations of tumor growth rates. *J. Urol.* **155**, 584A.

Breining, H., Helpac, B., Minderjahan, A., *et al.* (1974). Histologic and autoradiographic findings in cryonecrosis of the liver and kidney. *Cryobiology* **11**, 519–25.

Butler, B., Novick, A.C., Miller, D., *et al.* (1995). Management of small unilateral renal cell carcinomas: radical versus nephron sparing surgery. *Urology* **45**, 34–40.

Campbell, S.C., Novick, A.C., Herts, B., Fischler, D.F., Meyer, J., Levin, H.S., and Chen, R.N. (1997). Prospective evaluation of fine needle aspiration of small, solid renal masses: accuracy and morbidity. *Urology* **50** (1), 25–9.

Couillard, D.R. and deVere White, R.W. (1993). Surgery of renal cell carcinoma. *Urol. Clin. N. Am.* **20**, 263–75.

Delworth, M.G., Pisters, L.L., Fornage, B.D., *et al.* (1996). Cryotherapy for renal cell carcinoma and angiomyolipoma. *J. Urol.* **155**, 252–5.

Gill, I.S. (1998). Retroperitoneal laparoscopic nephrectomy. *Urol. Clin. N. Am.* **25**, 343–60.

Gill, I.S., McClennan, B.L., Kerbl, K., Carbone, J.M., Wick, M., and Clayman, R.V. (1994). Adrenal involvement from renal carcinoma: predictive value of computerized tomography. *J. Urol.* **152**, 1082–5.

Gill, I.S., Clayman, R.V., Ehrlich, R., Evans, R., Fuchs, G., Gersham, A., Hulbert, J.C., McDougal, E.M., Rosenthal, T., Schuessler, W.W., and Shepard, T. (1995). Complications of laparoscopic nephrectomy in 185 patients: a multi-institutional review. *J. Urol.* **154**, 479–83.

Gill, I.S., Novick, A.C., Soble, J.J., *et al.* (1998). Laparoscopic renal cryoablation: initial clinical series. *Urology* **52**, 543–51.

Giuliani, L., Gilberti, C., Matorana, G., and Rodovia, S. (1990). Radical extensive lymphadenectomy for renal cell carcinoma: long-term results and prognostic factors. *J. Urol.* **143**, 468–74.

Guillonneau, B., Ballanger, P., Lugagne, P.M., *et al.* (1996). Laparoscopic versus lumboscopic nephrectomy. *Eur. Urol.* **29**, 288–91.

Hafez, K.S., Novick, A.C., and Campbell, S.C. (1997). Patterns of tumor recurrence and guidelines for follow-up after nephron sparing surgery for sporadic renal cell carcinoma. *J. Urol.* **157**, 2067–70.

Hafez, K.S., Novick, A.C., and Butler, B. (1998). Management of small solitary, unilateral renal cell carcinomas: impact of central versus peripheral tumor location. *J. Urol.* **159**, 1156–60.

Herrlinger, A., Schrott, K.M., Schott, G., and Sigel, A. (1991). What are the benefits of extended dissection of the regional renal lymph nodes in the therapy of renal cell carcinoma. *J. Urol.* **146**, 1224–7.

Himpens, J., Cadiere, G.B., Vandewalle, J., *et al.* (1994). Operative strategy in laparoscopic nephrectomy. *Eur. Urol.* **26**, 276–80.

Kavoussi, L.R., Kerbl, K., Capelouto, C.C., *et al.* (1993). Laparoscopic nephrectomy for renal neoplasms. *Urology* **42**, 603–9.

Kerbl, K., Clayman, R.V., McDougall, E.M., *et al.* (1994). Trans-peritoneal nephrectomy for benign disease of the kidney: a comparison of laparoscopic and open surgical techniques. *Urology* **43**, 607–13.

Kigure, T., Harada, T., Yuri, Y., *et al.* (1996). Laparoscopic microwave thermotherapy on small renal tumors: experimental studies using implanted VX-2 tumors in rabbits. *Eur. Urol.* **30**, 337–82.

Lemer, S.E., Hawkins, C.A., Blute, M.L., *et al.* (1996). Disease outcome in patients with low stage renal cell carcinoma treated with nephron sparing or radical surgery. *J. Urol.* **155**, 1858–62.

Leveillee, R.J., Hoey, M.F., Mullier, P.M., *et al.* (1996). Radiofrequency interstitial renal ablation using a liquid electrolyte conductor: an *in vivo* model. *J. Endourol.* **10**, S61.

Licht, M.R. and Novick, A.C. (1993). Nephron sparing surgery for renal cell carcinoma. *J. Urol.* **149**, 1–7.

Licht, M.R., Novick, A.C., and Goormastic, M. (1994). Nephron sparing surgery in incidental versus suspected renal cell carcinoma. *J. Urol.* **152**, 39–42.

Marberger, M., Pugh, R.C.B., Auvert, J., *et al.* (1981). Conservation surgery of renal carcinoma: the EIRSS experience. *Br. J. Urol.* **53**, 528–32.

McDougall, E.M., Clayman, R.V., and Elashry, O.M. (1996). Laparoscopic radical nephrectomy for renal tumor: the Washington University experience. *J. Urol.* **155**, 1180–5.

McNichols, D.W., Segura, J.W., and DeWeerd, J.H. (1981). Renal cell carcinoma: long-term survival and late recurrence. *J. Urol.* **126**, 17–23.

Middleton, R.G. and Presto, A.J. III (1973). Radical thoracoabdominal nephrectomy for renal cell carcinoma. *J. Urol.* **110**, 36–3.

Moll, V., Becht, E., and Ziegler, M. Kidney preserving surgery in renal cell tumors: indications, techniques and results in 152. *J. Urol.* **150**, 319–23.

Morgan, W.R. and Zincke, H. (1990). Progression and survival after renal-conserving surgery for renal cell carcinoma: experience in 104 patients and extended follow-up. *J. Urol.* **144**, 852–7.

Nakada, S.Y., Moon, T.D., Gist, M., and Mahvi, D. (1997). Use of the pneumo sleeve as an adjunct in laparoscopic nephrectomy. *Urology* **49**, 612–16.

Nishiyama, T. and Terunuma, M. (1995). Laparoscopy-assisted radical nephrectomy in combination with minilaparotomy: report of initial 6 cases. *Int. J. Urol.* **2**, 124–8.

Novick, A.C. (1998). Nephron-sparing surgery for renal cell carcinoma. *Br. J. Urol.* **82**, 321–4.

Novick, A.C., Streem, S.B., Montie. J.E., *et al.* (1989). Conservative surgery for renal cell carcinoma: a single center experience with 100 patients. *J. Urol.* **141**, 835–9.

Parra, R.O., Perez, M.G., Bouillier, J.A., *et al.* (1995). Comparison between standard flank versus laparoscopic nephrectomy for benign renal disease. *J. Urol.* **153**, 1171–3.

Philips, P.E. and Messing, E.M. (1993). Role of lymphadenectomy in the treatment of renal cell carcinoma. *Urology* **41**, 9–15.

Provet, J., Tessler, A., Brown, J., Golimbu, M., Bosniak, M., and Morales, P. (1991). Partial nephrectomy for renal cell carcinoma: indications, results and implications. *J. Urol.* **145**, 472–6.

Rabinovitch, R.A., Zalefsky, M.J., Gaynor, J.J., and Fuks, Z. (1994). Patterns of failure following surgical resection of renal cell carcinoma: implications for adjuvant local and systemic therapy. *J. Clin. Oncol.* **12**, 206–12.

Robson, C.J., Churchill, B.M., and Anderson, W. (1969). The results of radical nephrectomy for renal cell carcinoma. *J. Urol.* **101**, 297–301.

Rodrigues, R., Bishoff, J.T., Chen, R.B., *et al.* (1998). Renal ablative cryosurgery in selected patients with peripheral renal masses [abstract]. *J. Urol.* **159**, 151.

Sagalowsky, A.I., Kadesky, K.T., Ewalt, D.M., and Kennedy, T.J. (1994). Factors influencing adrenal metastasis in renal cell carcinoma. *J. Urol.* **151**, 1181–4.

Selli, C., Hinshaw, W.M., Woodward, B.H., *et al.* (1983). Stratification of risk factors in renal cell carcinoma. *Cancer* **52**, 889–903.

Shalev, M., Cipolla, B., Guille, F., Staerman, F., and Lobel, B. (1995). Is ipsilateral adrenalectomy a necessary component of radical nephrectomy? *J. Urol.* **153**, 1415–17.

Skinner, D.G., Colvin, R.B., Vermillion, C.D., Pfister, R.C., and Ledbetter, W.F. (1971). Diagnosis and management of renal cell carcinoma: a clinical and pathologic study of 309 cases. *Cancer* **28**, 1165–77.

Skinner, D.G., Pfister, R.F., and Colvin, R. (1972). Extension of renal carcinoma into the vena cava: the rationale for aggressive surgical management. *J. Urol.* **107**, 711–15.

Steinbach, F., Stockle, M., Muller, S.C., *et al.* (1992). Conservative surgery of renal cell tumors in 140 patients: 21 years of experience. *J. Urol.* **148**, 24–9.

Steinbach, F., Stockle, M., and Hohenfellner, R. (1995). Current controversies in nephron-sparing surgery for renal cell carcinoma. *World J. Urol.* **13**, 163–5.

Suzuki, K., Masuda, H., Ushiyama, T., *et al.* (1995). Gasless laparoscopic-assisted nephrectomy without tissue morcellation for renal carcinoma. *J. Urol.* **154**, 1685–7.

Thrasher, J.B. and Paulson, D.F. (1993). Prognostic factors in renal cancer. *Urol. Clin. N. Am.* **20**, 247–62.

Thrasher, J.B., Robertson, J.E., and Paulson, D.F. (1994). Expanding indications for conservative renal surgery in renal cell carcinoma. *Urology* **43**, 160–8.

Uchida, M., Imaide, Y., Sugimoto, K., *et al.* (1995). Percutaneous cryosurgery for renal tumors. *Br. J. Urol.* **745**, 132–7.

Wolf, J.S. Jr, Moon, T.D., and Nakada, S.Y. (1998). Hand-assisted laparoscopic nephrectomy: comparison to standard laparoscopic nephrectomy. *J. Urol.* **160**, 22–7.

Zlotta, A.R., Wildschutz, T., Raviv, G., *et al.* Radiofrequency interstitial tumor ablation (RITA) is a possible new modality for treatment of renal cancer: *ex vivo* and *in vitro* experience. *J. Endourol.* **11**, 251–8.

27. Radical nephrectomy

Mark P. J. Wright and Alastair W. S. Ritchie

History

Gustav Simon performed the first nephrectomy in 1869 for treatment of a ureterovaginal fistula (Haeger 1988). He practiced the procedure on dogs before operating on humans. However, Morris first introduced the term 'nephrectomy' in 1881.

At the turn of the century there was controversy regarding the approach for exposure and removal of the kidney. Kocher (1878) advocated a transperitoneal approach via a midline incision but high rates of intraabdominal sepsis led most urologists to adopt a retroperitoneal approach during the first half of the twentieth century. Attempts to develop the procedure of partial nephrectomy were abandoned due to heavy intraoperative and postoperative haemorrhage.

In 1948 there were almost simultaneous case reports of large renal cell carcinomas (RCC) being removed through a thoracoabdominal approach. Robson (1963) published a paper describing the procedure of radical nephrectomy (RN) for renal tumours. In this procedure 'the entire envelope of peri-nephric fat, kidney and adrenal *en-bloc* and the lymphatic drainage field' are removed. The premise for performing this procedure for renal cancer was based on the retrospective analysis of previous nephrectomies performed at his institution where 28 per cent of cases had involvement of perinephric fat and 22 per cent had lymph node involvement. With the introduction of this new technique he reported a 5-year survival rate of 66 per cent compared to the then contemporary literature rate of 48 per cent. Radical nephrectomy thus became the 'gold standard' operation for RCC.

Preoperative preparation

Prior to embarking on surgery comprehensive counseling of the patient is required. Informed consent needs to be obtained and the topics covered in this process include a description of the procedure including: (1) the suspected diagnosis; (2) the need for removing the affected kidney, surrounding tissues, and ipsilateral adrenal gland if required; (3) the alternatives to the intended procedure such as cyroablation, partial nephrectomy, or laparoscopic RN; (4) the potential complications of the operation including hemorrhage, sepsis, pneumonia, and a deterioration in renal function; and (5) the need for long-term medical follow-up after surgery.

Thorough preparation preoperatively is necessary due to the potential compromise of respiratory function from the positioning of the patient and the extirpation of the tumour and kidney. A thorough cardiorespiratory history should be taken and physical examination performed. Patients should undergo a full blood count to exclude anemia or polycythemia, serum electrolyte and liver function analysis, and a 12-lead electrocardiogram. Chest X-ray can be used to assess the lung fields although thoracic computerized tomography (CT) is more sensitive at detecting tumour metastases. Global renal function is assessed by serum creatinine estimation and if there is any doubt about the differential function a MAG3 renogram should be performed. The extent and staging of the tumour with particular attention to the site, size, and involvement of the renal vein and inferior vena cava (IVC) is considered in Chapter 28.

Confirmation of the anatomy of the contralateral renal and ureteric unit is demonstrated by intravenous urography. Urinary tract infection must be excluded preoperatively and, if encountered on microscopy and culture of the urine, it should be treated with the appropriate antibiotics for at least 48 hours prior to the procedure.

Once this information has been obtained, careful consideration must be given as to whether or not surgery is possible. Contraindications include encasement of the great vessels with tumour, multiple co-morbidities or a high American Society of Anesthesiology (ASA) grade, and Jehovah's Witnesses if heavy blood loss is expected. Multiple metastases are another contraindication although RN may still be indicated in the context of a clinical trial (Flanigan *et al.* 2000) or in patients being treated with immunotherapy (Mickisch *et al.* 2000).

Radical nephrectomy

Standard technique

The principles of the technique involve the early ligation of the vessels and removal of the kidney outside of Gerota's fascia, ipsilateral adrenalectomy, and complete regional lymphadenectomy from the crus of the diaphragm to the origin of the inferior mesenteric artery.

Approaches

Several incisions are available for RN and no one approach is superior. The decision is usually a combination of surgeon preference and individual patient requirements. In a survey of urological surgeons undertaking RN, 46 per cent preferred the transperitoneal approach, 43 per cent a loin approach, and the rest a thoracoabdominal one (Ritchie and Chisholm 1983).

Anterior

A transperitoneal approach has the advantage of affording the surgeon access to assess the whole abdomen for metastatic disease and gives good access to the major vessels. Disadvantages include the probability of a postoperative ileus, potential complications in patients who have undergone previous extensive intraabdominal surgery, and problems in morbidly obese patients in whom access can be impaired from intra- and extraperitoneal fat deposits. Various incisions have been described including midline, paramedian, subcostal, and rooftop.

Thoracoabdominal

This approach can be useful for large upper pole tumours. A supra eighth or ninth rib incision is made, the pleura is entered, ipsilateral lung is deflated, and the diaphragm is divided peripherally, thus allowing the liver to be retracted cranially on the right and the spleen on the left. Although the amount of dissection and thus potential morbidity is greater, the superior exposure to the upper pole of the kidney and the inferior cava can be extremely useful for large upper pole tumours or level 2 caval dissections.

Flank

This approach can be utilized for small tumours, obese patients, and those patients who have had previous intraabdominal surgery. Contraindications include severe respiratory function and kyphosis of the spine. It is possible to mobilize Gerota's fascia posteriorly and anteriorly to gain access to the vascular pedicle and the great vessels. Lower rates of postoperative ileus have been reported with this approach (Sugao *et al.* 1991); however, access to the vessels is not as good as in a transperitoneal approach and exploratory laparotomy is not as easy to perform.

Extirpation

Good access is essential and one of the most important factors after approach to obtaining this is retraction. The authors recommend a self-retaining retraction system such as the Omni-Tract (Fig. 27.1) or Buck–Walter to afford good exposure.

On the right-hand side, the ascending colon is first reflected medially by incising along the line of Toldt and then the duodenum is Kocherized . This is followed by dissection of the renal pedicle. The right renal vein is short and care must be taken not to injure the IVC. The renal artery can then be mobilized lateral to the IVC or between the aorta and the IVC if there is a large medial tumour.

On the left-hand side the descending colon is mobilized and reflected medially. The left renal vein is much longer on this side and the gonadal and adrenal veins drain into it. These are mobilized and divided. The left renal vein can then be retracted to expose the renal artery posteriorly. Venous bleeding encountered whilst dissecting the renal pedicle is likely to be from one of three sources: (1) gonadal vein; (2) posterior lumbar vein entering the renal vein or IVC; (3) the IVC.

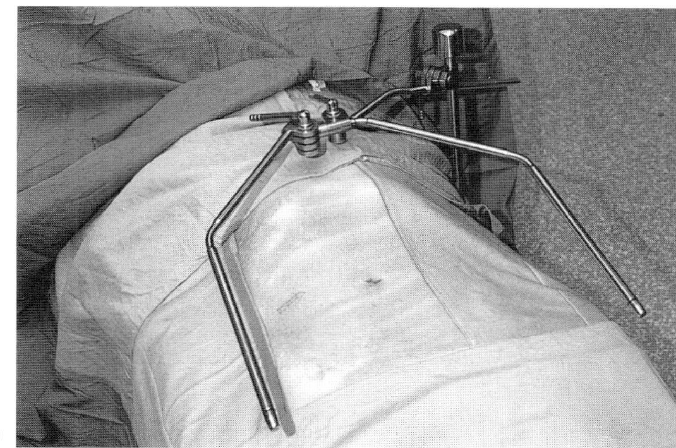

(a)

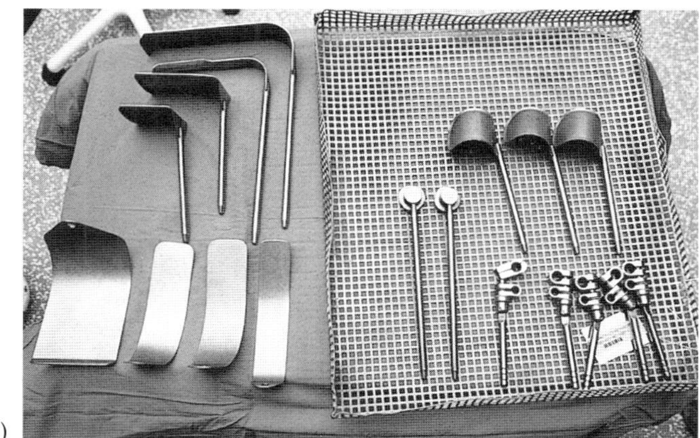

(b)

Fig. 27.1 Omni-Tract retractor system.

The renal artery is then skeletalized and triply ligated with O Vicryl ligatures and divided. Multiple renal arteries can occur in up to 38 per cent of patients (Fig. 27.2) and varying patterns are to be expected (Merklin and Michels 1958). The vein is then ligated and divided in a similar manner. The ureter is then ligated and divided. Suture ligation is then carried out to the adrenal vessels. The lymph nodes can be removed *en bloc* with the kidney and adrenal or removed separately. The lymph node dissection is initiated at the crus of the diaphragm and continued caudally to the origin of the inferior mesenteric artery.

Adrenalectomy

The standard procedure of radical nephrectomy involves excision of the ipsilateral adrenal gland *en bloc* with the kidney. However, with improved imaging systems there is now a move towards adrenal-sparing surgery. In a series of 285 consecutive patients undergoing radical nephrectomy including adrenalectomy (Shalev *et al.* 1995), 274 adrenal glands were free of disease. Of the eleven positive adrenals, seven were due to direct extension and four (1 per cent) had a metastasis. In all four of these cases there was advanced disease. Similar results have been obtained from other large series (Leibovitch *et al.* 1995; Wunderlich *et al.* 1999). Kletscher *et al.* (1995) reported on a series of 128 radical nephrectomies for T1 to T3N0M0 tumours and found that all four

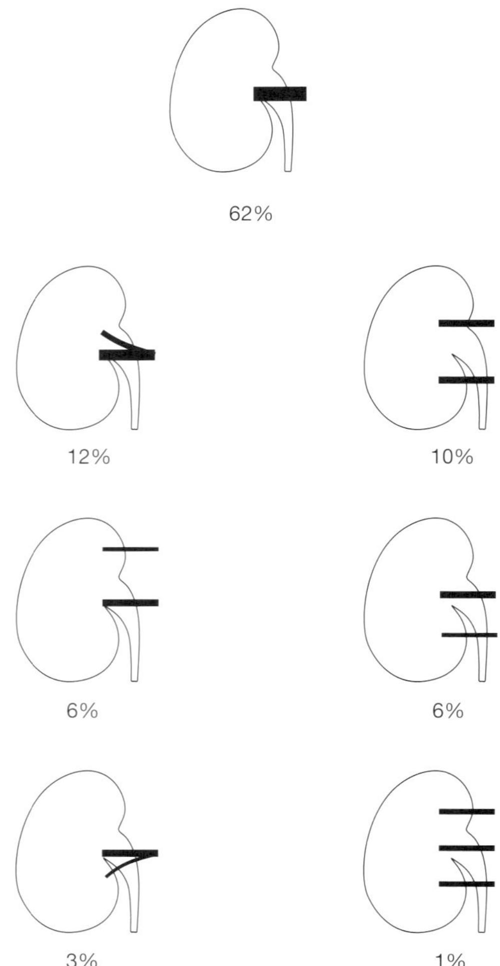

Fig. 27.2 Variations and incidence of the renal artery.

adrenal masses were identified on preoperative imaging (CT or magnetic resonance imaging (MRI)). The evidence therefore suggests that the rate of adrenal metastasis is low and that current imaging modalities are sensitive enough to pick up adrenal lesions. Simultaneous adrenalectomy at the time of radical nephrectomy should therefore be performed for large upper pole tumours or in patients with lesions visualized on preoperative scanning. These findings are confirmed in a contemporary prospective series of 511 nephrectomies from UCLA (Tsui *et al.*).

Lymphadenectomy

Preoperative CT has been found to be a good method of detecting enlarged lymph nodes in patients with RCC (Studer *et al.* 1990). In a series of 163 patients undergoing radical nephrectomy 95 per cent of enlarged lymph nodes were detected preoperatively. However, 58 per cent of patients with enlarged nodes were negative for tumor cells on subsequent histology. Thus enlarged lymph nodes on CT scan should not be interpreted as metastatic disease unless it has been proven cytologically on fine needle aspiration.

Although the procedure of radical nephrectomy classically includes the resection of hilar lymph nodes, there remains some debate as to the value of a retroperitoneal lymphadenectomy. A retrospective study on 95 lymph node dissections suggests that there is no benefit from this procedure (Ditonno *et al.* 1992). However, Giberti *et al.* (1997) have reported on a series of 328 patients who underwent a radical nephrectomy and regional retroperitoneal lymph node dissection. They reported positive lymph nodes in 6 per cent of pathologic (p)T1 tumors, 5 per cent for pT2, and 10 per cent for pT3 tumors. A 52 per cent 5-year survival for pN+M0N0 patients was reported and they concluded that the retroperitoneal lymph node dissection should be part of the radical nephrectomy procedure. Schafhauser *et al.* (1999) also showed a benefit in survival for patients undergoing a retroperitoneal lymph node dissection and radical nephrectomy versus radical nephrectomy alone. Herrlinger's group (1991) studied the effect of radical nephrectomy and retroperitoneal lymph node dissection prospectively on 320 patients and concluded that there were no increased operative risks. It would therefore appear that there is good evidence to suggest that there is a role for extended lymphadenectomy when performing a radical nephrectomy.

Closure

Once the specimen has been delivered, meticulous checks for hemorrhage and adjacent organ injury should be carried out. There exists some debate as to whether or not a drain should be placed after a RN. It is the author's view that the placement of a drain adds little to the potential morbidity of the procedure and can indicate postoperative hemorrhage. We usually place a fenestrated 20 French silastic drain.

Midline and subcostal incisions can be closed *en masse* with a loop suture of at least four times the length of the incision taking at least 1 cm bites of tissue (Leaper *et al.* 1977). Loin and thoraco-abdominal incisions should be closed in layers reapproximating the muscles and taking care not to damage the intercostals neurovascular bundles that run along the inferior border of each rib. If the pleural cavity has been opened, then a chest drain should be placed and connected to a sump containing sterile water before the lung is re-inflated and diaphragm repaired.

Postoperative management

Following radical nephrectomy there are reported complication rates of between 13 and 20 per cent (Swanson and Borges 1983). Results of a prospective audit of complications following RN over a 7–year period from our own hospital are presented in Table 27.1.

Table 27.1 Complications following radical nephrectomy.

Complication	Percentage
Death	1
Pneumonia	4
Wound infection	3
Urinary tract infection	2
Renal failure	1
Hemorrhage	1
Left ventricular failure	1

Systemic complications associated with any major intra-abdominal procedure include myocardial infarction, cerebrovascular accident, congestive cardiac failure, pulmonary embolus, atelectasis, and pneumonia. These can be reduced by appropriate preoperative preparation, avoidance of hypotension during the procedure, appropriate fluid/blood replacement, postoperative chest physiotherapy, early mobilization, and the use of antithrombotic compression stockings.

Intraoperative gastrointestinal injury should be carefully excluded before closing the abdominal wound. Hepatic tears can be repaired with mattress sutures, splenic lacerations often require splenectomy, and suspected pancreatic trauma requires a partial pancreatectomy with an omental patch onlay. Symptoms and signs of acute pancreatitis in the postoperative period should alert the surgeon to the possibility of a pancreatitis fistula. Drain fluid should be analysed for analyase levels and pH. Computerized tomography is the best form of imaging to demonstrate a retroperitoneal fluid collection. Management involves percutaneous or surgical drainage to avoid formation of a pancreatic abscess or pseudocyst. The majority of fistulae clear spontaneously with adequate drainage. Rarely, excision of the fistulous tract and then use of a Roux-en-Y jejunal loop anastomosed to the pancreas is required.

Gastrointestinal ileus is a common problem following transperitoneal surgery. Oral intake should be omitted until bowel sounds are present and flatus has been passed. Nasogastric tubes are particularly helpful where the duodenum has been mobilized for underlying right-sided renal tumours.

Secondary hemorrhage can occur following radical nephrectomy and bleeding may be from the renal pedicle or occasionally from an unrecognized injury to a neighboring structure during surgery. Resuscitation with intravenous fluids and blood should be given and, if the hemorrhage is significant, re-exploration and removal of hematoma and ligation of the bleeding point(s) should be carried out. Rarely, the wound will required packing and subsequent pack removal 48 hours later.

Pneumothorax may occur during loin or thoracoabdominal incisions. A formal check of the pleura should be made before closing by asking the anesthetist to hyperinflate the patient's lungs. Any defects should be directly repaired. A postoperative pneumothorax of > 10 per cent or a tension pneumothorax requires immediate insertion of a chest drain.

Laparoscopic radical nephrectomy

Recent advances in laparoscopic surgery have prompted surgeons to attempt radical nephrectomy as a minimally invasive procedure. The perceived benefits are a shorter hospital stay and decreased patient discomfort (Nakada *et al.* 1996), whereas concerns about the procedure include adequacy of surgical margins, tumor spillage, and trocar site seeding of tumor.

Caddeddu *et al.* (1998) report on a series of 157 laparoscopic radical nephrectomies for T1–2 renal cell cancers with a mean follow-up of 19 months. They found no evidence of port site or renal fossa recurrence. Similar results were obtained from Abbou's

group (1999) who also showed a significantly lower hospital stay and blood loss for laparoscopic compared to open radical nephrectomy.

It therefore appears that there may be a place for laparoscopic radical nephrectomy for patients with small organ-confined tumours.

References

Abbou, C.C., Cicco, A., Gasman, D., Hoznek, A., Antiphon, P., Chopin, D.K., and Salomon, L. (1999). Retroperitoneal laparoscopic versus open radical nephrectomy. *J. Urol.* **161** (6), 1776–80.

Cadeddu, J.A., Ono, Y., Clayman, R.V., Barrett, P.H., Janetschek, G., Fentie, D.D., McDougall, E.M., Moore, R.G., Kinukawa, T., Elbahnasy, A.M., *et al.* (1998). Laparoscopic nephrectomy for renal cell cancer: evaluation of efficacy and safety: a multicenter experience. *Urology* **52** (5), 773–7.

Ditonno, P., Traficante, A., Battaglia, M., Grossi, F.S., and Selvaggi, F.P. (1992). Role of lymphadenectomy in renal cell carcinoma. *Prog. Clin. Biol. Res.* **378**, 169–74.

Flanigan, F.L., Blumenstein, B.A., and Salmon, S. (2000). Cytoreduction in metastatic renal cancer: the results of the Southwest Oncology Group trial 8949. *J. Urol.* **163** (4 suppl.), abstr. 685.

Giberti, C., Oneto, F., Martorana, G., Rovida, S., and Carmignani, G. (1997). Radical nephrectomy for renal cell carcinoma: long-term results and prognostic factors on a series of 328 cases. *Eur. Urol.* **31** (1), 40–8.

Haeger, K. (1988). *The illustrated history of surgery*, 1st edn. Harold, Starke, London.

Herrlinger, A., Schrott, G., Schrott, K., and Sigel, A. (1991). What are the benefits of extended dissection of the regional renal lymph nodes in the therapy of renal cell carcinoma. *J. Urol.* **145** (5), 1224–7.

Kletscher, B.A., Qian, J., Bostwick, D.G., Andrews, P.E., and Zincke, H. (1995). Prospective analysis of multifocality in renal cell carcinoma: influence of histological pattern, grade, number, size, volume and deoxyribonucleic acid ploidy. *J. Urol.* **153** (3, part 2), 904–6.

Kocher, T. (1878). Nephrotome wegen Neirnsarkom. *Deut. Z. Chirc.* **9**, 312.

Leaper, D.J., Pollock, A.V., and Evans, M. (1977). Abdominal wound closure: a trial of nylon, polyglycolic acid and steel sutures. *Br. J. Surg.* **64**, 603–6.

Leibovitch, I., Raviv, G., Mor, Y., Nativ, O., and Goldwasser, B. (1995). Reconsidering the necessity of ipsilateral adrenalectomy during radical nephrectomy for renal cell carcinoma. *Urology* **46** (3), 316–20.

Merklin, R.J. and Michels, N.A. (1958). The variant renal and suprarenal blood supply with data on the ureteral and gonadal arteries. *J. Int. Coll. Surg.* **28** (1), 41–74.

Mickisch, G.H., Garin, A., and Madej, M. (2000). Tumour nephrectomy plus interferon-a is superior to interferon-a alone in metastatic renal cell carcinoma. *J. Urol.* **163** (4 suppl.), abstr. 778.

Nakada, S.Y., McDougall, E.M., and Clayman, R.V. (1996). Laparoscopic extirpation of renal cell cancer: feasibility, questions, and concerns [review; 34 references]. *Sem. Surg. Oncol.* **12** (2), 100–12.

Ritchie, A.W. and Chisholm, G.D. (1983). Management of renal carcinoma—a questionnaire survey. *Br. J. Urol.* **55**, 591–4.

Robson, C.J. (1963). Radical nephrectomy for renal cell carcinoma. *J. Urol.* **89** (1), 37–41.

Schafhauser, W., Ebert, A., Brod, J., Petsch, S., and Schrott, K. (1999). Lymph node involvement in renal cell carcinoma and survival chance by systemic lymphadenectomy. *Anticancer Res.* **19**, 1573–8.

Shalev, M., Cipolla, B., Guille, F., Staerman, F., and Lovel, B. (1995). Is ipsilateral adrenalectomy a necessary component of radical nephrectomy? *J. Urol.* **153** (5), 1415–17.

Studer, U.E., Scherz, S., Scheidegger, J., Kraft, R., and Sonntag, R. (1990). Enlargement of regional lymph nodes in renal cell carcinoma is often not due to metastases. *J. Urol.* **144** (2), 243–5.

Sugao, H., Matsuda, M., Nakano, E., Seguchi, T., and Sonoda, T. (1991). Comparison of lumbar flank approach and transperitoneal approach for radical nephrectomy. *Urologia Int.* **46** (1), 43–5.

Swanson, D.A. and Borges, P.M. (1983). Complications of trans-abdominal radical nephrectomy for renal cell carcinoma. *J. Urol.* **129**, 704.

Tsui, K., Shvarts, O., Barbaric, Z., Figlin, R., deKernion, J.B., and Belldegrun, A. Is adrenalectomy a necessary component of radical nephrectomy? UCLA experience with 511 radical nephrectomies. *J. Urol.* **163**, 437–41.

Wunderlich, H., Schlichter, A., Reichelt, O., Zermann, D.H., Janitzky, V., Kosmehl, H., and Schubert, J. (1999). Real indications for adrenalectomy in renal cell carcinoma. *Eur. Urol.* **35** (4), 272–6.

28. Inferior vena caval tumors

Andrea Sorcini and John A. Libertino

Renal cell carcinoma (RCC) has the propensity to infiltrate the surrounding parenchyma, to penetrate the capsule and extend into the perirenal adipose tissue and adjacent structures, and, in particular, to infiltrate the venous system and propagate into the inferior vena cava (IVC). Electron microscopy reveals renal tumor cells around thin-walled vessels and small fenestrations with the neoplastic process prolapsing into the lumen. These characteristics are consistent with RCC, but they have been described in conjunction with adrenocortical carcinomas and Wilms' tumors. An association with caval thrombi has been sporadically reported in association with renal sarcoma, retroperitoneal leiomyosarcoma, malignant histiocytoma, adrenal pheochromocytoma, paratesticular rhabdomyosarcoma, and transitional cell carcinoma of the renal pelvis (Rodriguez *et al.* 1997; Novick *et al.* 1990; Williams *et al.* 1996; Skinner *et al.* 1989).

RCC involves the renal vein 16–33 per cent of the time and the inferior vena cava 4–13 per cent of the time (Marshall *et al.* 1970; Skinner *et al.* 1972*a*; Novick and Cosgrove 1980; Ljungberg *et al.* 1995). Although the prognosis for patients with RCC is difficult to predict because of variations in clinical behavior, definite risk factors for relapse of disease and overall prognosis have been established. Tumor staging is the most important prognostic factor. It is based on size of the neoplasm, presence of tumor extension beyond the capsule of the kidney, invasion through Gerota's fascia, evidence of regional lymph node metastases, and the presence of distant metastatic disease.

Infiltration of vessels has been shown to be a highly negative prognostic predictor in many other tumors, such as testicular, colorectal, and breast carcinoma. The importance of venous invasion in RCC is still a controversial subject. Although some reports demonstrate that involvement of the venous system adversely affects survival, others have shown that venous extension alone, excluding capsular penetration and perirenal fat infiltration, does not have an adverse impact on survival (Golimbu *et al.* 1986; Hatcher *et al.* 1991; Libertino *et al.* 1987; Swierzewski *et al.* 1994). Moreover, there is no agreement on the prognostic value of the level of the intracaval tumor extension, capsular infiltration, and metastatic spread (Ljungberg *et al.* 1995; Hatcher *et al.* 1991; O'Donohoe *et al.* 1987; Giuliani *et al.* 1990; Clayman *et al.* 1980; Sosa *et al.* 1984; Montie *et al.* 1991).

Despite these controversies, great improvement has been achieved in the surgical treatment of this challenging clinical entity. Initial reports concerning the surgical therapy of patients with RCC with IVC extension were generally negative, except for a few sporadic reports of long-term survivors (Myers *et al.* 1968; McDonald and Priestley 1943; Marshall *et al.* 1970). Walters and Priestley (1934) were the first to report on the successful extraction of a large intravenous extension of RCC by opening the IVC. In 1956, the first long-term survivor after caval thrombectomy was reported (Skinner *et al.* 1972*b*). It was recognized that RCC with extension of tumor thrombus into the IVC was a potentially curable condition provided the entire lesion could be removed. Five- and 10-year survival rates of 55 and 43 per cent, respectively, were reported. Advances in surgical techniques and postoperative care have enhanced the safety of the operation and determined improved outcome. In the absence of metastatic disease, surgical extirpation represents the only possibility of prolonging survival rates and potential cure.

Clinical presentation and diagnosis

The clinical presentation of patients with retroperitoneal tumors and extension of thrombi into the IVC depends, for the most part, on the original neoplasm. RCC with caval extension affects the right side more frequently than the left (ratio 2:1) and men more often than women (ratio 2:1) in their fifth to sixth decade of life. If RCC is the original tumor, the lesion is usually not smaller than 5 cm in diameter.

Hematuria, weight loss, and flank pain are present in about 50 per cent of patients. Classically, signs strictly secondary to caval involvement are related to the rapidity of the development of venous obstruction. Bilateral edema of the lower extremities and, in men, acute onset of varicocele occur in 32–45 per cent of patients and are associated with recent caval occlusion. The presence of venous collateral on the abdominal wall (caput medusae) is present in 12–15 per cent of patients and this means that the obstruction has been present long enough to permit the development of a collateral venous network (Pritchett *et al.* 1986). The documented association of pulmonary embolism has been reported. When tumor thrombus occludes the contralateral renal vein, the clinical presentation could be characterized by renal failure. Similarly, involvement of the hepatic veins by the obstructing process could result in hepatic insufficiency.

Radiologic imaging is important for the initial diagnosis or suspicion of caval extension of the tumor. It also represents a fundamental aspect of the preoperative assessment. Renal or retroperitoneal tumors are typically diagnosed by excretory urography (intravenous pyelography, IVP), ultrasonography, or computerized tomography (CT) obtained because of some other clinical indication or, with increasing frequency, as an incidental finding. Usually, the suspicion of caval thrombi is raised by these initial tests (mainly ultrasonography or CT or both).

Unfortunately, these studies are not adequate to accurately complete clinical staging. The therapeutic approach is based on further imaging studies to rule out the presence of metastatic disease and to define the level of the tumor thrombus. A complete oncologic evaluation should include CT of the abdomen and pelvis with and without an intravenous contrast agent and chest x-ray followed by CT of the chest if indicated because of suspicious or positive findings on radiography of the chest. Bone scan and CT of the head are also obtained if clinically indicated.

Ultrasonography and conventional CT have demonstrated good specificity in detecting the presence of tumor thrombus in the renal vein and IVC. Their sensitivity has been reported to range from 65 to 90 per cent as single studies, reaching 87 per cent when used in combination (Kallman *et al.* 1992). The accuracy of detecting cranial extension of the thrombus ranges from 68 to 95 per cent. The main problems associated with CT are poor bolus injection of intravenous contrast media and that inaccurate timing of scanning may generate false-negative results. Sources of error usually are underopacification streaming, streak artifacts, and layering caused by the increased density of contrast material compared with blood. Large masses or diffuse lymphadenopathy may compress and obscure the IVC. Helical and electron beam CT scanning has the ability to pinpoint renal vein involvement with improved accuracy and may represent an important method of evaluating these tumors (Welch and LeRoy 1997). Doppler examination with ultrasonography is an excellent study of the proximal renal vein and the intrahepatic and suprahepatic portions of the IVC, but it is suboptimal in visualizing the distal renal vein and the infrahepatic vena cava. The accuracy of sonographic examinations is operator-dependent and may be influenced by the patient's body habitus.

Inferior venography with catheterization of the femoral vein has been preferred for many years and, in some institutions, is still considered the standard modality to determine the level of tumor thrombus. Venacavography has been demonstrated to be 100 per cent sensitive in many series (Kallman *et al.* 1992; Horan *et al.* 1989; Lang 1984; Hietala *et al.* 1988). False-positive results have been reported in instances of extrinsic compression of the cava, generally secondary to metastatic lymphadenopathy. Inferior venacavography is an accurate method to establish the extent of the tumor thrombus. A retrograde transatrial study from the basilic vein is often necessary to define the cranial level of the thrombus, particularly when the vena cava is completely obstructed (4–10 per cent of patients with vena cava involvement).

During the last decade, magnetic resonance imaging (MRI) has gained increasing importance in the evaluation of retroperitoneal masses, especially when the vessels are involved. Because flowing blood gives no signal, the tumor thrombus gives a relatively high signal within the low signal of the vascular lumen. T1-weighted spin echo images have a high resolution to vascular structures, are relatively free from motion artifact, and provide precise and clear anatomic depiction. When a gradient refocused echo technique is used, the blood vessels appear bright compared with surrounding soft tissues and intracaval thrombus. The use of gadolinium may be helpful in distinguishing tumor thrombus from bland thrombus without the need for an invasive procedure and without affecting renal function, which sometimes is already impaired in this group of patients.

Another advantageous characteristic of MRI is the possibility of obtaining images in multiple planes. Coronal and sagittal views are the most familiar to surgeons, resembling traditional cavography (Fig. 28.1). Sagittal views provide accurate information regarding the cranial extent of the thrombus even in the presence of complete caval obstruction (Fig. 28.2). Problematic differentiation between

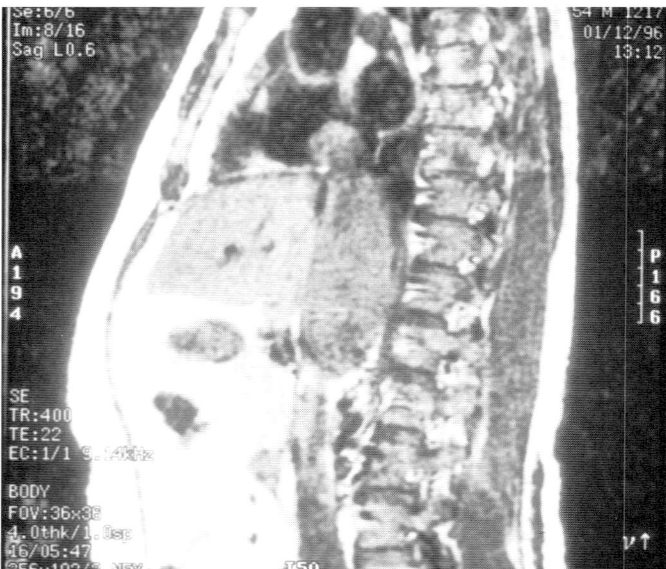

Fig. 28.1 Magnetic resonance image. Intraatrial tumor thrombus (sagittal view).

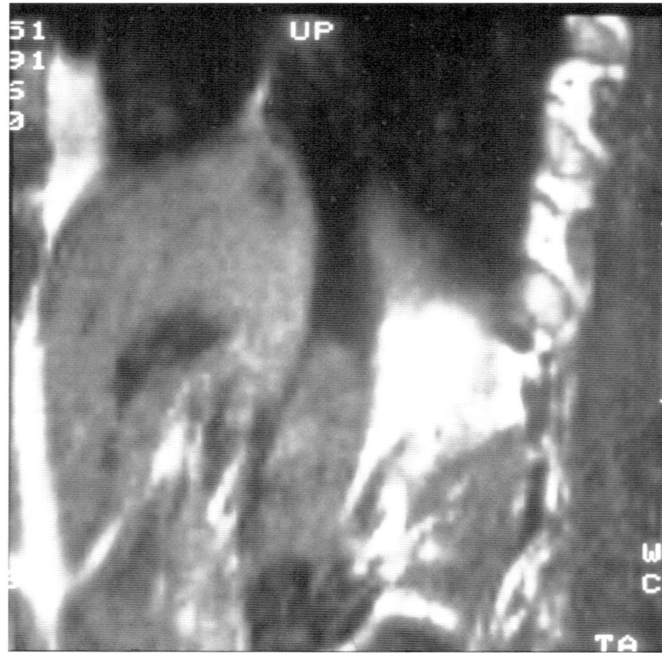

Fig. 28.2 Magnetic resonance image. Level II tumor thrombus.

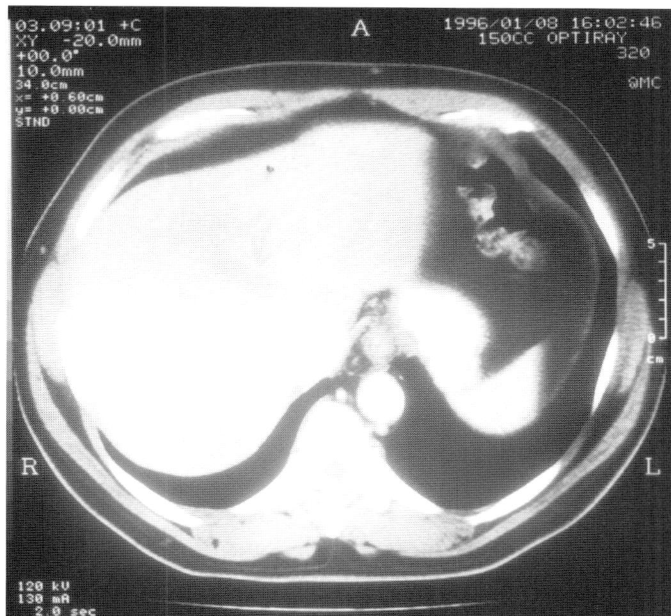

Fig. 28.3 Magnetic resonance image. Tumor thrombus at the level of the hepatic veins.

infrahepatic and suprahepatic tumor thrombi has been reported. Axial images are often useful to demonstrate the vascular patency of important structures, such as the contralateral vein or the hepatic veins (Fig. 28.3). In most of the reported series, the sensitivity of MRI has been reported to be between 98 and 100 per cent. False-positive results are mostly reported as a consequence of flow artifacts. Axial single-breath-hold gradient echo images are useful in excluding these artifacts. The most accurate detection of the extent of caval thrombus is obtained by complementary use of cavography and MRI (Straton *et al.* 1992).

Transesophageal echocardiography (TEE) is a relatively new technique for imaging the heart and great vessels. It may be useful preoperatively, particularly when it is not clear whether the cranial extent of the thrombus is infrahepatic or suprahepatic. Additional information that can be obtained by TEE concerns the presence of thrombus invading the hepatic veins, ventricular size and function, and the presence of valvular heart disease in patients who potentially may require cardiopulmonary bypass (Treiger *et al.* 1991). Furthermore, the presence of a patent foramen ovale can be excluded by TEE. This information is useful to assess the need for repair of the defect at the time of tumor thrombectomy to prevent paradoxical embolism to the brain in the presence of intraoperative or postoperative pulmonary embolism. In many institutions, TEE is used mainly intraoperatively to confirm the cephalad extent of the thrombus, to monitor the patency of the pulmonary artery, to monitor cardiac function, and to verify complete removal of the entire tumor thrombus (Glazer and Novick 1997).

Patients with tumor thrombi above the level of the hepatic veins are also evaluated with pulmonary function tests and ventilation/perfusion scans to exclude the presence of pulmonary embolus. All patients who are scheduled to have cardiopulmonary bypass and deep hypothermic circulatory arrest have coronary angiography to rule out the presence of significant ischemic disease. Finally, preoperative renal artery embolization has been proposed to facilitate nephrectomy of large renal masses, ligating the anteriorly located renal vein first and reducing the amount of blood loss. Other factors favoring preoperative angioinfarction are reported shrinkage of the tumor thrombus and improvement in the clinical status after angioinfarction (Craven *et al.* 1991). Decreased blood loss and thrombus shrinkage have not been confirmed, and occasional reports of pulmonary embolism after angioinfarction make the use of arterial embolization controversial and a matter of personal preference (Christensen *et al.* 1985).

Preoperative evaluation is of great importance in establishing the surgical strategy. The presence of metastatic disease should be ruled out with certainty. Metastatic dissemination represents a contraindication to surgery in asymptomatic patients.

The accurate assessment of the extent of the intraluminal tumor thrombus is of paramount importance (Fig. 28.4). The surgical approach, the position of the patient on the table, and the

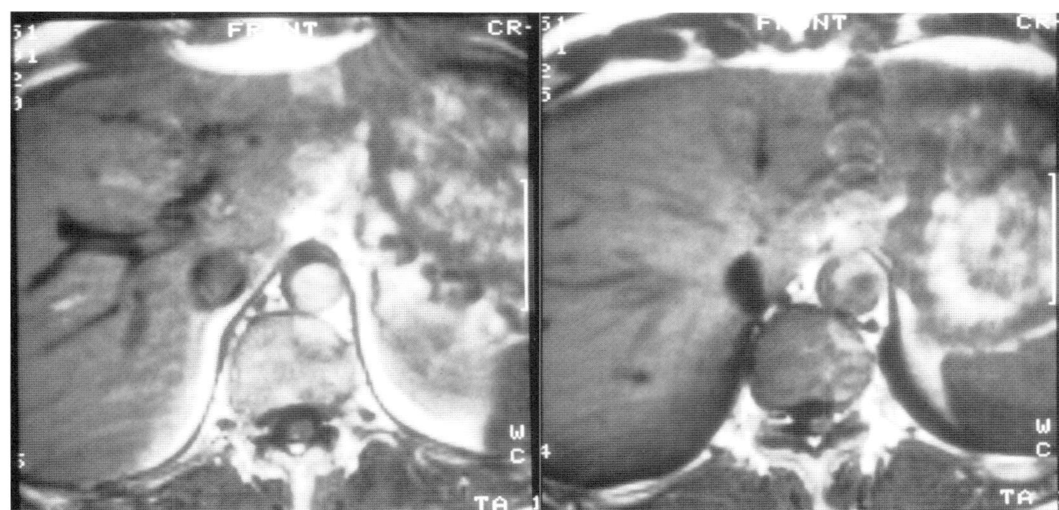

Fig. 28.4 Magnetic resonance image. Axial view of the cranial level of the tumor thrombus in the intrahepatic vena cava.

need for cardiopulmonary bypass are dependent on the level of the thrombus.

Classification and surgical approach

Regardless of the level of the tumor, the incision chosen, and the likelihood of needing cardiopulmonary bypass, the abdominal and retroperitoneal portions of the procedure are completed before any required thoracic procedure. The resectability of the tumor is initially assessed. The abdomen and retroperitoneum are carefully examined, with the goal of identifying any evidence of metastatic disease and excluding extension of the tumor beyond Gerota's fascia. The incidence of metastatic lesions incidentally found by surgical exploration ranges from 21 to 44 per cent, according to different series (Pritchett *et al.* 1986; Polascik *et al.* 1998).

After the initial assessment, the most critical aspects of procedures for retroperitoneal tumors with caval extension are control and dissection of the IVC regardless of the tumor level (Figs 28.5 and 28.6). Exposure of the vena cava is the critical step to prevent the two major complications associated with this procedure: pulmonary embolization and hemorrhage. For the right-sided lesion, the duodenum is mobilized medially by the Kocher maneuver, and the hepatic flexure of the colon, ascending colon, and root of small bowel mesentery are dissected to expose the IVC. For a left-sided tumor, additional dissection of the descending colon and splenic flexure is performed. If necessary, the vena cava is dissected from the caudate lobe of the liver, ligating the minor hepatic veins. Mobilization of the liver and dissection of the IVC just below the diaphragm are occasionally necessary for a tumor at a higher level (Fig. 28.7). The contralateral renal vein and the vena cava proximal and distal to the tumor thrombus are

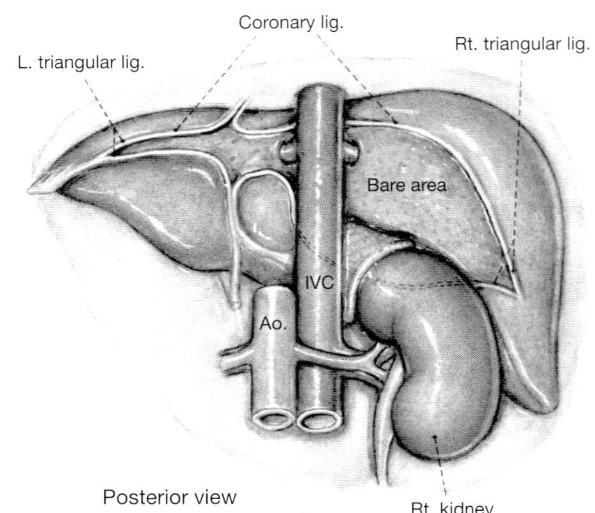

Fig. 28.6 Surgical anatomy of the upper abdomen: posterior view. (Reprinted with permission of Lahey Clinic, Burlington, Massachusetts.)

dissected and surrounded with Rummel tourniquets. The degree of caval dissection depends mainly on the level of the thrombus.

In the perioperative period, the major complication associated with tumor thrombectomy is pulmonary embolization. Excessive dissection and manipulation of the renal tumor or vena cava or both may cause dislodgment of the thrombus, with tragic consequences. Bland thrombus may be present distal or, more often,

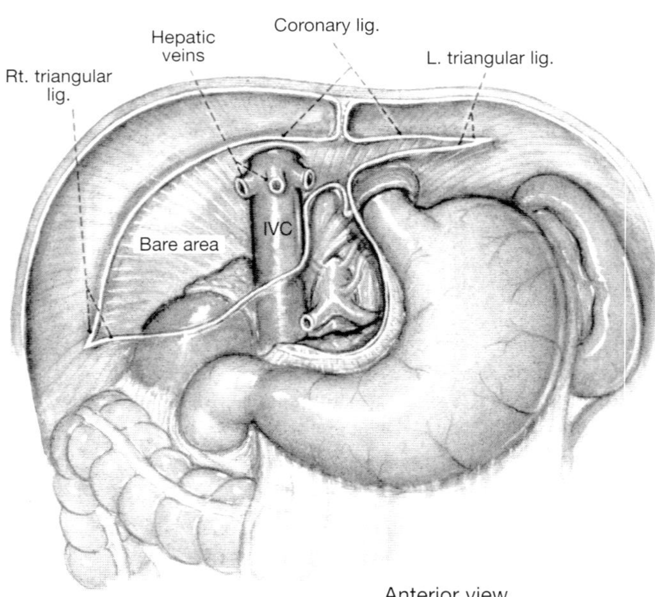

Fig. 28.5 Surgical anatomy of the upper abdomen: anterior view. (Reprinted with permission of Lahey Clinic, Burlington, Massachusetts.)

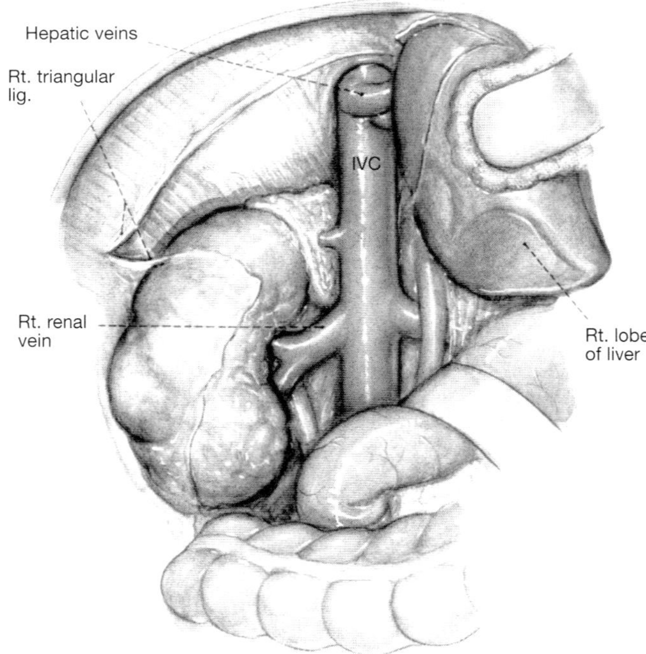

Fig. 28.7 Exposure of the intrahepatic inferior vena cava by incision of the right triangular ligament and medial mobilization of the right hepatic lobe. (Reprinted with permission of Lahey Clinic, Burlington, Massachusetts.)

proximal to the tumor thrombus. In a few instances, the proximal bland thrombus causes such a severe inflammatory reaction that complete removal of the thrombus is not possible without resection of the vena cava. In these instances, biopsy of the intracaval bland thrombus is accomplished to confirm the benign nature of the lesion and to place a Greenfield filter or a DeWeese clip below the ostia of the renal veins to prevent postoperative pulmonary embolization.

In the author's institution in the last 3 years, the surgical strategy for patients with caval thrombi above the level of the hepatic veins has also been changed. Thrombectomy is performed before performing any dissection of the kidney to minimize the chance of intraoperative embolization. As a general rule, an effort should be made to minimize maneuvers that could contribute to deterioration of renal function.

The left renal vein usually has a rich venous collateral network via the gonadal, adrenal, lumbar, inferior diaphragmatic, and ureteral veins. The right renal vein does not have such an abundant collateral system (Fig. 28.8). These considerations are important in situations in which, because of tumor infiltration of the vena cava, complete caval resection is warranted. Ligation of the proximal left renal vein can be tolerated well without long-term damage to the kidney even though transient elevation of the crea-

tinine level and permanent renal dysfunction have been reported in almost 50 per cent of patients (McCullough and Gittes 1975).

A simple way to predict whether ligation of the left renal vein is going to affect renal function is to clamp the left renal vein and the right ureter and administer intravenous indigo carmine dye. The appearance of Indigo blue dye in the urine within 12 minutes is a sign that ligation of the vein is tolerated fairly well, and resection of the vena cava can be performed. Evidence of a pressure less than 40 mm Hg in the ligated vein is another sign of collateral venous drainage (Clayman *et al.* 1980).

The presence of obstructing caval thrombus may be helpful paradoxically in stimulating the development of collaterals before the operation. When the extent of caval infiltration is such that complete resection and ligation of the renal vein are necessary (especially on the right side) and it appears that renal function is impaired, the only alternatives available are replacement of the vena cava with pericardium or synthetic tube grafts, renal autotransplantation, or reanastomosis of the renal vein to the portal or splenic vein. To preserve renal function as much as possible, attention should be paid to the placement of vascular clamps. Many times, the shape and position of the tumor thrombus into the vena cava permit partial occlusion of the vena cava with a long curved vascular clamp. This is feasible mainly for level I and, rarely, for level II thrombi. In other instances, the tumor configuration permits placement of the vascular clamp or tourniquet around the vena cava in an oblique fashion so that the contralateral vein is above the clamp and venous drainage into the proximal inferior vena cava is maintained.

The surgical approach is based on the distal level of the tumor thrombus (Fig. 28.9).

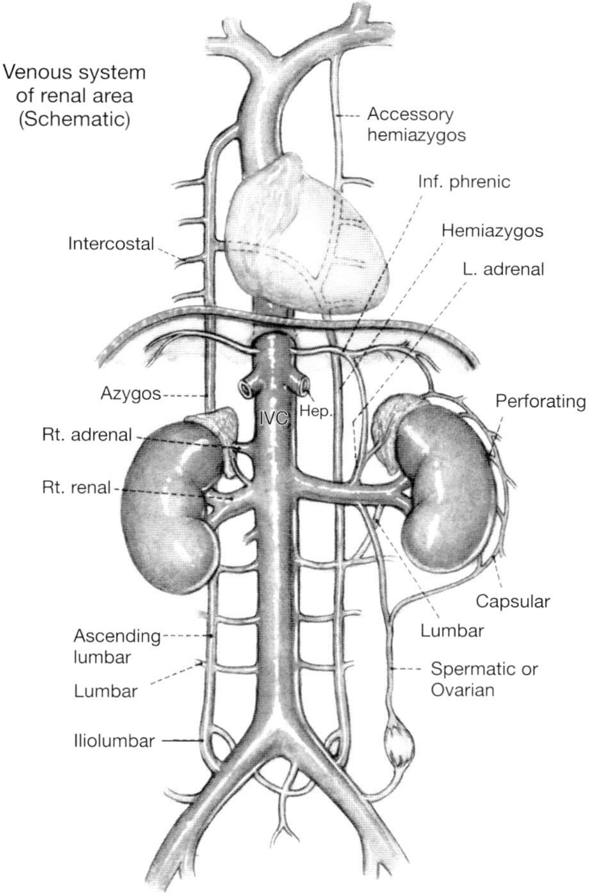

Fig. 28.8 Collateral venous drainage of left kidney compared with right kidney. (Reprinted with permission of Lahey Clinic, Burlington, Massachusetts.)

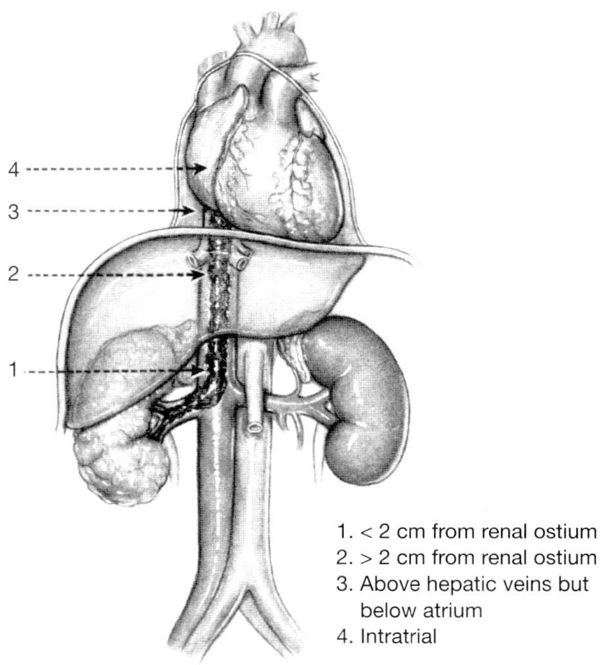

Fig. 28.9 Classification of inferior vena caval tumor by cranial level. (Reprinted with permission of Lahey Clinic, Burlington, Massachusetts.)

Level I thrombi (< 2 cm from renal venous ostium)

Level I tumor thrombi are limited to < 2 cm from the renal vein ostium. They are usually not adherent to the caval wall or adherent only at the level of the renal vein, and the vena cava is usually only partially obstructed. Most of the time, these tumor thrombi are 'floating' in the lumen of the IVC and can easily be 'milked' back into the renal vein.

These tumors are usually approached through a supracostal 11th rib incision. The retroperitoneum is entered through the lumbodorsal fascia, and the peritoneum is pushed medially. The kidney is dissected outside of Gerota's fascia. Anteriorly, the dissection is carried between Gerota's fascia and the peritoneum. The duodenum is Kocherized for right-sided tumors or the descending colon is mobilized medially for left-sided lesions. With this maneuver, the renal vein is exposed. The renal artery is ligated and divided posteriorly if arterial embolization has not previously been performed. Two DeBakey clamps are applied to permit a side bite of the vena cava after the thrombus has been 'milked' into the renal vein. With this technique, the flow into the vena cava and contralateral renal vein is preserved, but the thrombus is isolated and embolization is prevented. The vena cava is incised about 5 mm around the ostium of the renal vein. After the radical nephrectomy with tumor thrombectomy has been completed, the clamp close to the ostium is removed, and the vena cava is closed with a 4–0 Prolene running suture. The same technique can be applied using a midline longitudinal or a transverse abdominal incision.

Level II thrombi (> 2 cm from venous ostium, below the hepatic veins)

Excision of level II tumors requires more extensive dissection to achieve control of the vena cava above and below the thrombus and the contralateral renal vein. These tumors are approached through a right thoracoabdominal incision to permit optimal exposure of the infrahepatic and, when necessary, intrahepatic IVC (Fig. 28.10). After medial mobilization of duodenum and hepatic flexure, the IVC is exposed. When necessary, identification and ligation of minor hepatic veins to the caudate lobe of the liver facilitate exposure of most of the intrahepatic vena cava. When

the tumor thrombus is up to the level of the hepatic veins, incision of the coronary and right triangular ligament with medial mobilization of the right hepatic lobe permits excellent exposure of the entire intrahepatic vena cava (see Fig. 28.7).

Vascular control is ensured by placing Rummel tourniquets or vascular clamps sequentially on the infrarenal vena cava, contralateral renal vein, and suprarenal vena cava above the upper level of the thrombus (Fig. 28.11). Ligation of the lumbar veins entering the vena cava in the tract included in the tourniquets may be helpful to prevent bothersome bleeding at the time of cavotomy. When vascular control is achieved, a cavotomy is performed starting laterally, just below the renal ostium, and continuing on the lateral wall up to 1 to 2 cm below the tip of the thrombus. The thrombus is dissected and removed with the entire renal ostium (Fig. 28.12). A generous piece of vena cava may need to be removed when tumor infiltration is suspected. The lumen of the vena cava is flushed and inspected for residual thrombus infiltrating the wall or extending into lumbar or gonadal veins.

The cavotomy is closed using a 4–0 Prolene running suture (see Fig. 28.12). Before the suturing has been completed, the distal tourniquets are released to flush out residual air or clots or both. The tourniquets are removed, starting with the distal inferior vena cava, followed by the contralateral renal vein, and finally the proximal clamp (Libertino *et al.* 1998).

Traditionally, dissection of the entire kidney was performed before the cavotomy and thrombectomy. In the last 3 years, we have elected to postpone the dissection until after the vascular component of the operation has been completed to prevent tumor embolization associated with overaggressive manipulation of the kidney. The only dissection performed is to ligate the renal artery if it has not previously been embolized.

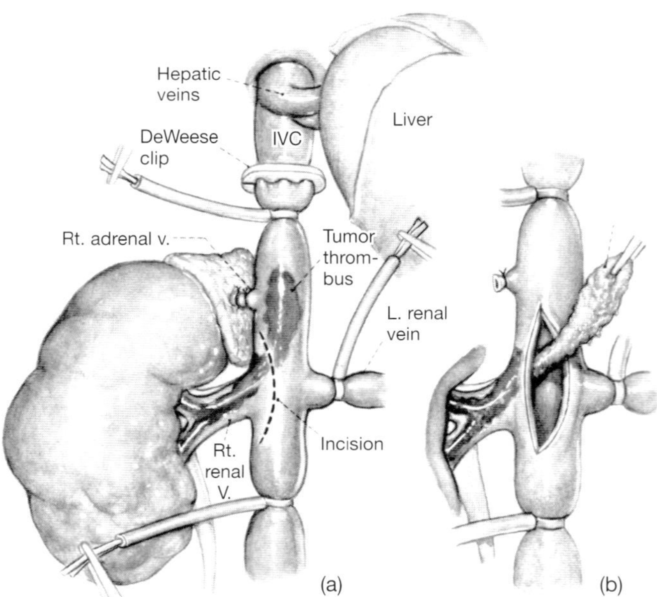

Fig. 28.11 Isolation of the inferior vena cava by proximal and distal clamping and clamping of the contralateral renal vein. (Reprinted with permission of Lahey Clinic, Burlington, Massachusetts.)

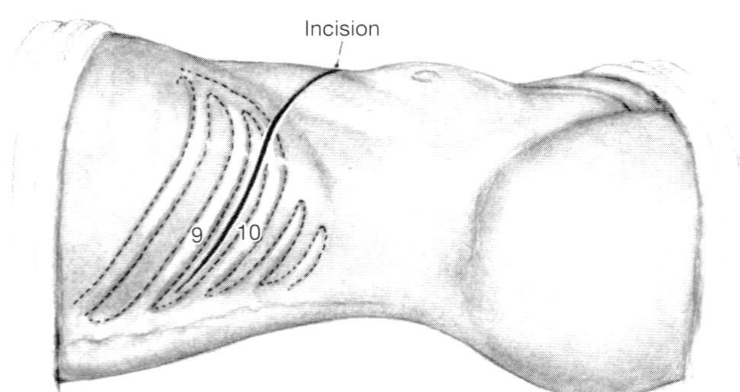

Fig. 28.10 Approach to level II tumor thrombi of the inferior vena cava. (Reprinted with permission of Lahey Clinic, Burlington, Massachusetts.)

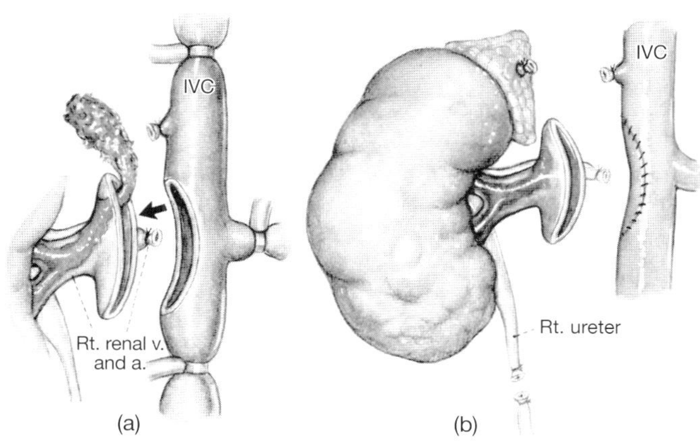

Fig. 28.12 (a), (b) *En bloc* removal of right kidney, tumor thrombus, and patch of inferior vena cava surrounding the venous ostium. (Reprinted with permission of Lahey Clinic, Burlington, Massachusetts.)

Level III thrombi (tumor above the hepatic veins but below the cavoatrial junction)

The approach to level III tumor thrombi is probably the most controversial, and a variety of surgical techniques to excise these tumors have been described. Intraoperative TEE is usually used for these tumors. Thrombi at this level can safely be excised with traditional technique, but with an increase risk of blood loss and complications. In some of these patients, additional exposure of the intrahepatic IVC may be achieved by incising the triangular and coronal ligaments and rotating the right hepatic lobe medially. Dissection to control the vena cava just below the diaphragm or in the intrapericardial portion is sometimes difficult and may cause dislodgment of the thrombus with disastrous consequences.

The main issues in resecting level III tumors include the fact that clamping the vena cava in its intrapericardial portion can compromise venous return to the heart. Subsequent decreased cardiac output, hemodynamic instability, and hypoperfusion of vital organs may occur unless the aorta is controlled as well. Cross-clamping the vena cava can also produce significant hemorrhage from venous collaterals that is often difficult to control. A trial of cross-clamping may be attempted to see how well the obstruction of the cava is tolerated hemodynamically.

Paradoxically, resection of a tumor that is completely obstructing is usually better tolerated: chronic obstruction probably leads to the development of a collateral network that is able to provide sufficient return of blood. Patients with partial obstruction have a sudden increase of venous pressure at the time of cross-clamping, with a subsequent increased chance of bleeding. Moreover, the hepatic veins are usually difficult to control and, to prevent excessive bleeding, dissection and temporary clamping of the porta hepatis (Pringle's maneuver) are generally necessary. Although this technique is often effective, prolonged clamping of the hepatic hilum (more than 20 minutes) may cause ischemic damage to the liver. Clamping of the portal vein leads to the accumulation of ischemic metabolites in the intestine. These are suddenly washed into the central circulation when the cross-clamp is released and

may lead to 'declamping' shock. Instances of spontaneous splenic rupture immediately following Pringle's maneuver have been described (Baniel *et al.* 1994).

Resection of level III tumors frequently requires some vascular bypass. Venovenous bypass is a method of avoiding the hemodynamic variations related to cross-clamping of the IVC that is often used during the anhepatic phase of liver transplantation. Bypass is initiated after careful dissection of the IVC and ligation of the lumbar veins. Venous drainage is established from the femoral vein or the IVC well below the caudal aspect of the tumor thrombus using a 20 to 28 French venous cannula. Cannulation of the vena cava in relation to the thrombus could increase the risk of dislodging the thrombus or part of it, with massive embolization. The outflow is returned either by direct cannulation of the auricle of the right atrium or by cannulation of the brachial or axillary veins (Fig. 28.13).

Portal decompression may be obtained by placing a 16 French venous cannula into the inferior mesenteric vein. Coated heparin-bonded tubing connects the cannulas to an electromagnetic centrifugal pump to establish venovenous bypass at 2 to 2.5 l/minute. With this technique, systemic heparinization (1 mg/kg) is necessary. The main advantage of venovenous bypass is that blood return to the heart is maintained. Unfortunately, the problems of bleeding from the hepatic veins and the necessity to dissect and control the intrapericardial vena cava with the risk of embolization are not obviated by this technique.

Cardiopulmonary bypass with deep hypothermic circulatory arrest, traditionally used for level IV tumors, is also a valid option for tumor thrombi above the level of the hepatic veins but not intraatrial. This technique requires specialized anesthesiology and neurology staff and is performed under continuous electroencephalographic monitoring.

Level IV thrombi (in the right atrium)

For tumors that extend to the right atrium, it is necessary to use cardiopulmonary bypass. TEE is routinely used. The abdomen is explored as usual to confirm the absence of metastatic disease and resectability of the tumor. The vena cava is exposed in its infrahepatic portion, and the minor hepatic veins to the caudate lobe are ligated. At this point, the thoracic portion of the operation can be started. Access to the right atrium and great vessels can be obtained through a median sternotomy combined with either a midline longitudinal or a transverse chevron abdominal incision (Fig. 28.14). We recently described a minimal access approach with a small right subclavicular incision to access the right subclavian artery for arterial access rather than the traditional aortic arch approach and a right parasternal incision to access the right atrium (Fitzgerald *et al.* 1998) (Fig. 28.15).

After venous access has been achieved, a two-stage venous cannula is placed into the auricle of the right atrium. An arterial cannula is placed into either the right subclavian artery or the aortic arch, and extracorporeal circulation is instituted. At this point, the patient is cooled down to 16–18°C. Circulatory arrest is achieved after metabolic suppression with thiopental. When electroencephalography monitoring shows an isoelectric pattern, circulatory arrest has been obtained (Belis *et al.* 1989). Topical

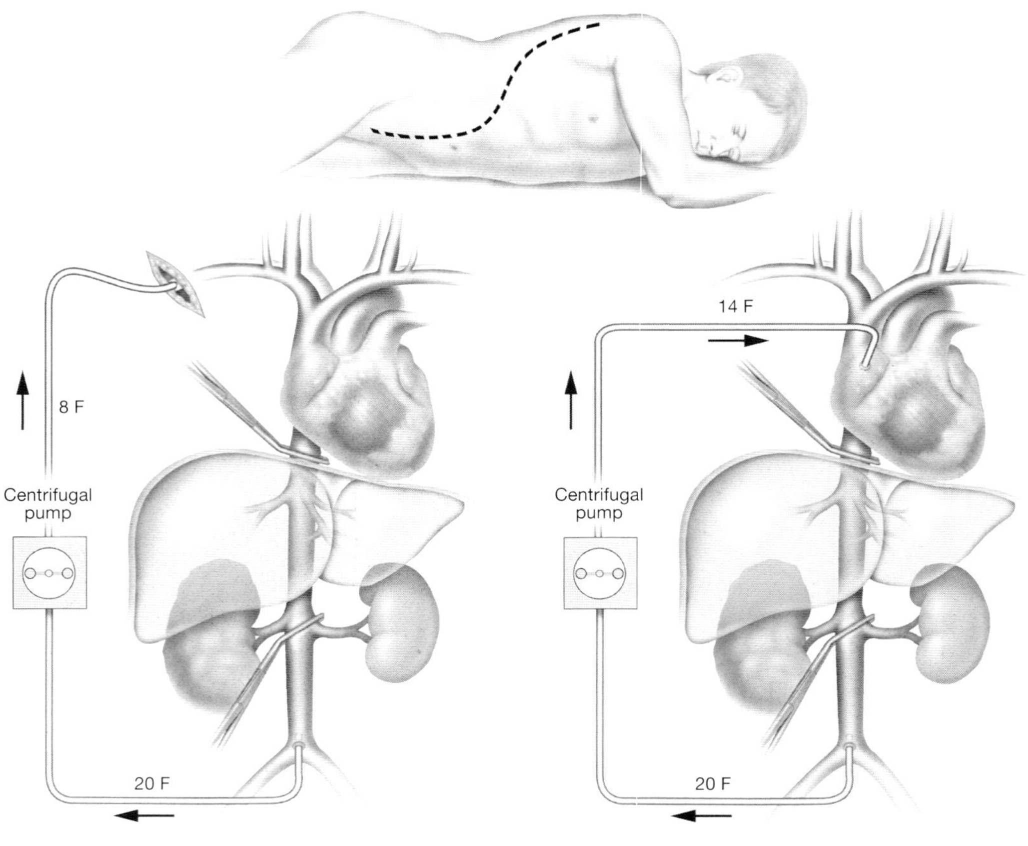

Fig. 28.13 Venovenous bypass between distal inferior vena cava and right subclavian vein or right atrium. (Reprinted with permission of Lahey Clinic, Burlington, Massachusetts.)

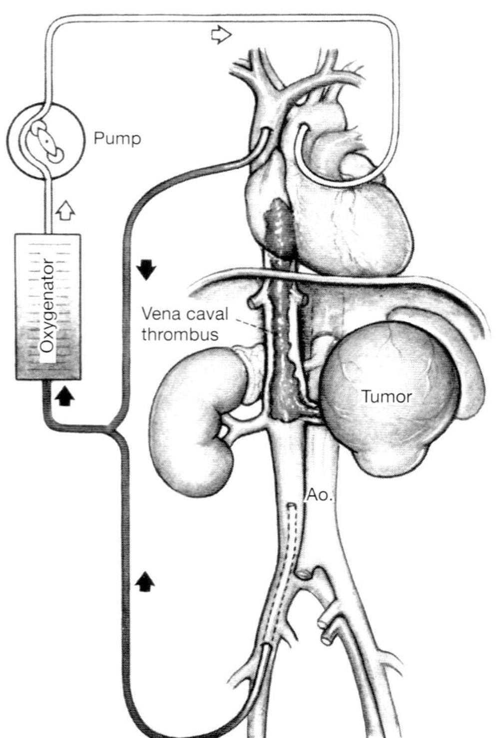

Fig. 28.14 Cardiopulmonary bypass for cavoatrial tumor thrombus using traditional technique. (Reprinted with permission of Lahey Clinic, Burlington, Massachusetts.)

hypothermia is maintained, placing physiologic slush saline solution around the heart and in the abdomen.

After cooling and cardiac arrest have been achieved, cardiopulmonary bypass is discontinued, the arterial line is clamped, and the patient is exsanguinated, draining all the blood into the oxygenator reservoir. The atrial venous cannula is removed. A longitudinal right atriotomy is performed simultaneously with the inferior venacavotomy. These two incisions provide complete visualization of the interior of the atrium and IVC and resection of the tumor thrombus. Careful examination of the atrial and caval lumen in a bloodless field permits accurate detection of residual tumor adherent to the wall or infiltrating the ostia of communicating vessels as hepatic veins, lumbar veins, gonadal vein, and contralateral renal vein. The tumor can usually be dissected off the caval wall and off these vessels or, sometimes, resection of a portion of the cava become necessary.

After excision of the tumor thrombus has been completed, the atriotomy and cavotomy are closed using a 4–0 Prolene running suture. Rarely, a Greenfield caval filter is positioned below the ostium of the remaining renal vein to prevent postoperative pulmonary embolization. After closure of vena cava and atrium, the venous cannula is reinserted, and cardiopulmonary bypass is reinstituted. If the aortic arch was cross-clamped, the clamp is removed and the patient warmed. At this point, the heparin is neutralized with protamine, based on activated whole blood clotting times and the anticoagulation corrected with blood products. When normal cardiac activity returns and the patient warms to

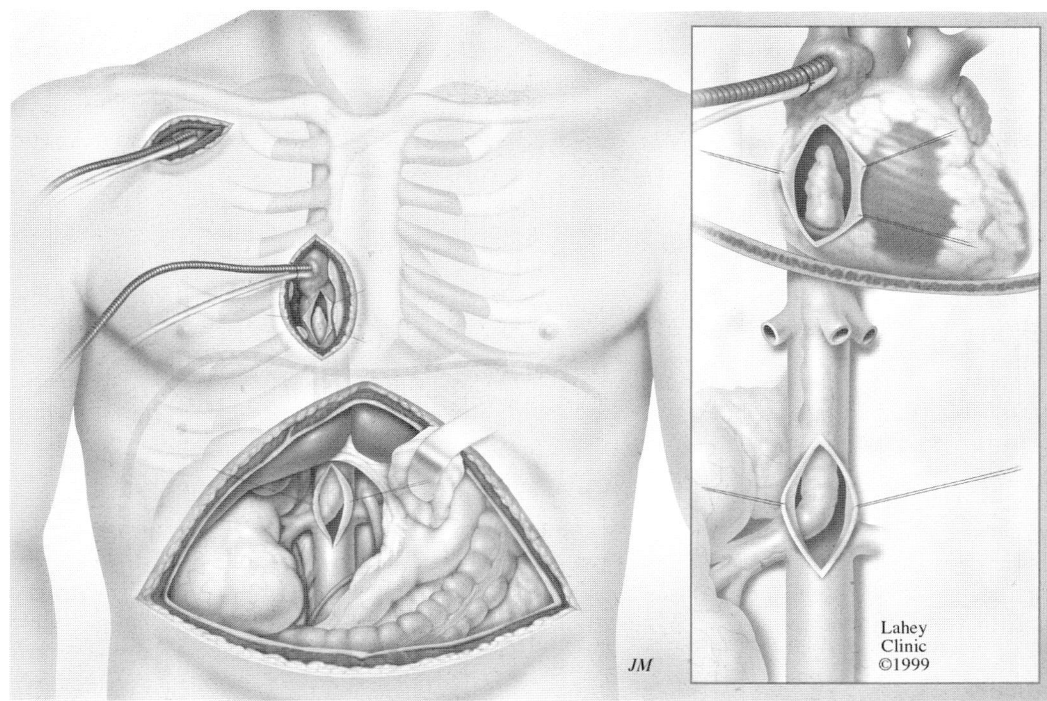

Fig. 28.15 Minimal access approach for cardiopulmonary bypass and deep hypothermic cardiocirculatory arrest. (Reprinted with permission of Lahey Clinic, Burlington, Massachusetts.)

37°C of nasopharyngeal temperature, cardiopulmonary bypass is slowly disconnected.

During this time, excision of the retroperitoneal tumor is completed. As previously mentioned, traditionally, mobilization of the kidney or adrenal gland was performed before the institution of cardiopulmonary bypass and the administration of heparin. The rationale was to minimize blood loss, avoiding an extensive dissection on an anticoagulated patient. A report from Hershey Medical Center (Belis *et al.* 2000) and our personal experience showed that the estimated blood loss with this new surgical approach is acceptable and comparable to our experience with traditional techniques. The reason to postpone dissection of the retroperitoneal mass until after the institution of cardiopulmonary bypass is to prevent tumor embolization secondary to excessive surgical manipulation.

The advantages of cardiopulmonary bypass and deep hypothermic circulatory arrest are the possibility of performing accurate resection of the tumor thrombus in a bloodless field and the ability to have complete control of the vascular structures and the thrombus.

The technique of deep hypothermia and circulatory arrest was initially introduced in pediatric patients with Wilms' tumors infiltrating the vena cava up to the right atrium (Belis *et al.* 2000; Murphy *et al.* 1973; Utley *et al.* 1973). The technique was then applied to adult patients. Maintaining a very low temperature of the head with topical ice bags and limiting as much as possible the time of circulatory arrest can minimize the occurrence of neurologic complications related to this technique. It is also important to suppress cerebral metabolic activity using either thiopental or isoflurane (Hirotani *et al.* 1999).

Studies have shown that the technique of retrograde cerebral perfusion during circulatory arrest may provide significant protection against neurologic complications (Raskin *et al.* 1996; Appoo *et al.* 1998; Beltz *et al.* 1999). There is a direct correlation between circulatory arrest time and the incidence of neurologic sequelae (Oates *et al.* 1995). It is generally believed, and it is our experience, that a circulatory arrest time shorter than 30–45 minutes is a safe limit to avoid ischemic damage (Hickey 1998; Jonas 1999). Cardiac protection is achieved as well with systemic and topical hypothermia and, in selected patients at risk for cardiac ischemia, with infusion of cold (4°C) potassium (20 mEq/l) cardioplegic solution. If surgical coronary artery disease is diagnosed preoperatively, coronary artery bypass can be performed after cardiopulmonary bypass has been started (Wickey *et al.* 1988; Zinman *et al.* 1989). Other organs have a tolerance to the 'protected' ischemia associated with deep hypothermia and circulatory arrest that can last for several hours (Bigelow and McBirnie 1953). The liver and kidney can tolerate up to 2 hours of hypothermic circulatory arrest without having functional sequelae. The use of cardiopulmonary bypass appears to have no influence on the prognosis.

Advancements in surgical techniques and the improved ability to correct coagulopathy after bypass play an important role in the perioperative management and overall outcome (Bidstrup *et al.* 1989.

Vena cava reconstruction

The prognosis of patients undergoing radical excision of retroperitoneal tumors and caval thrombectomy is influenced by the ability to extirpate the neoplastic process completely. In patients with complete resection of all tumor found at inspection of the vena cava, there is a 36 per cent 5-year actuarial survival rate compared with evidence of no survivors within 6 postoperative months if complete resection was not possible (Pritchett *et al.*

1986). Depending on the amount of vena cava that needs to be resected, the reconstruction technique may vary from patch reconstruction using either synthetic material or autogenous tissue to replacement entire segments of the vena cava with prosthetic tube grafts (Marshall and Reitz 1985; Bower *et al.* 1993; Huguet *et al.* 1995; Sarkar *et al.* 1998).

In asymptomatic patients with complete caval obstruction, the presence of venous collaterals that reconstitute the vena cava above the level of obstruction may be presumed, and this is often demonstrated with cavography or MRI. Unfortunately, these patients may not have signs or symptoms of obstruction preoperatively, but they become symptomatic postoperatively if resection of the tumor compromises the collateral network. This is particularly evident when extirpation of the tumor includes resection and ligation of the vena cava.

Partial reconstruction may be accomplished using a patch of pericardium that is readily available if the procedure is performed through a median sternotomy or a minimal access approach for cardiopulmonary bypass or through a right thoracoabdominal incision. Other options are the use of autologous vein (saphenous, umbilical; Motta *et al.* 1987) or the use of polytetrafluoroethylene patches.

Tube grafts of expanded polytetrafluoroethylene have been used in instances in which the extent of caval resection was extensive (Sarti 1970). The efficacy of synthetic tubes for venous grafts was experimentally documented in dogs. In a few instances, creation of femoral arteriovenous fistula was required to increase the venous pressure and maintain the patency. Clinically, there are only few small series of patients with vena cava replaced by a synthetic tube graft. It appears that an expanded polytetrafluoroethylene tubular vascular graft externally supported by stents to counteract the abdominal pressure represents the best option for synthetic material (Motta *et al.* 1987). A replaced vena cava that was patent at 96 months has been reported (Okada *et al.* 1996).

Prognosis

The prognosis of patients with retroperitoneal tumors with extension into the IVC or into the right atrium is dictated by the nature of the primary lesion. In the presence of adrenocortical carcinoma, the prognosis is very poor, with an overall survival rate of only 15 per cent at 5 years. The rarity of this neoplasm and the even more rare presence of tumor thrombus in the venous system do not permit any conclusions regarding the prognostic significance of caval invasion. Most of the patients sporadically reported did not survive for more than 2 years. Although much larger series of RCC have been published, the prognosis has been difficult to predict because of the wide variety of clinical behaviors that characterize these lesions. Only a few studies have reported cancer-specific survival rates after surgical treatment of RCC with caval invasion.

It is difficult to interpret studies on renal cell cancers with caval extension because of lack of long-term follow-up and, for the most part, because of the small number of patients. Only in a few studies has a multivariate analysis investigated the impact of different tumor characteristics on the prognosis. In fact, the wide variability in survival rates in the literature is probably a reflection of the different characteristics (that is, histology, staging) of the primary renal cancer rather than a consequence of caval extension.

Tumor stage is the most important prognostic factor. Histopathologic grading and DNA ploidy also have prognostic value. Other well-established risk factors are a sarcomatoid histologic presentation (spindle cells or irregular tissue pattern) or highly polymorphic nuclear or nucleolar configuration (Skinner *et al.* 1971; Fuhrman *et al.* 1982). It has been accepted that involvement of the vena cava does not worsen the prognosis of the patient with RCC in the absence of metastasis. The specific prognostic values of local and distant metastatic spread, capsular perforation, venous invasion, and level of tumor thrombus are still controversial.

Metastatic disease

The presence of lymphatic, visceral, or hematogenous metastatic disease at the time of presentation is an ominous sign. After complete removal of the primary tumor and resection of the thrombus, the 5-year survival rate for patients without metastases at the time of surgery has been reported to be between 30 and 72 per cent (Libertino *et al.* 1987; Glazer and Novick 1996; Belis and Kandzari 1990; Reissigl *et al.* 1995; Neves and Zincke 1987). Several studies (Libertino *et al.* 1987; Belis and Kandzari 1990; Heney and Nocks 1982) have demonstrated diminished 5-year survival rates for patients with metastases discovered at the time of surgery or by pathologic examination. Skinner and colleagues (1989) reported actuarial and actual 1-year survival rates of 37 and 26 per cent, respectively. Only 8 per cent of patients were alive at 1 year if complete excision of all grossly apparent tumor was not possible (Skinner *et al.* 1989). Although the prognostic value of metastatic disease is considered an ominous sign, reports (Nesbitt *et al.* 1997; Tongaonkar *et al.* 1995) showed that the presence of distant metastasis does not influence survival rates. These studies found that invasion of perirenal fat and spread to locoregional lymph nodes was a negative prognostic factor. Our experience and that of others (Hatcher *et al.* 1991; Swierzewski *et al.* 1994; Neves and Zincke 1987; Tongaonkar *et al.* 1995; Kuczyk *et al.* 1997) confirm that both lymph node and hematogenous metastases are associated with a poor prognosis.

Perirenal fat infiltration

RCC with caval infiltration tends to be large and to have extension beyond the renal capsule at presentation. Perirenal fat extension has been identified in 40–67 per cent of patients in different series (Hatcher *et al.* 1991; Polascik *et al.* 1998; Glazer and Novick 1996). The prognostic importance of perinephric extension is controversial. We (Swierzewski *et al.* 1994) did not find any statistically significant difference in survival in 29 patients with extracapsular disease compared with 43 patients with organ-confined disease. These finding have been supported by others and by a review of patients with tumor thrombi above the level of the hepatic veins (levels III and IV) (Skinner *et al.* 1989; Polascik *et al.* 1998). However, most of the other series reported have demonstrated improved long-term survival in patients without evidence of capsular penetration compared with patients with perinephric fat involvement (Hatcher *et al.* 1991; Glazer and Novick 1996).

Caval wall infiltration

The spread of tumor into the renal vein or vena cava is commonly and incorrectly defined as 'venous invasion'. In reality, tumor thrombi from RCC, adrenocortical carcinoma, or other rare neoplasms grow into the venous lumen and only occasionally are found to invade the venous wall if studied microscopically (Sosa *et al.* 1984). Invasion of the renal vein wall is common. Actual invasion of the wall of the vena cava is present in about 20 per cent of patients, but it is usually limited to the region of the renal vein ostium (Skinner *et al.* 1972b; Neves and Zincke 1987; Suggs *et al.* 1991). Invasion of the venous wall may be suggestive of poor prognosis, but this phenomenon has not been studied commonly (Hatcher *et al.* 1991). Intensive infiltration of the vena caval wall, precluding the possibility of complete resection of the entire tumor thrombus, is associated with decreased survival. Sosa and colleagues (1984) reported no survivors at the end of 1 year when only a nephrectomy was performed, leaving the tumor thrombus in the vena cava (Mrstik *et al.* 1992).

Level of tumor thrombus

The first surgical series reporting on prognosis of the patient suggested that there was an unfavorable correlation between tumors with a high level of caval extension and survival. Skinner *et al.* (1989) indicated a 5-year survival rate of 35 per cent after surgery for patients with subhepatic IVC thrombi compared with 18 per cent for patients with intrahepatic extension and 0 per cent for patients with atrial thrombi.

Even in recent sporadic reports, the level of vena caval invasion was found to be an important prognostic factor (Sosa *et al.* 1984). In particular, Montie *et al.* (1991), investigating 68 patients, noted that intraatrial extension of tumor thrombus indicated a significantly worse prognosis than at other levels of vena caval involvement. Currently, most studies (Ljungberg *et al.* 1995; Hatcher *et al.* 1991; Swierzewski *et al.* 1994; O'Donohoe *et al.* 1987; Giuliani *et al.* 1990; Clayman *et al.* 1980; Cherrie *et al.* 1982) suggest that the upper extent of tumor thrombus has no significant impact on survival. Glazer and Novick (1997) demonstrated extended cancer-free survival after surgical treatment of intraatrial tumor extension in 18 patients. The survival rates obtained were comparable to those reported for patients with RCC and infrahepatic or intrahepatic caval thrombi. Of these patients, 50 per cent had evidence of metastatic disease within the first 18 postoperative months. When the literature is analysed regarding the potential prognostic importance of higher versus lower cranial extent of caval thrombi, it is important to ascertain whether there is an increased incidence of metastatic disease at the initial presentation or whether there is an increased incidence of postoperative metastases in patients with local disease only at time of surgery. Despite controversies, it appears that neither the incidence of metastases at presentation nor postoperatively is increased in patients with tumor thrombi at higher levels (Novick *et al.* 1990; Hatcher *et al.* 1991; Swierzewski *et al.* 1994; Pagano *et al.* 1992).

Summary

Retroperitoneal tumors with extension into the vena cava present a challenging problem from an oncologic and surgical standpoint. Accurate definition of the cranial extent of the thrombus is of paramount importance in deciding the surgical approach. An aggressive surgical approach is the only treatment for patients with RCC and caval extension that may provide cure. In patients without metastatic disease at the time of surgery, long-term survival can be obtained. The surgical strategy is important in minimizing the incidence of pulmonary embolism and severe hemorrhage. The ability to perform accurate resection of the primary tumor and the thrombus has prognostic significance and depends on optimal exposure of the lumen of the vena cava. Cardiopulmonary bypass and deep hypothermic circulatory arrest are valuable methods of facilitating accurate resection of suprahepatic tumor thrombi.

References

Appoo, J.J., Ralley, F., Baslaim, G., and de Varennes, B. (1998). Anesthesia for deep hypothermic circulatory arrest in adults: experience with the first 50 patients. *J. Cardiothoracic Vasc. Anesth.* **12**, 260–5.

Baniel, J., Bihrle, R., Wahle, G.R., and Foster, R.S. (1994). Splenic rupture during occlusion of the porta hepatis in resection of tumors with vena caval extension. *J. Urol.* **151**, 992–4.

Belis, J.A. and Kandzari, S.J. (1990). Five-year survival following excision of renal cell carcinoma extending into inferior vena cava. *Urology* **35**, 228–30.

Belis, J.A., Pae, W.E. Jr, Rohner, T.J. Jr, *et al.* (1989). Cardiovascular evaluation before circulatory arrest for removal of vena caval extension of renal carcinoma. *J. Urol.* **141**, 1302–7.

Belis, J.A., Levinson, M.E., and Pae, W.E. Jr (2000). Complete radical nephrectomy and vena caval thrombectomy during circulatory arrest. *J. Urol.* **163**, 434–6.

Beltz, M.S., Pae, W.E. Jr, and Belis, J.A. (1999). Application of retrograde cerebral perfusion and moderate systemic hypothermic circulatory arrest for cavoatrial tumor resection. *Techn. Urol.* **5**, 87–91.

Bidstrup, B.P., Royston, D., Sapsford, R.N., and Taylor, K.M. (1989). Reduction in blood loss and blood use after cardiopulmonary bypass with high dose aprotinin (Trasylol). *J. Thoracic Cardiovasc. Surg.* **97**, 364–72.

Bigelow, W.G. and McBirnie, J.E. (1953). Further experiences with hypothermia for intracardiac surgery in monkeys and groundhogs. *Ann. Surg.* **137**, 361–5.

Bower, T.C., Nagorney, D.M., Toomey, B.J., *et al.* (1993). Vena cava replacement for malignant disease: is there a role? *Ann. Vasc. Surg.* **7**, 51–62.

Cherrie, R.J., Goldman, D.G., Lindner, A., and deKernion, J.B. (1982). Prognostic implications of vena caval extension of renal cell carcinoma. *J. Urol.* **128**, 910–12.

Christensen, K., Dyreborg, U., Andersen, J.F., and Nissen, H.M. (1985). The value of transvascular embolization in the treatment of renal carcinoma. *J. Urol.* **133**, 191–3.

Clayman, R.V., Jr., Gonzalez, R., and Fraley, E.E. (1980). Renal cancer invading the inferior vena cava: clinical review and anatomical approach. *J. Urol.* **123**, 157–63.

Craven, W.M., Redmond, P.L., Kumpe, D.A., Durham, J.D., and Wettlaufer, J.N. (1991). Planned delayed nephrectomy after ethanol embolization of renal carcinoma. *J. Urol.* **146**, 704–8.

Fitzgerald, J.M., Tripathy, U., Svensson, L.G., and Libertino, J.A. (1998). Radical nephrectomy with vena caval thrombectomy using a minimal access approach for cardiopulmonary bypass. *J. Urol.* **159**, 1292–3.

Fuhrman, S.A., Lasky, L.C., and Limas, C. (1982). Prognostic significance of morphologic parameters in renal cell carcinoma. *Am. J. Surg. Pathol.* **6**, 655–63.

Giuliani, L., Giberti, C., Martorana, G., and Rovida, S. (1990). Radical extensive surgery for renal cell carcinoma: long-term results and prognostic factors. *J. Urol.* **143**, 468–74.

Glazer, A.A. and Novick, A.C. (1996). Long-term followup after surgical treatment for renal cell carcinoma extending into the right atrium. *J. Urol.* **155**, 448–50.

Glazer, A. and Novick, A.C. (1997). Preoperative transesophageal echocardiography for assessment of vena caval thrombi: a comparative study with venacavography and magnetic resonance imaging. *Urology* **49**, 32–4.

Golimbu, M., Joshi, P., Sperber, A., Tessler, A., Al-Askari, S., and Morales, P. (1986). Renal cell carcinoma: survival and prognostic factors. *Urology* **27**, 291–301.

Hatcher, P.A., Anderson, E.E., Paulson, D.F., Carson, C.C., and Robertson, J.E. (1991). Surgical management and prognosis of renal cell carcinoma invading the vena cava. *J. Urol.* **145**, 20–4.

Heney, N.M. and Nocks, B.N. (1982). The influence of perinephric fat involvement on survival in patients with renal cell carcinoma extending into the inferior vena cava. *J. Urol.* **128**, 18–20.

Hickey, P.R. (1998). Neurologic sequelae associated with deep hypothermic circulatory arrest. *Ann. Thoracic Surg.* **65** (6 suppl.), S65–76.

Hietala, S.O., Ekelund, L., and Ljungberg, B. (1988). Venous invasion in renal cell carcinoma: a correlative clinical and radiologic study. *Urol. Radiol.* **9**, 210–16.

Hirotani, T., Kameda, T., Kumamoto, T., Shirota S., and Yamano, M. (1999). Protective effect of thiopental against cerebral ischemia during circulatory arrest. *Thorac. Cardiovasc. Surg.* **47**, 223–8.

Horan, J.J., Robertson, C.N., Choyke, P.L., *et al.* (1989). The detection of renal carcinoma extension into the renal vein and inferior vena cava: a prospective comparison of venacavography and magnetic resonance imaging. *J. Urol.* **142**, 943–8.

Huguet, C., Ferri, M., and Gavelli, A. (1995). Resection of the suprarenal inferior vena cava. The role of prosthetic replacement. *Arch. Surg.* **130**, 793–7.

Jonas, R.A. (1999). Deep hypothermic circulatory arrest and retrograde cerebral perfusion. *J. Thorac. Cardiovasc. Surg.* **117**, 196–7.

Kallman, D.A., King, B.F., Hattery, R.R., *et al.* (1992). Renal vein and inferior vena cava tumor thrombus in renal cell carcinoma: CT, US, MRI, and venacavography. *J. Comput. Assist. Tomogr.* **16**, 240–7.

Kuczyk, M.A., Bokemeyer, C., Kohn, G., *et al.* (1997). Prognostic relevance of intracaval neoplastic extension for patients with renal cell cancer. *Br. J. Urol.* **80**, 18–24.

Lang, E.K. (1984). Comparison of dynamic and conventional computed tomography, angiography, and ultrasonography in the staging of renal cell carcinoma. *Cancer* **54**, 2205–14.

Libertino, J.A., Zinman, L., and Watkins, E. Jr (1987). Long-term results of resection of renal cell cancer with extension into inferior vena cava. *J. Urol.* **137**, 21–4.

Libertino, J.A., Swierzewski, D.J., and Swierzewski, M.J. (1998). Renal cell carcinoma with extension into vena cava. In *Reconstructive urologic surgery*, 3rd edn (ed. J.A. Libertino), pp. 47–54. Mosby-Year Book, St Louis.

Ljungberg, B., Stenling, R., Osterdahl, B., Farrelly, E., Aberg, T., and Roos, G. (1995). Vein invasion in renal cell carcinoma: impact in metastatic behavior and survival. *J. Urol.* **154**, 1681–4.

Marshall, F.F. and Reitz, B.A. (1985). Supradiaphragmatic renal cell carcinoma tumor thrombus: indications for vena caval reconstruction with pericardium. *J. Urol.* **133**, 266–8.

Marshall, V.F., Middleton, R.G., Holswade, G.R., and Goldsmith, E.I. (1970). Surgery for renal cell carcinoma in the vena cava. *J. Urol.* **103**, 414–20.

McCullough, D.L. and Gittes, R.F. (1975). Ligation of the renal vein in the solitary kidney: effects on renal function. *J. Urol.* **113**, 295–8.

McDonald, J.R. and Priestley, J.T. (1943). Malignant tumors of the kidney: surgical and prognostic significance of tumor thrombosis of the renal vein. *Surg. Gynecol. Obstet.* **77**, 295–8.

Montie, J.E., el Ammar, R., Pontes J.E., *et al.* (1991). Renal cell carcinoma with inferior vena cava tumor thrombi. *Surg. Gynecol. Obstet.* **173**, 107–15.

Motta, G., Ratto, G.B., Sacco, A., *et al.* (1987). Healing and long-term viability of grafts in the venae cavae reconstruction. *Vasc. Surg.* **21**, 316.

Mrstik, C., Salamon, J., Weber, R., and Stogermayer, F. (1992). Microscopic venous infiltration as predictor of relapse in renal cell carcinoma. *J. Urol.* **148**, 271–4.

Murphy, D.A., Rabinovitch, H., Chevalier, L., and Virmani, S. (1973). Wilms tumor in right atrium. *Am. J. Dis. Childhood* **126**, 210–11.

Myers, G.H. Jr, Fehrenbaker, L.G., and Kelalis, P.P. (1968). Prognostic significance of renal vein invasion by hypernephroma. *J. Urol.* **100**, 420–3.

Nesbitt, J.C., Soltero, E.R., Dinney, C.P., *et al.* (1997). Surgical management of renal cell carcinoma with inferior vena cava tumor thrombus. *Ann. Thorac. Surg.* **63**, 1592–600.

Neves, R.J. and Zincke, H. (1987). Surgical treatment of renal cell cancer with vena cava extension. *Br. J. Urol.* **59**, 390–5.

Novick, A.C. and Cosgrove, D.M. (1980). Surgical approach for removal of renal cell carcinoma into the vena cava and the right atrium. *J. Urol.* **123**, 947–50.

Novick, A.C., Kaye, M.C., Cosgrove, D.M., *et al.* (1990). Experience with cardiopulmonary bypass and deep hypothermic circulatory arrest in the management of retroperitoneal tumors with large vena caval thrombi. *Ann. Surg.* **212**, 472–7.

Oates, R.K., Simpson, J.M., Turnbull, J.A., and Cartmill, T.B. (1995). The relationship between intelligence and duration of circulatory arrest with deep hypothermia. *J. Thorac. Cardiovasc. Surg.* **110**, 786–92.

O'Donohoe, M.K., Flanagan, F., Fitzpatrick, J.M., and Smith, J.M. (1987). Surgical approach to inferior vena caval extension of renal carcinoma. *Br. J. Urol.* **60**, 492–6.

Okada, Y., Kumada, K., Terachi T., Nishimura, K., Tomoyoshi, T., and Yoshida, O. (1996). Long-term followup of patients with tumor thrombi from renal cell carcinoma and total replacement of the inferior vena cava using an expanded polytetrafluoroethylene tubular graft. *J. Urol.* **155**, 444–7.

Pagano, F., Dal Bianco, M., Artibani, A.W., Pappagallo, G., and Prayer Galetti, T. (1992). Renal cell carcinoma with extension into the inferior vena cava: problems in diagnosis, staging and treatment. *Eur. Urol.* **22**, 200–3.

Polascik, T.J., Partin, A.W., Pound, C.R., and Marshall, F.F. (1998). Frequent occurrence of metastatic disease in patients with renal cell carcinoma and intrahepatic or supradiaphragmatic intracaval extension treated with surgery: an outcome analysis. *Urology* **52**, 995–9.

Pritchett, T.R., Lieskovsky, G., and Skinner, D.G. (1986). Extension of renal cell carcinoma into the vena cava: clinical review and surgical approach. *J. Urol.* **135**, 460–4.

Raskin, S.A., Fuselier, V.W., Reeves-Viets, J.L., and Coselli, J.S. (1996). Deep hypothermic circulatory arrest with and without retrograde cerebral perfusion. *Int. Anesthesiol. Clin.* **34**, 177–93.

Reissigl, A., Janetschek, G., Eberle, J., *et al.* (1995). Renal cell carcinoma extending into the vena cava: surgical approach, technique and results. *Br. J. Urol.* **75**, 138–42.

Rodriguez-Rubio, F.I., Abad, J.I., Sanz, G., *et al.* (1997). Surgical management of retroperitoneal tumors with vena caval thrombus in the inferior cava using cardiopulmonary bypass, arrested circulation and profound hypothermia. *Eur. Urol.* **32**, 194–7.

Sarkar, R., Eilber, F.R., Gelabert, H.A., and Quinones-Baldrich, W.J. (1998). Prosthetic replacement of the inferior vena cava for malignancy. *J. Vasc. Surg.* **28**, 75–83.

Sarti, L. (1970). Total prosthetic transplantation of inferior vena cava, with venous drainage restoration of the one remaining kidney on the graft, successfully performed on a child with Wilms' tumor. *Surgery* **67**, 851–5.

Skinner, D.G., Colvin, R.B., Vermillion, C.D., Pfister, R.C., and Leadbetter, W.F. (1971). Diagnosis and management of renal cell carcinoma: a clinical and pathologic study on 309 cases. *Cancer* **28**, 1165–77.

Skinner, D.G., Vermillion, C.D., and Colvin, R.B. (1972*a*). The surgical management of renal cell carcinoma. *J. Urol.* **107**, 705–10.

Skinner, D.G., Pfister, R.F., and Colvin, R. (1972*b*). Extension of renal cell carcinoma into the vena cava: the rationale for aggressive surgical management. *J. Urol.* **107**, 711–16.

Skinner, D.G., Pritchett, T.R., Lieskovsky, G., Boyd, S.D., and Stiles, O.R. (1989). Vena caval involvement by renal cell carcinoma: surgical resection provides meaningful long-term survival. *Ann. Surg.* **210**, 387–94.

Sosa, R.E., Muecke, E.C., Vaughan, E.D. Jr, and McCarron, J.P. Jr (1984). Renal cell carcinoma extending into the inferior vena cava: the prognostic significance of the level of vena caval involvement. *J. Urol.* **132**, 1097–100.

Straton, C.S., Libertino, J.A., and Larsen, C.R. (1992). Is magnetic resonance imaging alone accurate enough in staging renal cell carcinoma. *Urology* **40**, 351–3.

Suggs, W.D., Smith, R.B. III, Dodson, T.F., Salam, A.A., and Graham, S.D. Jr (1991). Renal cell carcinoma with inferior vena caval involvement. *J. Vasc. Surg.* **14**, 413–18.

Swierzewski, D.J., Swierzewski, M.J., and Libertino, J.A. (1994). Radical nephrectomy in patients with renal cell carcinoma with venous, vena caval, and atrial extension. *Am. J. Surg.* **168**, 205–9.

Tongaonkar, H.B., Dandekar, N.P., Dalal, A.V., Kulkarni, J.N., and Kamat, M.R. (1995). Renal cell carcinoma extending to the renal vein and inferior vena cava: results of surgical treatment and prognostic factors. *J. Surg. Oncol.* **59**, 94–100.

Treiger, B.F., Humphrey, L.S., Peterson, C.V. Jr, *et al.* (1991). Transesophageal echocardiography in renal cell carcinoma: an accurate diagnostic technique for intracaval neoplastic extension. *J. Urol.* **145**, 1138–40.

Utley, J.R., Mobin-Uddin, K., Segnitz, R.H., Belin, R.P., and Utley J.F. (1973). Acute obstruction of tricuspid valve by Wilms' tumor. *J. Thorac. Cardiovasc. Surg.* **66**, 626–8.

Walters, W. and Priestley, J.T. (1934). Survey of the inferior vena cava. Clinical and experimental studies. *Ann. Surg.* **99**, 167–72.

Welch, T.J. and LeRoy, A.J. (1997). Helical and electron beam CT scanning in the evaluation of renal vein involvement in patients with renal cell carcinoma. *J. Comput. Assist. Tomogr.* **21**, 467–71.

Wickey, G.S., Martin, D.E., Larach, D.R., Belis, J.A., Kofke, W.A., and Hensley, F.A. Jr (1988). Combined carotid endarterectomy, coronary revascularization, and hypernephroma excision with hypothermic circulatory arrest. *Anesthes. Analges.* **67**, 473–6.

Williams, J.H., Frazier, H.A. II, Gawith, K.E., Laskin, W.B., and Christenson, P.J. (1996). Transitional cell carcinoma of the kidney with tumor thrombus into the vena cava. *Urology* **48**, 932–5.

Zinman, L.M., Libertino, J.A., and Shahian, D.M. (1989). Editorial comments on cardiovascular evaluation before circulatory arrest for renal carcinoma. *J. Urol.* **141**, 1307.

29. Laparoscopic radical nephrectomy

David Y. Chan and Louis R. Kavoussi

Introduction

Radical nephrectomy is the standard of care for the management of renal tumors (Robson 1963). Over the years, technical modifications have focused on extent of dissection and addressed issues such as the removal of the ipsilateral adrenal gland and the role of lymphadenectomy (Sagalowsky *et al.* 1994; Sandock *et al.* 1997; Giuliani *et al.* 1990; Johnsen and Hellsten 1997; Kardar *et al.* 1998). Nephron-sparing or partial nephrectomy has also altered the management of small (< 4 cm) renal cell carcinoma (Novick *et al.* 1991; Polascik *et al.* 1995; Duque *et al.* 1998; Van Poppel *et al.* 1998; Wunderlich *et al.* 1998; Hafez *et al.* 1998). However, all these studies validate the point that surgical extirpation remains the only curative procedure for localized renal cell carcinoma (RCC).

Although standard open surgery is highly effective, it is associated with significant patient morbidity. Advances in laparoscopic dissection techniques and organ removal have allowed for the performance of more complex operations with less patient discomfort. Procedures once deemed impossible, such as laparoscopic nephrectomy, have now become an integral part of the urologic armamentarium.

In this chapter, the role of laparoscopic radical nephrectomy will be reviewed through the presentation of available data. Indications and controversies will be discussed. A description of our current surgical approach will be given.

The first laparoscopic nephrectomy was performed by Clayman and associates in 1990 (Clayman *et al.* 1991). A 3 cm incidentally discovered renal mass was morcellated and removed laparoscopically. Although the tumor was an oncocytoma, this initial experience demonstrated the feasibility of using laparoscopic techniques to treat patients with renal masses.

Over the past decade, numerous studies have demonstrated the benefits of laparoscopy, including shorter hospital stay, improved cosmesis, and quicker convalescence (Gill *et al.* 1995*a*; Hoenig *et al.* 1997; Chen *et al.* 1998; Elashry *et al.* 1996; Nogueira *et al.* 1999; Fabrizio *et al.* 1999; Abdulmaaboud *et al.* 1998). With these encouraging results, laparoscopy has also been applied to treat various urologic malignancies. Recent reports have demonstrated feasibility and short-term success with laparoscopic radical nephrectomy for the treatment of RCC (Barrett *et al.* 1998; Cadeddu *et al.* 1998; Ono *et al.* 1999; McDougall *et al.* 1996; Chan *et al.* 2000, Dunn *et al.* 1999; Gill *et al.* 1999). Although laparoscopic radical nephrectomy is technically equivalent to open radical nephrectomy, fear concerning tumor spillage and trocar site implantation has generated controversy regarding the role of laparoscopy in oncology (Vukasin *et al.* 1996; Lacy *et al.* 1998; Kruitwagen *et al.* 1996; Schaeff *et al.* 1998; Bangma *et al.* 1995; Stolla *et al.* 1994; Andersen and Steven 1995; Elbahnasy *et al.* 1998; Otani *et al.* 1999; Ahmed *et al.* 1998).

Basic surgical principles

Indications and contraindications

Laparoscopic radical nephrectomy is indicated in patients with organ-confined tumors (that is, clinical stage T1 and T2 tumors). More advanced disease can be approached as indicated (Walther and Gill, personal communication). The size limitation is dependent on the experience and comfort of the surgeon. Tumors as large as 20 cm in diameter have been successfully removed laparoscopically. However, it should be noted that the need for open specimen removal and intraoperative conversion may be higher for larger tumors.

Patients with renal vein or vena cava involvement currently are not considered for laparoscopic radical nephrectomy since there are limited laparoscopic techniques for obtaining control of the vena cava and complete laparoscopic extraction of tumor thrombi extension has not been well established. Individuals with tumors extending beyond Gerota's fascia undergoing laparoscopic radical nephrectomy have been approached. However, a higher level of technical expertise is needed. Caution should also be exercised in patients with history of previous ipsilateral renal surgery, pyelonephritis, obesity, or adhesions from previous intra-abdominal surgery. These factors can significantly increase the possibility of open conversion (Higashihara *et al.* 1998; Keeley and Tolley 1998).

Preoperative preparation

The preoperative evaluation and preparation required for laparoscopic nephrectomy are identical to those for patients undergoing standard open radical nephrectomy. Routine laboratory studies including serum electrolytes, hepatic panel, hematology panel, coagulation studies, and urinalysis are obtained prior to surgery as indicated. Metastatic evaluation should include a chest radiograph and computerized tomography (CT) scan of the abdomen. A bone scan should also be obtained if the serum calcium or alkaline phosphatase is elevated. Any questions concerning the involvement of renal vein or vena cava demand further evaluation. Doppler ultrasonography, helical CT, and magnetic resonance (MR) angiography are minimally invasive modalities that can accurately assess tumor thrombus extension into the renal veins and the inferior vena cava (Habboub *et al.* 1997; Kallman *et al.* 1992; Choyke *et al.* 1997; Welch *et al.* 1997).

Serum creatinine level and contrast-enhanced CT scan are usually sufficient to provide information regarding the contralateral renal function; however, if there is any question, further investigation with a dimercaptosuccinic acid (DMSA) renal scan can be undertaken. Partial nephrectomy should be considered in patients with diminished renal function.

Surgeons with limited technical experience may consider obtaining a three-dimensional CT (3D CT) reconstruction as it can also provide a road map for renal vascular anatomy. 3D CT reconstruction has been shown to provide similar arterial and superior venous vascular anatomy with less morbidity when compared with traditional angiographic studies (Del Pizzo *et al.* 1999; Kaynan *et al.* 1999).

Informed consent should be obtained from all patients and the potential risk for conversion to an open procedure discussed. In general, the conversion rate is typically less than 5 per cent, but it is dependent on the experience of the surgeon.

Mechanical and antibiotic bowel preparations are not routinely administered. However, if patients have a history of pyelonephritis or a large renal tumor, bowel preparation may be helpful in improving laparoscopic exposure. Patients are typed for blood and cross-matched if indicated.

Operative technique

Laparoscopic radical nephrectomy can be completed by either a transperitoneal or retroperitoneal approach. As such, advantages of the retroperitoneal approach include rapid access to the hilum and avoidance of intraperitoneal organs. The transperitoneal approach offers a larger working space and greater anatomical orientation. The transperitoneal route is our preferred technique and, as it is more widely employed, will be described here.

Left radical nephrectomy

After induction with general endotracheal anesthesia, a Foley catheter is inserted and the patient is placed in a modified 30 degree lateral decubitus position (Fig. 29.1). An oral-gastric tube is placed to drain gastric contents and minimize bowel distension during the procedure. Care is taken to prevent neuromuscular injury by padding and supporting all potential pressure points with pillows and foam. Particular attention is paid to the contralateral elbow and both legs and ankles. The arms are flexed and crossed over the chest hugging a pillow, and a soft roll is positioned under the axilla. Pneumatic compression stockings are applied to both legs. The lower leg is flexed while the upper leg is straight. Wide cloth tape is used to secure the patient, and the operating table is maximally rotated in both directions to ensure the patient is completely secured. The patient is widely prepped with betadine and draped in standard fashion from the xyphoid to

the pubis and from the contralateral rectus muscle to the paraspinous muscle.

The abdomen is insufflated by inserting a Veress needle or open trocar placement. The Veress needle can be inserted in the mid-clavicular line at the level of the umbilicus or directly into the base of the umbilicus. Proper placement is confirmed by observing that the initial abdominal pressure is less than 5 mm Hg. Once correct position is confirmed, the abdomen is insufflated with CO_2 to a pressure of 20 mm Hg.

Three trocars are usually sufficient to complete a radical nephrectomy. The first 12 mm trocar is placed at the level of the umbilicus lateral to the ipsilateral rectus muscle, using a Visiport trocar (US Surgical Corp., Norwalk, CT) (Fig. 29.1). The Visiport allows for endoscopic visualization as the trocar passes through the abdominal wall. After the first port is placed, the abdomen is inspected to ensure that no bowel injuries occurred during the initial Veress needle entry.

Secondary port placement is accomplished under direct vision. A 12 mm port is placed at the umbilicus and a 5 mm port is placed halfway between the umbilicus and xyphoid (Fig. 29.1). All trocars are secured in place with 2–0 sutures to prevent inadvertent removal while changing instruments. Additional trocars can be placed if the configuration does not provide optimal access. To allow additional retraction of the bowel medially, a 5 or 10 mm trocar can be placed in the midline 2 cm above the pubic symphysis. This port site can be extended as a Pfannenstiel incision if intact organ removal is preferable at the conclusion of the procedure. The laparoscope is placed at the umbilical port and instruments are placed as indicated through the remaining ports.

The trocar configuration may need to be modified to access patients with unique body habiti. In the morbidly obese patients, the trocars are shifted laterally to allow adequate visualization. When moving trocars laterally, care should always be taken to avoid epigastric vessel injury. Also, obese or tall patients may require the use of long instruments to access the upper pole.

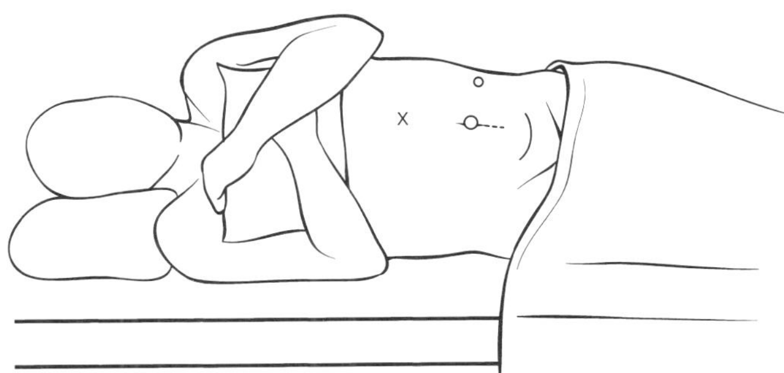

Fig. 29.1 Modified left flank position for left laparoscopic radical nephrectomy. Large circle, 10/12 mm umbilical port; small circle, 10/12 mm lateral port; ×, 5 mm subxyphoid midline port. Dashed and solid lines, respectively, denote periumbilical and Pfannenstiel incisions for intact specimen extraction.

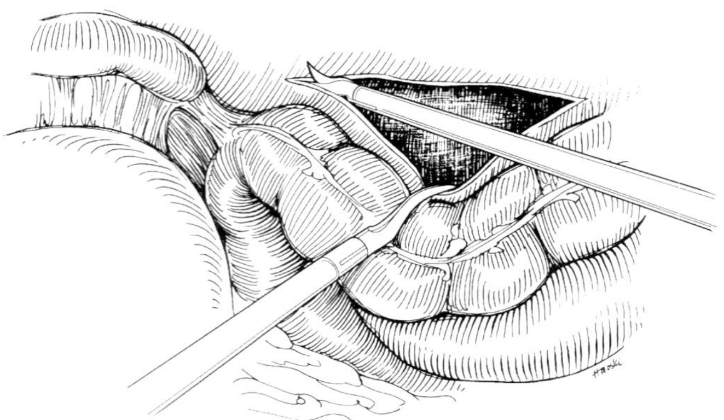

Fig. 29.2 Incision of the line of Toldt for left radical nephrectomy. The bowel is mobilized and reflected medially to expose Gerota's fasica. Reflection of the spleen markedly facilitates upper pole dissection.

Incision of the line of Toldt and mobilization of the colon

Left laparoscopic radical nephrectomy

The procedure begins by incising the line of Toldt with electrosurgical scissors and bluntly teasing the tissue medially with atraumatic forceps. The lateral colonic peritoneal reflection is incised from the level of the splenic flexure to the common iliac vessels (Fig. 29.2). Once the lateral peritoneal reflection is incised, the colon is reflected medially to expose Gerota's fascia. Care is taken to not enter Gerota's fascia. Early release of the posterior renal attachments will hamper the dissection of the hilum and should be avoided. The phrenocolic and splenorenal ligaments should be completely released. The colorenal attachments are also divided to complete the reflection of the descending colon and this maneuver will facilitate upper pole dissection. The medial boundary of the dissection on the left is the aorta.

Right laparoscopic radical nephrectomy

Certain modifications are required to perform the procedure on the right side. The lateral colonic peritoneal reflection is divided from the level of the right common iliac artery to the hepatic flexure (Fig. 29.3). The colorenal attachments are also released to allow mobilization of the colon medially. On the right side, after mobilizing the colon, the Kocher maneuver must be performed to allow the duodenum to fall medially. Judicious use of electrocautery is essential to avoid inadvertent bowel and pancreatic injury. The medial boundary of the dissection on the right is the medial border of the vena cava. Often, the take-off of the right gonadal vein is seen on this side.

The liver may overlie the kidney and retraction will be needed for adequate visualization. A 3 mm port can be placed halfway between the upper abdominal port and xyphoid to permit retraction. A locking grasper is passed under the liver to the side wall and used to lift the liver anteriorly.

Identification and securing of the ureter

Once the retroperitoneal space is entered and the superficial attachments to the kidney are released, attention is turned to locating of the renal hilum. This is facilitated by identification of the ureter (Fig. 29.4). By gently sweeping the retroperitoneal fat superficial and medial to the psoas muscle, the proximal ureter and gonadal vein can be identified. The ureter is isolated lateral to the gonadal vein, elevated, and traced proximally. The ureter should not be divided because the intact ureter can be tented and serve as a handle for traction.

Mobilization of the lower pole of the kidney

Tracing the ureter in a retrograde manner will guide the surgeon to the renal hilum. The lower pole within Gerota's fascia is freed by placing a grasper in the upper midline port, advancing it under the ureter to reach the sidewall and lifting superiorly. The inferior sidewall attachments are released sharply with electrosurgical scissors or bluntly with irrigator–aspirator. Care is taken to leave Gerota's fascia intact. This lower pole dissection facilitates the identification of the hilar vessels. The upper pole and the lateral posterior attachments are not dissected at this time to prevent renal rotation.

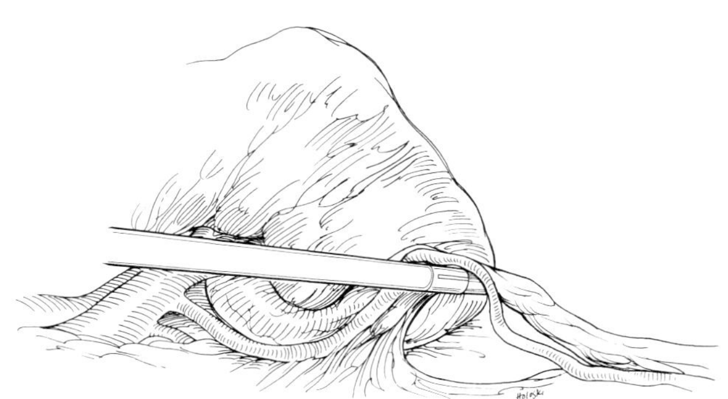

Fig. 29.3 Incision of line of Toldt for right radical nephrectomy. Similarly to the left radical nephrectomy, the bowel is mobilized and reflected medially. Often a fourth trocar is placed in the middle before the xyphoid to facilitate exposure assisting with liver retraction.

Fig. 29.4 Identification and mobilization of the ureter and gonadal vein. Posterior dissection medial to the ureter will reveal the posterior musculature.

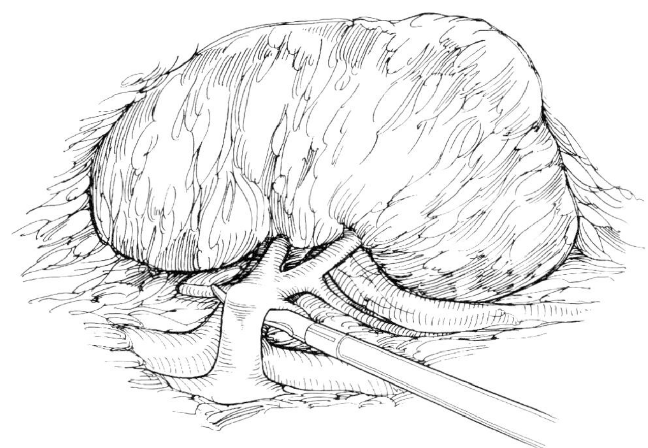

Fig. 29.5 Identification and isolation of the renal vein. After cephalad dissection of the ureter, the lower pole is mobilized and the renal hilum is identified. The renal vein is circumferentially dissected to expose the posterosuperior renal artery.

Identification and ligation of hilar vessels

The main goal in the hilar dissection is the early ligation of the renal artery and vein. This necessitates identification and careful dissection of the renal vein circumferentially (Fig. 29.5). On the left side, early ligation of gonadal and lumbar vein may facilitate exposure of the renal artery. Identification and ligation of these venous branches can also minimize bleeding and allows easier manipulation of the renal vein.

The renal artery is often encased in dense lymphatic tissue. Complete skeletonization of hilar vessels is not necessary since the endovascular stapler will occlude and transect perivascular lymphatic and fatty tissue. However, judicious use of vascular clips must be employed in this area as they can interfere with endovascular GIA stapler application and result in malfunction and the need for emergency open conversion (Fig. 29.6). The renal vein should be identified anterior to the artery and a space between the vessels carefully created. The GIA is then used to ligate and transect all the tissue surrounding the artery.

The tissue anterior to the renal vein is next dissected free. If the renal vein fails to collapse after renal artery ligation, accessory

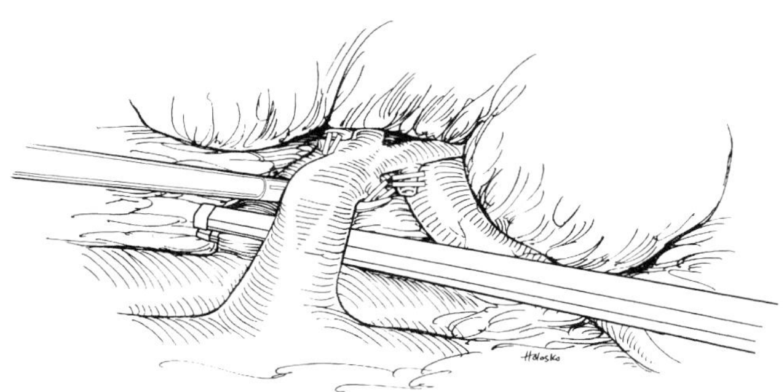

Fig. 29.6 Ligation of renal artery. The renal vein is carefully displaced superiorly to allow ligation of renal artery of endovascular GIA stapler.

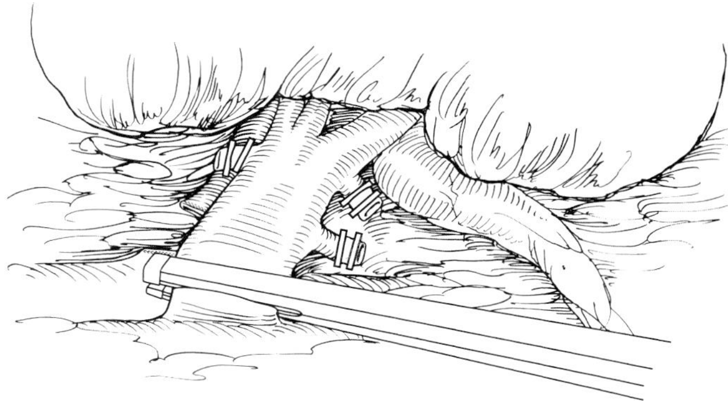

Fig. 29.7 After the renal artery is ligated, the renal vein should collapse. The renal vein is then ligated with the endovascular GIA stapler.

renal arteries or a renal vein thrombus must be suspected (Fig. 29.7). Care must be taken to ensure complete occlusion and division of each vessel separately. Attempts to divide the hilum using a single stapler risk the formation of an arteriovenous fistula and should be avoided. On the left side, if the decision to perform a concomitant ipsilateral adrenalectomy is made, the adrenal vein should be identified and the GIA stapler placed on the renal vein just distal to its take-off. If the adrenal gland is to be removed, the stapler is placed proximal to the take-off of the adrenal vein.

Dissection of the upper pole and adrenal gland

After the ligation of the renal hilum is complete, the posterior and lateral attachments are released from the side wall and psoas muscle. The superior margin of dissection is dependent on the need to remove the ipsilateral adrenal gland. In general, the ipsilateral adrenal gland is only removed in patients with upper pole tumors, advanced clinical stage, or multifocal disease. During dissection, constant vigilance is required to avoid injuring adjacent organs such as the pancreas, duodenum, or spleen.

If the adrenal gland is to remain intact, Gerota's fascia overlying the upper pole is incised and the kidney is freed in a circumferential fashion from attachments. If the adrenal gland is to be removed, the upper medial border of Gerota's fascia is teased away from surrounding tissue taking care to clip the perforating blood supply.

Release of lateral attachments

Following the ligation of the renal hilum and the dissection of the upper pole, lateral attachments are released. The ureter is used as the handle to facilitate the dissection of these attachments. The dissection is outside of Gerota's fascia and can be performed bluntly with the irrigator–aspirator or electrocautery scissors. At this point, the ureter should be the only remaining attachment.

Division of the ureter

Once the kidney is completely freed from surrounding attachments, the ureter can be divided between clips (Fig. 29.8). The ureter usually is not divided prior to the ligation of the renal

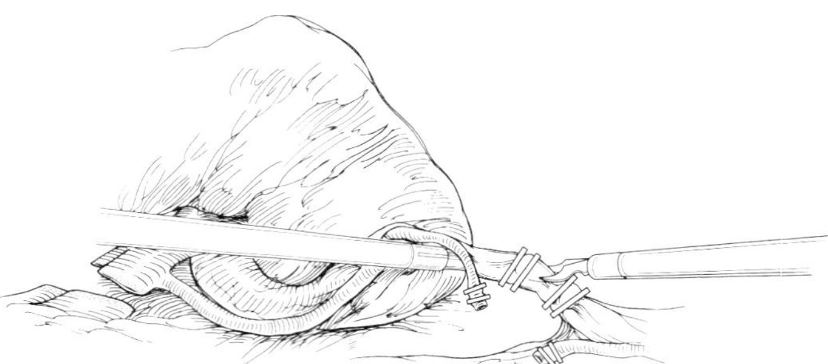

Fig. 29.8 Division of the ureter. After the kidney is completely freed from the lateral attachments, the ureter can be divided and used as a handle to place the kidney on top of the spleen or the liver for specimen entrapment.

hilum as it provides stability for specimen manipulation. On occasion, in order to adequately mobilize the upper pole of the kidney, the ureter must be ligated after the transection of the hilum. By grasping the ureter, the kidney can be rolled on top of the spleen or liver providing access to upper pole attachments.

Organ entrapment and removal

Specimen entrapment minimizes the risk of tumor spillage. Using atraumatic graspers, the specimen is positioned on top of the spleen or liver, depending on the side of the nephrectomy. If the specimen is to be removed intact, the 15 mm EndoCatch retrieval device and bag (US Surgical Corp, Norwalk, CT) is inserted through the 12 mm umbilical trocar site after the camera is moved to the lateral 12 mm trocar. After removing the umbilical trocar, the EndoCatch can be passed into the peritoneal cavity under direct vision. Once the EndoCatch device is deployed intraabdominally, the specimen is swept from atop of the spleen or liver and manipulated into the open bag (Fig. 29.9). The EndoCatch device and bag is withdrawn through the umbilical trocar site. Either a midline periumbilical trocar site extension or a lower Pfannenstiel incision can be used to extract the intact specimen (Fig. 29.1). A sufficient incision needs to be created to minimize the risk of bag rupture.

If the specimen is to be morcellated or fractionated, the EndoCatch bag should not be used to entrap the radical nephrectomy specimen. The EndoCatch bag can be easily perforated during morcellation. As such, the heavier LapSac entrapment bag (Cook Urological, Inc., Spencer, IN) should be used for morcellation.

The LapSac is technically more challenging to manipulate, as it does not open automatically. The LapSac must be wrapped around an atraumatic grasper and introduced independently through a trocar site. Once introduced, the LapSac is unwrapped and placed flat with the bag opening facing the specimen. An additional trocar and grasper can facilitate specimen retrieval by keeping the sack open. Similar to the EndoCatch, the specimen is swept from atop of the spleen or liver into the LapSac. Once the specimen is completely enclosed in the LapSac, the drawstrings are tightened and withdrawn through the 12 mm umbilical port. The neck of the bag is worked out through the skin and manual morcellation with a Kelly clamp, ring forceps, or high-speed electrical morcellation used to remove the specimen. The intra-abdominal portion of the LapSac must be under direct vision during the entire morcellation process to monitor for inadvertent bag perforation and injury to other organs. Once the specimen has been sufficiently reduced in size, the entire LapSac is withdrawn from the trocar site.

Wound closure

If the specimen was removed intact using the EndoCatch device, the incision should be closed in standard fashion and the abdomen reinsufflated to allow for inspection for bleeding and injury prior to port closures. All 10/12 mm ports are closed using the Carter–Thomsen device. All ports are removed sequentially under direct laparoscopic vision to rule out potential bleeding. The pneumoperitoneum is vented completely prior to removing the last trocar. The skin incision is closed using subcutaneous absorbable suture.

Postoperative management

On postoperative day one, patients' diets are advanced as tolerated and the urethral catheter removed. Patients are encouraged to ambulate and resume usual activities as indicated.

Clinical results

Since Clayman and associates (Clayman *et al.* 1991) performed the first laparoscopic nephrectomy, the applications of laparoscopy to urologic procedures have grown tremendously. The focus has shifted from feasibility of laparoscopy in benign conditions to improving safety and demonstrating efficacy of laparoscopy in the management of urologic malignancies. Studies have shown less postoperative pain and quicker convalescence when compared with open radical nephrectomy (Kavoussi *et al.* 1993). However, concerns regarding prolonged operative times, steep learning curve, patient morbidity, effective cancer control, and risk for potential port site metastases have emerged.

Cancer control

Laparoscopic radical nephrectomy has evolved to become a new alternative for the management of renal tumors. Many centers now employ this technique to treat most clinically localized renal tumors. At our institution, between February 1991 and July 1999, 67 laparo-

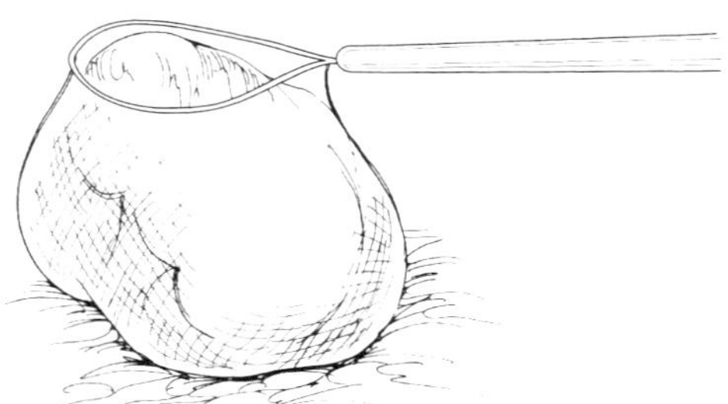

Fig. 29.9 Specimen entrapment using EndoCatch device for intact extraction.

Table 29.1 Comparison of a group of patients undergoing open radical nephrectomy with a contemporary group undergoing laparoscopic radical nephrectomy

| | Radical nephrectomy | | |
	Laparoscopic	Open	p value*
Number (n)	67	54	
Male/female	40/27	38/16	
Right/left	30/37	29/25	
Clinical stage, cT1/cT2	53/14	40/14	
Pathologic stage, pT1/pT2	NA	40/14	
Mean age (years)	61 (33–88)	59 (21–79)	NS
Mean size (cm)	5.1 (1–13)	5.4 (0.2–18)	NS
Median size (cm)	5.0	4.8	NS
Operating room time (min)			
Mean	256 (115–600)	193 (99–409)[†]	$p < 0.001$
Median	245	190	
Mean operating room time (min)			
Cases 1–34	289 (150–600)	NA	$p < 0.005$
Cases 35–67	222 (115–480)	NA	$p < 0.005$
Estimated blood loss (cm^3)			
Mean	289 (50–2000)	309 (1400–50)[†]	NS
Median	200	200	NS
Length of hospital stay (days)			
Mean	3.8 (2–14)	7.2 (4–28)	$p < 0.001$
Median	3	6	$p < 0.001$
Mean follow-up (months)	35.6	44.0	$p < 0.001$

* NA, not applicable; NS, not significant.
[†] Only 40 (74%) anesthesia records were available for review for the open radical nephrectomy series.

Table 29.2 Pathologic grade distribution in a group of patients undergoing open radical nephrectomy ($N = 54$) compared with that in a contemporary group undergoing laparoscopic radical nephrectomy ($N = 67$)

| | Radical nephrectomy (number) | |
Pathologic grade	Laparoscopic	Open
1	7	1
2	31	34
3	17	16
4	1	0
NA*	11	3

* NA, no specimen grading available.

scopic radical nephrectomies were performed for clinically (c) localized, cT1–2 pathologically confirmed RCC. We compared these patients' clinical outcome with a contemporary series of patients undergoing open radical nephrectomy with pathologically (p) confirmed pT1–2N0Mx RCC. In terms of patient demographics, there were no differences in the age of the patients, the size, grade, or distribution of the tumors. (Tables 29.1 and 29.2). Although, the operative time was consistently longer in the laparoscopic group, the patients benefited with a shorter length of hospitalization.

In the laparoscopic group the selection criteria were based on clinical stage. As such, a significant portion of the RCC were found to be pathologically T3 (13/17). In contrast all tumors in the open series were selected pathologically as T1 or T2. Despite this understaging in the laparoscopic group, there was no statistical difference in the Kaplan–Meier disease-free and actuarial survival analysis between the two groups (Figs 29.10 and 29.11).

The mean follow-up for the laparoscopic group was 35.6 months (range 12–111 months) with 35 patients followed up for at least 2 years and 10 followed for at least 4 years. Although the period of study was the same for the laparoscopic and open radical nephrectomy groups, the mean follow-up was shorter in the laparoscopic group. This was the result of the progressive acceptance of the new procedure. No laparoscopic trocar site implantations have been identified. To date, eight patients have expired in the laparoscopic group. Two patients died with metastatic disease to the lung and bone. One patient with renal hilar lymph node metastasis expired in an automobile accident. Five patients died of unrelated causes. Currently, 59 patients are alive without metastasis or tumor recurrences.

Early reports of laparoscopic radical nephrectomy from the literature have also demonstrated efficacy in the treatment of RCC (Barrett *et al.*1998; Cadeddu *et al.* 1998; Ono *et al.* 1999; McDougall *et al.* 1999; Chan *et al.* 2000). Our laparoscopic 5-year disease-free rates are analogous to other previously published results by Ono *et al.* (1999) and Cadeddu *et al.* (1998), 97.5 and 91 per cent, respectively. Despite likely understaging of the renal tumors in the laparoscopic group, the clinical results, as reflected by the 5-year disease-free and actuarial survival rates, 95 and 86 per cent, respectively, are comparable to those of the contemporary open radical nephrectomy series as well as to those of historic controls for stage I RCC, 86 and 76 per cent and 92 and 65–88 per cent, respectively (Ljungberg *et al.* 1998; Robson *et al.* 1969; Skinner *et al.* 1972; Siminovitch *et al.* 1983; Golimbu *et al.* 1986; Best 1987).

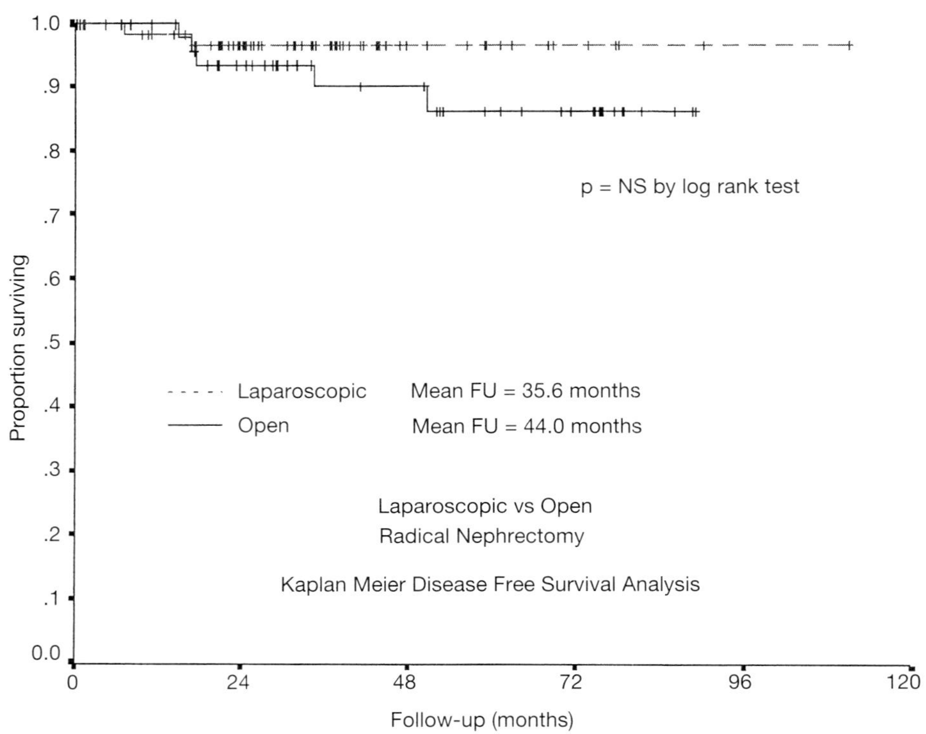

Fig. 29.10 Kaplan–Meier disease-free survival analysis for a group undergoing lapararoscopic (dashed line; mean follow-up 35.6 months) radical nephrectomy compared with that for a group undergoing open (solid line; mean follow-up 44.0 months) radical nephrectomy. *p* is not significant by log rank test.

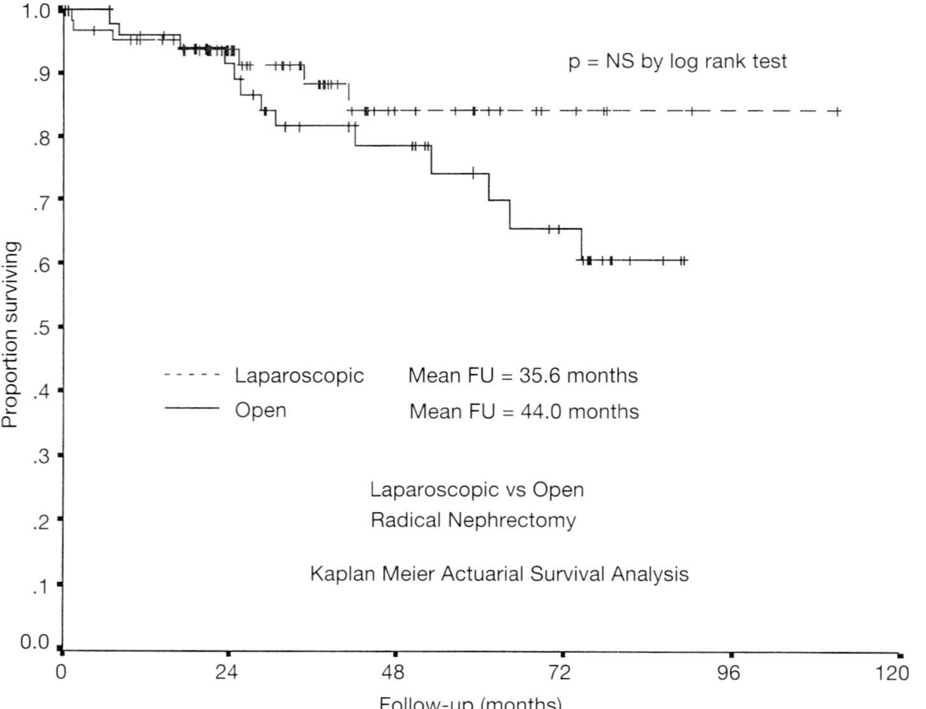

Fig. 29.11 Kaplan–Meier actuarial survival analysis for a group undergoing lapararoscopic (dashed line; mean follow-up 35.6 months) radical nephrectomy compared with that for a group undergoing open (solid line; mean follow-up 44.0 months) radical nephrectomy. *p* is not significant by log rank test.

Risk for port site metastases

Published reports of port site tumor recurrences have raised concern regarding the safety of utilizing laparoscopy to treat malignancies. A significant portion of literature on the etiology of port site recurrences derives from the laparoscopic-assisted resection of colorectal carcinoma. Over 60 cases of clinical tumor recurrences in laparoscopic port site wounds have been reported in patients after laparoscopic surgery for colorectal cancer (Melotti *et al.* 1999). The incidence of port site recurrence ranges from 0 to 21.4 per cent in series with a mean time between surgery and recurrence of 7 months. However, there is strong evidence that port site recurrences reflect the underlying biology of the disease, rather than the technique of laparoscopy. Pearlstone noted that, in many cases of port site recurrences, evidence of diffuse intraperitoneal disease was already present at the time of laparoscopy (Pearlstone *et al.* 1999). Port site recurrences are often harbingers of more insidious evidence of disseminated disease or multiple sites of metastasis and rarely occur as an isolated event. Undoubtedly, trocar site recurrences are real. However, they probably represent the natural history of the disease or deviation from standard oncologic surgical practice. Recent results of clinical trials comparing open and laparoscopic colectomy have suggested that the recurrence rates are similar and approach 1 per cent (Melotti *et al.* 1999; Pearlstone *et al.* 1999; Allardyce 1999; Lacy *et al.* 1998; Vukasin *et al.* 1996; Tomita *et al.* 1999; Leung *et al.* 1999).

In regard to port site recurrences to RCC, several groups have reported their experience with laparoscopic radical nephrectomy (Barrett *et al.* 1998; Cadeddu *et al.* 1998; Ono *et al.* 1999; Dunn *et al.* 1999; Gill *et al.* 1999; Chan *et al.* 2000). Most groups morcellate or fractionate their specimens. To date, two reports of port site recurrences associated with laparoscopic nephrectomy involved intact removal of renal transitional cell carcinoma (TCC) (Otani *et al.* 1999; Ahmed *et al.* 1998). In one case, a port site metastasis occurred after laparoscopic nephrectomy was performed for a nonfunctional, tuberculous, atrophic kidney, serendipitously found to contain an unsuspected TCC. During retrieval, the entrapment sack was torn and the specimen was removed directly through the trocar port without morcellation (Otani *et al.* 1999). In the second case report, laparoscopic nephroureterectomy with transurethral resection of ureteral orifice was performed for presumed renal pelvis TCC (Ahmed *et al.* 1998). The intact specimen was removed at the lateral port site. Eight months after surgery, the patient presented with a painful incisional hernia at periumbilical port site. Exploration revealed metastatic TCC. It was not stated whether an entrapment bag was used for tumor extraction and how the cystotomy was managed.

One case of RCC seeding a trocar site after laparoscopic radical nephrectomy has been reported from the University of Saskatchewan (Barret and Fentie 1999). The case involved a grade 4 RCC. The specimen was entrapped and morcellated without apparent complications. The etiology of this solitary port site metastasis at 25 months after surgery was unclear as no deviations from standard laparoscopic technique were noted.

Based on the potential for seeding, tumor entrapment is preferable where feasible. If the specimen is small enough to entrap, an attempt at fractionation is acceptable. This should be done under direct vision and only in entrapment sacs designed for this purpose. For larger tumors or instances where accurate pathological analysis is needed, the specimen can be removed intact through an expanded trocar site or Pfannenstiel incision. Of note, in our series, there was no difference in the length of hospitalization between the morcellation and intact specimen groups, 3.6 versus 3.9 days, respectively (unpublished data).

Prolonged operative times

Laparoscopic radical nephrectomy does require longer operative times than standard open nephrectomy. In our initial 67 patients, the mean operating time was 4.3 hours; however, a learning curve exists and times improve with experience. Significant difference between the first 34 and last 33 laparoscopic radical nephrectomies does exist as illustrated in Fig. 29.12. This is consistent with other large series (Table 29.3). Of note, there has been no increase in patient morbidity related to the longer operative times.

Complications

Complications are a part of surgical practice and laparoscopic renal surgery has defined potential risks that need to be discussed in details with patients. Basic preventive planning and prompt recognition are crucial to minimize patient morbidity.

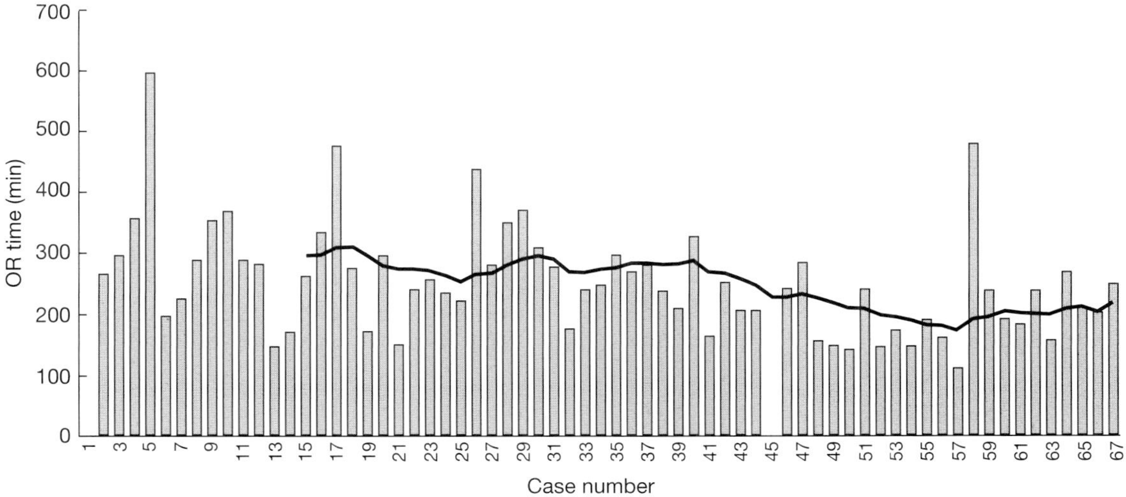

Fig. 29.12 Operating room (OR) time for our series of 67 cases undergoing laparoscopic radical nephrectomy. The OR time is significantly less for the last 33 cases, reflecting surgeons' increasing experience with the operation.

Table 29.3 Comparison of various series of laparoscopic radical nephrectomies

Study	N	Mean operating procedure time (hours)	Mean follow-up (months)	Complications rate (%)	5-year disease-free survival (%)
Cadeddu et al. 1998	157	—	19.2	10	91
Barrett et al. 1998	57	2.9	21.4	11	(0)*
Ono et al. 1999	60	5.2	24.0	13	96
Gill et al. 1999	40	3.1	6.5	13	–
Dunn et al. 1999	47	5.5	28.0	5/4[†]	(3)*
Chan et al. 2001	67	4.3	35.6	16	9

* Number of patients with tumor recurrence.
[†] Major/minor complications rate.

Table 29.4 Comparison of complication rates in our series of laparoscopic and open radical nephrectomies

Laparoscopic radical nephrectomy		Open radical nephrectomy	
Complication	Number	Complication	Number
Total	11 (16%)	Total	8 (15%)
Bowel injury during morcellation requiring open conversion and bowel resection	1	Retroperitoneal hematoma requiring re-exploration	1
		Pneumonia	1
Trocar site hernia	2	Congestive heart failure	1
Small bowel obstruction	1	Ileus requiring readmission	1
Congestive heart failure	1	Contact dermatitis	1
Pulmonary embolus	1	Flank hernia	1
Spleen laceration	1	Epididymal orchitis	1
Aspiration pneumonia	1	Urinary tract infection	1
C. difficile colitis	1		
Urinary tract infection	2		

In our experience, laparoscopic complication rates appear equivalent to those of open series. The overall complication rate in our laparoscopic group was 16 per cent (Table 29.4). A bowel injury was sustained in one case during morcellation of the kidney specimen. The LapSac perforated during morcellation and a segment of small bowel was injured. This required extended incision of the trocar site for bowel resection. The patient is alive and disease-free at 2 years. One patient developed small bowel obstruction secondary to an incisional hernia at the trocar site and required surgical intervention. A superficial spleen laceration was managed conservatively without sequelae. Six patients required blood transfusions (8 per cent). In the open series, complications were retrospectively identified in 8 patients (15 per cent) One patient developed a significant postoperative bleed and required surgical re-exploration. One patient was readmitted for ileus, and one patient was found to have an incisional flank hernia. There were no splenectomies, or liver injuries. Eleven patients received blood transfusions (20 per cent), which was not statistically different from laparoscopic approach ($p > 0.5$). Although chest tube placement is not considered a complication, it is a source of discomfort for patients and can delay patient recovery. Twelve patients (22 per cent) required intraoperative chest tube placement in the open group.

Our complication rate is similar to those of other laparoscopic series (Table 29.3) (Barrett *et al.* 1998; Cadeddu *et al.* 1998; Ono

et al. 1999; Dunn *et al.* 1999; Gill *et al.* 1999). However, the types of complications may differ between laparoscopic and open approaches. Pneumothoraces are rare with the laparoscopic approach. Although not addressed in this study, long-term pain, numbness, and abdominal wall laxity are more prevalent in open procedures than in the laparoscopic approach. In one study, 12 per cent of patients who underwent open radical nephrectomy continued to have significant wound-related symptoms (hernia, parasthesias, pain) at 1 year of follow-up (Kavoussi *et al.* 1993).

The pneumoperitoneum and novel laparoscopic access techniques can result in unique complications. Carbon dioxide insufflation can produce arrhythmias including bradycardia, atrioventricular (AV) dissociation, and nodal rhythms due to a vagal response to abdominal distension and peritoneal irritation (Reed and Nourse 1998; Myles 1991) The use of atropine prior to insufflation may prevent vagal reactions.

A rare but potentially fatal complication related to the pneumoperitoneum is a gas embolism (Gomar *et al.* 1985; Ostman *et al.* 1990; Kleppinger 1974; McKenzie 1971; Keith *et al.* 1974). Although intravasation of gas due to the increased intraabdominal pressure has been suggested as an etiology, the most common cause is direct insufflation into a vein. Patient survival depends upon rapid diagnosis and treatment. The diagnosis can be difficult as often there is no warning prior to acute cardiovascular collapse. A mill-wheel murmur may be auscultated just prior to the acute event. Also an acute decrease in measured end-tidal carbon dioxide measurements will be noted as the embolism occludes the pulmonary trunk.

Several potential pitfalls can occur during initial access as this is a relatively blind procedure and, therefore, bowel or major vascular structures may be perforated (Gill *et al.* 1995*b*). Vascular injuries during access account for the major portion of laparoscopic injuries. Most are due to incision of one of the abdominal wall vessels during trocar placement. These are diagnosed by visualizing blood dripping from the trocar sleeve or hematoma formation about the trocar site. Vascular injuries related to the upper urinary tract usually involve the branches of the renal vein or vena cava. Arterial injuries are also possible. Inadvertent vascular occlusion can occur through blind clip placement or vigorous retraction. Reports of compromise to major abdominal organs and the entire small bowel have also been reported.

Dissection and access injuries have been reported to the stomach, intestines, liver, spleen, pancreas, and mesentery. Unfortunately, bowel injuries are often not recognized at the time of initial laparoscopic surgery. Failure to recognize such an injury can result in significant morbidity. Patients usually present 3 to 7 days postoperatively with a persistent ileus, vague abdominal pain, trocar site pain, and nausea (Bishoff *et al.*1999). Many patients will only have a low-grade fever and leukocytosis may not be present. A plain abdominal film may reveal an ileus pattern and free air; however, this latter finding is not helpful as the insufflant from the pneumoperitoneum may be visible for several days following laparoscopy. If a postoperative patient does not rapidly respond to conservative measures, radiographic studies and laparotomy should be undertaken as indicated.

Conclusions

Laparoscopic radical nephrectomy is an effective alternative for the treatment of localized RCC. Although laparoscopic radical nephrectomy is a longer operative procedure with a significant learning curve, patients continue to benefit with shorter hospitalization and an acceptable complication rate. Initial data demonstrate effective cancer control with no statistically significant difference in disease-free and actuarial survival between laparoscopic and open radical nephrectomy when principles of surgical oncology are maintained. Longer follow-up will be helpful in comparing the long-term survival and disease-free rates with those of open surgery.

References

Abdulmaaboud, M.R., Shokeir, A.A., Farage, Y., Abd El-Rahman, A., El-Rakhawy, M.M., and Mutabagani, H. (1998). Treatment of varicocele: a comparative study of conventional open surgery, percutaneous retrograde sclerotherapy, and laparoscopy. *Urology* 52, 294–300.

Ahmed, I., Shaikh, N.A., and Kapadia, C.R. (1998). Track recurrence of renal pelvic transitional cell carcinoma after laparoscopic nephrectomy. *Br. J. Urol.* 81, 319.

Allardyce, R.A. (1999). Is the port site really at risk? Biology, mechanisms and prevention: a critical view. *Aust. NZ J. Surg.* 69, 479–85.

Andersen, J.R. and Steven, K. (1995). Implantation metastasis after laparoscopic biopsy of bladder cancer. *J. Urol.* 153, 1047–8.

Bangma, C.H., Kirkels, W.J., Chadha, S., and Schroder, F.H. (1995). Cutaneous metastasis following laparoscopic pelvic lymphadenectomy for prostatic carcinoma. *J. Urol.* 153, 1635–6.

Barrett, P.H. and Fentie, D.D. (1999). Longer follow-up for laparoscopic radical nephrectomy with morcellation for renal cell carcinoma. *J. Endourol.* 13 (S1), A62.

Barrett, P.H., Fentie, D.D., and Taranger, L.A. (1998). Laparoscopic radical nephrectomy with morcellation for renal cell carcinoma: the Saskatoon experience. *Urology* 52, 23–8.

Best, B.G. (1987). Renal carcinoma: a ten-year review 1971–1980. *Br. J. Urol.* 60, 100–2.

Bishoff, J., Kirkles, W., Moore, R., Kavoussi, L., and Schroder, F. (1999). Laparoscopic bowel injury: incidence and unique clinical presentation. *J. Urol.* 161, 887–90.

Cadeddu, J.A., Ono, Y., Clayman, R.V., Barrett, P.H., Janetschek, G., Fentie, D.D., McDougall, E.M., Moore, R.G., Kinukawa, T., Elbahnasy, A.M., Nelson, J.B., and Kavoussi, L.R. (1998). Laparoscopic nephrectomy for renal cell cancer: evaluation of efficacy and safety: a multicenter experience. *Urology* 52 (5),773–7.

Chan, D.Y., Cadeddu, J.A., Jarrett, T.W., Marshall, F.F., and Kavoussi, L.R. (2001). Laparoscopic radical nephrectomy for cancer control in renal cell carcinoma. *J. Urol.* 166, 2095–9.

Chen, R.N., Moore, R.G., and Kavoussi, L.R. (1998). Laparoscopic pyeloplasty: indications, technique, and long-term outcome. *Urol. Clin. N. Am.* 25 (2),323–30.

Choyke, P.L., Walther, M.M., Wagner, J.R., Rayford, W., Lyne, J.C., and Linehan, W.M. (1997). Renal cancer: preoperative evaluation with dual-phase three-dimensional MR angiography. *Radiology* 205 (3), 767–71.

Clayman, R.V., Kavoussi, L.R., Soper, N.J., Dierks, S.M., Meretyk, S., Darcy, M.D., Roemer, F.D., Pingleton, E.D., Thomson, P.G., and Long, S.R. (1991). Laparoscopic nephrectomy: initial case report. *J. Urol.* 146 (2), 278–82.

Del Pizzo, J.J., Sklar, G.N., You-Cheong, J.W., Levin, B., Krebs, T., and Jacobs, S.C. (1999). Helical computerized tomography arteriography for evaluation of live renal donors undergoing laparoscopic nephrectomy. *J. Urol.* 162 (1), 31–4.

Dunn, M.D., Portis, A.J., Shalhav, A.L., Elbahnasy, A.M., McDougall, E.M., and Clayman, R.V. (1999). Laparoscopic versus open radical nephrectomy for renal tumor: the Washington University experience [abstract 638]. *J. Urol.* 161 (4), 166.

Duque, J.L., Loughlin, K.R., O'Leary, M.P., Kumar, S., and Richie, J.P. (1998). Partial nephrectomy: alternative treatment for selected patients with renal cell carcinoma. *Urology* 52, 584–90.

Elashry, O.M., Nakada, S.Y., Wolf, J.S. Jr, Figenshau, R.S., McDougall, E.M., and Clayman, R.V. (1996). Ureterolysis for extrinsic ureteral obstruction: a comparison of laparoscopic and open surgical techniques. *J. Urol.* 156, 1403–10.

Elbahnasy, A.M., Hoenig, D.M., Shalhav, A., McDougall, E.M., and Clayman, R.V. (1998). Laparoscopic staging of bladder tumor: concerns about port site metastases. *J. Endourol.* 12, 55–9.

Fabrizio, M.D., Ratner, L.E., Montgomery, R.A., and Kavoussi, L.R. (1999). Laparoscopic live donor nephrectomy. *Urol. Clin. N. Am.* 26, 247–56.

Gill, I.S., Clayman, R.V., and McDougall, E.M. (1995*a*). Advances in urological laparoscopy. *J. Urol.* 154, 1275–94.

Gill, I.S., Kavoussi, L.R., Clayman, R.V., Erlich, R., Evans, R., Fuchs, G., Gersham, A., Hulbert, J., McDougal, E.M., Rosenthal, T., Schusler, W.W., and Shepard, T. (1995*b*). Complications of laparoscopic nephrectomy in 185 patients: a multiinstitutional review. *J. Urol.* 154, 479–83.

Gill, I.S., Hobart, M., Soble, J., Sung, G.T., Schweizer, D., and Novick, A.C. (1999). Retroperitoneal laparoscopic radical nephrectomy comparison with open surgery [abstract 637]. *J. Urol.* 161 (suppl. 1), 166.

Giuliani, L., Giberti, C., Martorana, G., and Rovida, S. (1990). Radical extensive surgery for renal cell carcinoma: long-term results and prognostic factors. *J. Urol.* 143, 468–73.

Golimbu, M., Joshi, P., Sperber, A., Tessler, A., Al-Askari, S., and Morales, P. (1986). Renal cell carcinoma: survival and prognostic factors. *Urology* 27, 291–301.

Gomar, C., Fernandez, C., Villalonga, A., and Nalda, M.A. (1985). Carbon dioxide embolism during laparoscopy and hysteroscopy *Ann. Fr. Anesth. Reanim.* **4**, 380–2.

Habboub, H.K., Abu-Yousef, M.M., Williams, R.D., See, W.A., and Schweiger, G.D. (1997). Accuracy of color Doppler sonography in assessing venous thrombus extension in renal cell carcinoma. *Am. J. Roentgenol.* **168**, 267–71.

Hafez, K.S., Novick, A.C., and Butler, B.P. (1998). Management of small solitary unilateral renal cell carcinomas: impact of central versus peripheral tumor location. *J. Urol.* **159**, 1156–60.

Higashihara, E., Baba, S., Nakagawa, K., Murai, M., Go, H., Takeda, M., Takahashi, K., Suzuki, K., Fujita, K., Ono, Y., Ohshima, S., Matsuda, T., Terachi, T., and Yoshida, O. (1998). Learning curve and conversion to open surgery in cases of laparoscopic adrenalectomy and nephrectomy. *J. Urol.* **159**, 650–3.

Hoenig, D.M., McDougall, E.M., Shalhav, A.L., Elbahnasy, A.M., and Clayman, R.V. (1997). Laparoscopic ablation of peripelvic renal cysts. *J. Urol.* **158**, 1345–8.

Johnsen, J.A. and Hellsten, S. (1997). Lymphatogenous spread of renal cell carcinoma: an autopsy study. *J. Urol.* **157**, 450–3.

Kallman, D.A., King, B.F., Hattery, R.R., Charboneau, J.W., Ehman, R.L., Guthman, D.A., and Blute, M.L. (1992). Renal vein and inferior vena cava tumor thrombus in renal cell carcinoma: CT, US, MRI and venacavography. *J. Comput. Assist. Tomogr.* **16** (2), 240–7.

Kardar, A.H., Arafa, M., Al Suhaibani, H., Pettersson, B.A., Lindstedt, E., Hanash, K.A., and Hussain, S. (1998). Feasibility of adrenalectomy with radical nephrectomy. *Urology* **52**, 35–7.

Kavoussi, L.R., Kerbl, K., Capelouto, C.C., McDougall, E.M., and Clayman, R.V. (1993). Laparoscopic nephrectomy for renal neoplasms: *Urology* **42**, 603–9.

Kaynan, A.M., Rozenblit, A.M., Figueroa, K.I., Hoffman, S.D., Cynamon, J., Karwa, G.L., Tellis, V.A., and Lerner, S.E. (1999). Use of spiral computerized tomography in lieu of angiography for preoperative assessment of living renal donors. *J. Urol.* **161**, 1769–75.

Keeley, F.X. and Tolley, D.A. (1998). A review of our first 100 cases of laparoscopic nephrectomy: defining risk factors for complications. *Br. J. Urol.* **82**, 615–18.

Keith, L., Silver, A., and Becker, M. (1974). Anesthesia for laparoscopy: *J. Reprod. Med.* **12**, 227–33.

Kleppinger, R.K. (1974). One thousand laparoscopies at a community hospital. *J. Reprod. Med.* **13**, 13–20.

Kruitwagen, R.F., Swinkels, B.M., Keyser, K.G., Doesburg, W.H., and Schijf, C.P. (1996). Incidence and effect on survival of abdominal wall metastases at trocar or puncture sites following laparoscopy or paracentesis in women with ovarian cancer. *Gynecol. Oncol.* **60**, 233–7.

Lacy, A.M., Delgado, S., Garcia-Valdecasas, J.C., Castells, A., Pique, J.M., Grande, L., Fuster, J., Targarona, E.M., Pera, M., and Visa, J. (1998). Port site metastases and recurrence after laparoscopic colectomy. A randomized trial. *Surg. Endosc.* **12**, 1039–42.

Leung, K.L., Yiu, R.Y., Lai, P.B., Lee, J.F., Thung, K.H., and Lau, W.Y. (1999). Laparoscopic-assisted resection of colorectal carcinoma: five-year audit. *Dis. Colon Rectum* **42**, 327–32.

Ljungberg, B., Alamdari, F.I., Holmberg, G., Granfors, T., and Duchek, M. (1998). Radical nephrectomy is still preferable in the treatment of localized renal cell carcinoma. A long-term follow-up study. *Eur. Urol.* **33**, 79–85.

McDougall, E., Clayman, R.V., and Elashry, O. (1996). Laparoscopic radical nephrectomy for renal tumor: the Washington University experience. *J. Urol.* **155**, 1180–5.

McKenzie, R. (1971). Laparoscopy. *NZ Med. J.* **74**, 87–91.

Melotti, G., Tamborrino, E., Lazzaretti, M.G., Bonilauri, S., Mecheri, F., and Piccoli, M. (1999). Laparoscopic surgery for colorectal cancer. *Sem. Surg. Oncol.* **16**, 332–6.

Myles, P.S. (1991). Bradyarrhythmias and laparoscopy: a prospective study of heart rate changes with laparoscopy. *Aust. NZ J. Obstet. Gynaecol.* **31**, 171–3.

Nogueira, J.M., Cangro, C.B., Fink, J.C., Schweitzer, E., Wiland, A., Klassen, D.K., Gardner, J., Flowers, J., Jacobs, S., Cho, E., Philosophe, B., Bartlett, S.T., and Weir, M.R. (1999). A comparison of recipient renal outcomes with laparoscopic versus open live donor nephrectomy. *Transplantation* 15 **67**, 722–8.

Novick, A.C., Gephardt, G., Guz, B., Steinmuller, D., and Tubbs, R.R. (1991). Long-term follow-up after partial removal of a solitary kidney. *New Engl. J. Med.* 10; **325**, 1058–62.

Ono, Y., Kinukawa, T., Hattori, R., Yamada, S., Nishiyama, N., Mizutani, K., and Ohshima, S. (1999). Laparoscopic radical nephrectomy for renal cell carcinoma: a five-year experience. *Urology* **53**, 280–6.

Ostman, P.L., Pantle-Fisher, F.H., Faure, E.A., and Glosten, B. (1990). Circulatory collapse during laparoscopy. *J. Clin. Anesthesiol.* **2**, 129–32.

Otani, M., Irie, S., and Tsuji, Y. (1999). Port site metastasis after laparoscopic nephrectomy: unsuspected transitional cell carcinoma within a tuberculous atrophic kidney. *J. Urol.* **162**, 486–7.

Pearlstone, D.B., Feig, B.W., and Mansfield, P.F. (1999). Port site recurrences after laparoscopy for malignant disease. *Sem. Surg. Oncol.* **16**, 307–12.

Polascik, T.J., Pound, C.R., Meng, M.V., Partin, A.W., and Marshall, F.F. (1995). Partial nephrectomy: technique, complications, and pathological findings. *J. Urol.* **154**, 1312–18.

Reed, D.N. Jr and Nourse, P. (1998). Untoward cardiac changes during CO_2 insufflation in laparoscopic cholecystectomies in low-risk patients. *J. Laparoendosc. Adv. Surg. Techn. A* **8**, 109–14.

Robson, C.B. (1963). Radical nephrectomy for renal cell carcinoma. *J. Urol.* **89**, 37–42.

Robson, C.J., Churchill, B.M., and Anderson, W. (1969). The results of radical nephrectomy for renal cell carcinoma. *J. Urol.* **101**, 297–301.

Sagalowsky, A.I., Kadesky, K.T., Ewalt, D.M., and Kennedy, T.J. (1994). Factors influencing adrenal metastasis in renal cell carcinoma. *J. Urol.* **151**, 1181–4.

Sandock, D.S., Seftel, A.D., and Resnick, M.I. (1997). Adrenal metastases from renal cell carcinoma: role of ipsilateral adrenalectomy and definition of stage. *Urology* **49**, 28–31.

Schaeff, B., Paolucci, V., and Thomopoulos, J. (1998). Port site recurrences after laparoscopic surgery. A review. *Dig. Surg.* **15**, 124–34.

Siminovitch, J.M., Montie, J.E., and Straffon, R.A. (1983). Prognostic indicators in renal adenocarcinoma. *J. Urol.* **130**, 20–3.

Skinner, D.G., Vermillion, C.D., and Colvin, R.B. (1972). The surgical management of renal cell carcinoma. *J. Urol.* **107**, 705–10.

Stolla, V., Rossi, D., Bladou, F., Rattier, C., Ayuso, D., and Serment, G. (1994). Subcutaneous metastases after coelioscopic lymphadenectomy for vesical urothelial carcinoma. *Eur. Urol.* **26**, 342–3.

Tomita, H., Marcello, P.W., and Milsom, J.W. (1999). Laparoscopic surgery of the colon and rectum. *World J. Surg.* **23**, 397–405.

Van Poppel, H., Bamelis, B., Oyen, R., and Baert, L. (1998). Partial nephrectomy for renal cell carcinoma can achieve long-term tumor control. *J. Urol.* **160**, 674–8.

Vukasin, P., Ortega, A.E., Greene, F.L., Steele, G.D., Simons, A.J., Anthone, G.J., Weston, L.A., and Beart, R.W. Jr (1996). Wound recurrence following laparoscopic colon cancer resection. Results of the American Society of Colon and Rectal Surgeons Laparoscopic Registry. *Dis. Colon Rectum* **39** (10 suppl.), S20–3.

Welch, T.J. and LeRoy, A.J. (1997). Helical and electron beam CT scanning in the evaluation of renal vein involvement in patients with renal cell carcinoma. *J. Comput. Assist. Tomogr.* **21**, 467–71.

Wunderlich, H., Reichelt, O., Schumann, S., Schlichter, A., Kosmehl, H., Werner, W., Vollandt, R., and Schubert, J. (1998). Nephron sparing surgery for renal cell carcinoma 4 cm. or less in diameter: indicated or undertreated? *J. Urol.* **159**, 1465–9.

30. Nephron-sparing surgery

Reza Ghavamian and Horst Zincke

Introduction

The curative management of renal cell carcinoma (RCC) remains surgical. Recent advances in preoperative staging, specifically modern imaging techniques, and improvements in surgical techniques have made nephron-sparing surgery (NSS) an attractive alternative to radical nephrectomy in select patients. Over the past decade, there has been an increasing body of literature regarding, not only the indications, but also the safety and efficacy of NSS for RCC. The goals of conservative resection of RCC are complete local surgical removal of the malignancy and preservation of adequate renal function. This is a delicate balance, which makes renal-preserving surgery at times both challenging and controversial.

Indications

Nephron-sparing surgery is generally an absolute indication for patients with synchronous bilateral tumors, tumors in a solitary kidney, or the presence of a poorly functional contralateral renal unit. The latter scenario could result from the concomitant presence of a unilateral RCC and a contralateral kidney that is afflicted with disease processes such as chronic pyelonephritis, renal arterial disease, calculus disease, or the presence of systemic diseases such as diabetes.

Recently, the indications for NSS for RCC have been expanded to include the setting of a normal contralateral renal unit, especially in the younger patient with an incidental, localized, single and small (≤ 4 cm) RCC (Butler *et al.* 1995; Lerner *et al.* 1996). Approximately 10 to 15 per cent of small (< 3 cm) solid renal tumors are oncocytomas (Smith *et al.* 1989; Levine *et al.* 1989). A recent study (Dechet *et al.* 1999) from the Mayo Clinic of 106 renal masses treated with surgical resection revealed that 14 per cent were benign (10 per cent were oncocytomas). When considering tumors smaller than 4 cm, the incidence of benign tumors increased to 22 per cent, of which, 18 per cent were oncocytomas. Considering these factors, NSS would prevent unwarranted removal of a kidney for a benign lesion.

In addition to size, the location of the lesion in the kidney is an important criterion when considering NSS. Admittedly, centrally located tumors that are close to the hilum and are adjacent to the collecting system are technically more difficult to remove than exophytic, peripheral lesions. In a recent study, treatment with NSS or radical nephrectomy was equally effective regardless of tumor location (Hafez *et al.* 1998). There were no differences in 5-year cancer-specific survival (100 versus 97 per cent), tumor recurrence (5.7 versus 4.5 per cent), postoperative renal function, or complications between centrally and peripherally located tumors, respectively.

The value of NSS is further realized when one considers the unreliability of current imaging studies in distinguishing between malignant and benign tumors of the kidney. The most clinically relevant scenario is that of a small Bosniak category 3 lesion that does not meet the criteria of clearly malignant or benign lesions (Bosniak 1995). Renal exploration and NSS is indicated and is the ideal form of treatment. Radical nephrectomy in this setting has to be considered excessive in the modern era.

Diagnosis

With the advent of modern imaging modalities, most RCC are detected incidentally during cross-sectional abdominal imaging or abdominal ultrasonography. If the renal mass was not originally detected by intravenous urography, there is no need to obtain an excretory urogram with the availability of cross-sectional imaging. The size, location, and characteristics of the renal mass (cystic versus solid) are adequately assessed with ultrasonography, computerized tomography (CT), and magnetic resonance imaging (MRI) of the abdomen. The latter two modalities can be beneficial to rule out metastatic or locally extensive disease. MRI also has a role in evaluating the inferior vena cava for presence of tumor thrombus and its proximal and distal extent. Inferior and superior venacavography are generally not needed in the era of modern cross-sectional imaging. Furthermore, preoperative imaging modalities must delineate the relationship of the tumor to the normal, surrounding parenchyma to allow for safe and adequate tumor excision while preserving maximal normal renal parenchyma.

Although not imperative in small peripherally located tumors, preoperative evaluation of the vasculature of the kidney and the tumor can aid in tumor excision. This is especially true of the larger lesions and those that occupy a more central position close to the renal hilum especially in a solitary kidney. In the past, renal angiography was routinely used to delineate the vasculature.

In the modern era alternative, less morbid and invasive modalities such as magnetic resonance angiography (MRA) can substitute for the classical renal angiography in the majority of cases. Also, recently, three-dimensional helical CT has provided important three-dimensional anatomical information on the vasculature and excretory function of the affected kidney (Coll *et al.* 1999). However, when the above studies fail to provide an adequate picture, conventional renal angiography can be of considerable value. Oblique views of the kidney may further delineate the segmental arteries. It should be noted that an important part of renal angiography is the venous phase of the study as the anatomy of the venous system is an equally important preoperative consideration especially when NSS is contemplated for an imperative indication. This complete delineation of the renal arterial and venous vasculature is especially mandatory in the setting of a centrally located tumor in a solitary kidney.

Further metastatic work-up can include a preoperative chest X-ray, liver function tests, and alkaline phosphatase. In the event of abnormal liver function tests or elevated serum alkaline phosphatase a bone scan can be performed.

Preoperative preparation

Patients being considered for NSS should be prepared for possible radical nephrectomy. Patients should be aware of the risk for possible temporary or permanent dialysis in the setting of a solitary functioning kidney. The optimal treatment is decided at the time of surgery. Patients should have optimal renal perfusion provided by a hydration regime of about ≥ 200 ml/h of crystalloids overnight. Alternatively, same-day admission and hydration with a 1 liter crystalloid bolus over an hour prior to the scheduled operation is acceptable. Ice slush in anticipation of arterial occlusion and regional hypothermia should be available.

Surgical considerations

In the vast majority of cases today using the correct preoperative imaging and employment of the correct incision, partial nephrectomies can be performed *in situ*. Temporary arterial occlusion and regional hypothermia is employed when necessary depending on the size, location, and number of the renal masses. Possible options include enucleation with a rim of normal parenchyma, wedge resection, polar nephrectomy, or bench surgery and autotransplantation (*ex vivo*).

Several principles should be kept in mind when performing NSS for RCC. Early vascular control, as well as the prompt utilization of renal hypothermia when necessary in cases where it was not originally planned, is the key to minimizing blood loss. Surface and core renal temperature cooling is achieved to minimize ischemic damage to the kidney. An important adjunct is employment of intraoperative frozen-section analysis of the margins of resection. Closure of the collecting system is mandatory to prevent fistula formation. In addition, the entire remaining surface of the kidney should be inspected to rule out multifocal RCC.

We do not hesitate to employ temporary renal artery occlusion and hypothermia, even for relatively small lesions. This approach decreases intraoperative bleeding and also, due to decreased tissue turgor, allows for palpation of the kidney for non-obvious intraparenchymal lesions that are not readily identifiable with the kidney perfused. It also allows for better dissection of especially centrally located tumors and assessment of the extent of involvement of contiguous intrarenal structures. Usually, only the renal artery is occluded except for a large centrally located tumor where renal vein occlusion can be attained to minimize bleeding and allow for easier dissection and reconstruction.

Some surgeons have utilized intraoperative ultrasonography for the evaluation of multifocality in select cases when preoperative imaging studies are equivocal or intraparenchymal nonpalpable tumors are suspected. In certain situations where complex cystic lesions are encountered, it can also serve a purpose to further characterize the lesion at the time of surgery. Ultrasonography can guide the incision in the renal capsule and find the shortest and easiest access to the lesion that would compromise and sacrifice the least amount of normal parenchyma. In one recent study, intraoperative ultrasonography did not add to preoperative CT or intraoperative inspection with regards to multifocality, but did aid in the nature of intraparenchymal mass and the surgical approach (Campbell *et al.* 1996).

Operative technique

According to the preference of the surgeon, a flank extraperitoneal or an anterior subcostal incision is used. A supine position with a tilt towards the contralateral side is our preferred approach (Fig. 30.1 (a), (b)). A rolled towel is placed underneath and lateral to the affected side and the table is flexed slightly. Alternatively, when a flank incision is contemplated, the lateral decubitus position is used. The kidney rest is raised halfway between the iliac crest and the costal margin and the table is flexed. The contralateral leg is flexed at the knee to provide stability and the ipsilateral lower extremity is kept straight. Pillows are placed in between to cushion bony prominences. The outermost arm is wrapped and placed on an armrest and an axillary roll is placed underneath the dependent axilla to avoid brachial plexus injuries.

Our preferred approach, in the absence of previous abdominal surgery, is the anterior subcostal incision starting at the tip of the 12th rib and coursing 3 cm below the costal margin and extending across the midline to the opposite side when necessary. The falciform ligament is divided after the peritoneum is entered. The advantage of this incision is evaluation of the intraabdominal viscera and excellent exposure of the renal vessels, especially in large or obese patients. The disadvantage is that the kidney is in the depth of the wound. It should be noted that the flank approach utilizing an extrapleural 11th or 12th rib incision also provides excellent and rapid exposure to the kidney and the hilum and is a reasonable approach. However, in older patients or those with poor respiratory reserve, pulmonary complications are more common. This is in part due to the increased pain that is associated with this incision compromising deep inspiration and subsequently leading to more atelectasis.

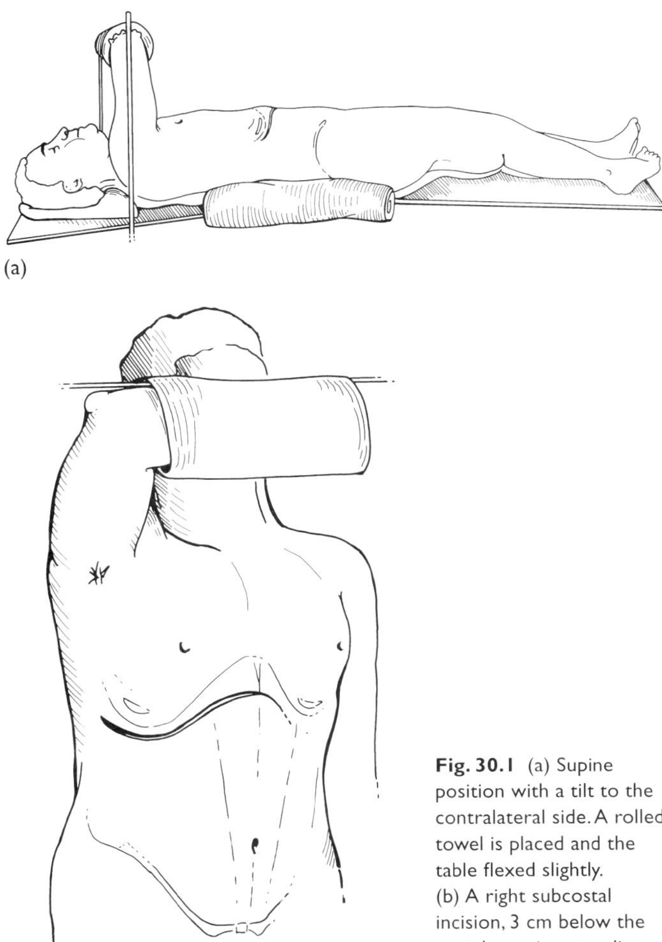

Fig. 30.1 (a) Supine position with a tilt to the contralateral side. A rolled towel is placed and the table flexed slightly. (b) A right subcostal incision, 3 cm below the costal margin extending just across the midline.

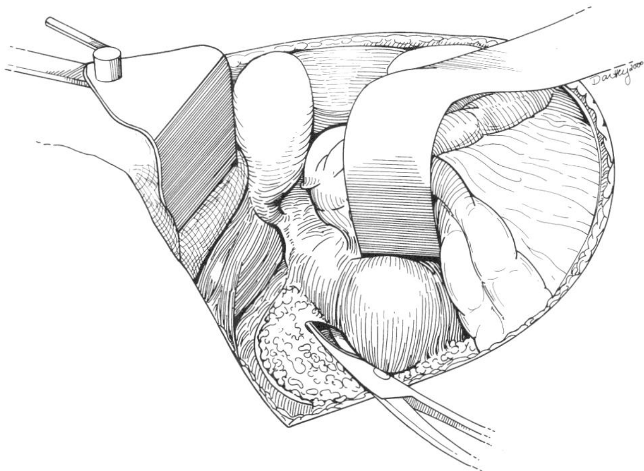

Fig. 30.2 On the right side, the ascending colon is mobilized and retracted. A Kocher maneuver is utilized to mobilize the duodenum, facilitating exposure to the renal hilum and inferior vena cava.

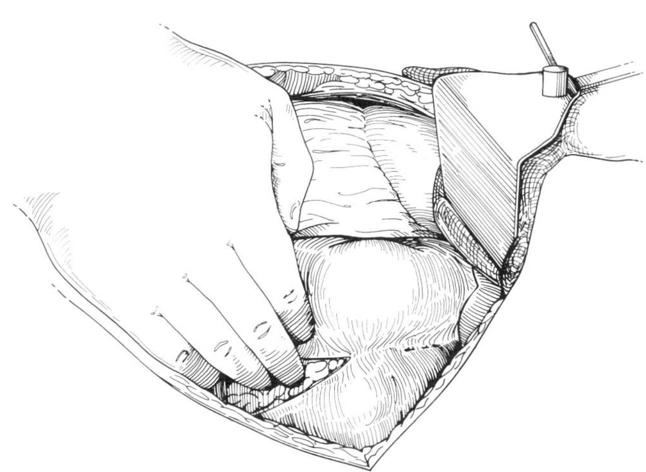

Fig. 30.3 On the left side the descending colon is gently mobilized and the splenorenal ligament is divided to avoid splenic capsular tears.

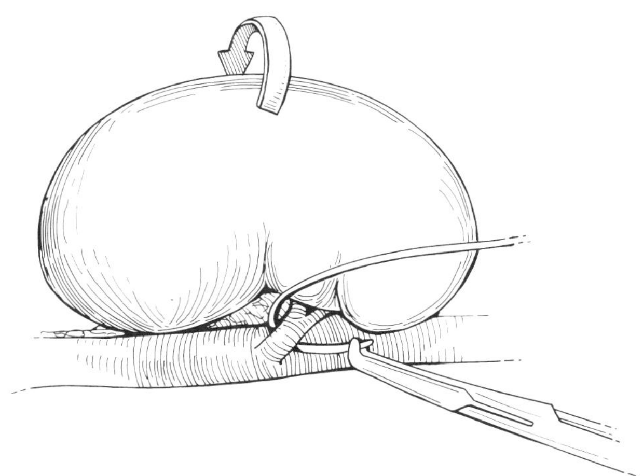

Fig. 30.4 The kidney is rotated medially and a vascular loop is placed around the renal artery.

Optimal renal exposure is the key to a successful outcome. The abdominal viscera are mobilized accordingly and the kidney is identified (Figs 30.2 and 30.3). The renal pedicle is identified and the vasculature defined. The renal artery is isolated and a vascular loop is placed (Fig. 30.4). Excessive dissection is avoided and surrounding perivascular adventitial layers are left intact to serve as a cushion if application of a vascular clamp is contemplated. This reduces the risk of intimal damage to the artery, which can result in arterial thrombosis. The perirenal fat is dissected free except the fat directly overlying the tumor. Enucleation with a rim of normal parenchyma can be utilized for smaller lesions (< 3 cm) (Fig. 30.5). Usually renal occlusion is not necessary. The capsule is scored with electrocautery and usually a plane is identified outside the pseudocapsule of the tumor and developed with the butt end of a scalpel handle or small Metzenbaum scissors. The tumor is then excised using a combination of blunt and sharp dissection. While the assisting surgeon is applying intermittent pressure, any bleeding vessel is suture-ligated utilizing 5.0 absorbable sutures. A frozen section is sent from the tumor crater bed, which represents the deep margin. The crater is then inspected for evidence of entry into the collecting system. If in doubt, 5 ml of indigo-carmine can be given intravenously or intrapelvic (collecting system) and the

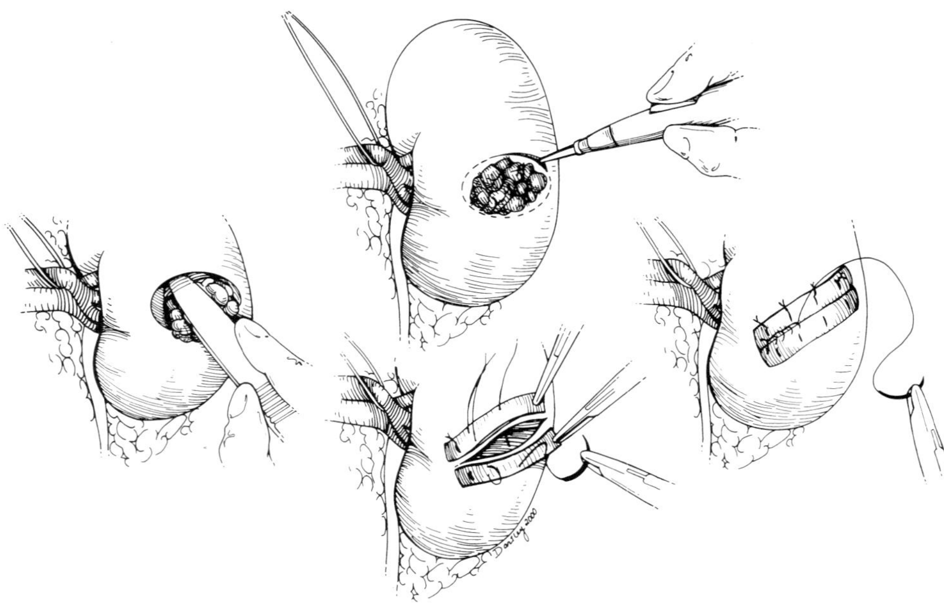

Fig. 30.5 Enucleation with a rim of normal tissue. Vascular occlusion is normally unnecessary. The renal capsule is scored with electrocautery and the tumor enucleated using the butt end of a scalpel handle. The defect is reconstructed with Gore-Tex.

tumor bed inspected for any leaks. Thrombin-soaked Surgicel is used liberally to aid in hemostasis. When the defect is small, the renal capsule is approximated to cover the defect utilizing Gelfoam or Surgicel bolsters. If the defect is relatively large, closure of the parenchymal defect is achieved by use of exogenous Gore-Tex bolsters (see next section) (Zincke and Ruckle 1995).

More sizeable lesions will need temporary arterial occlusion and hypothermia. Preoperative definition of the renal vasculature is more imperative if a larger partial resection is contemplated. When in doubt, the appropriate segmental artery supplying the tumor can be identified by injection of indigo carmine (Fig. 30.6). The areolar tissue is left intact at the junction of the renal vein and the vena cava to provide increased stability of the renal vein. Mannitol (12.5 g) is infused intravenously 5 and 10 minutes before anticipated renal occlusion. The renal artery is then occluded with an atraumatic vascular bulldog and a plastic sheet is wrapped around the kidney. We do not routinely occlude the renal vein, as we believe retrograde perfusion of the kidney might minimize the chance for acute tubular necrosis postoperatively. It also allows for easier identification of renal veins for ligature in the parenchyma and to differentiate them from small tangential cuts in the collecting system at the time of resection. Rigorous hydration is maintained throughout the procedure. Iced saline slush is applied and the kidney is cooled to allow for adequate core renal hypothermia (Fig. 30.7). The renal mass is then resected utilizing a combination of blunt and sharp dissection with a 1–2 cm margin of normal renal parenchyma (Fig. 30.8). Frozen sections are sent from the crater of the tumor bed. After the lesion is removed, the arterial bleeders and the visible bleeding veins are suture-ligated using 4–0 absorbable sutures. The collecting system, if entered, is closed with a 5–0 absorbable suture (Fig. 30.9). If the collecting system is not easily identified, indigo carmine can be injected into the renal pelvis directly, while occluding the ureter, to detect an obvious leak.

With the assistant approximating the edges of the parenchymal defect (Fig. 30.9), the defect is closed utilizing two 1.0–1.5 cm

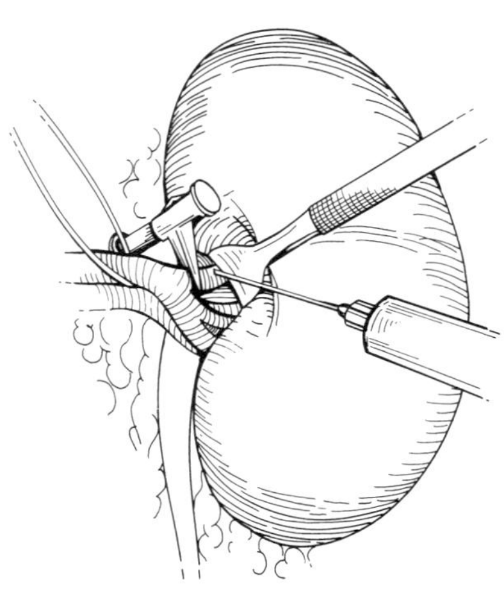

Fig. 30.6 Injection of indigo carmine to delineate the supply area of the appropriate segmental artery coursing towards the tumor.

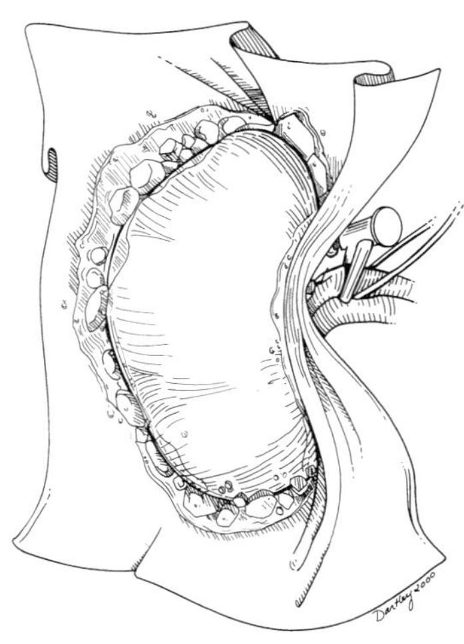

Fig. 30.7 Arterial occlusion and regional hypothermia utilizing plastic sheet and iced saline slush.

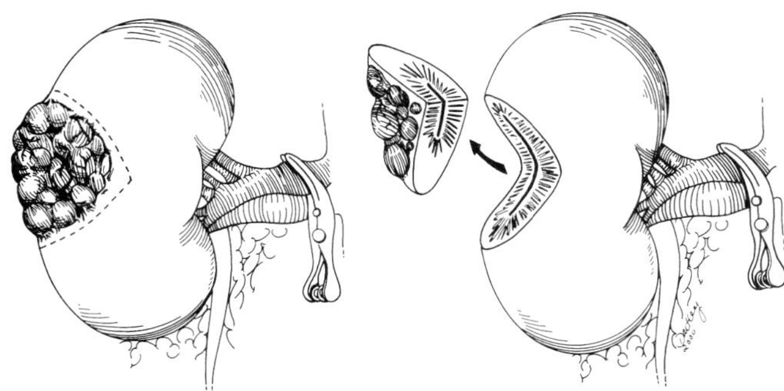

Fig. 30.8 Wedge resection utilizing a 1–2 cm margin of normal parenchyma utilizing blunt and sharp dissection.

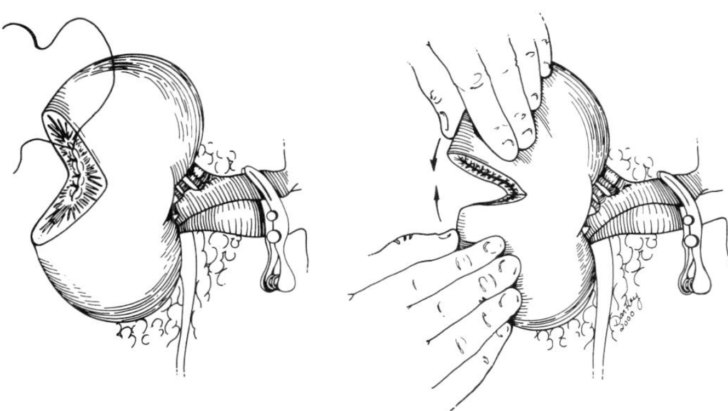

Fig. 30.9 The collecting system is closed utilizing 5.0 absorbable suture after which the assistant approximates the edges of the defect in preparation for closure.

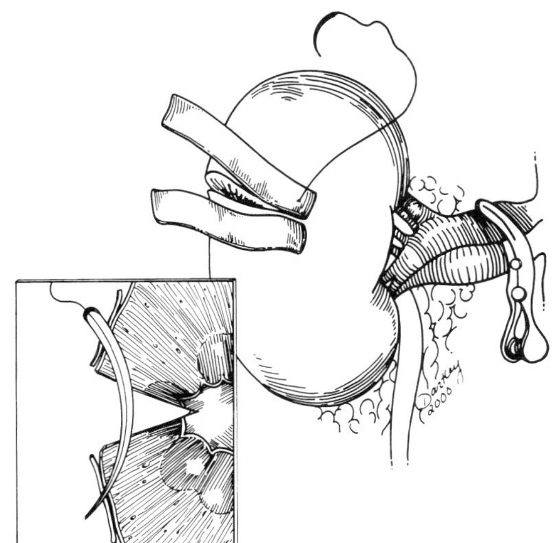

Fig. 30.10 Two 1.0–1.5 cm Gore-Tex strips are used to close the defect. Initially interrupted horizontal mattress sutures of 2.0 polyglycolic acid are passed through the bolster and incorporate the renal capsule 1.0 cm away from the edge of the defect. The suture is carried towards the opposite aspect of the defect incorporating parenchyma and the Gore-Tex bolster as shown (insert).

wide strips of Gore-Tex graft material. The two strips are laid along the length of the defect on each side. Several 2–0 polyglycolic acid horizontal mattress sutures are passed through the renal capsule, approximately 1 cm away from the edge of the parenchymal defect on each side, thereby incorporating the Gore-Tex strips along each side of the defect (Fig. 30.10). The parenchyma is malleable due to arterial occlusion and should be closed along whichever axis allows for an easier approximation. The interrupted sutures are then tied over the bolster. It is important to place all sutures in first, then have the assistant provide uniform and direct approximation while tying these sutures. The medial edges of the bolster material are sutured using a running locked 2–0 polyglycolic suture to provide complete closure of the bolster and a watertight closure (Fig. 30.11). The arterial clamp is then removed and the kidney perfused.

Large polar resections are approached in the same manner and are invariably performed best under regional hypothermia and arterial occlusion with core cooling. Usually, a transverse resection is required (Fig. 30.12). These are usually larger lesions and require ligation of the segmental arteries and veins supplying the tumor and the corresponding section of the kidney. The position of the ureter and the renal pelvis has to be carefully noted and the collecting system is closed with a running 5–0 absorbable suture. Due to the usually extensive resection, insertion of an indwelling double J ureteral stent, placed in an antegrade fashion, is advisable. The parenchymal defect is closed as depicted above.

In the modern era, most partial nephrectomies are amenable to *in situ* techniques. With adequate cooling and exposure, 3 hours of safe ischemia is ample time for nearly all renal tumors. An indication for *ex vivo* (bench) NSS in the past was a centrally located tumor, with concerns about adequate tumor excision and reconstruction. A recent study from a single center with extensive experience in NSS did not find the location of the tumor (central versus peripheral) to be a significant factor affecting outcome especially in single, small, unilateral, and incidentally detected RCC (Hafez *et al.* 1998). Today, in experienced hands, this approach is usually not necessary. The most perceivable indication is the presence of a large central tumor in a solitary kidney. The technique involves a standard radical nephrectomy with particular attention to preserving the maximum length on the renal artery and vein. Intravenous mannitol (total

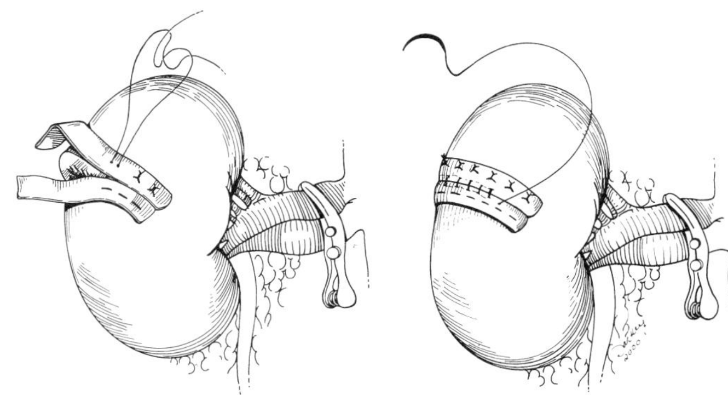

Fig. 30.11 Once all horizontal mattress interrupted sutures are laid, the medial edges of the bolster strips are approximated utilizing a running locked 2.0 polyglycolic acid suture.

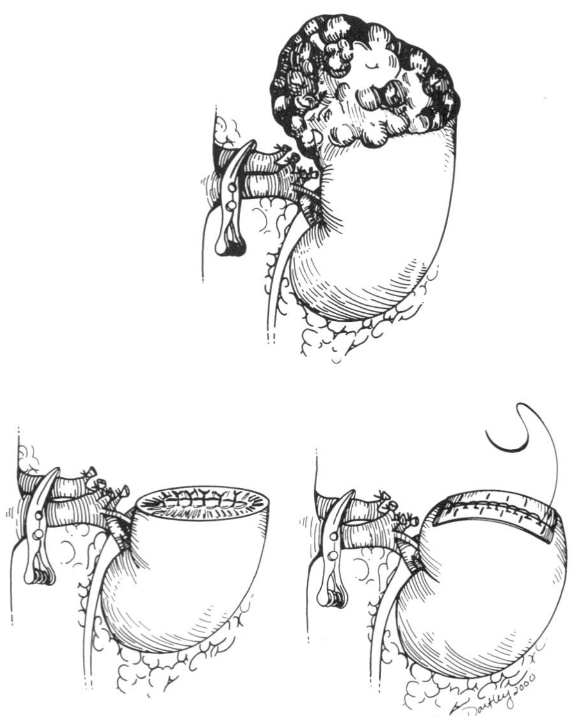

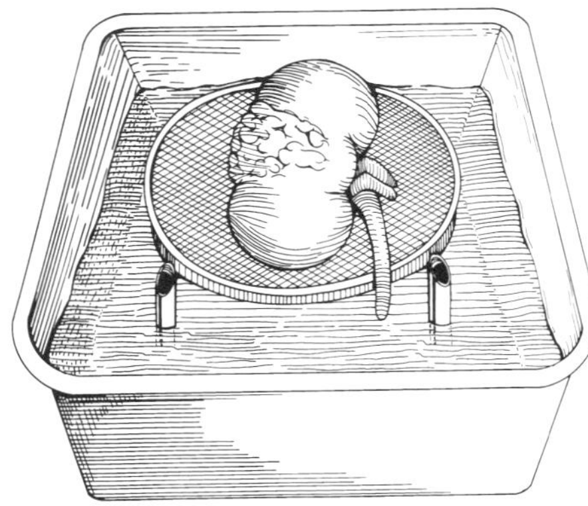

Fig. 30.12 Transverse resection. Entry into the collecting system is usually inevitable and, therefore, closure of the collecting system is required. Note individual ligation of segmental arteries and veins. Closure is with Gore-Tex bolsters as previously depicted.

25 g) is administered 5 and 10 minutes before removal and maximum ureteral length with adequate adventitia is achieved. Adequate hydration is provided and Furosemide is administered liberally to maintain diuresis. After removal, the kidney is perfused with the University of Wisconsin solution or Euro-Collin's solution at 7°C via the renal artery and the kidney is placed in a shallow basin filled with cold saline slush (Fig. 30.13). The tumor is resected and frozen-section analysis of the margins is obtained. The reconstruction is then carried out as depicted above (Fig. 30.14). Infusion of the artery and vein with Euro-Collin's solution before transplantation allows

Fig. 30.13 The kidney is perfused, placed in a shallow basin filled with cold saline slush, and prepared for excision of the tumor and *ex vivo* reconstruction.

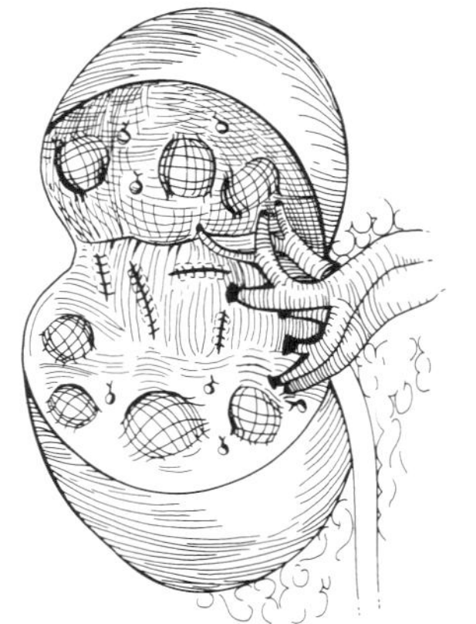

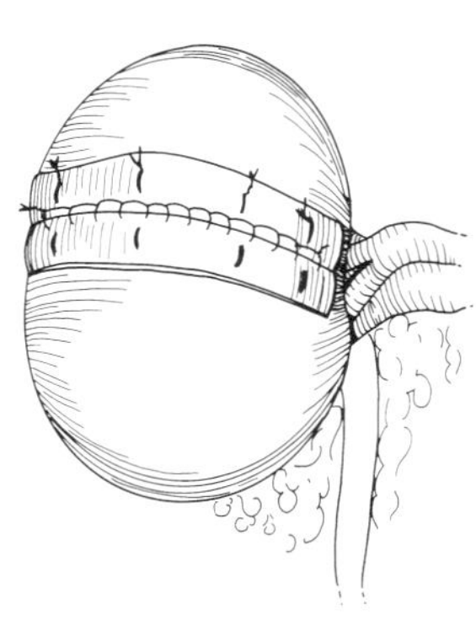

Fig. 30.14 The kidney after complete tumor resection, ligation of intraparenchymal vessels, closure of the collecting system, and, finally, closure of the parenchymal defect.

for the identification and closure of small leaking vessels. The reconstructed kidney is reimplanted in the contralateral iliac fossa, utilizing standard renal transplantation technique (Fig. 30.15). The ureter is stented and reimplanted using a modified Lich–Gregoire technique.

Nephron-sparing surgery in patients with hereditary RCC

Recently the role of NSS in hereditary renal cancer, namely, von Hippel–Lindau disease and hereditary papillary RCC, has been studied. These conditions are characterized by multiple, bilateral, usually (but not always) low-grade RCC that develop and may recur throughout the patient's lifetime. The spectrum of renal lesions includes lesions of various sizes ranging from cysts to cysts with hyperplastic clear cells to frank solid lesions. The concern with NSS in this population is the high recurrence rate due to the

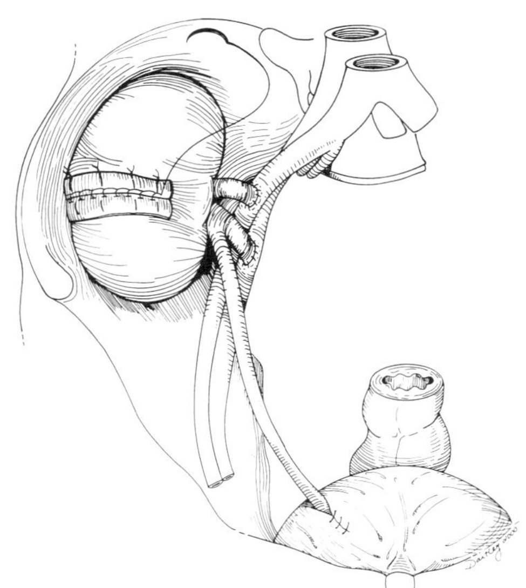

Fig. 30.15 The completed autotransplant. Ureteral reimplantation is carried out utilizing a modified Lich–Gregoire technique.

nature of the disease. A multicenter trial addressing this issue and the role of partial nephrectomy was conducted in 65 von Hippel–Lindau patients with bilateral (54) and unilateral (11) renal tumors (Steinbach *et al.* 1995). Forty-nine and 16 patients underwent partial nephrectomy and radical nephrectomy, respectively. The 5- and 10-year cancer-specific survival rates were 100 and 81 per cent, respectively, utilizing partial nephrectomy. Therefore, partial nephrectomy has a clear role in von Hippel–Lindau disease. However, no clear guidelines exist for the timing of surgical intervention and the optimal method of treatment. In order to answer this question, investigators at the US National Cancer Institute recently evaluated a 3 cm surgical threshold in this group of patients (Walther *et al.* 1999). Tumors were less than 3 cm in 52 patients and greater than 3 cm in 44 patients with von Hippel–Lindau disease. Patients in the former group underwent parenchymal-sparing surgery more frequently than the latter group. None of the patients with tumors less than 3 cm developed metastases as opposed to 25 per cent in the greater than 3 cm group. A total of 23 patients had hereditary papillary renal cell cancers; ten less than 3 cm and 13 had greater than 3 cm tumors. None of the patients with tumors less than 3 cm developed metastatic disease as opposed to 15 per cent with larger tumors. These investigators recommend careful follow-up of tumors less than 3 cm in size in this group of patients with prompt parenchymal-sparing surgery when this threshold is exceeded. Enucleation allows for maximal renal preservation in these patients who can have innumerable renal tumors and in whom standard partial nephrectomy with 1 cm normal parenchyma will invariably lead to significant cumulative parenchymal loss. Indeed, investigators at the US National Institutes of Health have noted patients with these hereditary conditions to have 1100 to 3400 microscopic lesions per kidney and have postulated frank tumor development to be related to clustering of microscopic tumors (Ornstein *et al.* 2000). These lesions are characteristically of lower grade and have a distinct pseudocapsule allowing for easy enucleation along this natural plane (Poston *et al.* 1994). Smaller, additional cysts and lesions can be fulgurated. Intraoperative ultrasound may be of value in the detection and removal of lesions deeper in the cortex. Even after meticulous removal of all identifiable renal lesions, these patients are not cured and careful follow-up is mandatory as tumors that were microscopic at the time of surgery can become clinically detectable.

Additional considerations

Using adequate preoperative planning, meticulous surgical technique, proper patient selection, and attention to detail, NSS can be performed with minimal morbidity and excellent outcomes for the majority of patients selected. The role of partial nephrectomy in the setting of metastatic disease and a solitary kidney is not clearly defined. Certainly, this operation is contraindicated in the presence of nodal metastases. The use of intraoperative adjuncts such as ultrasonography and especially frozen-section analysis are invaluable to the operating surgeon in prompt and effective decision-making.

The placement of a closed suction drain is imperative after NSS. The use of this technique provides a watertight closure of large parenchymal defects. Certainly there are other traditional methods of closure such as closure of the parenchyma with horizontal sutures over the length of the defect utilizing fat, Oxycel or closure using Gelfoam and Surgicel bolsters. These methods depend on the strength of the renal capsule. The use of Gore-Tex allows for an even distribution of tension along the length of the closure. Small bleeding vessels are easily tamponaded. It also allows for the ability to tie the sutures with the desired tension, without risking tear of the kidney capsule especially when the arterial clamp is removed in transverse resections carried out for larger tumors. One concern about use of exogenous material has been the postoperative tissue reaction that might occur, particularly when a repeat resection is contemplated in the future. In the authors' experience Gore-Tex is relatively unreactive and, although a pseudocapsule will form, the subsequent explorations have not been difficult and the inflammatory tissue reaction around the Gore-Tex has been minimal.

Complications

Most complications of nephron sparing surgery can be managed conservatively (Campbell *et al.* 1994). The risk of a significant complication, however, increases as the technical complexity of the case increases. There is a direct correlation between morbidity and the extent of the NSS. Morbidity is least in enucleation and *in situ* conservative surgery, where most tumors are smaller and peripherally located (Lerner *et al.* 1996). In these patients the morbidities of NSS parallel those of radical nephrectomy (Lerner *et al.* 1996; Campbell *et al.* 1994). Accordingly, complication rates are higher in larger tumor resections in patients who have multifocal or bilateral tumors or resections in patients with large tumors in a solitary kidney. Extracorporeal surgery is associated with an increased risk of major complications including renal vascular thrombosis and renal failure (Campbell *et al.* 1994; Stormont *et al.* 1992). These resections usually involve extensive manipulation of the renal vasculature and collecting system.

Hemorrhage

The most troublesome and common intraoperative complication of partial nephrectomy is excessive bleeding. In this respect meticulous dissection, attention to detail, and ligation of intraparenchymal vessels are of paramount importance. The easy access to the renal hilum, provided by early identification and isolation of the renal artery, provides the additional safety of prompt arterial occlusion when excessive bleeding precludes a clear surgical field and adequate visualization. Postoperative hemorrhage usually is self- resolving and may be confined to the retroperitoneum or present with gross hematuria, decreased hematocrit, or flank ecchymosis. Treatment is expectant consisting of volume resuscitation, serial hematocrits, and bedrest. Embolization is an option in the unusual case where bleeding persists after conservative management, requiring multiple transfusions. Re-exploration is the last resort for severe intractable bleeding.

Urinary fistula

Entry into the collecting system should be recognized intraoperatively and repaired. Failure to do so can result in a postoperative urinoma. Risk factors include central location, larger tumor size, and increased complexity of the nephron-sparing operation (Campbell *et al.* 1994). A small amount of urinary leakage is conceivably common and usually ceases spontaneously. Persistent drainage through the drain suggests a larger leak, which can still be managed expectantly. In the absence of ureteral obstruction, the majority of leaks seal as more tissue healing occurs. If a urinoma forms after the flank drain has been removed, placement of a percutaneous drainage catheter in the urinoma is indicated to prevent abscess formation. The collecting system should also be drained with a percutaneous nephrostomy tube or, preferably, with a ureteral stent to seal the leakage site in the collecting system.

Renal insufficiency

Most cases of renal insufficiency after NSS are the result of transient ischemia during surgery and usually resolve spontaneously. Intraoperative measures to decrease the possibility of this complication ,namely, preoperative hydration, correction of electrolyte abnormalities, use of Mannitol, maintaining the arterial clamp time to a minimum, and utilization of surface hypothermia, are preventive. Patients should be aware of the risk of postoperative acute tubular necrosis and the possibility of temporary or permanent dialysis especially in the setting of a solitary kidney. When recognized postoperatively, appropriate fluid and electrolyte management and the use of dialysis if necessary can aid in the return of renal function. Nephrotoxic medications should be stopped or the dosages altered. The risk of permanent renal failure utilizing modern techniques in NSS, even in the setting of complex resections, were 3.8 and 4.3 per cent, respectively, in two large referral centers (Stormont *et al.* 1992; Morgan and Zincke 1990). If *ex vivo* cases representing complex resections are excluded from these series, the risk of renal insufficiency in the *in situ* partial nephrectomy is on the order of 1 per cent (Stormont *et al.* 1992). The risk of chronic renal failure after partial nephrectomy versus radical nephrectomy with a normal contralateral kidney has been addressed by Lau *et al.* from the Mayo Clinic (Lau *et al.* 2000). This long-term study series included 328 patients who were optimally matched for year of surgery, age, sex, renal function, grade, stage, and size of tumor. Local recurrence was only 2%. Tumor in the contralateral kidney occurred in 1 per cent of the patients in each group. The 10- and 15-year cause-specific survival were 98 and 91 per cent, and 96 and 96 per cent for partial and radical nephrectomy, respectively, thus showing no difference in outcome. The need for renal replacement therapy (hemodialysis) occurred more often in the nephrectomy series than in the NSS group. Furthermore, patients in the radical nephrectomy group had significantly higher serum creatinine ($p = 0.003$; 1.6 versus 1.3 mg per cent) than in the nephron-preserving group. This series is particularly credible, because of its long-term follow-up (15 years) and presents the first evidence that partial nephrectomy is associated with significantly less renal failure than experienced by patients who undergo ipsilateral radical nephrectomy in the presence of a contralateral normal kidney.

Other complications including infections or those attributable to anesthesia such as atelectasis and pneumonia can occur. Appropriate antibiotic treatment and postoperative use of incentive spirometry can manage and decrease their incidence.

Results of nephron-sparing surgery

Nephron-sparing surgery is now associated with improved technical success rates and long-term disease-free survival rates comparable to those of radical nephrectomy especially in low-stage disease (Butler *et al.* 1995; Lerner *et al.* 1996; Hafez *et al.* 1998). Excluding hereditary renal tumors, the overall risks of local recurrence in modern partial nephrectomy series are on the order of 4–6 per cent (Lerner *et al.* 1996; Morgan and Zincke 1990; Hafez *et al.*1997). Local recurrence rates were reported to be higher in patients with suspected disease (6.6 per cent) versus incidental disease (1.1 per cent) (Licht *et al.* 1994). Incidental tumors are of lower size, grade, and stage. Local recurrence after NSS represents, in part, growth of multifocal RCC and not incompletely resected tumor. In a recent study of multifocality in RCC the incidence of true unknown multifocality (at the time of surgery) was 6 per cent, corresponding roughly to the local recurrence rates in the studies cited above (Kletscher *et al.* 1995). The inherent risk of multifocality dictates a thorough inspection of the entire surface of the kidney at the time of the operation. Certain pathologic patterns raise suspicion of multifocality, namely papillary RCC or a mixed cell histological pattern (Kletscher *et al.* 1995).

Nephron sparing surgery for RCC can achieve long-term tumor control especially in the setting of a primary tumor less than 4 cm. In a recent study of 76 patients who underwent NSS, only three patients developed metastatic disease at a mean follow-up of 75 months (Van Poppel *et al.* 1998). Of the 51 patients who had a normal contralateral kidney, tumors were generally small and 49 patients had pathologic T1 or T2 tumors. Review of nephron-sparing surgical data from two large centers reveal a 5-year cause-specific survival at 5 years approaching 90–95 per cent for pathologic stage I RCC (Lerner *et al.* 1996; Morgan and Zincke 1990; Hafez *et al.* 1997). As the pathologic stage of the renal lesion is increased, the risk of local recurrence and metastatic disease also increase (Hafez *et al.* 1997).

Recently, this was further confirmed when an analysis of the long-term results of NSS for localized RCC was published (Fergany *et al.* 2000). The review included 107 patients with RCC, 96 of whom (90 per cent) underwent surgery for imperative indications. The 10-year cancer-specific survival was 73 per cent. The results are remarkable given the proportion of patients who underwent the operation for imperative indications. More than a third had pathologic T3 disease and 17 per cent had high-grade cancer. The recurrence rate was 10 per cent, also probably due to unfavorable characteristics. When considering tumors less than 4 cm, a more representative population in this era of increased cross-sectional imaging and incidental tumor detection, the cancer-specific survivals at 5 and 10 years were 98 and 92 per cent respectively. Local recurrence was detected in only 4 per cent of cases, which were salvaged by surgical resection. Based on this long-term study from an institution at the forefront of NSS, excellent long-term cancer control can be attained and isolated local recurrences do not always lead to metastases or cancer death. Ninety three per cent of patients in this group with imperative indications maintained sufficient renal function to avoid dialysis, further confirming the safety and efficacy of NSS. An even longer follow-up study is that of Lau *et al.* from the Mayo Clinic (unpublished data) who described a 15-year cause-specific survival of 91 per cent in a group of 164 patients who underwent partial nephrectomy for tumors an average of < 4 cm in diameter and where the local recurrence rate was only 2 per cent at this time interval. These long-term data from two major institutions confirm the disposition to proceed with partial nephrectomy in patients with smaller tumors even in the presence of a normal contralateral kidney.

The impact of primary tumor size on postoperative tumor recurrence and survival after partial nephrectomy has been controversial. The recent change in the TNM (tumor–node– metastasis) staging system for RCC that increases the size of the T1 renal lesion to 7 cm presents an additional variable in this equation (Guinan *et al.* 1997). A recent study that addresses outcomes according to tumor size revealed that 5- and 10-year cause-specific survival rates were 96 and 90 per cent, respectively, for tumors 4 cm or less versus 86 and 66 per cent, respectively, for those greater than 4 cm ($p = 0.0001$) (Hafez *et al.* 1999). The tumor recurrences rates were also significantly lower when the original size of the tumor was less than 4 cm. In addition to recommending the substratification of T1 renal lesions in the new TNM system, this large single-center study also serves to confirm the excellent success rate with elective NSS in patients with a solitary small (< 4 cm) RCC.

Follow-up

After NSS, patients are advised to return in 4 to 6 weeks for serum creatinine measurement and intravenous pyelography. In the absence of obstruction, the patient will undergo 6-monthly CT for 2 years, then yearly for the next 5 years after which the frequency is decreased to every 2 years. Chest X-rays, measurements of serum calcium, alkaline phosphatase, liver function tests, and creatinine are obtained yearly for the initial 5 years and biannually thereafter. Some advocate the frequency of postoperative evaluation as dictated by the initial tumor stage with less rigorous structured follow-up for low-stage, small tumors (Poston *et al.* 1994).

References

Bosniak, M.A. (1995). Observation of small incidentally detected renal masses. *Sem. Urol. Oncol.* **13**, 267.

Butler, B.P., Novick, A.C., Miller, D.P., Campbell, S.A., and Licht, M.R. (1995). Management of small unilateral renal cell carcinomas: radical versus nephron-sparing surgery. *Urology* **45**, 34.

Campbell, S.C., Novick, A.C., Streem, S.B., Klein, E., and Licht, M. (1994). Complications of nephron sparing surgery for renal tumors. *J. Urol.* **151**, 1177–80.

Campbell, S.C., Fichtner, J., Novick, A.C., Steinbach, F., Stockle, M., Klein, E.A., Filipas, D., Levi, H.S., Storkel, S, Schweden, F., Obuchowski, N.A., and Hale, J. (1996). Intraoperative evaluation of renal cell carcinoma: a prospective study of the role of ultrasonography and histopathological frozen sections. *J. Urol.* **155**, 1191–5.

Coll, D.M., Uzzo, R.G., Herts, B.R., Davros, W.J., Wirth, S.L., and Novick, A.C. (1999). 3-dimensional volume rendered computerized tomography for preoperative evaluation and intraoperative treatment of patients undergoing nephron sparing surgery. *J. Urol.* **161**, 1097.

Dechet, C.B., Sebo, T., Farrow, G., Blute, M.L., Engen, D.E., and Zincke, H. (1999). Prospective analysis of intraoperative frozen needle biopsy of solid renal masses in adults. *J. Urol.* **162**, 1282.

Fergany, A.F., Hafez, K.S., and Novick, A.C. (2000). Long-term results of nephron sparing surgery for localized renal cell carcinoma: 10 year followup. *J. Urol.* **163**, 442–5.

Guinan, P., Sobin, L.H., Algaba, F., Badellino, F., Kameyama, S., MacLennan, G., and Novick, A. (1997). TNM staging of renal cell carcinoma: workup no.3. Union International Contre le Cancer (UICC) and the American Joint Committee on Cancer (AJCC). *Cancer* **80**, 992.

Hafez, K.S., Novick, A.C., and Campbell, S.C. (1997). Patterns of tumor recurrence and guidelines for followup after nephron sparing surgery for sporadic renal cell carcinoma. *J. Urol.* **157**, 2067–70.

Hafez, K.S., Novick, A.C., and Butler, B. (1998). Management of small, solitary, unilateral renal cell carcinoma: impact of central versus peripheral tumor location. *J. Urol.* **159**, 1156.

Hafez, K.S., Fergany, A.F., and Novick, A.C. (1999). Nephron sparing surgery for localized renal cell carcinoma: Impact of tumor size on patient survival, tumor recurrence and TNM staging. *J. Urol.* **162**, 1930–3.

Kletscher, B.A., Qian, J., Bostwick, D.G., Andrews, P.E., and Zincke, H. (1995). Prospective analysis of multifocality in renal cell carcinoma: influence of histological pattern, grade, number, size, volume and deoxyribonucleic acid ploidy. *J. Urol.* **153**, 904–6.

Lau, W., Blute, M.L., Weaver, A.L., Torres, V.E., and Zincke, H. (2000). Matched comparison of radical neprectomy vs nephron sparing surgery in patients with unilateral renal cell carcinoma and a normal contralateral kidney. *Mayo Clin. Proc.* **75**, 1236–1242.

Lerner, S.E., Hawkins, C.A., Blute, M.L., Grabner, A., Wollan, P.C., Eickholt, J.T., and Zincke, H. (1996). Disease outcome in patients with low stage renal cell carcinoma treated with nephron sparing or radical surgery. *J. Urol.* **155**, 1868.

Levine, E., Huntrakoon, M., and Wetzel, C.H. (1989). Small renal neoplasms: clinical, pathologic and imaging features. *Am. J. Roentgenol.* **153**, 69.

Licht, M.R., Novick, A.C., and Goormastic, M. (1994). Nephron-sparing surgery in incidental versus suspected renal cell carcinoma. *J. Urol.* **152**, 39–42.

Morgan, W.R. and Zincke, H. (1990). Progression and survival after renal-conserving surgery for renal cell carcinoma: experience in 104 patients and extended followup. *J. Urol.* **144**, 852–7.

Ornstein, D.K., Lebensky, I.A., Venzon, D., Zbar, B., Linehan, W.M., and Walther, M.M. (2000). Prevalence of microscopic tumors in normal appearing renal parenchyma of patients with hereditary papillary renal cancer. *J. Urol.* **163**, 431–3.

Poston, C.D., Jaffe, G.S., and Lubensky, I.A. (1994). Characterization of the renal pathology of a familial form of renal cell carcinoma associated with von Hippel Lindau disease: clinical and molecular genetic implications. *J. Urol.* **153**, 561.

Smith, S.J., Bosniak, M.A., Megibow, A.J., Hulnick, D.H., Horii, S.C., and Raghavendra, B.N. (1989). Renal cell carcinoma: earlier discovery and increased detection. *Radiology* **170**, 699.

Steinbach, F., Novick, A.C., and Zincke, H. (1995). Treatment of renal cell carcinoma in von Hippel Lindau disease; a multicenter study. *J. Urol.* **153**, 1812–16.

Stormont, T.J., Bilhartz, D.L., and Zincke, H. (1992). Pitfalls of "bench surgery" and autotransplantation for renal cell carcinoma. *Mayo Clin. Proc.* **67**, 621–8.

Van Poppel, H., Bamelis, B., Oyen, R., and Baert, L. (1998). Partial nephrectomy for renal cell carcinoma can achieve long-term tumor control. *J. Urol.* **160**, 674–8.

Walther, M.M., Choyke, P.L., Glenn, G., Lyne, C., Rayford, W., Venzon, D., and Linehan, W.M. (1999). Renal cancer in families with hereditary renal cancer: prospective analysis of a tumor size threshold for renal parenchymal sparing surgery. *J. Urol.* **161**, 1475–9.

Zincke, H. and Ruckle, H.C. (1995). Use of exogenous material to bolster closure of the parenchymal defect following partial nephrectomy. *Urology* **46**, 96–8.

31. Lymph node dissection

Amnon Zisman, Allan J. Pantuck, and Arie S. Belldegrun

Introduction

Pathological evidence of lymph node positive disease portends a striking decrease in life expectancy for patients with renal cell carcinoma (RCC) (deKernion *et al.* 1978). Intuitively speaking, the inclusion of retroperitoneal lymph node dissection (RPLND) during radical nephrectomy should add information relevant to the determination of prognosis, but more intriguing is whether it exerts a survival advantage and what is the trade-off for this benefit as compared to the potential additional morbidity and mortality. Lately, substantial evidence stemming from European Organization for Research and Treatment of Cancer (EORTC) studies as well as UCLA experience suggest that nephrectomy followed by immunotherapy provides a survival advantage over nephrectomy alone for metastatic patients (Fig. 31.1). Concurrently, a parallel trend, in which larger number of patients with small, incidental, T1 lesions are being diagnosed and as a result are eligible for expanded surgical options, is taking place worldwide. These expanded options include partial nephrectomy with a normal contralateral kidney, laparoscopic nephrectomy, and experimental tissue ablative procedures such as cryoablation ,high-intensity focused ultrasound (HIFU), and radiofrequency interstitial tissue ablation (RITA). Therefore, reviewing the role of lymphadnectomy is timely and a discussion of the technique employed and its extensiveness is warranted. This chapter will concentrate on these pertinent questions associated with the modern role of RPLND in the comprehensive treatment of RCC.

The incidence of positive retroperitoneal lymph node dissection

The overall incidence of positive nodes in Robson's classical studies was 22.7 per cent (Robson *et al.* 1969). However, more recently, the reported incidence in the nephrectomy arm of the EORTC 30881 prospective study was only 3.3 per cent (Mickisch, 1999). According to the UCLA experience with 661 nephrectomies in 1989–99, the overall frequency of node-positive (N+) disease was 28 per cent. In this subset of patients, 46 per cent presented with extranodal distant metastases. Therefore node-positive disease would be better looked at in patients presenting with M0 disease. According to the UCLA experience, the incidence of T1N+M0 and T2N+M0 disease was low and similar to that reported by Mickisch (1999) (Table 31.1) However, among T3/4M0 patients the incidence is much higher (19.3 per cent) using the 1997 American Joint Committee on Cancer (AJCC) TNM (tumor-node–metastasis) classification for the T stage. A selection bias is naturally present so, given the fact that the incidence of patients with unknown node state is 7 per cent in the UCLA series, it is possible that the true N+ disease incidence is slightly higher then reported herein (Zisman *et al.* 2000).

The distribution of positive nodes in RCC patients

Understanding the distribution of positive nodes in RCC patients is pertinent for the evaluation of the merit as well as the extent of RPLND. Behind a decision to perform RPLND lies the assumption that nodal involvement is an orderly, predictable, pattern of spread going from microscopic to macroscopic, from proximal to distal, and with a pattern of dissemination that correlates with the primary tumor burden and its biological aggressiveness. Chaotic tumor behavior leading to an unpredictable course would make RPLND less attractive for either diagnostic or curative pur-

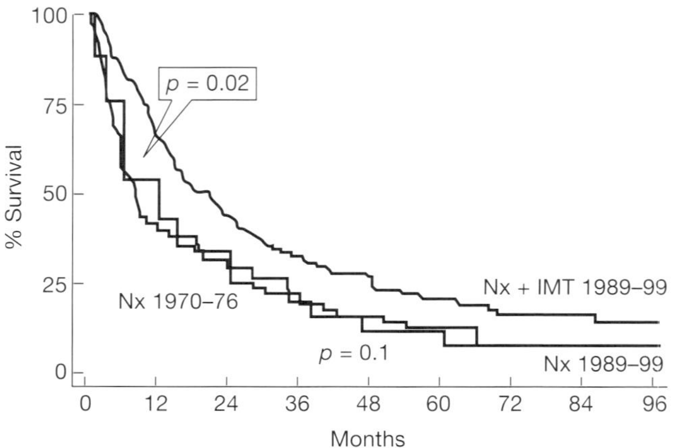

Fig. 31.1 UCLA experience (1988–99) with nephrectomy (Nx) + immunotherapy (IMT) versus nephrectomy alone and a comparison with compatible historical series (1970–76; deKernion *et al.* 1978).

Table 31.1 Incidence of N+ disease in different studies

Study	n/N	Group	N+ disease (%)
Robson *et al.* (1969)	16/70	Overall	23
Hülten *et al.* (1969)	6/22	Overall	27
Skinner *et al.* (1971a)	19/309	Overall	6
Carl *et al.* (1977)	40/270	Pathologic T1–2	9.3
		Pathologic T3–4	24
Sigel *et al.* (1981)	29/76	Formal RPLND	38
Giuliani *et al.* (1983)	15/104	Pathologic T1–2	5
		Pathologic T3–4	36
Herrlinger *et al.* (1990)	56/320	Formal RPLND in M0 patients	17.5
	19/191	No RPLND or limited RPLND	10
Zisman *et al.* (2000)*	156/510	T1	7
		T1N+M0	2
		T2	24
		T2N+M0	3
		T3/4N+M0	20

* In this study the AJCC's 1997 TNM classification for the T stage was used.

poses. The great interpatient variation in the anatomic structure of the lymphatic system and the complexity of the cellular events leading to the macroscopic phenomenon of metastasis probably contribute to some chaotic aspects in the progression of RCC within the retroperitoneal lymphatics. For example, Skinner *et al.* (1978) showed contralateral lymph node (LN) involvement in up to 25 per cent of patients who have regional and periaortic LN involvement. Therefore, when performed ipsilateral to the primary lesion, a unilateral RPLND would not be enough to provide the survival benefit expected with complete resection of the involved lymphatic tissue. Moreover, the asymmetry in the pattern of lymphatic drainage between the two sides of the retroperitoneum also results in a difference in the lymphatic progression of tumors originating from the right kidney and the left kidney.

The classic study in this field was published by Alice E. Parker (1935) of the University of Colorado School of Medicine. He injected Prussian blue into the kidneys of stillborn fetuses and looked at the distribution of the dye as it was carried proximally by the lymphatic system. He found three main vertical lymph channels: (1) left lateral lumbar; (2) interaortico-caval; (3) lateral caval. Channels 2 and 3 are the main vertical lymph pathways of the right lateral lumbar lymphatics. Other groups of lymph nodes and channels are the pre-aortic, post-aortic, pre-caval, post-caval, and sacral promontory lymph nodes all of whose related lymph vessels are engaged in cross-linking together the three vertical channels.

Parker noted that dye injection to the right kidney will immigrate through the efferent lymphatics to the regional LN (interaorto-caval, lateral caval, posterior caval, and pre-caval) and then superiorly to LN on the diaphragmatic crus as well as through the right roots of the thoracic duct into the blood circulation, inferiorly to the nodes of the sacral promontory and into the superior domains of the common iliac lymphatics, ipsilaterally as well as to the upper hypogastric LN and the external iliac chains. Medially the injected dye crosses to the posterior aortic and pre-aortic channels to the nodes of the left lateral lumbar chain and pre-aortic nodes. Laterally it is carried through post-caval channels to the lateral caval chain and thereafter it migrates inferiorly through

channels on the anterior surface of the right psoas muscle. Parker also demonstrated that, whenever the thoracic duct is filled by injection from the right kidney, it may extend in a retrograde fashion through the left roots of the thoracic duct and migrate as inferiorly as the common iliac vessels.

From the left kidney, dye may find its way to regional nodes: on the diaphragm superior or inferior to the renal blood vessels and from there to the thoracic duct or to intrathoracic nodes on the posterior wall of the thorax, to upper nodes in the left lateral lumbar chain in the vicinity of the inferior mesenteric artery outflow that drain to the thoracic duct, to preaortic LN, and occasionally to interaorto-caval nodes and inferiorly through the left lateral lumbar chain. When injection of the left kidney filled the thoracic duct with dye, a retrograde migration was noted through the right roots of the thoracic duct. Moreover, when the thoracic duct wad filled, there was a lateral flow to nodes in the chest cavity on both sides of the thoracic vertebrae below the level of the fourth intercostal space. Parker could not demonstrate any direct lymphatic connections between the right and left kidney. He noted that, although there are distinct lymph vessels anterior to the aorta that connect the right and left lateral lumbar lymph channels, a series of horizontal post-aortic lymph channels were commonly found and were more frequently functional than the pre-aortic lymph vessels in transporting an injection mass from one lateral abdominal lymph channel to the other. He also noted that an injection mass introduced into the parenchyma of either kidney will flow through lymph channels further than the regional nodes through the main posterior lymph channels of the abdomen and the thoracic duct.

This study, as well as others that documented the lymphatic drainage of normal kidneys, was extremely important in delineating the anatomic structure of the retroperitoneal lymphatics. However, it becomes apparent that tumor spread from advanced disease largely deviates from the aforementioned trails: the lymphatic channels from the perinephric fat drain into a more cranial and lateral position than described earlier for the renal parenchyma. Moreover, it would be expected that lymphatic drainage would follow the pathway of aberrant neovascularity known to emerge inside and in the vicinity of renal carcinomas. This, of course, potentially causes an unpredictable pattern of tumor spread to the retroperitoneal space, confounding attempts at surgical extirpation of all potential tumor-bearing lymphatics (deKernion 1980). Nevertheless, different tumor types as well as tumor–host relationships are probably of extreme importance: For example, although injection studies to the prostate could not demonstrate any lymphatic flow lateral to the obturator region (Raghavaiah and Jordan 1979), it is a well known fact that prostatic cancer metastasizes most commonly to the hypogastric and obturator LN (McLaughlin *et al.* 1976). Therefore injection studies provide the broad anatomical framework for understanding LN involvement and metastatic spread, but the actual events taking place are influenced by more complex interactions as yet not fully understood.

One of the most meticulous studies documenting the lymphatic involvement in RCC patients was published by Hülten *et al.* (1969). They found that the majority of the involved nodes were located adjacent to the ipsilateral renal hilum or near the junction between the renal vessels and the aorta and inferior vena cava but also on the opposite side of the great vessels and in the supraclavicular region. Confirmatory results were reported by others who all seem to agree that, in most cases, the regional ipsilateral nodes are primarily involved although occasionally chaotic nodal behavior is encountered (deKernion 1980; Giuliani *et al.* 1983; Pizzocaro 1986).

What is the benefit from improved staging offered by lymphadenectomy?

Does RPLND reflect the extent of the disease?

Blood-borne metastases of RCC are as common as lymphatic metastasis. Many patients without LN involvement die as a result of metastatic disease (deKernion 1980). As a group, 20 per cent of node-positive patients have negative regional nodes and only extraregional involvement (Giuliani *et al.* 1983). Therefore LN metastasis status has a limited significance in the prediction of the extent to which tumors escape the confines of the kidney. These arguments are supported by the UCLA experience, which shows that 86 per cent of patients with nodal involvement also had distant metastases (71, 91, 87, and 99 per cent of T1, T2, T3, and T4 patients, respectively), and 37 per cent of all the patients with distant metastasis had negative nodes at surgery (Zisman *et al.* 2000). Consequently, a positive RPLND may suggest a high risk for distant metastases, which may be T-stage-dependent, but a negative dissection does not necessarily assure a metastasis-free state. Therefore, as a diagnostic tool *per se*, the performance of RPLND adds only modestly and correlates poorly with the disease extent.

RPLND disclose pathological N+M0 disease in patients with clinically staged N0M0 disease

Immunotherapy is currently the preferred adjuvant therapy for metastatic RCC. The UCLA experience suggests that nephrectomy + immunotherapy has an advantage over nephrectomy alone in metastatic patients (Fig. 31.1). By using RPLND, patients otherwise staged as having clinical N– disease, may be histologically diagnosed as having a N+ disease and become candidates for immunotherapy or experimental protocols. Peters and Brown (1980) demonstrated that 24 out of 69 patients (35 per cent) staged as Robson's B had microscopic nodal involvement. A similar observation of 31 per cent was published by Waters and Richie (1977). Taking these values as rough estimates for the occurrence of microscopic nodal disease, it seems attractive to perform a RPLND in patients who preoperatively were staged as N0M0 since in some of them, in spite of imaging negative for nodal enlargement, finding a microscopic involvement in RPLND may cause pathological staging to become N+M0 and to turn this group of patients into immunotherapy candidates. From our perspective, the availability of immunotherapy in recent years is a major contributor to the relevance of this discussion on RPLND in RCC at general. However, as shown previously, the occurrence of N+M0 patients is extremely low among T1 and T2 patients. Only among T3 and T4 patients do we find a significant incidence of N+M0 patients (19 per cent). Peters and Brown (1980) reported that 77 per cent of 31 patients with stage III disease have microscopic nodal involvement. Therefore, these patients may benefit from RPLND in the sense of immediate diagnosis of an unexpected N+ disease and prompt administration of immunotherapy. Considering the opposite extreme, enlargement of regional lymph nodes in RCC detected by computerized tomography (CT) scan was shown not to be necessarily due to metastases in 31.2–42 per cent of cases (Studer *et al.* 1990; Phillips and Messing 1993). Therefore RPLND may supplement CT and magnetic resonance imaging (MRI) scans in this regard, and differentiate between patients who are candidates for immunotherapy and those who are falsely positive.

The therapeutic role of RPLND in RCC patients

Does lymphadenctomy plus radical nephrectomy provide an overall survival advantage over radical nephrectomy alone?

As far as we are aware, there is no prospective study published to answer this question. The only prospective study presented, and its results are not yet published, is the EORTC 30881. A preliminary analysis of the EORTC 30881 data could not demonstrate a survival advantage for patients having RPLND (Mickisch 1999). Although other retrospective publications on this matter suffer great limitations in terms of methodology and design, they provide substantial evidence to support an overall advantage for RPLND and radical nephrectomy as opposed to radical nephrectomy alone (Herrlinger *et al.* 1990). Peters and Brown (1980) reported on 13 patients who were staged as Robson C as a result of RPLND findings. These patients survived longer (5-year survival = 44 per cent) than patients staged as Robson C because of local extension or inferior vena cava (IVC) involvement who did not have RPLND (5-year survival = 26 per cent). They also demonstrated an improved survival in 59 out of 148 patients with systemic disease that had nephrectomy plus RPLND over patients who had nephrectomy alone (29 per cent 5-year survival, $n = 23$ versus 9 per cent, $n = 36$). For Robson's stage A and B a survival advantage was shown for 1 year of follow-up as well (100 versus 90 per cent and 92 versus 67 per cent, respectively). This advantage leveled off at 5 years.

Apart from being retrospective, these reports may be misleading since their results are subject to the influence of severe patient selection and surgeons' preference. Inaccuracies may also result from operator election not to undertake RPLND in patients who have very large nodes because of an assumption that they are positive, as a result of intraoperative conclusion of unresectability, or when an operator chooses not to perform RPLND because no enlargement is seen or palpated grossly.

This contradiction between many retrospective studies and the EORTC 30881 study does not solve the problem posed. There are still not enough data originating from controlled trials, particularly concerning the survival benefit of LN debulking in RCC patients and on differences in the response to immunotherapy and experimental therapies between patients who were given extensive LN debulking versus those who did not among N+M0 disease as well as N+M1 disease.

Our feeling is that, until the final results and conclusions of the EORTC 30881 study are available, it is possible that a survival benefit may result from RPLND and therefore in some centers extensive RPLND are being performed and may be justified.

Does RPLND lower the chance for local recurrence after nephrectomy?

Theoretically, RPLND should decrease the incidence of local recurrence since, in patients postnephrectomy; RPLND should eliminate residual disease in the vicinity of the renal bed. Local recurrence after radical nephrectomy without RPLND was reported to be 11 per cent (Parent *et al.* 1984; Phillips and Messing 1993), whereas after performance of extended RPLND the reported rates of local recurrence were shown to vary between 2.5 and 8 per cent (Giuliani *et al.* 1983; Skinner *et al.* 1971; Bassil *et al.* 1985). At UCLA we notice 2.8 per cent of local recurrence among 661 patients having radical nephrectomies and only limited RPLND. Nevertheless, the local recurrence rate for nephron-sparing surgery performed without RPLND is reported

to be only 4.1–5.8 per cent (Morgan and Zincke 1990; Steinbach *et al.* 1992; Licht *et al.* 1994). This low rate partially reflects selection of low-grade, low-stage patients for nephron-sparing surgery and gives some confidence that procedures such as laparoscopic radical nephrectomy and ablative measures (cryosurgery, HIFU, and RITA), currently performed without RPLND, will probably not result in higher incidence of local recurrence originating from LN in low-stage patients. However, since the data available on local recurrences is still controversial and primarily based on retrospective observations subjected to the influence of multiple biasing factors, the hypothesis that incompletely resected nodal metastases contribute substantially to local recurrence should be cautiously evaluated prospectively in the future.

Does RPLND add to radical nephrectomy morbidity?

Fundamental surgical concepts state that additional dissection always contributes to patient morbidity. The data available on RPLND morbidity is sparse, retrospective, and mainly refers to historical series approximately 20 years old (Table 31.2). These studies suggest a minimal increase in mortality for nephrectomy with RPLND over nephrectomy alone. However, these studies do not deal at all with more modern quality of life issues as we recognize them today, and also lack systemic stratification or multivariate analysis permitting identification of patients at risk for dying perioperatively as a result of the RPLND. Reported data on the morbidity of modified template RPLND performed for testicular tumors clearly demonstrate, even in much younger patients, that extended RPLND for RCC should have some additional morbidity. Although not exactly comparable, these data sets at least indicate that extensive RPLND is probably not lacking in morbidity. The current information, discussed earlier and in other chapters in this book, indicates that biological intervention in the form of immunotherapy integrated with extensive resection of the primary tumor has a survival advantage for metastatic patients (Franklin *et al.* 1996). This brings back the question as to what is the real morbidity associated with heroic nephrectomies and extensive RPLND. Other trends taking place in the last decades make judgement even more complicated. More patients are operated on with asymptomatic disease, the diagnosed tumors are smaller, and the number of patients with overt bulky node involvement is reduced (Mickisch 1999). At the same time resuscitative capabilities have expanded. This probably allows more

Table 31.2 Perioperative mortality rates for nephrectomy (Nx) and nephrectomy plus RPLND

Study	*n*	Procedure	Perioperative mortality (%)
Robson *et al.* (1969)	88	Radical Nx	3.4
Giuliani *et al.* (1983)	104	Radical Nx + extensive RPLND	10
Skinner *et al.* (1971a)	80	Simple Nx	2.75*
	149	Radical Nx + RPLND	
Herrlinger *et al.* (1990)	320	Radical Nx + extended RPLND	0.9

*This is the percentage increase in perioperative mortality for those experiencing radical nephrectomy + RPLND as compared with those experiencing simple nephrectomy alone.

extensive dissection with reduced biological price and broader safety margins and resuscitative back-up. It seems that it is increasingly difficult to address the morbidity question since the nature of the patients, the disease, and the supportive medical matrix has changed. It is our impression that these trends cause polarization of the morbidity question. On the one hand, there are low-stage, low-grade, asymptomatic patients who can better tolerate extensive RPLND but probably need it less and, on the other hand, there are metastatic and symptomatic patients requiring major interventions. Therefore prospective studies on the morbidity of RPLND are needed in order to weigh the potential morbidity versus the potential benefit of RPLND performed for the diagnosis of pathological N+M0 disease in patients with clinical presurgery N0M0 disease for the purpose of detecting potential candidates for adjuvant biological therapy and in order to weigh correctly any benefit in RPLND against increased morbidity in metastatic patients. Increased morbidity in metastatic patients is an extremely important issue since it may delay or even prevent the institution of immunotherapy.

The procedure

Extended RPLND is performed in order to remove all LN that are possibly affected by tumor. It is assumed that the primary nodes at the hilum are being taken as a part of the formal radical nephrectomy. When a right radical nephrectomy is supplemented with extended RPLND, it includes circumferential IVC dissection from the level of the right diaphragmatic crus inferiorly to the level of the IVC bifurcation (Marshall 1986) or to the lateral aspect of the common iliac artery (Pizzocaro 1986). The lateral border of the dissection includes the ipsilateral psoas muscle in order to include within the dissection the lymphatics, which often extend inferiorly on the anterior surface of the psoas muscle (Marshall 1986). Some also include within the right dissection the inter-aorto-caval lymphatics (Pizzocaro 1986). On the left side, the left lateral lumbar as well as the left diaphragmatic and the periaortic nodes are dissected superiorly from the level of the diaphragmatic crus and inferiorly to the level of the aortic bifurcation on both anterior and posterior aspect of the aorta (Marshall 1986) or even further to the level of the lateral aspect of the common iliac artery (Pizzocaro 1986).

Limited regional RPLND is advocated as well (deKernion 1980) as a reasonable and balanced procedure that recognizes, on the one hand, the potential survival benefit of excising all LN in the vast majority of cases and, on the other hand, limits the extent of the dissection and therefore lowers the rate and severity of the expected complications. Using this approach no extensive attempt is made to excise inter-aorto-caval, retro-caval or retro-aortic nodes. The dissection is limited inferiorly to the origin of the inferior mesenteric artery. Medially the dissection is carried to the ipsilateral side to the interface of the aorta or IVC. No attempt is made to dissect above the adrenal gland or on the anterior aspect of the psoas muscle (Fig. 31.2). Unless it is proven in future, prospective studies that extensive debulking of involved LN

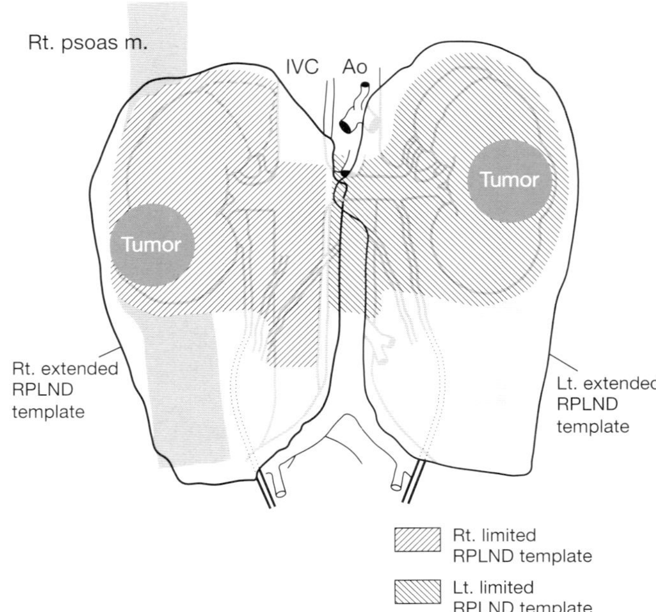

Fig. 31.2 Extended versus limited retroperitoneal lymph node dissection. (Modified with permission from deKernion (1980).)

provides a survival benefit for patients receiving adjuvant immunotherapy or other forms of adjuvant therapy, the limited RPLND approach seems attractive for most cases.

What to do and to whom?

Some authors are convinced that extended RPLND should be recommended for all patients (Marshall 1986). According to the studies presented herein as well as the UCLA experience, RPLND beyond the immediate nodes already included in the classical radical nephrectomy specimen in stage I patients (1997 TNM classification), has extremely low yield and therefore we are convinced that extended RPLND is not warranted in this subset of patients. According to the UCLA experience the risk for nodal involvement in patients with T1 tumors that are 4.5 cm in diameter or less and who do not have distant metastases at diagnosis is less then 1.6 per cent (Zisman *et al.* 2000*a*) and therefore should allow RPLND withholding.

Preoperatively there may be difficulty in distinguishing between pathological stage II and stage III tumors that extend beyond the renal capsule. It is our impression that this difficulty led to a lack of difference in survival between stage II and III patients at UCLA (Zisman *et al.* 2000*b*). There are a substantial number (19 per cent) of T3M0 patients who have nodal involvement. A significant part of them have only microscopic nodal disease. We, therefore, recommend performing RPLND in this subset of patient because it may lead in some of them to the diagnosis of nodal involvement that would have been overlooked if RPLND was withheld. This, of course, may lead to the earlier administration of immunotherapy or tumor vaccine. It may be possible that prospective studies will confirm that patients with only nodal involvement may have an increased benefit from immunotherapy over those with full-blown metastatic disease.

Although it seems that RPLND is extremely important for T2/3 patients with no evidence for distant metastasis, it is more difficult to recommend the appropriate extent of RPLND for these patients. As was suggested earlier (deKernion 1980), it may be possible that the spread of the tumor via the lymphatics in patients with large tumors may not follow the classical description of sequential tumor spread due to the development of parasitic lymphatics following tumor neovascularization and also due to different modes of drainage from the perinephric fat. It may be possible that extending the framework of the dissection in these cases may slightly increase the probability of making the diagnosis of nodal involvement in patients, who were otherwise diagnosed as pathological T2/3N0, but such an action would probably increase the morbidity of the procedure. Therefore our impression is that, as long as the benefit of extensive LN resection plus immunotherapy over limited RPLND plus immunotherapy is not established, there is not enough evidence to justify extended RPLND in patients who are preoperatively staged as T2/3N0M0.

For patients with preoperative evidence for nodal disease, resection of the suspected nodes is indicated in order to obtain a tissue diagnosis of nodal disease as well as to prevent leaving behind residual disease in the retroperitoneum and also to identify the large group of patients with enlarged but noncancerous nodes. There is some support for the meticulous surgical removal of tumoral tissues before and after immunotherapy (Franklin *et al.* 1996). However, the benefit of heroic efforts to perform a complete resection or massive retroperitoneal lymphadenopathy followed by immunotherapy is not yet proved to be superior in terms of patients' survival (Mickisch 1999), quality of life (Litwin *et al.* 1997), and complications. In the same fashion, there is currently not enough data to support a meticulous extended RPLND beyond the resection of grossly involved nodes as an adjunctive procedure to nephrectomy in patients with proven distant metastases who are candidates for postoperative immunotherapy or enrolment into experimental protocols.

References

Bassil, B., Dosoretz, D., and Prout, G.R. Jr (1985). Validation of the tumor, nodes and metastasis classification of renal cell carcinoma. *J. Urol.* **134** (3), 450–4.

Carl, P., Klein, U., *et al.* (1977). The value of lymphography for the TNM classification of renal carcinoma. *Eur. Urol.* **3**, 286–8.

deKernion, J. (1980). Lymphadenctomy for renal cell carcinoma. Therapeutic implications. *Urol. Clin. N. Am.* **7** (3), 697–703.

deKernion, J.B., Ramming, K.P., and Smith, R.B. (1978). The natural history of metastatic renal cell carcinoma: a computer analysis. *J. Urol.* **120**, 148–52.

Franklin, J.R., Figlin, R., Rauch, J., Gitlitz, B., and Belldegrun, A. (1996). Cytoreductive surgery in the management of metastatic renal cell carcinoma: the UCLA experience. *Sem. Urol. Oncol.* **14** (4), 230–6.

Giuliani, L., Martorana, G., *et al.* (1983). Results of radical nephrectomy with extensive lymphadenectomy for renal cell carcinoma. *J. Urol.* **130**, 664–8.

Herrlinger, A., Kuhn, R., *et al.* (1990). [What is the benefit of systematic regional lymph node dissection in tumor nephrectomy?]. *Helv. Chir. Acta* **57**, 477–81.

Hülten, L., Rosencrantz, M., *et al.* (1969). Occurrence and localization of lymph node metastases in renal carcinoma. A lymphographic and histopathological investigation in connection with nephrectomy. *Scand. J. Urol. Nephrol.* **3**, 129–33.

Licht, M.R., A. C. Novick, A.C., and Goormastic, M. (1994). Nephron sparing surgery in incidental versus suspected renal cell carcinoma. *J. Urol.* **152** (1), 39–42.

Litwin, M., Fine, J., *et al.* (1997). Health related quality of life outcomes in patients treated for metastatic kidney cancer: a pilot study. *J. Urol.* **157** (5), 1608–12.

Marshall, F. (1986). Lymphadenectomy for renal cell carcinoma. In *Tumors of the kidney. International perspectives in urology* (ed. J. Libertino), Vol. 13, pp 87–97. Williams and Wilkins, Baltimore.

McLaughlin, A., Saltzstein, S., *et al.* (1976). Prostatic carcinoma: incidence and location of unsuspected lymphatic metastases. *J. Urol.* **115** (1), 89–94.

Mickisch, G. (1999). Lymphatic metastasis in renal cell carcinoma. What is the value of operation and adjuvant therapy? *Urologe A* **38** (4), 326–31.

Morgan, W. and Zincke, H. (1990). Progression and survival after renal-conserving surgery for renal cell carcinoma: experience in 104 patients and extended follow-up. *J. Urol.* **144**, 852–7.

Parienty, R., Richard, F., *et al.* (1984). Local recurrence after nephrectomy for primary renal cancer: computerized tomography recognition. *J. Urol.* **132** (2), 246–9.

Parker, A. (1935). Studies on the main posterior lymph channels of the abdomen and their connections with the lymphatics of the genito-urinary system. *Am. J. Anat.* **56** (3), 409–43.

Peters, P. and Brown, G. (1980). The role of lymphadenectomy in the managment of renal cell carcinoma. *Urol. Clin. N. Am.* **7** (3), 705–9.

Phillips, E. and Messing, E. (1993). Role of lymphadenectomy in the treatment of renal cell carcinoma. *Urology* **41** (1), 9–15.

Pizzocaro, G. (1986). Lymphadenectomy in renal adenocarcinoma. In *Tumors of the kidney. International perspectives in urology* (ed. J. Libertino), Vol. 13, pp. 75–85. Williams and Wilkins, Baltimore.

Raghavaiah, N. and Jordan, W. (1979). Prostatic lymphography. *J. Urol.* **121**, 178–81.

Robson, C., Churchill, B., and Anderson, W. (1969). The results of radical nephrectomy for renal carcinoma. *J. Urol.* **101** (3), 297–301.

Sigel, A., Chlepas, S., *et al.* (1981). Die Operation des Nierentumors. *Chirurgerie* **52**, 545–52.

Skinner, D.G., Colvin, R.B., Vermillion, C.D., Pfister, R.C., and Leadbetter, W.F. (1971a). Diagnosis and management of renal cell carcinoma. A clinical and pathologic study of 309 cases. *Cancer* **28**, 1165–77.

Skinner, D.G., Vermillion, C.D., *et al.* (1971b). Renal cell carcinoma. *Am. Fam. Physcn* **4**, 89–94.

Skinner, D. G., Vermillion, C.D., and Colvin, R.B. (1972b). The surgical management of renal cell carcinoma. *J. Urol.* **107**, 705–10.

Skinner, D.G., Dekernion, J.B., *et al.* (1976). Advanced renal cell carcinoma: treatment with xenogeneic immune ribonucleic acid and appropriate surgical resection. *J. Urol.* **115**, 246–50.

Steinbach, F., Novick, A.C., and Zincke, H. (1995). Treatment of renal cell carcinoma in von Hippel–Lindau disease: a multicenter study. *J. Urol.* **153**, 1812–16.

Studer, U., S. Scherz, S., Scheidegger, J., Kraft, R., and Sonntag, R.. (1990). Enlargement of regional lymph nodes in renal cell carcinoma is not necessarily due to metastases. *J. Urol.* **144** (2), 243–5.

Waters, W. and Richie JP. (1977). Aggressive surgical approach to renal cell carcinoma: review of 130 cases. *J. Urol.* **122**, 306–9.

Zisman, A., Pantuck, A., *et al.* (2001a). Reevaluation of the 1997 TNM classification for renal cell carcinoma: T1 and T2 cutoff point at 4.5 rather then 7 cm better correlates with clinical outcome. *J. Urol.* **166**, 54–8.

Zisman, A., Pantuck, A., *et al.* (2001b). Improved prognostication of RCC using an integrated staging system *J. Clin. Oncol* **19**, 1649–57.

32. Surveillance strategies following surgery for renal cell carcinoma

Robert G. Uzzo and Andrew C. Novick

Introduction

Epithelial tumors of the kidney account for approximately 3 per cent of all solid neoplasms (Parker *et al.* 1997). Adenocarcinoma or renal cell carcinoma (RCC) represent nearly 85 per cent of newly diagnosed malignancies of the kidney occurring at an estimated rate of 4.4–11.1 per 100 000 person-years in the US (Chow *et al.* 2000). Recent data from the US Surveillance, Epidemiology, and End Results (SEER) program demonstrate a steady increase in RCC of 2.3–4.3 per cent annually between 1975 and 1995 (Chow *et al.* 2000). This rise can be attributed in part to early detection through the widespread use of non-invasive imaging techniques (Rodriguez *et al.* 1995), although this reason alone cannot fully explain the upward trend (Chow *et al.* 2000). Incidentally detected lesions tend to be lower-stage and -grade tumors, which, when resected, result in better patient survival with decreased risk of recurrence (Tsui *et al.* 2000). Paralleling this increased incidence is a small but significant improvement in overall 5-year survival for patients with RCC (Motzer *et al.* 1996). This is explained primarily by early detection, improved surgical and postoperative care, and routine follow-up with aggressive resection of isolated metastases, rather than by the development of an effective systemic therapy (Motzer and Russo 2000).

In properly selected patients, both radical nephrectomy (RN) and nephron-sparing surgery (NSS) yield excellent long-term patient survival free of cancer, particularly for low-stage disease. Yet, there has been no consensus on a standard surveillance protocol following these operations. When designing an effective surveillance strategy for monitoring patients after partial or radical nephrectomy, a number of fundamental issues must be addressed that focus on the natural history of RCC and stratifying those at risk for recurrence. Although treatment for patients with recurrent RCC continues to improve slowly, as with other solid malignancies where reliable curative therapy of advanced disease is unavailable, a balance must be achieved between reasonable studies aimed at identifying treatable disease and overly aggressive 'routine' follow-up. This must be done in an economically sensitive environment recognizing that although 'cost-efficient' guidelines may make sense on a broad medicosocial scale, this is not always the case when considering any individual patient.

The goals of surveillance after radical or partial nephrectomy can be easily summarized: to identify recurrences early, when they are still potentially surgically treatable; to preserve overall renal function; and to minimize the use of 'one size fits all' protocols while avoiding complex schedules that increase patient anxiety and expense. In order to achieve these goals, we must first understand the natural history of RCC and identify the most useful prognostic indicators of this disease. Integral to designing appropriate surveillance protocols is a fundamental understanding of *who* is at risk for recurrences, *when* are they likely to recur, *where* are they likely to recur, and *what* can be done in the event of a recurrence (Monte 1994). Finally, we must determine how these issues impact on designing effective surveillance guidelines.

The natural history of renal cell carcinoma

The natural history of RCC refers to its progression in the untreated individual. Since most patients will receive some form of surgical or systemic therapy during the course of their disease, the true natural history of RCC is difficult to quantitate accurately. Most RCC arise from the proximal tubular epithelium and grow in a local rather than infiltrating pattern. RCC develops as discrete, focal, mass lesions. Progression by local extension through the renal capsule and beyond Gerota's fascia may lead to involvement of contiguous retro- or intraperitoneal structures such as psoas, diaphragm, liver, bowel, or mesentery. Invasion into segmental branches of the renal vein is not uncommon. Subsequent extension into the main renal vein and inferior vena cava (IVC) allows hematogenous spread to the lungs, bones, and central nervous system (CNS). Metastases have been described in most soft tissues of the body including tongue (Aguirre *et al.* 1996), tonsils (Green *et al.* 1997), thyroid (Shimizu *et al.* 1995; Murakami *et al.* 1993), eye (Parnes *et al.* 1993; Mezer *et al.* 1997), breast (Pursner *et al.* 1997; Kannan 1998), gall bladder (Pagano *et al.* 1995; Golbey *et al.* 1991), pancreas (Fabre *et al.* 1995), stomach (Odori *et al.* 1998), heart (Bird *et al.* 1991), spermatic cord (Fallick *et al.* 1997), seminal vesicle (Yamamoto *et al.* 1998), bladder (Bolkier *et al.* 1993), vagina (Ovesen and Gerstenberg 1990), penis (Fallick *et al.* 1997), and most peripheral and axial skeletal muscles (Merimsky *et al.* 1990; Nakagawa *et al.* 1996; Linn *et al.* 1996). Symptomatic manifestations of metastatic or recurrent RCC are highly variable and may masquerade as more benign processes thereby delaying diagnosis. RCC can also metastasize through lymphatic channels to regional and mediastinal nodes. Nodal metastases do not always follow a predictable pattern due to variable lymphatic drainage in the upper abdomen thereby limiting the role of therapeutic lymphadenectomy (Ditonno *et al.* 1992).

The incidence of metastases typically increases with the size of the primary lesion (Fowler 1987; Hafez *et al.* 1999). Despite this tendency, metastases may occur from very small lesions and, conversely, the primary lesion may become quite large in the absence of identifiable extrarenal disease. Symptoms may be due to either local involvement of the tumor causing pain, hematuria, or a flank mass, or from manifestations of metastatic disease such as fever, weight loss, or other constitutional symptoms. Paraneoplastic syndromes occur in up to 30 per cent of patients with RCC and may include hypercalcemia, hypertension, pyrexia, erythrocytosis, and hepatic dysfunction (Sokoloff *et al.* 1996). In general, existing metastases progress and new lesions appear until, ultimately, cachexia, pain, persistent hematuria, venous thrombosis, pulmonary emboli, and other terminal manifestations arise in the setting of diffuse disease. The majority of patients presenting with metastatic disease die within 1 year of diagnosis due to complications arising from their metastases (Fowler 1987).

Confounding the management of patients with advanced disease is the unusual and unpredictable tendency of some lesions to remain quiescent or in rare instances regress (Ritchie *et al.* 1988; Vogelzang *et al.* 1992). The growth rate of individual metastases is not always uniform and specific lesions may remain stable while others expand. This may result in the unexpected survival of patients with metastatic disease for long periods. The literature is replete with reports of this unusual deviation from the predicted natural history of the disease (Bos and Mensink 1996; de la Figuera *et al.* 1985). Attempts to identify prognostic variables associated with progression have met with limited success and no single factor or marker of progression is currently available to guide the follow-up of patients with RCC.

The prognostic variables most useful in predicting progression of RCC can be divided into three broad categories: patient-related factors; tumor-related factors; and molecular or histologic markers. The most relevant and well-supported of these are patient- and tumor-related factors including extent of symptoms at presentation, objective performance status, disease-free interval, pathologic stage, histologic subtype, and nuclear grade (Bostwick and Murphy 1998). Unfortunately, most studies evaluating treatment strategies, outcomes, and survival are confounded by failure to control for these parameters and are therefore difficult to interpret and compare because of inherent selection bias. Clinicians are well aware that asymptomatic patients presenting with low-grade, low-stage disease and a good performance status generally fare well while those whose initial presentation is with locoregional symptoms, poor performance, and high-grade or -stage disease tend to have poor outcomes. Logic also predicts that patients who demonstrate a response to surgical or systemic therapy or who recur after a long disease-free interval have 'biologically favorable' tumors while non-responders or those who recur early do not. In the absence of effective systemic therapy, the basic biology of the tumor will dictate outcome. An understanding of the most fundamental cellular events involved in oncogenic transformation of the renal epithelium is imperative so that sensitive and specific

molecular markers of progression can be identified. Currently, investigation in the field focuses on genetic defects responsible for inherited forms of RCC. Recent identification, cloning, and mutational analysis of the von Hippel–Lindau gene (3p25–26) and its protein product (pVHL) (Linehan *et al.* 1995) have improved our understanding of the transcriptional events responsible for constitutive expression of pro-angiogenic proteins in RCC (Iliopoulos *et al.* 1996). Clear cell carcinomas are highly vascular and several investigators have evaluated tumor microvessel density as a potential marker of progression with very limited success (Nativ *et al.* 1998; Yoshino *et al.* 1995). Other recently evaluated markers of progression include nuclear morphometry (Carducci *et al.* 1999), measures of cellular mitosis (Ki-67 and proliferating cell nuclear antigen (PCNA)) (Delahunt *et al.* 1995; Cronin *et al.* 1994), tumor suppressor gene products such as p53 (Papadopoulos *et al.* 1997), nuclear matrix proteins (Nakagawa *et al.* 1998), and serum or intratumoral levels of cytokines, calcium, alkaline phosphatase, and others (Bostwick and Murphy 1998). To date, no single marker has proven useful enough to reliably predict disease recurrence and our best marker of progression remains pathologic and clinical stage. Surveillance protocols and follow-up recommendations are therefore primarily based on stage, which must be accurately determined clinically at presentation and pathologically after surgery using a standardized staging system such as the TNM (tumor–node–metastasis) system proposed by the International Union Against Cancer (Hermanek and Schrott 1990).

Who, when, where, and what of recurrent renal cell carcinoma

Clinically, pathologically, and biologically RCC represents a heterogeneous group of tumors. Patients with RCC surgically resected are not all at the same risk for recurrence, and those at highest risk require more frequent and intensive surveillance. Recent studies evaluating outcome after radical nephrectomy for localized RCC demonstrate that the risk of postoperative recurrence is largely stage-dependent (Levy *et al.* 1998; Ljungberg *et al.* 1999). In a study from the M.D. Anderson Cancer Center examining the incidence of recurrence following radical nephrectomy, 68 of 286 patients (23.8 per cent) developed metastases (Levy *et al.* 1998). Similar findings were reported by Ljungberg *et al.* (1999) where recurrence occurred in 56 of 187 patients (30 per cent) after curative radical nephrectomy for RCC. In these and other studies, the single best identified predictor of disease progression is pathological stage (Table 32.1). Patients with low pathological (p) stage (pT1) disease have a 4–7 per cent overall risk of recurrence while up to 25 per cent of those with pT2 tumors and nearly 45 per cent or more of patients with pT3 tumors recur (Fowler 1987; Sokoloff *et al.* 1996; Levy *et al.* 1998; Giulani *et al.* 1990; Klugo *et al.* 1977). Unfortunately, patients presenting with pT4 disease uniformly recur despite even the most aggressive surgical or systemic therapies (Motzer and Russo 2000). As recurrence rates rise, there is a predictable drop in both 5- and 10-year survival. These data indicate that surveillance for recurrent malignancy after surgical resection should be tailored according to the initial pathologic stage.

Table 32.1 Stage-specific recurrence rates, time interval to first recurrence, and 5- and 10-year disease-free survival for patients with RCC (Fowler 1987; Sokoloff *et al.* 1996; Ljungberg *et al.* 1999; Giuliani *et al.* 1990; Klugo *et al.* 1977)

| Pathologic stage | Recurrence rate (%) | Time to first recurrence (months) | Disease-free survival (%) | |
			5-year	10-year
pT1	4–7	38–45	90–98	85–90
pT2	7–27	32–40	75–85	70–75
pT3	22–45	17–28	37–70	35–50
pT4	> 85	< 12	5–15	< 5

As with most solid malignancies, the greatest risk of recurrence exists in the first 3–5 years after surgical resection. During this period, surveillance must be more frequent and the patient should understand the importance of appropriate follow-up. As the disease-free interval increases, the risk of recurrence diminishes gradually; however, late recurrences with RCC are not uncommon and all patients maintain a lifelong risk. When identified early, recurrent disease is typically amenable to surgical resection and potential cure. Patients and physicians must recognize the ability of RCC to recur late and include this in the differential diagnosis of unusual symptoms or soft-tissue lesions that develop years after surgery for RCC.

RCC can metastasize anywhere and symptomatic manifestations of metastatic or recurrent RCC are protean, making early diagnosis elusive. The most common sites of recurrence following radical nephrectomy are lung, bone, liver, and CNS (Levy *et al.* 1998; Ljungberg *et al.* 1999). Local retroperitoneal recurrences may involve the renal fossa, adrenal, or axial musculoskeletal structures. Node-positive (N+) patients appear to be at increased risk for developing local recurrence (Giuliani *et al.* 1990). Some authors believe that lymphadenectomy performed at the time of nephrectomy may help reduce the risk of local recurrence for patients with advanced tumors, but this has not been conclusively proven (Campbell and Novick 1994). Importantly, most patients with recurrent disease are asymptomatic, and periodic radiographic follow-up remains the cornerstone for early detection of metastatic disease following surgical resection.

Patients undergoing NSS present an additional challenge for surveillance—identifying recurrent disease in the renal remnant. Nephron-sparing approaches may theoretically increase the risk of local recurrence whereas Gerota's fascia is opened and complete tumor resection cannot be guaranteed (Campbell and Novick 1994). In addition, multicentric RCC is not uncommon, particularly in the setting of papillary tumors (Ornstein *et al.* 2000), and microscopic satellite lesions may become local recurrences. Despite these considerations, the risk of local recurrence following partial nephrectomy appears to be quite small (Table 32.2). Depending on the indication for NSS, the incidence of local recurrence is reported to be between 1 and 10 per cent (Licht *et al.* 1994; Moll *et al.* 1993; Steinbach *et al.* 1992). In patients with low-stage disease and those with elective indications, the risk is remarkably low (0–3 per cent) (Morgan and Zincke 1990; Provet *et al.* 1991; Carini *et al.* 1988) even as long as 10 years after surgery (Fergany *et al.* 2000). Treatment of locally recurrent RCC in the renal remnant involves removal of the remaining affected renal parenchyma (Campbell and Novick 1994). In situations where this would render the patient anephric, repeat partial nephrectomy has been successfully used with good results, depending on the size and stage of the recurrence. Recent data from the Cleveland Clinic Foundation on 327 patients undergoing NSS for sporadic RCC demonstrate that RCC recurred in 38 patients (11.6 per cent) overall including 13 (4 per cent) who had a local recurrence with or without concurrent metastatic disease and 25 (7.6 per cent) who developed metastatic disease without local recurrence. The incidences of postoperative local tumor recurrence and metastatic disease, respectively, according to the initial pathological tumor stage were as follows: 0 and 4.4 per cent for pT1N0M0 RCC; 2.0 and 5.3 per cent for pT2N0M0 RCC; 8.2 and 11.5 per cent for pT3aN0M0 RCC; and 10.6 and 14.9 per cent for pT3bN0M0 RCC. The peak postoperative intervals for developing local recurrence were 6–24 months in pT3 RCC patients and > 48 months in pT2 RCC patients (Hafez *et al.* 1997). The inci-

Table 32.2 Local recurrence following nephron-sparing surgery for RCC

| Reference | N | Recurrence in renal remnant (%) | | Mean follow-up (months) |
		Overall	After elective NSS	
Licht *et al.* 1994	216	4	0	50
Moll *et al.* 1993	143	1.4	0	36
Steinbach *et al.* 1992	140	3.6	3.3	> 36
Morgan and Zincke 1990	104	5.7	0	72
Provet *et al.* 1991	44	2.3	0	36
Carini *et al.* 1988	36	2.8	0	46
Hafez *et al.* 1997	327	4	NA	56

dence of both local recurrence and metastases increased with stage while the mean time to recurrence decreased. One-third of these patients were asymptomatic and detected only by surveillance on chest X-ray or computerized tomography (CT).

The efficacy of available therapeutic options for recurrent disease must also be considered when designing an effective surveillance strategy. The outlook for patients with advanced disease is generally poor, reflecting a lack of effective systemic therapy. There is currently no chemotherapeutic, hormonal, or immunologic agent that alone or in combination consistently achieves a response rate of more than 10–15 per cent (Motzer et al. 1999). The case for surgery in the setting of recurrent disease is therefore more compelling. Several studies demonstrate increased survival of well selected patients with recurrent RCC after surgical resection (Kavolius et al. 1998; O'Dea et al. 1978; Cerfolio et al. 1994). The data are however hampered by a lack of prospective randomized clinical trials and outcome analyses examining the issue. The wide spectrum of clinical scenarios and inherent selection bias reported in the literature make generalizations on this topic difficult. The most favorable setting for resection of recurrent disease is a patient with a high performance status and a solitary, metachronous, pulmonary lesion who presents after a long (> 3 year) disease-free interval. Conversely, the worst candidate is a patient with a poor performance status and multiple recurrent metastases presenting soon after initial treatment. This example underscores the confounding effect of patient selection in evaluating the role of surgery for recurrent RCC and may reflect the natural history of the individual's disease more than the intervention itself. The role of aggressive surgery for patients between these two clinical extremes is unclear and treatment decisions are often based on more subjective criteria due to lack of reliable data on the subject.

Middleton (1967) first reported on the role of surgery for metastatic and recurrent RCC (Table 32.3). He identified 503 cases from the New York Hospital and noted that only those who had excision of a lesion presenting metachronously gained a survival advantage. O'Dea et al. (1978) summarized the Mayo Clinic data on resection of solitary RCC metastasis and separated groups into those whose metastatic lesion presented synchronously versus those that presented at some time after the original nephrectomy. They found that 23 per cent with metachronous solitary lesions lived more than 5 years after resection while only 22 per cent of those whose solitary metastasis was resected at the time of nephrectomy survived more than 2 years. Subsequent studies by Golimbu et al. (1986), deKernion et al. (1978), and Kavolius et al. (1998) have corroborated the finding that favorable predictors of survival include a single, metachronous site of recurrence with a long disease-free interval.

The most 'favorable' site for recurrence appears to be in the lung. Cerfolio et al. (1994) reviewed the data from 96 consecutive patients treated at the Mayo Clinic who underwent complete pulmonary resection for metastatic RCC and noted a 45.6 per cent 5-year survival rate for patients with solitary metachronous lung lesions. Similarly, in a recent series from Memorial Sloan–Kettering, the 5-year survival rate was 54 per cent in 50 patients treated surgically for a solitary lung metastasis (Kavolius et al. 1998). Improved survival in patients with pulmonary metastasis may be due to earlier detection, less extensive surgical morbidity, and/or less associated functional impairment than with metastases to other organs such as the CNS (Kozlowski 1994). It remains to be determined whether RCC clones capable of metastasizing to the lung are biologically different than those that metastasize elsewhere.

In summary, the three primary determinants of success for surgery in the setting of metastatic RCC are: the length of the disease-free interval; the number and location of the lesions; and the patient's overall performance status. The incidence of subclinical, multifocal, microembolic disease is unknown but may explain early disease progression after aggressive surgery. A thorough clinical staging is mandatory before proceeding with any aggressive surgical resection. Whether the existing data on the topic are an actual reflection of the surgical intervention or simply a function of selecting less biologically aggressive tumors for surgery is debated. However, given that surgery for recurrence after radical nephrectomy or NSS provides the best chance for prolonged survival, surveillance strategies must attempt to identify recurrent disease early.

Table 32.3 Survival after resection of recurrent RCC

Reference	N	Metastatic site(s)*	Solitary (S) or multiple (M)	Median DFI[†] (months)	Overall 5-year survival (%)
Middleton 1967	4	Brain/lung	S	—	25
O'Dea et al. 1978	26	Bone/brain/lung/LN	S	34	23
Golimbu et al. 1986	13	Bone/lung/fossa	S (6); M (7)	29	25
Dineen et al. 1988	18	Bone/brain/lung/soft tissue/LN	S	38	13
Kierney et al. 1994	41	Bone/brain/lung/soft tissue	S	25	31
Cerfolio et al. 1994	48	Lung	S	41	46
	48	Lung	M[‡]		27
Kavolius et al. 1998	155	Bone/brain/lung/soft tissue/LN/fossa	S	25	54
	123	Bone/brain/lung/soft tissue/LN/fossa	M		29

* LN, lymph node.
[†] DFI, disease-free interval.
[‡] Includes four patients with synchronous lesions.

Stage-specific guidelines for surveillance following radical nephrectomy or nephron-sparing surgery

Based on these data, a stage-specific protocol for surveillance after radical or partial nephrectomy is proposed (Tables 32.4 and 32.5). Following radical nephrectomy, all patients should be evaluated with a medical history, physical examination, and selected blood studies on a yearly or twice yearly basis. Blood work should include serum calcium, liver function tests, alkaline phosphatase, blood urea nitrogen, creatinine, and electrolytes. For patients with pT1N0M0 RCC, routine postoperative radiographic imaging is not necessary due to the low risk of recurrent malignancy. For patients with pT2N0M0 RCC, a chest X-ray every year and an abdominal CT scan every 2 years are recommended. Patients with pT3N0M0 RCC have a higher risk of developing recurrent malignancy particularly during the first 3 years after radical nephrectomy and may benefit from more frequent laboratory and radiographic follow-up including an abdominal CT scan at 1 year, then every 2 years thereafter.

The need for postoperative surveillance after partial nephrectomy also varies according to the initial pathologic tumor stage. All patients should be evaluated with a medical history and physical examination and selected blood studies on a yearly or twice yearly basis. Patients who undergo partial nephrectomy for pT1N0M0 RCC do not require radiographic imaging postoperatively in view of the very low risk of recurrent malignancy. A yearly chest X-ray is recommended after partial nephrectomy for pT2N0M0 RCC since the lung is the most common site of postoperative metastasis. Abdominal or retroperitoneal tumor recurrence is uncommon in the latter group, particularly early after a partial nephrectomy, and these patients require only occasional follow-up abdominal CT scanning. We recommend that this be done every 2 years. Patients with pT3N0M0 have a high risk of

Table 32.4 Postoperative surveillance after radical nephrectomy for localized RCC

Months post-op	3	6	12	18	24	30	36	48	60
pT1									
History and examination			×		×			×	×
Blood			×		×			×	×
Chest X-ray									
Abdominal CT									
pT2									
History and examination			×		×		×	×	×
Blood			×		×		×	×	×
Chest X-ray			×		×		×	×	×
Abdominal CT					×			×	
pT3									
History and examination	×	×	×	×	×	×	×	×	×
Blood	×	×	×	×	×	×	×	×	×
Chest X-ray	×	×	×	×	×	×	×	×	×
Abdominal CT			×				×		×

Table 32.5 Postoperative surveillance after nephron-sparing surgery for localized RCC

Months post-op	3	6	12	18	24	30	36	48	60
pT1									
History and examination			×		×			×	×
Blood			×		×			×	×
Chest X-ray									
Abdominal CT									
pT2									
History and examination			×		×		×	×	×
Blood			×		×		×	×	×
Chest X-ray			×		×		×	×	×
Abdominal CT					×			×	
pT3									
History and examination		×	×	×	×	×	×	×	×
Blood		×	×	×	×	×	×	×	×
Chest X-ray		×	×	×	×	×	×	×	×
Abdominal CT		×	×	×	×	×	×		×

developing local tumor recurrence and metastatic disease, particularly during the first 2 years after partial nephrectomy. They may benefit from more frequent follow-up with chest X-ray and abdominal CT scanning. Initially, we recommend that these be done every 6 months during the first 3 years. Thereafter, a chest X-ray is done yearly and an abdominal CT scan done every 2 years.

Postoperative bone scans, bone plain films, and head or chest CT scans are necessary only in the presence of related symptoms. The role of abdominal ultrasound in evaluating recurrent lesions of the remnant kidney is unclear. Its use may decrease the overall cost of surveillance at the risk of potentially missing other intra-abdominal recurrences. Finally, periodic blood pressure checks and urinary screening for protein are important for patients with a solitary or remnant kidney. If urinary dip reveals proteinuria, a 24-hour quantitative urine protein should be obtained to screen for hyperfiltration nephropathy (Novick *et al.* 1991).

The surveillance schemes outlined here require identical follow-up for low-stage disease after radical or partial nephrectomy and neither surgical strategy will provide any cost disadvantage. The primary objective is to provide effective guidelines based on the likelihood of recurrence given the initial pathological stage of the tumor. The ultimate goal of cancer detection and surveillance is to identify sensitive molecular serum markers able to predict tumor recurrence at its most early stages. This will require a more fundamental understanding of the tumor's basic biology using the molecular tools that the future will inevitably bring.

References

Aguirre, A., Rinaggio, J., and Diaz-Ordaz, E. (1996). Lingual metastasis of renal cell carcinoma. *J. Oral Maxillofac. Surg.* **54**, 344–6.

Bird, D.J., Semple, J.P., and Seiler, M.W. (1991). Sarcomatoid renal cell carcinoma metastatic to the heart: report of a case. *Ultrastruct. Pathol.* **15**, 361–6.

Bolkier, M., Moskovitz, B., Munichor, M., Genesin, Y., and Levin, D.R. (1993). Metastatic renal cell carcinoma to the bladder. *Urol. Int.* **50**, 101–3.

Bos, S.D. and Mensink, H.J. (1996). Spontaneous caval tumor thrombus necrosis and regression of pulmonary lesions in renal cell cancer. *Scand. J. Urol. Nephrol.* **30**, 489.

Bostwick, D.G. and Murphy, G.P. (1998). Diagnosis and prognosis of renal cell carcinoma: highlights from an international consensus workshop. *Sem. Urol. Oncol.* **16** (1), 46–52.

Campbell, S.C. and Novick, A.C. (1994). Management of local recurrence following radical nephrectomy or partial nephrectomy. *Urol. Clin. N. Am.* **21** (4), 593–9.

Carducci, M.A., Piantadosi, S., Pound, C.R., Epstein, J.I., Simons, J. W., Marshall, F.F., and Partin, A.W. (1999). Nuclear morphometry adds significant prognostic information to stage and grade for renal cell carcinoma. *Urology* **53** (1), 44–9.

Carini, M., Selli, C., Barbanti, G., Lapini, A., Turini, D., and Constantini, A. (1988). Conservative surgical treatment of renal cell carcinoma: clinical experience and reprisal of indications. *J. Urol.* **140**, 725.

Cerfolio, R.J., Allen, M.S., Deschamps, C., Daly, R.C., Wallrichs, S.L., Trastek, V.F., and Pairolero, P.C. (1994). Pulmonary resection of metastatic renal cell carcinoma. *Ann. Thorac. Surg.* **57** (2), 339–44.

Chow, W.H., Devesa, S.S., Warren, J.L., and Fraumeni, J.F. Jr (2000). Rising incidence of renal cell cancer in the United States. *J. Am. Med. Assoc.* **281** (17), 1628–31.

Cronin, K.J., Williams, N.N., Kerin, M.J., Creagh, T.A., Dervan, P.A., Smith, J.M., and Fitzpatrick, J.M. (1994). Proliferating cell nuclear antigen: a new prognostic indicator in renal cell carcinoma. *J. Urol.* **152** (3), 834–6.

deKernion, J.B., Ramming, K.P., and Smith, R.B. (1978). The natural history of metastatic renal cell carcinoma: a computer analysis. *J. Urol.* **120**, 148–52.

de la Figuera, M., Biosca, M., and Garcia-Bragado, F. (1985). Spontaneous regression of bilateral hilar lymphadenopathy in renal cell carcinoma. *Eur. J. Resp. Dis.* **67**, 133.

Delahunt, B., Bethwaite, P.B., Thornton, A., and Ribas, J.L. (1995). Proliferation of renal cell carcinoma assessed by fixation-resistant polyclonal Ki-67 antibody labeling. Correlation with clinical outcome. *Cancer* **75** (11), 2714–19.

Dineen, M.K., Pastore, R.D., Emrich, L.J., and Huben, R.P. (1988). Results of surgical treatment of renal cell carcinoma with solitary metastasis. *J. Urol.* **140**, 277–9.

Ditonno, P., Traficante, A., Battaglia, M., Grossi, F.S., and Selvaggi, F.P. (1992). Role of lymphadenectomy in renal cell carcinoma. *Prog. Clin. Biol. Res.* **378**, 169–74.

Fabre, J.M., Rouanet, P., Dagues, F., Blanc, F., Baumel, H., and Domergue, J. (1995). Various features and surgical approach of solitary pancreatic metastasis from renal cell carcinoma. *Eur. J. Surg. Oncol.* **21**, 683–6.

Fallick, M.L., Long, J.P., and Ucci, A. (1997). Metachronous renal cell carcinoma metastases to spermatic cord and penis. *Scand. J. Urol. Nephrol.* **31**, 299–300.

Fergany, A.F., Hafez, K.S., and Novick, A.C. (2000). Long-term results of nephron sparing surgery for localized renal cell carcinoma: 10-year follow-up. *J. Urol.* **163**, 442–5.

Fowler, J.E. (1987). Nephrectomy in metastatic renal cell carcinoma. *Urol. Clin. N. Am.* **14** (4), 749–56.

Giuliani, L., Giberti, C., Martorana, G., and Rovida, S. (1990). Radical extensive surgery for renal cell carcinoma: long-term results and prognostic factors. *J. Urol.* **143** (3), 468–73.

Golbey, S., Gerard, P.S., and Frank, R.G. (1991). Metastatic hypernephroma masquerading as acute cholecystitis. *Clin. Imag.* **15**, 293–5.

Golimbu, M., Al-Askari, S., Tessler, A., and Morales, P. (1986). Aggressive treatment of metastatic renal cancer. *J. Urol.* **136**, 805–7.

Green, K.M., Pantelides, E., and de Carpentier, J.P. (1997). Tonsillar metastasis from a renal cell carcinoma presenting as a quinsy. *J. Laryngol. Otol.* **111**, 379–80.

Hafez, K.S., Novick, A.C., and Campbell, S.C. (1997). Patterns of tumor recurrence and guidelines for follow-up after nephron sparing surgery for sporadic renal cell carcinoma. *J. Urol.* **157**, 2067–70.

Hafez, K.S., Fergany, A.F., and Novick, A.C. (1999). Nephron sparing surgery for localized renal cell carcinoma: impact of tumor size on patient survival, tumor recurrence and TNM staging. *J. Urol.* **162** (6), 1930–3.

Hermanek, P. and Schrott, K.M. (1990). Evaluation of the new tumor, nodes and metastases classification of renal cell carcinoma. *J. Urol.* **144**, 238.

Iliopoulos, O., Levy, A.P., Jiang, C., Kaelin, W.G. Jr, and Goldberg, M.A. (1996). Negative regulation of hypoxia-inducible genes by the von Hippel–Lindau protein. *Proc. Natl Acad. Sci., USA* **93**, 10595–9.

Kannan, V. (1998). Fine-needle aspiration of metastatic renal-cell carcinoma masquerading as primary breast carcinoma. *Diag. Cytopathol.* **18**, 343–5.

Kavolius, J.P., Mastorakos, D.P., Pavlovich, C., Russo, P., Burt, M.E., and Brady, M.S. (1998). Resection of metastatic renal cell carcinoma. *J. Clin. Oncol.* **16** (6), 2261–6.

Kierney, P.C., van Heerden, J.A., Segura, J.W., and Weaver, A.L. (1994). Surgeon's role in the management of solitary renal cell carcinoma metastases occurring subsequent to initial curative nephrectomy: an institutional review. *Ann. Surg. Oncol.* **1** (4), 345–52.

Klugo, R.C., Detmers, M., and Stiles, R.E. (1977). Aggressive versus conservative management of stage IV renal cell carcinoma. *J. Urol.* **118**, 244–6.

Kozlowski, J.M. (1994). Management of distal solitary recurrence in the patient with renal cancer. *Urol. Clin. N. Am.* **21** (4), 601–24.

Levy, D.A., Slayton, J.W., Swanson, D.A., and Dinney, C.P. (1998). Stage specific guidelines for surveillance after radical nephrectomy for local renal cell carcinoma. *J. Urol.* **159** (4), 1163–7.

Licht, M.R., Novick, A.C., and Goormastic, M. (1994). Nephron sparing surgery in incidental versus suspected renal cell carcinoma *J. Urol.* **152** (1), 39–42.

Linehan, W.M., Lerman, M.I., and Zbar, B. (1995). Identification of the von Hippel–Lindau (VHL) gene. Its role in renal cancer. *J. Am. Med. Assoc.* **273**, 564–70.

Linn, J.F., Fichtner, J., Voges, G., Schweden, F., Storkel, S., and Hohenfellner, R. (1996). Solitary contralateral psoas metastasis 14 years after radical nephrectomy for organ confined renal cell carcinoma. *J. Urol.* **156**, 173.

Ljungberg, B., Alamdari, F.I., Rasmuson, T., and Roos, G. (1999). Follow-up guidelines for nonmetastatic renal cell carcinoma based on the occurrence of metastases after radical nephrectomy. *Br. J. Urol.* **84** (4), 405–11.

Merimsky, O., Levine, T., and Chaitchik, S. (1990). Recurrent solitary metastasis of renal cell carcinoma in skeletal muscles. *Tumor* **76**, 407–9.

Mezer, E., Gdal-On, M., and Miller, B. (1997). Orbital metastasis of renal cell carcinoma masquerading as Amaurosis fugax. *Eur. J. Ophthalmol.* **7**, 301–4.

Middleton, R.G. (1967). Surgery for metastatic renal cell carcinoma. *J. Urol.* **97**, 973–7.

Moll, V., Becht, E., and Ziegler, M. (1993). Kidney preserving surgery in renal cell tumors: indications, techniques and results in 152 patients. *J. Urol.* **150**, 319–23.

Montie, J.E. (1994). Follow-up after partial or total nephrectomy for renal cell carcinoma. *Urol. Clin. N. Am.* 21 (4), 589–92.

Morgan, W.R. and Zincke, H. (1990). Progression and survival after renal-conserving surgery for renal cell carcinoma: experience in 104 patients and extended follow-up. *J. Urol.* **144** (4), 852–7.

Motzer, R.J. and Russo, P. (2000). Systemic therapy for renal cell carcinoma. *J. Urol.* **163**, 408–17.

Motzer, R.J., Bander, N.H., and Nanus, D.M. (1996). Renal-cell carcinoma *New Engl. J. Med.* **335** (12), 865–75.

Motzer, R.J., Mazumdar, M., Bacik, J., Berg, W., Amsterdam, A., and Ferrara, J. (1999). Survival and prognostic stratification of 670 patients with advanced renal cell carcinoma. *J. Clin. Oncol.* **17** (8), 2530–40.

Murakami, S., Yashuda, S., Nakamura, T., Mishima, Y., Iida, H., Okano, H., and Nakano, M. (1993). A case of renal cell carcinoma with metastasis to the thyroid gland and concomitant early gastric cancer. *Surg. Today* **23**, 153–8.

Nakagawa, H., Mizukami, Y., Kimura, H., Watanabe, Y., and Kuwayama, N. (1996). Metastatic masseter muscle tumour: a report of a case. *J. Laryngol. Otol.* **110**, 172–4.

Nakagawa, Y., Tsumatani, K., Kurumatani, N., Cho, M., Kitahori, Y., Konishi, N., Ozono, S., Okajima, E., Hirao, Y., and Hiasa, Y. (1998). Prognostic value of nm23 protein expression in renal cell carcinoma. *Oncology* **55** (4), 370–6.

Nativ, O., Sabo, E., Reiss, A., Madjar, S., and Moskovitz, B. (1998). Clinical significance of tumor angiogenesis in patients with localized renal cell carcinoma. *Urology* **51** (5), 693–6.

Novick, A.C., Gephardt, G., Guz, B., Steinmuller, D., and Tubbs, R.R. (1991). Long-term follow-up after partial removal of a solitary kidney. *New Engl. J. Med.* **325** (15), 1058–62.

O'Dea, M.J., Zincke, H., Utz, D.C., and Bernatz, P.E. (1978). The treatment of renal cell carcinoma with solitary metastasis. *J. Urol.* **120**, 540–2.

Odori, T., Tsuboi, Y., Katoh, K., Yamada, K., Morita, K., Ohara, A., Kuroiwa, M., Sakamoto, H., and Sakata, T. (1998). A solitary hematogenous metastasis to the gastric wall from renal cell carcinoma four years after radical nephrectomy. *J. Clin. Gastroenterol.* **26**, 153–4.

Ornstein, D.L., Lubensky, I.A., Venzon, D., Zbar, B., Linehan, W.M., and Walther, M.M. (2000). Prevalence of microscopic tumor in normal appearing renal parenchyma of patients with hereditary papillary renal cancer. *J. Urol.* **163**, 431–3.

Ovesen, H. and Gerstenberg, T. (1990). Vaginal metastasis as the first sign of renal cell carcinoma. A case report and review of the literature. *Scand. J. Urol. Nephrol.* **24**, 237–8.

Pagano, S., Ruggeri, P., Franzoso, F., and Brusamolino, R. (1995). Unusual renal cell carcinoma metastasis to the gallbladder. *Urology* **45**, 867–9.

Papadopoulos, I., Rudolph, P., and Weichert-Jacobsen, K. (1997). Value of p53 expression, cellular proliferation, and DNA content as prognostic indicators in renal cell carcinoma. *Eur. Urol.* **32** (1), 110–17.

Parker, S.L., Tong, T., Bolden, S., and Wingo, P.A. (1997). Cancer statistics 1997. *CA Cancer J. Clin.* **47** (1), 5–27.

Parnes, R.E., Goldberg, S.H., and Sassani, J.W. (1993). Renal cell carcinoma metastatic to the orbit: a clinicopathologic report. *Ann. Ophthalmol.* **25**, 100–2.

Provet, J., Tessler, A., Brown, J., Golimbu, M., Bosniak, M., and Morales, P. (1991). Partial nephrectomy for renal cell carcinoma: indications, results and implications. *J. Urol.* **145** (3), 472–6.

Pursner, M., Petchprapa, C., Haller, J.O., and Orentlicher, R.J. (1997). Renal carcinoma: bilateral breast metastases in a child. *Pediatr. Radiol.* **27**, 242–3.

Ritchie, A.W., Layfield, L.J., and deKernion, J.B. (1988). Spontaneous regression of liver metastasis from renal cell carcinoma. *J. Urol.* **40**, 596.

Rodriguez, R., Fishman E.K., and Marshall, F. (1995). Differential diagnosis and evaluation of the incidentally discovered renal mass. *Sem. Urol. Oncol.* **13** (4), 246.

Shimizu, K., Nagahama, M., Kitamura, Y., Chin, K., Kitagawa, W., Shibuya, T., Mimura, T., Ozaki, O., Sugino, K., Ito, K., *et al.* (1995). Clinicopathological study of clear-cell tumors of the thyroid: an evaluation of 22 cases. *Surg. Today* **25**, 1015–22.

Sokoloff, M.H., deKernion, J.B., Figlin, R.A., and Belldegrun, A. (1996). Current management of renal cell carcinoma. *CA Cancer J. Clin.* **46** (5), 284–302.

Steinbach, F., Stockle, M., Muller, S. C., Thuroff, J. W., Melchior, S. W., Stein, R., and Hohenfellner, R. (1992). Conservative surgery of renal cell tumors in 140 patients: 21 years of experience. *J. Urol.* **148** (1), 24–9.

Tsui, K.H., Shvartz, O., Smith, R.B., Figlin, R., deKernion J.B., and Belldegrun, A. (2000). Renal cell carcinoma: prognostic significance of incidentally detected tumors. *J. Urol.* **163**, 426–30.

Vogelzang, N.J., Priest, E.R., and Borden, L. (1992). Spontaneous regression of histologically proved pulmonary metastases from renal cell carcinoma: a case with 5-year follow-up. *J. Urol.* **148**, 1247.

Yamamoto, S., Mamiya, Y., Noda, K., Samejima, T., Miki, M., and Akasaka, Y. (1998). A case of metastasis to the seminal vesicle of renal cell carcinoma. *Jpn J. Urol.* **89**, 563–6.

Yoshino, S., Kato, M., and Okada, K. (1995). Prognostic significance of microvessel count in low stage renal cell carcinoma. *Int. J. Urol.* **2** (3), 156–60.

33. Adjuvant therapy for renal cell carcinoma

Joseph Baar and Donald L. Trump

Introduction

It is estimated that there will be 31 200 new cases of renal cell carcinoma (RCC) diagnosed in the US in 2000, and 11 900 people will die from this disease (American Cancer Society). Approximately 70 per cent of patients present with localized or locally advanced disease (Golimbu *et al.* 1986) and are potentially curable by nephectomy alone. However, relapse rates are high in such patients, with 5-year survival rates of 56–100, 47–100, and 34–80 per cent in patients with stage I (that is, T1N0), stage II (that is, T2 N0), and stage III disease (that is, T1N1M0 to T3cN1M0), respectively. Studies have demonstrated that the most reliable predictor for poor outcome in locally advanced RCC is lymph node metastases. In most series, patients with lymph node involvement have a 5-year survival of 10–25 per cent (Robson *et al.* 1969; Skinner *et al.* 1971; Boxer *et al.* 1979; McNichols *et al.* 1981; Cherrie *et al.* 1982; Selli *et al.* 1983; Bassil *et al.* 1985; Golimbu *et al.* 1986). Therefore, studies have been undertaken to determine whether adjuvant therapy of RCC offers a benefit in terms of disease-free survival (DFS) and overall survival in patients at risk for relapse after radical nephrectomy. These adjuvant trials have tested postoperative adjuvant therapies such as radiation, hormonal therapy, vaccines, and interferon α (IFNα).

Adjuvant radiation therapy

Radiotherapy has been studied to determine whether the risk of local relapse could be decreased after radical nephrectomy. However, in a prospective study of postoperative radiotherapy versus observation in 72 patients who underwent nephrectomy for stages II and III RCC, no differences in relapse rate or survival were demonstrated (Kjaer *et al.* 1987). The treatments were also associated with a significant amount of morbidity to abdominal organs. The authors concluded from their study that post-nephrectomy radiotherapy was not warranted.

Adjuvant hormonal therapy

Hormonal agents such as medroxyprogesterone acetate (MPA) have been shown to block glucocorticoid receptors on some renal tumor cells (Bojar *et al.* 1979; Chen *et al.* 1980; Takenawa *et al.* 1995). Patients with metastatic RCC have had occasional responses to MPA and this has provided a rationale to test MPA in the adjuvant setting. In a prospective randomized study of adjuvant MPA after radical nephrectomy (Pizzocaro *et al.* 1987), 136 patients received either 500 mg MPA 3 times a week for 1 year or no treatment after radical nephrectomy. After a median follow-up of 5 years, 33.3 per cent of patients relapsed after a median disease-free interval of 17 months. Relapses occurred in 32.7 per cent of patients in the adjuvant treatment group and in 33.9 per cent of patients in the control group. Sex steroid hormone receptors were studied in 102 of the 120 evaluable patients, and no significant correlation was found among receptors, relapses, and treatment. Thus, the role of MPA in the adjuvant setting remains to be defined.

Adjuvant immunotherapy

Tumor cells express tumor antigens that are presented on the cell surface by major histocompatibility (MHC) class I or class II molecules and are capable of eliciting tumor-specific immune responses. These immune responses are mediated by CD8+ cytotoxic T lymphocytes (CTL), and the responses may be further amplified by cytokines secreted by CD4+ helper cells, such as interleukin 2 (IL-2) and IFNγ. A rationale therefore exists to immunize patients against antigens derived from tumor cells, either alone or in combination with hormones, cytokines, or immune adjuvants such as bacille Calmette–Guérin (BCG) to further enhance responses. Thus, several studies have tested adjuvant immunization of patients after nephrectomy.

In one prospective randomized trial, 43 patients were randomly allocated to either adjuvant hormonal-immunotherapy or hormonal therapy after nephrectomy (Adler *et al.* 1987). Immunotherapy consisted of autologous irradiated tumor cells admixed with BCG administered intradermally and endolymphatically. At a median follow-up of 30 months, while there was a trend for prolongation of DFS in patients with stages I–III RCC with localized disease and prolongation of survival in patients with metastatic disease ($p < 0.07$), these trends did not reach statistical significance.

Kirchner *et al.* (1995) studied 203 evaluable patients with either pT2–3a, N1–2, M0 ($n = 107$), pT3b-4 N0, M0 ($n = 68$), or pT3b–4, N1–2, M0 ($n = 23$) RCC, who received adjuvant vaccination with autologous, Newcastle disease virus-modified, irradiated tumor cells in combination with low-dose IL-2 and IFNα. Results revealed a median DFS of 21+ months. There was an 18 per cent relapse rate at a median follow-up of 39 months. While the authors concluded that these results were better than in analogous historical controls, only a randomized trial using an appropriate control group will address the efficacy of this approach.

Galligioni *et al* (1996) reported on a study in 120 patients randomized either to an untreated control group or to a group receiving autologous irradiated tumor cells mixed with BCG after radical nephrectomy. Patients were then tested at regular intervals for delayed-type hypersensitivity (DTH) responses to autologous tumor and autologous normal renal cells. Results revealed that baseline DTH responses were negative in all patients. One month after completing vaccination, 70 per cent of immunized patients showed a significant ($p < 0.01$) DTH response to autologous tumor but not to normal autologous renal cells. The DTH response persisted in 57 per cent of evaluable patients 12 months after vaccination. However, at a median follow-up of 61 months, there was no statistically significant difference in either 5-year DFS (63 per cent for treated patients and 72 per cent for control patients) or 5-year overall survival (69 and 78 per cent, respectively).

Repmann *et al.* (1997) treated 116 patients with an autologous tumor vaccine after radical nephrectomy for stage II and III RCC. However, because survival outcomes were compared to historical controls, conclusions are difficult to draw from this study.

Thus, while there is a rationale to test cancer vaccines in the adjuvant setting, optimal applications remain to be defined.

Adjuvant IFNα

Since patients with metastatic RCC can achieve a response rate of 12 per cent with IFNα therapy (Wirth 1993), these results have provided an impetus to evaluate IFNα in the adjuvant setting.

Takahashi *et al.* (1994) assessed the effect of recombinant IFNα2b therapy on natural killer cell (NK) activity and antibody-dependent cell-mediated cytotoxicity (ADCC) in 20 patients who had undergone a radical nephrectomy. Thirteen patients had stage I disease, one had stage II disease, and six had stage III disease. Three patients relapsed at 5, 7, and 32 months, respectively, after start of IFNα2b therapy. Results for all patients revealed that there was a significant increase in NK cell activity at 5 and 7 months after starting IFNα2b therapy, but there was no increase in ADCC. In the absence of an untreated control group, it is unclear whether adjuvant IFNα2b was of benefit to these patients.

In a retrospective analysis of 125 patients who underwent radical nephrectomy (Basting *et al.* 1999*a*), 33 patients received adjuvant IFNα for 1 year, whereas the other patients were untreated. Results revealed that there was no significant overall survival benefit to adjuvant IFNα in either the pT2 or the pT3/4 tumor cohorts. This study also investigated whether tumor ploidy could identify a group of patients who might benefit from the treatment (Basting *et al.* 1999*b*). Results revealed that 47 per cent

of tumors were diploid and 53 per cent were aneuploid, but adjuvant IFNα therapy did not provide a survival benefit to either of the two groups.

Pizzocaro *et al.* (1993) reported on 28 patients who underwent radical nephrectomy for Robson's stage II–III RCC and were treated with adjuvant IFNα2b, 5 MU subcutaneously 3 times a week for 6 consecutive months. A relapse rate of 26 per cent at a 16-month median follow-up was reported. However, in the absence of an untreated control group, the value of IFNα2b therapy in this study was unclear.

In an Eastern Cooperative Oncology Group/Intergroup randomized phase III trial (Trump *et al.* 1996), 258 patients who underwent radical nephrectomy and regional lymphadenectomy for stage pT3 or T4a, or N1, 2, 3, M0 RCC were randomized to receive up to 12 cycles of IFNα (3 MU/m^2 on day 1, 5 MU/m^2 on day 2, and 20 MU/m^2 on days 3, 4, and 5 by intramuscular injection, repeated every 3 weeks) or observation until recurrence. At a median follow-up of 5.3 years, there was no difference in recurrence-free survival or time to recurrence between groups. However, median survival of treated patients was 5.1 years but has not been reached in observed patients. Thus, in this study, survival was actually worsened by adjuvant treatment with IFNα.

Thus, on the basis of these studies, IFNα does not appear to have a benefit in the adjuvant therapy of locally advanced RCC.

Interleukin-2

While phase III adjuvant trials with IL-2 remain to be reported, the documented durable responses of high-dose bolus IL-2 in patients with metastatic RCC have led the Cytokine Working Group (CWG (USA)) to test IL-2 in the adjuvant setting. Patients with resected high-risk RCC (T3c, T4; N2 or N3 disease) or resected M1 disease will be randomized to either one full course of high-dose bolus intravenous IL-2 or to observation. The outcome of this trial is eagerly awaited.

Conclusion

In conclusion, optimal adjuvant therapy for resected RCC remains to be defined and the evaluation of adjuvant therapies will require properly controlled and adequately powered randomized trials. Observation alone after nephrectomy remains the standard of care. The CWG trial with high-dose IL-2 should provide insights into the efficacy of IL-2 in the adjuvant setting. Future adjuvant studies will undoubtedly incorporate combination cytokine regimens, new vaccines based on powerful tumor antigen-presenting cells, such as dendritic cells, and anti-angiogenic agents.

References

Adler, A., Gillon, G., Lurie, H., Shaham, J., Loven, D., Shachter, Y., Shani, A., Servadio, C., and Stein, J.A. (1987). Active specific immunotherapy of renal cell carcinoma patients: a prospective randomized study of hormono-immuno- versus hormonotherapy. Preliminary report of immunological and clinical aspects. *J. Biol. Response Mod.* **6**, 610–24.

Bassil, B., Dosoretz, D.E., and Prout, G.R. (1985). Validation of the tumor, nodes and metastasis classification of renal cell carcinoma. *J. Urol.* **134**, 450.

Basting, R., Corvin, S., Handel, D., Hinke, A., and Schmidt, D. (1999*a*). Adjuvant immunotherapy in renal cell carcinoma—comparison of interferon alpha treatment with an untreated control. *Anticancer Res.* **19**, 1545–8.

Basting, R., Corvin, S., Handel, D., Hinke, A., and Schmidt, D. (1999*b*). Adjuvant interferon alpha therapy in renal cell carcinoma (RCC): prognostic value of DNA cytophotometry. *Anticancer Res.* **19**, 1493–5.

Bojar, H., Maar, K., and Staib, W. (1979). The endocrine background of human renal cell carcinoma. IV. Glucocorticoid receptors as possible mediators of progestogen action. *Urol. Int.* **34**, 330–8.

Boxer, R.J., Waisman, J., Lieber, M.M., Mampaso, F.M., and Skinner, D.G. (1979). Renal carcinoma computer analysis of 96 patients treated by nephrectomy. *J. Urol.* **122**, 598.

Chen, L., Weiss, F.R., Chaichik, S., and Keydar, I.I. Sr (1980). Steroid receptors in human renal carcinoma. *J. Med. Sci.* **16**, 756–60.

Cherrie, R.J., Goldman, D.G., Lindner, A., and deKernion, J.B. (1982). Prognostic implications of vena caval extension of renal cell carcinoma. *J. Urol.* **128**, 910.

Galligioni, E., Quaia, M., Merlo, A., Carbone, A., Spada, A., Favaro, D., Santarosa, M., Sacco,C., and Talamini, R. (1996). Adjuvant immunotherapy treatment of renal carcinoma patients with autologous tumor cells and bacillus Calmette–Guerin: five-year results of a prospective randomized study. *Cancer* **77**, 2560–6.

Golimbu, M., Joshi, P., Sperber, A., Tessler, A., Al-Askari, S., and Morales, P. (1986). Renal cell carcinoma: survival and prognostic factors. *Urology* **27**, 291.

Kirchner, H. H., Anton, P., and Atzpodien, J. (1995). Adjuvant treatment of locally advanced renal cancer with autologous virus-modified tumor vaccines. *World J. Urol.* **13**,171–3.

Kjaer, M., Frederiksen, P.L., and Engelholm, S.A. (1987). Postoperative radiotherapy in stage II and III renal adenocarcinoma. A randomized trial by the Copenhagen Renal Cancer Study Group. *Int. J. Rad. Oncol. Biol. Physiol.* **13**, 665.

McNichols, D.W., Segura, J.W., and Deweerd, J. H. (1981). Renal cell carcinoma: long-term survival and late recurrence. *J. Urol.* **126**, 17.

Pizzocaro, G., Piva, L., Di Fronzo, G., Giongo, A., Cozzoli, A., Dormia, E., Minervini, S., Zanollo, A., Fontanella, U., Longo, G., *et al.* (1987). Adjuvant medroxyprogesterone acetate to radical nephrectomy in renal cancer: 5-year results of a prospective randomized study.*J. Urol.* **138**, 1379–81.

Pizzocaro, G., Piva, L., Faustini, M., Nicolai, N., Salvioni, R., Pisani, E., Maggioni, A., Mandressi, A., Dormia, E., Minervini, S., *et al.* (1993). Adjuvant interferon alpha in renal carcinoma with a high risk of recurrence. Multicenter pilot study. *Arch. Ital. Urol.* **65**, 173–6.

Repmann, R., Wagner, S., and Richter, A. (1997). Adjuvant therapy of renal cell carcinoma with active-specific-immunotherapy (ASI) using autologous tumor vaccine. *Anticancer Res.* **17**, 2879–82.

Robson, C.J., Churchill, B.M., and Anderson, W. (1969). The results of radical nephrectomy for renal cell carcinoma. *J. Urol.* **101**, 297.

Selli, C., Hinshaw, W.M., Woodard, B.H., and Paulson, D.F. (1983). Stratification of risk factors in renal cell carcinoma. *Cancer* **52**, 899.

Skinner, D.G., Calvin, R.B., Vermillion, C.D., Pfister, R.C., and Leadbetter, W.F. (1971). Diagnosis and management of renal cell carcinoma. *Cancer* **28**, 1165.

Takahashi, S., Tanigawa, T., Imagawa, M., Mimata, H., Nomura, Y., and Ogata, J. (1994).Interferon as adjunctive treatment for non-metastatic renal cell carcinoma. *Br. J. Urol.* **74**, 11–14.

Takenawa, J., Kaneko, Y., Okumura, K., Yoshida, O., Nakayama, H., and Fujita, J. (1995). Inhibitory effect of dexamethasone and progesterone *in vitro* on proliferation of human renal cell carcinomas and effects on expression of interleukin-6 or interleukin-6 receptor. *J. Urol.* **153**, 858–62.

Trump, D.L., Elson, P., Propert, K., Pontes, J., Crawford, E., Wilding, G., and Loehrer, P. (1996). Randomized, controlled trial of adjuvant therapy with lymphoblastoid inteferon (L-IFN) in resected, high-risk renal cell carcinoma (HR-RCC) [meeting abstract]. *Proceedings of the Annual Meeting of the American Society of Clinical Oncology*, Vol. 15, A648.

Wirth, P. (1993). Immunotherapy for metastatic renal cell carcinoma. *Urol. Clin. N. Am.* **20**, 283.

34. Complications of surgery for renal cell carcinoma

John M. Corman

Introduction

Renal cell carcinoma (RCC) is the most common malignancy of the human kidney and accounts for 3 per cent of all adult neoplasms (Landis *et al.* 1999). While radical nephrectomy remains the 'gold standard', modern diagnostic instruments, contemporary operative techniques, and advances in perioperative care have expanded treatment options for the disease. With earlier diagnosis of smaller tumors (Aso *et al.* 1992) and with an increased incidence of RCC (Chow *et al.* 1999) clinicians are faced with two important controversies. First, does nephron-sparing surgery offer cancer control rates that are similar to those of traditional open radical nephrectomy? Multiple reviews have addressed this first question (Lerner *et al.* 1996; Frydenberg *et al.* 1993; Hafez *et al.* 1999; Herr *et al.* 1994; Novick *et al.* 1989; Provet *et al.* 1991; Van Poppel *et al.* 1998). Second, do radical nephrectomy and nephron-sparing surgery have comparable morbidity and mortality? It is the second of these two issues that will be addressed in this chapter.

Radical nephrectomy and nephron-sparing surgery have common morbidities, such as the risk of complications related to anesthesia, positioning, and operative exposure. The surgical approach, whether transperitoneal or extraperitoneal, and operator experience are vital factors dictating the likelihood of exposure-related morbidities. Wound infections, incisional hernias, and anesthetic complications are often attributed to underlying predisposing factors and to technical errors rather than to the choice of procedure.

Radical nephrectomy

The mainstay of treatment of primary RCC is complete surgical excision. Radical nephrectomy via either an open or a minimally invasive approach remains the treatment of choice for large unilateral renal carcinoma (Novick *et al.* 1998*a*; Marshall *et al.* 1996). The classic radical nephrectomy includes removal of Gerota's fascia, adrenal gland, kidney, perinephric fat, and hilar lymph nodes (Robson *et al.* 1969). While modern diagnostic instruments, contemporary operative technique, and advances in perioperative care have made a great impact on the management of renal neoplasms, the largest studies reviewing morbidity and mortality from radical nephrectomy are drawn from older series

(Skinner *et al.* 1971; Schiff *et al.* 1977). The distinction between older series and more contemporary literature is vital because tumor size is the most significant independent predictor of outcome (cancer death and progression-free survival) and of intraoperative and postoperative morbidity. Thus, series published prior to the advent of modern diagnostic techniques and prior to the increased incidence of incidentally discovered renal masses tend to represent larger tumors with an attendant higher complication rate (Skinner *et al.* 1971; Scott *et al.* 1966; Schiff *et al.* 1977). Series with tumor volumes less than 5 cm have comparatively lower morbidity rates (Indudhara *et al.* 1997; Ljungberg *et al.* 1998; Swanson *et al.* 1983).

Intraoperative complications

Intraoperative morbidity from radical nephrectomies is most commonly related to issues of exposure. The most common morbidity associated with exposure is pneumothorax. This complication is not uncommon, particularly with flank approaches to renal masses. The choice of incision has a direct impact on the incidence of this complication: the higher the incision, the greater the risk of pleural injury. Transabdominal incisions are typically associated with lower risk of pneumothorax. Most small tears in the pleura can be repaired at the time of surgery without necessitating postoperative chest tube placement. Larger pleurotomies, as performed in thoracoabdominal incisions, often require postoperative drainage.

The second most common intraoperative morbidities are splenic and vascular injury. For large, left-sided renal masses splenic injuries are reported in up to 24 per cent of transabdominal cases (Swanson *et al.* 1983). Splenic injuries typically occur because large tumors may adhere closely to the spleen. Minor splenic rents are best treated conservatively using hemostatic agents (Avitene, thrombin, Surgicell). Closure of larger lacerations is accomplished using Gelfoam bolsters to facilitate splenorrhaphy. Because of the potential for postsplenectomy sepsis, the spleen should be preserved if at all possible. However, in the face of failed conservative measures or for severe injuries, splenectomy should be considered. Of note, because of the risk of developing pneumococcal infections, patients undergoing a splenectomy should receive prophylactic Pneumovax.

Pancreatic lacerations or hematomas can occur when the tail of the pancreas is mobilized to facilitate resection of left-sided tumors, or the head of the pancreas medialized during the Kocher maneuver to gain access to the right renal hilum. Unrecognized pancreatic injuries (particularly a laceration of the pancreatic duct) are associated with significant morbidity and mortality. When recognized intraoperatively, distal injuries are best treated by distal pancreatectomy and oversewing of the pancreatic duct. Lacerations of the pancreatic head are best treated by oversewing the affected area with interrupted 3–0 silk suture after ascertaining that the duct has not been injured (Hermann *et al.* 1985). For such injuries, general surgical consultation is recommended. A drain should be placed around the repaired pancreas in all circumstances.

Injury to the duodenum most commonly involves the second portion during mobilization to facilitate access to the right renal hilum. Lacerations are best repaired in two layers with omental wrapping and prolonged nasogastric suction. If the duodenal defect cannot be closed primarily without undue tension, a Roux-en-Y jejunal limb can be utilized to bridge the affected area (Hermann *et al.* 1985). Duodenal hematomas are best managed conservatively unless they become expansive. As in the case of pancreatic injury, general surgical consultation is recommended when a significant duodenal injury occurs.

Colonic injury may occur with either right- or left-sided tumors. Minimal injury can be primary repaired in two layers. More significant injury, particularly with direct tumor involvement, should be repaired with segmental resection or colostomy. Colonic mesenteric injury is an uncommon complication. However, when it occurs, a thorough evaluation of the viability of the affected colon must be performed. Following such injury, the possibilities of colonic resection, reanastomosis, and possible diversion should be entertained. Mesenteric defects that do not result in bowel ischemia should be closed to prevent herniation.

Adrenal injuries are common, especially in the course of adrenal-sparing nephrectomies. If salvage of the adrenal gland is necessary (for example, in the absence of the contralateral adrenal gland), adrenal parenchymal lacerations are best treated by oversewing the gland edges. Otherwise, torn edges of the adrenal gland are best managed by completing the adrenalectomy, as long as the contralateral gland is intact.

Renal vein avulsion is more common on the right side, where the short course of the vein as well as its direct insertion into the inferior vena cava can result in significant blood loss. This injury is best managed by optimizing exposure, by utilizing pressure to control the bleeding, by controlling the site of avulsion with an Allis clamp, and by using vascular suture for repair.

Specific complications

Intraoperative and perioperative complications described in series published since 1983 are reviewed in Table 34.1. The most common morbidity not directly associated with exposure remains retroperitoneal hemorrhage. Hemorrhage most commonly arises from injury of lumbar veins entering the vena cava, avulsion of the right gonadal vein as it enters the vena cava, tearing of the left lumbar vein as it enters into the left renal vein, or avulsion of the right adrenal vein as it enters into the vena cava. Intraoperative hemorrhage can best be controlled by direct pressure while maximizing exposure. Allis clamps are applied to the injured vessel until definitive hemostasis is obtained by oversewing the edges of the laceration or avulsion using 5–0 vascular suture.

The second most common morbidity associated with radical nephrectomy is perioperative cardiac or pulmonary complication (for example, myocardial infarction, congestive heart failure, pleural effusion, pulmonary embolus), which occurs in 2.9 per cent of cumulative cases. The etiology of cardiopulmonary morbidity often represents underlying medical disease in the face of anesthesia and fluid shifts. The morbidity is best avoided by meticulous intraoperative anesthesia and close monitoring of postoperative fluid changes. When cardiopulmonary complications arise, patients are best managed in an intensive care setting with appropriate specialist consultation.

Partial nephrectomy

Indications for nephron-sparing surgery initially evolved out of necessity when a malignancy was detected in a solitary kidney, in the presence of bilateral cancer, or in the setting of renal insufficiency (Zincke *et al.* 1985, 1988; Licht *et al.* 1994). Nephron-sparing surgery has now become an established effective treatment for renal masses in patients with solitary kidneys (Licht *et al.* 1993; Griffin *et al.* 1996). Some centers extend the indication for this procedure to include patients with small, unilateral tumors and

Table 34.1 Cumulative complications from radical nephrectomies in series published after 1983 (*N* = 604)*

Complication	n	%	Complication	n	%
Death	3	0.5	Sepsis	1	0.1
Pneumothorax	7	1.8	Vocal cord paralysis	1	0.1
Ileus	5	0.8	Hyperbilirubinemia	7	1.1
Hernia	4	0.6	Wound infection	4	0.6
Gastrointestinal bleed	7	1.1	Adrenal insufficiency	1	0.1
Acute renal failure	4	0.6	Re-operation/hemorrhage	21	3.4
Urinary tract infection	3	0.5	Mental confusion	2	0.3
Urinary retention	3	0.5	Cardiac/pulmonary event	18	2.9

* Studies in series: Butler *et al.* (1995), *n* = 193; Ljungberg *et al.* (1998), *n* = 89; Swanson *et al.* (1983), *n* = 71; Indudhara *et al.* (1997), *n* = 42; Lerner *et al.* (1996), *n* = 209.

Table 34.2 Cumulative complications from partial nephrectomies in series published after 1983 (*N* = 768)*

Complications	n	%	Complications	n	%
Death	4	0.5	Adrenal insufficiency	2	0.2
Urinoma	4	0.5	Arterial/venous thrombosis	7	0.9
Postoperative bleeding	16	2.1	UPJ obstruction	2	0.2
Cardiac/pulmonary event	5	0.7	Incidental splenectomy	3	0.4
Abscess	6	0.8	Wound infection	9	1.1
Urinary fistula	57	7.4	Re-exploration	3	0.4
Acute renal failure	40	5.2			

* Studies in series: Thrasher *et al.* (1994), *n* = 42; Campbell *et al.* (1994), *n* = 259; Lerner *et al.* (1996), *n* = 185; Duque *et al.* (1998), *n* = 66; Van Poppel *et al.* (1998), *n* = 76; Steinbach *et al.* (1998), *n* = 140.

normal, contralateral kidneys (Provet *et al.* 1991; Carini *et al.* 1988). The rationale is to preserve maximal renal function while conducting adequate cancer surgery. Many studies describe the complications of partial nephrectomy, including large series of patients from tertiary care centers (Novick *et al.* 1995; Campbell *et al.* 1994; Polascik *et al.* 1995). Table 34.2 lists the reported complications from contemporary series of partial nephrectomies from such institutions.

Many of the morbidities noted as associated with partial nephrectomy are not unique to this operation. Wound infection, re-exploration for hemorrhage, splenic injury, adrenal insufficiency, postoperative cardiac events, and postoperative mortality occur in both radical and nephron-sparing surgery. Other complications are more specific to partial nephrectomy: urinoma formation, urinary fistula, arterial and venous thrombosis, and postoperative renal hemorrhage. As partial nephrectomy has become more widely accepted as an alternative treatment for RCC, in addition to evaluation of cancer control rates, the surgeon must reconcile unique morbidities.

Urinary fistula is the most common procedure-specific complication noted in a review of the literature, occurring in 7.4 per cent of partial nephrectomies. In one series, significant risk factors for fistula formation include central tumor location, tumor size greater than 4.0 cm, the need for collecting system reconstruction, and extracorporeal surgery (Campbell *et al.* 1994). Urinary fistulas are commonly managed conservatively, sealing spontaneously or with outflow obstruction release (that is, urethral catheterization). When fistulas are more intractable, ureteral stent placement or percutaneous renal drainage can minimize caliceal pressure to facilitate fistula closure.

Patients with a solitary kidney undergoing partial nephrectomy are at much greater risk for developing acute renal failure as compared to patients with a normal contralateral renal unit. In one series, acute renal failure occurred in 26 per cent of partial nephrectomies performed on a solitary kidney versus 2 per cent when a contralateral kidney was present (Campbell *et al.* 1994). Additional risk factors for acute renal failure include: tumor size larger than 7 cm, greater than 50 per cent parenchymal excision, *ex vivo* surgery, and prolonged ischemia time. Significant postoperative factors resulting in acute renal failure include outflow obstruction (ureteral or urethral), vascular thrombosis, and urinoma formation. Duration of dialysis dependence varies depending upon the etiology of the renal failure. Resolution of ureteral obstruction and drainage of urine collections often result in improvement of renal function. Similarly, over time, ischemic nephrons may regain enough function to require only temporary dialytic support. To prevent acute renal failure renal perfusion should be maximized by using mannitol, intraoperative renal ischemia should be minimized, hypothermia should be used during ischemia, and meticulous postoperative fluid management must be employed.

Direct comparisons

Direct comparisons of nephron-sparing surgery with the classic radical nephrectomy include many reports of cancer recurrence rates (Novick *et al.* 1989; Morgan *et al.* 1990; Steinbach *et al.* 1995). Many now believe that radical and partial nephrectomies provide equally effective curative treatment for patients with single, small (< 4 cm), localized RCC (Novick *et al.* 1998*b*; Lerner *et al.* 1996). Other studies have reviewed complication and mortality rates in single-institution series (Campbell *et al.* 1994; Thrasher *et al.* 1994; Morgan *et al.* 1990). Others have directly compared morbidity and mortality retrospectively in consecutive patients undergoing the procedures (Indudhara *et al.* 1997; Butler *et al.* 1995).

Butler *et al.* (1995) reviewed their results in 64 patients undergoing radical and 60 patients undergoing partial nephrectomy. There were no significant differences between the two groups of patients in terms of age, sex, diabetes, hypertension, or renal function. There were no significant differences in length of hospitalization, blood transfusions, or perioperative morbidities. There were six perioperative complications in the radical nephrectomy group and seven complications in the nephron-sparing group. There was one perioperative death in the nephron-sparing group. Indudhara *et al.* (1997) similarly retrospectively compared 35 consecutive patients undergoing partial nephrectomy with 71 patients receiving a radical nephrectomy for T1 or T2 disease. In this study there were no significant differences in the patients' age, sex, tumor location, or bilaterality. There were no differences in major medical complications between the two groups. Urinoma and urinary fistula were seen in three patients in the nephron-sparing group.

National Veterans Affairs Surgical Quality Improvement Program

The National Veterans Affairs Surgical Quality Improvement Program (NSQIP), a large, population-based study, compared complication rates of these two common urologic procedures in risk-adjusted populations (Corman *et al.* 2000). In the NSQIP series, all patients undergoing a radical nephrectomy or partial nephrectomy were selected from the NSQIP database based upon current procedure terminology (CPT) coding . Mortality was defined as death within 30 days of the index surgery. Morbidity was defined as any of 20 complications within 30 days of surgery (Table 34.3). Because the NSQIP is designed to assess all surgical procedures, it does not include operation-specific complications (for example, urinary fistula, urinoma).

A risk-adjusted analysis was performed to adjust for possible baseline differences in preoperative patient characteristics between the two populations (Table 34.4). Multivariable logistic regression was then performed and stepwise selection techniques were used in model building. Separate models were developed using mortality and morbidity as the dependent variables. Indications for radical nephrectomy included: malignancy (86 per cent), infection (5 per cent), stone disease (3 per cent), renal cystic disease (2 per cent), and other (4 per cent). Partial nephrectomies were performed for malignancy (72 per cent), cystic disease (7 per cent), stone disease (3 per cent), and other (8 per cent).

Table 34.3 Outcome variables collected prospectively from 123 Veterans Administration medical centers

Postoperative length of stay	Respiratory occurrences	Cardiac occurrences
Wound occurrences	Pneumonia	Arrest requiring cardiopulmonary
Superficial wound infection	Unplanned intubation	resuscitation
Deep wound infection	Pulmonary embolism	Myocardial infarction
Wound disruption	Ventilator-dependent	Other occurrences
Urinary tract occurrences	Central nervous system occurrences	Ileus/bowel obstruction
Renal insufficiency	Stroke/cerebral vascular accident	Bleeding/transfusions
Acute renal failure	Coma > 24 hours	Graft/prosthesis/flap failure
Urinary tract infection	Peripheral nerve injury	Deep venous thrombosis/thrombophlebitis
		Systemic sepsis

Table 34.4 Preoperative patient characteristics collected in NSQIP

General	Other
Sex	Disseminated cancer
Race	Wound classification
Diabetes mellitus	Open wound
Smoker within 1 year	Steroid use for chronic condition
Smoking, pack-years	Weight loss > 10%
ETOH > 2 drinks/day	Bleeding disorders
ASA classification	Transfusion > 4 RBC units
Do not resuscitate status	Chemotherapy within 30 days
Functional status	Radiotherapy within 90 days
Central nervous system	Preoperative sepsis
Impaired sensorium	Urgency status: emergency case
Coma	Pulmonary
Hemiplegia	Dyspnea
History of transient ischemic attacks	Ventilator-dependent
Cerebral vascular accident	Chronic obstructive pulmonary disease
with deficit	Pneumonia
without deficit	Preoperative laboratory tests
Tumor involving central nervous system	Albumin
Hepatobiliary: ascites	Bilirubin
Cardiac: congestive heart failure within 1 month	Sodium
Renal	Creatinine
Acute renal failure	Blood urea nitrogen
Currently on dialysis	White blood cell count
	Aspartate aminotransferase
	Alkaline phosphatase
	Hematocrit
	Platelet count
	Partial thromboplastin time
	Prothrombin time

Table 34.5 Selected characteristics of 1885 patients treated with radical or partial nephrectomy

	Nephrectomy		
Characteristic	Radical (*n* = 1373)	Partial (*n* = 512)	*p*-value
Patient characteristic			
Gender			
Male, number (%)	1353 (98.5)	497 (97.1)	0.053
Female, number (%)	20 (1.5)	15 (2.9)	
Race			
White, number (%)	1001 (72.9)	372 (72.7)	0.907
Non-White, number (%)	372 (27.1)	140 (27.3)	
Age ± standard deviation, years	62.4 ± 11.0	62.6 ± 11.4	0.770
Smokers, number (%)	474 (34.5)	160 (31.3)	0.189
Disseminated cancer, number (%)	66 (4.8)	18 (3.5)	0.260
Serum creatinine ± standard deviation, mg/dl			
Preoperative	1.40 ± 1.44	1.45 ± 0.81	0.409
Postoperative	2.18 ± 2.08	2.16 ± 1.81	0.80
Process of care characteristic			
Operative time ± standard deviation, hours	3.42 ± 1.48	3.64 ± 1.77	0.013

Patient characteristics and unadjusted outcomes

The characteristics of patients treated with radical or partial nephrectomy are summarized in Table 34.5. None were significantly different between the two groups, except for mean operative time, which was slightly higher for the patients undergoing partial nephrectomy. There were no significant differences between radical and partial nephrectomy in unadjusted 30-day mortality, 30-day morbidity, or in specific complication rates.

Preoperative patient characteristics and mortality

Preoperative patient characteristics predictive of mortality in univariate analyses included: 10 per cent weight loss within 6 months prior to surgery ($p = 0.002$); congestive heart failure ($p < 0.001$); preoperative acute renal failure ($p < 0.001$); American Society of Anesthesiology (ASA) classification 3 or 4 and 5 ($p = 0.001$); albumin ≤ 3.5 g/dl ($p < 0.001$); blood urea nitrogen > 20 mg/dl ($p = 0.013$); creatinine > 1.2 mg/dl ($p = 0.039$); total bilirubin > 1.0 mg/dl ($p = 0.036$); and platelet count < 150 000/μL ($p = 0.004$). Patient characteristics that independently predicted mortality in the multivariable model included: greater than 10 per cent weight loss (odds ratio = 3.30); albumin ≤ 3.5 g/dl (odds ratio = 3.27); blood urea nitrogen > 20 mg/dl (odds ratio = 2.07); and platelet count < 150 000 000/μL (odds ratio = 3.77). After adjusting for other risk factors, the type of surgery (radical versus partial nephrectomy) did not predict mortality ($p = 0.561$).

Preoperative patient characteristics and morbidity

Patient characteristics predictive of morbidity included: diabetes ($p = 0.001$); previous cerebral vascular accident (CVA) with neurologic sequela ($p = 0.002$); ASA classification 3 or 4 and 5 ($p = 0.001$); abnormal sodium (< 135 or > 146 meq/l; $p = 0.02$); blood urea nitrogen > 20 mg/dl ($p < 0.001$); abnormal hematocrit (<3 8 or > 46 per cent; ($p = 0.001$); and albumin ≤ 3.5 g/dl ($p < 0.001$). Patient characteristics that independently predicted morbidity in the multivariable model included: greater than 10 per cent weight loss (odds ratio = 1.7); albumin ≤ 3.5 g/dl (odds

ratio = 1.42); dependent functional status (odds ratio = 1.79); ASA classification 4 and 5 (odds ratio = 2.57); ASA classification 3 (odds ratio=1.84); blood urea nitrogen > 20 mg/dl (odds ratio = 1.35); and billirubin > 1.0 mg/dl (odds ratio = 1.60). After adjusting for other risk factors, the type of surgery (radical versus partial nephrectomy) did not predict morbidity ($p = 0.348$).

Summary of the NSQIP study

The NSQIP study compared morbidity and mortality rates after 1373 radical nephrectomies and 512 partial nephrectomies. To control for preoperative patient characteristics, including renal dysfunction, the entire population was risk-adjusted utilizing multivariable logistic regression modeling. The operative and perioperative mortality rates for the radical and partial nephrectomy series were 2.04 and 1.56 per cent, respectively and the morbidity rates were 15.0 and 16.2 per cent respectively. These differences were not statistically significant. After risk adjustment, there were still no statistically significant differences in the overall mortality or morbidity between partial and radical nephrectomy. In addition, no statistically significant differences in the incidence of progressive renal failure, acute postoperative renal failure, urinary tract infection, prolonged ileus, transfusion requirement, deep wound infection, postoperative creatinine, or postoperative hospital stay were noted.

The NSQIP study has limitations. Because the database tracks all operations performed under general, spinal, or epidural anesthesia, the preoperative, intraoperative, and perioperative variables apply to all surgical patients. Specific complications associated with individual operations (for example, urinoma, urinary fistula, and postoperative ureteral stent requirements after a partial nephrectomy), pathologic staging, and cancer recurrence rates are not recorded. This is a limitation because several studies have shown that urinary leaks are a major risk factor after partial nephrectomy, particularly for central tumors (Lerner *et al.* 1996). Because the NSQIP lacks operation-specific perioperative morbidities, surrogate markers were utilized. For example, urinary fistula, urinoma formation, and perinephric abscess contribute to extended hospitalization; thus prolonged postoperative hospital stay was utilized as a surrogate for these complications. Arterial and venous thrombosis result in renal insufficiency; thus renal insufficiency and renal failure were utilized as surrogates. Delayed hemorrhage increases postoperative transfusion requirements; thus significant transfusion was used as a surrogate. Arguably, these surrogates may underestimate the operation-specific complications.

Conclusion

Selection of the optimal surgical approach for management of RCC remains an area of intense controversy. Cancer control and potential complications are the two primary areas of debate. When preservation of renal function is a relevant clinical issue, most agree that nephron-sparing surgery is the best choice. Such procedures provide cancer-survival rates that are comparable to those of radical nephrectomy. When the contralateral kidney is normal, however, radical nephrectomy has remained the treatment of choice for management of unilateral RCC. Recently, some centers, ours included, have advocated partial nephrectomy for patients with normal contralateral kidneys. This approach might be appropriate because more than one-third of all renal masses are now discovered incidentally. These tumors tend to be smaller (< 4.0 cm) and more amenable to nephron-sparing surgery.

References

Aso, Y. & Homma, Y. (1992). A survey on incidental adrenal tumors in Japan. *Journal of Urology*, **147**, 1478–81.

Butler, B.P., Novick, A.C., Miller, D.P., Campbell, S.A. & Licht, M.R. (1995). Management of small unilateral renal cell carcinomas: radical versus nephron-sparing surgery. *Urology*, **45**, 34–40; discussion 40–1.

Campbell, S.C., Novick, A.C., Streem, S.B., Klein, E. & Licht, M. (1994). Complications of nephron sparing surgery for renal tumors. *Journal of Urology*, **151**, 1177–80.

Carini, M., Selli, C., Barbanti, G., Lapini, A., Turini, D. & Costantini, A. (1988). Conservative surgical treatment of renal cell carcinoma: clinical experience and reappraisal of indications. *Journal of Urology*, **140**, 725–31.

Chow, W.H., Devesa, S.S., Warren, J.L. & Fraumeni, J.F., Jr. (1999). Rising incidence of renal cell cancer in the United States. *Jama*, **281**, 1628–31.

Corman, J., Penson, D., Hur, K., Khuri, S., Daley, J., Henderson, W. & Kriger, J. (2000). Comparison of Complications After Radical and Partial Nephrectomy: Results from the National VA Surgical Quality Improvement Program. American Urologic Association: Atlanta.

Duque, J.L., Loughlin, K.R., MP, O.L., Kumar, S. & Richie, J.P. (1998). Partial nephrectomy: alternative treatment for selected patients with renal cell carcinoma. *Urology*, **52**, 584–590.

Frydenberg, M., Malek, R.S. & Zincke, H. (1993). Conservative renal surgery for renal cell carcinoma in von Hippel-Lindau's disease. *Journal of Urology*, **149**, 461–4.

Griffin, J.H. & Flanigan, R.C. (1996). Nephron-sparing surgery for renal cell carcinoma. *Techniques in Urology*, **2**, 43–7.

Hafez, K.S., Fergany, A.F. & Novick, A.C. (1999). Nephron sparing surgery for localized renal cell carcinoma: impact of tumor size on patient survival, tumor recurrence and TNM staging. *Journal of Urology*, **162**, 1930–3.

Hermann, R.E. (1985). Intraoperative consultation for the liver, biliary system, pancreas, duodenum, and spleen. *Urologic Clinics of North America*, **12**, 469–76.

Herr, H.W. (1994). Partial nephrectomy for renal cell carcinoma with a normal opposite kidney. Cancer, **73**, 160–2.

Indudhara, R., Bueschen, A.J., Urban, D.A., Burns, J.R. & Lloyd, L.K. (1997). Nephron-sparing surgery compared with radical nephrectomy for renal tumors: current indications and results. *Southern Medical Journal*, **90**, 982–5.

Landis, S.H., Murray, T., Bolden, S. & Wingo, P.A. (1999). Cancer statistics, 1999. *Ca: a Cancer Journal for Clinicians*, **49**, 8–31, 1.

Lerner, S.E., Hawkins, C.A., Blute, M.L., Grabner, A., Wollan, P.C., Eickholt, J.T. & Zincke, H. (1996). Disease outcome in patients with low stage renal cell carcinoma treated with nephron sparing or radical surgery. *Journal of Urology*, **155**, 1868–73.

Licht, M.R. & Novick, A.C. (1993). Nephron sparing surgery for renal cell carcinoma. *Journal of Urology*, **149**, 1–7.

Licht, M.R., Novick, A.C. & Goormastic, M. (1994). Nephron sparing surgery in incidental versus suspected renal cell carcinoma [see comments]. *Journal of Urology*, **152**, 39–42.

Ljungberg, B., Alamdari, F.I., Holmberg, G., Granfors, T. & Duchek, M. (1998). Radical nephrectomy is still preferable in the treatment of localized renal cell carcinoma. A long-term follow-up study. *European Urology*, **33**, 79–85.

Marshall, F.F. (1996). Is nephron-sparing surgery appropriate for a small renal-cell carcinoma? *Lancet*, **348**, 72–3.

Morgan, W.R. & Zincke, H. (1990). Progression and survival after renal-conserving surgery for renal cell carcinoma: experience in 104 patients and extended followup. *Journal of Urology*, **144**, 852–7; discussion 857–8.

Novick, A. & Streem, S. (1998). Surgery of the Kidney. In *Campbell's Urology*, Walsh PC, R.A., Vaughan ED and Wein AJ (ed), Vol. 1. pp. 2993–2995. Saunders: Philadelphia, PA.

Novick, A.C. (1995). Partial nephrectomy for renal cell carcinoma [editorial]. *Urology*, **46**, 149–52.

Novick, A.C. (1998). Nephron-sparing surgery for renal cell carcinoma. *British Journal of Urology*, **82**, 321–4.

Novick, A.C., Streem, S., Montie, J.E., Pontes, J.E., Siegel, S., Montague, D.K. & Goormastic, M. (1989). Conservative surgery for renal cell carcinoma: a single-center experience with 100 patients. *Journal of Urology*, **141**, 835–9.

Polascik, T.J., Pound, C.R., Meng, M.V., Partin, A.W. & Marshall, F.F. (1995). Partial nephrectomy: technique, complications and pathological findings [see comments]. *Journal of Urology*, **154**, 1312–8.

Provet, J., Tessler, A., Brown, J., Golimbu, M., Bosniak, M. & Morales, P. (1991). Partial nephrectomy for renal cell carcinoma: indications, results and implications. *Journal of Urology*, **145**, 472–6.

Robson, C.J., Churchill, B.M. & Anderson, W. (1969). The results of radical nephrectomy for renal cell carcinoma. *Journal of Urology*, **101**, 297–301.

Schiff M, J., Glazier WB. (1977). Nephrectomy: Indications and complications in 347 patients. *Journal of Urology*, **118**, 930–931.

Scott, R.F., Jr. & Selzman, H.M. (1966). Complications of nephrectomy: review of 450 patients and a description of a modification of the transperitoneal approach. *Journal of Urology*, **95**, 307–12.

Skinner DG, C.R., Vermillion CD *et al.* (1971). Diagnosis and management of renal cell carcinoma: A clinical and pathologic study of 309 cases. *Cancer*, **28**, 1165–1169.

Steinbach, F., Stockle, M. & Hohenfellner, R. (1995). Current controversies in nephron-sparing surgery for renal-cell carcinoma. *World Journal of Urology*, **13**, 163–5.

Steinbach, F., Stockle, M., Muller, S.C., Thuroff, J.W., Melchior, S.W., Stein, R. & Hohenfellner, R. (1992). Conservative surgery of renal cell tumors in 140 patients: 21 years of experience. *Journal of Urology*, **148**, 24–9; discussion 29–30.

Swanson, D.A. & Borges, P.M. (1983). Complications of transabdominal radical nephrectomy for renal cell carcinoma. *Journal of Urology*, **129**, 704–7.

Thrasher, J.B., Robertson, J.E. & Paulson, D.F. (1994). Expanding indications for conservative renal surgery in renal cell carcinoma. *Urology*, **43**, 160–8.

Van Poppel, H., Bamelis, B., Oyen, R. & Baert, L. (1998). Partial nephrectomy for renal cell carcinoma can achieve long-term tumor control. *Journal of Urology*, **160**, 674–8.

Zincke, H., Engen, D.E., Henning, K.M. & McDonald, M.W. (1985). Treatment of renal cell carcinoma by in situ partial nephrectomy and extracorporeal operation with autotransplantation. *Mayo Clinic Proceedings*, **60**, 651–62.

Zincke, H. & Sen, S.E. (1988). Experience with extracorporeal surgery and autotransplantation for renal cell and transitional cell cancer of the kidney. *Journal of Urology*, **140**, 25–7.

Part 1, Section 4

Renal cell carcinoma: metastatic disease

35. Immunologic therapy for renal cell carcinoma

Allan J. Pantuck, Amnon Zisman, and Arie Belldegrun

Introduction

Conventional therapy for metastatic renal cell carcinoma (RCC) is associated with a poor response rate and few patients are long-term survivors. Patients with advanced disease have an average survival of less than a year from the time of diagnosis (Elson *et al.* 1988). Although quite controversial and being challenged by recent studies, traditionally it has been felt that nephrectomy does not benefit survival when metastases are present (deKernion *et al.* 1978) and the objective response rate to conventional chemotherapy is only 6 per cent and of very short duration (Yagoda *et al.* 1995). However, up to 1–5 per cent of RCC patients will experience spontaneous tumor regression, mainly involving their pulmonary metastases (Papac 1996). The reason for this is not well understood, but the occurrence of spontaneous tumor regression and the prolonged latency period between primary tumor removal and the appearance of metastases in some patients suggest the existence of important host immune responses to autologous tumor cells. With this in mind, diverse treatment strategies have been sought to enhance the immune system's ability to fight metastatic tumors. With the advent of molecular gene transfer techniques and increased knowledge of the basic pathways of immune activation, the field of cancer immunotherapy has finally begun to develop novel and effective approaches for harnessing the immune system as a therapeutic agent. These diverse strategies are generally termed 'immunotherapy'.

Historical perspective

For at least 100 years, immunologists have proposed activating the immune system to specifically target and eradicate autologous tumor cells. The idea that tumor cells may possess properties that can be recognized as foreign by the host's immune system is a fundamental concept of tumor immunology. This concept of tumor cell recognition was first postulated by Paul Ehrlich at the turn of the century.

In 1943, Gross noted that, when tumor cells were injected subcutaneously into syngeneic mice, the cells were capable of forming nodules that grew for a few days but then regressed (Gross 1943). When the same mice were challenged a second time by tumor reinjection, the tumors subsequently failed to produce nodules or grow. This failure of the tumor to grow in previously exposed mice was interpreted to mean that the tumor cells had failed to grow as a result of the mice becoming immunologically resistant to the tumor, suggesting the existence of tumor-associated antigens. In 1954, Billingham introduced the term adoptive immunity to describe the acquisition of immunity as a result of the transference of immunologically competent cells (Billingham *et al.* 1954). Prehn and Main (1957) demonstrated, further, that immunization of syngeneic mice with a given tumor protected the mice against a second challenge with the same tumor, but did not protect them from other tumors. In the same year, Isaacs and Lindenmann (1957) first described the class of immunomodulators known as the interferons, named for their ability to interfere with viral infection of untreated tissues.

In 1959, Lewis Thomas suggested that the immune response might be able to rid the body of abnormal cells (Thomas *et al.* 1959). His theories were later refined into the immune surveillence hypothesis of Burnet (1970), which suggests that the immune system could recognize malignant cells as foreign and generate a response against them and that only tumors capable of evading the body's surveillance would be able to grow. In 1972, Borberg successfully documented the ability of adoptively transferred immune cells to cause regression of established tumors (Borberg *et al.* 1972). In the 1980s, progress was made in the use of cytokines for patients with metastatic RCC (deKernion *et al.* 1983). Finally, the first successful clinical application of cellular therapy in man was performed at the US National Cancer Institute by Rosenberg *et al.* (1985) in patients with metastatic melanoma and RCC. Peripheral blood lymphocytes of patients were activated *ex vivo* with interleukin 2 (IL-2), previously known as T-cell growth factor, to generate lymphokine-activated killer cells (LAK) that were capable of non-(major histocompatibility complex; MHC)-restricted tumor lysis when reinfused into patients.

Components of the immune response

The immune system comprises a complex network that protects the host from foreign biologic substances, accomplishing this task with mechanisms that depend on the system's ability to recognize these factors as foreign, to recall prior recognition, and to mount an enhanced response when re-exposure occurs. In tumor immunology, tumor cells are recognized as foreign by the host's immune system, and are attacked by the immune system's effector mechansims, which include humoral (antibody-mediated) and cell-mediated components. The development of an immune response against a tumor requires changes in the surface components of the tumor cell that do not occur in its nonmalignant counterpart and that give rise to structures that may be antigenic. Tumor-associated antigens are epitopes that allow the host immune system to recognize tumor cells as foreign. Tumor-associated antigens on the surfaces of malignant cells may be unique to the cancerous cells and therefore absent from their normal, benign counterparts. On the other hand, tumor antigens may be present on normal cells but merely become unmasked on the malignant cell. Finally, they may represent products that are present during embryonic development but are absent in the normal adult tissue. A description of the main cellular and humoral components of the immune system and their proposed mechansims of action in tumor immunity will follow.

Cellular immunity

The immune system is thought to contribute to the surveillance and destruction of tumor cells primarily via its cellular arm, which refers to the function of thymus-derived lymphocytes also known as T cells. Delayed-type hypersensitivity and rejection of foreign grafts are some of the functions of cellular immunity. Cellular mediators include MHC-restricted cytotoxic and helper T cells, non-specific natural killer (NK) cells, and antigen-presenting cells (including monocytes, macrophages, and dendritic cells). Antigen-presenting cells (APC) continually sample the host's molecular environment by phagocytosis or endocytosis of viral, bacterial, and cellular elements, which are then enzymatically digested into peptide fragments. These processed fragments bind to the individual's polymorphic MHC class molecules and are transported back to the APC's cell surface where they put on display for other immune cells to inspect.

When peptide antigens are displayed with the appropriate MHC molecule, T cells are able to examine the peptides via binding with their T-cell receptors (TCR). The TCR (Marrack and Kappler 1987) is capable of tolerating an individual's 'self' molecules while recognizing and reacting against foreign peptides. A T-cell immune response is triggered by the interaction of the TCR with the MHC/peptide complex on the surface of the APC when it is accompanied by binding of co-stimulatory molecules on the APC such as the B7 molecule. A complex intracellular cascade known as signal transduction is initiated that results in activation and proliferation (Jenkins and Johnson 1993) of T cells that are capable of lysing cells that express the peptide antigen and the appropriate MHC molecule.

The functional T-cell population can be divided into distinct subsets having unique cell surface markers and activities. Cells expressing the CD4 molecule are associated with T-cell helper activity, while those expressing the CD8 molecule are associated with T-cell cytotoxic or suppressor activity. Helper T cells predominantly interact with foreign antigens originating outside the cell in association with MHC class II molecules, whereas cytotoxic T cells predominantly interact with cells displaying antigens that have been actively synthesized within the cell in association with MHC class I products. CD8+, MHC I restricted T cells that can lyse and kill appropriate target cells such as cultured tumor cells are called cytotoxic T lymphocytes (CTL). CTL must not only be stimulated by coming into contact with a specific antigen on target cells but must also be able to receive signals from helper T cells.

Helper (CD4+, MHC II restricted) T cells typically secrete cytokines in response to antigen binding. There appear to be two distinct populations of helper cells (Th1 and Th2), which can be distinguished by the types of immunostimulatory cytokines they produce. Th1 cells secrete interferon γ (IFNγ) and tumor necrosis factor α (TNFα), which mediate responses to bacteria, viruses, and protozoans. Th2 cells secrete cytokines such as IL-4 and IL-10 that help B cells proliferate and differentiate (Constant and Bottomly 1997).

Natural killer (NK) cells are another class of immune cells whose functional mechanisms are poorly understood. NK cells differ from the classic T lymphocytes in that their cytolytic activity is nonspecific. They recognize target cells in a non-MHC-restricted manner, and their development is non-thymic-dependent. NK cells, which are CD56+, are thought to be involved in tumor surveillance (Lanier *et al.* 1983) and it is thought that one function of NK cells is to eliminate cells that have somehow lost expression of MHC molecules. Loss of MHC expression by tumor cells is thought to represent one way in which tumors can circumvent immune surveillance. NK cells exposed to high concentrations of IL-2 become LAK cells, which are capable of lysing Daudi cells, a LAK target, as well as fresh tumor (Lotze *et al.* 1981).

Cells involved in the processing and presentation of antigens are called antigen-presenting cells (APC), which include dendritic cells (DC), Langerhans cells, and cells of the monocyte and macrophage lineage. DC are considered the most potent APC in the immune system. They are capable of triggering powerful T-cell responses when exposed to antigens and possess the unique ability to stimulate naïve T cells (Steinman 1991). DC function as the immune system's sentinels, capturing microorganisms for presentation to immune cells as they are found in the skin, respiratory system, gastrointestinal system, and interstitial regions of solid organs (Austyn 1996). Furthermore, DC express high levels of co-stimulatory molecules such as CD80 and CD86, which are required for full T-cell activation (Steinman 1991). DC can be obtained from an individual's bone marrow or peripheral blood by *ex vivo* culture and isolation in the presence of cytokines such as granulocyte–macrophage colony stimulating factor (GM-CSF) and IL-4 (Bender *et al.* 1996) producing large numbers of DC for use in tumor vaccination strategies. Tumor lysate, individual tumor peptides, or tumor-derived RNA can be fed or 'pulsed' *ex vivo* directly to DC where they associate with MHC molecules and are presented by DC to initiate an antitumoral T-cell res=ponse when reinfused to the patient. In effect, the patient's own immune system is used as a bioreactor to educate and expand tumor-specific CTL *in vivo* (Celluzzi *et al.* 1996).

Humoral immunity

Humoral immunity refers to the system of immune recognition that takes place through B lymphocytes and is mediated by the production and function of antibodies. Antibody production is unique to B lymphocytes, which are derived from hematopoietic stem cells in the bone marrow. These cells mature in the bone marrow where they acquire the ability to synthesize membrane-bound immunoglobulin molecules. Immunoglobulin molecules on the surface of B cells can directly recognize foreign molecules without the need for MHC presentation. Mature B cells proliferate and differentiate into antibody-secreting cells when they encounter and bind foreign antigen in the peripheral circulation. T helper cells can provide further stimulation to B cells through the release of cytokines. Release of antibodies systemically allows for binding and neutralization of foreign molecules. In the past, the role of antibodies in tumor immunology was limited. However, with the development of hybridoma technology, unlimited quantities of pure monoclonal antibody can be produced against single antigens. Monoclonal antibodies have proven to have multiple applications, including their use in *in vitro* diagnostics such as immunohistochemistry, to *in vivo* diagnostic imaging using radioactive labeling (for example, Prostascint scan for prostate cancer) and, most recently, to their use as therapeutic agents (for example, Rituxan for lymphomas).

Cytokines and adoptive immunotherapy

Cytokines are biologically active soluble factors that are responsible for communication between cells of the immune system. They are produced by cells of the immune system and they generate direct tumoricidal effects as well as causing further activation of effector responses by components of the immune system. Cytokines are generated during the effector phases of natural immunity and they serve to mediate and regulate subsequent immune and inflammatory responses. Cytokines, like other natural polypeptide hormones, initiate their action by binding to specific receptors on the surface of target cells. Most cellular responses to cytokines are slow and require new mRNA and protein synthesis. For many target cells, cytokines act as growth factors and as regulators of cell division. The cytokines that have been the most extensively studied include tumor necrosis factor, the interferons, and the interleukins.

IFNα and IL-2 have been the focus of the majority of immunotherapy trials for RCC and have the greatest follow-up. The interferon family of proteins produces numerous effects on immune stimulation. IFNα induces a marked increase in the surface expression of Fc (crystallizable fragment) receptors and MHC class I and tumor-associated antigens in addition to possessing direct antitumor activity. IFNγ causes a marked increase in the surface expression of both the MHC I and MHC II antigens, enhances the presentation of antigenic peptides to T helper cells, can directly inhibit tumor growth in a variety of cell lines, and, like IFNα< modulates B-cell function.

The initial reports that recombinant IFNα produced responses of 15–20 per cent with duration up to 10 months provided early enthusiasm for the use of immunotherapy for RCC (deKernion *et al.* 1983; Quesada *et al.* 1985). These reports suggested an important role for IFNα in select patients, namely, those with a good performance status, prior nephrectomy, long disease-free interval, and lung-predominant metastatic disease. A large review

of 1042 patients treated with IFNα monotherapy reported a response rate of 12 per cent (Wirth 1993). Response durability has remained problematic, however, and few long-term survivors have been reported with time to disease progression rarely exceeding 2 years (Minasian *et al.* 1993). An open label, prospective, multicenter trial that used low-dose, subcutaneously administered IFNγ-1b showed an overall response rate of only 3 per cent with a complete response rate of only 1.5 per cent (Small *et al.* 1998). To date, it remains unclear whether interferon's mechanism of action involves direct anti-proliferative effects or whether it works via stimulation of host immune response.

In 1965 it was determined that soluble factors were present in the supernatant from mixed lymphocyte cultures grown in conditioned media (Kasakura and Lowenstein 1965) and, later, that these factors could maintain normal human T cells in culture (Morgan *et al.* 1976). Ultimately, it has been determined that IL-2, formerly known as this T-cell growth factor, is produced by activated T cells and causes proliferation of CTL and NK capable of lysing autologous, syngeneic, or allogeneic tumor cells. Unlike IFN, Il-2 has no intrinsic, direct antitumoral action. In addition to activation of cytotoxic responses, IL-2 is chemotactic for T cells, and causes proliferation and differentiation of B cells.

Recombinant human Il-2 monotherapy has well documented activity in metastatic RCC and was approved by the US Food and Drug Administration (FDA) for use in this disease in 1992. A recent update on the use of high-dose, bolus IL-2 in RCC was presented using the 255-patient database that resulted in IL-2's approval by the US FDA. Patients were treated with 600 000 or 720 000 IU/kg by intravenous bolus infusion every 8 hours for as many as 14 doses during a 5-day hospitalization, followed by a second, identical cycle of treatment after a 10-day resting interval. This study demonstrated 7 per cent complete responders and 8 per cent partial response rates (Fisher 1999). Median duration for all objective responders was 54 months and more, significantly, median duration of response for all complete responders has still not been reached but is now at least 80 months (range 3 to 126+ months). Median survival was 16 months and overall 10 per cent of treated patients remain alive; however, some responding patients have remained alive for 11 years following treatment. Of the original 37 responding patients, 49 per cent (18) have not yet progressed. Patient selection remains of paramount importance and should focus on patients with low Eastern Cooperative Oncology Group (ECOG) status, no concomitant underlying diseases, as well as good cardiac, respiratory, and renal function. The use of high-dose IL-2 is associated with significant dose-related side-effects, including azotemia, hypotension, pulmonary edema, renal failure, fluid retention, myocardial infarction, gastrointestinal bleeding, and death. The toxicity of IL-2 makes a case for treatment at specialized centers by skilled physicians and nurses capable of optimizing therapy while minimizing potential morbidity and mortality. Although interferon-based therapy generates similar overall response rates to IL-2, with both in the range of 15–20 per cent (Bukowski 1997), it is generally believed that IL-2 monotherapy generates a higher frequency of complete remission and more durable response times.

The toxicity of IL-2 has led to alternative doses and schedules in an attempt to reduce morbidity. Unfortunately, without randomized trials it is difficult to compare the various regimens described. At the National Cancer Institute, an ongoing randomized trial is being performed with three arms comparing high-dose, low-dose, and outpatient subcutaneous schedules of IL-2. Only with trials such as these will we be able to adequately compare the results of alternate regimens with the FDA-approved schedule of high-dose, bolus IL-2. Interim results have been presented (Yang and Rosenberg 1999). In a comparison of concurrently randomized patients, the response rates are 18 per cent for high-dose intravenous IL-2, 7 per cent for low-dose intravenous IL-2, and 11 per cent for subcutaneous IL-2. Significant follow-up after full accrual will be necessary to detect meaningful differences in long-term survival between treatments.

When cytokines are given systemically to a patient to stimulate an immune response, they are given as active immunotherapy. Active immunotherapy refers to immunization of patients with agents that increase the host's immune response against a tumor. Other examples of active immunotherapy include the development of tumor vaccines that are transfected *in vitro* with cytokine-producing genes prior to reinfusion to the patient, and *in vivo* intralesional injection of genetic elements that will enhance MHC expression, or stimulate local cytokine production. Alternatively, cytokines may be used in a strategy of adoptive (passive) immunotherapy. Adoptive immunotherapy refers to the transfer of cells that themselves possess antitumor activity. The activated cell populations studied to date have principally included T lymphocytes and activated NK cells.

The first attempts to apply adoptive immunotherapy utilized nonspecific LAK cells that were lymphocytes isolated from the patient's peripheral blood, incubated *in vitro* with IL-2, and re-infused into the patient. A number of clinical trials demonstrated an average response rate of 21 per cent (Bukowski 1997). Despite promising preclinical murine data and these encouraging early-phase human studies, three separate phase III trials failed to show superiority of LAK plus IL-2 over IL-2 alone in the treatment of metastatic RCC (Rosenberg *et al.* 1991; McCabe *et al.* 1991; Bajorin *et al.* 1990).

A more specific application is the combination of IL-2 with tumor-infiltrating lymphocytes (TIL). TIL are lymphoid cells infiltrating solid tumors that can be cultured and expanded *ex vivo* in IL-2 and are assumed to have immunologic memory to tumor antigens. IL-2 cultivation of TIL induces growth, cytotoxicity, and multicytokine synthesis (Belldegrun *et al.* 1996). TIL isolated from primary RCC include a heterogeneous population of CTL that mediate antitumor activity via both MHC-restricted and MHC-non-restricted pathways. On a cellular basis, TIL are 50–100 times more potent than LAK cells in mediating tumor regression in animal immunotherapy models (Rosenberg *et al.* 1986). Few clinical studies have been undertaken with TIL. At UCLA, TIL are isolated from fresh nephrectomy specimens of RCC patients, expanded *in vitro* with IL-2 in the presence of tumor extract, and then re-infused to the patient. In a recent report on 55 patients treated with cytokine-primed or CD8-selected TIL combined with an outpatient regimen of IFN and IL-2 following radical nephrectomy, there was an objective response of 35 per cent and a 9.1 per cent complete response rate (Figlin *et al.* 1997). These responses appeared durable, with a

mean duration of response of 14 months and a median survival for all patients of 22 months. Median survival for responders has not yet been reached. However, a multicenter, randomized, phase III trial comparing IL-2 alone versus CD8+ TIL in combination with low-dose IL-2 failed to demonstrate additional efficacy with the addition of TIL (Figlin *et al.* 1999). Unfortunately, though, among 72 eligible patients, 41 per cent were not able to receive TIL because of an inability to generate sufficient numbers of viable TIL in *ex vivo* culture.

Regardless of the specific immunotherapy regimen used, patients included in immunotherapy clinical trials have experienced improved prognosis when compared to patients treated by other clinical protocols in which no immunotherapy was given (Motzer *et al.* 1999). The overall outcome of high-dose intravenous recombinant IL-2 alone appears to be superior to other regimens. However, this treatment is accompanied by very high toxicity and other adverse reactions. Therefore, newer, innovative strategies for immunotherapy are continuously being sought.

New approaches in immunotherapy for RCC

Molecular-based therapeutic strategies have evolved beyond the above-described immunotherapeutic techniques, to include a variety of genetic and cell signaling-based strategies. Examples of new innovative approaches in immunotherapy for RCC include gene therapy, monoclonal antibody therapy, and vaccine therapy. Classification of these diverse therapies based on their strategic approach to eliminate tumor cells is provided in Table 35.1. Many of these strategies will be discussed fully in other chapters; however, a brief overview is presented here.

Immune-based gene therapy

The overall goal of gene therapy is the transfer of a new genetic material into cells with the hope of leading to a therapeutic benefit. Gene therapy approaches utilize three main concepts for creation of tumor vaccines: (1) *in vitro* transformation of autologous tumor with genes producing cytokines; (2) generation of super TIL via transfection of autologous T cells with cytokine genes; and (3) *in vivo* transfer of MHC or other genes by intralesional injection. One rationale for this approach is to preserve the antitumor activity of cytokines while minimizing their systemic adverse effects by local introduction and confined production of high levels of the gene products within the tumor vicinity. The gene products that are produced locally in high concentrations may directly alter neoplastic properties associated with invasion and metastasis. This approach carries significant advantage in that it is associated with lower toxicity than systemic administration of cytokines (Saffran *et al.* 1998). Animal studies using this technique have demonstrated prevention of tumor growth, decreased metastatic spread, and prolonged immunologic memory, resulting in rejection of subsequent tumor challenges.

At UCLA we have transfected the genes for IL-2 and IFNα into human RCC lines. When these cells were implanted subcutaneously into nude mice, their cytokine secretion inhibited

Table 35.1 Approaches to immune- and gene-based therapies for RCC

Immunotherapy
- Systemic cytokine administration (e.g. IL-2, IFN, IL-4, GM-CSF, IL-12)
- Adoptive immunotherapy: *ex vivo* activation of autologous immune effector cells (e.g. LAK, TIL) using recombinant cytokines followed by passive, reinfusion of immune-competent cells
- Antigen-presenting cell therapy alone or in combination with cytokines (e.g. tumor cell lysate pulsed dendritic cells)

Immune-based gene therapy (cancer vaccines)
- Autologous tumor cells transfected with cytokine or growth factors genes (e.g. IL-2, GM-CSF, IL-12) injected into the tumor site
- Viral vectors/gene carriers (e.g. adenoviruses, retroviruses, vaccinia virus)
- Direct transfection of naked DNA/genes

Cytoreductive therapies
- Suicide genes (e.g. thymidine kinase gene therapy, which converts inactive pro-drug such as gancyclovir into toxic metabolite)
- Drug-activated suicide genes
- Oncolytic viruses (e.g. adenovirus such as ONYX-015 capable of replication and lysis only in *p53*-deficient cells)
- Toxic gene therapy (necrosis and apoptosis induction by diphtheria toxin)

Corrective gene therapy
- Introduction of wild-type suppressor genes (e.g. p53, VHL gene) into tumor cells with defective or inactive tumor suppressors
- Modulation of tumor growth and survival using antisense oligonucleotides (e.g. antisense bcl-2, antisense TGFβ)

local tumor growth in a more effective manner than achieved by systemic administration of IL-2 and IFNα (Belldegrun *et al.* 1993). In addition to IL-2 and IFNα< various other genes of immune system modulators, including GM-CSF (Seigne *et al.* 1999) and the co-stimulatory molecule B7 (Jung *et al.* 1999), were tested as possible tumor vaccines for RCC (Gitlitz *et al.* 1996). One of the options used to confine the cytokines to the tumor site is by transfecting TIL with the cytokine genes (Mulders *et al.* 1998). The rationale is that the TIL will home back to tumor deposits. In this way secretion of the relevant gene product may be localized and continuous, leading to augmented killing. A phase I clinical trial using irradiated RCC cells transfected *ex vivo* with human GM-CSF gene was performed to test the safety and the induction of immune responses in patients with metastatic RCC (Simons 1997). No significant toxicity or autoimmune responses were reported, and one of 16 patients had a partial response. Furthermore, recent studies using modified dendritic cells (Mulders *et al.* 1999) and studies directly introducing the cytokines into the tumor have been performed at UCLA as well as at other centers. At this time, tumor vaccine-based gene therapy appears to be safe but its efficacy in metastatic RCC has yet to be proved.

Cytoreductive therapy

This therapeutic approach shares with the previous one the concept of introducing specific genes into the tumor site. However, in cytoreductive therapy a suicide gene is introduced into the tumor that encodes for an enzyme capable of converting an otherwise benign medication (pro-drug) into a highly cytotoxic one. Administration of the pro-drug produces a high concentration of the cytotoxic metabolite in the tumor area, but not in normal tissues that did not receive the gene, resulting in reduced systemic toxicity. The most commonly used system in this group is herpes simplex virus thymidine kinase gene (HSV-tk). HSV-tk phosphorylates gancyclovir to gancyclovir monophosphate, which is converted to gancyclovir triphosphate by cellular kinases. The resulting triphosphate acts as a false base, inhibiting DNA polymerase and DNA synthesis, leading to cell death. Other examples of cytoreductive strategies include: (1) replication competent, oncolytic virus systems that target only p53-deficient cells and (2) diphtheria toxin gene whose product induces necrosis and apoptosis.

Corrective gene therapy

This therapeutic approach attempts to correct a specific genetic alteration such as over expression of an oncogene or inactivation of a tumor-suppressor gene (for example, p53 gene) by a mutation. The logic for corrective gene therapy is that its restoration should result in normal growth control. Corrective gene therapy uses the same vectors as immunotherapy and cytoreductive therapy in order to introduce the relevant wild-type gene into the tumor cells.

Genetic studies of families with hereditary RCC, in the presence or absence of von Hippel–Lindau (VHL) syndrome contributed to our current view of the tumorogenetic pathways of RCC, possibly leading to the design of future gene-targeted therapies. These studies identified a loss of chromosome 3p in many sporadic and familial RCC patients (Glenn *et al.* 1992) and localized the VHL gene on chromosome 3p25–26 (Glenn *et al.* 1992; Linehan *et al.* 1995). The wild-type VHL gene is a tumour suppressor protein that regulates angiogenesis, extracellular matrix formation, and hypoxia-inducible mRNA such as the mRNA encoding vascular endothelial growth factor (VEGF). More than half of the patients with sporadic RCC have a detectable mutation in one allele of the VHL gene (Shui *et al.* 1994) and allelic loss in the other allele is seen in up to 98 per cent of tumors (Gnarra *et al.* 1994). Therefore, the VHL gene and gene products may serve as potential targets for corrective gene therapy.

Initial studies have been performed to replace the defective tumor suppressor product by the wild-type gene in an attempt to reverse the cancer phenotype. Wild-type VHL gene was transfected into RCC cell lines lacking the normal expression of the gene and attached to a constitutively activated cytomegalovirus promoter and via a liposome vehicle (Chen *et al.* 1995). Transfection of the wild-type VHL gene resulted in growth suppression of the RCC cell line. In addition, it was recently shown that loss of VHL gene was associated with increased expression of TGFβ and TGFβ1, and transfection of RCC cell lines with wild-type VHL substantially decreased TGFβ and TGFβ1 mRNA and protein by shortening their mRNA half-life (Ananth *et al.* 1999). Thus, gene replacement therapy using the wild-type VHL gene may have a role in treating patients with RCC, although the safety and efficacy of this treatment is yet to be defined.

Alternatively, corrective gene therapy can be achieved by introducing the complementary stretch of mRNA for a protein whose function is undesired. This complementary stretch, called 'antisense mRNA' binds to the sense mRNA and blocks the translation of its protein. This has been attempted using oligodeoxynucleotides against oncogenes like bcl-2 and growth factor genes like TGFβ (Morelli *et al.* 1997).

G250

G250 is a new tumor marker that has been recently introduced for RCC. This protein is detected on the majority of primary and metastatic RCC but is absent from kidney and other normal tissues with the exception of gastric mucosal cells and cells of the larger bile ducts (Bander *et al.* 1997). G250 is a transmembrane protein identical to the tumor-associated antigen MN/CA IX that was previously identified in cervical carcinoma. Its function and association to cancer development are unclear; however, its unique expression on RCC tissues makes it a potential candidate for both tumor diagnosis and therapy (Oosterwijk *et al.* 1993). Therapeutic studies are underway to determine whether G250 is immunogenic and has potential for use in a kidney cancer vaccine. Various potential therapeutic approaches can be considered, including targeting the tumors using radiolabeled antibodies to G250 (Divgi *et al.* 1998).

A list of current clinical trials using molecular-based therapies for RCC is presented in Table 35.2.

Conclusions

In the past 20 years, there has been impressive progress in the application of immunotherapy to treating RCC. There is no doubt that current immunotherapeutic protocols produce alterations in the natural history of this disease and cause significant and lasting remissions in select patients. At UCLA we have seen a progressive increase in responses to treatment as therapy has evolved from systemic IFNα administration (16 per cent), to combination IFN + IL-2 (25 per cent), to the current method of bulk TIL (33 per cent) and CD8+ TIL (40 per cent). The reinsertion of inactivated tumor suppressor genes, the inactivation of oncogenes, the insertion of immunomodulatory genes, and the insertion of suicide genes have all been used to treat genitourinary malignancies *in vitro* and in animal models. Progress is being made in better understanding the genetic and cellular mechanisms that underlie tumorigenesis. Patient characteristics that predict improved responsiveness to therapy have been identified, and treatment protocols that decrease toxicity have been developed. The most encouraging results have been the improved rates of complete clinical response, most of which are durable and longlasting.

Table 35.2 Current clinical trials for renal cell cancer using molecular-based approaches*

Basic principle	Principal investigator	Site
Intratumoral injection of Leuvectin (phase II)	Belldegrun	UCLA
TIL + INF + IL-2	Belldegrun	UCLA
Liposome IL-2	Figlin	UCLA
HLA-B7 and IL-2 gene	Figlin	UCLA
Multiantigen loaded dendritic cell vaccine (adoptive immunotherapy—phase I)	Gitlitz	UCLA
HLA-B7 and IL-2	Antonia	University of South Florida
IL-4	Lotze	University of Pittsburgh
TNFα	Rosenberg	National Institutes of Health
IL-2	Rosenberg	National Institutes of Health
Liposome HLA-B7/beta-2 microglobulin	Chang	Multicenter
Autologous tumor cell vaccine + IFN/GM-CSF (phase II)	Dillman	Multicenter
IL-2 (allogeneic)	Gansbacher	Memorial Sloan-Kettering Cancer Center
GM-CSF	Simons	Johns Hopkins
HLA-B7/beta-2 microglobulin	Fox	Chiles Research Institute

* Adapted with changes from National Cancer Institute Web Site: www.cancernet.nci.nih.gov and from Rodriguez and Simons (1999).

References

Ananth, S., Knebelmann, B., Gruning, W., *et al.* (1999). Transforming growth factor beta 1 is a target for the von Hippel Lindau tumor suppressor and a critical growth factor for clear cell renal carcinoma. *Cancer Res.* **59**, 2210–16.

Austyn, J.M. (1996). New insights into the mobilization and phagocytic activity of dendritic cells. *J. Exp. Med.* **183**, 1287–92.

Bajorin, D., Sell, K.W., Richards, J.M., *et al.* (1990). A randomized trial of interleukin-2 plus lymphokine activated killer cells versus interleukin-2 alone in renal cell carcinoma. *Proc. Am. Assoc. Cancer Res.* **31**, 1106.

Bander, N.H., Carroll, P.R., and Russo, P. (1997). Summary of immuno-histologic dissection of the human kidney using monoclonal antibodies. *Sem. Urol. Oncol.* **15**, 123–9.

Belldegrun, A., Tso, C.L., Sakata, T., *et al.* (1993). Human renal cell carcinoma line transfected with interleukin-2 and/or interferon-gamma genes: implications for live cancer vaccines. *J. Natl Cancer Inst.* **85**, 207–16.

Belldegrun, A., Tso, C.L., Kaboo, R., *et al.* (1996). Natural immune reaction-associated therapeutic response in patients with metastatic renal cell carcinoma receiving tumor-infiltrating lymphoctyes and interleukin-2 based therapy. *J. Immunother.* **19**, 149–61.

Bender, A., Sapp, M., Schuler, G., *et al.* (1996). Improved methods for the generation of dendritic cells from non-proliferating progenitors in human blood. *J. Immunol. Methods* **196**, 121–35.

Billingham, R.E., Brent, L., and Medawar, P.B. (1954). Quantitative studies on tissue transplantation immunity, Vol. II: the origin, strength and duration of activity and adoptively acquired immunity. *Proc. R. Soc. Biol.* **143**, 58–80.

Borberg, H., Oettgen, H.F., Choudry, K., *et al.* (1972). Inhibition of established transplants of chemically induced sarcomas in syngeneic mice by lymphocytes from immunized donors. *Int. J. Cancer* **10**, 539–47.

Bukowski, R.M. (1997). Natural history and therapy of metastatic renal cell carcinoma. *Cancer* **80**, 1198–220.

Burnet, F.M. (1970). The concept of immunological surveillance. *Prog. Exp. Tumor Res.* **13**, 1–27.

Celluzzi, C.M., Mayordomo, J.I., Storkus, W.J., *et al.* (1996). Peptide pulsed dendritic cells induce antigen-specific CTL mediated protective tumor immunity. *J. Exp. Med.* **183**, 283–98.

Chen, F., Kishida, T., Yao, M., Hustad, T., *et al.* (1995). Germline mutations in the von Hippel–Lindau gene: correlations with phenotype. *Hum. Mutat.* **5**, 66–75.

Constant, S.L. and Bottomly, K. (1997). Induction of Th1 and Th2 CD4+ T cell responses: the alternative approach. *Ann. Rev. Immunol.* **15**, 297–322.

deKernion, J.B., Ramming, K.P., and Smith, R.B. (1978). The natural history of metastatic renal cell carcinoma: a computer analysis. *J. Urol.* **120**, 148–52.

deKernion, J.B., Sarna, G., Figlin, R., Lindner, A., and Smith, R.B. (1983). The treatment of renal cell carcinoma with human leukocyte alpha-interferon. *J. Urol.* **130**, 1063–6.

Divgi, C.R., Bander, N.H., Scott, A.M., *et al.* (1998). Phase I/II radio-immunotherapy trial with iodine-131-labeled monoclonal antibody G250 in metastatic renal cell carcinoma. *Clin. Cancer Res.* **4**, 2729–39.

Elson, P.J., Witte, R.S., and Trump, D.L. (1988). Prognostic factors for survival in patients with recurrent or metastatic renal cell carcinoma. *Cancer Res.* **48**, 7310–13.

Figlin, R., Pierce, W.C., Kaboo, R., Tso, C.L., Moldawer, N., Gitlitz, B., deKernion, J., and Belldegrun, A. (1997). Treatment of metastatic renal cell carcinoma with nephrectomy, interleukin-2 and cytokine primed or CD8+ selected tumor infiltrating lymphocytes from primary tumor. *J. Urol.* **158**, 740–5.

Figlin, R.A., Thompson, J.A., Bukowski, R.M., Vogelzang, N.J., Novick, A.C., Lange, P., Steinberg, G.D., and Belldegrun, A.S. (1999). Multicenter, randomized, phase III trial of CD8+ tumor-infiltrating lymphocytes in combination with recombinant interleukin-2 in metastatic renal cell carcinoma. *J. Clin. Oncol.* **17**, 2521–9.

Fisher, R.I., Rosenberg, S.A., Fyfe, G: Long term survival update for high dose recombinant interleukin-2 in patients with renal cell carcinoma. *Cancer J. Sci. Am.* **1**, 555–7, 2000.

Gitlitz, B., Belldegrun, A., and Figlin, R.A. (1996). Immunotherapy and gene therapy. *Sem. Urol. Oncol.* **14**, 237–43.

Glenn, G.M., Linehan, W.M., Hosoe, S., *et al.* (1992). Screening for von Hippel–Lindau disease by DNA polymorphism analysis. *J. Am. Med. Assoc.* **267**, 1226–31.

Gnarra, J.R., Tory, K., Weng, Y., *et al.* (1994). Mutations of the VHL tumor suppressor gene in renal carcinoma. *Nat. Genet.* **7**, 85–90.

Gross, L. (1943). Intradermal immunization of C3H mice against a sarcoma that originated in an animal of the same line. *Cancer Res..* **3**, 326–33.

Isaacs, A. and Lindenmann, J. (1957). Viral interference. *Proc. R. Soc.* **147**, 258–67.

Jenkins, M.K. and Johnson, J.G. (1993). Molecules involved in T-cell costimulation. *Curr. Opin. Immunol.* **5**, 361–7.

Jung, D., Hilnes, C., Knuth, A., Jaeger, E., Huzer, C., and Seliger, B. (1999). Gene transfer of the co-stimulatory molecules B7-1 and B7-2 enhances the immunogenicity of human renal cell carcinoma to different extents. *Scand. J. Immunol.* **50**, 242–9.

Kasakura, S. and Lowenstein, L. (1965). A factor stimulating DNA synthesis derived from the medium of leucocyte cultures. *Nature* **206**, 794–5.

Lanier, L.L., Le, A.M., Phillips, J.H., *et al.* (1983). Subpopulations of human natural killer cells defined by expression of the Leu-7 (HNK-1) and Leu-11 (HNK-15) antigens. *J. Immunol.* **131**, 1789–96.

Linehan, W.M., Lerman, M.I., and Zbar, B. (1995). Identification of the von Hippel–Lindau gene. Its role in renal carcinoma. *J. Am. Med. Assoc.* **273**, 564–70.

Lotze, M.T., Grimm, E.A., Mazumbar, A., *et al.* (1981). Lysis of fresh and cultured autologous tumor by human lymphocytes cultured in T-cell growth factor. *Cancer Res.* **41**, 4420–5.

Marrack, P. and Kappler, J. (1987). The T cell receptor. *Science* **238**, 1073–9.

McCabe, M., Stablein, D., and Hawkins, M.J. (1991). The modified group C experience—phase III randomized trials of IL-2 versus IL-2/LAK in advanced renal cell carcinoma and advanced melanoma. *Proc. Am. Soc. Clin. Oncol.* **10**, 213.

Minasian, L.M., Motzer, R.J., Gluck, L., *et al.* (1993). Interferon alpha-2a in advanced renal cell carcinoma: treatment results and survival in 159 patients with long-term follow up. *J. Clin. Oncol.* **11**, 1368–77.

Morelli, S., Delia, D., Capaccioli, S., Quattrone, A., *et al.* (1997). The antisense bcl-2-IgH transcript is an optimal target for synthetic oligonucleotides. *Proc. Natl Acad. Sci., USA* **94**, 8150–5.

Morgan, D.A., Ruscetti, F.W., and Gallow, R.G. (1976). Selective *in vitro* growth of T lymphocytes from normal bone marrows. *Science* **193**, 1007–8.

Motzer, R.J., Mazumdar, M., Bacik, J., Berg, W., Amsterdam, A., and Ferrara, J. (1999). Survival and prognostic stratification of 670 patients with advanced renal cell carcinoma. *J. Clin. Oncol.* **17**, 2530–40.

Mulders, P., Tso, C.L., Pang, S., Kaboo, R., Mcbride, W.H., Hinkel, A., Gitlitz, B., Dannull, J., Figlin, R., and Belldegrun, A. (1998). Adenovirus mediated interleukin-2 production by tumors induced growth of cytotoxic tumor-infiltrating lymphocytes against human renal cell carcinoma. *J. Immunother.* **21**, 170–80.

Mulders, P., Tso, C.L., Gitlitz, B., Kaboo, R., Hinkel, A., Frand, S., Kiertscher, S., Roth, M.D., deKernion, J., Figlin, R., and Belldegrun, A. (1999). Presentation of renal tumor antigens by human dendritic cells activates tumor infiltrating lymphocytes against autologous tumor: implications for live cancer vaccines. *Clin. Cancer Res.* **5**, 445–54.

Oosterwijk, E., Bander, N.H., Divgi, C.R., Welt, S., *et al.* (1993). Antibody localization in human renal cell carcinoma: a phase I study of monoclonal antibody G250. *J. Clin. Oncol.* **11**, 738–50.

Papac, R.J. (1996). Spontaneous regression of cancer. *Cancer Treatment Rev.* **22**, 395–423.

Prehn, R.T. and Main, J.M. (1957). Immunity to methylcholanthrene-induced sarcomas. *J. Natl Cancer Inst.* **18**, 769–78.

Quesada, J.R., Swanson, D.A., and Gutterman, J.U. (1985). Phase II study of interferon alpha in metastatic renal cell carcinoma: a progress report. *J. Clin. Oncol.* **3**, 1086–92.

Rodriquez, R. and Simons, J.W. (1999). Urologic applications of gene therapy. *Urology* **54**, 401–6.

Rosenberg, S.A., Lotze, M.T., Muul, L.M., *et al.* (1985). Observations on the systemic admininstration of autologous lymphokine-activated killer cells and recombinant interleukin-2 in patients with metastatic cancer. *New Engl. J. Med.* **313**, 1485–92.

Rosenberg, S.A., Speiss, P., and Lafreniere, R. (1986). A new approach to the adoptive immunotherapy of cancer with tumor-infiltrating lymphocytes. *Science* **233**, 1318–21.

Rosenberg, S.A., Lotze, M.T., Yang, J.C., *et al.* (1991). Prospective randomized trial of high dose interleukin-2 alone or in combination with lymphokine activated killer cells for the treatment of patients with advanced cancers. *J. Natl Cancer Inst.* **85**, 622–32.

Saffran, D.C., Horton, H.M., Yankauckas, M.A., Anderson, D., Barnhart, K.M., Abai, A.M., Hobart, P., Manthorpe, M., Norman, J.A., and Parker, S.E. (1998). Immunotherapy of established tumors in mice by intra-tumoral injection of interleukin-2 plasmid DNA: induction of CD8+ T-cell immunity. *Cancer Gene Ther.* **5**, 321–30.

Seigne, J., Turner, J., Diaz, J., Hackney, J., Pow-Sang, J., Helal, M., Lockhart, J., and Yu, H. (1999). A feasibility study of gene gun mediated immuno-therapy for renal cell carcinoma. *J. Urol.* **162**, 1259–63.

Shui, T., Kondo, K., Torigoe, S., *et al.* (1994). Frequent somatic mutation and loss of heterozygosity of the von Hippel–Lindau tumor suppressor gene in primary human renal cell carcinoma. *Cancer Res.* **54**, 2852–5.

Simons, J.W. (1997). Bioactivity of human GM-CSF gene therapy in metastatic renal cell carcinoma and prostate cancer. *Hinyokika Kiyo* **43**, 821–2.

Small, E.J., Weiss, G.R., Malik, U.M., *et al.* (1998). The treatment of metastatic renal cell carcinoma patients with gamma interferon. *Cancer J. Sci. Am.* **4**, 162–7.

Steinman, R.M. (1991). The dendritic cell system and its role in immuno-genicity. *Ann. Rev. Immunol.* **9**, 271–96.

Thomas, L. and Lawrence, H.C. (1959). *Cellular and humoral aspects of the hypersensitive states.* Hoeber-Harper, New York.

Wirth, M.P. (1993). Immunotherapy for metastatic renal cell carcinoma. *Urol. Clin. N. Am.* **20**, 283–94.

Yagoda, A., Abi-Rached, B., and Petrylak, D. (1995). Chemotherapy for advanced renal cell carcinoma: 1983–1993. *Sem. Oncol.* **22**, 42–60.

Yang, J.C. and Rosenberg, S.A. (1999). A randomized comparison of IL-2 dosing regimens in the treatment of patients with metastatic renal cell carcinoma. Presented at Proleukin Second International Congress. San Francisco.

36. Natural history and prognostic factors associated with metastatic renal cell carcinoma

David M.J. Hoffman and Robert A Figlin

General description

With approximately 38 500 new cases and 16 600 deaths expected in the US in the year 2002, renal cell carcinoma (RCC) is the seventh leading cause of cancer, accounting for 3 per cent of malignancies in men (Greenlee *et al.* 2000). Males are affected twice as frequently as females, with RCC most commonly developing in the fifth and sixth decades of life. There has been a steady increase in the incidence of RCC since the 1970s, which is only partly explained by incidentally discovered tumors found by widespread use of modern imaging techniques (Chow *et al.* 1999). Worldwide mortality is predicted to exceed 100 000 in 2000 (Motzer *et al.* 1996).

The cell of origin is the epithelial proximal convoluted renal tubule (Cotran *et al.* 1979). Tumors typically arise in the renal cortex, and occur sporadically in either kidney at similar frequency.

The primary therapeutic modality for localized tumors remains surgical resection. Advanced disease is resistant to standard cytotoxic chemotherapy, and the majority of patients with metastases prove refractory to systemic treatments, eventually succumbing to the disease. However, a significant minority of patients benefit from immunotherapeutic approaches. The clinical observations that RCC can often have a long treatment-free interval even in the face of metastatic disease and the knowledge that there are well-documented cases of spontaneous regressions in patients with widespread metastases have pointed to the importance of the immune system in the regulation of this disease (Figlin 1999).

Approximately one-third of cases of RCC present initially with metastases, and up to 50 per cent of patients resected for cure will relapse during the course of the disease. Patients with metastases at initial presentation exhibit an average survival rate of 6 to 12 months, and only 10 per cent survive more than 2 years (Vogelzang and Stadler 1998). Patients who develop metachronous metastases after nephrectomy have a slightly more favorable prognosis (Maldazys and deKernion 1986; Middleton 1967; Skinner *et al.* 1971). Autopsy studies demonstrate frequent sites of metastases including lung (76 per cent), lymph nodes (64 per cent), bone (43 per cent), liver (41 per cent), ipsilateral and contralateral adrenal (19 and 11 per cent, respectively), contralateral kidney (25 per cent), and brain (11.2 per cent) (Saitoh *et al.* 1982*a*, *b*; Hajdu and Thomas 1967). Other unusual sites of metastases include ureter, penis, vagina, thyroid, heart, intestines, uterus, orbit, thyroid, gall bladder, and pancreas.

Symptoms

Often referred to as the internist's tumor because of the diversity of its presentation and pathophysiology, advanced RCC produces a spectrum of systemic symptoms. Early in its natural history, RCC is usually asymptomatic. Although the classic triad of flank pain, hematuria, and palpable abdominal mass is well-described, it is seen in only 10–20 per cent of patients and indicates advanced (and usually metastatic) disease (deKernion 1986).

While systemic symptoms are common, their frequency in reported series is variable. Gross hematuria is seen in 40–50 per cent of all cases of renal cell cancer (McDougal and Garnick 2000). Anemia, often hypochromic and microcytic, has been described in 21–88 per cent of patients (Skinner *et al.* 1971; Linehan *et al.* 1993). Frequently reported findings include fever, weight loss, hypercalcemia, erythrocytosis, and hepatomegaly. Elevation of hepatic transaminases (known as Stauffer's syndrome if accompanied by concomitant hepatomegaly) is seen in up to 40 per cent of patients (Utz *et al.* 1970; Hanash *et al.* 1971). Polycythemia, a reflection of endogenous production of erythropoietin by the tumor cells, is seen in fewer than 5 per cent of cases. Hypercalcemia may be seen in the absence of bony metastases and results from the production of a parathyroid hormone (PTH)-like hormone produced by the tumor. Other paraneoplastic syndromes described with RCC include hypertension (24 per cent), amyloidosis (3–5 per cent), enteropathy (3 per cent), and neuromyopathy (3 per cent).

Systemic involvement with metastases can produce symptoms referable to the affected site. Pulmonary metastases are usually silent until they have achieved sufficient size to cause airway compression or irritation. Cough, hemoptysis, and dyspnea usually reflect large-volume pulmonary parenchymal involvement or pleural-based disease with resultant malignant effusion. Skeletal involvement is heralded by bone pain and/or swelling of an affected extremity. Epidural cord compression can be seen from extension of vertebral bony disease, and usually presents with back pain or neurologic deficit. Headache can be secondary to skull- or dural-based metastases or frank involvement of cortical brain. Any space-occupying lesion within the cranium can lead to signs of increased intracranial pressure.

It is noteworthy that, in a minority of patients, metastatic disease is clinically silent, and is discovered incidentally. Most commonly this subgroup of patients has small-volume pulmonary parenchymal metastases found on a preoperative chest radiograph prior to nephrectomy.

Histologic types

Clear cell carcinoma is the most common histologic type of RCC, and is seen in 75 per cent of cases. These tumors largely arise from the proximal convoluted tubule, and are associated with the von Hippel–Lindau (VHL) gene inactivation on the short arm of chromosome 3. Papillary carcinoma, also termed chromophilic, occurs in 10 per cent of patients. These tumors are not associated with inactivation of VHL gene, but arise from the same origin as clear cell carcinoma, and portend a better prognosis. Sarcomatoid RCC, associated with p53 inactivation, has a poorer prognosis stage for stage than clear cell carcinoma.

Tumor grade is an important biologic feature. Well-differentiated nuclear grade I tumors, even in the metastatic setting, may grow slowly and have an indolent natural history. Patients who survive with metastatic disease beyond 10 years invariably have grade I lesions (Zisman et al., in press).

Other less common neoplasms include Bellini (collecting duct) tumors, oncocytoma, sarcoma, lymphoma, adult Wilms' tumor, and transitional cell carcinoma. These tumors are distinctly different in terms of prognosis and management from classical RCC.

Prognostic factors

Untreated, overall 5-year survival in metastatic RCC is < 2 percent. Identification of characteristics that predict response to treatment would allow identification of subgroups that could be spared ineffective therapy.

Poor performance status

Patients with Eastern Cooperative Oncology Group (ECOG) status of 2 or greater have a significantly shorter survival compared to patients with ECOG status of 0 or 1 (Maldazys and deKernion 1986; Stenzl et al. 1989).

Poor nutritional status

Unintentional weight loss of 10 percent or more below ideal body weight is indicative of aggressive tumor biology.

Tumor stage

Stage, based on the 1997 TNM (tumor–node–metastasis) system, is the most important prognostic factor for overall survival.

Stage I   60–90 percent overall survival.

Stage II 50–60 percent overall survival.

Stage III 20–40 percent overall survival. Within stage III, microscopic renal vein involvement compared to no venous involvement was found to have a worse 5-year survival for patients with T2 disease in one study (Hermanek and Schrott 1990). Macroscopic renal vein invasion is worse than absence of invasion and portends a prognosis similar to that for inferior vena cava (IVC) involvement (Hermanek and Schrott 1990; Giuliani et al. 1990; Tongaonkar et al. 1995; Giberti et al. 1997). Despite the negative impact of vessel involvement, long-term survival rates approaching 50 percent have been reported after removal of IVC tumor thrombus in the absence of nodal involvement or distant metastases (Giuliani et al. 1990).

Lymph node involvement is an indicator of adverse prognosis. The number, size, and location of involvement are important considerations. Large-volume (> 5 cm in one dimension) disease is worse than smaller-volume disease (Hermanek and Schrott 1990). If surgically accessible, nodal involvement may be curatively resected. The most reliable method of determining extent of nodal involvement is to perform a lymph node dissection during radical nephrectomy. Evidence suggests a small survival advantage with extended lymphadenectomy, perhaps from cure of patients with localized nodal involvement (Golimbu et al. 1990).

Stage IV 0–10 percent overall survival. Patients who develop metastatic disease less than 1 year following nephrectomy for localized disease have a 2-year survival approaching zero. On the opposite side of the spectrum, metastatic disease occurring longer than 2 years after nephrectomy is more indolent, with 20 percent of patients alive at 5 years. Additionally, patients with metastases confined to the lung have a better prognosis than patients with disease involving other sites (Maldazys and deKernion 1986; Stenzl et al. 1989)

High Fuhrman grade

Increasing grade of clear cell carcinoma is defined by more prominent, larger, and more irregular nucleoli. The area of poorest differentiation determines the prognosis. Many, if not all, of the patients who survive for protracted periods in the face of metastatic disease have well-differentiated, low-grade tumors (Skinner et al. 1971; Zisman et al., in press; Rini and Vogelzang 2000; Fuhrman et al. 1982).

Sarcomatoid features

Sarcomatoid growth is a pattern of spindle-shaped cells and arises in various histologic subtypes of renal carcinoma. It is associated with overexpression of mutated p53, and signifies poor prognosis (Medeiros et al. 1988; Lanigan 1995; Mani et al. 1995). Sarcomatoid features imply a high rate of intratumoral proliferation.

Tumor proliferation

Silver-stained nucleolar organizing regions mark mitotic activity. A mean score of 4.4 per nucleus has been shown in one study to be a significant independent prognostic indicator (Yasunaga *et al.* 1998). Other markers of proliferative activity, such as proliferating cell nuclear antigen (PCNA) (Hofmockel *et al.* 1995; Tanoika *et al.* 1993; Cronin *et al.* 1994; Delahunt *et al.* 1993) and Ki-67 (Gerdes *et al.* 1983), have been found in isolated studies to be prognostically valuable, but the results have also been criticized because of intratumoral variability and high degree of subjectivity in interpretation (Tannapfel *et al.* 1996).

Tumor size

It is generally accepted that, the larger the tumor, the greater the metastatic potential. In a retrospective analysis of 326 patients treated at New York University Medical Center, tumor size < 5 cm was correlated with improved survival (Golimbu *et al.* 1986)

Tumor ploidy

Flow cytometry of the nephrectomy specimen to analyze tumor DNA ploidy may add prognostic information in early-stage disease. Preliminary studies have suggested a difference in survival rates and incidence of disease progression favoring diploid rather than aneuploid tumors. These studies have yet to be confirmed, and tumor ploidy is not routinely used as a means of risk stratification (Ljungberg *et al.* 1991; Currin *et al.* 1990).

Tumor metastases

Solitary metastases are better prognostically compared to multiple metastases. Between 1.5 and 3.5 percent of patients with solitary metastases are candidates for surgical resection of metastatic deposits. Resection of both primary tumor and solitary site of metastatic disease confers a 5-year survival rate of 34 to 59 percent (McDougal and Garnick 2000; Ljungberg *et al.* 1991).

Cytogenetics

Both sporadic and hereditary forms of RCC have partial or complete loss of chromosome 3, or a genetic mutation on the short arm of chromosome 3, resulting in loss of one or more tumor suppressor genes such as the VHL gene at 3p25–26 (Currin *et al.* 1990; Pathak *et al.* 1982; Zbar *et al.* 1987). Other tumor suppressor genes in sporadic cases may be located at 3p21–22 and 3p13–14 (Storkel 2000). In clear cell carcinomas with evidence of dedifferentiation, chromosomes 7, 5q, and 10 have been overexpressed (Morita *et al.* 1991). Metastasis is associated with 1q segment amplification. *p53* expression has been associated with poor rate of survival (Uhlman *et al.* 1994).

Symptoms

Patients who present with symptoms have a poorer prognosis than patients with incidentally discovered disease. This is ex- plained by the overall volume of disease, which tends to be greater in those who are symptomatic (Tsukamoto *et al.* 1991).

Serum studies

Patients with humoral hypercalcemia of malignancy at the time of presentation with metastases have a very poor prognosis (Bukowski and Novick 1997). An analysis of 170 unselected RCC patients from Sweden looked at several serum markers as potential correlative parameters of prognosis (Ljungberg *et al.* 1995). Included among these were erythrocyte sedimentation rate (ESR), haptoglobin, ferritin, C-reactive protein, orosomucoid, and alpha-1-antitrypsin (all acute-phase reactants). Using a multivariate Cox analysis, only ESR was an independent prognostic variable.

Immunotherapy

The use of immune-based therapy, most notably interleukin 2 (IL-2) and interferon alpha (IFNa), has revolutionized the treatment of metastatic RCC. Once a disease believed to be refractory to all therapy, immunotherapy has not only defined a subset of patients who achieve durable remissions, but has also opened the door to the greater understanding of tumor immunology. Innovative approaches manipulating host immunity are in clinical development, with a clear trend toward a favorable change in the natural history of the disease.

Patterns of spread

A retrospective report from Memorial Sloan–Kettering Cancer Center examined the patterns of failure of 172 patients with unilateral, non-metastatic RCC treated with definitive surgery alone (Rabinovitch *et al.* 1994). There was a minimum follow-up duration of 1 year, and the distribution of lesions was predominantly early-stage (T1/T2 65 percent, T3/T4 35 percent). Approximately 6 percent of patients had either positive surgical margins or lymph node involvement. Local failure developed in only six patients, with a 7-year actuarial incidence of 5 percent. Four of these six patients developed distant metastases. Overall, distant spread developed in 30 patients, with a 7-year actuarial incidence of 26 percent. Significant independent predictors of distant failure included positive lymph nodes and renal vein extension. The investigators concluded that local failure is rare and is not the cause of mortality. Patients die of distant metastases, and there is no role for adjuvant radiation therapy to the tumor bed.

Spontaneous regression

The observation that (rarely) metastases may regress after nephrectomy led to the finding that manipulation of the immune system has therapeutic value in the treatment of metastatic RCC (Fairlamb 1981). Future therapies, including non-myeloablative allogeneic bone marrow transplantation, are being developed as the role of the immune system in tumor surveillance and destruction is better understood (Childs *et al.* 2000).

Disease stabilization

Defined as lack of growth of established lesions and no appearance of new lesions, stable disease can be achieved in a minority of patients treated with immunotherapy, or may occur spontaneously. Unlike many other solid tumors, RCC has an intermittent pattern of growth, and may remain dormant or quiescent for months or years. This may reflect host immunity or other poorly understood aspects of the unique biology of this tumor.

Site-specific disease therapy

Central nervous system (CNS)

Metastatic deposits in the brain occur in 4–13 per cent of patients with RCC (Gay *et al.* 1987). Patients who are treated for solitary metastasis at any site have a 25–35 per cent probability of 5-year survival. The optimum management for intracranial disease is not known. As most brain metastases are well-circumscribed, they are amenable to focal therapeutic strategies. RCC is classically considered to be radioresistant, and the concern regarding radiation-induced morbidity has tempered any enthusiasm toward utilizing high-dose-fractions or large total-dose whole-brain radiation therapy (WBRT). However, stereotactic radiosurgery can deliver a tightly focused beam of high-dose radiation to a target lesion within the brain, sparing normal tissue. This approach maintains the integrity of the cranial vault and is associated with shorter hospitalization and lower cost compared to metastasectomy. Recently, investigators at the University of California at San Francisco reviewed their experience with radiosurgery in metastatic RCC (Dave *et al.* 1998). Fourteen patients with 32 lesions were treated. Freedom from local failure was 96 per cent at 6 months and 91 per cent at 1 year. The freedom from development of new brain metastases was 92 per cent at 6 months and 67 per cent at 1 year. Three patients with new brain metastases were successfully re-treated. Two of 14 patients developed symptomatic radionecrosis treated with steroids. Median survival was 14.1 months. Only 1 patient died of uncontrolled brain metastases.

Skeletal metastases (Joyce 2000)

Skeletal metastases from RCC are usually lytic rather than blastic. Orthopedic evaluation, along with radiographic assessment with plain films to correlate symptomatic areas or abnormalities on a nuclear bone scan, should be obtained early in the disease course. Bony destruction is the result of humorally mediated osteoclast activation. The treatment of lesions involving the appendicular skeleton is rigid fixation, with intramedullary placement of fixative hardware, often accompanied by methylmethacrylate for immediate cementing. Early radiotherapy, in concert with orthopedic fixation, can prevent growth of large destructive lesions and further cortical bone loss.

Lesions involving the cervical spine must be recognized before neurologic impairment is severe or permanent. Imaging with magnetic resonance imaging (MRI), computerized tomography (CT), and plain films should be used together to best define epidural masses, bone lesions, and the structural integrity and stability of the spine. Surgical intervention via an anterior approach is the standard during attempts at decompression and stabilization. Likewise, anterior approaches are employed for thoracic spine lesions, whereas either posterior or anterior approaches are utilized for lumbar lesions.

The hypervascular nature of RCC raises the concern of excessive intraoperative blood loss. Preoperative non-absorbable embolization can significantly reduce bleeding when vessels feeding the tumor are identified and treated (Roscoe *et al.* 1989; Olerud *et al.* 1993; Miller *et al.* 1995). Caution must be taken to avoid embolization of a critical lesion near the spinal cord, as these lesions present risk of spinal cord infarction.

Lesions near the end of the bone or adjacent to the joint are difficult to repair with fixation and fracture techniques. Lesions involving the lesser trochanter, greater trochanter, and femoral neck should be replaced rather than fixed.

The presentation of an isolated bony metastasis raises the consideration of an intralesional curettage or *en bloc* resection for cure. Unfortunately, new skeletal mestastases often appear within 2 years, signifying that the original skeletal lesion was not an isolated focus of disease. While there are incidental reports of favorable long-term outcomes in the literature, there are no large series of isolated renal cell metastases to bone resected for cure.

Anecdotal reports describe spontaneous regression of metastatic lesions following palliative nephrectomy, with evidence of reversal of established bone destruction.

Reports of survivorship after skeletal metastases vary widely among published series (Maldazys and deKernion 1986; Skinner *et al.* 1971; Thompson *et al.* 1975; deKernion *et al.* 1978; Tobisu *et al.* 1989; Smith *et al.* 1992). Median 1-year survival ranges from 21.5 to 77 per cent and 5-year survival ranges from 0 to 55 per cent. Clearly, a fraction of these patients will survive for an extended period. Good prognostic indicators include initial presentation without bony metastases, long disease-free interval following nephrectomy, and solitary mestastasis.

Pulmonary metastases (Rice 2000)

The lung is the most common site of metastatic involvement in RCC, and lung metastasis can be seen in up to 75 per cent of patients (Maldazys and deKernion 1986; Pastorino 1997; Patel and Lavengood 1978). At initial diagnosis, 25 to 40 per cent will have pulmonary involvement (Patel and Lavengood 1978; Kierney *et al.* 1994). As many as 50 per cent of patients undergoing nephrectomy for presumably organ-confined disease will develop lung metastastases (Kierney *et al.* 1994), 70 per cent within the first year (deKernion *et al.* 1978). As mentioned previously, lung metastases are associated with improved survival compared to other sites of spread (Maldazys and deKernion 1986).

The first patient with metastatic RCC to benefit from pulmonary metastesectomy was described in 1939 (Barney and Churchill 1939). Despite the increased frequency of this therapeutic modality over the past two decades, the ability to identify which patients will derive significant benefit remains a challenge. Most cases of pulmonary spread are the result of hematogenous spread, with an estimated 6–8 per cent due to dissemination via lymphatics (Yang and Lin 1972). Interestingly, lymphatic drainage from an established pulmonary metastasis, rather than from abdominal lymphatics, is the primary source of lymphatic pulmonary involvement (Janower and Blennerhassett 1971).

Due to their predilection for a peripheral location, 85–90 per cent of pulmonary lesions are asymptomatic, and are often discovered incidentally by routine radiographs. However, because of lack of sensitivity of plain films, CT examination of the chest should be performed prior to scheduled nephrectomy (Ren *et al.* 1989), and postoperative screening imaging with CT scans should be routinely scheduled every 3 to 6 months for the first 2 to 3 years following resection.

Only 50 to 70 per cent of pulmonary nodules will represent metastatic deposits. Second primary lung cancers and benign nodules comprise the remainder (McCormack 1990; Nakamoto *et al.* 1995). Multiple nodules (Johnson *et al.* 1982), or nodules developing within 39 months of nephrectomy (Nakamoto *et al.* 1995), are more likely to be metastatic but, among a group of resected malignant lesions, occasionally a proportion will be benign.

Candidates for surgical resection must have a controlled primary tumor, no other sites of distant spread, resectability of all pulmonary lesions, adequate pulmonary reserve, and no medical contraindication to surgery. Survivorship following resection is determined by adequacy of resection, presence of a single metastatic focus, and disease-free interval of at least 3 years (Pastorino *et al.* 1997). Characteristics of a metastasis that is amenable to successful extirpation include a solitary lesion that is asymptomatic, less than 3 cm, metachronous, slow-growing, without lymphatic involvement, and of similar or lesser grade than the original tumor.

Preoperative assessment should include spirometry and arterial blood gas determination. Diffusing capacity of the lung for carbon monoxide DL_{CO} should be added for patients who have received chemotherapy. In patients with marginal lung function, quantitative perfusion scanning can provide an estimate of functional pulmonary parenchyma that will remain after resection.

If preoperative diagnosis is desired, tissue may be obtained via sputum cytology, bronchoscopy with bronchial washings and brushings, transbronchial biopsy, percutaneous needle biopsy, or thoracoscopy. Bronchoscopy is also valuable to evaluate for the presence of endobronchial lesions or direct involvement of bronchi (Oshikawa *et al.* 1998; Yim *et al.* 1996; Salud *et al.* 1996). Thoracoscopy should be used with diagnostic rather than therapeutic intent (McCormack *et al.* 1993, 1996; Amos *et al.* 1997).

The standard resection is a non-anatomical wedge excision. A segmentectomy or lobectomy may be required for deeper lesions. Solitary hilar metastasis requiring pneumonectomy is associated with increased operative mortality. Sampling of hilar and mediastinal nodes should always be perfomed during metastasectomy. Operative mortality ranges from 0 to 2.2 per cent, and increases with age greater than 70 years (Cerfolio *et al.* 1994; Cozzoli *et al.* 1995; Fourquier *et al.* 1997). Five-year survival postresection

ranges from 21 to 44 per cent (Fourquier *et al.* 1997; Dernnevik *et al.* 1985). Re-resection of recurrent pulmonary metastases is generally not indicated but has been successful in selected patients (Cerfolio *et al.* 1994; Fourquier *et al.* 1997)

Solitary metastatic deposits

The incidence of a solitary metastasis, either synchronous or metachronous, ranges from 1.6 (Middleton 1967) to 3.6 per cent (Skinner *et al.* 1971). Solitary metastses occur most commonly in the lung (30 per cent), followed by bone (15 per cent), lymph node (14 per cent), CNS (8 per cent), liver (5 per cent), adrenal (2.7 per cent), contralateral kidney (1.4 per cent), and skin (1.4 per cent) (Saitoh *et al.* 1982*a*, *b*; Hajdu and Thomas 1967). Surgical metastectomy has resulted in 5-year overall survival rates of 35–50 per cent. In patients with excellent performance status and long disease-free interval from nephrectomy to systemic relapse, 50 per cent overall survival at 3 years has been documented following the resection of a solitary pulmonary metastatic lesion (Maldazys and deKernion 1986).

Radiation therapy

RCC is a relatively radioresistant tumor, leaving little role for radiation therapy as a palliative modality. Indications for radiation include uncontrolled pain and/or bleeding from the primary tumor, and symptomatic involvement of CNS or bone (Halperin and Harisiadis 1983; Onufrey and Mohiuddin 1985). Additionally, focused radiation such as stereotactic radiosurgery may be employed as an alternative to surgical resection of brain metastases.

Role of nephrectomy

The role of nephrectomy in metastatic disease continues to evolve. Traditionally, the indications for nephrectomy in a patient with synchronous metastases were limited to intractable pain, refractory hypercalcemia, or significant ongoing hematuria with profound anemia or passage of clots. However, recent data has supported a benefit to cytoreductive therapy in combination with standard immune-based systemic therapy. Theoretically, a decreased tumor burden may improve the immunologic parameters needed for a meaningful response to treatment. A recent retrospective analysis of 679 patients with all stages of RCC reports that, for metastatic RCC, cytoreductive nephrectomy prior to IL-2-based immunotherapy may result in significantly improved survival compared to that in patients treated with IL-2 alone (Pantuck *et al.* 2000). Patients with metastatic RCC with primary tumors intact treated only with IL-2 immunotherapy demonstrated 1- and 2-year survival rates of 29 and 4 per cent, respectively, compared to 1- and 2-year survival rates of 67 and 44 per cent, respectively, for patients treated with nephrectomy followed by systemic IL-2. In patients treated with nephrectomy/TIL/IL-2, 38 per cent were alive at 3 years in contrast to 4 per cent treated with IL-2 without prior nephrectomy.

Recently, investigators from the Southwest Oncology Group reported results from a randomized trial of nephrectomy followed by systemic therapy with interferon alpha 2b versus immediate monotherapy with interferon in 246 patients with metastatic renal cell cancer (Flanigan *et al.* 2000) Patients in both arms received interferon at 5 MU/m^2 on Monday, Wednesday, and Friday each week until progression. Median survival was 12.5 months for patients who received nephrectomy compared to 8.1 months in patients who did not have the primary tumor resected ($p = 0.033$). The authors concluded that nephrectomy prior to systemic therapy yields a statistically significant survival benefit.

Conclusion

The natural history of metastatic RCC is varied and challenging, involving disparate organs and causing a panoply of symptoms. Metastases can be spread hematogenously, via lymphatics, or by direct extension, and can involve any site in the body. Paraneoplastic syndromes are common and are often difficult to manage effectively. The majority of patients presenting with metastatic disease die within 1 year of diagnosis because of complications arising from their metastases (Fowler 1987). To add to the complexity, there is an unpredictable tendency for some lesions to remain quiescent or, rarely, regress and this may result in extended survival. Attempts to identify important prognostic factors point to various patient characteristics such as extent of symptoms at presentation, performance status, disease-free interval, and tumor characteristics such as pathologic stage, histology, and nuclear grade (Zisman *et al.* in press; Bostwick and Murphy 1998). There continue to be advances in the systemic as well as the local management strategies for metastatic RCC. The ability to surgically resect primary tumors as well as metastatic lesions is contributing to the improvement of patients with widespread disease, and is having a positive impact on the formerly dismal natural history and biology of this disease.

References

Amos, A.M., Kim, F.H., and McRoberts, J.W. (1997). The utility of video-assisted thoracic surgery in the diagnosis of pulmonary metastases from renal carcinoma. *Urology* **49**, 123–7.

Barney, J.D. and Churchill, E.J. (1939). Adenocarcinoma of the kidney with metastasis to the lung cured by nephrectomy and lobectomy. *J. Urol.* **42**, 269–76.

Bostwick, D.G. and Murphy, G.P. (1998). Diagnosis and prognosis of renal cell carcinoma: highlights from an international consensus workshop. *Sem. Urol. Oncol.* **16**, 46–52.

Bukowski, R.M. and Novick, A.C. (1997). Clinical practice guidelines: renal cell carcinoma. *Cleveland Clin. J. Med.* **64** (SI), 1–48.

Cerfolio, R.J., Alles, M.S., Deschamps, C., Daly, R.C., Wallrichs, S.L., Trastek, V.F., and Pairolero, P.C. (1994). Pulmonary resection of metastatic renal cell carcinoma. *Ann. Thorac. Surg.* **57**, 339–44.

Childs, R., Chernoff, A., Contentin, N., *et al.* (2000). Regression of metastatic renal cell carcinoma after nonmyeloablative allogeneic peripheral-blood stem-cell transplantation. *New Engl. J. Med.* **343**, 750–8.

Chow, W.H., Devesa, S.S., Warren, J.L., *et al.* (1999). The rising incidence of renal cell cancer in the United States. *J. Am. Med. Assoc.* **281**, 1628–31.

Cotran, R.S., Kumar, V., and Robbins, S.L. (editors) (1979). The kidney. In *Robbins pathologic basis of disease*, 2nd edn, pp. 1011–81. W.B. Saunders Company, Philadelphia.

Cozzoli, A., Milano, S., Cancarini, G., Zanotelli, A., and Cosciani Cunico, S. (1995). Surgery of lung metastases in renal cell carcinoma. *Br. J. Urol.* **75**, 445–7.

Cronin, K.J., Williams, N.N., Kerin, M.J., *et al.* (1994). Proliferating cell nuclear antigen: a new prognostic indicator in renal cell carcinoma. *J. Urol.* **152**, 834–6.

Currin, S.M., Lee, S.E., and Walther, P.J. (1990). Flow cytometric assessment of deoxyribonucleic acid content in renal adenocarcinoma: does ploidy status enhance prognostic stratification over stage alone? *J. Urol.* **143**, 458–63.

Dave, G.V., Sneed, P.K., McDermott, M.W., Lamborn, K.R., Wara, W.M., and Larson, D.A. (1998). Low failure rate after radiosurgery for brain metastases from renal cell carcinoma. *Cancer Therapeut.* **1**, 27–32.

deKernion, J.B. (1986). Renal tumors. In *Campbell's urology* (ed. P.C. Walsh, R.F. Gittes, and A.D. Perlmutter), pp. 1294–342. W.B. Saunders, Philadelphia.

deKernion, J.B., Ramming, K.P., and Smith, R.B. (1978). The natural history of metastatic renal cell carcinoma: a computer analysis. *J. Urol.* **120**, 148–52.

Delahunt, B., Bethwaite, P.B., Nacey, J.N., *et al.* (1993). Proliferating cell nuclear antigen (PCNA) expression as a prognostic indicator for renal cell carcinoma: comparison with tumor grade, mitotic index, and silver-staining nucleolar organizing region numbers. *J. Pathol.* **170**, 471–7.

Dernnevik, L., Berggren, H., Larsson, S., *et al.* (1985). Surgical removal of pulmonary metastases from renal cell carcinoma. *Scand. J. Urol. Nephrol.* **19**, 133–7.

Fairlamb, D.J. (1981). Spontaneous regression of metastases of renal cancer: a report of two cases including the first recorded regression following irradiation of a dominant metastasis and review of the world literature. *Cancer* **47**, 2102–6.

Figlin, R.A. (1999). Renal cell carcinoma: management of advanced disease. *J. Urol.* **161**, 381–7.

Flanigan, R.C., Blumenstein, B.A., Salmon, S., *et al.* (2000). Cytoreductive nephrectomy in metastatic renal cancer: the results of Southwest Oncology Group trial 8949. *Proc. Am. Soc. Clin. Oncol.* **19**, 163 [abstract 685].

Fowler, J.E. (1987). Nephrectomy in metastatic renal cell carcinoma. *Urol. Clin. N. Am.* **14**, 749–56.

Fourquier, P., Regnard, J.F., Rea, S., Levi, J.F., and Levasseur, P. (1997). Lung metastases of renal cell carcinoma: results of surgical resection. *Eur. J. Cardiothorac. Surg.* **11**, 17–21.

Fuhrman, S.A., Lasky, L.C., and Limas, C. (1982). Prognostic significance of morphologic parameters in renal cell carcinoma. *Am. J. Surg. Pathol.* **6**, 655–63.

Gay, P.C., Litchy, W.J., and Cacino, T.L. (1987). Brain metastases in hypernephroma. *J. Neurooncol.* **5**, 51–6.

Gerdes, J., Schwab, U., Lemke, H., *et al.* (1983). Production of a mouse monoclonal antibody reactive with a human nuclear antigen associated with cell proliferation. *Int. J. Cancer* **31**, 13–20.

Giberti, C., Oneto, E., Martorana, G., *et al.* (1997). Radical nephrectomy for renal cell carcinoma: long-term results and prognostic factors on a series of 328 cases. *Eur. Urol.* **31**, 40–8.

Giuliani, L., Giberti, C., Martorana, G., *et al.* (1990). Radical extensive surgery for renal cell carcinoma: long-term results and prognostic factors. *J. Urol.* **143**, 468–73.

Golimbu, M., Joshi, P., Sperber, A., Tessler, A., Al-Askari, S., and Morles, P. (1986). Renal cell carcinoma: survival and prognostic factors. *Urology* **27**, 291–301.

Golimbu, M., Tessler, A., Joshi, P., *et al.* (1990). Renal cell carcinoma: survival and prognostic factors. *Urology* **27**, 291–301.

Hajdu, S.I. and Thomas, A.G. (1967). Renal cell carcinoma and autopsy. *J. Urol.* **97**, 978.

Halperin, E.C. and Harisiadis, L. (1983). The role of radiation therapy in the management of metastatic RCC. *Cancer* **51**, 614–17.

Hanash, K.A., Utz, D.C., Ludwig, J., Wakim, K.G., Ellefson, R.D., and Kelalis, P.P. (1971). Syndrome of reversible hepatic dysfunction associated with hypernephroma: an experimental study. *Invest. Urol.* **8**, 399–404.

Hermanek, P. and Schrott, K.M. (1990). Evaluation of the new tumor, nodes, and metastases classification of renal cell carcinoma. *J. Urol.* **144**, 238–42.

Hofmockel, G., Tsatalpas, P., Muller, H., *et al.* (1995). Significance of conventional and new prognostic factors for locally confined renal cell carcinoma. *Cancer* **76**, 296–306.

Janower, M.L. and Blennerhassett, J.B. (1971). Lymphatic spread of metastatic cancer to the lung. *Radiology* **101**, 267–73.

Jemal, A., Thomas, A., Murray, T., Thun, M. (2002). Cancer Statistics, 2002. *CA Cancer J. Clin.* **52**, 23–47.

Johnson, H. Jr, Fantone, J., and Flye, M.W. (1982). Histological evaluation of the nodules resected in the treatment of pulmonary metastatic disease. *J. Surg. Oncol.* **21**, 1–4.

Joyce, M.J. (2000). Management of skeletal metastases in renal cell carcinoma patients. In *Current clinical oncology: renal cell carcinoma: molecular biology, immunology, and clinical management* (ed. R.M. Bukowski and A.C. Novick), pp. 239–67. Humana, Totowa, New Jersey.

Kierney, P.C., van Heerden, J.A., Segura, J.W., Segura, J.W., and Weaver, A.L. (1994). Surgeon's role in the management of solitary renal cell carcinoma metastases occurring subsequent to initial curative nephrectomy: an institutional review. *Ann. Surg. Oncol.* **1**, 345–52.

Lanigan, D. (1995). Prognostic factors in renal cell carcinoma. *Br. J. Urol.* **75**, 565–71.

Linehan, W.M., Shipley, W., and Parkinson, D. (1993). Cancer of the kidney and ureter. In *Cancer: principles and practice of oncology* (ed. V.T. DeVita Jr, S. Hellman, and S.A. Rosenberg), pp. 1023–51. J.B. Lippincott, Philadelphia.

Ljungberg, B., Larsson, P., Stenling, R., and Roos, G. (1991). Flow cytometric deoxyribonucleic acid analysis in stage I renal cell carcinoma. *J. Urol.* **146**, 697–9.

Ljungberg, B., Grankvist, K., and Rasmuson, T. (1995). Serum acute phase reactants and prognosis in renal cell carcinoma. *Cancer* **76**, 1435–9.

Maldazys, J.D. and deKernion, J.B. (1986). Prognostic factors in metastatic renal cell carcinoma. *J. Urol.* **136**, 376–9.

Mani, S., Todd, M.B., Katz, K., *et al.* (1995). Prognostic factors for survival in patients with metastatic renal cancer treated with biologic response modifiers. *J. Urol.* **154**, 35–40.

McCormack, M. (1990). Surgical resection of pulmonary metastases. *Sem. Surg. Oncol.* **6**, 297–302.

McCormack, P.M., Ginsberg, K.B., Bains, M.S., *et al.* (1993). Accuracy of lung imaging in metastases with implication for the role of thoracoscopy. *Ann. Thorac. Surg.* **56**, 863–6.

McCormack, P.M., Bains, M.S., Begg, C.B., *et al.* (1996). Role of video-assisted thoracic surgery in the treatment of pulmonary metastases: results of a prospective trial. *Ann. Thorac. Surg.* **62**, 213–17.

McDougal, W.S. and Garnick, M.B. (2000). Clinical signs and symptoms of renal cell carcinoma. In *Genitourinary oncology* (ed. N.J. Vogelzang, P.T. Scardino, W.U. Shipley, and D.S. Coffey), pp. 111–15. Lippincott Williams & Wilkins, Philadelphia.

Medeiros, L.J., Gelb, A.B., and Weiss, L.M. (1988). Renal cell carcinoma: prognostic significance of morphologic parameters in 121 cases. *Cancer* **61**, 1639–51.

Middleton, R.G. (1967). Surgery for metastatic renal cell carcinoma. *J. Urol.* **97**, 973.

Miller, D., Haines, G., Juliano, P., and Ghoshs, B. (1995). Preoperative embolization of osseous metastases from hypervascular cancers. *J. Surg. Oncol.* **60**, 133–4.

Morita, G., Saito, S., Ishijawa, J., *et al.* (1991). Common regions of deletions on chromosomes 5q, 6q and 10q in renal cell carcinoma. *Cancer Res.* **51**, 5817–20.

Motzer, R.J., Bander, N.H., and Nanus, D.M. (1996). Renal cell carcinoma—review article. *New Engl. J. Med.* **12**, 865–75.

Nakamoto, T., Igawa, M., Mitani, S., Usui, A., Yoshioka, S., Nishiki, M., and Usui, T. (1995). Pulmonary nodules in patients with a history of radical nephrectomy for renal cell carcinoma. *Int. J. Urol.* **2**, 229–31.

Olerud, C., Jonsson, H., Lofberg, A., *et al.* (1993). Embolization of spinal metastases reduces preoperative bone loss. 21 patients operated on for renal cell carcinoma. *Acta Ortho. Scand.* **64**, 9–12.

Onufrey, V. and Mohiuddin, M. (1985). Radiation therapy in the treatment of metastatic RCC. *Int. J. Radiat. Oncol. Biol. Phys.* **11**, 2007–9.

Oshikawa, K., Ohno, S., Ishii, Y., *et al.* (1998). Evaluation of bronchoscopic findings in patients with metastatic pulmonary tumor. *Int. Med.* **37**, 349–53.

Pantuck, A.J., Zisman, A., Shvarts, O., Gitlitz, B.J., deKernion, J.B., Figlin, R.A., and Belldegrun, A.S. (2000). Natural history and the role of nephrectomy in the biology of RCC: the UCLA experience. *Proc. Am. Soc. Clin. Oncol.* **19**, 343 [abstract 1348].

Pastorino, U. (1997). Lung metastasectomy: why, when, how. *Crit. Rev. Oncol. Hematol.* **26**, 137–45.

Pastorino, U., Buyse, M., Friedel, G., *et al.* (The International Registry of Lung Metastases) (1997). Long-term results of lung metastasectomy: prognostic analyses based on 5206 cases. *J. Thorac. Cardiovasc. Surg.* **113**, 37–49.

Patel, N.P. and Lavengood, R.W. (1978). Renal cell carcinoma: natural history and results of treatment. *J. Urol.* **119**, 722–6.

Pathak, S., Strong, L.C., Ferrell, R.E., and Trinidad, A. (1982). Familial renal cell carcinoma with a 3;11 chromosome translocation limited to tumor cells. *Science* **217**, 939–41.

Rabinovitch, R.A., Zelefsky, M.J., Gaynor, J.J., and Fuks, Z. (1994). Patterns of failure following surgical resection of renal cell carcinoma: implications for adjuvant local and systemic therapy. *J. Clin. Oncol.* **12** (1), 206–12.

Ren, H., Hruban, R.H., Kuhlman, J.E., *et al.* (1989). Computed tomography of inflated fixed lungs: the beaded spectrum sign of pulmonary metastases. *J. Comput. Assist. Tomogr.* **13**, 411–16.

Rice, T.W. (2000). Management of pulmonary metastases in renal cell carcinoma patients. In *Current clinical oncology: renal cell carcinoma: molecular biology, immunology, and clinical management* (ed. R.M. Bukowski and A.C. Novick), pp. 229–38. Humana, Totowa, New Jersey.

Rini, B. and Vogelzang, N. (2000). Prognostic factors in renal carcinoma. *Sem. Oncol.* **27** (2), 213–20.

Roscoe, M., McBloom, R., St. Louis, E., *et al.* (1989). Preoperative embolization in treatment on osseous metastasis from renal cell carcinoma. *Clin. Orth. Rel. Res.* **238**, 302–7.

Saitoh, H., Hida, M., Nakamura, K., *et al.* (1982*a*). Metastatic processes and a potential indication of treatment from metastatic lesions of renal adenocarcinoma. *J. Urol.* **128**, 916.

Saitoh, H., Nakayama, M., Nakamura, K., and Satoh, T. (1982*b*). Distant metastases of renal adenocarcinoma in nephrectomized cases. *J. Urol.* **127**, 1092.

Salud, A., Porcel, J.M., Rovirosa, A., *et al.* (1996). Endobronchial metastatic disease: analysis of 32 cases. *J. Surg. Oncol.* **62**, 249–52.

Skinner, D.G., Colvin, R.D., Vermillion, C.D., *et al.* (1971). Diagnosis and management of renal cell carcinoma. A clinical and pathologic study of 309 cases. *Cancer* **28**, 1165–77.

Smith, E., Kursh, E., Makley, J., and Resnick, M. (1992). Treatment of osseous metastases secondary to renal cell carcinoma. *J. Urol.* **184**, 784–7.

Stenzl, A. and deKernion, J.B. (1989). Pathology, biology, and clinical staging of renal cell carcinoma. *Sem. Oncol.* **16** (suppl. 1), 3–11.

Storkel, S.F. (2000). Classification of renal cancer: correlation of morphology and cytogenetics. In *Genitourinary oncology* (ed. N.J. Vogelzang, P.T. Scardino, W.U. Shipley, and D.S. Coffey), pp. 136–42. Lippincott Williams & Wilkins, Philadelphia.

Tannapfel, A., Hahn, H.A., Katalinic, A., *et al.* (1996). Prognostic value of ploidy and proliferation markers in renal cell carcinoma. *Cancer* **77**, 164–71.

Tanoika, F., Hiroi, M., Yamane, T., *et al.* (1993). Proliferating cell nuclear antigen (PCNA), immunostaining and flow cytometric DNA analysis of renal cell carcinoma. *Zentralbl. Pathol.* **139**, 185–93.

Thompson, I.M., Shannon, H., Ross, J., and Montie, J. (1975). An analysis of factors affecting survival of 150 patients with renal cell carcinoma. *J. Urol.* **114**, 694–6.

Tobisu, K., Kakizoe, T., Takai, K., and Tanaka, Y. (1989). Prognosis in renal cell carcinoma: analysis of clinical course following nephrectomy. *Jpn J. Clin. Oncol.* **19**, 142–8.

Tongaonkar, H.B., Dandekar, N.P., Dalal, A.V., *et al.* (1995). Renal cell carcinoma extending to the renal vein and inferior vena cava: results of surgical treatment and prognostic factors. *J. Surg. Oncol.* **59**, 94–100.

Tsukamoto, T., Kumamoto, Y., Yamazaki, K., *et al.* (1991). Clinical analysis of incidentally found renal cell carcinomas. *Eur. Urol.* **19**, 109–13.

Uhlman, D.L., Nguyen, P.L., Manivel, J.C., *et al.* (1994). Association of immunohistochemical staining for p53 with metastatic progression and poor survival in patients with renal cell carcinoma. *J. Natl Cancer Inst.* **86**, 1470–5.

Utz, D.W., Warren, M.M., and Gregg, J.A. (1970). Reversible hepatic dysfunction associated with hypernephroma. *Mayo Clin. Proc.* **45**, 161.

Vogelzang, J.H. and Stadler, W.M. (1998). Kidney cancer. *Lancet* **352**, 1691.

Yang, S.P. and Lin, C.C. (1972). Lymphangitic carcinomatosis of the lungs: the clinical significance of its roentgenologic classification. *Chest* **62**, 179–87.

Yasunaga, Y., Shin, M., Miki, T., *et al.* (1998). Prognostic factors in renal cell carcinoma: a multivariate analysis. *J. Surg. Oncol.* **68**, 11–18.

Yim, A.P.C., Abdullah, V.J., and Chan, H.S. (1996). A case of bronchial obstruction by metastatic renal cell carcinoma. *Surg. Endosc.* **10**, 855–6.

Zbar, B., Brach, H., Talmage, C., and Linehan, M. (1987). Loss of alleles of loci on the short arm of chromosome 3 in renal cell carcinoma. *Nature* **327**, 721–4.

Zisman, A., Pantuck, A.J., Dorey, F., Shvarts, O., Figlin, R.A., Quintana, D., Gitlitz, B.J., deKernion, J.B., and Belldegrun, A.S. (2001). Improved prognostication of RCC using an integrated staging system (UISS). *J. Clin. Oncol.* **19** 1649–1657.

37. Radiation therapy: basic sciences

Jesse Aronowitz, Peter Hahn, and Gabriel Haas

Historical perspective

X-rays were incorporated into the practice of medicine soon after Wilhelm Roentgen reported his discovery in December 1895. Within a year of Roentgen's report, physicians and dentists on both sides of the Atlantic began utilizing 'skiagraphy' (diagnostic radiology) (Brecher and Brecher 1969), and literature appeared devoted to the new modality (Morton and Hammer 1896; Williams 1901). Roentgenotherapy soon followed. Within 5 years of Roentgen's discovery over 100 maladies were being treated by X-rays (Grubbe 1949, p. 111), and radiotherapy texts were published (Pusey and Caldwell 1903; Freund 1904). Dermatologists were among the first to appreciate the utility of X-rays and radiation therapy remained a pillar of dermatologic therapeutics for more than 50 years. Ionizing radiation was applied to inflammatory, infectious, as well as neoplastic conditions. Particular benefit was noted in the treatment of lupus vulgaris (cutaneous tuberculosis) and epithelioma (squamous cell carcinoma). The therapeutic use of radioactive substances lagged because of their scarcity and expense. Even so, radium therapy was practised in the first decade of the century (Abbe 1906; Wickham and Degrais 1910). By 1915, new sources of radium were developed, and the element was adopted by surgeons. By 1920, intracavitary radium had largely replaced surgery for gynecological malignancies, and the prostate was being implanted transperineally with 'radium emanation' (radon) seeds (Janeway and Barringer 1917, pp. 233–42).

Knowledge expanded empirically, but science lagged. In an era before institutional review boards, treatment was attempted for almost any malady, without comprehension of either the physical nature or the biologic impact of the modality. An understanding of radiation physics came first. Early discoveries by Lord Rayleigh and Ernest Rutherford provided insight into the physical basis of X- and gamma-rays, as well as nuclear transformations. Engineering advances increased beam penetration, so that subsurface tissues could be treated. The quantification of radiation 'dose' was a necessary step in the progress of the modality.

Initially, X- and gamma-rays were thought to be harmless; soon, their darker side emerged. Both patients and physicians suffered painful dermatitis and ulcers from overexposure. Early researchers and practitioners typically calibrated their equipment on their own anatomy; many developed chronic dermatitis, skin atrophy, or radiation-induced malignancy. In 1902, Holzknecht severely injured a patient and was the target of a successful lawsuit (*Lancet* 1906); he later developed the radiometer to quantify dose, improving the safety of radiation therapy (del Regato 1993, p. 26). His appreciation of the destructive power of X-rays came too late; like many pioneers, he lost appendages to sequelae of chronic radiation exposure. It became evident that X- and gamma-rays were double-edged swords. The challenge then, as it is today, was to maximize therapeutic benefit while minimizing toxicity. An understanding of radiation biology was needed to optimize the 'therapeutic ratio'.

Radiation physics and treatment planning

X-rays and gamma rays are electromagnetic radiations of greater energy and shorter wavelength than radiowaves, microwaves, and light. Electromagnetic radiations have a dual nature; in addition to their wave characteristics, they are particles of energy, called photons. These particles have no mass or charge. The photons of X- and gamma rays are called 'ionizing radiations' because they contain enough energy to ionize (dislodge an electron from) atoms with which they collide.

X-rays are produced by X-ray tubes and linear accelerators. In both devices, electrons are hurtled through a vacuum toward a positively charged anode target (Fig. 37.1). Upon impact, most of the electrons' kinetic energy is converted to heat; a smaller fraction is released as photons. The resultant photons have a spectrum of energies, up to the voltage that generated the electron stream.

Gamma rays differ from X-rays in that they are emitted during the nuclear transformation of radionuclides, atoms with unstable nuclei. Radionuclides may be naturally occurring (for example, radium) or man-made (for example, cobalt-60). They decay at characteristic immutable rates, releasing energy as accelerated subatomic particles (alpha or beta particles) and/or gamma rays. Unlike X-rays, gamma rays have specific energy levels characteristic of the radionuclide from which they were released. In all other ways (including interaction with matter), they are identical to X-rays.

Photons transfer energy to tissues they traverse upon collision with tissue molecules. Atoms and molecules consist of dense nuclei and tiny orbiting electrons; most of their volume is empty space. A photon, which has no charge, is far more likely to pass

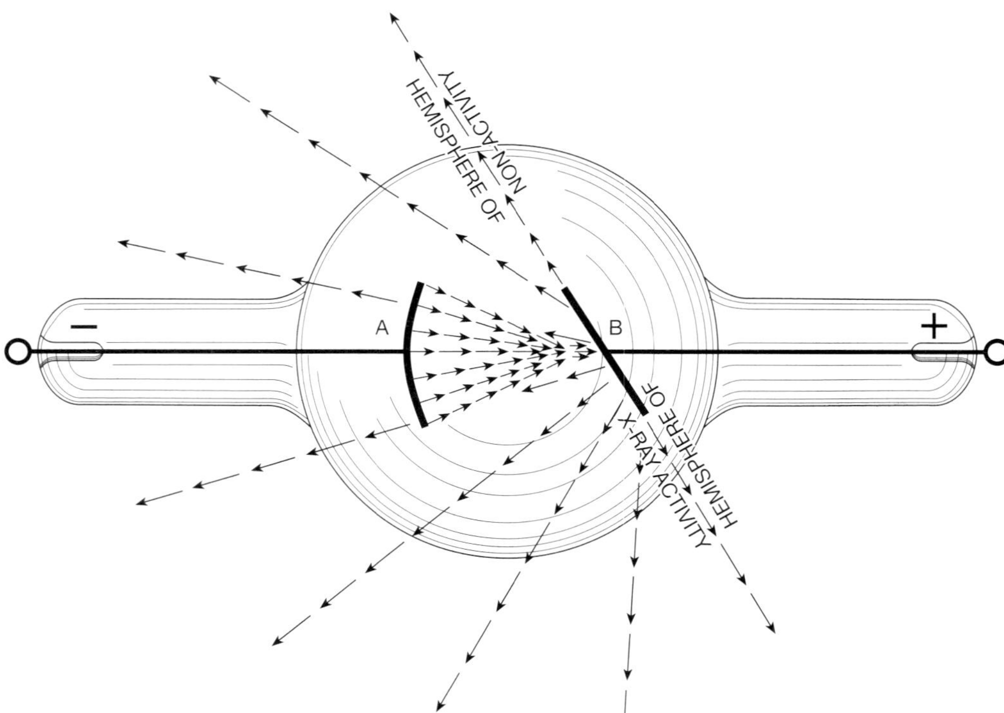

Fig. 37.1 Production of X-rays in an early X-ray tube. Electrons ('cathode rays') stream from the cathode toward the anode; upon collision their kinetic energy is converted to heat and X-rays. (From the frontispiece of Morton and Hammer (1896).)

through an atom than to collide with it. It may travel great distances through tissue without collision. The likelihood of an interaction between a photon and the matter it is traversing is defined by a constant, the linear attenuation coefficient, which is characteristic for the photon beam's energy and the material it is transiting. Weaker beams and denser materials interact more frequently, leading to greater beam attenuation per thickness of material. In other words, higher energy photons have greater penetrating power. When a photon *does* collide with a molecule, it may dislodge and accelerate an electron (ionization), to which it imparts some of its energy. As water is the most common molecule in living tissue, most photon interactions are with water. Photons of low energy are far more likely to interact with tissues of greater atomic number (such as bone). They are rarely used in therapy, as they have low penetrating power (useful only for treating surface lesions) and are inordinately absorbed by bone (which may be overdosed). Low photon energy beams, however, are the cornerstone of diagnostic radiology, where marked differences in beam attenuation are used to define tissues of different density.

The high-energy photons used in radiotherapy dislodge and accelerate electrons; the remaining (less energetic) photons, as well as the accelerated electron, interact with other atoms, accelerating still more electrons. Due to their charge, electrons travel shorter distances between interactions, and so are more densely ionizing than photons. In fact, almost the entire effect of radiation is due to the cascade of energetic electrons. They ionize water molecules, creating free radicals (Fig. 37.2). Free radicals are highly reactive, interacting with other molecules within nanoseconds. These reactions can break chemical bonds.

In summary, photons accelerate electrons in tissue. Accelerated electrons ionize water, creating free radicals, which in turn break chemical bonds. Photons are not the direct cause of biological effects, but rather the instrument by which energy is delivered deeply into tissue.

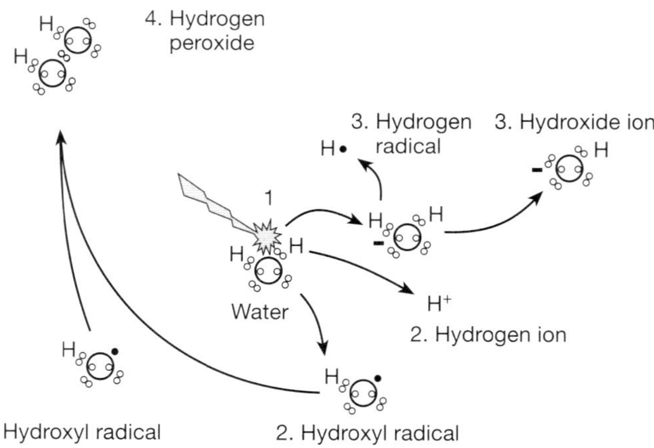

Fig. 37.2 Free radical formation. Most of the damage caused by ionizing radiation is indirect, with free radicals as the intermediary agent. Free radicals are molecular species with unpaired electrons (shown in red). They are highly reactive, causing damage by interacting with chromosomal DNA. (1) Collision of an accelerated electron with a water molecule produces (2) hydroxyl radicals and (3) hydrogen radicals. (4) Hydrogen peroxide, which is cytotoxic, is formed when two hydroxyl radicals join.

Particles are also used in radiotherapy. Linear accelerators can generate electron beams. Because of the limited penetration of charged particle beams, their energy is deposited within a short distance of the skin surface, and they are particularly useful for treating superficial tumors. A novel use of electron beams is intraoperative radiotherapy (IORT). The surgeon's dissection exposes an unresectable tumor or the soiled tumor bed. Radio-sensitive organs (for example, bowel) can be retracted, allowing the radiation oncologist to direct an electron or low-energy photon beam to the now isolated target, minimizing exposure to neighboring normal tissue.

Dosimetry is the process by which radiation is quantified and delivery is planned. The quantity of energy deposited in tissue is 'dose'. Indirect measurements of dose, such as elapsed treatment time, proved inadequate as the radiation output and quality of different apparatus varied widely. The dose necessary to cause skin erythema was a simple gauge of dose. Holzknecht introduced the first device to quantify dose, the chemoradiometer. A major advance was development of the ionization chamber, capable of measuring ionization of air by X-rays. A unit of exposure, the Roentgen (R), was established in 1928 to measure ion production, and was used for decades. Exposure of an ionization chamber submerged in a water bath (phantom) is a reflection of the dose delivered to a tumor at the same depth in a patient. Exposure, however, is not applicable to the high-energy beams generated by linear accelerators. The modern conception of dose is energy deposited per unit of matter; its unit is the rad (radiation absorbed dose), defined as 100 erg deposited per gram of material. The metric unit, the gray (Gy), is equal to 1 joule deposited in a kilogram of material. One gray = 100 rad (1 centigray = 1 rad).

As each X-ray apparatus produces a beam with a characteristic spectrum of photon wavelengths, it is important to also quantify beam quality. A simple technique was to describe the beam by measuring its ability to penetrate metal filters. The thickness of a given metal necessary to reduce a beam's exposure by 50 per cent was defined as that beam's 'half value thickness'. In modern practice, linear accelerators undergo an exhaustive commissioning process, whereby beam characteristics are measured across the beam's breadth at varying depths in a water phantom. These data are entered into the treatment planning computer for use in preparation of actual patient treatment plans. The equipment is recalibrated at intervals.

Most tumors are located at a depth below the skin surface. Photon beams must transit through normal tissue *en route* to the tumor; these tissues attenuate the beam, absorbing dose that can cause tissue injury. Avoidance of injury in traversed tissue may require limitation of the prescribed dose. The introduction of high-energy megavoltage equipment has ameliorated this difficulty. Modern treatment plans utilize multiple beams converging at the tumor; each individual beam delivers only a fraction of the prescribed dose to the tissues they traverse, but there will be summation of dose from all the beams at the point of intersection. It is the aim of the radiation oncologist to position the tumor at the intersection. Modern therapy units rotate around a point in space, called the 'isocenter' so that, no matter how the equipment is configured, beams will always pass through the isocenter. The patient is positioned on the treatment table such the tumor is located at the isocenter.

Sophisticated treatment plans require the collaboration of the radiation oncologist, medical physicist, and radiation dosimetrist, aided by high-powered computers running sophisticated dosimetry programs. An essential part of the treatment planning equipment is the simulator, a fluoroscopy unit that mimics the geometry of the therapy unit. The simulator helps localize the patient's anatomy, allowing positioning of the patient such that the tumor is at the isocenter. When this is achieved, the skin is marked so that the patient can be positioned exactly the same way on the treatment table. Treatment beams are modified by wedges and blocks to shape and contour them to best advantage, so that the prescribed dose is distributed homogeneously across the tumor volume and neighboring normal tissue is relatively spared. A major advance in treatment planning has been the development of three-dimensional conformal radiation therapy (3DCRT). A computerized tomography (CT) or magnetic resonance imaging (MRI) scanner is utilized as the simulator, taking advantage of its capacity to better delineate organs in a three-dimensional fashion. High-powered computers can then devise complex treatment plans utilizing an array of intricately shaped beams so that the volume receiving the prescribed dose conforms to the shape of the target.

Classical radiobiology

Comprehension of the interaction between ionizing radiation and biological systems has evolved more slowly than our understanding of radiation physics. Many basic questions remain unanswered.

The impact of radiation on a population of cells can be assessed by irradiating a cell culture. A known quantity of cells (either cultured tumor cells or fibroblasts) is irradiated and then incubated. Cells that retain reproductive capacity (clonogens) will form colonies within a few days. Those that are killed or rendered sterile are 'non-clonogenic' (will not form colonies). The quotient of clonogens divided by the number of irradiated cells is the surviving fraction. This assay became an important research tool in the mid-twentieth century. 'Cell survival curves' were generated to quantify clonogen survival after irradiation to varying doses (Fig. 37.3). Clearly, the number of clonogens falls with escalating doses. Careful examination of the curve, however, reveals two distinct sections joined by a bend (descriptively termed the

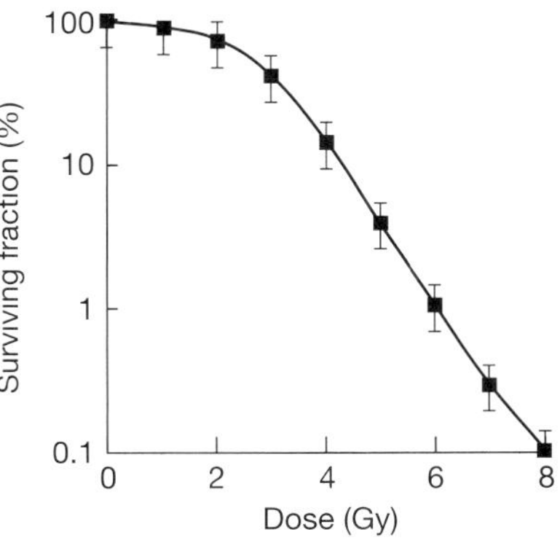

Fig. 37.3 Survival curve. When the log of the surviving fraction of irradiated cells is plotted as a function of dose, the typical shouldered survival curve results.

'shoulder'). Although increasing doses of radiation lead to greater cell kill along the entire curve, the steeper slope after the 'shoulder' suggests more efficient killing at higher doses. Prior to the shoulder, cell kill is linearly related to dose; beyond the shoulder, the relationship is exponential.

A given dose of radiation will kill fewer cells if it is split into two fractions, separated by a time interval. The reduction in lethality is related to the interval between the partial doses; the longer the interval, the greater the proportion of surviving clonogens. If the interval is long enough, the 'split dose' has effectively become two individual doses, with no impact of the first dose on the effectiveness of the second. Essentially, the 'shoulder' is recapitulated. This finding suggests that, given adequate time, cells have the capacity to repair 'sublethal' radiation-induced damage.

The quantity of energy imparted to tissue from even lethal doses of radiation is minuscule; physical destruction cannot account for the profound biological effects. It is deduced that injury is inflicted upon a vital structure. The vital structure is believed to be chromosomes, and the injury is breakage of DNA strands. Indirect evidence supporting this deduction includes the following.

- Microbeam experiments have localized the nucleus as the site where radiation induces cell death.
- Chromosomes are essential and unique molecules; in a cell with trillions of molecules, there are only a handful of chromosomes, which are unique and indispensable. The loss of a single chromosome would have a profound effect.
- Chromosomes are long and thin, and are therefore large, fragile targets.

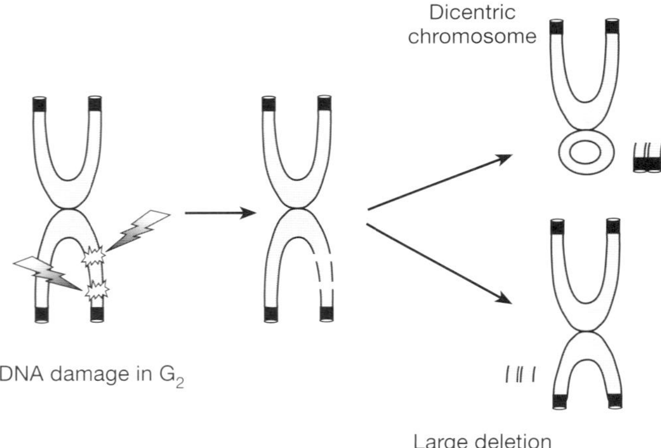

Fig. 37.4 Chromosome aberrations. Ionizing radiation can fracture cellular DNA, but most of the damage is repaired. Occasionally, DNA breaks are misrepaired, leading to chromosome aberrations. For example, two breaks in a single chromosome can lead to the formation of large interstitial deletions wherein the wrong fragments are joined together. The result is that the damaged chromosome is shorter than before, with the missing material contained in an acentric chromosome fragment that would be lost following cell division. Alternatively, the broken chromosome might be replicated, and the replicated broken end joined to the original break. When the fused sister chromatids attempt to segregate during mitosis, they form an anaphase bridge, which leads to further chromosome breakage as the two centromeres are pulled in opposite directions.

- Cell lines with defective DNA repair mechanisms are especially radiosensitive.
- Radiation-induced chromosomal aberrations can be seen in otherwise healthy cells that have become sterile or will die during mitosis.

Both normal and malignant cells have mechanisms to rapidly repair the large majority of simple DNA strand breaks. Death is due to *misrepaired* breaks. Misrepair occurs when nearby breaks are rejoined incorrectly (Fig. 37.4). Misjoining can often be identified microscopically as chromosomal aberration. For such misrepair to occur, the chromosomal breaks must be very close together, both spatially and temporally. Either a single accelerated electron can cause nearby breaks ('one-hit' phenomenon), or two electrons may cause nearby breaks simultaneously ('two-hit'). This theoretical construct is compatible with the cell survival data. The incidence of one-hit phenomena should increase linearly with dose, whereas two-hit phenomena (which require two separate events) would be exponentially related to dose. If the likelihood of a lethal one-hit event is represented by the constant α, and if the likelihood of a lethal two-hit event is represented by the constant β, then the percentage of surviving cells, S, would be reflected by the binomial equation

$$S = \exp(-\alpha D - \beta D^2)$$

where the cell kills from one hit and two hits are additive and where D is the dose. At lower doses, the one-hit cell kill predominates, but at higher doses (beyond the cell survival curve shoulder) two-hit events would kill a greater proportion of cells.

Fractionation, or the delivery of a course of radiation in multiple treatments over elapsed days or weeks, has been with us since the inception of radiation therapy. Initially, fractionation was a necessity, as early equipment delivered radiation so slowly that treatment had to be broken into daily sessions. In the first two decades of the twentieth century there was much disagreement among researchers as to whether fractionation was beneficial or detrimental to treatment outcome. By the 1920s it was recognized that fractionation allowed normal tissue to repair and regenerate between treatments, so that toxicity became a less limiting factor. Tumor cells can also repair and regenerate between fractions, so daily dose and overall treatment time must be skillfully manipulated to favor tissue recovery over tumor recovery.

Several theories have been posited as to why fractionated radiation relatively spares normal tissue. There may be subtle differences in the shape of cell survival curves favoring normal tissue. If alpha cell kill is relatively more damaging to tumor cells, then irradiation to lower dosages (before the shoulder of normal cells' survival curve) would kill more tumor cells than normal cells; at higher doses, this normal-tissue 'sparing' effect would be lost. In fact, typical treatment fractions (approximately 200 rad) correspond to the shoulder region. Although the magnitude of the survival benefit from a single fraction may be modest, following a 7-week course of therapy (five treatments a week), the benefit would be elevated to the 35th power; the cell kill differential increases exponentially. Other explanations for the benefit of fractionated therapy are that tissue has the capacity to regenerate between fractions faster than the tumor can, and that irradiated tissue can recruit stem cells from nearby unirradiated tissue. In many cases, radiation destroys both tumor and normal parenchyma, which are replaced by sterile scar.

There are other benefits of dose fractionation. Oxygen increases radiation lethality, perhaps by binding with the broken DNA strands and preventing their repair. Tumors tend to outgrow their vascular supply, and develop hypoxic sectors. Hypoxic tumor is relatively radioresistant. Fractionated radiotherapy can overcome this difficulty by progressively reducing the number of oxic clonogens, thereby making more oxygen available to portions of tumor further removed from blood supply. The ischemic portion of the tumor becomes re-oxygenated, and radiosensitivity is restored.

It has been determined that a cell's radiosensitivity is largely dependent upon its position in the cell cycle. Generally, cells in mitosis or late G_2 phase are radiosensitive, whereas those in S phase are relatively radioresistant. In a typical tumor, cells are distributed throughout the cell cycle. Those in mitosis are likely to be destroyed by the first fraction; subpopulations in more radioresistant phases of the cycle will probably survive. With multiple fractions over many weeks, however, surviving cells will progress through the cycle, eventually entering the more radiosensitive phases (reassortment).

Tumors repopulate during radiotherapy, sometimes regenerating at increased rates during the latter part of a treatment course (accelerated repopulation). This is particularly problematic when therapy is protracted over longer than 4 weeks. To overcome this difficulty, overall treatment time can be shortened by reducing the interval between fractions. Accelerated hyperfractionation is a treatment schedule whereby small fractions (to reduce normal tissue toxicity) are delivered several times daily (to shorten overall treatment time). Although demonstrated to be effective, such schedules are resource-intensive and wearing on patients.

Increasing the efficacy of therapy

Eradication of tumor without destruction of the normal tissue that harbors it is the challenge of effective radiotherapy. Maneuvers that overcome tumor radioresistance without increasing tissue toxicity are said to improve the 'therapeutic ratio'. Fractionation is used to achieve 'therapeutic gain'; other maneuvers have been sought.

Hypoxia may be overcome by delivering hyperbaric oxygen, utilizing vasoactive agents (carbogen, nicotinamide), or administering chemotherapy that is especially toxic to hypoxic cells (mitomycin). It has long been recognized that anemic patients have worse prognosis, possibly due to tumor hypoxia. There is evidence that transfusion of anemic patients improves outcome.

Agents that sensitize tumor to the effects of irradiation have been sought. Several chemotherapeutic drugs, at low doses, have been found to do so. Platinum compounds inhibit sublethal damage repair, and taxol is thought to arrest tumor cells in a radiosensitive portion of the cell cycle. In clinical practice fluorouracil, platinum compounds, and taxenes are often infused concomitantly with radiation. Improved cure rates have been demonstrated in carcinoma of the lung, esophagus, cervix, bladder, and anus. Although tissue toxicity is acutely increased, the negative effects are largely reversible.

Another approach is to utilize agents that selectively protect normal tissue from the effects of irradiation. It was discovered in the 1940s that molecules with a thiol moiety have radioprotectant effects, probably by scavenging free radicals. One such agent, amifostine, has recently become available for clinical use. The drug is dephosphorylated to WR 1065, which is radioprotective. The prodrug is converted to the active metabolite by alkaline phosphatase, which is present in normal tissue capillaries but relatively lacking in tumor. Amifostine has been demonstrated to reduce toxicity of both radiotherapy and cisplatin without compromising treatment effectiveness.

Perhaps the most basic way to enhance therapeutic ratio is to selectively irradiate tumor while avoiding normal tissue. Some normal tissue is always irradiated, however, for the following reasons.

- Malignancy arises in, and generally infiltrates, normal tissue. It spreads to neighboring organs and, distantly, through lymphatics. Radiotherapy treats these organs without amputation.
- Unless the tumor is on the skin surface, beams must pass through normal tissue to reach the target (entry dose); they will also continue past the target (exit dose).
- Standard therapy planning, based on diagnostic radiographs, is hampered by the uncertainty of imprecise tumor localization. To avoid a geographical miss of tumor with the treatment beam, the radiation oncologist irradiates a margin of normal tissue.
- An additional margin must be added to compensate for small errors of positioning, which occur randomly on a daily basis.

Much of the technological advancement of the past few decades has been directed at minimizing injury to normal tissues. High-energy (megavoltage) beams reduce entry dose. The use of multiple intersecting beams limits the volume of tissue irradiated to the full prescription dose. Advanced imaging capabilities better localize and define the target, and powerful planning computers allow precise beam shaping to conform the high-dose region more tightly around the target. Custom-fabricated immobilization cradles and wall-mounted localization lasers improve the accuracy and reproducibility of daily patient positioning. By reducing the volume of irradiated tissue, dose can be escalated without incurring prohibitive toxicity.

Radiation pathology and radiation carcinogenesis

Ionizing radiation damages the chromosomes of normal tissue as well as tumor. Functionally mature cells do not undergo mitosis and therefore survive even if radiation-induced damage is misrepaired. Injury of normal tissue is due to depletion of stem cells, which are radiosensitive. Stem cells are necessary for repletion of functionally mature cells; tissue injury becomes apparent when mature parenchymal cells, lost to senescence, are not replaced because of a depleted stem cell population. Tissues that have rapid cell turnover exhibit *acute* injury, which occurs during treatment. Gut epithelium, for example, is normally replaced every 4–5 days. If mature epithelial cells are not constantly replaced, the lumen will soon become denuded. Symptoms of malabsorption (gaseousness, diarrhea) become apparent during therapy. The stem cell compartment is repleted (either from surviving stem cells in irradiated tissue or migrating stem cells from outside the treated volume) within weeks after treatment is completed, and most (if not all) of the 'early' toxicity is reversed.

Injury to more slowly proliferating tissue may not be apparent for months or years after treatment is completed. Classic late injury occurs in small vasculature (arterioles, capillaries). Endothelial cell turn-over is slow, and depopulation of the stem cell compartment eventually leads to reactive hyperplasia, vessel constriction, and thrombosis. Resulting ischemia causes classic 'late' toxicity: atrophy and fibrosis. Unlike 'early' toxicity, 'late' effects are usually not reversible.

It is understood that acutely reacting tissues have kinetics similar to that of tumor, so that techniques that reduce acute toxicity often spare tumor also. As acute toxicity is reversible, it is generally managed (supportive measures) rather than avoided. Chronic toxicity is of greater concern, and attempts are made to prevent or minimize it.

The degree to which late toxicity occurs is quite variable. Certainly, some tissues and some patients are more radiosensitive than others. It is unclear what factors determine an individual's radiosensitivity; assays may someday direct clinical decision-making in a manner analogous to antibiotic-sensitivity testing. We do know, however, that certain parameters influence the likelihood of development of late toxicity:

- Total dose.
- Fraction size: smaller fraction sizes favor normal tissue preservation. Hyperfractionation schemes seek to profit from this effect.
- Tissue volume: a small volume of normal tissue can tolerate a higher dose than a larger volume can. Also, a small portion of an organ (for example, lung) may often be sacrificed without significant impact on the patient's well-being.
- Other treatments: chemotherapy also depletes stem cells, potentiating the effects of radiotherapy to both tumor and tissue.
- Coexisting morbidity: patients with maladies that damage vasculature (hypertension, diabetes) are at higher risk to develop late radiation toxicity.

Kidneys are particularly radiosensitive organs. A single kidney will tolerate treatment to a dose of 2000 to 3000 rad before clinically significant irreparable damage occurs; as this dose is well below that necessary to sterilize even microscopic deposits of renal carcinoma, radiotherapy cannot replace nephrectomy (or supplement partial nephrectomy).

Two organs that are typically irradiated by adjuvant therapy following nephrectomy are small bowel and liver. As noted above, irradiated small bowel develops acute toxicity within weeks of initiation of therapy. Symptoms are largely reversed within weeks of delivery of moderate doses of irradiation, although mild bowel

dysfunction may persist. Potential late complications include malabsorption, ulceration, and fibrosis. Stenosis of even a small portion of a 'serial' organ like bowel leads to dysfunction of the entire organ (obstruction). Fortunately, resection or bypass of the affected portion may reverse severe toxicity. Serious late effects rarely occur at doses below 4500 rad, but are highly likely at doses greater than 6000 rad. The usually prescribed adjuvant radiation dose is between these two extremes. Limitation of the irradiated bowel volume is essential in reducing the impact of malabsorption; communication between surgeon and radiation oncologist is therefore essential. The surgeon should leave clips at the site of gross or suspected microscopic residual disease to direct the radiation oncologist, allowing more tightly focused treatment.

The liver is irradiated during treatment of the right renal bed. Hepatocytes are 'reverting mature cells'; they do not cycle unless recruited by injury, in which case they can dedifferentiate and proliferate. Irradiated liver may show no acute radiation toxicity (because the hepatocytes are not undergoing mitosis) but, if later disturbed (by resection of a metastasis, for example), hepatocytes will attempt proliferation and necrosis may result. If more than half the liver is spared, clinically useful doses of irradiation (4500 rad) can be delivered; if larger doses are delivered or most of the liver is irradiated, hepatomegaly and ascites may ensue due to veno-occlusive disease. In a randomized trial of postnephrectomy adjuvant radiation in which large volumes of liver were treated to 5000 rad in large fractions, several patients developed radiation hepatitis (Kjaer *et al.* 1987).

Most abdominal organs are extremely radiosensitive, whereas renal carcinoma is radioresistant. Postnephrectomy irradiation should be limited to situations where there is high likelihood of local recurrence and treatment can be directed to a small target. Advanced treatment planning techniques and carefully selected dose and fractionation may limit toxicity.

Radiation-induced chromosomal breakage may repair correctly or incorrectly. Misjoining may lead to cell death or sterilization. Cells that survive misrepair contain aberrant chromosomes and, if not rendered sterile, will pass the mutation to daughter cells. Certain mutations can induce cancer by activating oncogenes or disabling tumor suppressor genes.

Radiation-induced cancers are clinically identical to spontaneous cancers. Radiation seems to increase the natural incidence of naturally occurring cancers. Risk appears linearly related to dose, perhaps without a threshold; theoretically, even a single photon may induce cancer, although the incidence of carcinogenesis following small incidental exposure is minimal. Carcinogenesis declines at high doses due to the reduction of the number of surviving stem cells. Overall, radiation probably increases the natural occurrence of cancer by less than 5 per cent (Hall 1994, p. 336). A latent period exists between radiation exposure and the onset of malignancy; for leukemia and lymphoma, latency is typically 5–10 years and, for solid tumors, it is greater than 10 years.

Radiation was used to treat many benign diseases in the first half of the twentieth century. Certainly, the potential for induction of cancer should limit the use of ionizing radiation to serious disorders. For most patients with cancer, however, the benefit of treating an existing cancer outweighs the small risk of inducing a second malignancy in the distant future.

Molecular radiation biology

Molecular biology originated with the discovery that genes are encoded by chromosomal DNA. Its central principle is that DNA makes RNA, which, in turn, makes protein. Southern, Northern, and Western blots are techniques that were developed to study DNA, RNA, and proteins, respectively. Combined with genetic techniques that transfer genes among different organisms, fundamental biological processes can be studied in molecular detail. We now have a deeper understanding of the biological effects of ionizing radiation. The effects of radiation on the cell cycle and radiation-induction of apoptosis have both received considerable attention in the past few years. Tumor cells have been found to respond differently from normal cells in this regard.

The cell cycle

The mammalian cell cycle is divided into periods of DNA replication (S phase) or division (mitosis, or M phase). The intervening periods, or gaps, occur either before (G_1) or after (G_2) DNA replication (Fig. 37.5). In the 1950s and 1960s, radiation biologists noted that irradiation of mammalian cells in G_1 delayed their entry into S phase. It was concluded that this delay allows the irradiated cell to repair damaged DNA damage prior to replication, thereby avoiding destructive mutation. The mechanism by which this protective delay is induced has recently been elucidated.

Check-point controls

The molecular explanation came from an unlikely source. Scientists working with yeast isolated mutants defective in the ability to delay the cell cycle progression in response to DNA damage. Two classes of proteins were found to play key roles: cyclins and protein kinases (which phosphorylate proteins). Cyclins complex with specific protein kinases (cyclin-dependent kinases, or CDK) to regulate the cell cycle. The phosphate moieties provided by the kinases act as on–off switches, and increasing cyclin concentrations reflect the phase of the cell cycle.

The cyclin–CDK complexes function as the controlling elements in a complex signal transduction system that determines whether the cell is ready to progress in the cycle. When cyclin levels have built up sufficiently, the CDK transfers its phosphate to the retinoblastoma protein (Rb), which, in turn, releases bound transcription factor E2F, initiating S phase. Any radiation-induced DNA damage will result in a signal being sent to the cyclin–CDK complex preventing it from allowing the cell to proceed to S phase. Other members of the cyclin family of proteins complex with different members of the CDK family of kinases to control other stages of the cell cycle in an analogous manner.

p53, the key to signal transduction

p53 is a protein central to the cell cycle signal transduction pathway (Fig. 37.6). DNA damage activates p53, which in turn induces the cyclin–CDK complex to prohibit the transition to S phase. p53 induces synthesis of many proteins in response to DNA damage, including the synthesis of p53 itself. ATM is the protein that is deficient in the radiosensitive people suffering from the genetic disease ataxia telangectasia. The protein signals (through p53) that DNA damage has occurred, halting DNA synthesis in S phase so that repair can occur.

Apoptosis: programmed cell death

Within the past 20 years it has become understood that mammalian cells can die by a necrotic cell death or a programmed, 'apoptotic' death. Normal mammalian cells possess the ability to respond to chromosomal damage by undergoing a genetically controlled series of events that result in self-digestion followed by engulfment by macrophages. This process, referred to as 'apoptosis', prevents the production of mutated cells avoiding necrosis, which would elicit an injurious inflammatory response. Ionizing radiation is a potent inducer of apoptosis.

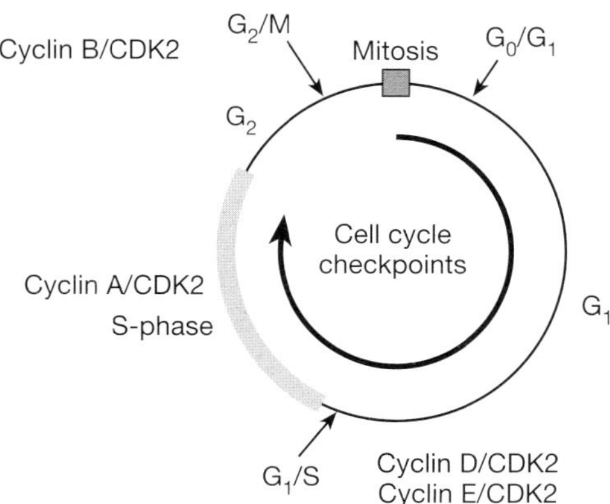

Fig. 37.5 The cell cycle is divided into three periods defined in relation to DNA replication. The period of DNA replication is referred to as S phase for DNA synthesis. During the 'gap' in DNA synthesis immediately prior to S phase the cells are said to be in the G_1 phase, whereas immediately after S phase the cells are said to be in G_2 phase. During G_2 phase, the cells contain twice as much DNA than in G_1 phase. Mitosis separates G_2 from G_1. Non-cycling cells are said to be in G_0 phase. Transition from one phase of the cell cycle to another is controlled by cyclins and cyclin-dependent kinases. For example, the G_1/S transition is controlled by the cyclin D/CDK4 heterodimer. When the cell is ready to proceed, the Rb protein is phosphorylated releasing the transcription factor E2F, which initiates DNA replication.

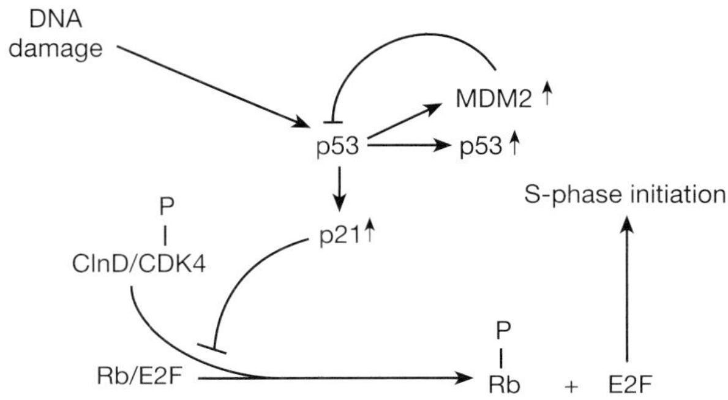

Fig. 37.6 DNA damage results in the elevation of levels of the key cell cycle regulating protein p53. Increased p53 inhibits the ability of cyclins and cyclin-dependent kinases to permit transition to the next phase of the cell cycle. This is referred to as checkpoint control.

The signal to undergo apoptosis in response to DNA damage also passes through p53. Inactivation of p53 is one of the early events of tumorigenesis. When p53 functions normally, damaged DNA triggers the synthesis of apoptotic proteins. One such protein, Bax, signals the mitochondria to execute apoptosis. The related protein Bcl-2 inhibits apoptosis by protecting mitochondria from Bax. When p53 is defective, DNA damage is ignored, and cells may survive injury that should initiate apoptosis. The surviving defective cell may undergo subsequent mutations, eventually progressing to oncogenesis.

p53-independent apoptosis

Many cells undergo apoptosis in response to stimuli that have nothing to do with DNA damage. For example, thymocytes immediately undergo apoptosis when exposed to FasL, the ligand for one of the so-called death-receptors, even in the absence of the p53 gene. These cells are responding to a signal transduction network that permits different cells to respond to the same signal by either more rapid growth, or by death, dependent upon the needs of the organism. There is increasing evidence that ionizing radiation can trigger these pathways.

Following activation of these pathways, for example, by binding of FasL to the Fas receptors, a cascade of cysteine proteases is activated. The individual proteases are referred to as 'caspases'. Following binding of FasL to the Fas receptor in thymocytes, caspase-8 is activated. It activates other caspases, and also activates sphingomyelinase. Ultimately, mitochondrial membranes are affected, resulting in the activation of caspase-9 and caspase-3. Caspase-3 activation is associated with irreversible commitment to apoptosis. Active caspase-3 inactivates the DNA repair enzymes PARP and DNA-PK, simultaneously activating a DNase to digest chromosomal DNA. Active caspase-3 also inactivates Bcl-2, permitting other mitochondria to activate caspase-3. Active caspase-3 also sets in motion the digestion of structural lamins that control the shape of the nuclear membrane.

The productive use of radiotherapy in renal cancer

Adjuvant radiotherapy for renal cell carcinoma is challenging because the tumor extension may have been incompletely resected. Irradiation should be considered only for cases in which there is a significant risk of local recurrence, such as extracapsular tumor that was dissected from nearby muscle. Treatment should be focused to the smallest possible volume. Three-dimensional or intensity-modulated techniques should be utilized. A dose fractionation scheme that respects the tolerance of surrounding tissue should be devised; it may require hyperfractionation. Radiosensitizers and radioprotectants may be part of the treatment plan. If the skills and equipment are available, intraoperative radiotherapy or brachytherapy can selectively spare normal tissue.

Close communication between surgeon and radiation oncologist is necessary to safely and effectively focus treatment to tissues at risk. It is inadequate to simply file a written request for radiotherapy in the patient's chart. Instead, the surgeon should graphically relate the specific site of concern, either intraoperatively (by the placement of marker clips) or postoperatively (by reviewing treatment planning CT scans with the radiation oncologist).

References

Abbe, R. (1906). Radium in surgery. *J. Am. Med. Assoc.* **47**, 183–5.

Brecher, R. and Brecher, E. (1969). Putting the X-rays to work. In *The X-rays*, pp. 59–69. Williams and Wilkins, Baltimore.

del Regato, J.A. (1993). *Radiation oncologists: unfolding of a medical specialty*. Radiology Centennial, Reston, Virginia.

Freund, L. (1904). *Elements of general radio-therapy for practitioners*. Rebman, New York.

Grubbe, E.H. (1949). *X-ray treatment, its origin, birth and early history*. Bruce, St. Paul, Minnesota.

Hall, E.J. (1994). *Radiobiology for the radiologist*. Lippincott, Philadelphia.

Janeway, H.H. and Barringer, B. (1917). *Radium therapy in cancer at the Memorial Hospital*. Hoebner, New York.

Kjaer, M., Frederiksen, P.L., and Engelholm, S.A. (1987). Postoperative radiotherapy in stage II and III renal carcinoma: a randomized trial of the Copenhagen Renal Cancer Study Group. *Int. J. Radiat. Oncol. Biol. Phys.* **13**, 665.

Lancet (1906). X-ray treatment resulting in action for damages. *Lancet* 13 January 1906, p. 127.

Morton, W.J. and Hammer, E.W. (1896). *The X-ray or photography of the invisible and its value in surgery*. American Technical Book, New York.

Pusey, W.A. and Caldwell, E.W. (1903). *Practical application of the Roentgen rays in therapeutics and diagnosis*. W.B. Saunders, Philadelphia.

Wickham, L. and Degrais (1910). *Radiumtherapy*. Cassell, London.

Williams, F.H. (1901). *The Roentgen rays in medicine and surgery*. MacMillan, New York.

38. The use of systemic chemotherapy in the treatment of metastatic renal cell carcinoma

Lucy A. Godley and Nicholas J. Vogelzang

Introduction

The treatment of metastatic renal cell cancer has remained a challenge for clinicians despite the many chemotherapy agents that are now available. Renal cell cancer is highly resistant to traditional cytotoxic chemotherapeutic drugs, and few are useful in the management of metastatic disease. An approach utilizing immunological agents, especially interleukin-2 and interferon alpha, along with selected chemotherapeutic agents has proven to be the most effective, with response rates averaging about 20 per cent. This chapter will review the use of chemotherapy, hormonal agents, and combination regimens that include immunotherapy to treat advanced renal cell cancer.

Chemotherapy

Chemotherapy alone has yielded disappointing responses in patients with renal cell carcinoma (RCC). In a review of 161 publications involving 4093 evaluable patients, Yagoda *et al.* (1995) summarized the results of chemotherapy trials from 1983 until 1993. Overall, only 6 per cent of patients obtained a measurable response. In another summary of the literature from 1975 until 1994, 143 responses were seen out of 3951 evaluable patients, an overall response rate of only 4 per cent (Motzer and Vogelzang 1997). These figures do not reflect a wide range of responses among agents. Rather, all classes of agents yield a similarly poor response to chemotherapy (Table 38.1). Among all of the chemotherapy agents tested, the best responses have been seen with gemcitabine, 5-fluorouracil (5-FU), and vinblastine, with response rates of 10, 11, and 16 per cent, respectively (Table 38.1). Based on this observation, many of the combination regimens tested have included one or more of these drugs (see below).

The key to understanding the extreme chemoresistance of renal carcinoma cells may lie in their overexpression of proteins that confer the ability to detoxify cells: the multidrug resistance (MDR) or p170 glycoprotein and glutathione-S-transferase (Mickisch 1994; Mickisch *et al.* 1990*a*). In normal kidney, MDR is most highly expressed by the proximal tubule cells, the cell that gives rise to RCC (Fojo *et al.* 1987*a*; Thiebaut *et al.* 1987). Not surprisingly, the *mdr1* gene, which encodes the MDR protein, is overexpressed in RCC and in cell lines derived from them (Fojo *et al.* 1987*a*, *b*; Thiebaut *et al.* 1987; Goldstein *et al.* 1989; Mickisch *et al.* 1990*b*; Yu *et al.* 1998). The MDR protein functions as a transmembrane transporter, which extrudes xenobiotic and hydrophobic compounds from the cytoplasm. Interestingly, 5-FU, the most active single chemotherapeutic agent, is not extruded from the cell by an MDR-like mechanism. Several agents have been used to try to inhibit the activity of MDR: calcium channel blockers, especially verapamil, quinidine, cyclosporine A, and tamoxifen. *In vitro* experiments using these agents to block the activity of the MDR protein are successful in restoring chemosensitivity to cell lines (Fojo *et al.* 1987*b*; Tsuruo *et al.* 1982, 1984; Ramu *et al.* 1984; Slater *et al.* 1986; Twentyman *et al.* 1987; Fine *et al.* 1991; Kirk *et al.* 1993; Foster *et al.* 1988; Zamora *et al.* 1988; Kanamaru *et al.* 1989). Some of these agents have been tested in patients with metastatic RCC. Unfortunately, they have proven disappointing. In 33 patients assigned to receive vinblastine followed by vinblastine with high-dose cyclosporine A, no responses were observed (Samuels *et al.* 1997). Furthermore, in 35 patients who received vinblastine followed by vinblastine combined with tamoxifen, only one complete response was seen, a response rate of only 3 per cent (Samuels *et al.* 1997). The activity of glutathione-S-transferase (GST) within cells further contributes to chemoresistance by providing a source of reducing potential with which to detoxify drugs. There is a linear relationship between the degree of chemoresistance of renal carcinoma cell lines and the amount of GST activity, which is independent of cellular MDR levels (Mickisch *et al.* 1990*b*).

One of the most exciting new areas of drug research involves the use of novel cytostatic agents, including angiogenesis inhibitors (Folkman 1996). Multiple studies of patients with RCC have shown higher expression levels of angiogenic factors, such as basic fibroblast growth factor (bFGF), hepatocyte growth factor/scatter factor, vascular endothelial growth factor (VEGF), and angiogenin (AG) (Dosquet *et al.* 1997; Nakagawa *et al.* 1997; Nicol *et al.* 1997; Takahashi *et al.* 1999; Thelen *et al.* 1999; Tomisawa *et al.* 1999; Wechsel *et al.* 1999). Furthermore, VEGF may be particularly important for the development of the highly vascular renal tumors that develop in von Hippel–Lindau (VHL) disease, since renal cancer cells that lack expression of VHL show deregulated expression of VEGF (Siemeister *et al.* 1996). Studies to test the clinical efficacy of anti-angiogenesis drugs are ongoing, although the first such analysis yielded no objective responses, merely long-term stabilization of disease (Stadler *et al.* 1999).

Table 38.1 Response rates of RCC to single-agent chemotherapy

Agent	Reference	N	CR	PR	Overall response (%)
			Number of patients		
Acivicin	Elson *et al.* 1988	27	0	1	4
Aclacinomycin	Decker *et al.* 1984	15	0	0	0
L-Alanosine	Elson *et al.* 1988	36	1	0	3
Altretamine	McLean *et al.* 1994	30	0	0	0
6-Aminonicatinamide	Cowan and Alison 1970	19	1	0	5
Ametantrone	Hansen *et al.* 1985	25	0	2	8
Aminothiazide	Elson *et al.* 1988	46	0	1	2
Amonafide	Higano *et al.* 1991	24	0	0	0
	Witte *et al.* 1996	17	0	0	0
Ampligen	Strayer *et al.* 1992	31	1	1	7
Amsacrine	Schneider *et al.* 1980	21	0	0	0
	Van Echo *et al.* 1980	16	0	0	0
	Amrein *et al.* 1983	42	0	1	2
	Earhart *et al.* 1983	61	0	1	2
5'-Aza-2-deoxycytidine	Abele *et al.* 1987	12	0	0	0
Bisantrene	Myers *et al.* 1982	37	0	2	3
	Scher *et al.* 1982	26	0	0	0
	Evans *et al.* 1985	20	0	0	0
	Spicer *et al.* 1985	14	0	0	0
	Elson *et al.* 1987	29	1	2	10
Bleomycin	Johnson *et al.* 1975	15	0	0	0
	Haas *et al.* 1976	8	0	3	37
	Hahn *et al.* 1977	7	0	0	0
Caracemide	Witte *et al.* 1996	17	0	0	0
Carboplatin	Tait *et al.* 1988	19	0	0	0
	Trump and Elson 1990	18	0	0	0
Chlorozotocin	Gralla and Yagoda 1979	21	0	0	0
CI-980 (NSC 613862)	Stadler *et al.* 1998*b*	12	0	0	0
Cisplatin	Rodriguez and Johnson 1978	23	0	0	0
	Merrin 1979	10	0	0	0
Cyclophosphamide	Kiruluta *et al.* 1975	10	0	0	0
	Hahn *et al.* 1979	44	0	2	4
	Wajsman *et al.* 1980	12	0	0	0
+ misonidazole	Glover *et al.* 1986	30	0	1	3
Cystemustine	Chauvergne *et al.* 1995	54	1	0	2
Dactinomycin	Hahn *et al.* 1981	61	0	1	2
10-Deazaaminopterin	Scher *et al.* 1984	12	0	0	0
2-Deoxycoformycin (Pentostatin)	Venner *et al.* 1991	18	0	0	0
	Witte *et al.* 1992*a*	25	0	0	0
4'-Deoxydoxorubicin (Esorubicin)	Braich *et al.* 1986	12	0	0	0
	van Oosterom *et al.* 1986	27	0	0	0
	Carlson *et al.* 1987	24	0	0	0
	Hurteloup *et al.* 1989	19	1	1	10
	Kish *et al.* 1990	15	0	1	7
4-Demethoxydaunorubicin	Scher *et al.* 1985	19	0	0	0
Dexniguldipine	Herrmann *et al.* 1994	29	0	4	14
Dianhydrogalactitol	Hahn *et al.* 1979	53	0	0	0
	Ratanatharathorn *et al.* 1982	41	0	1	2
Diaziquone	Nichols *et al.* 1982	20	0	0	0
	Hansen *et al.* 1984	29	0	0	0
	Decker *et al.* 1986	15	0	0	0
	Stephens *et al.* 1986	55	0	1	2
Dibromodulcitol (Mitolactol)	Mischler *et al.* 1981	13	0	1	8
	Brubaker *et al.* 1986*a*	31	1	2	10
Didemnin B	Motzer *et al.* 1990	21	0	1	5
	Taylor *et al.* 1992	22	0	0	0
Docetaxel	Bruntsch *et al.* 1994	32	0	1	3
	Mertens *et al.* 1994	18	0	0	0
Doxorubicin	O'Bryan *et al.* 1977	38	0	2	5
Liposomal	Murray Law *et al.* 1994*a*	14	0	0	0

Table 38.1 Response rates of RCC to single-agent chemotherapy—*cont'd*

Agent	Reference	N	CR	PR	Overall response (%)
			Number of patients		
Echinomycin	Marshall *et al.* 1993	47	0	1	2
	Chang *et al.* 1994	17	0	0	0
Edatrexate	Dreicer *et al.* 1997	37	0	2	5.4
Elliptinium	Caille *et al.* 1985	38	2	3	13
	Sternberg *et al.* 1985	8	0	0	0
	Piot *et al.* 1988	14	0	0	0
4'-Epi-adriamycin (Epirubicin)	Fossa *et al.* 1982	20	0	0	0
	Benedetto *et al.* 1983	19	0	0	0
Estramustine	Swanson and Johnson 1981	16	0	0	0
Etoposide	Hahn *et al.* 1979	43	1	0	2
Flavopiridol	Senderowicz *et al.* 1998	NA	0	1	NA
Floxurine	Damascelli *et al.* 1990	42	3	3	14
	Hrushesky *et al.* 1990	56	4	7	20
	Dexeus *et al.* 1991	40	0	4	10
	Merrouche *et al.* 1991	14	0	0	0
	Richards *et al.* 1991	29	0	0	0
	Budd *et al.* 1992	26	0	2	8
	Conroy *et al.* 1993	28	0	4	14
	Poorter *et al.* 1993	15	0	1	7
	Wilkinson *et al.* 1993	29	1	5	21
	Baiocchi *et al.* 1996	15	0	2	13
	Aveta *et al.* 1997	50	1	5	11
+ folinic acid	Raminski *et al.* 1992	15	0	0	0
Fludarabine	Balducci *et al.* 1987	30	0	0	0
	Shevrin *et al.* 1989	15	0	0	0
5-Fluorouracil	Schulof *et al.* 1991	27	0	2	7
	Ahlgren *et al.* 1993	35	0	4	11
	Kish *et al.* 1994	61	1	2	5
+ folinic acid	Zaniboni *et al.* 1989	14	0	0	0
Fosquidone	Kaye *et al.* 1992	21	0	0	0
Fotemustine	Chevallier *et al.* 1991	62	1	3	7
	Lasset *et al.* 1993	16	0	0	0
Ftorafur	Esteban *et al.* 1993	14	0	0	0
Gallium nitrate	Schwartz and Yagoda 1984	10	0	0	0
	Vugrin *et al.* 1987	25	0	1	4
Gemcitabine	Mertens *et al.* 1993	18	0	1	6
	De Mulder *et al.* 1996	37	1	2	8
	Rohde *et al.* 1996	37	1	2	8
Homoharringtonine	Witte *et al.* 1996	14	0	0	0
Hydroxyurea	Stolbach *et al.* 1981	19	0	1	5
ICRF-187	Brubaker *et al.* 1986b	40	0	0	0
Ifosfamide	Fossa and Talle 1980	11	0	1	9
	Heim *et al.* 1981	10	0	2	20
	DeForges *et al.* 1987	16	0	0	0
	Bodrogi *et al.* 1988	9	0	0	0
Irinotecan	Escudier *et al.* 1997	17	0	2	11
Iscador	Kjaer 1989	14	0	0	0
Lomustine	Hahn *et al.* 1977	9	0	0	0
	Presant *et al.* 1986	5	0	0	0
Lonidamine	Weinerman *et al.* 1986	25	0	2	8
	Stahl *et al.* 1991	19	1	1	10
Mafosfamide	Schomburg *et al.* 1992	16	1	0	6
Melphalan	Falkson 1993	8	0	0	0
Menogaril	Stephens *et al.* 1990	56	0	3	5
	Long *et al.* 1991	15	0	0	0
Merbarone	Flanigan *et al.* 1994	36	0	1	3
Methodichlorophen	Hindmarsh *et al.* 1979	10	0	3	30
Methotrexate	Baumgartner *et al.* 1980	8	0	2	25
Mitoguazone (methyl-GAG)	Fuks *et al.* 1981	14	0	0	0
	Todd *et al.* 1981	25	1	3	16

Table 38.1 Response rates of RCC to single-agent chemotherapy—*cont'd*

Agent	Reference	N	CR	PR	Overall response (%)
	Zeffren *et al.* 1981	31	0	0	0
	Child *et al.* 1982	30	0	3	10
	Knight *et al.* 1983	87	1	3	4
Mitomycin	Stewart *et al.* 1987	12	0	3	25
Mitotane	Hogan *et al.* 1981	12	0	0	0
Mitoxantrone	De Jager *et al.* 1984	20	0	0	0
	Taylor *et al.* 1984	49	0	0	0
	van Oosterom *et al.* 1984	29	0	0	0
	Gams *et al.* 1986	48	0	0	0
Mitozolomide	van Oosterom *et al.* 1989*a*	17	0	0	0
N-methylformamide	Sternberg *et al.* 1986	16	0	0	0
	Abrams *et al.* 1989	14	0	0	0
Navelbine	Canobbio *et al.* 1991	14	0	0	0
	Wilding *et al.* 1993	24	1	0	4
Paclitaxel	Einzig *et al.* 1991	18	0	0	0
PALA (sparfosic acid)	Natale *et al.* 1982	15	0	0	0
	Earhart *et al.* 1983	52	0	2	4
PCNU	Harvey *et al.* 1984	34	0	1	3
	Elson *et al.* 1987	45	0	0	0
Pirarubicin	DeVassal *et al.* 1987	16	0	1	6
	Roche *et al.* 1993	34	0	1	3
Piperazinedione	Pasmantier *et al.* 1977	23	0	0	0
Piroxantrone	Allen *et al.* 1992	32	0	0	0
	Shevrin *et al.* 1993	31	0	1	3
Pyrazine diazohydroxide	Vogelzang *et al.* 1998	15	0	0	0
Razoxane	O'Byrne *et al.* 1997	31	0	0	0
13-*cis*-retinoic acid	Berg *et al.* 1997	25	0	0	0
Spirogermanium	Schulman *et al.* 1984	36	0	0	0
	Saiers *et al.* 1987	26	0	0	0
Streptozocin	Licht and Garnick 1987	18	0	1	6
Sulofenur	Weinerman *et al.* 1992	18	0	0	0
	Mahjoubi *et al.* 1993	16	1	0	6
Suramin	La Rocca *et al.* 1991	10	0	0	0
	Motzer *et al.* 1992	26	0	1	4
Tauromustine	van Oosterom *et al.* 1989*b*	33	0	0	0
Teniposide	Hire *et al.* 1979	12	0	0	0
	Pfiefle *et al.* 1984	32	0	3	9
	Oishi *et al.* 1987	51	0	1	2
6-Thioguanine	Shevrin *et al.* 1994	39	0	3	8
Thiotepa	Hahn *et al.* 1977	7	0	1	14
TNP-470	Stadler *et al.* 1999	33	0	1	3
Topotecan	Murray Law *et al.* 1994*b*	14	0	0	0
Triazinate	Hahn *et al.* 1981	59	1	2	5
1,2,4-Triglycidyl-urazol	Bruntsch *et al.* 1986	14	0	0	0
	Wagner *et al.* 1987	16	0	0	0
Trimetrexate	Sternberg *et al.* 1989	14	0	0	0
	Witte *et al.* 1992*b*	34	0	1	3
Vinblastine	Hahn *et al.* 1977	10	0	0	0
	Kuebler *et al.* 1984	19	0	3	16
	Zeffren *et al.* 1984	10	0	0	0
	Tannock and Evans 1985	14	0	0	0
	Crivellari *et al.* 1987	21	1	1	9
	Elson *et al.* 1988	35	0	3	9
	Pyrhonen *et al.* 1999	79	1	1	2
	Fossa *et al.* 1992*a*	26	1	0	4
Vindesine	Wong *et al.* 1977	17	0	0	0
	Fossa *et al.* 1983	24	0	0	0
Yoshi-864	Altman *et al.* 1982	30	0	2	6

N, number of evaluable patients; CR, complete response; PR, partial response; NA, not applicable.

Hormonal therapy

Early studies demonstrated the presence of progesterone receptors in human RCC as well as hormone-dependence of renal tumors in Syrian hamsters (Kirkman and Bacon 1952; Bloom 1964), prompting studies of hormonal agents in human RCC (Table 38.2). For many years, medroxyprogesterone acetate (MPA) was the main hormone used, although, in review, the literature does not strongly support its use (Kjaer 1988). Response rates with the anti-estrogens tamoxifen and toremifene, as high as 13 and 17 per cent, respectively (Table 38.2), have prompted further studies combining hormonal agents with chemotherapy and immunologic agents (see below). In general however, regimens utilizing multiple hormonal therapies have not been successful (Papac and Keohane 1993) and are not currently in clinical use.

Immunotherapy

Since chemo- and hormonal therapy for RCC yield response rates of less than 10 per cent in most cases, many groups have tested the use of agents that stimulate a patient's immune system to eradicate cancer. Both interleukins and interferons have proven useful in the treatment of RCC. Interleukin 2 (IL-2) is a secreted protein produced by activated helper T cells and is known to stimulate the secretion of other lymphokines as well as the activity of antigen-specific T cells and nonspecific cytotoxic lymphocytes (lymphokine-activated killer cells; LAK cells) (Morgan *et al.* 1976; Strotter *et al.* 1980; Wagner *et al.* 1980; Gillis and Smith 1977; Yamamoto *et al.* 1982; Howard *et al.* 1983; Grimm *et al.* 1982). Animal models have established the ability of high-dose IL-2 to cause regression of murine pulmonary and hepatic metastases (Rosenberg *et al.* 1985; Sondel *et al.* 1986; Lafreniere and Rosenberg 1985). The precise mechanism of action of interferon alpha (IFNα) is unclear, but may involve its role in upregulating the expression of class I major histocompatibility complex (MHC) molecules and thereby increasing the presentation of tumor antigens. Overall, treatment of patients with metastatic RCC with IL-2 and/or IFNα yields response rates between 10 and 20 per cent (see the accompanying chapters, 'Immunologic therapy' and 'Immunotherapy').

Other interleukins have been studied in the context of advanced renal cell cancer, especially IL-4, since IL-4 also mediates regres-

Table 38.2 Response rates of RCC to single-agent hormonal therapy

Agent	Reference	N	Number of patients		Overall response (%)
			CR	PR	
Androgens	Talley *et al.* 1969	11	0	0	0
	Wagle and Murphy 1971	27	0	2	7
	Alberto and Senn 1974	23	0	0	0
	Morales *et al.* 1975	20	0	0	0
Flutamide	Ahmed *et al.* 1984	25	0	1	4
Nafoxidine	Feun *et al.* 1979	20	0	1	5
	Stolbach *et al.* 1981	19	2	1	16
Progestins	Talley *et al.* 1969	8	0	2	13
	Paine *et al.* 1970	15	0	2	13
	Bloom 1971	60	0	9	15
	Wagle and Murphy 1971	35	0	6	17
	Werf-Messing and Gilse 1971	21	0	2	10
	Talley 1973	61	5	2	11
	Alberto and Senn 1974	17	0	0	0
	Tirelli *et al.* 1980	23	1	2	13
	Pearson *et al.* 1981	9	0	0	0
	Nakano *et al.* 1984	13	0	0	0
	Gottesman *et al.* 1985	18	0	0	0
	Samuels *et al.* 1968	21	1	2	14
Tamoxifen	Glick *et al.* 1980	15	0	0	0
	Ferrazzi *et al.* 1980	12	0	0	0
	Al-Sarraf *et al.* 1981	79	2	3	6
	Weiselberg *et al.* 1981	10	0	0	0
	Lanteri *et al.* 1982	15	0	2	13
	Stahl *et al.* 1991	25	2	1	12
	Stahl *et al.* 1992	34	1	3	12
	Papac and Keohane 1993	20	1	0	5
	Schomburg *et al.* 1993	59	0	1	2
	Henriksson *et al.* 1998	63	2	ND	3
Toremifene	Gershanovich *et al.* 1993	25	0	3	12
	Gershanovich *et al.* 1997	35	1	5	17

N, number of evaluable patients; CR, complete response; PR, partial response; ND, not done.

sion of pulmonary metastases in mouse models (Hillman *et al.* 1995). *In vitro*, IL-4 has been shown to inhibit the proliferation of renal carcinoma cell lines (Cheon *et al.* 1996). However, when tested in patients with metastatic renal cell cancer, IL-4 has not proven to have clinical efficacy in the dosages tested (Margolin *et al.* 1994; Stadler *et al.* 1995).

Attempts at stimulating the immune system with granulocyte–macrophage colony-stimulating factor (GM-CSF) have yielded meek responses. In one study of 26 patients, 3 μg/kg GM-CSF was administered subcutaneously for 14 days out of a 28 day cycle, for at least three cycles. Two patients had a partial response, a response rate of 8 per cent (Wos *et al.* 1996). In another phase II trial, 24 patients received 10 μg/kg subcutaneous GM-CSF per day for 14 days out of a 28 day cycle, and half of them received pentoxifylline, an inhibitor of tumor necrosis factor release. One patient had stable disease (4 per cent response) and two other patients had slowing of their disease progression (Rini *et al.* 1998).

A full discussion of the use of immune therapy in metastatic RCC is given in the accompanying chapters, 'Immunologic therapy' and 'Immunotherapy'.

Combination chemo/hormonal/ immunotherapy

The best response rates have been reported in phase II trials of combinations using all of the previously described modalitites (Table 38.3) and recently reviewed (Motzer and Russo 2000). Some combinations, like IFNα/ floxurine, have a wide range of response rates among studies—a low of 0 per cent (Stadler *et al.* 1992; Sori *et al.* 1999) to a high of 33 per cent (Falcone *et al.* 1993)—whereas other combinations are more universally successful.

Most studies involving the use of IFNα and vinblastine have shown response rates greater than 15 per cent (Table 38.3). However, of the published studies, again there is a wide range of response rates observed, from 0 (Merimsky *et al.* 1991) to 44 per cent (Ceto *et al.* 1986). The reason for such disparity among studies is not clear, but may involve patient selection, study size, and the specifics of each dosing regimen. Recently, Pyrhonen *et al.* (1999) compared single-agent vinblastine to vinblastine/IFNα and showed a nearly complete lack of effect of vinblastine versus a significant survival advantage for the IFNα arm. Out of 79 evaluable patients receiving vinblastine alone, one complete response and one partial response were seen (2 per cent response rate) versus seven complete responses and six partial responses observed in 77 evaluable patients (17 per cent response rate) receiving both vinblastine and IFNα (see Pyrhonen *et al.* (1999) and Tables 38.1 and 38.3). This study strongly suggests that IFNα has a life-prolonging capacity, whereas vinblastine has no role in metastatic RCC. Combinations of IL-2/ IFNα/ vinblastine, Tegafur/ tamoxifen, and Tegafur/ tamoxifen/ doxorubicin/ methotrexate have all yielded response rates of greater than 35 per cent, but have so far been published only from single-institution

phase II studies and therefore have not been validated in multi-center trials.

The combination that demonstrates the most consistent response rates in multiple analyses is IL-2/IFNα/5-FU (Table 38.3). Three studies involving 19–35 patients each have yielded response rates from 38 to 49 per cent (Atzpodien *et al.* 1993; Sella *et al.* 1994a; Hofmockel *et al.* 1996). In these regimens, subcutaneous injections of IL-2 and IFNα are given along with intravenous 5-FU. The IFNα is given for 8 consecutive weeks, while the IL-2 and 5-FU are given for 4 out of 8 weeks. So far, these regimens have yielded encouraging responses on an outpatient basis with minimal toxicity, but will require phase III trials for validation.

One of the newest modalities to be applied to metastatic renal cell cancer is the use of non-myeloablative allogeneic peripheral stem cell transplant. In this case, the donor's transplanted immune system provides *in vivo* immunotherapy aimed at exploiting the graft versus tumor effect demonstrated for leukemia, lymphoma, and multiple myeloma. Thus far, non-myeloablative chemotherapy has been used along with the re-infusion of allogeneic peripheral blood stem cells to create full donor lymphoid chimerism. These so-called 'minitransplants' have the advantage of minimal morbidity and mortality and are much better tolerated than complete allogeneic bone marrow transplantation in which myeloablative dosages of chemotherapy are employed. This technique was recently successful in the treatment of one patient who had complete resolution of pulmonary metastases and has remained without detectable disease for more than 1 year after transplant (Childs *et al.* 1999). Obviously, the usefulness of this approach will depend on the outcome of other patients, but it provides an exciting option for the future.

Conclusions

Advanced RCC remains a challenge for clinicians with promising combination regimens currently under development. Single-agent chemotherapy has proven ineffective in controlling metastatic disease with response rates less than 20 per cent. Such findings have prompted studies of aggressive combination treatments utilizing hormonal and immunological approaches. The most successful of these involves the use of IL-2/ IFNα/ 5-FU, and promising results have been obtained in single-institution studies of gemcitabine plus 5-FU (Rini *et al.*, unpublished data), IFNα/ 13-*cis*-retinoic acid (with or without IL-2) (Stadler *et al.* 1998a), and Tegafur/tamoxifen (Wada *et al.* 1995). Although some of these combination regimens have shown response rates of greater than 35 per cent, no randomized phase III trials have documented a survival or response rate advantage. The future will bring further analysis of such combinations as well as more novel approaches such as the use of cytostatic chemotherapies as well as non-myeloablative peripheral stem cell transplantation, which exploits a graft versus tumor effect. Although clinically difficult to manage currently, metastatic RCC presents an exciting field of investigation with encouraging results from aggressive immunotherapy/ chemotherapy regimens.

Table 38.3 Response rates of RCC to combination chemo-/hormonal/immunotherapy regimens

Agent	Reference	N	Number of patients		Overall response (%)
			CR	PR	
Gemcitabine/5-FU	Rini et al., unpublished data	39	0	7	17
IFNα/floxurine	Dimopoulous et al. 1991	13	0	4	31
	Stadler et al. 1992	20	0	0	0
	Falcone et al. 1993	15	1	4	33
	Soori et al. 1999	14	0	0	0
IFNα/5-FU	Murphy et al. 1992	14	0	0	0
	Schuth et al. 1993	21	0	5	24
	Haarstad et al. 1994	31	1	6	23
	Gebrosky et al. 1997	21	4	5	43
IFNα/5-FU/mitomycin C	Sella et al. 1992	20	0	7	35
IFNα/13-*cis*-retinoic acid	Motzer et al. 1995	43	3	10	30
IFNα/IL-2/13-*cis*-retinoic acid	Stadler et al. 1998a	47	1	7	17
IFNα/all-*trans*-retinoic acid	Escudier et al. 1998	31	0	1	3
IFNα/vinblastine	Figlin et al. 1985	23	0	3	13
	Ceto et al. 1986	18	1	7	44
	Fossa et al. 1986	16	0	5	31
	Otto et al. 1987	24	1	8	37
	Fossa and deGaris 1987	13	0	3	23
	Bergerat et al. 1988	40	1	16	42
	Rizzo et al. 1989	18	1	4	28
	Schornagel et al. 1989	56	0	9	16
	Palmeri et al. 1990	11	0	2	18
	Kellokumpu-Lehtinen et al. 1990	22	3	3	30
	Trump et al. 1990	15	0	1	7
	Massidda et al. 1991	42	1	5	14
	Merimsky et al. 1991	9	0	0	0
	Neidhart et al. 1991	83	3	4	8
	Fossa et al. 1992b	66	1	15	24
	Kriegmair et al. 1995	41	4	5	22
	Pyrhonen et al. 1999	77	7	6	17
IFNα/vinblastine/doxorubicin	Jekunen and Pyrhonen 1996	11	0	2	18
IL-2/IFNα/5-FU	Atzpodien et al. 1993	35	4	13	49
	Sella et al. 1994a 19	3	6	47	
	Sella et al. 1994b	21	1	1	10
	Gitlitz et al. 1996	23	0	6	26
	Hofmockel et al. 1996	34	3	10	38
	Joffe et al. 1996	38	0	9	24
	Olencki et al. 1996	18	0	0	0
	Dutcher et al. 1997	50	1	7	16
	Ellerhorst et al. 1997	52	4	12	31
	Kirchner et al. 1998	246	26	54	33
	Ravaud et al. 1998	111	0	5	2
	Tourani et al. 1998	62	1	11	19
IL-2/IFNα/tamoxifen	Henriksson et al. 1998	65	5	ND	7
IL-2/IFNα/vinblastine	Pectasides et al. 1998	31	4	8	39
Tegafur/tamoxifen	Wada et al. 1995	10	1	3	40
Tegafur/tamoxifen/doxorubicin/ methotrexate	Wada et al. 1993	8	2	2	50
Tegafur/uracil	Esteban et al. 1993	14	0	0	0
Vinblastine/tamoxifen	Samuels et al. 1997	35	1	0	3
Vinblastine/toremifene	Vallis et al. 1994	18	2	0	11

N, number of evaluable patients; CR, complete response; PR, partial response; ND, not done.

References

Abele, R., Clavel, M., Dodion, P., *et al.* (1987). The EORTC early clinical trials cooperative group experience with 5 -aza-deoxycytidine (NSC 127716) in patients with colorectal, head and neck, renal carcinomas, and malignant melanomas. *Eur. J. Cancer Clin. Oncol.* **23** (12), 1921–4.

Abrams, J.S., Tait, N., Silva, H., *et al.* (1989). Phase II trial of *N*-methylformamide in advanced renal cancer. *Am. J. Clin. Oncol.* **12** (1), 41–2.

Ahlgren, J.D., Lokich, J., Auerbach, M., *et al.* (1993). Protracted infusional 5FU (PIF): a well tolerated regimen in metastatic renal carcinoma (MRC): a Mid-Atlantic Oncology Program (MOAP) study [abstract]. *Proc. Am. Soc. Clin. Oncol.* **12**, 244.

Ahmed, T., Benedetto, P., Yagoda, A., *et al.* (1984). Estrogen, progesterone, and androgen-binding sites in renal cell carcinoma: observations obtained in phase II trial of flutamide. *Cancer* **54** (3), 477–81.

Alberto, P. and Senn, H.J. (1974). Hormonal therapy of renal carcinoma alone and in association with cytostatic drugs. *Cancer* **33** (5), 1226–9.

Allen, A., Wolf, M., Crawford, E.D., Davis, M.P., Natale, R.B., and Barnett, M.L. (1992). Phase II evaluation of piroxantrone in renal cell carcinoma: a Southwest Oncology Group Study. *Invest. New Drugs* **10** (2), 129–32.

Al-Sarraf, M., Eyre, H., Bonnet, J., *et al.* (1981). Study of tamoxifen in metastatic renal cell carcinoma and the influence of certain prognostic factors: a Southwest Oncology Group Study. *Cancer Treat. Rep.* **65** (5–6), 447–51.

Altman, S.J., Stephens, R.L., and Bonnet, J.D. (1982). Yoshi 864 plus medroxyprogesterone acetate in adenocarcinoma of the kidney: a Southwest Oncology Group Study. *Cancer Treat. Rep.* **66** (9), 1781–2.

Amrein, P.C., Coleman, M., Richards, F. II, *et al.* (1983). Phase II study of amsacrine in metastatic renal cell carcinoma: a Cancer and Leukemia Group B study. *Cancer Treat. Rep.* **67** (11), 1043–4.

Atzpodien, J., Kirchner, H., Hanninen, E.L., Deckert, M., Fenner, M., and Poliwoda, H. (1993). Interleukin-2 in combination with interferon-alpha and 5-fluorouracil for metastatic renal cell cancer. *Eur. J. Cancer* **29A** (suppl. 5), S6–S8.

Aveta, P., Terrone, C., Neira, D., Cracco, C., and Rocca Rossetti, S. (1997). Chemotherapy with FUDR in the management of metastatic renal cell carcinoma. *Ann. Urol. (Paris)* **31** (3), 159–63.

Baiocchi, C., Landonio, G., Cacioppo, C., *et al.* (1996). Continuous non-chronomodulated infusion of floxuridine in metastatic renal cell carcinoma (MRCC); report of 17 cases. *Tumori* **82** (3), 225–7.

Balducci, L., Blumenstein, B., Van Hoff, D.D., *et al.* (1987). Evaluation of fludarabine phosphate in renal cell carcinoma: a Southwest Oncology Group Study. *Cancer Treat. Rep.* **71** (5), 543–4.

Baumgartner, G., Heinz, R., Arbes, H., Lenzhofer, R., Pridun, N., and Schuller, J. (1980). Methotrexate-citrovorum factor used alone and in combination chemotherapy for advanced hypernephromas. *Cancer Treat. Rep.* **64** (1), 41–6.

Benedetto, P., Ahmed, T., Needles, B., Watson, R.C., and Yagoda. A. (1983). Phase II trial of 4´epi-adriamycin for advanced hypernephroma. *Am. J. Clin. Oncol.* **6** (5), 553–4.

Berg, W.J., Schwartz, L.H., Amsterdam, A., *et al.* (1997). A phase II study of 13-*cis*-retinoic acid in patients with advanced renal cell carcinoma. *Invest. New Drugs* **15**, 353–5.

Bergerat, J.P., Herbrecht, R., Dufour, P., *et al.* (1988). Combination of recombinant interferon alpha-2a and vinblastine in advanced renal cell cancer. *Cancer* **62** (11), 2320–4.

Bloom, H.J. (1964). Hormone treatment of renal tumours: experimental and clinical observations. In *Tumours of the kidney and ureter* (ed. E. Riches), p. 311. E.S. Livingstone, Edinburgh.

Bloom, H.J. (1971). Medroxyprogesterone acetate (Provera) in the treatment of metastatic renal cancer. *Br. J. Cancer* **25** (2), 250–65.

Bodrogi, I., Baki, M., Sinkovics, I., and Eckhardt, S. (1988). Ifosfamide chemotherapy of metastatic renal cell cancer. *Sem. Surg. Oncol.* **4** (2), 95–6.

Braich, T.A., Salmon, S.E., Robertone, A., *et al.* (1986). Phase II trial of esorubicin (4´-deoxydoxorubicin) in cancers of the breast, colon, kidney, lung and melanoma. *Invest. New Drugs* **4** (3), 269–74.

Brubaker, L.H., Nelson, M.O. Jr, Birch, R., and Williams, S. (1986*a*). Treatment of advanced adenocarcinoma of the kidney with mitolactol: a Southeastern Cancer Study Group Trial. *Cancer Treat. Rep.* **70** (2), 305–6.

Brubaker, L.H., Vogel, C.L., Einhorn, L.H., and Birch, R. (1986*b*). Treatment of advanced adenocarcinoma of the kidney with ICRF-187: a Southwestern Cancer Study Group Trial. *Cancer Treat. Rep.* **70** (7), 915–16.

Bruntsch, U., Dodion, P., ten Bokkel Huinink, W.W., *et al.* (1986). Primary resistance of renal adenocarcinoma to 1,2,4-triglycidylurazol (TGU, NSC332488), a new triexpoxide cytostatic agent—a phase II study of the EORTC early clinical trials group. *Eur. J. Cancer Clin. Oncol.* **22** (6), 697–9.

Bruntsch, U., Heinrich, B., Kaye, S.B., *et al.* (1994). Docetaxel (Taxotere) in advanced renal cell cancer. A phase II trial of the EORTC Early Clinical Trials Group. *Eur. J. Cancer* **30A** (8), 1064–7.

Budd, G.T., Murthy, S., Klein, E., *et al.* (1992). Time-modified infusion of floxuridine in metastatic renal cell carcinoma (RCC) [abstract]. *Proc. Am. Assoc. Cancer Res.* **33**, 220.

Caille, P., Mondesir, J.M., Droz, J.P., *et al.* (1985). Phase II elliptinium in advanced renal cell carcinoma. *Cancer Treat. Rep.* **69** (7–8), 901–2.

Canobbio, L., Boccardo, F., Guarneri, D., *et al.* (1991). Phase II study of navelbine in advanced renal cell carcinoma. *Eur. J. Cancer* **27** (6), 804–5.

Carlson, R.W., Williams, R.D., Billingham, M.E., Kohler, M., and Torti, F.M. (1987). Phase II trial of esorubicin in the treatment of metastatic carcinoma of the kidney: a study of the Northern California Oncology Group. *Cancer Treat. Rep.* **71** (7–8), 767–8.

Ceto, G.L., Franceschi, T., Bassetto, M.A., Molino, A.M., and Capelli, C. (1986). Phase I/II trial of recomninant alpha-2 interferon (IFN) and vinblastine (VBL) in metastatic renal cell cancer (MRCC) [abstract]. *Proc. Am. Soc. Clin. Oncol.* **5**, 110.

Chang, A.Y., Tu, Z.N., Bryan, G.T., Kirkwood, J.M., Oken, M.M., and Trump, D.L. (1994). Phase II study of echinomycin in the treatment of renal cell carcinoma ECOG study E2885. *Invest. New Drugs* **12** (2), 151–3.

Chauvergne, J., Kerbrat, P., Adenis, A., *et al.* (1995). Phase II study of cystemustine in advanced renal cancer. *Eur. J. Cancer* **31A** (1), 130–1.

Cheon, J., Chung, D.J., Kim, J.J., Koh, S.K., and Sohn, J. (1996). Inhibitory effects of interleukin-4 on human renal cell carcinoma cells *in vitro*: in combination with interferon-alpha, tumor necrosis factor-alpha or interleukin-2. *Int. J. Urol.* **3** (3), 196–201.

Chevallier, B., Toussaint, C., Kerbrat, P., *et al.* (1991). Final report: phase II study of fotemustine in advanced renal cell carcinoma (RCC): an assessment of Elson prognostic factors [abstract]. *Proc. Am. Soc. Clin. Oncol.* **10**, 180.

Child, J.A., Bono, A.V., Fossa, S.D., ten Bokkel Huinink, W.W., De Pauw, M., and Stoter, G. (1982). An EORTC phase II study of methyl-glyoxal bis-guanyl-hydrazone in advanced renal cell cancer. *Eur. J. Cancer Clin. Oncol.* **18** (1), 85–7.

Childs, R., Clave, E., Tisdale, J., Plante, M., Hensel, N., and Barrett, J. (1999). Successful treatment of metastatic renal cell carcinoma with a nonmyeloablative allogeneic peripheral-blood progenitor-cell transplant: evidence for a graft-versus-tumor effect. *J. Clin. Oncol.* **17** (7), 2044–9.

Conroy, T., Geoffrois, L., Guillemin, F., *et al.* (1993). Simplified chronomodulated continuous infusion of floxuridine in patients with metastatic renal cell carcinoma. *Cancer* **72** (7), 2190–7.

Cowan, D.H. and Alison, R.E. (1970). Evaluation of 6-aminonicotinamide (NSC 21206) in the treatment of metastatic hypernephroma; part 1. *Cancer Chemother. Rep.* **54** (3), 175–9.

Crivellari, D., Tumolo, S., Frustaci, S., *et al.* (1987). Phase II study of five-day continuous infusion of vinblastine in patients with metastatic renal-cell carcinoma. *Am. J. Clin. Oncol.* **10** (3), 231–3.

Damascelli, B., Marchiano, A., Spreafico, C., *et al.* (1990). Circadian continuous chemotherapy of renal cell carcinoma with an implantable, programmable infusion pump. *Cancer* **66** (2), 237–41.

Decker, D.A., Drelichman, A., Opipari, M.I., and Al-Sarraf, M. (1984). Phase II evaluation of aclacinomycin-A (NSC 208734) in adenocarcinoma of the kidney. *Am. J. Clin. Oncol.* **7** (5), 527–8.

Decker, D.A., Kish, J., Al-Sarraf, M., and Goldfarb, S. (1986). Phase II clinical evaluation of AZQ in renal cell carcinoma. *Am. J. Clin. Oncol.* **9** (2), 126–8.

DeForges, A., Droz, J.P., Ghosn, M., and Theodore, C. (1987). Phase II trial of ifosfamide/mesna in metastatic adult renal carcinoma. *Cancer Treat. Rep.* **71** (11), 1103.

De Jager, R., Cappelaere, P., and Armand, J.P. (1984). An EORTC phase II study of mitoxantrone in solid tumors and lymphomas. *Eur. J. Cancer Clin. Oncol.* **20** (11), 1369–75.

De Mulder, P.H.M., Weissbach, L., Jakse, G., Osieka, R., and Blatter, J. (1996). Gemcitabine: a phase II study in patients with advanced renal cancer. *Cancer Chemother. Pharmacol.* **37**, 491–5.

Dexeus, F.H., Logothetis, C.J., Sella, A., *et al.* (1991). Circadian infusion of floxuridine in patients with metastatic renal cell carcinoma. *J. Urol.* **146** (3), 709–13.

DeVassal, F., Misset, J.L., Brienza, S., *et al.* (1987). A phase II trial of 4′-O-tetrahydropyranyl-adriamycin (THP-ADM) in advanced solid tumors. *Invest. New Drugs* **5**, 123.

Dimopoulous, M.A., Dexeus, F.H., Jones, E., Amato, R.J., Sella, A., and Logothetis, C.J. (1991). Evidence for additive anti-tumor activity and toxicity for the combination of FUDR and interferon alpha2B in patients (pts) with metastatic renal cell carcinoma (RCC) [abstract]. *Proc. Am. Assoc. Cancer Res.* **32**, 186.

Dosquet, C., Coudert, M.-C., Lepage, E., Cabane, J., and Richard, F. (1997). Are angiogenic factors, cytokines, and soluble adhesion molecules prognostic factors in patients with renal cell carcinoma? *Clin. Cancer Res.* **3**, 2451–8.

Dreicer, R., Propert, K.J., Kuzel, T., Kirkwood, J.M., O'Dwyer, P.J., and Loehrer, P.J. (1997). A phase II trial of edatrexate in patients with advanced renal cell carcinoma. *Am. J. Clin. Oncol.* **20** (3), 251–3.

Dutcher, J., Atkins, M., Fisher, R., *et al.* (1997). IL-2-based therapy for metastatic renal cell cancer: the Cytokine Working Group experience, 1989–1997. *Cancer J. Sci. Am.* **3** (suppl. 1), S73–S78.

Earhart, R.H., Elson, P.J., Rosenthal, S.N., Hahn, R.G., and Slayton, R.E. (1983). Phase II study of PALA and AMSA in advanced renal cell carcinoma. *Am. J. Clin. Oncol.* **6** (5), 555–60.

Einzig, A.I., Gorowski, E., Sasloff, J., and Wiernik, P.H. (1991). Phase II trial of taxol in patients with metastatic renal cell carcinoma. *Cancer Invest.* **9** (2), 133–6.

Ellerhorst, J.A., Sella, A., Amato, R.J., *et al.* (1997). Phase II trial of 5-fluorouracil, interferon-alpha and continuous infusion interleukin-2 for patients with metastatic renal cell carcinoma. *Cancer* **80** (11), 2128–32.

Elson, P.J., Earhart, R.H., Kvols, L.K., *et al.* (1987). Phase II studies of PCNU and bisantrene in advanced renal cell carcinoma. *Cancer Treat. Rep.* **71** (3), 331–2.

Elson, P.J., Kvols, L.K., Vogl, S.E., *et al.* (1988). Phase II trials of 5-day vinblastine infusion (NSC 49842), L-alanosine (NSC 153353), acivicin (NSC 163501), and aminothiadiazole (NSC 4728) in patients with recurrent or metastatic renal cell carcinoma. *Invest. New Drugs* **6** (2), 97–103.

Escudier, B., Fizazi, K., Rolland, F., *et al.* (1997). Phase II study of irinotecan (CPT-11) in pretreated or not pretreated patients with advanced renal cell carcinoma [abstract]. *Proc. Am. Soc. Clin. Oncol.* **16**, 33a.

Escudier, B., Ravaud, A., Berton, D., Chevreau, C., Douillard, J.-Y., and Dietrich, P.-Y. (1998). Phase II study of interferon-α and all-*trans* retinoic acid in metastatic renal cell carcinoma. *J. Immunother.* **21** (1), 62–4.

Esteban, E., Buesa, J.M., Cueva, J., *et al.* (1993). Phase II study of oral ftorafur and uracil in patients with advanced renal cell carcinoma. *Eur. J. Cancer* **29A** (9), 1354.

Evans, W.K., Shepherd, F.A., and Blackstein, M.E. (1985). Phase II evaluation of bisantrene in patients with renal cell carcinoma. *Cancer Treat. Rep.* **69** (6), 727–8.

Falcone, A., Cianci, C., Ricci, S., Brunetti, I., Bertuccelli, M., and Conte, P.F. (1993). Alpha-2B-interferon plus floxuridine in metastatic renal cell carcinoma: a phase I–II study. *Cancer* **72** (2), 564–8.

Falkson, C.I. (1993). New formulation intravenous melphalan in the treatment of patients with metastatic renal cancer. *Invest. New Drugs* **11** (1), 93.

Ferrazzi, E., Salvagno, L., Fornasiero, A., Cartei, G., and Fiorentino, M. (1980). Tamoxifen treatment for advanced renal cell cancer. *Tumori* **66** (5), 601–5.

Feun, L.G., Drelichman, A., Singhakowinta, A., Vaitkevicius, V.K., and Oishi, N. (1979). Phase II study of nafoxidine in the therapy for advanced renal carcinoma. *Cancer Treat. Rep.* **63** (1), 149–50.

Figlin, R.A., deKernion, J.B., Maldazys, J., and Sarna, G. (1985). Treatment of renal cell carcinoma with alpha (human leukocyte) interferon and vinblastine in combination: a phase I–II trial. *Cancer Treat. Rep.* **69** (3), 263–7.

Fine, R., Saachs, C., Albers, M., and Williams A. (1991). Tamoxifen potentiates the cytotoxocity of vinblastine by increasing intracellular drug accumulation. *Proc. Am. Assoc. Cancer Res.* **32**, 375.

Flanigan, R.C., Saiers, J.H., Wolf, M., *et al.* (1994). Phase II evaluation of merbarone in renal cell carcinoma. *Invest. New Drugs* **12** (2), 147–9.

Fojo, A.T., Ueda, K., Slamon, D.J., Poplack, D.G,. Gottesman, M.M., and Pastan, I. (1987*a*). Expression of a multidrug-resistance gene in human tumors and tissues. *Proc. Natl Acad. Sci., USA* **84**, 265–9.

Fojo, A.T., Shen, D.-W., Mickley, L.A., Pastan, I., and Gottesman, M.M. (1987*b*). Intrinsic drug resistance in human kidney cancer is associated with expression of a human multidrug-resistance gene. *J. Clin. Oncol.* **5** (12), 1922–7.

Folkman, J. (1996). New perspectives in clinical oncology from angiogenesis research. *Eur. J. Cancer* **32A** (14), 2534–9.

Fossa, S.D. and de Garis, S.T. (1987). Further experience with recombinant alfa-2a with or without vinblastine in metastatic renal cell carcinoma: a progress report. *Int. J. Cancer* **1**, 36–40.

Fossa, S.D. and Talle, K. (1980). Treatment of metastatic renal cancer with ifosfamide and mesnum with and without irradiation. *Cancer Treat. Rep.* **64** (10–11), 1103–8.

Fossa, S.D., Wik, B., Bae, E., and Lien, H.H. (1982). Phase II study of 4′-epidoxorubicin in metastatic renal cancer. *Cancer Treat. Rep.* **66** (5), 1219–21.

Fossa, S.D., Denis, L., van Oosterom, A.T., De Pauw, M., and Stoter, G. (1983). Vindesine in advanced renal cancer: a study of the EORTC Genito-urinary Tract Cancer Cooperative Group. *Eur. J. Cancer Oncol.* **19** (4), 473–5.

Fossa, S.D., de Garis, S.T., Heier, M.S., *et al.* (1986). Recombinant interferon with or without vinblastine in metastatic renal cell carcinoma. *Cancer* **57** (8 suppl.), 1700–4.

Fossa, S.D., Droz, J.P., Pavone-Macaluso, M.M., Debruyne, F.J., Vermeylen, K., and Sylvester, R. (1992*a*). Vinblastine in metastatic renal cell carcinoma: EORTC phase II trial 30882: the EORTC Genitourinary Group. *Eur. J. Cancer* **28A**, 878–80.

Fossa, S.D., Martinelli, G., Otto, U., *et al.* (1992*b*). Recombinant interferon alfa-2a with or without vinblastine in metastatic renal cell carcinoma: results of a European multi-center phase III study. *Ann. Oncol.* **3** (4), 301–5.

Foster, B., Grotzinger, K., McKoy, W., Rubinstein, L., and Hamilton, T. (1988). Modulation of induced resistance to adriamycin in two human breast cancer cell lines with tamoxifen or perhexiline maleate. *Cancer Chemother. Pharmacol.* **22**, 147–52.

Fuks, A.Z., Van Echo, D.A., and Aisner, J. (1981). Phase II trial of methyl-G (methyl-glyoxal bis-guanylhydrazone) in patients with metastatic renal cell carcinoma. *Cancer Clin. Trial* **4** (4), 411–14.

Gams, R.A., Nelson, O., and Birch, R. (1986). Phase II evaluation of mitoxantrone in advanced renal cell carcinoma: a Southeastern Cancer Study Group Trial. *Cancer Treat. Rep.* **70** (7), 921–2.

Gebrosky, N.P., Koukol, S., Nseyo, U.O., Carpenter, C., and Lamm, D.L. (1997). Treatment of renal cell carcinoma with 5-fluorouracil and alfa-interferon. *Urology* **50**, 863–8.

Gershanovich, M.M., Moisevenko, V., Kapyla, H., *et al.* (1993). High dose of new antiestrogen toremifene in advanced renal cell carcinoma [abstract]. *Eur. J. Cancer* **29A**, S233.

Gershanovich, M.M., Moiseyenko, V.M., Vorobjev, A.V., Kapyla, H., Ellmen, J., and Anttila, M. (1997). High-dose toremifene in advanced renal-cell carcinoma. *Cancer Chemother. Pharmacol.* **39**, 547–51.

Gillis, S. and Smith, K. (1977). Long-term culture of tumour-specific cytotoxic T-cells. *Nature* **268**, 154–5.

Gitlitz, B.J., Dolan, N., Pierce, W., *et al.* (1996). Fluoropyrimidines plus interleukin-2 and interferon-alpha in the treatment of metastatic renal cell carcinoma: the UCLA Kidney Cancer Program [abstract]. *Proc. Am. Soc. Clin. Oncol.* **15**, 248.

Glick, J.H., Wein, A., Torri, S., Alavi, J., Harris, D., and Brodovsky, H. (1980). Phase II study of tamoxifen in patients with advanced renal cell carcinoma. *Cancer Treat. Rep.* **64** (6–7), 813–18.

Glover, D., Trump, D., Kvols, L., Elson, P., and Vogl, S. (1986). Phase II trial of misonidazole (MISO) and cyclophosphamide (CYC) in metastatic renal cell carcinoma. *Int. J. Radiat. Oncol. Biol. Phys.* **12** (8), 1405–8.

Goldstein, L., Galski, H., Fojo, A., *et al.* (1989). Expression of a multidrug resistance gene in human tumors. *J. Natl Cancer Inst.* **81**, 116–24.

Gottesman, J.E., Crawford, E.D., Grossman, H.B., Scardino, P., and McCracken, J.D. (1985). Infarction-nephrectomy for metastatic renal carcinoma. *Urology* **25** (3), 248–50.

Gralla, R.J. and Yagoda, A. (1979). Phase II evaluation of chlorozotocin in patients with renal cell carcinoma. *Cancer Treat. Rep.* **63** (6), 1007–8.

Grimm, E.A., Mazumder, A., Zhang, H.Z., *et al.* (1982). Lymphokine-activated killer cell phenomenon: lysis of natural killer-resistant fresh solid tumor cells by interleukin-2-activated autologous human peripheral blood lymphocytes. *J. Exp. Med.* **155**, 1823–41.

Haarstad, H., Jacobsen, A.B., Schjolseth, S.A., Risberg, T., and Fossa, S.D. (1994). Interferon-alpha, 5-FU and prednisone in metastatic renal cell carcinoma: a phase II study. *Ann. Oncol.* **5** (3), 245–8.

Haas, C.D., Coltman, C.A., Gottlieb, J.A., *et al.* (1976). Phase II evaluation of bleomycin. *Cancer* **38** (1), 8–12.

Hahn, D.M., Schimpff, S.C., Ruckdeschel, J.C., and Wiernik, P.H. (1977). Single-agent therapy for renal cell carcinoma: CCNU, vinblastine, thioTEPA, or bleomycin. *Cancer Treat. Rep.* **61** (8), 1585–7.

Hahn, R.G., Bauer, M., Wolter, J., Creech, R., Bennett, J.M., and Wampler, G. (1979). Phase II study of single-agent therapy with megestrol acetate, VP-16–213, cyclophosphamide, and dianhydrogalactitol in advanced renal cell cancer. *Cancer Treat. Rep.* **63** (3), 513–15.

Hahn, R.G., Begg, C.B., and Davis, T. (1981). Phase II study of vinblastine-CCNU, triazinate, and dactinomycin in advanced renal cell cancer. *Cancer Treat. Rep.* **65** (7–8), 711–13.

Hansen, M., Gallmeier, W.M., Vermorken, J., Hansen, H.H., Renard, J., and Rozencweig, M. (1984). Phase II trial of diaziquone in advanced renal adenocarcinoma. *Cancer Treat. Rep.* **68** (7–8), 1055–6.

Hansen, M., Clavel, M., Zonnenberg, B.A., Bruntsch, U., Knobf, M.K., and Rozencweig, M. (1985). Phase II study of ametantrone (NSC 287513) in advanced renal cell carcinoma [abstract]. *Proc. Am. Soc. Clin. Oncol.* **4**, 99.

Harvey, J.H., Smith, F.P., Bowers, M.W., *et al.* (1984). Phase II trial of PCNU in advanced renal cell carcinoma and malignant mesothelioma. *Cancer Treat. Rep.* **68** (7–8), 1049–50.

Heim, M.E., Fiene, R., Schick, E., Wolpert, E., and Queisser, W. (1981). Central nervous side effects following ifosfamide monotherapy of advanced renal carcinoma. *J. Cancer Res. Clin. Oncol.* **100** (1), 113–16.

Henriksson, R., Nilsson, S., Colleen, S., *et al.* (1998). Survival in renal cell carcinoma—a randomized evaluation of tamoxifen vs. interleukin-2, alfa-interferon (leucocyte) and tamoxifen. *Br. J. Cancer* **77** (8), 1311–17.

Herrmann, R., Manegold, C., Keliner, S., *et al.* (1994). The MDR1 modulator dexniguldipine (DNIG) has antineoplastic activity in metastatic renal cell cancer [abstract]. *Proc. Am. Soc. Clin. Oncol.* **13**, 158.

Higano, C.S., Goodman, P., Craig, J.B., *et al.* (1991). Phase II evaluation of amonafide in renal cell carcinoma: a Southwest Oncology Group study. *Invest. New Drugs* **9** (4), 361–3.

Hillman, G.G., Younes, E., Visscher, D., *et al.* (1995). Systemic treatment with interleukin-4 induces regression of pulmonary metastases in a murine renal cell carcinoma model. *Cell Immunol.* **160** (2), 257–63.

Hindmarsh, J.R., Hall, R.R., and Kulatilake, A.E. (1979). Renal cell carcinoma: a preliminary clinical trial of methodichlorophen (D.D.M.P.). *Clin. Oncol.* **5** (1), 11–15.

Hire, E.A., Samson, M.K., Fraile, R.J., and Baker, L.H. (1979). Use of VM-26 as a single agent in the treatment of renal carcinoma. *Cancer Clin. Trial* **2** (4), 293–5.

Hofmockel, G., Langer, W., Theiss, M., Gruss, A., and Frohmuller, H.G.W. (1996). Immunochemotherapy for metastatic renal cell carcinoma using a regimen of interleukin-2, interferon-alfa, and 5-fluorouracil. *J. Urol.* **156**, 18–21.

Hogan, T.F., Citrin, D.L., and Freeberg, B.L. (1981). A preliminary report of mitotane therapy of advanced renal and prostate cancer. *Cancer Treat. Rep.* **65** (5–6), 539–40.

Howard, M., Matis, L., Malek, T.R., *et al.* (1983). Interleukin-2 induces antigen-reactive T cell lines to secrete BCGF-1. *J. Exp. Med.* **158**, 2024–34.

Hrushesky, W.J., van Roemeling, R., Lanning, R.M., and Rabatin, J.T. (1990). Circadian-shaped infusions of floxuridine for progressive metastatic renal cell carcinoma. *J. Clin. Oncol.* **8** (9), 1504–13.

Hurteloup, P., Chollet, P., Roche, H., *et al.* (1989). Phase II trial of esorubicin in advanced renal carcinoma: Clinical Screening Group of the EORTC. *Eur. J. Cancer Clin. Oncol.* **25** (6), 995–6.

Jekunen, A. and Pyrhonen, S. (1996). A combination of vinblastine and doxorubicin with interferon alpha. *Am. J. Clin. Oncol.* **19** (4), 384–5.

Joffe, J.K, Banks, R.E., Forbes, M.A., *et al.* (1996). Phase II study of interferon-alpha, interleukin-2 and 5-fluorouracil in advanced renal carcinoma. Clinical data and laboratory evidence of protease action. *Br. J. Urol.* **77** (5), 638–49.

Johnson, D.E., Chalbaud, R.A., Holoye, P.Y., and Samuels, M.L. (1975). Clinical trial of bleomycin (NSC-125066) in the treatment of metastatic renal carcinoma: part 1. *Cancer Chemother. Rep.* **59** (2, Pt. 1), 433–5.

Kanamaru, H., Kakehi, Y., Yoshida, O., Nakanishi, S., Pastan, I., and Gottesman, M. (1989). MDR1 RNA levels in human renal cell carcinomas: correlation with grade and prediction of reversal of doxorubicin resistance by quinidine in tumor explants. *J. Natl Cancer Inst.* **81**, 844–9.

Kaye, S.B., Brampton, M., Harper, P., *et al.* (1992). Phase II trials of fosquidone (GR63178A), in colorectal, renal and non-small cell lung cancers: CRC Phase II Clinical Trials Committee. *Br. J. Cancer* **65** (4), 624–5.

Kellokumpu-Lehtinen, P. and Nordman, E. (1990). Recombinant interferon-alpha 2a and vinblastine in advanced renal cell cancer: a clinical phase I–II study. *J. Biol. Resp. Mod.* **9** (4), 439–44.

Kirchner, H., Buer, J., Probst-Kepper, M., *et al.* (1998). Risk and long-term outcome in metastatic renal cell carcinoma patients receiving SC interleukin-2, SC interferon-alfa2a and IV fluoruracil [abstract]. *Proc. Am. Soc. Clin. Oncol.* **17**, 310.

Kirk, J., Houlbrook, S., Stuart, N., Stratford, I., Harris, A., and Carmichael, J. (1993). Selective reversal of vinblastine resistance in multidrug resistant cell lines by tamoxifen, toremifene and their metabolites. *Eur. J. Cancer* **29A**, 1152–7.

Kirkman, H. and Bacon, R.L. (1952). Estrogen-induced tumors of the kidney I. Incidence of renal tumors in intact and gonadectomized male golden hamsters treated with diethylstilbestrol. *J. Natl Cancer Inst.* **13**, 745.

Kiruluta, G., Morales, A., and Lott, S. (1975). Response of renal adeno-carcinoma to cyclophosphamide. *Urology* **6** (5), 557–8.

Kish, J.A., Ensley, J.F., and Al-Sarraf, M. (1990). Phase II evaluation of 4′deoxy-doxorubicin in advanced renal cell carcinoma. *Am. J. Clin. Oncol.* **13** (1), 17–18.

Kish, J.A., Wolf, M., Crawford, E.D., *et al.* (1994). Evaluation of low dose continuous infusion 5-fluorouracil in patients with advanced and recurrent renal cell carcinoma: a Southwest Oncology Group Study. *Cancer* **74** (3), 916–19.

Kjaer, M. (1988). The role of medroxyprogesterone acetate (MPA) in the treatment of renal adenocarcinoma. *Cancer Treat. Rev.* **15**, 195–209.

Kjaer, M. (1989). Mistletoe (Iscador) therapy in stage 4 renal adenocarcinoma: a phase II study in patients with measurable lung metastases. *Acta Oncol.* **28**, 489–94.

Knight, W.A., Drelichman, A., Fabian, C., and Bukowski, R.M. (1983). Mitoguazone in advanced renal carcinoma: a phase II trial of the Southwest Oncology Group. *Cancer Treat. Rep.* **67** (12), 1139–40.

Kriegmair, M., Oberneder, R., and Hofstetter, A. (1995). Interferon alfa and vinblastine versus medroxyprogesterone acetate in the treatment of metastatic renal cell carcinoma. *Urology* **45**, 5758–62.

Kuebler, J.P., Hogan, T.F., Trump, D.L., and Bryan, G.T. (1984). Phase II study of continuous 5-day vinblastine infusion in renal adenocarcinoma. *Cancer Treat. Rep.* **68** (6), 925–6.

Lafreniere, R. and Rosenberg, S.A. (1985). Successful immunotherapy of experimental hepatic metastases with lymphokine-activated killer cells and recombinant interleukin-2. *Cancer Res.* **45**, 3735–41.

Lanteri, V.J., Dragone, N., Choudhury, M., Beckley, S., Wajsman, Z., and Pontes, J.E. (1982). High-dose tamoxifen in metastatic renal cell carcinoma. *Urology* **XIX** (6), 623–5.

La Rocca, R.V., Stein, C.A., Danesi, R., Cooper, M.R., Uhlrich, M., and Myers, C.E. (1991). A pilot study of suramin in the treatment of metastatic renal cell carcinoma. *Cancer* **67** (6), 1509–13.

Lasset, C., Merrouche, Y., Negrier, S., *et al.* (1993). Phase II study of fotemustine as second-line treatment after failure of immunotherapy in metastatic renal cell carcinoma. *Cancer Chemother. Pharmacol.* **32** (4), 329–31.

Licht, J.D. and Garnick, M.B. (1987). Phase II trial of streptozocin in the treatment of advanced renal cell carcinoma. *Cancer Treat. Rep.* **71** (1), 97–8.

Long, H.J., Hauge, M.D., Therneau, T.M., Buckner, J.C., Frytak, S., and Hahn, R.G. (1991). Phase II evaluation of menogaril in patients with advanced hypernephroma. *Invest. New Drugs* **9** (3), 261–2.

Mahjoubi, M., Kattan, J., Bonnay, M., Schmitt, H., and Droz, J.P. (1993). Phase II trial of LY 186641 in advanced renal cancer. *Invest. New Drugs* **11** (4), 323–8.

Margolin, K., Aronson, F.R., Sznol, M., *et al.* (1994). Phase II studies of recombinant human interleukin-4 in advanced renal cancer and malignant melanoma. *J. Immunother. Emphasis Tumor Immunol.* **15** (2), 147–53.

Marshall, M.E., Wolf, M.K., Crawford, E.D., *et al.* (1993). Phase II trial of echinomycin for the treatment of advanced renal cell carcinoma: a Southwest Oncology Group study. *Invest. New Drugs* **11** (2–3), 207–9.

Massidda, B., Migliari, R., Padovani, A., *et al.* (1991). Metastatic renal cell cancer treated with recombinant alpha 2a interferon and vinblastine. *J. Chemother.* **3** (6), 387–9.

McLean, J., Loehrer, P., Picus, J., *et al.* (1994). A phase II study of altretamine for the treatment of metastatic renal cell carcinoma: a Hoosier Oncology trial [abstract]. *Proc. Am. Soc. Clin. Oncol.* **13**, 244.

Merimsky, O., Shnider, B.I., and Chaitchik, S. (1991). Does vinblastine add to the potency of alpha interferon in the treatment of renal cell carcinoma? *Mol. Biother.* **3** (1), 34–7.

Merrin, C.E. (1979). Treatment of genitourinary tumors with *cis*-dichlorodiammineplatinum (II): experience in 250 patients. *Cancer Treat. Rep.* **63** (9–10), 1579–84.

Merrouche, Y., Negrier, S., and Lanier, F., *et al.* (1991). Phase II study of continuous circadian infusion FUDR in metastatic renal cell cancer (RCC) [abstract]. *Eur. J. Cancer Clin. Oncol.* **27**, S102.

Mertens, W.C., Eisenhauer, E.A., Moore, M., *et al.* (1993). Gemcitabine in advanced renal cell carcinoma: a phase II study of the National Cancer Institute of Canada Clinical Trials Group. *Ann. Oncol.* **4**, 331–2.

Mertens, W.C., Eisenhauer, E.A., Jolivet, J., Ernst, S., Moore, M., and Muldal, A. (1994). Docetaxel in advanced renal carcinoma: a phase II trial of the National Cancer Institute of Canada Clinical Trials Group. *Ann. Oncol.* **5** (2), 185–7.

Mickisch, G.H. (1994). Chemoresistance of renal cell carcinoma: 1986–1994. *World J. Urol.* **12**, 214–23.

Mickisch, G.H., Roehrich, K., Koessig, J., Forster, S., Tschada, R.K., and Alken, P.M. (1990*a*). Mechanisms and modulation of multidrug resistance in primary human renal cell carcinoma. *J. Urol.* **144**, 755–9.

Mickisch, G., Bier, H., Bergler, W., Bak, M., Tschada, R., and Alken, P. (1990*b*). P-170 glycoprotein, glutathione and associated enzymes in relation to chemoresistance of primary human renal cell carcinomas. *Urol. Int.* **45**, 170–6.

Mischler, N.E., Tormey, D.C., Klotz, J., *et al.* (1981). Phase II study of dibromodulcitol in colorectal, kidney, and other carcinomas. *Cancer Clin. Trials* **4** (4), 407–10.

Morales, A., Kiruluta, G., and Lott, S. (1975). Hormones in the treatment of metastatic renal cancer. *J. Urol.* **114** (5), 692–3.

Morgan, D.A., Ruscetti, F.W., and Gallo, R. (1976). Selective *in vitro* growth of T lymphocytes from normal human bone marrows. *Science* **193**, 1007–8.

Motzer, R.J. and Russo, P. (2000). Systemic therapy for renal cell carcinoma. *J. Urol.* **163**, 408–17.

Motzer, R.J. and Vogelzang, N.J. (1997). Chemotherapy for renal cell carcinoma. In *Principles and practice of genitourinary oncology* (ed. D. Raghavan, H.I. Scher, S.A. Leibel, and P.H. Lange), pp. 885–96. Lippincott–Raven Publishers, Philadelphia.

Motzer, R., Scher, H., Bajorin, D., Sternberg, C., and Bosl, G.J. (1990). Phase II trial of Didemnin B in patients with advanced renal cell carcinoma. *Invest. New Drugs* **8** (4), 391–2.

Motzer, R.J., Nanus, D.M., O'Moore, P., *et al.* (1992). Phase II trial of suramin in patients with advanced renal cell carcinoma: treatment results, pharmacokinetics, and tumor growth factor expression. *Cancer Res.* **52** (20), 5775–9.

Motzer, R.J., Schwartz, L., Murray Law, T., *et al.* (1995). Interferon alfa-2a and 13-*cis*-retinoic acid in renal cell carcinoma: antitumor activity in a phase II trial and interactions *in vitro*. *J. Clin. Oncol.* **13** (8), 1950–7.

Murphy, B.R., Rynard, S.M., Einhorn, L.H., and Loehrer, P.J. (1992). A phase II trial of interferon alpha-2A plus fluorouracil in advanced renal cell carcinoma: a Hoosier Oncology Group Study. *Invest. New Drugs* **10** (3), 225–30.

Murray Law, T., Mencel, P., and Motzer, R.J. (1994*a*). Phase II trial of liposomal encapsulated doxorubicin in patients with advanced renal cell carcinoma. *Invest. New Drugs* **12** (4), 323–5.

Murray Law, T., Ilson, D.H., and Motzer, R.J. (1994*b*). Phase II trial of topotecan in patients with advanced renal cell carcinoma. *Invest. New Drugs* **12** (2), 143–5.

Myers, J.W., Von Hoff, D.D., and Coltman, C.A. (1982). Phase II evaluation of bisantrene in patients with renal cell carcinoma. *Cancer Treat. Rep.* **66** (10), 1869–71.

Nakagawa, M., Emoto, A., Hanada, T., Nasu, N., and Nomura, Y. (1997). Tubulogenesis by microvascular endothelial cells is mediated by vascular endothelial growth factor (VEGF) in renal cell carcinoma. *Br. J. Urol.* **79**, 681–7.

Nakano, E., Tada, Y., Fujioka, H., *et al.* (1984). Hormone receptor in renal cell carcinoma and correlation with clinical response to endocrine therapy. *J. Urol.* **132** (2), 240–5.

Natale, R.B., Yagoda, A., Kelsen, D.P., Gralla, R.J., and Watson, R.C. (1982). Phase II trial of PALA in hypernephroma and urinary bladder cancer. *Cancer Treat. Rep.* **66** (12), 2091–2.

Neidhart, J.A., Anderson, S.A., Harris, J.E., *et al.* (1991). Vinblastine fails to improve response of renal cancer to interferon alfa-n1: high response rate in patients with pulmonary metastases. *J. Clin. Oncol.* **9** (5), 832–6.

Nichols, W.C., Kvols, L.K., and Richardson, R.L. (1982). A phase II study of azirinylbenzoquinone (AZQ) in advanced genitourinary (GU) cancer [abstract]. *Proc. Am. Soc. Clin. Oncol.* **1**, 117.

Nicol, D., Hii, S.-I., Walsh, M., *et al.* (1997). Vascular endothelial growth factor expression is increased in renal cell carcinoma. *J. Urol.* **157**, 1482–6.

O'Bryan, R.M., Baker, L.H., and Gottlieb, J.E. (1977). Dose response evaluation of adriamycin in human neoplasia. *Cancer* **39** (5), 1940–8.

O'Byrne, K.J., Propper, D., Braybooke, J., *et al.* (1997). Razoxane: a phase II trial in renal cell cancer evaluating anti-angiogenic activity [abstract]. *Proc. Am. Soc. Clin. Oncol.* **16**, 325a.

Oishi, N., Berenberg, J., Blumenstein, B.A., *et al.* (1987). Teniposide in metastatic renal and bladder cancer: a Southwest Oncology Group Study. *Cancer Treat. Rep.* **71** (12), 1307–8.

Olencki, T., Bukowski, R.M., Budd, G.T., *et al.* (1996). Phase I/II trial of simultaneously administered rIL-2/rHuIFN and 5-FU in patients with metastatic renal cell carcinoma [abstract]. *Proc. Am. Soc. Clin. Oncol.* **15**, 263.

Otto, U., Schneider, A., Conrad, S., *et al.* (1987). Treatment of patients with metastatic renal cell carcinoma: results of two clinical phase II studies with alpha-2-interferon plus vinblastine or gamma interferon in 55 patients [abstract]. *J. Urol.* **137**, 327a.

Paine, C.H., Wright, F.W., and Ellis, F. (1970). The use of progestogen in the treatment of metastatic carcinoma of the kidney and uterine body. *Br. J. Cancer* **24** (2), 277–82.

Palmeri, S., Gebbia, V., Russo, A., Gebbia, N., and Rausa, L. (1990). Vinblastine and interferon-alpha-2a regimen in the treatment of metastatic renal cell carcinoma. *Tumori* **76** (1), 64–5.

Papac, R.J. and Keohane, M.F. (1993). Hormonal therapy for metastatic renal cell carcinoma combined androgen and provera followed by high dose tamoxifen. *Eur. J. Cancer* **29A** (7), 997–9.

Pasmantier, M.W., Coleman, M., Kennedy, B.J., *et al.* (1977). Piperazinedione in metastatic renal carcinoma. *Cancer Treat. Rep.* **61** (9), 1731–2.

Pearson, J., Friedman, M.A., and Hoffman, P.G. Jr (1981). Hormone receptors in renal cell carcinoma: their utility as predictors of response to endocrine therapy. *Cancer Chemother. Pharmacol.* **6** (2), 151–4.

Pectasides, D., Varthalitis, J., Kostopoulou, M., *et al.* (1998). An outpatient phase II study of subcutaneous interleukin-2 and interferon-alpha-2b in combination with intravenous vinblastine in metastatic renal cell cancer. *Oncology* **55**, 10–15.

Pfiefle, D., Renter, N., and Hahn, R. (1984). Phase II trial of VM-26 in advanced measurable renal cell carcinoma [abstract]. *Proc. Am. Soc. Clin. Oncol.* **3**, 162.

Piot, G., Droz, J.P., Theodore, C., Ghosn, M., Rouesse, J., and Amiel, J.L. (1988). Phase II trial with high-dose elliptinium acetate in metastatic renal cell carcinoma. *Oncology* **45** (5), 371–2.

Poorter, R.L., Bakker, P.J.M., Kurth, K.H., Rietbroek, R.C., Biermans-van Leeuwe, D.M.J., and Veenhof, C.H.N. (1993). Circadian modulated continuous infusion of FUDR in patients with disseminated renal cell cancer (RCC). *Eur. J. Cancer* **29**, 116.

Presant, C.A., Kennedy, P., Wiseman, C., *et al.* (1986). Pilot phase II trial of amphotericin B and CCNU in renal and colorectal carcinomas. *Eur. J. Cancer Clin. Oncol.* **22** (3), 329–30.

Pyrhonen, S., Salminen, E., Ruutu, M., *et al.* (1999). Prospective randomized trial of interferon alfa-2a plus vinblastine versus vinblastine alone in patients with advanced renal cell cancer. *J. Clin. Oncol.* **17** (9), 2859–67.

Raminski, D., Creaven, P.J., Rustum, Y.M., *et al.* (1992). Phase I clinical trial of floxuridine (FUdr) with leucovorin (LV) in patients (PTS) with advanced genitourinary cancer (AGC) [abstract]. *Proc. Am. Soc. Clin. Oncol.* **11**, 206.

Ramu, A., Glaubiger, D., and Fuks, Z. (1984). Reversal of acquired resistance to doxorubicin in P388 murine leukemia cells by tamoxifen and other triparanol analogues. *Cancer Res.* **44**, 4392–5.

Ratanatharathorn, V., Baker, L.H., Balducci, L., Talley, R.W., and Hoogstraten, B. (1982). Phase II trial of dianhydrogalactitol in advanced renal cell carcinoma: a Southwest Oncology Group study. *Cancer Treat. Rep.* **66** (5), 1231–2.

Ravaud, A., Audhuy, B., Gomez, F., *et al.* (1998). Subcutaneous interleukin-2, interferon alfa-2a, and continuous infusion fluorouracil in metastatic renal cell carcinoma: a multicenter phase II trial. Groupe Francais d'Immunotherapie. *J. Clin. Oncol.* **16** (8), 2728–32.

Richards, F. III, Cooper, M.R., Jackson, D.V., *et al.* (1991). Continuous 5-day (D) intravenous (IV) FUDR infusion for renal cell carcinoma (RCC): a phase I–II trial of the Piedmont Oncology Association [abstract]. *Proc. Am. Soc. Clin. Oncol.* **10**, 170.

Rini, B.I., Stadler, W.M., Spielberger, R.T., Ratain, M.J., and Vogelzang, N.J. (1998). Granulocyte–macrophage-colony stimulating factor in metastatic renal cell carcinoma: a phase II trial. *Cancer* **82** (7), 1352–8.

Rizzo, M., Bartoletti, R., Selli, C., Sicignano, A., and Criscuolo, D. (1989). Interferon alpha-2a and vinblastine in the treatment of metastatic renal carcinoma [review]. *Eur. Urol.* **16** (4), 271–7.

Roche, H., Guiochet, N., Kerbrat, P., *et al.* (1993). Phase II trials of tetrahydropyranyl-adriamycin (Pirarubicin) on renal and colon carcinoma, melanoma, and soft tissue sarcoma. *Am. J. Clin. Oncol.* **16** (2), 137–9.

Rodriguez, L.H. and Johnson, D.E. (1978). Clinical trial of cisplatinum (NSC 119875) in metastatic renal cell carcinoma. *Urology* **11** (4), 344–6.

Rohde, D., De Mulder, P.H.M., Weissbach, L., Osieka, R., Blatter, J., and Jakse, G. (1996). Experimental and clinical efficacy of 2′,2′-difluorodeoxycytidine (Gemcitabine) against renal cell carcinoma. *Oncology* **53**, 476–81.

Rosenberg, S.A., Mule, J.J., Spiess, P.J., *et al.* (1985). Regression of established pulmonary metastases and subcutaneous tumor mediated by the systemic administration of high-dose recombinant interleukin-2. *J. Exp. Med.* **161**, 1169–88.

Saiers, J.H., Slavik, M., Stephens, R.L., and Crawford, E.D. (1987). Therapy for advanced renal cell cancer with spirogermanium: a Southwest Oncology Group Study. *Cancer Treat. Rep.* **71** (2), 207–8.

Samuels, M.L., Sullivan, P., and Howe, C.D. (1968). Medroxyprogesterone acetate in the treatment of renal cell carcinoma (hypernephroma). *Cancer* **22** (3), 525–32.

Samuels, B.L., Hollis, D.R., Rosner, G.L., *et al.* (1997). Modulation of vinblastine resistance in metastatic renal cell carcinoma with cyclosporine A or tamoxifen: a Cancer and Leukemia Group B study. *Clin. Cancer Res.* **3**, 1977–84.

Scher, H.I., Schwartz, S., and Yagoda, A. (1982). Phase II trial of 9, 10 antracenedicarboxaldehyde bis (4,5 dihydro-1 H imidazol-2-yl) hydrazone) dichloride (CL 216.942). *Cancer Treat. Rep.* **66** (8), 1653–5.

Scher, H.I., Yagoda, A., Ahmed, T., Hollander, P., and Watson, R.C. (1984). Phase II trial of 10-deazaaminopterin for advanced hypernephroma. *Anticancer Res.* **4** (6), 409–10.

Scher, H.I., Yagoda, A., Ahmed, T., Budman, D., Sordillo, P., and Watson, R.C. (1985). Phase II trial of 4-demethoxydaunorubicin (DMDR) for advanced hypernephroma. *Cancer Chemother. Pharmacol.* **14** (1), 79–80.

Schneider, R.J., Woodcock, T.M., and Yagoda, A. (1980). Phase II trial of 4′-(9-acridinylamino)methanesulfon-m-anisidide (AMSA) in patients with metastatic hypernephroma. *Cancer Treat. Rep.* **64** (1), 183–5.

Schomburg, A., Menzel, T., Hadam, M., *et al.* (1992). Biological and therapeutic efficacy of mafosfamide in patients with metastatic renal cell carcinoma. *Mol. Biother.* **4** (2), 58–65.

Schomburg, A., Kirchner, H., Fenner, M., Menzel, T., Poliwoda, H., and Atzpodien, J. (1993). Lack of therapeutic efficacy of tamoxifen in advanced renal cell carcinoma. *Eur. J. Cancer* **29A** (5), 737–40.

Schornagel, J.H., Verweij, T., ten Bokkel Huinink, W.W., *et al.* (1989). Phase II study of recombinant interferon alpha-2a and vinblastine in advanced renal cell carcinoma. *J. Urol.* **142** (2, Pt. 1), 253–6.

Schulman, P., Davis, R.B., Rafla, S., Green, M., and Henderson, E. (1984). Phase II trial of spirogermanium in advanced renal cell carcinoma: a Cancer and Leukemia Group B study. *Cancer Treat. Rep.* **68** (10), 1305–6.

Schulof, R., Lokich, J., Wampler, G., Schultz, J., and Ahgren, J. (1991). Phase II trial of protracted infusional 5-FU (PIF) for metastatic renal cell carcinoma [abstract]. *Proc. Am. Soc. Clin. Oncol.* **10**, 170.

Schuth, J., Goldschmidt, J.W., and Tunn, U.V. (1993). Response in patients with metastatic renal cell carcinoma (RCC) during the treatment with alpha interferon in combination with 5-fluorouracil [abstract]. *Eur. J. Cancer* **29**, 234.

Schwartz, S. and Yagoda, A. (1984). Phase I–II trial of gallium nitrate for advanced hypernephroma. *Anticancer Res.* **4** (4–5), 317–18.

Sella, A., Logothetis, C.J., Fitz, K., *et al.* (1992). Phase II study of interferon-alpha and chemotherapy (5-fluorouracil and mitomycin C) in metastatic renal cell cancer. *J. Urol.* **147** (3), 573–7.

Sella, A., Zukiwski, A., Robinson, E., *et al.* (1994*a*). Interleukin-2 (IL-2) with interferon-alpha (IFN-alpha) and 5-fluorouracil (5-FU) in patients with metastatic renal cell cancer (RCC) [abstract]. *Proc. Am. Soc. Clin. Oncol.* **13**, 237.

Sella, A., Kilbourn, R.G., Gray, I., *et al.* (1994*b*). Phase I study of interleukin-2 combined with interferon-alpha and 5-fluorouracil in patients with metastatic renal cell cancer. *Cancer Biother.* **9** (2), 103–11.

Senderowicz, A.M., Headlee, D., Stinson, S.F., *et al.* (1998). Phase I trial of continuous infusion flavopiridol, a novel cyclin-dependent kinase inhibitor, in patients with refractory neoplasms. *J. Clin. Oncol.* **16** (9), 2986–99.

Shevrin, D.H., Lad, T.E., Kilton, L.J., *et al.* (1989). Phase II trial of Fludarabine phosphate in advanced renal cell carcinoma: an Illinois Cancer Council Study. *Invest. New Drugs* **7** (2–3), 251–3.

Shevrin, D., Wade, J., Mullane, M., *et al.* (1993). Phase II study of piroxantrone in advanced renal cell cancer (RCC): an Illinois Cancer Center study [abstract]. *Proc. Am. Soc. Clin. Oncol.* **12**, 240.

Shevrin, D.H., Kilton, L.J., Lad, T.E., *et al.* (1994). Phase II trial of 6-thioguanine in advanced renal cell carcinoma. An Illinois Cancer Center study. *Invest. New Drugs* **12** (4), 345–6.

Siemeister, G., Weindel, K., Mohrs, K., Barleon, B., Martiny-Baron, G., and Marme, D. (1996). Reversion of deregulated expression of vascular endothelial growth factor in human renal carcinoma cells by von Hippel–Lindau tumor suppressor protein. *Cancer Res.* **56** (10), 2299–301.

Slater, L., Sweet, P., Stupecky, M., and Gupta, S. (1986). Cyclosporin A reverses vincristine and daunorubicin resistance in acute lymphatic leukemia *in vitro. J. Clin. Invest.* **77**, 1405–8.

Sondel, P.M., Hank, J.A., Kohler, P.C., *et al.* (1986). Destruction of autologous human lymphocytes by interleukin-2-activated cytotoxic cells. *J. Immunol.* **137**, 502–11.

Soori, G., Schulof, R., Stark, J., *et al.* (1999). Continuous infusion floxuridine and alpha interferon in metastatic renal cancer: a national biotherapy study group phase II study. *Cancer Invest.* **17** (6), 379–84.

Spicer, D., Daniels, J., Skinner, D., *et al.* (1985). Phase II study of bisantrene administered weekly in patients with advanced renal cell carcinoma. *Proc. Am. Soc. Clin. Oncol.* **4**, 101.

Stadler, W.M., Vogelzang, N.J., Vokes, E.E., Charette, J., and Whitman, G. (1992). Continuous-infusion fluorodeoxyuridine with leucovorin and high-dose interferon: a phase II study in metastatic renal-cell cancer. *Cancer Chemother. Pharmacol.* **31** (3), 213–16.

Stadler, W.M., Rybak, M.E., and Vogelzang, N.J. (1995). A phase II study of subcutaneous recombinant human interleukin-4 in metastatic renal cell carcinoma. *Cancer* **76** (9), 1629–33.

Stadler, W.M., Kuzel, T., Dumas, M., and Vogelzang, N.J. (1998*a*). Multicenter phase II trial of interleukin-2, interferon-alpha, and 13-*cis*-retinoic acid in patients with metastatic renal cell carcinoma. *J. Clin. Oncol.* **16** (5), 1820–5.

Stadler, W.M., Vogelzang, N.J., Hoffman, P., *et al.* (1998*b*). CI-980 in renal cell and non-small cell lung cancer. *Cancer Therapeut.* **1** (5), 318–20.

Stadler, W.M., Kuzel, T., Shapiro, C., Sosman, J., Clark, J., and Vogelzang, N.J. (1999). Multi-institutional study of the angiogenesis inhibitor TNP-470 in metastatic renal carcinoma. *J. Clin. Oncol.* **17** (8), 2541–5.

Stahl, M., Schmoll, E., Becker, H., *et al.* (1991). Lonidamine versus high-dose tamoxifen in progressive, advanced renal cell carcinoma: results of an ongoing randomized phase II study. *Semin. Oncol.* **18** (2, suppl. 4), 33–7.

Stahl, M., Wilke, H., Schmoll, H.-J., *et al.* (1992). A phase II study of high dose tamoxifen in progressive, metastatic renal cell carcinoma. *Ann. Oncol.* **3** (2), 167–8.

Stephens, R.L., Kirby, R., Crawford, E.D., Bukowski, R., Rivkin, S.E., and O'Bryan, R.M. (1986). High dose AZQ in renal cancer: a Southwest Oncology Group phase II study. *Invest. New Drugs* **4** (1), 57–9.

Stephens, R.L., Goodman, P., Crawford, E.D., *et al.* (1990). Evaluation of menogaril in renal cell carcinoma: a Southwest Oncology Group phase II study (8504). *Invest. New Drugs* **8** (suppl. 1), S69–S71.

Sternberg, C.N., Yagoda, A., Casper, E., Scoppetuolo, M., and Scher, H.I. (1985). Phase II trial of elliptinium in advanced renal cell carcinoma and carcinoma of the breast. *Anticancer Res.* **5** (4), 415–17.

Sternberg, C.N., Yagoda, A., Scher, H.I., and Hollander, P. (1986). Phase II trial of *N*-methylformamide for advanced renal cell carcinoma. *Cancer Treat. Rep.* **70** (5), 681–2.

Sternberg, C.N., Yagoda, A., Scher, H., *et al.* (1989). Phase II trial of trimetrexate in patients with advanced renal cell carcinoma: Clinical Community Oncology Program. *Eur. J. Cancer Clin. Oncol.* **25** (4), 753–4.

Stewart, D.J., Futter, N., Irvine, A., Danjoux, C., and Moors, D. (1987). Mitomycin-C and metronidazole in the treatment of advanced renal-cell carcinoma. *Am. J. Clin. Oncol.* **10** (6), 520–2.

Stolbach, L.L., Begg, C.B., Hall, T., and Horton, J. (1981). Treatment of renal carcinoma: a phase III randomized trial of oral medroxyprogesterone (Provera), hydroxyurea, and nafoxidine. *Cancer Treat. Rep.* **65** (7–8), 689–92.

Strayer, D.R., Hubbell, H.R., Carter, W.A., *et al.* (1992). A phase I–II study of ampligen treatment of metastatic renal cell carcinoma: comparison of treatment with low dose versus high dose [abstract]. *Proc. Am. Soc. Clin. Oncol.* **11**, 210.

Strotter, H., Rude, E., and Wagner, H. (1980). T-cell factor (interleukin-2) allows *in vivo* induction of T helper cells against heterologous erythrocytes in athymic (*nu/nu*) mice. *Eur. J. Immunol.* **10**, 719–22.

Swanson, D.A. and Johnson, D.E. (1981). Estramustine phosphate (Emcyt) as treatment for metastatic renal carcinoma. *Urology* **17** (4), 344–6.

Tait, N., Abrams, J., Egorin, M.J., Cohen, A.E., Eisenberger, M., and Van Echo, D.A. (1988). Phase II carboplatin (CBDCA) for metastatic renal cell cancer with a standard dose (SD) and a calculated dose (CD) according to renal function [abstract]. *Proc. Am. Soc. Clin. Oncol.* **7**, 125.

Takahashi, A., Sasaki, H., Kim, S.J., *et al.* (1999). Identification of receptor genes in renal cell carcinoma associated with angiogenesis by differential hybridization technique. *Biochem. Biophys. Res. Commun.* **257** (3), 855–9.

Talley, R.W. (1973). Chemotherapy of adenocarcinoma of the kidney. *Cancer* **32** (5), 1062–5.

Talley, R.W., Moorhead, E.I., Tucker, W.G., San Diego, E.L., and Brennan, M.J. (1969). Treatment of metastatic hypernephroma. *J. Am. Med. Assoc.* **207** (2), 322–8.

Tannock, I.F. and Evans, W.K. (1985). Failure of 5-day vinblastine infusion in the treatment of patients with renal cell carcinoma. *Cancer Treat. Rep.* **69** (2), 227–8.

Taylor, S.A., Von Hoff, D.D., Baker, L.H., and Balcerzak, S.P. (1984). Phase II clinical trial of mitoxantrone in patients with advanced renal cell carcinoma: a Southwest Oncology Group study. *Cancer Treat. Rep.* **68** (6), 919–20.

Taylor, S.A., Goodman, P., Crawford, E.D., Stuckey, W.J., Stephens, R.L., and Gaynor, E.R. (1992). Phase II evaluation of didemnin B in advanced adenocarcinoma of the kidney: a Southwest Oncology Group study. *Invest. New Drugs* **10** (1), 55–6.

Thelen, P., Hemmerlein, B., Kugler, A., *et al.* (1999). Quantification by competitive quantitative RT-PCR of VEGF121 and VEGF165 in renal cell carcinoma. *Anticancer Res.* **19** (2C), 1563–5.

Thiebaut, F., Tsuruo, T., Hamada, H., Gottesman, M., Pastan, I., and Willingham, M. (1987). Cellular localization of the multidrug resistance gene product P-glycoprotein in normal human tissues. *Proc. Natl Acad. Sci., USA* **84**, 7735–8.

Tirelli, U., Frustaci, S., Galligioni, E., *et al.* (1980). Medical treatment of metastatic renal cell carcinoma. *Tumori* **66** (2), 235–40.

Todd, R.F. III, Garnick, M.B., Canellos, G.P., *et al.* (1981). Phase I–II trial of methyl-GAG in the treatment of patients with metastatic renal adenocarcinoma. *Cancer Treat. Rep.* **65** (1–2), 17–20.

Tomisawa, M., Tokunaga, T., Oshika, Y., *et al.* (1999). Expression pattern of vascular endothelial growth factor isoform is closely correlated with tumour stage and vascularisation in renal cell carcinoma. *Eur. J. Cancer* **35** (1), 133–7.

Tourani, J.M., Pfister, C., Berdah, J.F., *et al.* (1998). Outpatient treatment with subcutaneous interleukin-2 and interferon alfa administration in combination with fluorouracil in patients with metastatic renal cell carcinoma: results of a sequential nonrandomized phase II study. Subcutaneous Administration Propeukin Program Cooperative Group. *J. Clin. Oncol.* **16** (7), 2505–13.

Trump, D.L. and Elson, P. (1990). Evaluation of carboplatin (NSC 241240) in patients with recurrent or metastatic renal cell carcinoma. *Invest. New Drugs* **8** (2), 201–3.

Trump, D.L., Ravdin, P.M., Borden, E.C., Magers, C.F., and Whisnant, J.K. (1990). Interferon-alpha and continuous infusion vinblastine for the treatment of advanced renal cell carcinoma. *J. Biol. Resp. Mod.* **9** (1), 108–11.

Tsuruo, T., Iida, H., Tsukagoshi, S., and Sakurai, Y. (1982). Increased accumulation of vincristine and adriamycin in drug resistant P388 tumor cells following incubation with calcium antagonists and calmodulin inhibitors. *Cancer Res.* **42**, 4730–3.

Tsuruo, T., Iida, H., Kitatani, Y., Yokota, K., Tsukagoshi, S., and Sakurai, Y. (1984). Effects of quinidine and related compounds on cytotoxicity and cellular accumulation of vincristine and adriamycin in drug-resistant tumor cells. *Cancer Res.* **44**, 4303–7.

Twentyman, P., Fox, N., and White, D. (1987). Cyclosporin A and its analogues as modifiers of adriamycin and vincristine resistance in a multidrug resistant human lung cancer cell line. *Br. J. Cancer* **56**, 55–7.

Vallis, K., Philip, P., Rockett, H., *et al.* (1994). Multidrug resistance reversal with toremifine in renal cell cancer [abstract]. *Proc. Am. Soc. Clin. Oncol.* **69**, 23.

Van Echo, D.A., Markus, S., Aisner, J., and Wiernik, P.H. (1980). Phase II trial of 4′-(9-acridinylamino)methanesulfon-m-aniside (AMSA) in patients with metastatic renal cell carcinoma. *Cancer Treat. Rep.* **64** (8–9), 1009–10.

van Oosterom, A.T., Fossa, S.D., Pizzocaro, G., *et al.* (1984). Mitoxantrone in advanced renal cancer: a phase II study in previously untreated patients from the EORTC Genito-Urinary Tract Cancer Cooperative Group. *Eur. J. Cancer Clin. Oncol.* **20** (10), 1239–41.

van Oosterom, A.T., Bono, A.V., Kaye, S.B., *et al.* (1986). 4′Deoxydoxorubicin in advanced renal cancer: a phase II study in previously untreated patients from the EORTC Genito-Urinary Tract Cancer Cooperative Group [letter]. *Eur. J. Cancer Clin. Oncol.* **22** (12), 1531–2.

van Oosterom, A.T., Stoter, G., Bono, A.V., *et al.* (1989*a*). Mitozolomide in advanced renal cancer: a phase II study in previously untreated patients from the EORTC Genito-Urinary Tract Cancer Cooperative Group. *Eur. J. Cancer Clin. Oncol.* **25** (8), 1249–50.

van Oosterom, A.T., Droz, J.P., Fossa, S.T., *et al.* (1989*b*). TCNU in advanced renal cancer: phase II study in previously untreated patients from the EORTC Genito-Urinary Tract Cancer Cooperative Group. *Eur. J. Cancer Clin. Oncol.* **25** (12), 1889–90.

Venner, P., Eisenhauer, E.A., Wierzbicki, R., and Johnston, J. (1991). Phase II study of 2′-deoxycoformycin in patients with renal cell carcinoma. A National Cancer Institute of Canada Clinical Trials Group study. *Invest. New Drugs* **9** (3), 273–5.

Vogelzang, N.J., Mani, S., Schilsky, R.L., *et al.* (1998). Phase II and pharmaco-dynamic studies of pyrazine diazohydroxide (NSC 361456) in patients with advanced renal and colorectal cancer. *Clin. Cancer Res.* **4**, 929–34.

Vugrin, D., Einhorn, L.H., and Birch, R. (1987). Phase II trial of gallium nitrate in patients with metastatic renal cell carcinoma [abstract]. *Proc. Am. Soc. Clin. Oncol.* **28**, 203.

Wada, T., Houjou, T., Kubo, R., Yasutomi, M., and Kurita, T. (1993). A combined chemo-endocrine treatment with tegafur, adriamycin, methotrexate and tamoxifen for advanced renal cell carcinoma. *Anticancer Res.* **13**, 2465–8.

Wada, T., Nishiyama, K., Maeda, M., *et al.* (1995). Combined chemoendocrine treatment with tegafur and tamoxifen for advanced renal cell carcinoma. *Anticancer Res.* **15**, 1581–4.

Wagle, D.G. and Murphy, G.P. (1971). Hormonal therapy in advanced renal cell carcinoma. *Cancer* **28** (2), 318–21.

Wagner, H., Hardt, C., Heeg, K., *et al.* (1980). T-cell derived helper factor allows *in vivo* induction of cytotoxic T cells in *nu/nu* mice. *Nature* **284**, 278–80.

Wagner, H., Possinger, K., Bremer, K., Donhujsen-Ant, R., Peukert, M., and Queisser, W. (1987). Phase II trials of 1,2,4-triglycidylurazol in patients with metastasized renal cell carcinoma. *Cancer Treat. Rep.* **71** (2), 209–10.

Wajsman, Z., Beckley, S., and Madajewicz, S. (1980). High dose cyclophosphamide in metastatic renal cell cancer [abstract]. *Proc. Am. Soc. Clin. Oncol.* **21**, 423.

Wechsel, H.W., Bichler, K.H., Feil, G., Loeser, W., Lahme, S., and Petri, E. (1999). Renal cell carcinoma: relevance of angiogenetic factors. *Anticancer Res.* **19** (2C), 1537–40.

Weinerman, B.H., Eisenhauer, E.A., Besner, J.G., Coppin, C.M., Stewart, D., and Band, P.R. (1986). Phase II study of lonidamine in patients with metastatic renal cell carcinoma: a National Cancer Institute of Canada Clinical Trials Group Study. *Cancer Treat. Rep.* **70** (6), 751–4.

Weinerman, B., Eisenhauer, E., Stewart, D., *et al.* (1992). Phase II study of sulofenur (LY186641) in measurable metastatic renal cancer. *Ann. Oncol.* **3** (1), 83–4.

Weiselberg, L., Budman, D., Vinciguerra, V., Schulman, P., and Degnan, T.J. (1981). Tamoxifen in unresectable hypernephroma: a phase II trial and review of the literature. *Cancer Clin. Trial* **4** (2), 195–8.

Werf-Messing, B. and Gilse, H.A. (1971). Hormonal treatment of metastases of renal carcinoma. *Br. J. Cancer* **25** (3), 423–7.

Wilding, G., Kirkwood, J., Clamon, G., *et al.* (1993). Phase II trial of navelbine in metastatic renal cancer [abstract]. *Proc. Am. Soc. Clin. Oncol.* **12**, 253.

Wilkinson, M.J., Frye, J.W., Small, E.J., *et al.* (1993). A phase II study of constant-infusion floxuridine for the treatment of metastatic renal cell carcinoma. *Cancer* **71** (11), 3601–4.

Witte, R.S., Walsh, C., Fisher, H., Okem, M.M., Reding, D.J., and Trump, D.L. (1992*a*). Evaluation of deoxycoformycin in patients with advanced renal cell carcinoma. An ECOG pilot study. *Invest. New Drugs* **10** (1), 49–50.

Witte, R.S., Elson, P., Bryan, G.T., and Trump, D.L. (1992*b*). Trimetrexate in advanced renal cell carcinoma: an ECOG phase II trial. *Invest. New Drugs* **10** (1), 51–4.

Witte, R.S., Hsieh, P., Elson, P., Oken, M.M., and Trump, D.L. (1996). A phase II trial of amonafide, caracemide, and homoharringtonine in the treatment of patients with advanced renal cell carcinoma. *Invest. New Drugs* **14** (4), 409–13.

Wong, P.P., Yagoda, A., Currie, V.E., and Young, C.W. (1977). Phase II study of vindesine sulfate in the therapy for advanced renal carcinoma. *Cancer Treat. Rep.* **61** (9), 1727–9.

Wos, E., Olencki, T., Tuason, L., *et al.* (1996). Phase II trial of subcutaneously administered granulocyte–macrophage colony-stimulating factor in patients with metastatic renal cell carcinoma. *Cancer* **77** (6), 1149–53.

Yagoda, A., Abi-Rached, B., and Petrylak, D. (1995). Chemotherapy for advanced renal-cell carcinoma: 1983–1993. *Sem. Oncol.* **22** (1), 42–60.

Yamamoto, J.K., Farrar, W.L., and Johnson, H.M. (1982). Interleukin 2 regulation of mitogen induction of immune interferon (IFN gamma) in spleen cells and thymocytes. *Cell Immunol.* **66**, 333–41.

Yu, D.-S., Chang, S.-Y., and Ma, C.-P. (1998). The expression of mdr-1-related gp-170 and its correlation with anthracycline resistance in renal cell carcinoma cell lines and multidrug-resistant sublines. *Br. J. Urol.* **82**, 544–7.

Zamora, J., Pearce, H., and Beck, W. (1988). Physical–chemical properties shared by compounds that modulate multidrug resistance in human leukemic cells. *Mol. Pharmacol.* **33**, 454–62.

Zaniboni, A., Simoncini, E., Marpicati, P., Montini, E., Ferrari, V., and Marini. G. (1989). Phase II trial of 5-fluorouracil and high-dose folinic acid in advanced renal cell cancer. *J. Chemother.* **1** (5), 350–1.

Zeffren, J., Yagoda, A., Watson, R.C., *et al.* (1981). Phase II trial of methylgloxal bis-guanylhydrazone in advanced renal cancer. *Cancer Treat. Rep.* **65** (5–6), 525–7.

Zeffren, J., Yagoda, A., Kelsen, D., and Winn, R. (1984). Phase I–II trial of a 5-day continuous infusion of vinblastine sulfate. *Anticancer Res.* **4** (6), 411–13.

39.   Interferon for renal cell carcinoma

Eric J. Small and Robert J. Motzer

Introduction

The outlook for patients with metastatic renal cell carcinoma (RCC) is poor. Overall survival for patients presenting with metastatic disease has not changed in the last decade, with less than 10 per cent of patients surviving 5 years after diagnosis (Motzer *et al.* 1996). RCC is largely resistant to chemotherapy. Only the fluoropyrimidines have modest antitumor activity (Yagoda *et al.* 1983). Immunologic manipulations clearly play an important role in the systemic therapy of RCC, and the use of interferons is one of the cornerstones of immunologic therapy for RCC.

The interferons were first described by Isaacs and Lindenaman in 1957. These cytokines were named for their ability to mediate viral interference, where one virus interferes with replication of a second (Pfeffer and Donner 1990). In addition to antiviral activity, interferons modulate immune response and cell proliferation. Many cells have the capacity to produce these proteins, which may function as local paracrine and autocrine factors in influencing cell growth and function.

More than 20 homologous interferons have been identified. These are divided into distinct antigen subtypes according to differences in antigenic, biologic, and chemical properties. Three subtypes (α, β, γ) have been described and characterized in humans; all are commercially available. Interferon α (IFNα) and interferon β (IFNβ) are encoded on chromosome 9, share homology, and are collectively referred to as type I interferons. Interferon γ (IFNγ) is encoded on chromosome 12, is dissimilar to the other two interferons in structure, binds to a distinct cell membrane receptor, and is referred to as type II.

Lymphocytes and macrophages produce IFNα, whereas fibroblasts and mesenchymal cells produce IFNβ. Both IFNα and IFNβ are produced and secreted in response to viruses, double-stranded RNA, or other inducers. IFNγ is produced by T lymphocytes and, to a lesser extent, by natural killer (NK) cells. IFNγ is induced during activation of lymphocytes, and has greater immuno-modulatory but less antiviral properties than the type I interferons. In fact, activated T cells can be classified functionally by whether IFNγ is produced (T helper (Th)1 cell type) or interleukins (IL) IL-4 and IL-10 are produced (Th2 cell type).

Potential mechanisms for antitumor effects of interferons include enhanced tumor immunogenicity, decreased virulence, inhibition of angiogenesis, and inducement of immune response.

Activities on the immune system include stimulation of cytotoxic T lymphocytes (CTL) capable of recognizing and lysing foreign cells based on major histocompatibility complex (MHC) class I antigens, upregulation of MHC antigens, and augmentation of antibody-dependent cellular cytotoxicity. Interferons act as positive and negative regulators of NK cells and modify the susceptibility of target cells to lysis. IFNγ, in particular, is a potent regulator of macrophage activity.

Interferons, and in particular IFNα, have direct effects on tumor cells and surrounding tissues. Antiproliferative effect has been correlated to degree of downregulation of the interferon receptor following interaction with the ligand *in vitro* (Pfeffer and Donner 1990) and *in vivo* (Bartsch *et al.* 1989). The inhibitory effect is not specific to one phase of the cell cycle, but cells in G_0 have been observed to be the most sensitive (Sreevalsan 1995). Antiproliferative effects on endothelial cells and fibroblasts may contribute to anti-angiogenic properties, and are evidenced by the successful treatment of hemangiomas with IFNα (Ezekowitz *et al.* 1992).

Interferons also appear to have the capacity of affecting cellular differentiation. This property may contribute to the therapeutic efficacy of IFNα against hairy cell leukemia (Grossberg and Taylor 1985). Interferon genes and interferon-induced genes have been shown *in vitro* to demonstrate tumor suppressor properties, and are considered a class of tumor suppressor genes (Lengyel 1993). In summary, interferons have a broad range of effects that could potentially induce clinical responses in patients with RCC. The precise mechanism(s) responsible for clinical response against RCC has not been defined, but almost certainly includes cellular immunologic effects as well as possibly more directly cytotoxic effects.

Response assessment in renal cell carcinoma

For virtually any agent used for the treatment of RCC, it is important to recognize that a variety of pretreatment variables may impact significantly on clinical outcomes (including response proportion). Consequently, an overview of the literature such as this one should be cautiously interpreted. Implicit in the reports summarized is a wide variability in inclusion criteria and pretreatment risk factors.

For example, longer survival following treatment with IFNα has been associated with high performance status, prior nephrectomy, long disease-free interval between initial diagnosis and relapse, and lung-predominant metastases (Minasian *et al.* 1993; Fossa *et al.* 1992). A reasonably high response proportion of 30 per cent has been reported for patients with prior nephrectomy and lung-only metastasis (Neidhart *et al.* 1991). However, others have found pretreatment features to be less predictive of response, and suggest a 2-month trial of therapy to identify patients who will experience tumor reduction (Fossa *et al.* 1990). An overview of series with more than 100 patients each summarizing pretreatment prognostic variables in patients with metastatic RCC has been reported (Small *et al.* 1998). Features most commonly predictive of increased survival included performance status, prior nephrectomy, and metastasis-free interval. Some series also found the number of metastatic sites, pulmonary versus extrapulmonary disease, hemoglobin (Hgb), and lactate dehydrogenase (LDH) to be significant.

More recently, the relationship between pretreatment clinical features and survival in 670 patients with advanced RCC treated in 24 Memorial Sloan–Kettering Cancer Center clinical trials of immunotherapy and chemotherapy between 1975 and 1996 was reported (Motzer *et al.* 1999*a*). This included 328 patients treated with IFNα. The median overall survival time was 10 months. Fifty-seven (8 per cent) of 670 patients remained alive and the median follow-up time for the survivors was 33 months. The proportion of patients surviving at 1 year was 42 per cent; the 2- and 3-year survival proportions were 20 and 11 per cent, respectively. Survival was greater for patients treated with immunotherapy versus chemotherapy.

In a multivariate analysis, pretreatment features associated with a shorter survival were low Karnofsky performance status (< 80 per cent), high lactate dehydrogenase (> 1.5 upper limit of normal), low hemoglobin (< lower limit of normal), high corrected serum calcium (> 10 mg/dl), and absence of nephrectomy. These prognostic factors were used to categorize patients by risk into three different groups. The median time to death in the 25 per cent of patients with zero risk factors (favorable risk) was 20 months. Fifty-three per cent of the patients had one or two of these prognostic features (intermediate risk), and the median survival in this group was 10 months. Patients with three or more risk factors (poor risk), comprising 22 per cent of the patients, had a median survival of 4 months.

Monotherapy with interferon

IFNα

Antitumor activity of interferon against RCC was initially reported in 1983, using partially purified human IFNα preparation, or a partially purified lymphoblastoid IFN. Response proportions in the 10 to 20 per cent range were reported (Quesada *et al.* 1983; deKernion *et al.* 1983; Neidhart *et al.* 1984). Subsequently, recombinant technology has resulted in the development of highly purified preparations that can be produced in bulk quantities.

Two preparations, recombinant IFNα-2a (Roferon®, Hoffman LaRoche), and recombinant IFNα -2b (Intron®, Schering Plough Laboratories) are commercially available, and have been extens-

Table 39.1 Results with recombinant IFNα

Reference	N[†]	Dose ($\times 10^6$ IU), schedule[◊]	IFNα type	Number of*[ ]		
				CR	PR	CR + PR (%)
Minassian *et al.* 1993	39	50, 3× weekly IM	2a	0	7	18
Minassian *et al.* 1993	59	3 to 36, QD IM	2a	2	5	11
Quesada *et al.* 1985	41	20/m², daily IM	2a	1	11	29
	15	2/m², daily IM	2a	0	0	0
Umeda and Niijima 1986	108	3 to 36/m², QD IM	2a	2	13	14
Schnall *et al.* 1986	22	3 to 36 QD IM	2a	0	1	5
Kempf *et al.* 1999	10	2/m², 3× weekly SC	2a	0	0	0
Kempf *et al.* 1999	10	30/m², 3× weekly IV	2a	0	1	10
Fossa 1988	17	18 to 36/m², 3× weekly IM	2a	0	2	11
Foon *et al.* 1988	21	2/m², SQ 3× weekly	2b	0	1	5
Steineck *et al.* 1990	30	10 to 20/m², 3× weekly IM	2a	1	1	6
Marshall *et al.* 1989	17	1, QD SC	2a	0	4	24
Umeda and Niijima 1986	45	3 to 36, QD IM	2b	1	7	18
Muss *et al.* 1987	46	30 to 50/m², 5× weekly Q 3 weeks IV	2b	1	2	7
Muss *et al.* 1987	51	2–10/m², 3× weekly SC	2b	1	4	10
Levens *et al.* 1989	15	10, QD SC	2b	1	3	27
Bono *et al.* 1991	61	3/m², 3× weekly SC	2b	2	3	8
Buzaid *et al.* 1987	22	3 to 36, IM QD	2a	0	5	23
Figlin *et al.* 1988	19	3 to 36, IM QD 5 days/wk	2a	1	4	26

* CR, complete response; PR, partial response.

[†] N, number of evaluable patients.

[◊] IM, intramuscular; SC, subcutaneous; IV, intravenous; QD, every day; SQ, ; Q, every.

Table 39.2 Randomized trials evaluating effect of IFNα on survival in patients with metastatic RCC

Reference	Treatment	N	Response (%)	Median survival (months)	Survival benefit? (p value)
Steineck et al. 1990	IFNα vs.	30	6	7	No (not given)
	Medroxyprogesterone	30	3	7	
Kriegmar et al. 1998	IFNα + vinblastine vs.	41	35	16	No (0.19)
	Medroxyprogesterone	35	0	10	
Pyrhonen et al. 1996	IFNα + vinblastine vs.	79	16	17	Yes (0.0049)
	Vinblastine	81	2	10	
Ritchie et al. 1998	IFNα vs.	167	16	8.5	Yes (0.011)
	Medroxyprogesterone	168	2	6	

ively evaluated in patients with metastatic RCC (Table 39.1). There is no immediately apparent difference in efficacy between the two preparations, although direct comparisons have not been undertaken. Response proportions range between 0 and 30 per cent, and the overall response proportion is 14.5 per cent (95 per cent confidence interval (CI); 12–17 per cent: 13 complete and 81 partial responses) in 648 patients (Minasian *et al.* 1993; Quesada *et al.* 1985; Umeda and Niijima 1986; Schnall *et al.* 1986; Kempf *et al.* 1999; Fossa 1988; Foon *et al.* 1988; Steineck *et al.* 1990; Marshall *et al.* 1989; Muss *et al.* 1987; Levens *et al.* 1989; Bono *et al.* 1991).

Efforts to define the optimal dose of IFNα have taken the form of both randomized trials and retrospective analyses. One randomized trial compared treatment with 2 MU/m^2 to treatment with 20 MU/m^2 (Quesada *et al.* 1985). None of 15 patients responded to the lower dose and this arm of the trial was closed, while the higher dose yielded a response proportion of 29 per cent (Quesada *et al.* 1985). A second trial compared IFNα dosed from 2 MU/m^2 subcutaneously (SC) escalated to 10 MU/m^2 SC versus 30 MU/m^2 intravenously (IV) and was unable to demonstrate any difference in response proportion (Muss *et al.* 1987). However, the higher dose clearly resulted in excessive toxicity requiring frequent dose attenuation.

Retrospective analyses have categorized IFNα regimens on the basis of the dose utilized; for example, low dose (less than 5 MU/day), intermediate dose (5–20 MU/day), and high dose (> 20 MU/day) (Krown 1987). One retrospective analysis (Wirth 1993) reported higher response proportions in patients treated at the medium dose (5–20 MU/day), while a second (Savage and Muss 1995) found the highest response proportions in patients treated at between 5 and 10 MU/day. It is likely that significant attenuation of dosing in the high-dose regimens was required because of toxicity, and this may have accounted for lower response proportions in these groups. Since toxicity is dose-dependent, a dose of between 5 and 10 MU three to five times a week could be considered optimal.

The mean time to objective response is 3 to 4 months and most responses are evident following 2 months of therapy. However, the response can be characterized by a slow regression of tumor masses, with criteria for a partial response not being met as long as 12 months after initiation of therapy. The median response duration is approximately 6 months and rarely exceeds 2 years (Savage and Muss 1995). However, long-term survivors following treatment with IFNα have, rarely, been reported (Minasian *et al.* 1993).

Four randomized trials have compared IFNα with either medroxyprogesterone or vinblastine (Table 39.2). Two trials (Steineck *et al.* 1990; Kriegmar *et al.* 1998) failed to show a survival benefit, but both were comprised of a small number of patients, and one study design included a provision for cross-over to interferon (Steineck *et al.* 1990). The two larger, more recent randomized trials reported a small but significant improvement in survival with IFNα therapy (Pyrhonen *et al.* 1996; Ritchie *et al.* 1998). In one, IFNα was compared to medroxyprogesterone and resulted in an improvement in median survival of 3 months (Ritchie *et al.* 1998). In the other, IFNα plus vinblastine was compared to vinblastine alone, and the combination showed a benefit in median survival of 6 months for IFNα therapy (Pyrhonen *et al.* 1996). The addition of vinblastine to IFNα has not been shown to improve survival compared to IFNα alone (Minasian *et al.* 1993; Neidhart *et al.* 1991; Fossa *et al.* 1992) and many trials of vinblastine have failed to demonstrate single-agent activity in RCC (Yagoda *et al.* 1983). Therefore, the improvement in survival in the interferon/vinblastine versus vinblastine trial can be attributed to treatment with IFNα. While these two studies suggested a survival benefit, the response proportion observed with IFNα monotherapy remains low, and long-term survival is rare. Moreover, the impact of interferon on quality of life needs to be investigated.

IFNβ

IFNβ and IFNγ have been evaluated in phase II trials (Tables 39.3 and 39.4). The overall response to IFNβ was 11 per cent in four small trials comprising a total of 71 patients (Rinehart *et al.* 1987a; Kish *et al.* 1986; Nelson *et al.* 1989; Kinney *et al.* 1990). Since three of these four trials had minimal response proportions

Table 39.3 Results with recombinant human IFNβ treatment for RCC

		Number of*		
Source	N[†]	CR	PR	CR + PR (%)
Rinehart et al. 1987a	15	0	2	13
Kish et al. 1986	16	0	1	6
Nelson et al. 1989	15	0	0	0
Kinney et al. 1990	25	1	4	20

* PR, partial response; CR, complete response.
[†] N, number of evaluable patients.

Table 39.4 Results with IFNγ treatment for RCC

Reference	N[†]	Dose ($\times$ 10^6 IU), schedule[◊]	Number of*		
			CR	PR	CR + PR (%)
Quesada et al. 1987	14	5 to 20/m^2, IM	0	1	7
Quesada et al. 1987	16	0.2 to 1/m^2, IV	0	1	6
Koiso 1987	32	8 to 12/m^2, QD IV or IM	0	2	6
Koiso 1987	39	40, IV	1	5	20
Machida et al. 1987	32	8–12/m^2, IV or IM QD	0	2	6
Machida et al. 1987	30	40/m^2, IV QD ×5, Q 2 wks	1	5	20
Rinehart et al. 1987b	13	0.01 to 75/m^2, IV twice weekly	0	0	0
Garnick et al. 1988	41	0.2 to 60/m^2, IV QD	1	3	10
Kuebler et al. 1989	27	0.25/m^2, CIV QD Q 4 wks	0	0	0
Aulitzky et al. 1989	20	2, SC tiw, Q 2 weeks	2	4	30
Grups and Frohmuller 1989	9	5, IM QD 8×, Q 4 wks	0	3	33
Bruntsch et al. 1999	40	2/m^2, IV tiw, Q 2 wks	0	1	2
Foon et al. 1988	21	1/m^2, SC 3×/wk	0	1	5
Ellerhorst et al. 1994	34	100 μg, SC weekly	1	3	15
Small et al. 1998	202	60 μg/m^2, SC weekly	3	3	3
Gleave et al. 1998	91	60 μg/m^2, SC weekly	3	1	4

* CR, complete response; PR, partial response.

[†] N, number of evaluable patients.

[◊] IM, intramuscular; SC, subcutaneous; IV, intravenous; CIV, continuous intravenous; QD, every day; Q, every; tiw, twice weekly.

(0, 6, and 13 per cent), there has been limited interest in further evaluation of this agent.

IFNγ

IFNγ was more extensively investigated, with a response range of 0 to 30 per cent in 15 trials including a total of 570 patients (Small *et al.* 1998; Quesada *et al.* 1987; Koiso 1987; Machida *et al.* 1987; Rinehart *et al.* 1987b; Garnick *et al.* 1988; Kuebler *et al.* 1989; Aulitzky *et al.* 1989; Grups and Frohmuller 1989; Bruntsch *et al.* 1999; Foon *et al.* 1988; Ellerhorst *et al.* 1994). Interest in IFNγ was generated by two reports showing responses of 15 and 30 per cent, respectively (Aulitzky *et al.* 1989; Ellerhorst *et al.* 1994). These earlier studies had defined the optimal IFNγ dose utilizing biological endpoints, (β_2 microglobulin and neopterin levels) and had reached the conclusion that the optimal IFNγ dose was not the maximum tolerated dose, but rather a lower 'biologically active' dose. This dose (60 μg/m^2) was the dose used in both a large multicenter phase II study and a placebo-controlled phase III study (Small *et al.* 1998; Gleave *et al.* 1998). Eligibility for the multicenter, phase II trial required prior nephrectomy or tumor embolization. The response proportion in 202 patients was a disappointing 3 per cent and median survival was 13.4 months (range: 5.5–29.2+ months) (Small *et al.* 1998).

A subsequent randomized trial compared IFNγ to placebo injections in 197 patients with advanced RCC. The response to placebo was 7 per cent compared to 4 per cent in the group treated with IFNγ ΣGleave *et al.* 1998). Although there are issues with how responses were assessed in this study (for example, the use of chest X-rays to assess pulmonary disease), these are nevertheless startling data, as they suggest that a full 7 per cent of

responses reported in other series could potentially represent 'background' noise, that is, placebo effect or spontaneous remissions. There was no significant difference in median time to progression (1.9 months for both groups) or in median survival (12 months with IFNγ, 16 months with placebo) (Gleave *et al.* 1998). The results of this study and the low response proportion in the multicenter phase II trial of 3 per cent in 202 patients (Small *et al.* 1998) indicate that IFNγ has no role as single-agent therapy in the treatment of metastatic RCC.

Interferon as part of combination therapy programs

As previously noted, the combination of IFNα plus vinblastine showed a high response proportion in several single-arm phase II trials. However, randomized trials failed to show improved survival in the combination arms compared with IFNα alone, and the addition of vinblastine to interferon contributed gastrointestinal and hematologic toxicity (Fossa *et al.* 1992; Neidhart *et al.* 1991).

The combination of IFNα plus interleukin-2 (IL-2) was supported by preclinical studies that suggested a synergistic interaction. A large number of regimens have studied this combination, with wide variation in doses, schedules, and routes of administration. A review of 607 patients treated with IFNα plus IL-2 on 23 clinical trials showed a 19 per cent response, similar to that achieved with IL-2 alone (Vogelzang *et al.* 1993). The toxicities of these two agents in combination were additive, and a therapeutic benefit for the combination compared to IL-2 alone was not immediately apparent.

A randomized phase II trial of high-dose IL-2 with IFNα versus high-dose IL-2 alone showed no difference in response proportion (Atkins *et al.* 1993). Moreover, in this randomized trial, increased toxicity was seen with the addition of IFNα to IL-2. A second randomized trial (the French CRECY trial) reported a higher response proportion for the combination of IL-2 plus IFNα compared to either agent given alone (Negrier *et al.* 1998). However, there was no benefit in survival associated with the combination therapy compared to interferon or IL-2 monotherapy, and the toxicity was more severe. It is not entirely clear why the higher response proportion in the combination arm did not translate into a survival advantage, although the effect of cross-over cannot be excluded.

Combination therapy with 5-fluorouracil (5-FU)/interferon, with/without IL-2, has been given in various schedules as in- and out-patient therapy. In several of these regimens, high responses of between 30 and 40 per cent were reported (Hanninen *et al.* 1996; Ellerhorst *et al.* 1997; Kirchner *et al.* 1998). However, the same combination studied by others has shown a response rate of less than 20 per cent, characterized by a relatively short duration of response and formidable toxicity (Dutcher *et al.* 1997; Olencki *et al.* 1996; Tourani *et al.* 1998; Ravaud *et al.* 1998). The three-drug 5-FU-containing combination is currently being compared to interferon plus IL-2 in two randomized phase III trials underway in Europe. Preliminary results from one showed no improvement in response to the combination of interferon, IL-2 plus 5-FU compared to interferon plus IL-2 (Negrier *et al.* 1997). In this trial, the response to the three-drug regimen was 8 per cent. Inclusion of 5-FU with IFNα and IL-2 contributes toxicity, and a conclusive statement on efficacy awaits further study in randomized trials.

Several series have investigated the combination of a 5-FU derivative, floxuridine (FUDR), with IFNα. While single-institution series have reported response rates as high as 33 per cent (Reese *et al.* 1999; Falcone *et al.* 1996), survival does not seem to be appreciably affected and other studies of this combination have reported negligible activity (Sori *et al.* 1999). Definite conclusions as to the efficacy of this regimen cannot be made without a randomized trial. Similarly, results of phase II trials suggested that retinoids augmented the antitumor effect of IFNα against RCC (Motzer *et al.* 1995; Paule *et al.* 1997; Stadler *et al.* 1996; Atzpodien *et al.* 1996). However, a recently completed phase III trial failed to show a benefit for the combination compared to IFNα alone (Motzer *et al.* 1999*b*). In summary, to date there has been no sufficiently powered randomized phase III trial showing a survival benefit for combination therapy compared to single-agent interferon (Table 39.5). The promise shown in any number of phase II trials has yet to be realized in the form of prolonged survival and emphasizes the necessity for phase III trials to prove efficacy of novel treatment programs.

Second-line therapy

A recent trial addressed the potential role for treatment with IFNα in patients with advanced RCC following progression to treatment with IL-2 (Escudier *et al.* 1999). Patients were selected from the CRECY trial, a randomized comparison of IFNα, IL-2, or combination therapy (Negrier *et al.* 1998). Forty-eight patients were treated with IFNα as salvage therapy following treatment with IL-2. A single patient achieved a partial response (2 per cent) of 18 months duration, with toxicity similar to that observed in first-line treatment (Escudier *et al.* 1999). The authors concluded that monotherapy with IFNα after failure of IL-2 is not effective therapy in patients with advanced RCC. Conversely, in the same report, the use of IL-2 following front-line therapy with IFNα in 65 patients yielded a partial response in only 3 patients (4.6 per cent).

Adjuvant therapy

Twenty to 30 per cent of patients with completely resected RCC relapse after a radical nephrectomy. Predictors of relapse include renal vein involvement and nodal involvement (Sandock *et al.* 1995; Rabinovitch *et al.* 1994; Levy *et al.* 1998). IFNα given as adjuvant therapy following complete resection of RCC with renal vein or nodal involvement has been compared to observation in three randomized trials (Trump *et al.* 1996; Porzsolt 1992; Pizzocaro *et al.* 1997). None showed a delay in time to relapse or overall survival, although these trials were underpowered to detect anything but a very large impact on survival. A phase II trial of IL-2 given as adjuvant therapy is underway but no results have been reported. Therefore, outside of a clinical trial, standard care remains observation following nephrectomy, since no recognized systemic therapy reduces the likelihood of relapse.

Future directions

Metastatic RCC remains a disease highly resistant to systemic therapy. Small numbers of patients exhibit complete or partial

Table 39.5 Phase III trials of interferon monotherapy against interferon combination programs

Reference	Treatment	N	Survival benefit for combination?
Fossa *et al.* 1992	IFNα vs. IFNα + vinblastine	178	No
Neidhart *et al.* 1991	IFNα vs. IFNα + vinblastine	165	No
Negrier *et al.* 1998	IFNα vs. IL-2 vs. IFN + IL-2	425	No
Motzer *et al.* 1999*b*	IFNα vs. IFNα + 13-*cis*-retinoic acid	283	No
Sagaster *et al.* 1995	IFN vs. IFNα + coumarin and cimetidine	148	No
DeMulder *et al.* 1995	IFNα vs. IFNα + IFNγ	102	No
Creagan *et al.* 1991	IFNα vs. IFNα + aspirin	176	No

responses to interferon and/or IL-2, but most patients do not respond and there are few long-term survivors. Therefore, the identification of new agents with better antitumor activity against metastases remains the highest priority of clinical investigation in this refractory tumor. Efforts of continued investigation for interferon focus on studies of combination therapy. As noted, randomized trials are under way to assess the relative efficacy of IFNα in combination with IL-2 and 5-FU, and it is possible that novel agents in combination with IFNα will demonstrate increased activity. Second-generation IFNα compounds are currently in clinical trials as well. For example, polyethylene glycol conjugated to IFNα (pegylated IFNα) is currently being studied. The prolonged half-life of elimination associated with pegylated IFNα-2a allows for weekly administration, which may represent an advantage over the more frequent administration required for currently available preparations. The relative efficacy and toxicity compared to standard recombinant preparations is being investigated.

References

Atkins, M.B., Sparano, J., Fisher, R.I., *et al.* (1993). Randomized phase II trial of high-dose interleukin-2 either alone or in combination with interferon alfa-2b in advanced renal cell carcinoma. *J. Clin. Oncol.* **11**, 661–70.

Atzpodien, J., Buer, J., Probst, M., *et al.* (1996). Clinical and pre-clinical role of 13-*cis*-retinoic acid in renal cell carcinoma: Hannover experience. *Proc. Am. Soc. Clin. Oncol.* **15**, 247.

Aulitzky, W., Gastl, G., Aulitzky, W.E., *et al.* (1989). Successful treatment of metastatic renal cell carcinoma with a biologically active dose of recombinant interferon-gamma. *J. Clin. Oncol.* **7**, 1875–84.

Bartsch, H.H., Pfizenmaier, K., Hamusch, A., *et al.* (1989). Sequential therapy with recombinant interferon gamma and alpha in patients with unfavorable prognosis of chronic myelocytic leukemia: clinical responsiveness to recombinant IFN-alpha correlates with the degree of receptor down-regulation. *Int. J. Cancer* **43**, 235–40.

Bono, A.V., Reali, L., Benvenuti, C., *et al.* (1991). Recombinant alpha interferon in metastatic renal cell carcinoma. *Urology* **38**, 60–3.

Bruntsch, U., de Mulder, P.H., ten Bokkel Huinink, W.W., *et al.* (1999). Phase II study of recombinant human interferon-gamma in metastatic renal cell carcinoma. *J. Biol. Resp. Mod.* **9**, 335–8.

Buzaid, A.C., Robertone, A., Kisala, C., *et al.* (1987). Phase II study of interferon alfa-2a, recombinant (Roferon-A) in metastatic renal cell carcinoma. *J. Clin. Oncol.* **5**, 1083–9.

Creagan, E.T., Twito, D.I., Johansson, S.L., *et al.* (1991). A randomized prospective assessment of recombinant leukocyte A human interferon with or without aspirin in advanced renal adenocarcinoma. *J. Clin. Oncol.* **9**, 2104–9.

deKernion, J.B., Sarna, J.B., Figlin, R., *et al.* (1983). The treatment of renal cell carcinoma with human leukoctye alpha-interferon. *J. Urol.* **130**, 1063–6.

de Mulder, P., Oosterhof, G., Bouffioux, C., *et al.* (1995). EORTC (30885) randomised phase III study with recombinant interferon alpha and recombinant interferon alpha and gamma in patients with advanced renal cell carcinoma. *Br. J. Cancer* **71**, 371–5.

Dutcher, J., Atkins, M., Fisher, R., *et al.* (1997). Il-2-based therapy in metastatic renal cell cancer: Cytokine Working Group experience. *Proc. Am. Soc. Clin. Oncol.* **16**, 327a.

Ellerhorst, J.A., Kilbourn, R.G., Amato, R.J., *et al.* (1994). Phase II trial of low dose gamma-interferon in metastatic renal cell carcinoma. *J. Urol.* **152**, 841–5.

Ellerhorst, J.A., Sella, A., Amato, R.J., *et al.* (1997). Phase II trial of 5-fluorouracil, interferon-alfa and continuous infusion interleukin-2 for patients with metastatic renal cell carcinoma. *Cancer* **80**, 2128–32.

Escudier, B., Chevreau, C., Tasset, C., Douillard, J.Y., *et al.* (1999). Cytokines in metastatic renal cell carcinoma: is it useful to switch to interleukin-2 or interferon after failure of a first treatment? *J. Clin. Oncol.* **17**, 2039–43.

Ezekowitz, H.A., Mulliken, J.B., and Folkman, J. (1992). Interferon alpha-2a therapy for life-threatening hemangiomas of infancy. *New Engl. J. Med.* **326**, 1456–63.

Falcone, A., Cianci, C., Pfanner, E., Ricci, S., Lencioni, M., *et al.* (1996). Treatment of metastatic renal cell carcinoma with constant-rate floxuridine infusion plus recombinant alpha 2b-interferon. *Ann. Oncol.* **7**, 601–5.

Figlin, R.A., deKernion, J.B., Mukamel, E., *et al.* (1988). Recombinant interferon alfa-2a in metastatic renal cell carcinoma: assessment of antitumor activity and anti-interferon antibody formation. *J. Clin. Oncol.* **6**, 1604–10.

Foon, K., Doroshow, J., Bonnem, E., *et al.* (1988). A prospective randomised trial of alpha 2B-interferon/gamma-interferon or the combination in advanced metastatic renal cell carcinoma. *J. Biol. Resp. Mod.* **7**, 540–5.

Fossa, S.D. (1988). Is interferon with or without vinblastine the "treatment of choice" in metastatic renal cell carcinoma. *Sem. Surg. Oncol.* **4**, 178–83.

Fossa, S.D., Nesland, J.M., Melvik, J.E., *et al.* (1990). Prediction of objective response to recombinant interferon-alpha with or without vinblastine in metastatic renal cell carcinoma. *Acta Oncol.* **29**, 303–6.

Fossa, S.D., Martinelli, G., Otto, U., *et al.* (1992). Recombinant interferon alfa-2a with or without vinblastine in metastatic renal cell carcinoma: results of a European multi-center phase III study. *Ann. Oncol.* **3**, 301–5.

Garnick, M.B., Reich, S.D., Maxwell, B., *et al.* (1988). Phase I/II study of recombinant interferon gamma in advanced renal cell carcinoma. *J. Urol.* **139**, 251–5.

Gleave, M.E., Elhilali, M., Fradet, Y., *et al.* (1998). Interferon gamma-1b compared with placebo in metastatic renal-cell carcinoma. *New Engl. J. Med.* **338**, 1265–71.

Grossberg, S.E. and Taylor, J.L. (1985). Interferon effects on cell differentiation In *Interferon* (ed. R.M. Friedman), pp. 299–317. Elsevier, Amsterdam.

Grups, J.W. and Frohmuller, G. (1989). Cyclin interferon gamma treatment of patients with metastatic renal cell carcinoma. *Br. J. Urol.* **64**, 218–20.

Hanninen, E.J., Kirchner, H., and Atzpodien, J. (1996). Interleukin-2 based home therapy of metastatic renal cell carcinoma: risks and benefits in 215 consecutive patients. *J. Urol.* **155**, 19–25.

Isaacs, A. and Lindenman, J. (1957). Virus interference I. The interferon. *Proc. R. Soc.* **147**, 258–67.

Kempf, R.A., Grunberg, S.M., Daniels, J.R., *et al.* (1999). Recombinant interferon alpha-2 (intron A) in a phase II study of renal cell carcinoma. *J. Biol. Resp. Mod.* **5**, 27–35.

Kinney, P., Triozzi, P., Young, D., *et al.* (1990). Phase II trial of interferon-beta-serine in metastatic renal cell carcinoma. *J. Clin. Oncol.* **8**, 881–5.

Kirchner, H., Buer, J., Probst-Kepper, M., *et al.* (1998). Risk and long-term outcome in metastatic renal cell carcinoma patients receiving SC interleukin-2, SC interferon-alfa2a and IV 5-fluoruracil. *Proc. Am. Soc. Clin. Oncol.* **17**, 310a.

Kish, J., Ensley, J., Al-Sarraf, M., *et al.* (1986). Activity of serine inhibited recombinant DNA beta interferon (IFN beta) in patients with metastatic and recurrent renal cell carcinoma. *Proc. Am. Assoc. Cancer Res.* **27**, 184.

Koiso, K. (1987). Recombinant Human Interferon Gamma Research Group: phase II study of recombinant human interferon gamma on renal cell carcinoma. *Cancer* **60**, 929–33.

Kriegmar, M., Oberneder, R., and Hofstetter, A. (1998). Interferon alfa and vinblastine versus medroxyprogesterone acetate in the treatment of metastatic renal cell carcinoma. *Urology* **45**, 758–62.

Krown, S.E. (1987). Interferon treatment of renal cell carcinoma: current status and future prospects. *Cancer* **59**, 647–51.

Kuebler, J., Brown, T., Goodman, P., *et al.* (1989). Continuous infusion recombinant gamma interferon (Clr-GIFN) for metastatic renal cell carcinoma. *Proc. Am. Soc. Clin. Oncol.* **8**, 140.

Lengyel, P. (1993). Tumor-suppressor genes: news about the interferon connection. *Proc. Natl Acad. Sci., USA* **90**, 5893–5.

Levens, W., Ruebben, H., and Ingenhag, W. (1989). Long-term interferon treatment in metastatic renal cell carcinoma. *Eur. Urol.* **16**, 378–81.

Levy, D.A., Slaton, J.W., Swanson, D.A., *et al.* (1998). Stage specific guidelines for surveillance after radical nephrectomy for local renal cell carcinoma. *J. Urol.* **159**, 1163–7.

Machida, T., Koiso, K., Takaku, F., *et al.* (1987). Phase II study of recombinant human interferon gamma (S-6810) in renal cell carcinoma. *Gan to Kagaku Ryoho* **14**, 440–5.

Marshall, M.E., Simpson, W., Butler, K., *et al.* (1989). Treatment of renal cell carcinoma with daily low-dose alpha-interferon. *J. Biol. Resp. Mod.* **8**, 453–61.

Minasian, L.M., Motzer, R.J., Gluck, L., *et al.* (1993). Interferon alfa-2a in advanced renal cell carcinoma: treatment results and survival in 159 patients with long-term follow-up. *J. Clin. Oncol.* **11**, 1368–75.

Motzer, R.J., Schwartz, L., Murray Law, T., *et al.* (1995). Interferon alfa-2a and 13-*cis*-retinoic acid in renal cell carcinoma: antitumor activity in a phase II trial and interactions *in vitro*. *J. Clin. Oncol.* **13**, 1950–7.

Motzer, R.J., Bander, N.H., and Nanus, D.M. (1996). Renal-cell carcinoma. *New Engl. J. Med.* **335**, 865–75.

Motzer, R.J., Mazumdar, M., Bacik, J., Berg, W., *et al.* (1999*a*). Survival and prognostic stratification of 670 patients with advanced renal cell carcinoma. *J. Clin. Oncol.* **17**, 2530–40.

Motzer, R.J., Murphy, B.A., Mazumdar, M., *et al.* (1999*b*). Randomized phase III trial of interferon alfa-2a (IFN) versus IFN plus 13-*cis*-retinoic acid in patients with advanced renal cell carcinoma. *Proc. Am. Soc. Clin. Oncol.* **18**, 330.

Muss, H.B., Costanzi, J.J., Leavitt, R., *et al.* (1987). Recombinant alfa interferon in renal cell carcinoma: a randomized trial of two routes of administration. *J. Clin. Oncol.* **5**, 286–91.

Negrier, S., Escudier, B., Douillard, J.Y., *et al.* (1997). Randomized study of interleukin-2 and interferon with or without 5-FU (FUCY study) in metastatic renal cell carcinoma. *Proc. Am. Soc. Clin. Oncol.* **16**, 326a.

Negrier, S., Escudier, B., Lasset, C., *et al.* (1998). Recombinant human interleukin-2, recombinant human interferon alfa-2a, or both in metastatic renal-cell carcinoma. *New Engl. J. Med.* **338**, 1273–8.

Neidhart, J., Gagan, M., and Young, D. (1984). Interferon-alpha therapy of renal cancer. *Cancer Res.*. **44**, 4140–3.

Neidhart, J.A., Anderson, S.A., Harris, J.E., *et al.* (1991). Vinblastine fails to improve response of renal cancer to interferon alfa-n1: high response rate in patients with pulmonary metastases. *J. Clin. Oncol.* **9**, 832–6.

Nelson, K.A., Wallenberg, J.C., and Todd, M.B. (1989). High-dose intravenous therapy with beta-interferon in patients with renal cell cancer. *Proc. Am. Assoc. Cancer Res.* **30**, 260.

Olencki, T., Bukowski, R.M., Budd, G.T., *et al.* (1996). Phase I/II trial of simultaneously administered rIL-2/rHuIFN and 5-FU in patients with metastatic renal cell carcinoma. *Proc. Am. Soc. Clin. Oncol.* **15**, 263.

Paule, B., Bonhomme-Faivre, L., Rudant, E., *et al.* (1997). Interferon alfa-2a plus tretinoin in patients with metastatic renal cell carcinoma: a pilot study. *Am. J. Health-Syst. Pharmacol.* **54**, 190–2.

Pfeffer, L.M. and Donner, D.B. (1990). The down regulation of alpha-interferon receptors in human lymphoblastoid cells: relation of cellular responsiveness to the antiproliferative action of alph-interferon. *Cancer Res.* **50**, 2654–8.

Pizzocaro, G., Piva, L., Costa, A., *et al.* (1997). Adjuvant interferon to radical nephrectomy in Robson's stage II and III renal cell cancer, a multicenter randomized study with some biological evaluations. *Proc. Am. Soc. Clin. Oncol.* **16**, 318a.

Porzsolt, F. (1992). Adjuvant therapy of renal cell cancer with interferon alfa-2a. *Proc. Am. Soc. Clin. Oncol.* **11**, 202.

Pyrhonen, S., Salminen, E., Lehtonen, T., *et al.* (1996). Recombinant interferon alfa-2a with vinblastine vs. vinblastine alone in advanced renal cell carcinoma. A phase III study. *Proc. Am. Soc. Clin. Oncol.* **15**, 244.

Quesada, J.R., Swanson, D.A., Trindade, A., *et al.* (1983). Renal cell carcinoma: antitumor effects of leukocyte interferon. *Cancer Res.* **43**, 940–3.

Quesada, J.R., Swanson, D.A., and Gutterman, J.U. (1985). Phase II study of interferon alpha in metastatic renal-cell carcinoma: a progress report. *J. Clin. Oncol.* **3**, 1086–92.

Quesada, J.R., Kurzrock, R., Sherwin, S.A., *et al.* (1987). Phase II studies of recombinant human interferon gamma in metastatic renal cell carcinoma. *J. Biol. Resp. Mod.* **6**, 20–7.

Rabinovitch, R.A., Zelefsky, M.J., Gaynor, J.J., *et al.* (1994). Patterns of failure following surgical resection of renal cell carcinoma: implications for adjuvant local and systemic therapy. *J. Clin. Oncol.* **12**, 206–12.

Ravaud, A., Audhuy, B., Gomez, F., *et al.* (1998). Subcutaneous interleukin-2, interferon alfa-2a, and continuous infusion of fluorouracil in metastatic renal cell carcinoma: a multicenter trial. *J. Clin. Oncol.* **16**, 2728–32.

Reese, D.M., Corry, M., and Small, E.J. (1999). Infusional floxuridine-based therapy for metastatic renal cell carcinoma. *Cancer* in press.

Rinehart, J.J., Young, D., Laforge, J., *et al.* (1987*a*). Phase I/II trial of interferon-beta-serine in patients with renal cell carcinoma: immunological and biological effects. *Cancer Res.* **47**, 2481–5.

Rinehart, J.J., Young, D., Laforge, J., *et al.* (1987*b*). Phase I/II trial of recombinant gamma-interferon in patients with metastatic renal cell carcinoma: immunologic and biologic effects. *J. Biol. Resp. Mod.* **6**, 302–12.

Ritchie, A.W.S., Griffiths, G., Cook, P., *et al.* (1998). Alpha interferon improves survival in patients with metastatic renal cell carcinoma—preliminary results of an MRC randomised trial. *Proc. Am. Soc. Clin. Oncol.* **17**, 310a.

Sagaster, P., Micksche, M., Flamm, J., *et al.* (1995). Randomised study using IFN-alpha plus coumarin and cimetidine for treatment of advanced renal cell cancer. *Ann. Oncol.* **6**, 999–1003.

Sandock, D.S., Seftel, A.D., and Resnick, M.I. (1995). A new protocol for the followup of renal cell carcinoma based on pathological stage. *J. Urol.* **154**, 28–31.

Savage, P.D. and Muss, H.B. (1995) Renal cell cancer. In *Biological therapy of cancer* (ed. V.T. De Vita, S. Hellman, and S.A. Rosenberg), pp. 373–87. J.B. Lippincott, Philadelphia.

Schnall, S.F., Davis, C., Ziyadeh, T., *et al.* (1986). Treatment of metastatic renal cell carcinoma with intramuscular (IM) recombinant interferon alpha A (IFN, Hoffmann-LaRoche). *Proc. Am. Soc. Clin. Oncol.* **5**, 227.

Small, E.J., Weiss, G.R., Malik, U.K., *et al.* (1998). The treatment of metastatic renal cell carcinoma patients with recombinant human gamma interferon. *Cancer J. Sci. Am.* **4**, 162–7.

Sori, G.S., Schulof, R.S., Stark, J.J., Wieman, M.C., Honeycutt, P.J., *et al.* (1999). Continuous-infusion floxuridine and alpha interferon in metastatic renal cancer: a National Biotherapy Study Group phase II study. *Cancer Invest.* **17**, 379–84.

Sreevalsan, T. (1995). Biologic therapy with interferon-alfa and beta: preclinical studies. In *Biological therapy of cancer* (ed. V.T. De Vita, S. Hellman, and S.A. Rosenberg), pp. 347–64. J.B. Lippincott, Philadelphia.

Stadler, W.M., Talabay, K., and Vogelzang, N.J. (1996). Interleukin-2, interferon-alpha, and *cis*-retinoic acid: an effective outpatient regimen for metastatic renal cell carcinoma. *Proc. Am. Soc. Clin. Oncol.* **15**, 241.

Steineck, G., Strander, H., Carbin, B.E., *et al.* (1990). Recombinant leukocyte interferon alpha-2a and medroxyprogesterone in advanced renal cell carcinoma. A randomized trial. *Acta Oncol.* **29**, 155–62.

Tourani, J.M., Pfister, C., Berdah, J.F., *et al.* (1998). Outpatient treatment with subcutaneous interleukin-2 and interferon alfa administration in combination with fluorouracil in patients with metastatic renal cell carcinoma: results of a sequential nonrandomized phase II study. *J. Clin. Oncol.* **16**, 2505–13.

Trump, D.L., Elson, P., Propert, K., *et al.* (1996). Randomized, controlled trial of adjuvant therapy with lymphoblastoid interferon (L-IFN) in resected, high-risk renal cell carcinoma. *Proc. Am. Soc. Clin. Oncol.* **15**, 253.

Umeda, T. and Niijima, T. (1986). Phase II study of alpha interferon on renal cell carcinoma. Summary of three collaborative trials. *Cancer* **58**, 1231–5.

Vogelzang, N.J., Lipton, A., and Figlin, RA. (1993). Subcutaneous interleukin-2 plus interferon alfa-2a in metastatic renal cancer: an outpatient multicenter trial. *J. Clin. Oncol.* **11**, 1809–16.

Wirth, M.P. (1993). Immunotherapy for metastatic renal cell carcinoma. *Urol. Clin. N. Am.* **20**, 283–95.

Yagoda, A., Bassam, A.R., and Petrylak, D. (1983). Chemotherapy for advanced renal cell carcinoma. *Sem. Oncol.* **22**, 42–60.

40. The role of interleukin in metastatic renal cell carcinoma

Ronald M. Bukowski

Introduction

The treatment of metastatic renal cell carcinoma (RCC) presents a therapeutic challenge to the medical oncologist. The traditional modality of chemotherapy has minimal activity, with most agents demonstrating response rates less than 5 per cent (Yagoda 1990). The recognition of an antitumor immune response (Finke *et al.* 1994) and the occurrence of spontaneous regression in patients with this neoplasm (Oliver *et al.* 1988; Gleave *et al.* 1998) led to studies investigating a variety of biologic agents in this patient population. These have included the cytokines, both natural and recombinant molecules. One class of cytokines that has been widely investigated is the interleukins. Interleukin 2 has been shown to have a limited, but reproducible antitumor activity in RCC. This chapter will review several interleukins that have been employed in metastatic RCC, including the rationale and clinical results for these agents.

Interleukin-2

Rationale

Interleukin 2 (IL-2) is a 15 kDa glycoprotein that functions as a growth factor for T cells and natural killer (NK) cells (Grimm *et al.* 1982; Baker *et al.* 1979). It was first described by Morgan *et al.* (1976) as a soluble factor in medium from phyto-hemagglutin-stimulated mononuclear cells that sustained the proliferation of antigen-specific cytolytic T lymphocytes (CTL) (Gillis *et al.* 1979). The primary source of IL-2 is CD4+ T-cells, and it is produced during a T helper type 1 (Th1) type of immune response (Mosmann *et al.* 1986). Molecularly, it resembles granulocyte–macrophage colony stimulating factor (GM-CSF) and IL-4 (Morgan *et al.* 1976), and is comprised of four parallel alpha helices. Initial studies with IL-2 utilized purified protein produced by the Jurkat T-cell tumor line (Lotze *et al.* 1985). Recombinant IL-2 (rIL-2) then became available and has been utilized subsequently. Several rIL-2 muteins produced in *E. coli* (Bukowski *et al.* 1996) have been used clinically, with the Chiron preparation being most widely employed (Proleukin, Chron, Emeryville, CA).

IL-2 is produced when T lymphocytes are activated (Kroemer *et al.* 1991). Two signals are required for IL-2 gene expression,

including ligation of the T-cell receptor (TCR)/CD3 complex, with a second signal provided by cells expressing B7, a ligand for CD28 or CTL-A that is present on T cells (Linsley *et al.* 1990). The biologic effects of IL-2 occur following its binding to the interleukin-2 receptor (IL-2R). This complex contains three discrete chains (α, β, γ). The IL-2R with the highest affinity contains all three chains (Smith 1993; Takeshita *et al.* 1992). Signaling via IL-2R requires both the β and γ chains (Oliver *et al.* 1988; Kroemer *et al.* 1991).

The biologic effects produced by IL-2 include clonal expansion of antigen-specific CTL (Baker *et al.* 1979), enhancement of T-cell and NK-cell cytotoxicity (Kroemer *et al.* 1991; Baker *et al.* 1978), enhanced expression of proteins such as granzyme B and perforin (Liu *et al.* 1989), and induction of cytokine secretion, for example, interferon gamma (IFNγ) (Kroemer *et al.* 1991). All of these may play a role in the development of host immunity, and an antitumor response. Preclinical studies in murine tumor models demonstrated the antineoplastic effects of this cytokine (Rosenberg *et al.* 1985), and it was then utilized in patients as therapy for various malignancies including metastatic RCC.

The possibility that RCC is a tumor sensitive to the immunologic response is suggested by the series of observations outlined in Table 40.1. Clinically, the development of renal cancer in immunosuppressed transplant patients (Kliem *et al.* 1997) and the finding of spontaneous regression of metastatic RCC (Oliver *et al.* 1988; Gleave *et al.* 1998) were reported. The role of T lymphocytes as effectors in these patients was suggested by their presence in renal tumors (Finke *et al.* 1988; Kowalczyk *et al.* 1997), demonstrated immunohistologically. Clonal expansion of the T-lymphocyte population was also found. It has been difficult to culture major histocompatibility complex (MHC)-restricted CTL from

Table 40.1 Evidence suggesting an immunologic response in renal cell carcinoma (RCC)

Clinical observations
   Spontaneous regressions
   Development of RCC in immunosuppressed patients
   Infiltrates of T lymphocytes in RCC

Laboratory observations
   Clonal expansion of T cells in RCC tumors
   Tumor-specific CTL lines and clones
   Identification of T-cell defined antigens

---

these tumors, but several investigators have reported their presence (Finke *et al.* 1994; Angevin *et al.* 1997; Schendel *et al.* 1993). Finally, tumor-associated antigens recognized by patient T cells have been reported (Brossart *et al.* 1998; Neumann *et al.* 1998). These observations and laboratory findings suggest that IL-2 may be of therapeutic value in RCC patients.

Recent observations, however, also suggest the presence of T-lymphocyte dysfunction in cancer patients (Finke *et al.* 1993). Abnormalities of the TCR including decreases in TCRζ (Finke *et al.* 1993), abnormal NFκB activation (Li *et al.* 1994), and enhanced apoptosis of T lymphocytes (Uzzo *et al.* 1999) both in peripheral blood and tumor have been noted. NFκB is a transcription factor that translocates to the nucleus and regulates transcription of genes important for T-cell function (Baeverde and Baltimore 1996). Reports indicate that NFκB activation is abnormal in over 60 per cent of patients with renal cell cancer (Bukowski *et al.* 1998).

Tumors may also escape immune recognition through induction of T-lymphocyte apoptosis. The interactions between the Fas receptor (APO-1/CD95) and its ligand (Fas-L/CD95-L) may regulate a number of normal and pathologic events controlling T-cell function. Fas-L on lymphocytes may induce apoptosis in Fas-expressing targets (Hahne *et al.* 1996). Tumor cells including RCC can express Fas-L, and possibly utilize this mechanism to escape destruction, with tumor-infiltrating lymphocytes (TIL) being targets. Uzzo *et al.* (1999) reported that RCC tumor cells expressing Fas-L can induce apoptosis in activated T cells from RCC patients. Over 90 per cent of tumors examined expressed significant levels of Fas-L, and only minimal levels of Fas. The possibility that immune dysregulation may negatively impact on results with IL-2 in RCC patients therefore exists.

Clinical results: single-agent rIL-2

The clinical use of rIL-2 has been extensively explored in patients with metastatic RCC. A review of single-agent rIL-2 activity (Bukowski 1997; Bukowski and Dutcher 2000) indicates an overall response rate of 15 per cent in over 1900 patients treated in a series of trials employing various dose levels and schedules of rIL-2 (see Table 40.2). Complete responses have been noted in from 3 to 5 per cent of patients. The routes and scheduled of rIL-2 utilized have been quite variable, and have included intravenous bolus, continuous intravenous infusion (CIV), and subcutaneous

(SC) administration. Overall response rates do not appear to differ between these routes.

The possibility that complete regressions are more frequent and durable with high doses of rIL-2 has been suggested (Fyfe *et al.* 1995), but randomized data are not available to confirm this. In view of this, selection of therapy is guided by multiple factors, which include patient expectations, co-morbid factors, and prognostic factors.

Bolus IL-2

A review by Fyfe *et al.* (1995) of 255 patients treated with high-dose rIL-2 (600 000 to 720 000 IU/kg as a 15 minute IV infusion every 8 hours over 5 days) reported a response rate of 14 per cent with a 5 per cent complete response (regression) (CR) rate. The CRs were durable with median response duration not yet reached. The toxicity with this regimen is substantial and a 4 per cent treatment-related death rate was noted, with over 50 per cent of patients requiring vasopressors.

It is unclear if this dose and schedule are required to produce the complete and durable responses noted. A recent randomized trial from the US National Cancer Institute (Yang *et al.* 1994) investigated two doses of rIL-2 (720 000 versus 72 000 IU/kg IV every 8 hours for 5 days). Response rates to both regimens were similar (15 versus 20 per cent, respectively), and complete responses were found in 7 compared to 3 per cent of patients, respectively. The rigorous patient eligibility criteria in the high-dose treatment regimens vary from those utilized in the majority of trials in RCC patients. In view of this, randomized trials are required to document improved response rates and durations in patients treated with high-dose bolus rIL-2. Data available presently do not confirm the superiority of this approach.

The toxicity of bolus IL-2 depends upon the dose utilized. A flu-like syndrome that includes fever, chills, and myalgias is experienced by most patients. Cardiovascular, pulmonary, and central nervous system (CNS) toxicity are associated with high-dose rIL-2 (Yang *et al.* 1994). Cardiovascular toxicity includes hypotension requiring vasopressors, cardiac arrhythmias, myocardial infarction, and myocarditis. Pulmonary toxicity secondary to the capillary leak syndrome may develop and require mechanical ventilation. Grade 3 renal toxicity with oliguria can occur in over 20 per cent of treated patients, with creatinine levels > 8 mg/dl reported in 2 per cent (Yang *et al.* 1994). Confusion and neuropsychiatric complaints are also common. Careful patient

Table 40.2 Single-agent IL-2 in metastatic renal cell carcinoma: summary

Schedule	Number of patients	Number of responses (%)		Overall response rate (%)
		Complete	**Partial**	
IV bolus*	733	38 (5)	83 (11)	16
CIV[†]	922	25 (2.5)	98 (10.6)	13.3
Subcutaneous[†]	290	8 (3)	40 (13.8)	16.8
Totals	1945	71 (3.6)	221 (11.4)	15.0

* Source: Bukowski (1997).
[†] Source: Bukowski and Dutcher (2000).

selection is required to minimize the morbidity and mortality associated with high-dose rIL-2 (Yang *et al.* 1994).

Continuous infusion IL-2

The short half-life of intravenous bolus IL-2 prompted the use of CIV of this cytokine. Various administration schedules and doses have been utilized. The majority of reports have employed 18.0 MIU/m^2/day. Reported response rates vary but, in a group of 922 patients recently reviewed (Table 40.2), the overall rate was 13.3 per cent (Bukowski and Dutcher 2000). Complete regressions occur, and in some series (Escudier *et al.* 1994) are similar to those reported with high-dose bolus rIL-2.

A single randomized trial utilizing CIV rIL-2 has been reported. In this study (Negrier *et al.* 1998) patients were randomized to either CIV rIL-2, SC IFNα, or the combination. The response rate in 138 patients receiving rIL-2 was 6.5 per cent, with 94/138 individuals developing hypotension resistant to vasopressor agents. The toxicity of single-agent rIL-2 given as a CIV at doses > 18 MIU/m^2 is, therefore, significant. At this dose level hospitalization is required, and outcomes do not appear different from those experienced with single-agent IFNα. Lower doses of CIV rIL-2 are associated with less toxicity. Caliguri (1994) utilized 0.05 to 0.6 MIU/m^2/day as a CIV for up to 90 days. The clinical activity of this approach in RCC patients is however unclear.

Subcutaneous rIL-2

SC rIL-2 also has been used in RCC patients, but published experience is limited. The majority of reports involve less than 25 patients and, in a group of 290 patients recently reviewed (Bukowski and Dutcher 2000), a response rate of 16.8 per cent was found. In several series (Lissoni *et al.* 1992; Buter *et al.* 1993*a*), SC rIL-2 is initially administered at a higher dose level for 2 to 5 days followed by maintenance rIL-2. Buter *et al.* (1993*a*) noted two complete responses lasting for 29.0 and > 35.0 months, respectively, suggesting that some of these responses may be durable. Yang and Rosenberg (1997) are conducting a prospective randomized trial to determine the effectiveness of SC rIL-2 compared to bolus rIL-2. Regimens utilized include the following: high-dose bolus (720 000 IU/kg); low-dose bolus (72 000 IU/kg); and SC (week one, 250 000 IU/kg/day for 5 of 7 days, followed by 125 000 IU/kg/day for 5 of 7 days in weeks two to six). One hundred and sixty-four patients have been randomized, and the preliminary response rates are 16, 4, and 11 per cent, respectively. The lower-dose regimens were associated with less severe toxicity. The response frequency and duration, and median survival remain preliminary.

The SC route is associated with less toxicity; however, it does produce significant fatigue, fever, and malaise. Development of subcutaneous nodules at injection sites has also been noted. Hypotension and the capillary leak syndrome are uncommon with this administration route.

Inhalation IL-2

Administration of nebulized medications has been investigated for numerous pulmonary disorders. Administration of proteins such as IL-2 via this route has also been undertaken. Aerosol therapy produces high pulmonary drug concentrations and low systemic drug levels, thereby enhancing the therapeutic index (Newman and Clark 1983). Huland *et al.* (1992) have reported the use of natural IL-2 administered via nebulizer. 100 000 units were delivered five times daily, and it was combined with systemic IL-2 and IFNα. The toxicity of inhaled IL-2 was reported as minimal, permitting outpatient administration. Antitumor responses were reported; however, the contribution of inhaled IL-2 is unclear in view of the concurrent administration of IFNα and systemic rIL-2.

Huland *et al.* (1997) have recently updated their results in 116 patients with pulmonary and/or mediastinal metastatic disease of whom 11 per cent received only inhaled rIL-2, 33 per cent concomitant SC rIL-2, and 56 per cent concomitant rIL-2 and IFNα. In 105 patients with pulmonary metastases, 16 patients responded (15.2 per cent), with 3 individuals having complete responses. The median response duration was 15.5 months. The authors note that the toxicity of this approach appears less than that produced by systemic administration of rIL-2. In order to assess the value of inhalational rIL-2, randomized trials comparing patients receiving only inhaled cytokine with those receiving systemic therapy with/without inhaled cytokine are required.

Pegylated IL-2

Conjugation of proteins to polyethylene glycol (PEG) increases their half-life and permits retention of biologic activity. One such preparation is pegylated IL-2 (PEG IL-2). Clinically, the use of PEG IL-2 has been limited. The maximum tolerated dose (MTD) for IV PEG IL-2 is 20 × 10^6 IU/m^2 when administered weekly (Meyers *et al.* 1991). The toxicity of this preparation is similar to that of rIL-2 and includes hypotension and cardiopulmonary complications. Patient numbers receiving PEG IL-2 are limited, and response rates preliminary. In a group of 62 patients receiving this preparation, in various phase I and II reports (Meyers *et al.* 1991; Bukowski *et al.* 1993; Yang *et al.* 1995), 7 per cent (4/64) had partial responses. The role of this IL-2 preparation is unclear but, in view of the increased half-life, less frequent administration may be possible.

Interleukin-2 combination therapy

Therapeutic trials in patients with metastatic RCC have utilized a variety of IL-2-based regimens that have combined this cytokine with other biologic agents and/or chemotherapy. The combination of rIL-2 with IFNα represents the most widely used approach.

IL-2 and IFNα

Rationale

Preclinical investigations in a variety of murine tumor models established the rationale for employing rIL-2 and IFNα in combination. The antitumor effects of rIL-2 and the pleiotropic immunomodulatory actions of IFNα provided a rationale for initiating these investigations. A number of studies (Chikkala *et al.* 1990; Camerin *et al.* 1988) demonstrated synergistic antitumor effects when rIL-2 and rIFNα A/D were co-administered. Investigators have also utilized other interferon types, for example, IFNγ (Mule and Rosenberg 1991); however, combinations of

Table 40.3 Summary of reported clinical results with rIL-2 and IFNα in metastatic renal cell carcinoma*

rIL-2 Schedule	Number of patients	Number of responses (%)		Overall response rate (%)
		Complete	Partial	
Subcutaneous	920	47 (5.1)	127 (13.8)	18.9
CIV	556	20 (3.6)	91 (16.4)	20.0
IV bolus	194	10 (5.1)	28 (14.4)	19.5
Total	1670	77 (4.6)	245 (14.7)	19.3

* Adapted from Bukowski and Dutcher (2000).

rIL-2 and a type 1 interferon (IFNα, IFNβ) appear to be the most effective (Mule and Rosenberg 1991).

The operative mechanisms remain unclear, but studies suggest these are multifactorial. The actions of IFNα include direct suppression of tumor growth, modulation of the host immune response, and upregulation of MHC antigens (Witt *et al.* 1996). In contrast, rIL-2 mediates its antitumor effects by nonspecifically enhancing the proliferation of various lymphocyte subsets. It is possible IFNα increases the *in vivo* expression of class I MHC molecules on tumor cells, increasing their susceptibility to rIL-2 (Wan *et al.* 1987). The lack of synergy between IL-2 and IFNγ, however, suggests other factors also play a role. Additionally, the mechanisms found in these models may be dependent on the tumor utilized (Mule and Rosenberg 1991). Finally, the effects of immune dysregulation on the antitumor effects of combination therapy remain to be defined.

Clinical results

The phase I and II clinical trials conducted with rIL-2 and IFNα were initiated on the basis of the preclinical observations noted previously. A variety of administration routes, schedules, and doses have been utilized and, when viewed collectively, the studies suggest a response rate to this cytokine combination of approximately 20 per cent. Table 40.3 reviews recent data from over 1600 patients treated with rIL-2 and IFNα (Bukowski and Dutcher 2000). No differences in overall response rates between regimens utilizing bolus, CIV, or SC administration of rIL-2 are apparent. Complete regressions have been seen in from 3 to 5 per cent of patients. The durability of these responses and survival rates are variable, and in many of the trials were not specified.

Palmer *et al.* (1993) have reviewed European data for 425 patients who were treated with either CIV rIL-2 (225 patients) or SC rIL-2 and IFNα (200 patients) in four different protocols. The response rates were 15 per cent (95 per cent confidence limits 10–20 per cent) and 20 per cent (95 per cent confidence limits 14–20 per cent), respectively. Four per cent of patients had complete responses. Median survivals were 9.1 and 13.0 months, respectively, and median time to progression was 3.4 and 3.5 months. The regression rates were similar ($p = 0.13$), but median survival was improved in patients receiving the cytokine combination ($p = 0.01$). This study was retrospective and recently a series of randomized trials have been reported investigating the efficacy of rIL-2 and IFNα.

In view of the importance of prognostic factors in predicting the outcome in patients with metastatic RCC, randomized trials are required to demonstrate improvement with a regimen, such as rIL-2 and IFNα. Six such trials have been reported (Negrier *et al.* 1998; Henriksson *et al.* 1998; Atkins *et al.* 1993; Jayson *et al.* 1998; Lissoni *et al.* 1993; Lümmen *et al.* 1996), and the majority are small phase II studies. The two largest studies (Negrier *et al.* 1998;

Table 40.4 Phase III trials involving rIL-2 and IFNα in metastatic renal cell carcinoma*

Regimen	Number of patients	Response rate (%)			1-year progression-free survival (%)	Median survival (months)
		Complete	Partial	Overall		
Results of Negrier *et al.* 1998						
rIL-2 (CIV)	138	1.5	5.0	6.5[†]	13.8[‡]	12.0[§]
IFNα (SC)	147	0	7.5	7.5[†]	9.7[‡]	13.0[§]
rIL-2 (CIV) + IFNα	140	1.0	17.6	18.6[†]	20.9[‡]	17.0[§]
Results of Henriksson *et al.* 1998						
rIL-2 (SC) + IFNα (SC) + TMX	65	NS	NS	NS	NS	11.8[§]
TMX	63	NS	NS	NS	NS	13.3[§]

* CIV, continuous intravenous; SC, subcutaneous; TMX, tamoxifen; NS, not stated.
[†] $p < 0.04$.
[‡] $p < 0.01$.
[§] No significant differences reported within trial.

Henriksson *et al.* 1998) are summarized in Table 40.4. They utilized different regimens with rIL-2 given as a CIV in one (Negrier *et al.* 1998) and SC in the second (Henriksson *et al.* 1998). The study reported by Negrier *et al.* (1998) allocated patients to three arms, and results demonstrated that the combination of CIV rIL-2 and IFNα produced a significantly higher response rate than either cytokine alone and also improved 1-year progression-free survival. Henriksson *et al.* (1998) reported a study in which patients with evaluable or measurable disease were randomized to either rIL-2, IFNα and tamoxifen, or tamoxifen alone. Response rates were not reported, and no differences in survival were seen. In all studies, comparing an rIL-2/IFNα regimen with another treatment arm, where median survivals have been reported, no significant differences between patients receiving the combination or other therapy has been found.

The available data suggest that the response rate to rIL-2 and IFNα is approximately 20 per cent, and may be higher than that produced by CIV rIL-2 (Negrier *et al.* 1998) as a single agent. Adequate comparisons of the combination to high-dose rIL-2 or SC rIL-2 have not been performed, however. The survival data reported do not demonstrate differences; however, in the report by Negrier *et al.* (1998) patient cross-over at progression was permitted, potentially obscuring a survival benefit. The duration of response in these reports was generally not mentioned. In the randomized phase II study by Atkins *et al.* (1993), patients receiving high-dose rIL-2 had response durations lasting from 4.0 to 25+ months (10/12 > 12+ months). In contrast, patients who received rIL-2 and IFNα had response durations from 7.0 (18) to 13.0 ± 5.0 months (Atkins *et al.* 1993). Complete response rates in the phase III trials have been low (< 2 per cent), and no differences between rIL-2 and the combination regimen are apparent.

A second rationale for development of the rIL-2 and IFNα combination was to reduce the systemic toxicity associated with high-dose rIL-2 therapy. Administration of rIL-2 as a CIV or intravenous bolus is associated with severe dose-dependent side effects including hypotension, acute respiratory distress, and fluid retention secondary to capillary leak syndrome, which require inpatient treatment. Subcutaneous rIL-2 is associated with less toxicity, even when combined with IFNα. Fewer grade 3 or 4 side effects occur with SC rIL-2 and IFNα compared to other regimens (Bukowski and Dutcher 2000; Yang *et al.* 1994). All these approaches, however, produce constitutional toxicity such as fever, chills, malaise, and myalgias.

Interleukin-2 and other interferons

Interferon-beta (IFNβ) is a type I interferon with potent *in vitro* activity against selected solid tumor cell lines (Borden *et al.* 1982). The reports with rIL-2 and IFNα resulted in studies with rIL-2 and IFNβ. A single-institution phase II trial (Krigel *et al.* 1988) and a subsequent randomized phase II study (Witte *et al.* 1995) have been reported. The latter trial randomized patients to bolus rIL-2 alone or the combination. rIL-2 was administered as a bolus three times weekly via IV bolus at doses of 6.0 or 5.0 MIU/m² in the two arms, respectively. In both studies, patients received rIL-2 and IFNβ, and 16 per cent responded. Witte *et al.* (1995) suggested that the response rates to this combination resemble those reported with rIL-2 alone.

Interferonγ (IFNγ) is a type II interferon and *in vitro* synergizes with rIL-2 (Findley *et al.* 1990). *In vivo* studies in murine tumor models (Mule and Rosenberg 1991) have not, however, demonstrated synergistic antitumor effects of the combination. Several phase I trials of rIL-2 and IFNγ have been performed (Redman *et al.* 1990; Viens *et al.* 1992; Taylor *et al.* 1992). Escudier *et al.* (1993) reported a phase II study combining CIV rIL-2 (24 MIU/m²) and IFNγ (5 × 10² U/m² SC days 1 and 2), in which 7/33 patients (21 per cent) responded. The lack of activity (response rate < 5 per cent) for IFNγ reported in recent studies (Gleave *et al.* 1998; Small *et al.* 1998) suggests that further investigations with this combination are not warranted.

Miscellaneous combinations

Preclinical observations of synergistic activity and/or single-agent activity have prompted investigators to explore rIL-2 in combination with a variety of other cytokines. Examples include IL-4 (Olencki *et al.* 1996), GM-CSF (Schiller *et al.* 1996), tumor necrosis factor (TNFα) (Markowitz *et al.* 1989), levamisole (Ahmed *et al.* 1996), and OKT3 (Buter *et al.* 1993b). These studies have been phase I or phase II trials in which small numbers of RCC patients were treated, and results do not suggest differences from results obtained with single-agent rIL-2.

Interleukin-2 and chemotherapy

Rationale

The synergism of chemotherapy and rIL-2 has been explored. The preclinical and clinical reports of IFNα in combination with the fluorinated pyrimidines in colorectal carcinoma (Houghton *et al.* 1993) and subsequently in RCC patients (Gegrosky *et al.* 1997) suggest improved efficacy. The basis for combining rIL-2 with chemotherapy varies depending upon the agent involved (Mitchell 1992). The use of cyclophosphamide with rIL-2 is based on the finding that cyclophosphamide enhances cell-mediated immunity presumably by inhibition of suppressor cells (Mitchell 1992). The combination or rIL-2 and vinblastine utilized two agents with some antitumor activity in RCC patients. Finally, the rationale for combining rIL-2, IFNα, and a fluorinated pyrimidine was based on the clinical activities of rIL-2 and IFNα, and the possible synergy of IFNα and 5-fluorouracil (5-FU).

Several chemoimmunotherapy regimens employing these agents were developed. Atzpodien *et al.* (1993) reported a phase II trial with SC IL-2 and IFNα plus IV 5-FU. Thirty-five patients with metastatic RCC were treated. An overall response rate of 48.6 per cent (11.4 per cent complete response) was reported and generated significant interest. Since 1993, multiple trials have been conducted in which these three agents were combined. Table 40.5 summarizes data from phase II and phase III (Atzpodien *et al.* 1997; Negrier *et al.* 1997) trials employing 5-FU, rIL-2, and IFNα. In most studies, rIL-2 was administered SC. The doses and schedule of 5-FU are variable, with from 200 to 1000 mg/m² administered either as a continuous ambulatory infusion (Ravaud *et al.* 1998), 5-day CIV (Ellerhorst *et al.* 1997), or intravenous bolus (Kirchner *et al.* 1998). Overall response rates range from 1.8 to 39 per cent and, for the 836 patients reviewed, was 25.3 per cent. Complete response rates and median survival data are also vari-

Table 40.5 Summary of phase II/III trials utilizing fluorouracil, rIL-2, and IFNα in metastatic renal cell carcinoma*

Reference	Number of patients	Number of response (%)		Overall response rate (%)	Median survival[†] (months)
		Complete	Partial		
Kirchner et al. 1998	246	26 (10.5)	54 (22.0)	32.6	21.0
Lopez Hänninen et al. 1996	120	13 (10.8)	34 (28.2)	39.1	NS
Atzpodien et al. 1997	41	7 (17.0)	9 (22.0)	39.0	> 42.0
Savage et al. 1996	24	1 (4.0)	3 (13.0)	17	NS
Ravaud et al. 1998	105	0 (0)	2 (1.8)	1.8	11.9
Joffe et al. 1996	38	0 (0)	9 (23.6)	23.6	11.9
Hofmockel et al. 1996	34	3 (9.0)	10 (29.0)	38	12.6[‡]
Ellerhorst et al. 1997	55	4 (7.2)	12 (21.8)	31	22.9
Negrier et al. 1997[‡]	61	0 (0)	5 (8.2)	8.2	NS
Dutcher et al. 1997	50	2 (4.0)	6 (12.0)	16.0	16.7
Tourani et al. 1998	62	1 (1.6)	11 (17.7)	19.3	16.0
Totals	836	57 (6.8)	155 (18.5)	25.3	

* Adapted from Bukowski and Dutcher (2000).
[†] NS, not stated.
[‡] Mean survival.
[§] Randomized trial comparing rIL-2 + IFNα ± fluorouracil.

able. These observations suggest that patient selection and prognostic factors may be responsible for these differences. A randomized trial by Negrier *et al.* (1997) compared rIL-2 and IFNα to the same combination plus 5-FU. One hundred and thirty-one patients were treated, and response rates were 1.4 and 8.2 per cent, respectively. The authors concluded that this regimen was inactive. In the trial reported by Ravaud *et al.* (1998), only 1.8 per cent of patients responded. The toxicity of the combination was significant. Tourani *et al.* (1998) report delays and/or dose reductions in over 50 per cent of treated individuals. In the absence of randomized trials demonstrating enhanced response and/or survival, the value of this chemoimmunotherapy regimen remains unclear.

Empiric combination of rIL-2 and vinblastine and rIL-2 plus IFNα and vinblastine have also been reported. The results of studies in which rIL-2 and vinblastine are combined (Guida *et al.* 1997; Taberno *et al.* 1998) appear unremarkable. The study (Indrova *et al.* 1994; Pectasides *et al.* 1998) that utilized rIL-2, IFNα, and vinblastine appears to have a higher response rate, but the contribution of the chemotherapy is unclear. The toxicity of these programs reflects the cytokine dose and schedule, with vinblastine producing increased myelosuppression (Kuebler *et al.* 1993).

The effects of cyclophosphamide (CTX) at low doses on cellular and humoral inhibitors of the immune response have been reported (Berd and Mastrangelo 1987; Askenase *et al.* 1975). The combination of rIL-2 and CTX was initially administered in conjunction with the adoptive transfer of immune cells such as lymphokine-activated killer cells (LAK) (Rosenberg *et al.* 1989) or TIL (Oldham *et al.* 1991*a*). The dose of CTX used was 1000 mg/m². Lower doses of CTX can also reportedly inhibit generation of 'suppressor cells' and thereby augment immunity (Berd *et al.* 1984). The combination of rIL-2 and CTX has also been reported with CTX administered 72 hours before rIL-2 (Mitchell 1992). Bolus (Mitchell 1992) and CIV (Oldham *et al.* 1991*b*) rIL-2 have also been employed, and one investigation utilized rIL-2, IFNα, and CTX (Wersall *et al.* 1993). Reported results do not appear

different from those with single-agent rIL-2 (see Table 40.2). The toxicity resembles that produced by single agent rIL-2. Wersall *et al.* (1993) reported increased NK and LAK activity in responding patients receiving CTX, rIL-2, and IFNα, but the role of CTX was unclear. Overall, the available studies do not suggest that CTX enhances the antitumor effects of rIL-2.

Preclinical studies have also reported variable immunologic effects of other chemotherapeutic agents. Doxorubicin (Orsimi *et al.* 1977) and flavone-8-acetic acid (FAA; Wiltrout *et al.* 1988; Ching and Baguley 1987) appear to augment the induction of NK and LAK activity and/or cytokine production when combined with rIL-2. These combinations have been investigated in phase I and II trials. Holmlund *et al.* (1995) evaluated FAA (3.4–10.0 g/m²) in combination with rIL-2 (1.0–3.0 MIU/m² via CIV) and, among 10 patients with RCC, no responses were noted. The experience with rIL-2 and doxorubicin is similar. Several phase I trials combining these agents have been conducted (Bukowski *et al.* 1991; Margolin *et al.* 1993; Paciucci *et al.* 1991). The number of RCC patients treated (3) was small, and no responses were reported. Naglieri *et al.* (1998) combined 4-epirubicin with SC rIL-2 (9.0 MIU days 1 and 2, followed by 4.5 MIU days 3–5, and days 1–5 of weeks 2–6), and compared it to subcutaneous rIL-2 and IFNα. Thirty-eight RCC patients were randomized, with 20 receiving chemoimmunotherapy. Two responses (1 complete, 1 partial) in each arm were noted. The information available does not suggest that addition of an anthracycline enhances the clinical activity of rIL-2.

Interleukin-4

Rationale

Interleukin-4 (IL-4) is a pleiotropic cytokine that was first described in 1982 (Howard *et al.* 1982; Isakson *et al.* 1982) as a T-cell-derived factor with B-lymphocyte stimulatory activity.

Since its initial description, IL-4 has been reported to affect a wide variety of cell types (Yokota *et al.* 1986) and to have both stimulatory and suppressive effects on various responses. IL-4 is a glycoprotein with a molecular weight between 15 and 19 kDa. The IL-4 gene is on chromosome 5 at band q 23–31 (Le Beau *et al.* 1989). It is located in the vicinity of the genes encoding IL-3 and GM-CSF (van Leeuween *et al.* 1989). The human IL-4 gene has been expressed in *E. coli* (Schering-Plough), and milligram quantities are available. Recombinant IL-4 has a molecular weight of 14.9 kDa and contains 129 amino acids.

IL-4 produces its effects by interaction with cell surface receptors (IL-4R), which are present on various hematopoietic (Ohara and Paul 1987) and non-hematopoietic cells. IL-4R is upregulated by cytokines such as IL-2, IL-4 (Ohara and Paul 1988; Wagteveld *et al.* 1991), IFNγ, and IL-6 (Feldman and Finbloom 1990). IL-4 signaling depends on binding to the IL-4 receptor (IL-4R), which is composed of two chains. IL-4 actually binds to the 140 kDa IL-4R α chain with high affinity (Park *et al.* 1987; Galizzi *et al.* 1989).

This cytokine is produced by activated T helper cells (Mossmann *et al.* 1986) and mast cells (Plaut *et al.* 1989) and has pleiotropic effects. Stimulation of B- and T-cell functions has been recognized, and a wide range of effects on diverse cell populations has also been reported. Recently, the effects of IL-4 on dendritic cell maturation have been reported (Sallusto and Langavecchia 1994). This cell population is diverse, including both lymphoid and myeloid precursors (Hsu *et al.* 1997). They function as antigen-processing cells, which present peptide fragments of antigens to T lymphocytes during an immune response (Flamand *et al.* 1994).

Antitumor activity of IL-4 is suggested by a series of observations. Various murine epithelial tumor cells express IL-4R (Puri *et al.* 1991, and *in vivo* administration has antineoplastic effects. Tepper (1989) demonstrated that IL-4 gene transfection into murine tumor cells results in their rejection. In another model, IL-4-producing tumor cells (Golumbek *et al.* 1991) induced systemic immunity against murine spontaneous renal carcinoma cells (RENCA). Studies with human tumors have demonstrated that rhuIL-4 inhibits the *in vitro* growth of various tumor cells (Defrance *et al.* 1992; Tungekar *et al.* 1991; Toi *et al.* 1992). In view of these observations, clinical trials with systemic IL-4 were conducted in patients with malignancy, including RCC.

Clinical results

In the phase I trials of single-agent IL-4 reported to date, no responses in patients with RCC have been reported (Bukowski *et al.* 1996). IL-4 has been combined with rIL-2 in a phase I trial (Olencki *et al.* 1996). In this study, no responses in 14 patients with metastatic RCC were reported.

Interleukin-12

Rationale

IL-12 was first isolated as a molecule secreted by Epstein–Barr virus (EBV)-transformed B-cell lines. Early characterization revealed that this protein synergized with IL-2 to augment CTL responses (Gately *et al.* 1986), enhanced the proliferation of mitogen-activated peripheral blood lymphoblasts (Gately *et al.* 1992), and induced IFNγ secretion by resting lymphocytes (Gately *et al.* 1991; Chan *et al.* 1991). Upon purification, IL-12 was found to be a 70 kDa heterodimeric protein composed of two polypeptide chains with molecular weights of 35 and 40 kDa (Podlaski *et al.* 1992).

A number of different cell types can produce IL-12. Among normal peripheral blood mononuclear cells, monocytes and monocyte-derived macrophages are significant producers of this cytokine (Stern *et al.* 1990; D'Andrea *et al.* 1992). Dendritic cells can also produce IL-12 during antigen presentation (Trinchieri 19??; Snijders *et al.* 1998).

The IL-12 receptor is a heterodimer containing beta 1 and beta 2 chains. IL-12R beta 1 is the polypeptide that binds IL-12 (Gubler and Presky 1996; Presky *et al.* 1996), and the beta 2 chain is the component that transduces the IL-12 signal to the nucleus (Presky *et al.* 1996; Thibodeaux *et al.* 1999).Normal T helper type 1 (Th1) cells express both chains and hence are fully IL-12 responsive, whereas Th2 cells express only the IL-12R beta 1 chain.

The antitumor effects of IL-12 have been demonstrated in a number of murine models (Brunda *et al.* 1993; Tannenbaum *et al.* 1998). IL-12 therapy results in inhibition of tumor growth, reduction of metastatic lesions, increased survival time, and, in some models, regression and resistance to secondary challenge with the same tumor (Brunda *et al.* 1993; Tannenbaum *et al.* 1998). IL-12 is distinctive among cytokines displaying antitumor activity in that it often has proven effective even when therapy is initiated weeks after establishment of a significant tumor burden (Brunda *et al.* 1993; Tannenbaum *et al.* 1998; Martinotti *et al.* 1995).

Since IL-12 has no direct cytotoxicity or anti-proliferative effect on cultured tumor cells, antitumor effect is mediated indirectly through IL-12-inducible cellular and molecular intermediates (Martinotti *et al.* 1995; Tannenbaum *et al.* 1996). One molecule induced by and central to IL-12 activity is IFNγ. While IFNγ is required for the antitumor effects of IL-12, exogenous IFNγ does not mediate this activity (Brunda *et al.* 1995). These observations resulted in clinical trials of IL-12 in solid tumor patients, especially those with metastatic RCC.

Clinical results

Phase I trials utilizing either IV or SC administration of IL-12 have been performed. Motzer *et al.* (1998) performed a phase I trial in which IL-12 was administered SC at a fixed dose weekly for 3 weeks to patients with RCC. An MTD of 0.5 μg/kg/week was identified, with hepatic, leukopenia, and pulmonary toxicity being dose-limiting. Other toxicities seen with IL-12 included constitutional symptoms, anemia, and myelosuppression. A second phase of this trial involved gradual escalation of the IL-12 dose level following an initial dose of 0.1 μg/kg. In this portion of the trial, an MTD of 1.25 μg/kg/week was identified.

IV IL-12 has also been investigated in a phase I trial. Forty patients (20 with renal cancer) were enrolled (Atkins *et al.* 1997). Two weeks after a single injection of IL-12 (3–1000 ng/kg), patients received an additional 6-week course of IV IL-12 therapy, administered on 5 consecutive days every 3 weeks. The MTD was

0.5 μg/kg/day, and toxicities included fever/chills, fatigue, nausea, and headaches. Laboratory findings included anemia, neutropenia, lymphopenia, hyperglycemia, thrombocytopenia, and hypoalbuminemia.

A phase II trial of IV IL-12 was then initiated in RCC patients utilizing 0.5 μg/kg/day for 5 days (Mier *et al.* 1998). Seventeen patients were entered and, due to unexpectedly severe toxicity, the study was abandoned. The data from both the SC and IV phase I trials suggest a single predose of IL-12 may be associated with a decrease in toxicity and permit escalation of high doses.

In the reported phase I and II trials with IL-12, 118 patients with metastatic RCC were treated (Motzer *et al.* 1998; Atkins *et al.* 1997; Mier *et al.* 1998; Berg *et al.* 1998). Four responses were noted, two partial and two complete. In view of this limited activity, combinations of IL-12 with rIL-2 or IFNα are under investigation. These results remain preliminary.

References

Ahmed, F.Y., Leonard, G.A., A'Hern, R., Taylor, A.E., Lorentzos, A., Atkinson, H., *et al.* (1996). A randomized dose escalation study of subcutaneous interleukin-2 with and without levamisole in patients with metastatic renal cell carcinoma or malignant melanoma. *Br. J. Cancer* **74**, 1109.

Angevin, E., Kremer, F., Gaudin, C., Hercend, T., and Triebel, F. (1997). Analysis of T-cell immune response in renal cell carcinoma: polarization of type I-like differentiation pattern, clonal T-cell expansion and tumor-specific cytotoxicity. *Int. J. Cancer* **72**, 431–40.

Askenase, P.W., Hayden, B., and Gershon, R.K. (1975). Augmentation of delayed-type hypersensitivity by dose of cyclophosphamide which does not affect antibody synthesis. *J. Exp. Med.* **141**, 697.

Atkins, M.B., Sparano, J., Fisher, R.I., Weiss, G.R., Margolin, K.A., Fink, K.I., *et al.* (1993). Randomized phase Ii trial of high-dose interleukin-2 either alone or in combination with interferon alfa-2b in advanced renal cell carcinoma. *J. Clin. Oncol.* **11**, 661–70.

Atkins, M.B., Robertson, M.J., Gordon, M., Lotze, M.T., Decosta, M., DuBois, J.S., *et al.* (1997). Phase I evaluation of intravenous recombinant human interleukin-12 in patients with advanced malignancies. *Clin. Cancer Res.* **3**, 409–17.

Atzpodien, J., Kirchner, H., Hänninen, E., Deckert, M., Fenner, M., and Poliwada, H. (1993). Interleukin-2 in combination with interferon-α and 5-fluorouracil for metastatic renal cell carcinoma. *Eur. J. Cancer* **29A**, 56.

Atzpodien, J., Kirchner, H., Franzke, A., Wandert, T., Probst, M., Buer, J., *et al.* (1997). Results of a randomized clinical trial comparing SC interleukin-2, SC alpha-2a-interferon, and IV bolus 5-fluorouracil against oral tamoxifen in progressive metastatic renal cell carcinoma patients [abstract]. *Proc. Am. Soc. Clin. Oncol.* **16**, 326a.

Baeverde, P.A. and Baltimore, D. (1996). NfκB: ten years after. *Cell* **87**, 13.

Baker, P.E., Gillis, S., Ferm, M.M., and Smith, K.A. (1978). The effect of T cell growth factor on the generation of cytolytic T cells. *J. Immunol.* **121**, 2168.

Baker, P.E., Gillis, S., Smith, and K.A. (1979). Monoclonal cytolytic T-cell lines. *J. Exp. Med.* **1429**, 273.

Berd, D. and Mastrangelo, M. (1987). Effect of low-dose cyclophosphamide on the immune system of cancer patients: reduction of T-suppressor function without depletion of the CD8+ subset. *Cancer Res.* **47**, 3317–23.

Berd, D., Maguire H.C. Jr, and Mastrangelo, M.J. (1984). Potentiation of human cell-mediated and humoral immunity by low-dose cyclophosphamide. *Cancer Res.* **44**, 5439–45.

Berg, W.J., Bukowski, R., Thompson, J., Neumanitis, J., Murphy, B., Ellerhorst, J., *et al.* (1998). A randomized phase II trial of recombinant human interleukin-12 (IL-12) versus interferon alpha 2A (IFN) in advanced renal cell carcinoma (RCC) [abstract]. *Proc. Am. Soc. Clin. Oncol.* **17**, 318a.

Borden, E.C., Hogan, T.F., and Voelkel, J. (1982). The comparative antiproliferative activity *in vitro* of natural interferons alpha and beta for diploid and transformed human cells. *Cancer Res.* **42**, 4948–53.

Brossart, P., Stuhler, G., Flad, T., Stevanovic, S., Rammensee, H.G., Kanz, L., *et al.* (1998). Her-2/neu-derived peptides are tumor-associated antigens expressed by human renal cell and colon carcinoma lines and are recognized by *in vitro* induced specific cytotoxic T lymphocytes. *Cancer Res.* **58**, 732–6.

Brunda, M.J., Luistro, L., Warrier, R.R., Wright, R.B., Hubbard, B.R., Murphy, M., *et al.* (1993). Antitumor and antimetastatic activity of interleukin 12 against murine tumors. *J. Exp. Med.* **178**, 280–8.

Brunda, M.J., Luistro, L., Hendrzak, J.A., Fountoulakis, M., Garotta, G., and Gately, M.K. (1995). Role of interferon-gamma in mediating the antitumor efficacy of interleukin-12. *J. Immunother. Emphasis Tumor Immunol.* **17**, 71–7.

Bukowski, R.M. (1997). Natural history and therapy of metastatic renal cell carcinoma: role of interleukin 2. *Cancer* **80**, 1198–220.

Bukowski, R.M. and Dutcher, J.P. (2000). Low-dose interleukin-2. In *Genitourinary oncology.* (ed. N.J. Vogelzang, P.T. Scardino, W.W. Shipley, and D.S. Coffey), pp. 218–33. Lippincott, Williams and Wilkins, Philadelphia.

Bukowski, R.M., Sergi, J.S., Budd, G.T., Murthy, S., Tubbs, R., Gibson, V., *et al.* (1991). Phase I trial of continuous infusion interleukin-2 and doxorubicin in patients with refractory malignancies. *J. Immunother.* **10**, 432–9.

Bukowski, R.M., Young, J., Goodman, G., Meyers, F.J., Issell, B.F., Sergi, J.S., *et al.* (1993). Polyethylene glycol conjugated interleukin 2: clinical and immunologic effects in patients with advanced renal cell carcinoma. *Invest. New Drugs* **11**, 211.

Bukowski, R.M., McLain, D., and Finke, J.F. (1996). Clinical pharmacokinetics of interleukin-1, -2, -4, tumor necrosis factor and macrophage colony-stimulating factor. In *Cancer chemotherapy and biotherapy: principles and practice* (ed. B. Chabner and D. Longo), pp. 612–19. Lippincott–Raven, Philadelphia.

Bukowski, R.M., Rayman, P., Uzzo, R., Bloom, T., Sandstrom, K., Peereboom, D., *et al.* (1998). Signal transduction abnormalities in T-lymphocytes from patients with advanced renal cell carcinoma: clinical relevance and effects of cytokine therapy. *Clin. Cancer Res.* **4**, 2337.

Buter, J., Sleijfer, D.T., van der Graaf, W.T.A., de Vries, E.G., Willemse, P.H., and Mulder, N.H. (1993*a*). A progress report on the outpatient treatment of patients with advanced renal cell carcinoma using subcutaneous recombinant interleukin-2. *Sem. Oncol.* **20**, 16.

Buter, J., Janssen, R.A., Martens, A., Sleijfer, D.T., de Leij, L., Mulder, N.M. (1993*b*). Phase I/Ii study of low-dose intravenous OKT3 and subcutaneous interleukin 2 in metastatic cancer. *Eur. J. Cancer* **28**, 2108.

Caligiuri, M.A. (1994). Low-dose recombinant interleukin-2 therapy: rationale and potential clinical applications. *Am. J. Clin. Oncol.* **17**, 199.

Camerin, R.B., McIntosh, J., and Rosenberg, S.A. (1988). Synergistic antitumor effects of combination immunotherapy with recombinant interleukin-2 and recombinant hybrid interferon or the treatment of established hepatic metastasis. *Cancer Res.* **48**, 5819–27.

Chan, S.H., Perussia, B., Gupta, J.W., Kobayashi, M., Pospisil, M., Young, H.A., *et al.* (1991). Induction of interferon gamma production by natural killer cell stimulatory factor: characterization of the responder cells and synergy with other inducers. *J. Exp. Med.* **173**, 869–70.

Chikkala, N.F., Lewis I., Ulchaker, J., Stanley, J., Tubbs, R., and Finke, J.H. (1990). Interactive effects of α-interferon A/D and interleukin-2 on murine lymphokine-activated killer activity: analysis at the effector and precursor level. *Cancer Res.* **50**, 1176–82.

Ching, L.M. and Baguley, B.C. (1987). Induction of natural killer activity by the antitumor compound flavone acetic acid (NSC 347 512). *Eur. J. Cancer Clin. Oncol.* **23**, 1047–50.

D'Andrea, A., Rengaraju, M., Valiante, N.M., Chehimi, J., Kubin, M., Aste, M., *et al.* (1992). Production of natural killer cell stimulatory factor (interleukin 12) by peripheral blood mononuclear cells. *J. Exp. Med.* **176**, 1387–98.

Defrance, T., Fluciger, A.C., Rossi, J.F., Magaud, J.P., Sotto, J.J., and Banchereau, J. (1992). Antiproliferative effects of IL-4 on freshly isolated non-Hodgkin malignant B-lymphoma cells. *Blood* **79**, 990–6.

Dutcher, J.P., Atkins, M., Fisher, R., Weiss, G., Margolin, K., Aronson, F., *et al.* (1997). Interleukin-2 based therapy for metastatic renal cell cancer: the cytokine working group experience, 1989–1997. *Cancer J. Sci. Am.* **3**, 572.

Ellerhorst, J.A., Sella, A., Amato, R.J., Tu, S.M., Milliken, R.E., Finn, L.D., *et al.* (1997). Phase II trial of 5-fluorouracil, interferon-α and continuous infusion interleukin-2 for patients with metastatic renal cell carcinoma. *Cancer* **80**, 2128.

Escudier, B., Farace, F., Angevin, E., Triebel, F., Antoun, S., Leclercq, B., *et al.* (1993). Combination of interleukin-2 and gamma interferon in metastatic renal cell carcinoma. *Eur. J. Cancer* **29A**, 724–28.

Escudier, B., Ravaud, A., Fabbro, M., Douillard, J.Y., Negrier, S., Chevreau, C., *et al.* (1994). High-dose interleukin-2 two days a week for metastatic RCC: a FNCLCC multicenter study. *J. Immunother.* **27**, 1583.

Feldman, G.M. and Finbloom, D.S. (1990). Induction and regulation of IL-4 receptor expression on murine macrophage cell lines and bone marrow-derived macrophages by IFN-γ. *J. Immunol.* **145**, 854–9.

Findley, H.W., Nasr, S., Afify, Z., and Ragab, A.H. (1990). Effects of recombinant interferon-gamma and interleukin-2 on the generation of lymphokine-activated killed cells *in vitro*. *Cancer Invest.* **8**, 493–500.

Finke, J.H., Connelly, B., Tubbs, R., Connelly, B., Pontes, E., and Montie, J. (1988). Tumor-infiltrating lymphocytes in patients with renal cell carcinoma. *Ann. NY Acad. Sci.* **532**, 287–94.

Finke, J.H., Zea, A.H., Stanley, J., Longo, D.L., Mizogucki, H., Tubbs, R.R., *et al.* (1993) Loss of T-cell receptor zeta chain and p561ck in T-cells infiltrating human renal cell carcinoma. *Cancer Res.* **53**, 5613.

Finke, J.H., Rayman, P., Hart, L., Alexander, J.P., Edinger, M.G., Tubbs, R.R., *et al.* (1994). Characterization of tumor-infiltrating lymphocyte subsets from human renal cell carcinoma: specific reactivity defined by cytotoxicity, interferon-γ secretion, and proliferation. *J. Immunother. Emphasis Tumor Immunol.* **15**, 91–104.

Flamand, V., Sornasse, T., Thielemans, K., Demanet, K., Bakkus, C., Bozin, M., *et al.* (1994). Murine dendritic cells pulsed *in vitro* with tumor antigen induce tumor resistance *in vivo*. *Eur. J. Immunol.* **24**, 605–10.

Fyfe, G., Fisher, R.I., Rosenberg, S.A., Sznol, M., Parkinson, D.R., and Louie, A.C. (1995). Results of treatment of 255 patients with metastatic renal cell carcinoma who receive high dose recombinant interleukin-2 therapy. *J. Clin. Oncol.* **13**, 688–96.

Galizzi, J.P., Zuber, C.E., Cabrillat, H., Djossou, O., and Banchereau, J. (1989). Internalization of human interleukin-4 receptor and transient down-regulation of its receptor in the CD23-inducible jijoye cells. *J. Biol. Chem.* **264**, 6984–9.

Gately, M.K., Wilson, D.E., and Wong, H.L. (1986). Synergy between recombinant interleukin 2 (rIL 2) and IL 2-depleted lymphokine-containing supernatants in facilitating allogeneic human cytolytic T lymphocyte responses *in vitro*. *J. Immunol.* **136**, 1274–82.

Gately, M.K., Desai, B.B., Wolitzky, A.G., Quinn, P.M., Dwyer, C.M., Podlaski, F.J., *et al.* (1991). Regulation of human lymphocyte proliferation by a heterodimeric cytokine, IL-12 (cytotoxic lymphocyte maturation factor). *J. Immunol.* **147**, 874–82.

Gately, M.K., Wolitzky, A.G., Quinny, P.M., and Chizzonite, R. (1992). Regulation of human cytolytic lymphocyte responses by interleukin-12. *Cell. Immunol.* **143**, 127–42.

Gegrosky, N.P., Koukol, S., Nseyo, U.O., Carpenter, C., and Lamm, D.L. (1997). Treatment of renal cell carcinoma with 5-fluorouracil and alfa-interferon. *Urology* **50**, 863–8.

Gillis, S., Union, N.A., and Gallo, R.C. (1979). The *in vitro* generation and sustained culture of nude mouse cytolytic T-lymphocytes. *J. Exp. Med.* **149**, 1460.

Gleave, M.E., Elhilali, M., Frodet, Y., David, I., Venner, P., Saad, F., *et al.* (1998). Interferon gamma-1b compared with placebo in metastatic renal cell carcinoma. *New Engl. J. Med.* **338**, 1265–71.

Golumbek, P.T., Lazenby, A.J., Levitsky, H.I., Jaffe, L.M., Karasuyama, H., Baker, M., *et al.* (1991). Treatment of established renal cancer by tumor cells engineered to secrete interleukin-4. *Science*, **254**, 713–16.

Grimm, E.A., Mazumder, A., Zhang, H.Z., and Rosenberg, S.A. (1982). Lymphokine-activated killer cell phenomenon. Lysis of natural killer-resistant fresh solid tumor cells by interleukin-2 activated autologous human peripheral blood lymphocytes. *J. Exp. Med.* **155**, 1823–41.

Gubler, U. and Presky, D.H. (1996). Molecular biology of interleukin-12 receptors. *Ann. NY Acad. Sci.* **795**, 36–40.

Guida, M., Lattoree, A., and Selvaggi, F.P. (1997). Subcutaneous recombinant interleukin-2 plus α-interferon and vinblastine in metastatic renal cell carcinoma: a phase II study. *Int. J. Oncol.* **10**, 487–90.

Hahne, M., Rimoldi, D., Schroter, M., Romero, P., Schrier, M., French, L.E., *et al.* (1996). Melanoma cell expression of Fas (APO 1/CD95) ligand: implications for tumor immune escape. *Science* **274**, 1363.

Henriksson, R., Nilsson, S., Colleen, S., Wersall, P., Helsing, M., Zimmerman, R., *et al.* (1998). Survival in renal cell carcinoma—a randomized evaluation of tamoxifen vs interleukin-2, α interferon (leukocyte) and tamoxifen. *Br. J. Cancer* **77**, 1311–17.

Hofmockel, G., Langer, W., Theiss, M., Gruss, A., and Frohmuller, H.G. (1996). Immunochemotherapy for metastatic renal cell carcinoma using a regimen of interleukin-2, interferon-α and 5-fluorouracil. *J. Urol.* **156**, 18.

Holmlund, J.T., Kopp, W.C., Wiltrout, R.H., Longo, D.L., Urba, W.J., Janick, J.E., *et al.* (1995). A phase I clinical trial of flavone-8-acetic acid in combination with interleukin-2. *J. Natl Cancer Inst.* **87**, 134–6.

Houghton, J.A., Morton, C.L., Adkins, D.A., and Rahman, A. (1993). Locus of the interaction among 5-fluorouracil, leucovorin, and interferon-α2a in colon carcinoma cells. *Cancer Res.* **53**, 4243.

Howard, M., Farrar, J., Hilfiker, M., Johnson, B., Takatsu, K., Hamaoka, T., *et al.* (1982). Identification of a T cell-derived B cell stimulatory factor distinct from IL-2. *J. Exp. Med.* **155**, 914–23.

Hsu, F., Engleman, E.G., and Levy, R. (1997). Dendritic cells and their application in immunotherapeutic approaches to cancer therapy. In *Updates principles and practice of oncology* (ed. V.T. De Vita, S. Hellman, and S.A. Rosenberg), Vol. 11, pp. 1–14. Lippincott–Raven Healthcare, New Jersey.

Huland, E., Huland, H., and Heinzer, H. (1992). Interleukin-2 by inhalation: local therapy for metastatic renal cell carcinoma. *J. Urol.* **147**, 344.

Huland, E., Heinzer, H., Mir, T.S., and Huland, H. (1997). Inhaled interleukin-2 therapy in pulmonary metastatic renal cell carcinoma: six years of experience. *Cancer J. Sci. Am.* **3**, S98.

Indrova, M., Bubenik, J., Jakoubkova, J., Simova, J., Jandlova, T., Helmichova, E., *et al.* (1994) Subcutaneous interleukin-2 in combination with vinblastine for metastatic renal cancer: cytolytic activity of peripheral blood lymphocytes [abstract]. *Neoplasma* **41**, 197.

Isakson, P.C., Pure, E., Vitetta, S., and Krammer, P.H. (1982). T cell-derived B cell differentiation factor(s). Effect on the isotype switch of murine B cells. *J. Exp. Med.* **155**, 734–48.

Jayson, G.C., Middleton, M., Lee, S.M., Ashcroft, L., Thatcher, N. (1998). A randomized phase II trial of interleukin 2 and interleukin 2-interferon alpha in advanced renal cancer. *Br. J. Cancer* **78**, 366–9.

Joffe, J.K., Banks, R.E., Forbes, M.A., Hallam, S., Jenkins, A., Patel, P.M., *et al.* (1996). A phase II study of interferon-α, interleukin-2 and 5-fluorouracil in advanced renal carcinoma: clinical data and laboratory evidence of protease activation. *Br. J. Urol.* **77**, 638–43.

Kirchner, H., Buer, J., Probst-Kepper, M., Franzke, A., Hoffman, R., Wittke, F., *et al.* (1998). Risk and longer-term outcome in metastatic renal cell carcinoma patients receiving SC interleukin-2, SC interferon-alfa 2A, and IV 5-fluorouracil [abstract]. *Proc. Am. Soc. Clin. Oncol.* **17**, 310a.

Kliem, V., Kolditz, M., Behrend, M., Ehlending, G., Pichlmayr, R., Koch, K.M., *et al.* (1997). Risk of renal cell carcinoma after kidney transplantation. *Clin. Transplant.* **11**, 255–8.

Kowalczyk, D., Skorupski, W., Kwias, Z., and Nowak, J. (1997). Flow cytometric analysis of tumor-infiltrating lymphocytes in patients with renal cell carcinoma. *Br. J. Urol.* **80**, 543–7.

Krigel, R.L., Padvec-Shaller, K.A., Rudolph, A.R., Litvin, S., Konrad, M., Bradley, E.C., *et al.* (1988). A phase I study of recombinant interleukin 2 plus recombinant β-interferon. *Cancer Res.* **48**, 3875–8.

Kroemer, G., Andreu, J.L., Gonzale, J.A., Gutierrez-Ramos, J.C., and Martinez, C. (1991). Interleukin 2, autotolerance and autoimmunity. *Advan. Immunol.* **50**, 147.

Kuebler, J.P., Whitehead, R.P., Ward, D.L., Hemstreet, G.P., and Bradley, E.C. (1993). Treatment of metastatic renal cell carcinoma with recombinant interleukin-2 in combination with vinblastine or lymphokine activated killer cells. *J. Urol.* **150**, 814–20.

Le Beau, M.M., Lemons, R.S., Espinoza R. III, Larson, R.A., Arai, N., and Rowley, J.D. (1989). Interleukin-4 and interleukin-5 map to human chromosome 5 in a region encoding growth factors and receptors are deleted in myeloid leukemias with del (5q). *Blood* **73**, 647–50.

Li, X., Liu, J., Park, J.K., *et al.* (1994). T cells from renal carcinoma patients exhibit an abnormal pattern of kappa B-specific DNA binding activity: a preliminary report. *Cancer Res.* **54**, 5424.

Linsley, P.S., Clark, E.A., and Ledbetter, J.A. (1990). T-cell antigen CD28 mediates adhesion with B cells by interacting with activation antigen B7/BB-1. *Proc. Natl Acad. Sci., USA* **238**, 75.

Lissoni, P., Barni, S., Ardizzoia, A., Grispono, S., Paolorossi, F., Archili, C., *et al.* (1992). Second line therapy with low-dose subcutaneous interleukin-2 alone in advanced renal cancer patients resistant to interferon-alpha. *Eur. J. Cancer* **51**, 59.

Lissoni, P., Barni, S., Ardizzoia, A., Andres, M., Scardino, E., Cardellini, P., *et al.* (1993). A randomized study of low-dose interleukin-2 plus interferon-alpha first line therapy for metastatic RCC. *Tumor* **79**, 397–400.

Liu, C.C., Rafi, S., Granelli-Piperno, A., Trapani, J.A., and Young, J.D. (1989). Perforin and serine esterase gene expression in stimulated human T cells: kinetics, mitogen requirements, and effects of cyclosporin. *J. Exp. Med.* **170**, 2105.

Lopez Hänninen, E., Kirchner, H., and Atzpodien, J. (1996). Interleukin-2 based home therapy of metastatic renal cell carcinoma: risks and benefits in 215 consecutive single institution patients. *J. Urol.* **155**, 19.

Lotze, M.T., Frana, L.W., Sharrow, S.O., Robb, R.J., and Rosenberg, S.A. (1985). *In vivo* administration of purified human interleukin 2. I. Half-life and immunologic effects of the Jurkat cell line-derived interleukin 2. *J. Immunol.* **134**, 157.

Lümmen, G., Goepel, M., Möllhof, S., Hinke, A., Otto, T., and Rubben, H. (1996). Phase II study of interferon γ versus interleukin-2-interferon–$2\alpha b$ in metastatic renal cell carcinoma. *J. Urol.* **155**, 455–58.

Margolin, K.A., Doroskow, J.H., Akman, S.A., Leong, L.A., Morgan, R., Raschko, J., *et al.* (1993). Phase I trial of interleukin-2 plus doxorubicin. *J. Immunother.* **14**, 70–6.

Markowitz, A., Parkinson, D., Miller, L., Levitt, D., Saks, S., and Gutterman, J. (1989). Phase I study of recombinant tumor necrosis factor (rTNF) and recombinant interleukin-2 (rIL-2) [abstract]. *Proc. Am. Soc. Clin. Oncol.* **8**, 195.

Martinotti, A., Stoppacciaro, A., Vagliani, M., Melani, C., Spreafico, F., Wysocka, M., *et al.* (1995). CD4 T cells inhibit *in vivo* the CD8-mediated immune response murine colon carcinoma cells transduced with interleukin-12 genes. *Eur. J. Immunol.* **25**, 137–46.

Meyers, F.J., Paradise, C., Scudder, S.A., Goodman, G., and Konrad, A. (1991). A phase I study including pharmacokinetics of polyethylene glycol conjugated interleukin 2. *Clin. Pharmacol. Therapeut.* **49**, 307.

Mier, J.W., Gollob, J.A., and Atkins, M. (1998). Interleukin 12, a new antitumor cytokine. *Int. J. Immunopathol. Pharmacol.* **11**, 109–15.

Mitchell, M.S. (1992). Chemotherapy in combination with biomodulation: a 5-year experience with cyclophosphamide and interleukin-2. *Sem. Oncol.* **19** (Suppl. 4), 80–8.

Morgan, D.A., Ruscetti, F.W., and Gallo, R.C. (1976). Selective *in vitro* growth of T lymphocytes from normal bone marrows. *Science* **193**, 1007.

Mossmann, T.R., Cherwinski, H., Bond, M.W., Giedlin, M.A., and Coffman, R.L. (1986). Two types of murine helper T cell clones. Definition according to profiles of lymphokine activities and secreted proteins. *J. Immunol.* **136**, 2348–57.

Motzer, R.J., Rakhit, A., Schwartz, L.H., Olencki, T., Malone, T., Sandstrom, K., *et al.* (1998). Phase I trial of subcutaneous recombinant human interleukin-12 on patients with advanced renal cell carcinoma. *Clin. Cancer Res.* **4**, 1183–91.

Mule, J.J. and Rosenberg, S.A. (1991). Combination cytokine therapy: experimental and clinical trials. In *Biologic therapy of cancer* (ed. V. DeVita, S. Hellman, and S. Rosenberg), pp. 142–58. Lippincott, Philadelphia.

Naglieri, E., Gebbra, V., Durini, E., Lelli, E., Albate, I., Selvaggi, F.P., *et al.* (1998). Standard interleukin-2 (IL-2) and interferon-α immunotherapy versus an IL-2 and 4-epirubicin immunochemotherapeutic association in metastatic renal cell carcinoma. *Anticancer Res.* **18**, 2021–6.

Negrier, S., Escudier, B., Douillard, J.Y., Lesimple, T., Rossi, J.F., Viens, F., *et al.* (1997). Randomized study of interleukin-2 (IL2) and interferon (IFN) with or without 5-FU (FUCY study) in metastatic renal cell carcinoma (MRCC) [abstract]. *Proc. Am. Soc. Clin. Oncol.* **16**, 326a.

Negrier, S., Escudier, B., Lasset, C., Douillard, J.Y., Savary, J., Chevreau, C., *et al.* (1998). Recombinant human interleukin-2, recombinant interferon alfa-2a, or both in metastatic renal cell carcinoma. *New Engl. J. Med.* **338**, 1272.

Neumann, E., Engelberg, A., Decker, J., Storkel, S., Jaeger E., Huber, C., *et al.* (1998). Heterogenous expression of the tumor-associated antigens RAGE-1, PRAME, and glycoprotein 75 in human renal cell carcinoma: candidates for T-cell-based immunotherapies? *Cancer Res.* **58**, 4090–5.

Newman, S.P. and Clarke, S.W. (1983). Therapeutic aerosols: practical considerations. *Thorax* **38**, 881.

Ohara, J. and Paul, W.E. (1987). Receptors for B-cell stimulatory factor-1 expressed on cells of hematopoietic lineage. *Nature* **325**, 537–40.

Ohara, J. and Paul, W.E. (1988). Upregulation of interleukin 4/B cell stimulatory factor-1 receptor expression. *Proc. Natl Acad. Sci., USA* **85**, 8221–5.

Oldham, R.K., Dillman, R.O., Yannelli, J.R., Barth, N.M., Maleckar, J.R., Sferuzza, A., *et al.* (1991*a*). Continuous infusion interleukin-2 and tumor-derived activated cells as treatment of advanced solid tumors: a national biotherapy study group trial. *Mol. Biother.* **3**, 68–73.

Oldham R.K., Stark, J., Barth, N.M., Hoogstraten, B., Brown, C.H., O'Connor, T., *et al.* (1991*b*). Continuous infusion of interleukin-2 and cyclo-phosphamide as treatment of advanced cancers: a national biotherapy study group trial. *Mol. Biother.* **3**, 74–8.

Olencki, T., Finke, J., Tubbs, R., Tauson, L., Greene, T., Mc Lain, D., *et al.* (1996). Phase IA/IB trial of interleukin-2 and interleukin-4 in patients with refractory malignancies. *J. Immunother. Emphasis Tumor Immunol.* **19**, 69–80.

Oliver, R.T.D., Mehta, A., and Barnett M.J. (1988). A phase 2 study of sur-veillance in patients with metastatic renal cell carcinoma and assessment of response of such patients to therapy on progression. *Mol. Biother.* **1**, 14–20.

Orsini, F., Pavelic, Z., and Mihich, E. (1977). Increased primary cell mediated immunity in culture subsequent to adriamycin or doxorubicin treatment of spleen donor mice. *Cancer Res.* **37**, 1719–24.

Paciucci, P.A., Bekesi, G., Ryder, J.S., Odchimar, R., Chahinian, P.A., and Holland, J.F. (1991). Immunotherapy with IL-2 by constant infusion and weekly doxorubicin. *Am. J. Oncol.* **14**, 341–8.

Palmer, P.A., Atzpodien, J., Philip, T., Negrier, S., Kirchner, H., von der Mass, H., *et al.* (1993). A comparison of 2 modes of administration of recom-binant interleukin-2: continuous intravenous infusion alone versus sub-cutaneous administration plus interferon alpha in patients with advanced renal cell carcinoma. *Cancer Biother.* **8**, 123–36.

Park, L.S., Friend, D., Sassenfeld, H.M., and Urdal, D.L. (1987). Charac-terization of the human B cell stimulatory factor 1 receptor. *J. Exp. Med.* **166**, 476–88.

Pectasides, D., Varthalitis, J., Kostopoulou, M., Mylonakis, A., Triantaphyllis, D., Papadopoulou, M., *et al.* (1998). An outpatient phase II study of subcutaneous interleukin-2 and interferon-alpha-2b in combination with intravenous vinblastine in metastatic renal cell cancer. *Oncology* **55**, 10–15.

Plaut, M., Pierce, J.H., Watson, C.J., Hanley-Hyde, J., Nordan, R.P., and Paul, W.E. (1989). Mast cell lines produce lymphokines in response to cross lineage of FC_FR1 or to calcium ionophores. *Nature* **6219**, 64–7.

Podlaski, F.J., Naduri, V.B., Hulmes, J.D., Pan, Y.C., Levin, W., Danho, W., *et al.* (1992). Molecular characterization of interleukin 12. *Arch. Biochem. Biophys.* **294**, 230–7.

Presky, D.H., Yang, H., Minetti, L.J., Chua, A.O., Nabavi, N., Wu, C.Y., *et al.* (1996). A functional interleukin 12 receptor complex is composed of two beta-type cytokine receptor subunits. *Proc. Natl Acad. Sci., USA* **93**, 15002–7.

Puri, R.K., Ogata, M., Leland, P., Feldman, G.M., Fitzgerald, D., and Paston, I. (1991). Expression of high affinity IL-4 receptors on murine sarcoma cells and receptor mediated cytotoxicity of tumor cells to chimeric protein between IL-4 and pseudomonas exotoxin. *Cancer Res.* **51**, 3011–17.

Ravaud, A., Audhuy, B., Gomez, F., Escudier, B., Lesimple, T., Chevreau, C., *et al.* (1998). Subcutaneous interleukin-2, interferon alfa-2a, and continuous infusion of fluorouracil in metastatic renal cell carcinoma: a multicenter phase II trial. *J. Clin. Oncol.* **16**, 2728.

Redman, B.G., Flaherty, L., Chou, T.H., al-Katib, A., Kraut, M., Martino, S., *et al.* (1990). A phase I trial of recombinant interleukin-2 combined with recombinant interferon-gamma in patients with cancer. *J. Clin. Oncol.* **8**, 1269–76.

Rosenberg, S.A., Mule, J.S., Speiss, P.J., Reichert, C.M., and Schwarz, S.L. (1985). Regression of established pulmonary metastases and subcutaneous tumor mediated by the systemic administration of high-dose recombinant interleukin 2. *J. Exp. Med.* **161**, 1169.

Rosenberg, S.A., Lotze, M.T., Yang, J.C., Aebersold, P.M., Linehan, W.M., Seipp, C.A., *et al.* (1989). Experience with the use of high dose interleukin-2 in the treatment of 652 cancer patients. *Ann. Surg.* **210**, 474–84.

Sallusto, F. and Langavecchia, A. (1994). Efficient presentation of soluble antigen by cultured human dendritic cells is maintained by granulocyte/macrophage colony- stimulating factor plus interleukin-4 and down-regulated by tumor necrosis factor alpha. *J. Exp. Med.* **179**, 1109–14.

Savage, P., Costelna, D., Moore, J., and Gore, M.E. (1996). A phase II study of continuous infusional 5-fluorouracil (5-FU) and subcutaneous interleukin-2 (IL-2) in metastatic renal cancer. *Eur. J. Cancer* **33**, 1149.

Schendel, D.J., Gansbacher, B., Oberneder, R., Kriegmair, M., Hofstetter, A., Riethmuller, G., *et al.* (1993). Tumor-specific lysis of human renal cell carcinomas by tumor-infiltrating lymphocytes. I. HLA-A2-restricted recognition of autologous and allogeneic tumor lines. *J. Immunol.* **151**, 4209–20.

Schiller, J.H., Hank, J.A., Khorsand, M., Storer, B., Borchert, A., Huseby-Moore, K., *et al.* (1996). Clinical and immunological effects of granulocyte–macrophage colony stimulating factor co-administered with interleukin-2: a phase IB study. *Clin. Cancer Res.* **2**, 319–30.

Small, E.J., Weiss, G.R., Malik, U.K., Walther, P.J., Johnson, D., Wilding, G., *et al.* (1998). The treatment of metastatic renal cell carcinoma patients with recombinant human gamma interferon. *Cancer J. Sci. Am.* **4**, 162–7.

Smith, K.A. (1993). Lowest dose interleukin 2 immunotherapy. *Blood* **81**, 1414.

Snijders, A., Kalinski, P., Hilkens, C.M., and Kapsenberg, M.L. (1998). High-level IL 12 production by human dendritic cells requires two signals. *Int. Immunol.* **10**, 1593–8.

Stern, A.S., Podlaski, F.J., Holmes, J.D., Pan, Y.C., Quinn, P.M., Wolitzky, A.G., *et al.* (1990). Purification to homogeneity and partial characterization of cytotoxic lymphocyte maturation factor from human B-lymphoblastoid cells. *Proc. Natl Acad. Sci., USA* **87**, 6808–12.

Taberno, J., Pazares, L., Cubedo, R., Carles, J., Blanco, R., Nogue, M., *et al.* (1998). Phase II study of subcutaneous (SC) recombinant interleukin-2 (RIL-2) and intravenous (IV) vinblastine (VBL) in advanced renal cell carcinoma (RCC) [abstract]. *Proc. Am. Soc. Clin. Oncol.* **17**, 345a.

Takeshita, T., Asao, H., Ohtani, K., Ishii, N., Kumaki, S., Tanaka, N., *et al.* (1992). Cloning of the γ chain of the human IL-2 receptor. *Science* **257**, 379.

Tannenbaum, C.S., Wicker, N., Armstrong, D., Tubbs, R., Finke, J., Bukowski, R.M., *et al.* (1996). Cytokine and chemokine expression in tumors of mice receiving systemic therapy with IL-12. *J. Immunol.* **156**, 693–9.

Tannenbaum, C.S., Tubbs, R., Armstrong, D., Finke, J.H., Bukowski, R.M., and Hamilton, T.A. (1998). The CXC chemokines IP-10 and Miq are necessary for IL-12-mediated regression of the mouse RENCA tumor. *J. Immunol.* **161**, 927–32.

Taylor, C.W., Chase, E.M., Whitehead, R.P., Rinehart, J.J., Neidhart, J.A., Gonzalez, R., *et al.* (1992). A Southwest Oncology Group phase I study of the sequential combination of recombinant interferon-γ and recombinant interleukin-2 in patients with cancer. *J. Immunother.* **11**, 176–83.

Tepper, R.I. (1989). Murine interleukin-4 displays potent antitumor activity *in vivo*. *Cell* **57**, 503–12.

Thibodeaux, D.K., Hunter, S.E., Waldburger, K.E., Bliss, J.L., Tropicchio, W.L., Sypek, J.P., *et al.* (1999). Autocrine regulation of IL-12 receptor expression is independent of secondary IFN-gamma secretion and not restricted to T and NK cells. *J. Immunol.* **163**, 5257–64.

Toi, M., Bicknel, R., and Harris, A.L. (1992). Inhibition of colon and breast carcinoma cell growth by interleukin-4. *Cancer Res.* **52**, 275–9.

Tourani, J.M., Pfister, C., Berdah, J.F., Benhammouda, A., Salze, P., Monnier, A., *et al.* (1998). Outpatient treatment with subcutaneous interleukin-2 and interferon alfa administration in combination with fluorouracil in patients with metastatic renal cell carcinoma: results of a sequential nonrandomized phase II study. *J. Clin. Oncol.* **16**, 2505–10.

Trinchieri, G. (1994). Interleukin-12: a cytokine produced by antigen-presenting cells with immunoregulatory functions in the generation of T-helper cells type 1 and cytotoxic lymphocytes. *Blood* **84**, 4008–27.

Tungekar, M.F., Turley, H., Dunnill, M.S., Gotter, K.C., Ritter, M.A., and Harris, A.L. (1991). Interleukin-4 receptor expression on human lung tumors and normal lung. *Cancer Res.* **51**, 261–5.

Uzzo, R.G., Rayman, P., Kolenko, V., Clark, P.E., Bloom, T., Ward, A.M., *et al.* (1999). Mechanisms of apoptosis in T cells from patients with renal cell carcinoma. *Clin. Cancer Res.* **5**, 1219–29.

van Leeuween, B.H., Martinson, M.E., Webb, G.C., and Young, I.G. (1989). Molecular organization of the cytokine gene cluster, involving the human IL-3, IL-4, IL-5 and GM-CSF genes, on human chromosome 5. *Blood* **73**, 1142–8.

Viens, P., Blaise, D., Stoppa, A.M., Brandley, M., Baume, D., Olive, P., *et al.* (1992). Interleukin-2 in association with increasing doses of interferon-gamma in patients with advanced cancer. *J. Immunother.* **11**, 218–23.

Wagteveld, A.J., Zanten, A.K.V., Esselink, M.T., Halie, M.R., and Vellenga, E. (1991). Expression and regulation of IL-4 receptors on human monocytes and acute myeloblastic leukemia cells. *Leukemia* **5**, 782–8.

Wan, Y.J., Orrison, B.M., Lieberman, R., Lazarovici, P., and Ozato, K. (1987). Induction of major histocompatibility class I antigens by interferons in undifferentiated F9 cells. *J. Cell. Physiol.* **130**, 276–83.

Wersall, J.P., Masucci, G., Hjelm, A.L., Ragnhammer, P., Fagerberg, J., Frodin, J.E., *et al.* (1993). Low dose cyclophosphamide, alpha interferon and continuous infusions of interleukin-2 in advanced renal cell carcinoma. *Med. Oncol. Tumor Pharmacother.* **10**, 103–11.

Wiltrout, R.H., Boyd, M.R., Back, T.C., Salup, R.R., Arthur, J.A., and Hornung, R.L. (1988). Flavone-8-acetic acid augments systemic natural killer activity and synergizes with IL-2 for the treatment of murine renal cancer. *J. Immunol.* **140**, 3261–5.

Witt, P.L., Lindner, D.J., D'Ainha, J., Cunha, J., and Borden, E.C. (1996). Pharmacology of interferons: induced proteins, cell activations, and antitumor activity. In *Cancer chemotherapy and biotherapy: principles and practice*. (ed. B. Chabner and D Longo), pp. 585–608. Lippincott–Raven, Philadelphia.

Witte, R.S., Leong, T., Ernstoff, M.S., Krigel, R.L., Oken, M.M., Harris, J., *et al.* (1995). A phase II study of interleukin-2 with and without beta-interferon in the treatment of advanced renal cell carcinoma. *Invest. New Drugs* **13**, 241–7.

Yagoda, A. (1990). Phase II cytotoxic chemotherapy trials in RCC; 1983–1988. *Prog. Clin. Biol. Res.* **350**, 227–41.

Yang, J.C. and Rosenberg, S.A. (1997). An ongoing prospective randomized comparison of interleukin-2 regimens for the treatment of metastatic renal cell cancer. *Cancer J. Sci. Am.* **3**, 579.

Yang, J.C., Topalian, S.L., Parkinson, D., Schwartzentruber, D.J., Weber, J.S., Ettinghause, S.E., *et al.* (1994). Randomized comparison of high-dose and low-dose intravenous interleukin-2 for the therapy of metastatic RCC: an interim report. *J. Clin. Oncol.* **12**, 1572–6.

Yang, J.C., Topalian, S., Schwartzentruber, D.J., Parkinson, D.R., Marincola, T.M., Weber, J.S., *et al.* (1995). The use of polyethylene glycol-modified interleukin-2 (PEG IL-2) in the treatment of patients with metastatic renal cell carcinoma and melanoma. A phase I study and a randomized prospective study comparing IL-2 alone versus IL-2 combined with PEG-IL-2. *Cancer* **76**, 687.

Yokota, T., Otsuka, T., Mosmann, T., Banchereau, J., De France, T., Blanchard, D., *et al.* (1986). Isolation and characterization of a mouse interleukin cDNA that expresses B-cell stimulatory factor 1 activities, and T cell and mast cell stimulating activities. *Proc. Natl Acad. Sci., USA* **83**, 2061–5.

41. Adoptive immunotherapy of renal cell cancer

Alfred E. Chang, Qiao Li, Guihua Jiang, Donna M. Sayre, and Bruce G. Redman

Introduction

The passive transfer of immune lymphocytes into the tumor-bearing host or cancer patient is known as 'adoptive immunotherapy'. The requirements for successful adoptive immunotherapy in animal models involve the ability to generate tumor-reactive cells in sufficient quantities to cause tumor rejection *in vivo* (Greenberg 1991; Chang and Shu 1992). Compared with other immunotherapeutic modalities, such as cytokines, vaccines, or antibodies, adoptive immunotherapy has been significantly more effective in mediating regression of advanced tumor burdens in animal models (Chou *et al.* 1988*a*; Rosenberg *et al.* 1986). The translation of animal studies to the clinical setting required the development of methods to culture lymphocytes in bulk quantities. This was made possible by the discovery of interleukin 2 (IL-2) in 1976 (then known as T-cell growth factor) (Morgan *et al.* 1976). This chapter will review the experience of adoptive immunotherapy for renal cell cancer and summarize the clinical studies being performed at the University of Michigan.

Lymphokine-activated killer (LAK) cells

The culture of lymphocytes with high concentrations of IL-2 results in the activation of these lymphocytes to become non-specifically reactive to tumor cells. These lymphokine-activated killer (LAK) cells were described by Grimm *et al.* (1983) as lysing tumor cells, but not normal 'self'-lymphocytes, in a non-major histocompatibility (MHC) manner. Animal studies conducted by Mulé *et al.* (1984) demonstrated that the adoptive transfer of LAK cells can result in regression of established tumor; and that the concomitant administration of IL-2 will enhance the antitumor effect. LAK cells can be reliably generated from peripheral blood lymphocytes (PBL) of cancer patients and cultured in bulk culture conditions (Rayner *et al.* 1985; Muul *et al.* 1987).

Rosenberg *et al.* (1988) reported dramatic responses in patients with metastatic renal cell carcinoma (RCC) with an initial overall response rate (complete response (CR) + partial response (PR)) in 12 of 36 (33 per cent) patients. This therapy was evaluated by several other groups as summarized in Table 41.1 (Rosenberg 1988; West *et al.* 1987; Schoof *et al.* 1988; Thompson *et al.* 1989; Paciucci *et al.* 1989; Wang *et al.* 1989; Fisher *et al.* 1988; Parkinson *et al.* 1990). Utilizing different regimens of IL-2 along with LAK cell infusions, the overall response rate (CR + PR) in 198 patients was 22 per cent. Since high-dose IL-2 given by itself is associated with significant responses in RCC, it was critical to evaluate LAK plus IL-2 versus IL-2 alone in a prospective randomized trial. Such a study was performed by the US National Cancer Institute (NCI), which entered 54 melanoma and 97 RCC patients (Rosenberg *et al.* 1993). Overall, there was no significant difference in response rates between IL-2 alone versus IL-2 plus LAK cells, although there was a trend for increased survival in the melanoma patients

Table 41.1 Adoptive immunotherapy of renal cell cancer with LAK cells plus IL-2

				Tumor response*		
Reference	Number of patients	Number[†] of LAK[‡] cells (× 10^{10})	IL-2 infusion[§]	CR	PR	CR + PR
Rosenberg 1988	54	7.9	Bolus	7	10	17
West *et al.* 1987	6	6.8–9.1	CI	0	3	3
Schoof *et al.* 1988	10	4.3	Bolus	0	5	5
Thompson *et al.* 1989	8	3.4–4.3	Bolus/CI	1	0	1
Wang *et al.* 1989	32	4.9–6.1	CI	2	5	7
Paciucci *et al.* 1989	9	3.4	CI	0	1	1
Fisher *et al.* 1988	32	7.0	Bolus	2	3	5
Parkinson *et al.*1990	47	92	CI	2	2	2
Totals	198			14	29	43 (22%)

* CR, complete response: regression of all evaluable tumor; PR, partial response: ≥ 50 per cent regression of all evaluable tumor.
[†] Represents mean or median number of cells.
[‡] Modified LAK generated by periodate and IL-2.
[§] IL-2 infusion with the administration of LAK cells; CI, continuous infusion.

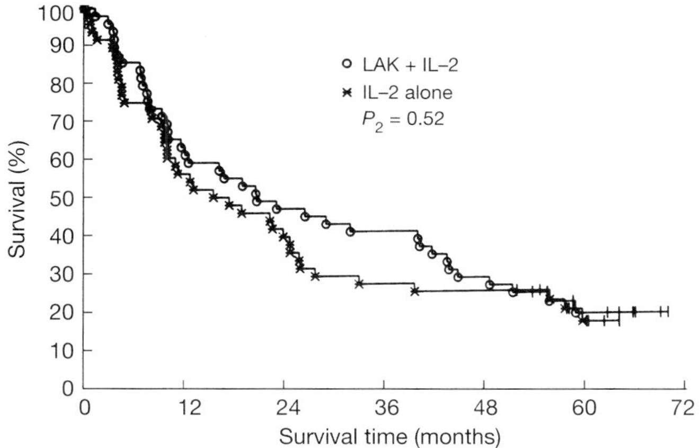

Fig. 41.1 Overall survival of patients with metastatic RCC randomly assigned to receive either IL-2 or LAK/IL-2. ($P_2 = 0.52$; reprinted with permission from Rosenberg, *et al.* (1993).)

who received cell therapy. Among the RCC patients, 87 were evaluable for response (CR + PR), which was observed in 15 of 46 (32 per cent) and 10 of 41 (24 per cent) patients who received LAK plus IL-2 versus IL-2 alone, respectively (not significantly different). The overall survival between the randomized RCC patient groups was not statistically different (Fig. 41.1). This study essentially eliminated LAK cell therapy as a superior therapy since IL-2 alone appeared to be equivalent in efficacy.

Tumor-infiltrating lymphocytes (TIL)

In contrast to LAK cells, which can be generated from the PBL of cancer patients, there have been no reliable methods to generate large quantities of tumor-reactive T cells from circulating lymphocytes due to their low frequency. An alternative source of lymphoid cells has been from within the tumor. It is possible that the lymphoid infiltrate within a tumor may represent a select population of cells that have preferentially migrated to the tumor and are retained there due to the presence of tumor antigen (Yron *et al.* 1980). Animal studies reported by Rosenberg and co-workers (1986) have demonstrated that TIL are highly efficient in mediat-

ing regression of bulky, advanced tumor burdens. TIL are generated by the *in vitro* culture of dissociated tumor cell preparations placed in conditioned media supplemented with IL-2. In direct comparative experiments, TIL were found to be more potent than LAK cells in eradicating established metastases (Spiess *et al.* 1987). IL-2 is routinely administered with TIL to enhance their proliferation and survival *in vivo*. In addition, agents such as cyclophosphamide or interferon alpha (IFNα) have been administered with TIL to improve their antitumor efficacy (Rosenberg *et al.* 1986; Cameron *et al.* 1988). Cyclophosphamide has been reported to reduce tumor-induced immune suppression and may also act by reducing tumor burden (Berd *et al.* 1986). IFNα is thought to enhance cellular therapies by upregulating MHC class I or II molecules on tumor cells and/or tumor antigens, thus allowing easier recognition of the tumor cells by immune T cells.

The application of TIL to patients with metastatic RCC is summarized in Table 41.2 (Topalian *et al.* 1988; Kradin *et al.* 1989; Bukowski *et al.* 1991; Figlin *et al.* 1997). The experience is varied with respect to the method of IL-2 administration, cell dose, and the use of other immunomodulatory agents. Hence, the overall response rate of 24 per cent may be misleading. The best results were reported by the UCLA group with the largest experience and a response rate of 34 per cent (Figlin *et al.* 1997). In this study, IFNα was administered in conjunction with TIL plus IL-2. In an attempt to determine if TIL plus IL-2 was superior to IL-2 alone in metastatic RCC, a prospective multicenter randomized trial was conducted by Figlin *et al.* (1999). Patients with stage IV RCC underwent nephrectomy and were randomized to receive TIL plus IL-2 or IL-2 only by continuous infusion. TIL were cultured to promote expansion of CD8[+] T cells. In this study, 160 were randomized; however, 20 received no therapy due to surgical complications or ineligibility. Among 72 patients eligible for TIL/IL-2, 33 (41 per cent) received no TIL therapy because of insufficient numbers of viable cells. Intent-to-treat analysis demonstrated response rates of 9.9 versus 11.4 per cent for the TIL/IL-2 and IL-2 control groups, respectively. This trial documents the difficulty in performing adoptive cellular therapies in a multicenter setting. The question as to whether TIL/IL-2 was better than IL-2 alone could not be adequately assessed due to the difficulty in getting patients into therapy. Furthermore, the generation of TIL was not consistently reliable despite a centralized facility set up to perform this task.

Table 41.2 Adoptive immunotherapy of renal cell cancer with TIL plus IL-2*

| Reference | Number[†] of | | IL-2 infusion[§] (n) | Other agents (n) | Tumor response |
	patients	TIL ($\times 10^{10}$)			
Topalian *et al.* 1988	4	4.8	Bolus	CYT (2)	1 (PR)
				No CYT (2)	0
Kradin *et al.* 1989	7	1	CI	None	2 (PR)
Bukowski *et al.* 1991	18	0.12–320	CI (15)	CYT (4)	0
			No IL-2 (3)	No CYT (14)	
Figlin *et al.* 1997	56	NS	CI	± IFNα	19 (7 CR, 12 PR)
Totals	85	21 (24%)			

* CI, continuous infusion; *n*, number of patients experiencing a particular treatment; CYT, cytoxan; CR, complete response; PR, partial response; NS, not stated.

The difficulty in reliably generating TIL cells for clinical therapy is a significant impediment. Until methods are developed that can ensure the culture of TIL in a majority of RCC tumor specimens, this therapy should be confined to institutions with the expertise to perform these procedures. The UCLA experience with TIL therapy in RCC indicates that this approach is feasible and may be enhanced by the concomitant administration of IFNα.

Vaccine-primed lymph node (VPLN) cells

Our laboratory has focused on the use of vaccine-primed lymph nodes (VPLN) as a source of immune lymphoid cells for adoptive immunotherapy. Based upon extensive animal studies, lymph nodes draining growing tumors harbor 'pre-effector' lymphoid cells that can be secondarily activated *ex vivo* to mature into competent effector cells (Chou *et al.* 1988*b*; Yoshizawa *et al.* 1991, 1992). These effector cells can mediate potent tumor regression of advanced tumor burdens in adoptive immunotherapy animal studies (Chang and Shu 1992). The method of secondary activation can be performed with autologous tumor cells or with a pan-T-cell activating antibody, anti-CD3 (Yoshizawa *et al.* 1991). The advantage of utilizing anti-CD3 monoclonal antibody (mAb), anti-CD3, is the avoidance of the need to have sufficient quantities of tumor cells for *in vitro* stimulation. The VPLN cells are also expanded in numbers utilizing low concentrations of IL-2. The use of a bacterial immune adjuvant admixed with irradiated tumor cells and inoculated as a vaccine in animals can elicit VPLN cells that can reject poorly immunogenic metastases (Geiger *et al.* 1993). In these animal models, the secretion of IFNγ and granulocyte–macrophage colony stimulating factor (GM-CSF) by the VPLN cells has been found to be an important mechanism in mediating tumor regression (Aruga *et al.* 1997*a*). By contrast, the secretion of IL-10 by the adoptively transferred cells has been suppressive in attaining tumor rejection (Aruga *et al.* 1997*b*).

On the basis of the animal model, we have been investigating the antitumor activity of anti-CD3 activated VPLN in the treatment of patients with metastatic cancer. Our preliminary studies included patients with metastatic melanoma and RCC (Chang *et al.* 1997). In that study 23 patients were treated (11 melanoma and 12 RCC). A mean of 8.4×10^{10} activated cells were infused along with the concomitant administration of IL-2 (360 000 IU/kg intravenous (IV) bolus every 8 hours for 15 doses). A majority of the activated lymph node (LN) cells showed specific release of IFNγ and GM-CSF to autologous tumor cells, but not allogeneic tumor stimulation (Fig. 41.2). This tumor-specific cytokine release was MHC class I restricted. Among 11 melanoma patients, there was one partial response. Among the 12 RCC patients, there were two complete and two partial responses.

Our preliminary experience prompted us to initiate a phase II clinical trial in patients with metastatic RCC for the adoptive transfer of anti-CD3 activated VPLN. All eligible patients had a nephrectomy either before protocol consideration or to obtain tumor tissue for vaccine generation. Each vaccine consisted of autologous tumor cells ($1–2 \times 10^7$ cells) irradiated with 2500 cGy

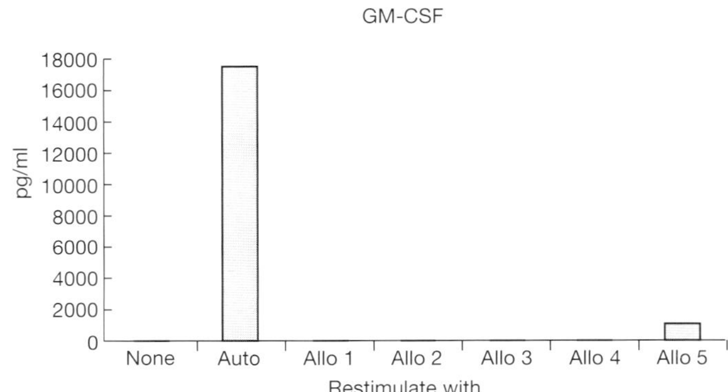

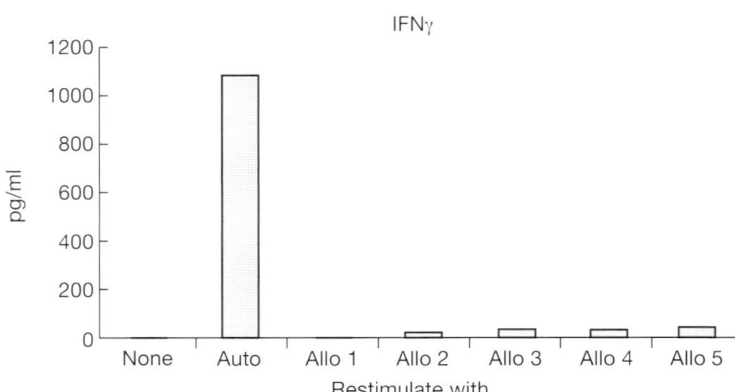

Fig. 41.2 GM-CSF and IFNγ release by anti-CD3 activated VPLN cells from an RCC patient. The cytokine release was specific to autologous (Auto) tumor, but not to five unrelated allogeneic (Allo) RCC tumors. This patient underwent a complete response to VPLN cell infusion therapy plus IL-2.

and admixed with 10^7 colony-forming units of Tice Bacille Calmette–Guérin (BCG; Organon Technika Corp., Durham, NC). Two vaccines were inoculated intradermally into separate thighs. Approximately 7–10 days later, the VPLN were identified by their hyperplastic appearance in each groin and removed. An aliquot of VPLN cells (approximately 5×10^8) were placed into the anti-CD3/IL-2 activation protocol as described in our preliminary report (Chang *et al.* 1997). After a period of approximately 15 days, the anti-CD3 activated cells were harvested and infused via a central line along with the concomitant infusion of IL-2 (360 000 IU/kg every 8 hours for 15 doses). After completion of therapy, patients were re-assessed 1 and 2 months later by radiological studies to evaluate for tumor response. If the tumor was stable or responding, the patient would undergo another cell infusion with VPLN cells cryopreserved from the initial harvest. A third infusion of cells would be given in patients continuing to respond. If cells were not available for this third infusion, then IL-2 only would be administered.

In a subgroup of patients, we evaluated what BCG was contributing to the vaccine (Li *et al.* 2000*a*). Patients underwent vaccination with the BCG-containing vaccine in one thigh, and autologous tumor cells only in the contralateral thigh. The VPLN cells were removed as described above. The VPLN draining

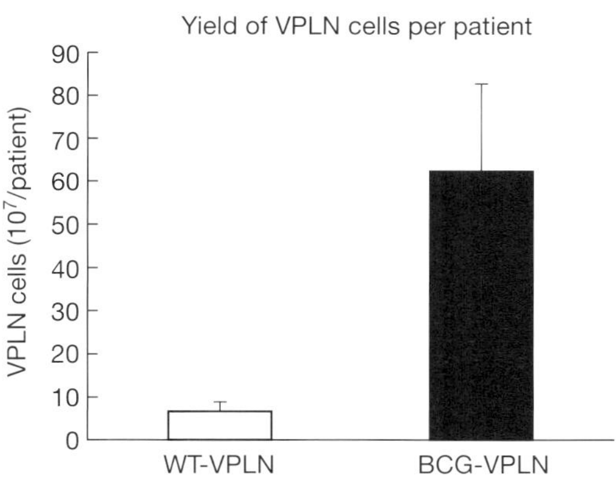

Fig. 41.3 Cell yield after vaccination with autologous tumor cells alone (WT-VPLN) or autologous tumor cells admixed with BCG (BCG-VPLN).

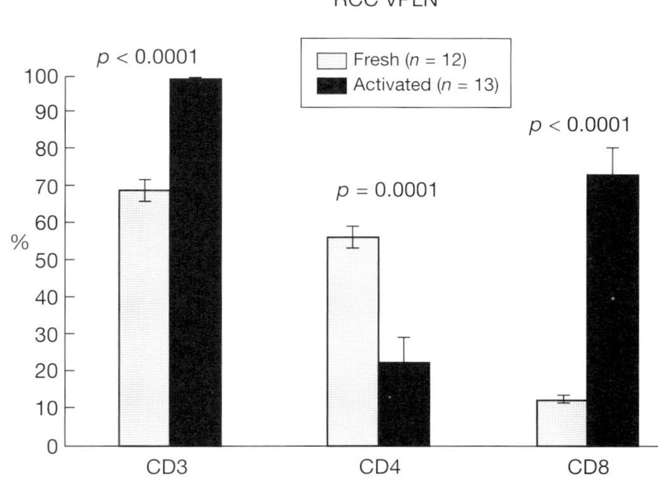

Fig. 41.5 Flow cytometry analysis of VPLN cells before and after activation with anti-CD3/IL-2; CD8⁺ cells are preferentially expanded.

the BCG-contvaccine was labelled BCG-VPLN, and the VPLN draining the autologous tumor cell vaccine was labelled the wild-type (WT)-VPLN. The presence of BCG significantly enhanced the number of VPLN cells harvested by 10-fold as shown in Fig. 41.3. There was no alteration in the phenotype of the T cells with respect to CD4 or CD8 markers between the two groups of VPLN cells. However, after anti-CD3 activation we observed a relatively consistent increase in the amount of IFNγ released by the BCG-VPLN cells as compared to the WT-VPLN cells in response to autologous tumor antigen (Fig. 41.4). Neither GM-CSF nor IL-10 cytokines were enhanced in their release (data

not shown). It was concluded that BCG was an effective immune adjuvant in enhancing type 1 responses of VPLN cells.

Analysis of the phenotype of the BCG-VPLN cells, activated for infusion was also performed. The mean percentages (SEM) of CD3⁺, CD4⁺, and CD8⁺ cells of the freshly harvested VPLN were 69 (3), 56 (3), and 12 (1), respectively. After activation, CD8⁺ were preferentially expanded as shown in

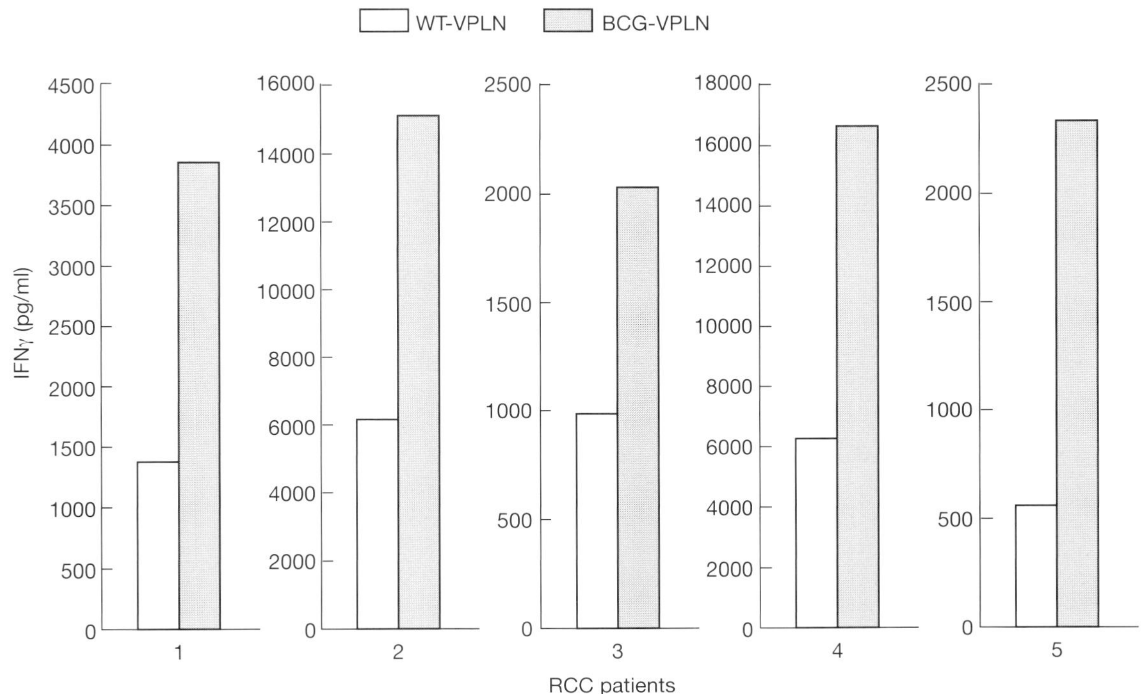

Fig. 41.4 Release of IFNγ from BCG-VPLN versus WT-VPLN in response to autologous tumor cells.

Table 41.3 Summary of variables between responders and non-responders after adoptive immunotherapy with anti-CD3 activated VPLN cells

Variable	Responders	Non-responders
Mean number of cells (SEM)*	3.4 (0.5)	4.2 (1.0)
Number of IL-2 doses (SEM)*	13 (1.3)	14 (0.2)
CD4(%)/CD8(%) cells	22/74	17/74
Median IFNγ release (pg/ml)	2829	957
Median GM-CSF release (pg/ml)	3246	999
Median IL-10 release (pg/ml)	262	171

* For first course of therapy.

Fig. 41.5 with the percentage of $CD3^+$, $CD4^+$, and $CD8^+$ cells being 99 (0.3), 21 (7), and 75 (7), respectively. For the first course of therapy, a mean (SEM) of 4.1 (0.8) × 10^{10} cells were infused with a mean (SEM) of 14 (1) doses of IL-2.

To date, a total of 37 patients have been entered into the phase II protocol. Thirty-two have gone on to receive cell infusions, while five did not. Among these five patients, three rapidly progressed after vaccination and could not proceed to cell infusion, one did not meet eligibility criteria, and one was found to undergo spontaneous remission of pulmonary disease after nephrectomy and vaccination. Of the 32 treated patients, 28 were evaluable for response with the other four still in the midst of evaluation. There have been seven responding patients with 3 CR and 4 PR for a response rate of 25 per cent. We have compared several parameters between responding and nonresponding patients to see if there are any indicators predictive of response (Table 41.3). We have not identified any significant differences between responding and non-responding patients, although the median values of IFNγ and GM-CSF release were higher for the responding group compared to the non-responding group. It will require larger numbers of patients to try and draw any correlates of immune function with response. We are planning to accrue a total of 40 evaluable patients in this phase II study.

Discussion

Renal cell cancers have proven to be immunogenic tumors capable of being rejected by cell-mediated mechanisms. The first line of therapy for metastatic disease should be IL-2 if the patient has no medical contraindications. So far, the use of adoptive cellular therapy has not shown a distinct advantage over IL-2 alone. Almost all reported clinical trials of adoptive cell transfer in RCC have been with the concomitant use of IL-2. Shu and co-workers have utilized VPLN cell therapy wherein the cells are activated by an alternative strategy involving superantigen activation and expansion in IL-2 (Plautz *et al.* 1999). Utilizing this protocol, they have treated metastatic RCC patients without the concomitant use of IL-2 and have observed tumor responses (Shu, personal communication). This observation is important, since it does indicate that the combination of tumor-reactive cells plus IL-2 should offer therapeutic advantages as has been reported in several animal models.

There are several directions being pursued in attempts to make adoptive cellular therapy more effective. One area is the enhancement of host T-cell sensitization to tumor antigen, which can improve the ability to isolate T cells *ex vivo* for bulk expansion and subsequent transfer. We have previously reported that the intratumoral inoculation of an allogeneic class I gene will result in enhanced TIL reactivity to tumor antigen (Nabel *et al.* 1996). Other investigators have been exploring the use of gene-modified tumor cells as more effective vaccines (Miller *et al.* 1994). These vaccines can be useful in generating VPLN cells for successful adoptive immunotherapy.

Another area where this therapy can be improved is in the development of more effective methods to expand tumor-reactive T cells. We have begun to examine the use of stimulating VPLN cells with antibodies mimicking co-stimulatory ligands in addition to anti-CD3. We have reported that the combination of anti-CD28 (which mimics CD80) with anti-CD3 leads to significantly enhanced proliferation compared to anti-CD3 alone (Li *et al.* 1999). The combination of antibodies also resulted in enhanced $CD4^+$ T cell proliferation. These $CD4^+$ T cells responded to autologous tumor cells with cytokine release that was MHC class II restricted. In animal studies, a direct comparison between anti-CD3 and anti-CD3/CD28 activated tumor-draining lymph node (TDLN) cells has revealed that the doubly activated cells were more effective in eradicating established tumor compared to anti-CD3 activated cells on a per cell basis (Li *et al.* 2000*b*). After completion of the current phase II trial, we plan to conduct a phase II trial of anti-CD3/CD28 activated VPLN in renal cell cancer patients.

Another area of potential improvement of adoptive cellular therapy is to purify and select out tumor-reactive T cells prior to bulk expansion. One approach is to utilize adhesion markers expressed by T cells. Shu and co-workers have reported that L-selectin[low]-expressing TDLN cells appear to enrich for the tumor-reactive cell population in animal models (Kagamu and Shu 1998). Stoolman and co-workers have similarly shown that P-selectinL[high] TDLN cells are also enriched for the tumor-reactive cells (Tanagawa *et al.* 2000). It appears that the P-selectinL[high] fraction of cells is a subpopulation of the L-selectin[low] cells and may represent a highly potent group of cells with antitumor reactivity (Stoolman, personal communication). In the future, it is anticipated that purification of T cells based on these approaches may prove more efficacious in eliciting tumor responses in clinical trials.

The generation of T cells with specific reactivity to tumor in patients who go on to respond to cellular therapy has provided opportunities to clone tumor-associated antigens (TAA) (Rosenberg 1996). Melanoma has been the prototype tumor in which this has been done. For known TAA, identifying the genetic constructs of T-cell receptors that can identify peptide epitopes offers the opportunity to genetically engineer T cells to recognize tumor cells (Clay *et al.* 1999). This may allow the generation of tumor-reactive T cells from a pool of naive lymphocytes.

In summary, the adoptive transfer of appropriately reactive T cells can result in significant tumor regression. The identification of the methods to generate and expand these cells *ex vivo* has given us insights into the critical mechanisms involved in establishing a therapeutic immune reaction response. Renal cell cancer has been a useful paradigm in this regard. It is predicted that TAA for RCC will be identified in the future and that immunotherapeutic approaches to RCC will become more established.

References

Aruga, A., Aruga, E., Cameron, M.J., and Chang, A.E. (1997*a*). Different cytokine profiles released by CD4+ and CD8+ tumor-draining lymph node cells involved in mediating tumor regression. *J. Leuk. Biol.* **61**, 1–10.

Aruga, A., Aruga, E., *et al.* (1997*b*). Type 1 versus type 2 cytokine release by Vb T cell subpopulations determines *in vivo* antitumor reactivity: IL-10 mediates a suppressive role. *J. Immunol.* **159** (2), 664–73.

Berd, D., Maguire, H.C. Jr, and Mastrangelo, M.J. (1986). Induction of cell-mediated immunity to autologous melanoma cells and regression of metastases after treatment with a melanoma cell vaccine preceded by cyclophosphamide. *Cancer Res.* **46**, 2572–7.

Bukowski, R.M., Sharfman, W., Murthy, S., Rayman, P., Tubbs, R., Alexander, J., *et al.* (1991). Clinical results and characterization of tumor-infiltrating lymphocytes with or without recombinant interleukin 2 in human metastatic renal cell carcinoma. *Cancer Res.* **51**, 4199–205.

Cameron, R.B., Macintosh, J.K., and Rosenberg, S.A. (1988). Synergistic antitumor effects of combination immunotherapy with recombinant interleukin-2 and a recombinant hybrid α-interferon in the treatment of established murine hepatic metastases. *Cancer Res.* **48**, 5810–17.

Chang, A.E. and Shu, S. (1992). Immunotherapy with sensitized lymphocytes. *Cancer Invest.* **10** (5), 357–69.

Chang, A.E., Aruga, A., Cameron, M.J., Sondak, V.K., Normolle, D.P., Fox, B.A., and Shu, S. (1997). Adoptive immunotherapy with vaccine-primed lymph node cells secondarily activated with anti-CD3 and interleukin-2. *J. Clin. Oncol.* **15** (2), 796–807.

Chou, T., Bertera, S., Chang, A.E., and Shu, S.Y. (1988*a*). Adoptive immunotherapy of microscopic and advanced visceral metastases with *in vitro* sensitized lymphoid cells from mice bearing progressive tumors. *J. Immunol.* **141**, 1775–81.

Chou, T., Chang, A.E., and Shu, S. (1988*b*). Generation of therapeutic T lymphocytes from tumor-bearing mice by *in vitro* sensitization: culture requirements and characterization of immunologic specificity. *J. Immunol.* **140**, 2543–61.

Clay, T.M., Custer, M.C., Sachs, J., Hwu, P., Rosenberg, S.A., and Nishimura, M.I. (1999). Efficient transfer of a tumor antigen-reactive TCR to human peripheral blood lymphocytes confers anti-tumor reactivity. *J. Immunol.* **163** (1), 507–13.

Figlin, R., Gitlitz, B., Franklin, J., Dorey, F., Moldawer, N., Rausch, J., *et al.* (1997). Interleukin-2-based immunotherapy for the treatment of metastatic renal cell carcinoma: an analysis of 203 consecutively treated patients. *Cancer J. Sci. Am.* **3**, S92–S97.

Figlin, R.A., Thompson, J.A., Bukowski, R.M., Vogelzang, N.J., Novick, A.C., Lange, P., *et al.* (1999). Multicenter, randomized, phase III trial of CD8^{+} tumor-infiltrating lymphocytes in combination with recombinant interleukin-2 metastatic renal cell carcinoma. *J. Clin. Oncol.* **17** (8), 2521–9.

Fisher, R.I., Coltman, C.A., Doroshow, J.H., Rayner, A.A., Hawkins, M.J., Mier, J.W., *et al.* (1988). Metastatic renal cancer treated with interleukin-2 and lymphokine-activated killer cells. A phase II clinical trial. *Ann. Intern. Med.* **108**, 518–23.

Geiger, J.D., Wagner, P.D., Cameron, M.J., Shu, S., and Chang, A.E. (1993). Generation of T cells reactive to poorly immunogenic B16–BL6 melanoma with efficacy in the treatment of spontaneous metastases. *J. Immunother.* **13**, 153–65.

Greenberg, P.D. (1991). Adoptive T cell therapy of tumors: mechanisms operative in the recognition and elimination of tumor cells. *Advan. Immunol.* **49**, 281–355.

Grimm, E.A., Robb, R.J., Roth, J.A., Neckers, L.M., Lachman, L.B., Wilson, D.J., and Rosenberg S.A. (1983). Lymphokine-activated killer cell phenomenon. III: Evidence that IL-2 is sufficient for direct activation of peripheral blood into lymphokine-activated killer cells. *J. Exp. Med.* **158** (4), 1356–61.

Kagamu, H. and Shu, S. (1998). Purification of L-selectin^{low} cells promotes the generation of highly potent CD4 antitumor effector T lymphocytes. *J. Immunol.* **160**, 3444–52.

Kradin, R.L., Lazarus, D.S., Dubinett, S.M., Kurnick, J.T., Preffer, F.I., Dubinett, S.M., *et al.* (1989). Tumour-infiltrating lymphocytes and interleukin-2 in treatment of advanced cancer. *Lancet* **1**, 577–80.

Li, Q., Furman, S.A., Bradford, C.R., and Chang, A.E. (1999). Expanded tumor-reactive CD4+ T-cell responses to human cancers induced by secondary anti-CD3/anti-CD28 activation. *Clin. Cancer Res.* **5**, 461–9.

Li, Q., Normolle, D.P., Sayre, D.M., Zeng, X., Sun, R., Jiang, G., *et al.* (2000*a*). Immunological effects of BCG as an adjuvant in autologous tumor vaccines. *Clin. Immunol.* **94** (1), 64–72.

Li, Q., Zeng, X., Grover, A., and Chang, A.E. (2000*b*). Antitumor reactivity of unfractionated tumor-draining lymph node (TDLN) cells vs. CD3 purified TDLN cells activated with anti-CD3/anti-CD28 mAb [abstract 1845]. *Proc. Am. Assoc. Cancer Res.* **41**, 290.

Miller, A.R., McBride, W.H., Hunt, K., and Economou, J.S. (1994). Cytokine-mediated gene therapy for cancer. *Ann. Surg. Oncol.* **1** (5), 436–50.

Morgan, D.A., Ruscetti, F.W., and Gallo R. (1976). Selective *in vitro* growth of T lymphocytes from normal human bone marrows. *Science* **193** (4257), 1007–8.

Mulé, J.J., Shu, S.Y., Schwarz, S.L., and Rosenberg, S.A. (1984). Adoptive immunotherapy of established pulmonary metastases with LAK cells and recombinant interleukin-2. *Science* **225**, 1487–9.

Muul, L.M., Nason-Burchenal, K., Carter, C.S., Cullis, H., Slavin, D., Hyatt, C., *et al.* (1987). Development of an automated closed system for generation of human lymphokine-activated killer (LAK) cells for use in adoptive immunotherapy. *J. Immunol. Methods* **101**, 171–81.

Nabel, G., Gordon, D., Bishop, D.K., Nickoloff, B.J., Yang, Z.Y., Aruga, A., *et al.* (1996). Immune response in human melanoma after transfer of an allogeneic class I major histocompatibility complex gene with DNA–liposome complexes. *Proc. Natl Acad. Sci., USA* **93**, 15388–93.

Paciucci, P.A., Holland, J.F., Glidewell, O., and Odchimar, R. (1989). Recombinant interleukin-2 by continuous infusion and adoptive transfer of recombinant interleukin-2 activated cells in patients with advanced cancer. *J. Clin. Oncol.* **7**, 869–78.

Parkinson, D.R., Fisher, R.I., Rayner, A.A., Paietta, E., Margolin, K.A., Weiss, G.R., *et al.* (1990). Therapy of renal cell carcinoma with interleukin-2 and lymphokine-activated killer cells: phase II experience with a hybrid bolus and continuous infusion interleukin-2 regimen. *J. Clin. Oncol.* **8**, 1630–6.

Plautz, G.E., Bukowski, R.M., Novick, A.C., Klein, E.A., Kursh, E.D., Olencki, T.E., *et al.* (1999). T-cell adoptive immunotherapy of metastatic renal cell carcinoma. *Urology* **54** (4), 617–23.

Rayner, A.A., Grimm, E.A., Lotze, M.T., Wilson, D.J., and Rosenberg, S.A. (1985). Lymphokine-activated killer (LAK) cell phenomenon. IV. Lysis by LAK cell clones of fresh human tumor cells from autologous and multiple allogeneic tumors. *J. Natl Cancer Inst.* **75** (1), 67–75.

Rosenberg, S.A. (1988). The development of new immunotherapies for the treatment of cancer using interleukin-2. *Ann. Surg.* **208**, 121–35.

Rosenberg, S.A. (1996). The immunotherapy of solid cancers based on cloning the genes encoding tumor-rejection antigens. *Ann. Rev. Med.* **47**, 481–91.

Rosenberg, S.A., Spiess, P., and Lafreniere, P. (1986). A new approach to the adoptive immunotherapy of cancer with tumor-infiltrating lymphocytes. *Science* **233**, 1318–21.

Rosenberg, S.A., Packard, V.S., Aebersold, P.M., Solomon, D., Topalian, S.L., Toy, S.T., *et al.* (1988). Use of tumor-infiltrating lymphocytes and interleukin-2 in the immunotherapy of patietns with metastatic melanoma: a preliminary report. *New Engl. J. Med.* **80**, 1393–7.

Rosenberg, S.A., Lotze, M.T., Yang, J.C., Topalian, S.L., Chang, A.E., Schwartzentruber, D.J., *et al.* (1993). Prospective randomized trial of high-dose interleukin-2 alone or in conjunction with lymphokine-activated killer cells for the treatment of patients with advanced cancer. *J. Natl Cancer Inst.* **85** (8), 622–32.

Schoof, D.D., Gramolini, B.A., Davidson, D.L., Massaro, A.F., Wilson, R.E., and Eberlein, T.J. (1988). Adoptive immunotherapy of human cancer using low-dose recombinant interleukin-2 and lymphokine-activated killer cells. *Cancer Res.* **48**, 5007–10.

Spiess, P.J., Yang, J.C., and Rosenberg, S.A. (1987). *In vivo* antitumor activity of tumor-infiltrating lymphocytes expanded in recombinant interleukin-2. *J. Natl Cancer Inst.* **79**, 1067–75.

Tanagawa, K., Phillips, K., Craig, R.A., Knibbs, R.N., Chang, A.E., and Stoolman, L.M. (2000). Tumor-specific responses in lymph nodes draining murine sarcomas are concentrated in cells expressing P-selectin binding sites [abstract 517]. *Proc. Am. Assoc. Cancer Res.* **41**, 81.

Thompson, J.A., Lee, D.J., Lindgren, C.G., Benz, L.A., Collins, C., and Shuman, W.P. (1989). Influence of schedule of interleukin-2 administration on therapy with interleukin-2 and lymphokine activated killer cells. *Cancer Res.* **49**, 235–40.

Topalian, S.L., Solomon, D., Avid, F.P., Chang, A.E., Freerkson, D.L., Linehan, W.M., *et al.* (1988). Immunotherapy of patients with advanced cancer using tumor-infiltrating lymphocytes and recombinant interleukin-2: a pilot study. *J. Clin. Oncol.* **6**, 839–53.

Wang, J.C.L., Walle, A., Novogrodsky, A., Suthanthiran, M., Silver, R.T., and Bander, N.H. (1989). A phase II clinical trial of adoptive immunotherapy for advanced renal cell carcinoma using mitogen-activated autologous leukocytes and continuous infusion interleukin-2. *J. Clin. Oncol.* **7**, 1885–91.

West, W.H., Tauer, K.W., Yannelli, J.R., Marshall, G.D., Orr, D.W., Thurman, G.B., *et al.* (1987). Constant-infusion recombinant interleukin-2 in adoptive immunotherapy of advanced cancer. *New Engl. J. Med.* **316**, 898–905.

Yoshizawa, H., Chang, A.E., and Shu, S. (1991). Specific adoptive immunotherapy mediated by tumor-draining lymph node cells sequentially activated with anti-CD3 and IL-2. *J. Immunol.* **147**, 729–37.

Yoshizawa, H., Chang, A.E., and Shu, S. (1992). Cellular interactions in effector cell generation and tumor regression mediated by anti-CD3/interleukin 2-activated tumor-draining lymph node cells. *Cancer Res.* **52**, 1129–36.

Yron, I., Wood, T.A. Jr, Spiess, P.J., and Rosenberg, S.A. (1980). *In vitro* growth of murine T cells. V. The isolation and growth of lymphoid cells infiltrating syngeneic solid tumors. *J. Immunol.* **125** (1), 238–45.

42. Immunotherapy for metastatic disease— the French experience

Sylvie Négrier and the Groupe Français d'Immunothérapie

By the end of the 1980s, Dr Steve Rosenberg (Surgical Branch, National Cancer Institute, Bethesda, Maryland, USA) had opened up the field of immunotherapy in oncology by reporting the first results of trials of interleukin-2 (IL-2) in the treatment of advanced cancers (Rosenberg *et al.* 1985, 1987). Melanoma and renal cell carcinoma (RCC) had already been identified as the tumors most sensitive to this newly available agent. The enthusiastic clinical development of this cytokine, despite its severe side-effects, was explained by the repeated failures observed with conventional cytotoxic drugs in metastatic renal cancer (Yagoda *et al.* 1995).

As in most European countries, French investigators actively participated in the clinical development program of IL-2 in metastatic RCC. As a consequence, IL-2 was registered for the treatment of metastatic RCC in 1990 in France. At this time, the enthusiasm for IL-2 had weakened, especially in view of the efficacy/toxicity ratio, which appeared disappointing. Questions were raised about the future use of this agent and became critical when the cost of the treatment was known. These were the main reasons for the birth of the Groupe Français d'Immunothérapie. French oncologists met and decided to pursue the clinical evaluation of IL-2 in patients with metastatic RCC. Investigators representing 25 centres (19 cancer centres and 6 university hospitals) designed and conducted several successive trials between 1991 and 1998. We will try to give an overview of the results of these trials and to bring out practical issues for the patients.

The CRECY trial

The results of this trial have been previously reported in detail (Negrier *et al.* 1998). Briefly, this multicenter randomized trial compared three different treatments: intravenous IL-2 versus α interferon (IFNα) versus a combination of both cytokines in patients with metastatic RCC. In case of failure of the initial treatment, a cross-over treatment was planned between the two cytokines given alone. Because of the dramatic and durable tumor regressions observed in some patients, the adjunction of a non-treated control group was judged unethical by the investigating group. However, the group was aware of the patient selection that will occur in conducting such a trial. The group decided to register ineligible patients, as well as the main reason for their ineligibility.

Four hundred twenty-five patients were randomized into the CRECY trial, but 722 patients were considered ineligible during the same period of time. The main reasons of ineligibility are detailed in Table 42.1. Notably, the most frequent reason was an impaired performance status which is known to be correlated with a poor outcome.

In terms of results, the combination of the two cytokines seems to have additive effects. Indeed, the response rate and the event-free survival at 1 year obtained with this combination were significantly improved when compared to those of each cytokine alone (Table 42.2). However, this additive effect was not maintained over time and the overall survivals of patients according to the treatment group were similar (Fig. 42.1). These last results

Table 42.1 Reasons for ineligibility of patients in the CRECY trial*

Reason	Patients ineligible for that reason (%)
ECOG PS score $\geq$ 2	25
Age < 18 or > 65 years	17
Organ dysfunction	13
Brain metastases	12
Previous treatment	11
Patient's refusal	6
Miscellaneous	16

*The total number of ineligible patients was 722.

Table 42.2 Results for the three treatment groups in the CRECY trial

	IL-2	IFNα	IL-2 + IFNα	*p*-value
Response rate (%)	6.5	7.5	18.6	< 0.01
Event-free survival at 1 year (%)	15	12	20	0.01
Overall median survival time (months)	12	13	17	0.55*

* Log rank test value.

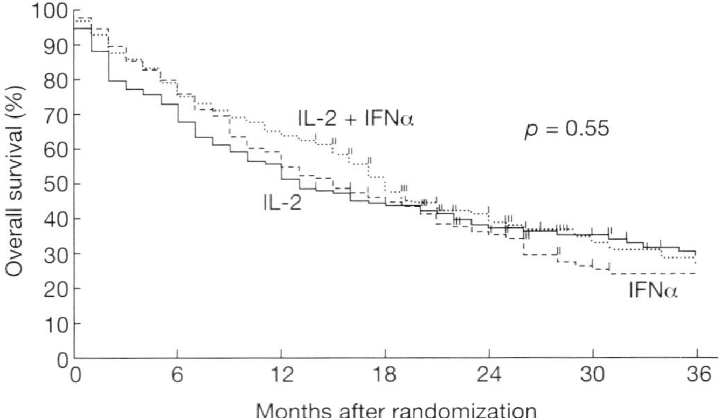

Fig. 42.1 Kaplan–Meier curves for overall survival of patients in the IL-2 + IFNα (gray dashed line), IL-2 alone (solid line), and IFNα alone (black dashed line) groups. Tick marks represent censored data. The data are based on an intention-to-treat analysis.

could be in part due to the cross-over treatment effect. Nevertheless, the results obtained with the cross-over treatments were negative and the absence of gain in survival with the combination of IL-2 and IFNα versus each cytokine alone appears quite reliable. Indeed, patients who failed to respond under one cytokine, either IL-2 or IFNα, have no chance of benefiting from the other cytokine as second-line treatment (Escudier *et al.* 1999).

Our conclusions were: (1) significant tumor regressions occur in a small minority of patients treated with IL-2 and/or IFNα; (2) these regressions are more likely to occur under the combination of the two cytokines than under one cytokine alone; (3) the combination of cytokines does not confer any overall survival advantage.

On a routine daily basis, the question of treating or not treating with cytokines a particular individual suffering from metastatic RCC remained; the crude results of our trial did not throw

any light on this point. This is the reason why we analyzed different types of prognostic factors with the aim of obtaining valuable information to help the physicians in their decisions. Univariate and multivariate analyses were performed to detect factors influencing the occurrence of a treatment-related death, the achievement of a tumor response, and the progression of the disease under treatment. Correlations were found between the occurrence of a treatment-related death and some well known prognostic factors of the disease (Table 42.3). These results show that patients with aggressive tumors that rapidly develop are not able to tolerate intravenous IL-2 treatment, which may cause their anticipated death.

Table 42.4 indicates the results of the multivariate analysis of factors predicting response or progression under cytokine treatment. The probability of obtaining a significant tumor regression was only correlated with two independent factors: (1) receiving the combination of IL-2 and IFNα and (2) having a metastatic involvement of one organ site only. The different probabilities of response corresponding to these factors are shown on Fig. 42.2. In the case of patient selection, predictive factors of progression under treatment may be more useful. Five different independent

Table 42.3 Parameters correlated with death related to treatment during the CRECY trial*

Factor	p-value
Performance status score at beginning of treatment	
ECOG 0	
ECOG I	0.001
ECOG 2	
Recent weight loss > 10%	0.004
Time from diagnosis to metastases	0.01
Dose of cytokines > median dose given in the trial	0.03

* 22/425 patients died during treatment of different causes not related to the disease.

Table 42.4 Multivariate analysis of predictive factors for response and rapid progression

Characteristic	Logistic relative risk*	95% Confidence interval
Predictive factors of response[†]		
Treatment arm (3 versus 1 or 2 treatments)	3.5	[1.9; 6.5]
Number of metastatic sites (1 versus ≥ 2)	3.0	[1.5; 5.6]
Predictive factors of rapid progression[††]		
Number of metastatic sites (1 versus ≥ 2)	2.8	[1.7; 4.8]
Metastasis-free interval (≤ 12 versus > 12 months)	2.5	[2.1; 3.9]
Liver metastases (yes versus no)	2.1	[1.2; 5.0]
Treatment arm (1 or 2 versus 3 treatments)	1.8	[1.1; 2.8]
Mediastinum involvement (yes versus no)	1.7	[1.0; 2.7]

* The odds ratios provided from the logistic model are defined as the exponential values of the beta coefficients.
[†] The following factors that were statistically significant during univariate analysis were included in the model: treatment arm (1 or 2 versus 3 treatments); number of metastatic sites (1 versus ≥ 2); ECOG status (0 versus 1 or 2); bone involvement (yes versus no); lung involvement (yes versus no); liver involvement (yes versus no); other site involvement (yes versus no).
[††] The following factors that were statistically significant during univariate analysis were included in the model: treatment arm (1 or 2 versus 3 treatments); number of metastatic sites (1 versus ≥ 2); ECOG status (0 versus 1 or 2); bone involvement (yes versus no); lung involvement (yes versus no); liver involvement (yes versus no); mediastinum involvement (yes versus no); metastasis-free interval ≤ 12 months (yes versus no); weight loss ≥ 10% (yes versus no).

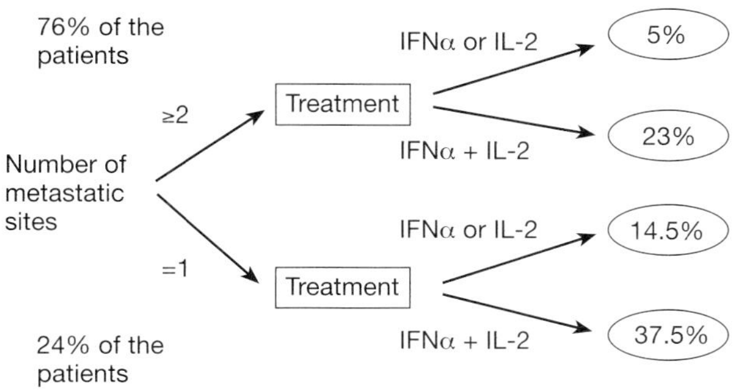

Fig. 42.2 Probabilities of response according to the different combined factors.

factors were identified and are detailed in Table 42.4. The different combinations of these clinical factors give different probabilities of disease progression as illustrated in Fig. 42.3. We identified a subset of patients with a probability of progression of at least 70 per cent under a combined treatment. These patients have two or more metastatic organ sites, liver involvement, and an interval between the primary tumor to the appearance of metastases of less than 1 year. This subgroup of patients represented 20 per cent of the patients enrolled in the study and they had a poor outcome with a median survival of 6 months. After the report of this analysis, the investigators, on a consensus basis, decided not to consider any longer these patients as candidates for cytokine treatment.

Studies of subcutaneous cytokine regimens

After the recruitment of patients in the CRECY trial was completed, and before the results were reported, the Groupe Français d'Immunothérapie investigated the effect of different regimens given subcutaneously and combining IL-2 and IFNα. Indeed, IL-2 had become commonly used via this route of administration after the publication of different phase II trials (Atzpodien *et al.* 1990; Sleijfer *et al.* 1992). These regimens were obviously less toxic than

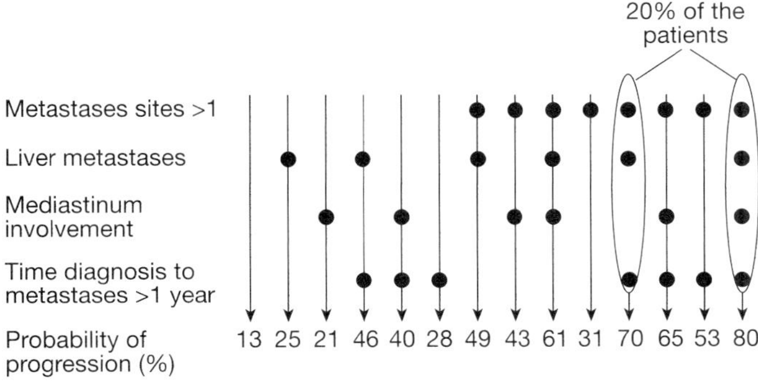

Fig. 42.3 Probabilities of progression according to the different parameters in patients receiving thecombination of IL-2 and IFNα.

those using intravenous IL-2, and the effect against the tumor appeared interesting. In addition, the highest response rates were obtained when these cytokines were associated with 5-fluorouracil (5-FU) (Hofmockel *et al.* 1996; Atzpodien *et al.* 1993).

The Groupe Français d'Immunothérapie conducted two successive trials (one phase II and a randomized trial) testing the triple combination of IL-2, IFNα, and 5-FU. The same subcutaneous regimen was administered in both trials but 5-FU was not given in one of the groups of the randomized trial. The results were very disappointing: the response rate observed in the phase II trial was 1.8 per cent (Ravaud *et al.* 1998). No differences in response rate, disease-free progression, or overall survival were detected between the groups of the randomized trial, whether patients received 5-FU or not (Negrier *et al.* 1998) (response rates: 1.8 per cent with IL-2 + IFNα versus 8.2 per cent with IL-2 + IFNα + 5-FU [$p = 0.1$]). Our conclusions were that 5-FU did not add any activity against metastatic renal carcinoma, and that this combined subcutaneous regimen of cytokines had a very limited efficacy.

Because of the unexpectedly low response rate observed in these studies, a new phase II trial was conducted. We tested the combined regimen we had used in the CRECY trial but IL-2 was given subcutaneously instead of intravenously (Negrier *et al.* 1999). The results obtained in 67 patients were again disappointing with a 7 per cent response rate and a relatively severe toxicity when compared to other subcutaneous regimens.We concluded that the doses of cytokines, which were rather high in this treatment regimen, may be more important than the route of administration in inducing toxic symptoms and that, again, these subcutaneous cytokine regimens have a very limited activity.

Discussion and perspectives

At the end of 1998, the investigators of the group met and discussed their work. The overall conclusion was that the major and most critical question remains: are IL-2 and/or IFNα useful for patients with metastatic RCC? A proposal to set up a trial with a non-treated group in order to answer this question was made and the discussion was left open for some months. During this period of time, two randomized trials were published, bringing some positive results in favor of the use of IFNα. The UK Medical Research Council Group on Renal Carcinoma reported a limited but significant advantage in survival with moderate doses of IFNα versus medroxyprogesterone acetate (Medical Research Council Renal Cancer Collaborators 1999). A few months later, a group from Finland also reported a significant advantage in survival with the combination of IFNα and vinblastine versus vinblastine alone (Pyrhonen *et al.* 1999).

Meanwhile, the Groupe Français d'Immunothérapie and another French collaborative group, the SCAPP Group, merged, to enlarge the potential accrual of patients. Together, we decided to interview the investigators, a number of referring physicians, and patients on the feasibility of a randomized trial comparing a cytokine treatment arm versus a no-treatment arm or a placebo arm.

The large majority of patients answered that they would not agree to participate in such a trial. A majority of investigators and referring physicians answered that they would agree to randomize patients in such a trial, with the exception of those patients with a high probability of tumor regression under treatment.

The selection of patients was again at the centre of the debate. As a consequence, we decided to use the prognostic factors identified in the CRECY trial, and to base our clinical trial strategy on patient selection. The first point of consensus was that patients with a bad prognosis would not be candidates for any cytokine trial. These patients were defined as those with an impaired performance status (Karnofsky score < 80 per cent) and the sub-group of patients with a high probability of progression identified from the CRECY study. The second point was to define which patients were considered to have a high probability of response. We used the predictive factor identified in the CRECY trial: patients having one metastatic organ site only. Indeed, these patients, who represent 25 per cent of all the patients enrolled in the study, had a probability of 37.5 per cent of achieving a significant tumor regression under the combined treatment with intravenous IL-2. The idea was to compare the effect of this regimen to that of a combination of cytokines given sub-cutaneously, in these highly selected patients. The remaining patients, identified as the intermediate prognostic group, would enter into a randomized trial testing subcutaneous cytokines and including a control arm with medroxyprogesterone acetate. These two complementary trials are developed within a new French evaluation programme called the PERCY program.

Conclusions

If we are asked what has changed in the treatment of patients suffering from metastatic renal carcinoma at the end of the twentieth century, we are forced to admit that no dramatic changes have occurred in the outcome of most patients. It is true, however, that a very small percentage of patients have been able to achieve important and durable remissions with IL-2 and/or IFNα. It is also true, unfortunately, that all other agents have failed to have any proven reproducible activity against this tumor. Therefore, we think it is important to use what we have learned from our previous experience. We must find sound arguments for the future to be able to decide whether or not to treat a patient with drugs that always give inconvenience and alter the quality of life. The study of relevant prognostic factors that allow effective patient selection is one important means of achieving this. Moreover, the continued study of novel treatment strategies or the identification of new agents must remain the highest priorities for the future.

References

Atzpodien, J., Korfer, A., Franks, C.R., Poliwoda, H., and Kirchner, H. (1990). Home therapy with recombinant interleukin-2 and interferon-alpha 2b in advanced human malignancies. *Lancet* **335**, 1509–12.

Atzpodien, J., Kirchner, H., Hanninen, E.L., Korfer, A., Fenner, M., Menzel, T., *et al.* (1993). European studies of interleukin-2 in metastatic renal cell carcinoma. *Sem. Oncol.* **20** (6, Suppl. 9), 22–6.

Escudier, B., Chevreau, C., Lasset, C., Douillard, J.Y., Ravaud, A., Fabbro, M., *et al.* (1999). Cytokines in metastatic renal cell carcinoma: is it useful to switch to interleukin-2 or interferon after failure of a first treatment? *J. Clin. Oncol.* **17**, 2039–43.

Hofmockel, G., Langer, W., Theiss, M., Gruss, A., and Frohmuller, H.G. (1996). Immunochemotherapy for metastatic renal cell carcinoma using a regimen of interleukin-2, interferon-alpha and 5-fluorouracil. *J. Urol.* **156**, 18–21.

Medical Research Council Renal Cancer Collaborators (1999). Interferon-alpha and survival in metastatic renal carcinoma: early results of a randomised controlled trial.. *Lancet* **353**, 14–17.

Negrier, S., Escudier, B., Lasset, C., Douillard, J.Y., Savary, J., Chevreau, C., *et al.* (1998). Recombinant human interleukin-2, recombinant human interferon alfa-2a, or both in metastatic renal-cell carcinoma. Groupe Francais d'Immunotherapie. *New Engl. J. Med.* **338**, 1272–8.

Negrier, S., Ravaud, A., Delva, R., Chevreau, C., Douillard, J.V., Fargeot, P., *et al.* (1999). Combination of cytokines in metastatic renal cell carcinoma (MRCC); is the subcutaneous (SC) route less active than the intravenous (iv) route? [abstract 1273] *Proc. Am. Soc. Clin. Oncol.* **18**, 331a.

Negrier, S., Caty, A., Lesimple, T., Gomez, F., Douillard, J.Y., Escudier, B., *et al.* (2000). Treatment of patients with metastatic renal carcinoma with a combination of subcutaneous interleukin-2 and Alpha-interferon with or without 5 fluorouracil. *J. Clin. Oncol.* **18**, 4009–15.

Pyrhonen, S., Salminen, E., Ruutu, M., Lehtonen, T., Nurmi, M., Tammela, T., Juusela, H., Rintala, E., Hietanen, P., and Kellokumpu-Lehtinen, P.L. (1999). Prospective randomized trial of interferon alfa-2a plus vinblastine versus vinblastine alone in patients with advanced renal cell cancer. *J. Clin. Oncol.* **17**, 2859–67.

Ravaud, A., Audhuy, B., Gomez, F., Escudier, B., Lesimple, T., Chevreau, C., *et al.* (1998). Subcutaneous interleukin-2, interferon alfa-2a, and continuous infusion of fluorouracil in metastatic renal cell carcinoma: a multicenter phase II trial. Groupe Francais d'Immunotherapie. *J. Clin. Oncol.* **16**, 2728–32.

Rosenberg, S.A., Lotze, M.T., Muul, L.M., Leitman, S., Chang, A.E., Ettinghausen, S.E., *et al.* (1985). Observations on the systemic administration of autologous lymphokine-activated killer cells and recombinant interleukin-2 to patients with metastatic cancer. *New Engl. J. Med.* **313**, 1485–92.

Rosenberg, S.A., Lotze, M.T., Muul, L.M., Chang, A.E., Avis, F.P., Leitman, S., *et al.* (1987). A progress report on the treatment of 157 patients with advanced cancer using lymphokine-activated killer cells and interleukin-2 or high-dose interleukin-2 alone. *New Engl. J. Med.* **316**, 889–97.

Sleijfer, D.T., Janssen, R.A., Buter, J., de Vries, E.G., Willemse, P.H., and Mulder, N.H. (1992). Phase II study of subcutaneous interleukin-2 in unselected patients with advanced renal cell cancer on an outpatient basis. *J. Clin. Oncol.* **10**, 1119–23.

Yagoda, A., Abi-Rached, B., and Petrylak, D. (1995). Chemotherapy for advanced renal-cell carcinoma: 1983–1993. *Sem. Oncol.* **22**, 42–60.

43. Cell-based therapy in the treatment of renal cell carcinoma

Barbara J. Gitlitz, Arie S. Belldegrun, and Robert A. Figlin

Introduction

Over the last 50 years, considerable advances have been made in our knowledge of tumor immunology. This encompasses concepts such as antigen processing and presentation via the major histo-compatability complex (MHC) (Bjorkman and Parham 1990; Bjorkman *et al.* 1987); regulation of the immune response by cytokines, the influence of secondary signals such as co-stimulatory molecules, any, most notably, the characterization of a variety of genes encoding tumor-associated antigens (TAA). For many tumor types, the DNA and amino acid sequences of TAA have been elucidated including MHC-restricted immunodominant peptide sequences. This basic research has formed the basis for the exploration of more targeted clinical immunotherapies. The ultimate goal of most immunotherapeutic strategies is the sensitization of immune effector cells to tumor antigens. As a result of this immune education, these effector cells can ultimately mediate the destruction of antigen-bearing tumor cells either directly (cytolysis) or indirectly (via cytokine mediators).

T lymphocytes are the effectors of the cellular immune system and recognize antigen via the T-cell receptor (TCR). The TCR is formed by recombination of germline genes enabling a wide diversity of receptors. In all mature human T cells, the TCR is associated with a glycoprotein complex called CD3. There are two major T-cell subsets based on TCR-restricted recognition of class I or class II molecules. The TCR binds to a small antigenic peptide located in a groove of the MHC molecule (Boon *et al.* 1994). The CD8+ subset of T cells shows affinity for recognition of antigen in association with class I molecules (Salter *et al.* 1990). The CD4+ subset of T cells shows affinity for recognition of antigen in association with class II molecules (Cammarota *et al.* 1992). The binding of the TCR to the MHC–antigen complex is crucial to the generation of effector cell function, including target cell lysis, clonal cell expansion, and secretion of cytokines.

The transfer of immune cells with antitumor reactivity to the tumor-bearing host is termed adoptive immunotherapy. Adoptively transferred T cells have been shown to bring about regression in animal tumor models (Mule *et al.* 1985; Ettinghausen *et al.* 1985; Speiss *et al.* 1987) and demonstrate durable responses in human cancers, most notably renal cell carcinoma (RCC) and melanoma. Interleukin 2 (IL-2) supports the clonal expansion and survival of lymphocyte populations and has been the key component underlying much of the research advancing our knowledge of rejection of cancer via immune effector cells. Enhanced therapeutic efficacy is observed when cultured immune cells used for adoptive transfer are accompanied by exogenous IL-2 administration (Cheever *et al.* 1982; Donohue *et al.* 1984). This exogenous use of IL-2 is also shown to cause *in vivo* proliferation and prolonged survival of cells used for adoptive immunotherapy (Cheever *et al.* 1984). IL-2 is manufactured predominantly by activated T cells. When a mature T cell encounters its specific antigen–MHC complex, signals transduced across the plasma membrane result in the transcriptional activation of the IL-2 gene and genes encoding for the IL-2 receptor (McGuire *et al.* 1998). Ligation of IL-2 to its membrane receptor results in cell cycle progression of the activated T lymphocyte and subsequent antigen-specific T-cell clonal expansion (Cantrell and Smith 1984). On the basis of these observations, exogenous IL-2 is often administered with the adoptive transfer of cultured immune effector cells.

More recently, vaccines have been used in an attempt to activate an antitumor T-cell response *in vivo*. These strategies include dendritic cells (DC) or other APC loaded with antigenic peptides, tumor lysates (TuLy), or other molecules such as cytokines that enhance their effectiveness. The goal of these vaccine therapies is to sensitize immune effector cells (T lymphocytes) to tumor antigens. As a result of this immune education, these effector cells can ultimately mediate the destruction of antigen-bearing tumor cells either directly (cytolysis) or indirectly (via cytokine mediators).

Adoptive immunotherapy

Autolymphocyte therapy (ALT)

Autolymphocyte therapy uses autologous lymphocytes from a tumor-bearing host activated *ex vivo* by anti-CD3 monoclonal antibody (mAb) and a mixture of previously prepared autologous cytokines (T3CS). Triggering the CD3 component of the TCR results in clonal T-cell proliferation through an IL-2 dependent autocrine pathway (Herzberg and Smith 1987). The theoretical basis of ALT relies on the activation of memory T lymphocytes by T3CS in the tumor-bearing host. These T lymphocytes presumably have been exposed *in vivo* to tumor antigens and may possess the potential for mediating tumor regression following nonspecific activation. Preclinical murine studies involved the adoptive infusion of donor memory cells (splenocytes) prepared *ex vivo* using and anti-CD3 mAb and T3CS (Gold and Osband 1994; Gold *et al.* 1995). Expansions of CD44+ (memory T cells) were the principal mediators of antitumor effects and protection from subsequent tumor challenge. Unfortunately however, these preclinical studies were retracted as based on inaccurate data (Gold and Osband 1994; Gold *et al.* 1995).

The preparation of ALT for immunotherapy is a multistep process. First, patients undergo pheresis to harvest peripheral blood mononuclear cells. These cells are incubated for 3 days in the presence of anti-CD3 mAb, and their supernatant, termed T3CS, is collected. This supernatant contains various cytokines including IL-l-α, IL-l-β, IL-6, gamma interferon (IFNγ), tumor necrosis factor beta (TNFβ), granulocyte–macrophage colony-stimulating factor (GM-CSF), and both the soluble IL-2 receptor and anti-CD3 mAb (Sawczuk 1993).

Two weeks after the initial pheresis, patients undergo repeat pheresis for the collection of peripheral blood lymphocytes (PBL) for activation. The cells are incubated for 5 days at 39°C in media containing 25 per cent T3CS, indomethacin, and cimetidine. Cimetidine is used in an attempt to blockade histamine 2 (H2) receptors expressed by suppressor T-lymphocyte subpopulations in the hope of preventing expansion of these clones during CD3-induced activation (Khan *et al.* 1985). Indomethacin is used to block prosglandin E-mediated inhibition of IL-2 mediated T-cell proliferation (Waymack *et al.* 1989). Following the 5-day incubation, activated cells are irradiated to 50 cGy to reduce the activity of suppressor T lymphocytes (Wasserman *et al.* 1982) and the cells are then infused into patients. Patients continue to receive oral high-dose cimetidine during ALT, and infusions are given on an outpatient basis every 4 weeks over a 6 month course.

In 1990, an initial report of a 90 patient randomized trial of ALT versus high-dose cimetidine alone for the treatment of metastatic RCC was published (Osband *et al.* 1990). ALT was safely administered without dose-limiting toxicity. Statistically significant findings included a 2.5-fold survival advantage in patients receiving ALT (21 versus 8.5 months) over cimetidine alone. In addition, those patients with > 500 pg of IL-l in their T3CS had a sixfold survival advantage. Unexpected findings in the report included an improved response rate in patients receiving ALT (21 per cent), but a lack of correlation between objective tumor response and survival. Furthermore, males who received ALT had a fourfold survival advantage, whereas females receiving ALT demonstrated no survival advantage.

This initial report has been updated (Lavia *et al.* 1992; Graham *et al.* 1993), and over 300 patients with metastatic RCC have been accrued into this multi-institutional clinical trial, with a persistent survival advantage being reported in the ALT arm. The early success of ALT in the treatment of metastatic RCC led to the establishment of a number of proprietary ALT treatment centers. Currently, there is a phase III trial comparing ALT to single-agent IFNα. A randomized trial comparing ALT to single-agent IL-2 therapy, the only US Food and Drugs Administration (FDA)-approved therapy for metastatic RCC, would be a valid test of the ability of ALT to improve survival inpatients with metastatic RCC.

There has been a small, randomized trial of ALT versus observation for the adjuvant treatment of RCC (Sawczuk *et al.* 1997). Forty-five patients were randomized according to stage, gender, time from nephrectomy, and serum IL-1 level. A significant difference in favor of ALT over observation for overall median time to progression was found. In subgroup analysis, there was an advantage in median time to recurrence in patients with node-positive disease, and T3 stage. This should form the basis for larger confirmatory trials. Currently, there is an ongoing phase II study of adjuvant ALT for non-metastatic RCC (US National Cancer Institute (NCI)/Physicians Data Query (PDQ)).

Lymphokine-activated killer cells (LAK)

LAK are peripherally circulating lymphoid cells activated *in vitro* by exposure to pharmacologically high concentrations of IL-2 (500 to 1000 IU/ml).

In the original description of the LAK phenomenon by Grimm *et al.* (1982, 1983), lymphokine activation of PBL from cancer patients or normal individuals led to MHC non-restricted cytotoxicity toward a variety of natural killer (NK) cell resistant, autologous and allogeneic solid tumor targets. The capacity to distinguish between tumor cells and normal cells is a hallmark of LAK activity, although the antigen receptors expressed on cells mediating MHC non-restricted cytotoxicity are largely unknown. Once target cell adhesion takes place, a number of calcium-dependent phases of LAK cell lytic function occur. These include granule reorientation, granule exocytosis, and perforation of the target cell membrane by granule-associated pore-forming proteins (Ortaldo and Hiserodt 1989). In addition to cytotoxic granule release, LAK cells express a membrane-associated toxin called M-CTX, which also mediates lytic activity against nucleated tumor targets (Hiserodt 1991).

When generated from human PBL, LAK precursors are contained primarily in the large granular lymphocyte population containing virtually all active NK cells (Herberman *et al.* 1987). These precursors express surface markers characteristic of NK cells, including CD56+ (Leu-19) and CD 16+ (Leu-11), and rarely express the T-cell-associated markers CD3 or CD5 (Hiserodt 1993). DM1 is another surface marker expressed by the majority of human LAK precursors (Morris and Pross 1989).

Murine models with experimentally induced metastases demonstrate that the adoptive transfer of LAK plus IL-2 leads to the regression of established lung, liver, or subcutaneous metastases from a variety of cancer types (Mule *et al.* 1985; Lafreniere and Rosenberg 1985; Papa *et al.* 1986). In most of these studies, the combined administration of LAK cells plus IL-2 led to improved efficacy over IL-2 alone. These animal studies also demonstrated the trophic effect of IL-2, causing *in vivo* expansion and proliferation of LAK cells, and LAK cell death when discontinued (Ettinghausen *et al.* 1985).

Initial human clinical trials using activated killer cells alone showed no clinical efficacy but demonstrated the tolerability of multiple infusions of up to 2×10^{11} cells with minimal side-effects (Rosenberg 1984; Mazumdar *et al.* 1984). In the first reported trial combining LAK plus IL-2 in patients with advanced solid tumors, 11 of 25 patients experienced objective tumor response (1 complete response (CR), partial responses (PR)) (Rosenberg *et al.* 1985). These responses occurred in patients with four histologic tumor types: renal cell, melanoma, lung, and colon

Table 43.1 Phase II trials of combination IL-2/LAK in the treatment of metastatic renal cell carcinoma

Reference	Number of patients	Objective response, number (%)
Weiss *et al.* 1992	94	16 (17)
Rosenberg 1992	72	25 (35)
Parkinson *et al.* 1990	47	4 (9)
Dillman *et al.* 1993	50	7 (14)
Palmer *et al.* 1992	102	17 (18)
Foon *et al.* 1992	23	6 (26)
Thompson *et al.* 1992	42	14 (33)
Gramata *et al.* 1996	72	23 (32)
Total	502	112 (22)

carcinoma. These landmark studies demonstrated the feasibility of adoptive immunotherapy of human cancers. A summary of clinical trials combining IL-2 plus LAK in 180 consecutively treated advanced cancer patients showed responses predominantly in patients with metastatic RCC and metastatic melanoma. Of 72 assessable patients with metastatic RCC, a CR was seen in 8 patients and a PR in 17 patients, for an overall response rate of 35 per cent (Rosenberg 1992). Based on these promising results, various institutions conducted phase II studies using LAK cells plus IL-2 in the treatment of metastatic RCC. A summary of the results of these trials is given in Table 43.1 (Rosenberg 1992; Weiss *et al.* 1992; Parkinson *et al.* 1990; Dillman *et al.* 1993; Palmer *et al.* 1992; Foon *et al.* 1992; Thompson *et al.* 1992; Gramata *et al.* 1996). These trials used a variety of preparative and treatment regimens, and response rates in metastatic RCC ranged from 9 to 35 per cent, with a combined objective response rate of 23 per cent in 502 patients.

To generate LAK cells, patients are initially treated with IL-2 and undergo leukopheresis 48 to 72 hours following the discontinuation of IL-2. Treatment with IL-2 induces an initial lymphopenia, followed by rebound lymphocytosis. Leukopheresis is performed at the peak of the rebound lymphocytosis. Both systemic low-dose and high-dose IL-2 regimens have been used for the generation of LAK (Sznol *et al.* 1992; Rosenberg *et al.* 1993). The PBL from the leukopheresis product are then cultured *in vitro* in high concentrations of IL-2 (400 to 1000 IU/ml), and approximately 10^{10} to 10^{11} LAK are generated. Both high-dose IL-2 regimens (6 to 7.2 $\times$ 10^5 IU/kg administered by intravenous bolus infusion every 8 hours for 4 to 5 days) and low-dose IL-2 regimens (1 to 6 $\times$ 10^6 IU/m^2/day administered by continuous intravenous infusion over 4 or more days) have been used concomitantly with the adoptive transfer of LAK. The optimal dose and schedule of IL-2 administration with LAK is not defined. Studies have found less clinical toxicity with lower-dose IL-2 infusion regimens when compared with bolus IL-2 infusions (Clark *et al.* 1990). Moreover, some studies have found an improved response rate using a low-dose continuous-infusion IL-2 schedule (Schoof *et al.* 1988). A randomized phase II trial by the NCI Extramural Working Group found equivalent anticancer activity and toxicity using high-dose IL-2 as a bolus versus high-dose continuous infusion IL-2 in the treatment of patients with metastatic RCC (Weiss *et al.* 1992).

The goal of combined therapy with LAK plus IL-2 is to improve on the objective response rates of IL-2 when used as a single agent. There have been three randomized trials comparing LAK/IL-2 to IL-2 alone. The first was performed by investigators of the Modified Group C Program, entering a total of 167 patients from 13 institutions, including 69 patients with metastatic RCC (McCabe *et al.* 1991). In metastatic RCC patients, the response rates for LAK/IL-2 and IL-2 were 13 and 8 per cent respectively. These results suggested that LAK cells did not contribute to higher response rates over IL-2 alone. The Surgery Branch of the NCI conducted a prospective randomized trial of 181 patients with advanced cancer, including 96 patients with metastatic RCC (Rosenberg *et al.* 1993). The high-dose bolus IL-2 regimen was used for both the induction of lymphocytosis for LAK harvest and in both treatment arms. There was no statistical difference in response rates (33 per cent LAK plus IL-2 versus 24 per cent IL-2 alone) or in survival (48-month survival: 29 per cent LAK plus IL-2 versus 25 per cent IL-2 alone). In the third trial, performed by investigators sponsored by Hoffman LaRoche (Bajorin *et al.* 1990), 49 patients were randomized to receive Roche IL-2 (3 $\times$ 10^6 U/m^2/day on days 1 through 5, 13 through day 17, 21 through day 24, and 28 through day 32) with or without LAK cells reinfused on days 13 through 15. There was no difference in the response rates between the arms of the trial. Although the power of each individual study is relatively low, the combined studies strongly suggest that the combination of LAK cells plus IL-2 has not demonstrated superiority over therapy with IL-2 alone for the treatment of metastatic RCC.

Tumour-infiltrating lymphocyes (TIL)

In 1980, NCI investigators reported a new technique to isolate and grow infiltrating lymphoid cells from solid tumors in large numbers by using IL-2 (Yron *et al.* 1980). Lymphocytes comprise a small proportion of cells in a neoplastic nodule, some of which contain IL-2 receptors, presumably because of interactions with tumor antigens. Under the influence of exogenous IL-2, these lymphocytes can grow in single-cell suspensions with tumor and appear to mediate the destruction of tumor cells, leaving relatively pure cultures of TIL. Murine TIL studies demonstrate significant cytotoxicity for syngeneic tumor cells. When compared to the adoptive transfer of LAK, TIL (both with accompanying IL-2) were found to be 50 to 100 times more potent on a per cell basis in the treatment of established lung micrometastases (Rosenberg *et al.* 1986). In addition, TIL can eliminate murine pulmonary metastases in the absence of IL-2 administration, although low doses of IL-2 enhanced their effectiveness by two- to fivefold (Speiss *et al.* 1987).

Numerous investigators have successfully established TIL cultures from hundreds of different human tumors, including RCC, melanoma, colon and breast cancer, lymphoma, and other tumor types (Yanelli *et al.* 1996). Some of these human TIL cultures have shown *in vitro* antitumor reactivity (Schwartzentruber *et al.* 1991).

The specificity of TIL antitumor activity is presumably mediated through tumor antigen–TCR interaction and is thus MHC-restricted. Some TIL cultures secrete cytokines, such as

GM-CSF, IFNγ, and TNFα in response to autologous tumor stimulation. This provides further evidence for immune recognition of tumor antigen (Schwartzentruber *et al.* 1991). IL-2-expanded TIL derived from melanoma and ovarian cancer patients have been shown to contain CTL that are primarily CD8+, recognize tumor cells via the TCR, and are MHC class I restricted (Ferrini *et al.* 1985; Itoh *et al.* 1988). Unlike the case in melanoma, autologous tumor-specific cytotoxicity has been difficult to demonstrate in RCC. There have been reports however identifying CTL with specificity for autologous human RCC (Yannelli *et al.* 1996; Koo *et al.* 1991; Finke *et al.* 1994; Schendel *et al.* 1993). Phenotypically, these TIL are mainly CD3+CD8+ T cells that are grown in the presence of low-dose IL-2 (20 U/ml) and irradiated autologous tumor stimulation (Koo *et al.* 1991). The autologous cytotoxicity can be inhibited by anti-CD3 antibody and anti-class I MHC, suggesting that recognition of tumor is via the TCR/CD3 complex. Other studies have demonstrated restricted TCR V$_\beta$ use in *ex vivo* IL-2-expanded TIL obtained from patients with RCC, suggesting the plausibility of a specific interaction between TIL-cell TCR and tumor antigen (Halapi *et al.* 1993). Furthermore, when compared to CD3+ PBL, TIL have higher expression levels of Th1 and Th2 cytokines reflecting *in vivo* activation at the tumor level (Elssasser-Beile *et al.* 1999).

The preparation of TIL for human adoptive cellular immunotherapy in the treatment of metastatic RCC occurs as follows (Belldegrun *et al.* 1993). Under aseptic conditions, radical nephrectomy specimens containing the primary tumor are first mechanically and subsequently enzymatically digested (collagenase, hyaluronidase, DNAse) to obtain a single cell suspension containing both viable mononuclear cells and tumor cells. These cells are expanded *ex vivo* under sterile conditions in the presence of IL-2. After approximately 2 weeks in culture, there is an absence of tumor cells, whereas TIL continue to proliferate. Following 5 to 6 weeks in culture, 10^8 to 10^9 initial mononuclear cells proliferate to approximately 10^{11} TIL, which can be adoptively transferred to the tumor-bearing host.

There have been several clinical trials using TIL in the adoptive immunotherapy of advanced human cancers. A pilot trial from the NCI used TIL with varying doses of IL-2, with and without cyclophosphamide, to treat 12 patients (Topalian *et al.* 1988). Two partial responses were observed among the 12 patients, occurring in a patient with metastatic melanoma and in another with metastatic RCC. Both responders were among the groups that received cyclophosphamide, IL-2, and TIL doses above the study median. The two responders were also among the group of nine patients whose TIL showed *in vitro* autologous tumor killing. This study established the feasibility of using TIL in combination therapy for human cancer. Another small study using TIL and low-dose IL-2 without cyclophosphamide in patients with advanced cancer reported an objective response rate in 18 per cent of 28 evaluable patients (Kraden *et al.* 1989). Responses were again seen in patients with metastatic melanoma and metastatic RCC, with responses lasting from 3 to 14 months. The response rate was similar to that seen in the NCI study but with low-dose IL-2 and without the use of cyclophosphamide.

In comparison to the number of patients treated with LAK/IL-2 few patients with metastatic RCC have received therapy with TIL.

Table 43.2 Phase I–II trials of combination IL-2/TIL in the treatment of metastatic renal cell carcinoma

Reference	Number of patients	Objective response, number (%)
Dillman *et al.* 1993	6	0
Topalian *et al.* 1988	4	1 (25)
Kradin *et al.* 1989	7	2 (29)
Bukowski *et al.* 1991; Olenki *et al.* 1994	34	4 (12)
figlin *et al.* 1997	55	19 (35)
Goedegebuure *et al.* 1995	8	0
Total	114	26 (23)

Table 43.2 shows the results of these trials (Dillman *et al.* 1993; Topalian *et al.* 1988; Kradin *et al.* 1989; Bukowski *et al.* 1991; Olencki *et al.* 1994; Figlin *et al.* 1997; Goedegebuure *et al.* 1995). The two larger studies, that at the Cleveland Clinic (Bukowski *et al.* 1991; Olencki *et al.* 1994), and that at UCLA (Figlin *et al.* 1997), demonstrate differing response rates (12 per cent in 34 patients versus 35 percent in 55 patients). This disparity may be explained by differences in protocol design. At the Cleveland Clinic, patients were treated in two clinical trials. In the first trial (Bukowski *et al.* 1991), 18 patients were treated with TIL isolated from primary tumor and metastatic sites. Patients were treated with one of four IL-2 dose levels, including level I, in which patients received no IL-2. Four patients received cyclophosphamide as part of their therapy. There were no responses among these 18 patients. In the second trial (Olencki *et al.* 1994), 16 patients were treated with TIL obtained from primary tumor and expanded in IL-2 and IL-4. The response rate for this trial was 25 per cent (4 of 16). At UCLA, patients received TIL isolated from primary tumor only. All patients received 3- or 4-week IL-2 infusions using a low-dose IL-2 regimen with demonstrable activity in the treatment of metastatic RCC (Figlin *et al.* 1992). The results obtained at UCLA (Figlin *et al.* 1997) can be summarized as follows (Table 43.3). Sixty-two patients with metastatic RCC presenting with their primary tumor in place underwent nephrectomy. Following radical nephrectomy, seven patients did not receive further therapy, including five who no longer met protocol requirements to safely receive systemic IL-2, one patient with failure of TIL culture and one patient found to have transitional cell carcinoma. Thirty-two of the patients received biologically

Table 43.3 UCLA trials of TIL/IL-2 immunotherapy for metastatic renal cell carcinoma ($N = 55$)*

Response, number (%)	
Overall	19 (34.6)
Complete	5 (9.1)
Partial	14 (25.5)
Median response duration (months)	
All	14 (range: 0.8+–64+)
Median survival (months)	
All	22 (range: 2–70+)
Responders	Not applicable (range: 2–63+)

* From Figlin *et al.* (1997).

active doses of cytokine prior to radical nephrectomy (IFNα, 15 patients; TNFα, 4 patients; IL-2, 4 patients; IL-2, 4 patients; IL-6, 4 patients; IFNγ, 5 patients) resulting in the generation of *in vivo* primed TIL. Twenty-three patients received CD84 selected TIL obtained by capture in anti-CD8 mAb coated flasks, and 32 patients received bulk TIL cultures. All patients received 96-hour repetitive weekly infusions of IL-2; 48 of the patients received IFNα administered subcutaneously on days 1 and 4 of the IL-2 infusion. A single treatment cycle consisted of 3 or 4 consecutive weeks of IL-2 therapy followed by 2 or 3 weeks of rest off all therapy. Thirty-four per cent of patients had an US Eastern Cooperative Oncology Group (ECOG) performance status of 0, and the remaining 66 per cent were ECOG 1. The clinical responses to treatment are demonstrated in Table 43.3. Overall, at the time of publication, there has been an objective of 34.6 per cent including 9 per cent CR, and an overall median duration of response of 14 months, (range 8+–64+ months). The actuarial survival was 65 per cent at 1 year, and 43 per cent at 2 years with an overall median survival of 22 months (range 2–70+). This compares favorably to the predicted survival without immuno-therapy of the patients based on ECOG performance status, prior nephrectomy, number of metastatic sites, weight loss, and prior cytotoxic therapy (Elson *et al.* 1988).

Cellular immunotherapy with TIL plus IL-2, has demonstrated promise in single-institution trials. The overall response rate of 34.6 per cent seen in 55 patients treated at UCLA compares favor-ably with the overall response rate of 15 per cent with high-dose IL-2 alone. This has formed the basis for a phase III trial random-izing patients to low-dose IL-2 plus CD8+ selected TIL (Figlin *et al.* 1999) (prepared at a centralized Good Manufacturing Practice (GMP) facility) versus low-dose IL-2 alone. All patients underwent radical nephrectomy to obtain tumor for TIL expan-sion. 160 patients were randomized (81 TIL/IL-2; 79 IL-2 alone); however, 20 of these patients received no treatment postnephrec-tomy because of surgical complications (4), operative mortality (2), or ineligibility for IL-2 therapy (14). Intent-to-treat analysis demonstrated objective response rates of 9.9 per cent versus 11.4 per cent and 1-year survival rates of 55 per cent versus 47 per cent respectively, and was unaffected by TIL treatment. However, it should be noted that, of the 72 patients randomized to TIL/IL-2, 33 (41 per cent) received no TIL because of cell-.processing failure. This inability prepare TIL compares quite unfavorably to other single-institution experience (Figlin *et al.* 1997), and leaves the question of the benefit of the addition of TIL to IL-2 based therapy still quite unanswered. At the present time, it may not be technically feasible to consistently and effectively deliver TIL-based treatment in a multiinstitutional fashion.

Having patients undergo nephrectomy in order to prepare adoptive immunotherapy brings forth controversy in the manage-ment of metastatic RCC. There have been single-institution reports of up to 40 per cent of patients with metastatic RCC who undergo nephrectomy subsequently failing to receive planned sys-temic immunotherapy due to perioperative morbidity/mortality or deterioration of performance status due to progressive disease (Walter *et al.* 1993; Flanigan 1996). In our experience, 89 per cent of 62 patients received their planned systemic therapy (TIL/IL-2) post-radical-nephrectomy despite some of these patients having to

undergo complicated operations including resection of caval thrombus, partial hepatectomy and splenectomy (Figlin *et al.* 1997; Franklin *et al.* 1996). Other single-institution experience supports these more favorable outcomes (Wolf *et al.* 1994; Fallick *et al.* 1997). The phase III multiinstitutional TIL trial likewise showed a 12.5 per cent postoperative failure to receive planned therapy (Figlin *et al.* 1999). It should be noted, however, that in these series patients are carefully selected for this 'aggres-sive' approach on the basis of such parameters as performance status and lack of brain metastases. However, these are some of the same selection criteria for patients to safely receive IL-2 alone for the treatment of metastatic RCC. At the present time, remov-ing the primary tumor prior to planned systemic immunotherapy can be considered in selected patients with good performance status, especially when part of investigational trials.

Therapy with TIL/IL-2 in the adjuvant setting after meta-stasectomy has been explored in a small feasibility trial of 22 patients including one with RCC (Ridolfi *et al.* 1998). TIL were successfully prepared for all participants and this ongoing trial will now focus on subjects rendered disease-free post-metastasectomy.

Attempts have been made to understand the biologic basis of response to TIL/IL-2 therapy in patients with metastatic RCC. *In vitro* studies show that the immune status of the patients as measured by the pretreatment CD56+ cell population and a serum factor able to augment *in vitro* PBL proliferation and cytotoxicity identified patients responding to immunotherapy (Belldegrun *et al.* 1996). These data strongly suggest that the immune status of the patient before immunotherapy may in part determine the outcome of therapy. Among various factors tested, responders did not differ significantly from non-responders in number of TIL infused, TIL phenotype, TIL cytokine mRNA expression, or *in vitro* cytotoxicity.

Further measures to better understand the biologic basis of response to adoptive immunotherapy need to be defined. The future role of TIL for the treatment of metastatic RCC will depend on improvements in our understanding of the immune process in the cancer-bearing host, specifically immunosuppressive factors. For example, TIL anti-tumor activity has been shown to be hindered by impaired TCR signaling function and immuno-suppressive cytokines (Finke *et al.* 1993; Reichert *et al.* 1998). Interleukin-6 secretion by RCC tumor cells has been specifically shown to protect these cells from TIL cytotoxicity (Steiner *et al.* 1999). When compared to PBL, TIL from patients with metastatic RCC have been shown to express increased Fas (CD95) receptors, possibly contributing to tumor escape from surveillance via Fas-induced apoptosis (Cardi *et al.* 1998). There are several poss-ible avenues of improvement of TIL therapy, the most important of which may rely on reversing the immunosuppressive environ-ment and the identification of tumor-associated antigen (TAA) targets.

The demonstration that some RCC lines express antigenic determinants that can be recognized by MHC-restricted CTL has led to efforts aimed at identifying TAA in human RCC. One recently cloned candidate RCC-TAA is G250 (Grabmaier *et al.* 2000). Studies using immunohistochemical techniques and radiolabeled antibody imaging reveal that mAb G250 reacts with

> 75 per cent of primary and metastatic RCC while no cross-reactivity exists with normal kidney. Studies of the imaging and biodistribution of iodine 131-labeled chimeric mAb G250 in patients with RCC revealed several areas of previously unrecognized metastases and that it has excellent tumor localization (Steffens *et al.* 1997). These characteristics strongly suggest that mAb G250 recognizes an RCC-TAA and is potentially an attractive therapeutic target. This same group has recently assessed whether the G250 antigen can be recognized by TIL derived from RCC patients (Grabmaier *et al.* 2000). The initial characterization of 18 different TIL cultures, however, suggests that anti-G250 reactivity is rare. However, using a system of DC loaded with G250 peptide and cultured with autologous T cells, they were able to generate human CTL capable of lysing a G250-expressing targets (Vissers *et al. 1999).* This suggests the possibility of TAA-based immunotherapeutic strategies for a proportion of patients with RCC.

TIL-based gene therapy

Gene therapy is a technique that generally involves the insertion of a functioning gene into a cell to correct an inborn genetic error, replace a defective/mutant gene, or to provide a new or improved function to the cell.

Antigen-specific lymphocytes have attributes that make them attractive as vehicles for the delivery of a beneficial molecule to a targeted site. It is possible to expand them by many orders of magnitude *in vitro* in response to IL-2 or antigen or both. The use of IL-2 *in vivo* can lead to further proliferation of transfected cells and to prolonged cell survival. Most promising of all is their ability to express recombinant protein (Kantoff *et al.* 1986).

Cytokine genes have been selected for TIL transduction in the hope of delivering high concentrations of cytokine to the local tumor environment, presumably increasing efficacy and decreasing systemic toxicity. There are numerous possibilities for the introduction of cytokine genes into TIL. The first cytokine gene selected by investigators at the NCI was that for TNF (Rosenberg 1992). This cytokine is effective in the treatment of established murine tumors (Asher *et al.* 1987), but highly toxic in human trials when used as an infusion. Investigators have found that retinoic acid (RA) can lead to upregulation of gene expression in human TIL retrovirally transduced with TNF gene (Treisman *et al.* 1994). Production of TNF was increased about twofold after treatment with RA, which has implications for TIL-based gene therapy.

Investigators have transduced T lymphocytes with the gene for IL-2 (Treisman *et al.* 1995). These cells were able to proliferate in the absence of exogenous IL-2 and still maintain effector function. This constitutive production of IL-2 by T lymphocytes may be an alternative method to prolong cell survival and possibly augment antitumor response of adoptively transferred cells.

Labeling a cell with a marker gene allows for the tracking of that cell in the body after its infusion. There have been studies using two gene-marked TIL for the treatment of metastatic RCC (Merrouche *et al.* 1995; Economou *et al.* 1996). Neither demonstrated selective homing of at the tumor site. In the study at UCLA (Economou *et al.* 1996), both TIL and activated PBL were genetically marked using vectors that differed in their nucleotide sequences. Both marked TIL and PBL could be detected in peripheral blood up to 99 days postinfusion. Both cell populations were detected in 6 of 9 tumor biopsies. There was no preference seen in tumor trafficking of TIL, which could be found in biopsies of muscle, fat, and skin at greater accumulation than in tumor. These labeling studies, however, demonstrated that a gene could be inserted and expressed in TIL that went on to have long-term survival in the circulation.

We have recently reported the use of an autologous RCC tumor line infected with the IL-2 gene via an adenoviral vector (RCC-Ad-IL-2) as a potent immune stimulant to propagate cytotoxic TIL *in vivo* (Mulders *et al.* 1998). Compared to standard TIL growth conditions in exogenous IL-2, TIL grown in the presence of the RCC-Ad-IL-2 had enhanced CD4+ CD8+ populations, enhanced TCR use, augmented HLA-restricted and tumor-specific cytotoxicity, and a unique cytokine profile with upregulation of IL-6 and GM-CSF. This work has implications for trials utilizing TIL propagated *in vitro* in the presence of RCC-Ad-IL-2.

Other therapeutic cell populations

Activated T cells from tumour-draining lymph nodes

Tumor-draining lymph nodes (TDLN) presumably contain sensitized precursor, but not fully functional effector T cells that can generate antigen-specific CTL. Prelinical murine models have shown therapeutic efficacy against established metastases using the adoptive transfer of TDLN that had been cultured *ex vivo* in low-dose IL-2, and anti-CD3 (Yoshizawa *et al.* 1991). Crosslinking of the TCR with anti-CD3 triggers a signaling cascade resulting in T-cell proliferation and cytokine synthesis (Meuer *et al.* 1983). These lymphocytes demonstrate nonspecific cytotoxicity against tumor and secrete GM-CSF and IFNγ when restimulated *in vitro* with tumor cells (Aruga *et al.* 1995). Patients with metastatic RCC have participated in early-phase clinical trials using *in vivo* tumor-vaccine-primed TDLN, harvested and then activated/ expanded *in vitro* with anti-CD3 mAb and IL-2 (Chang *et al.* 197). Lymphocytes were infused intravenously (IV) with concomitant administration of IL-2. Of 12 patients with RCC, there were two complete and two partial responses. The majority of activated lymphocytes released GM-CSF and IFNγ in an MHC-restricted manner in response to autologous but not allogeneic tumor. This approach has demonstrated encouraging results in small numbers of patients with metastatic RCC.

T-cell receptor-activated T cells (TRAC)

T-cell receptor-activated T cells (TRAC), are manufactured by the *ex vivo* stimulation of PBL by anti-CD3 mAb and high-dose IL-2 (100 IU/ml). They possess both NK- and LAK-type cytotoxicity patterns (non-MHC-restricted) and produce Th1 type cytokines (Sosman *et al.* 1989). In murine models TRAC were found to be more effective in the reduction of liver metastases than a similar number of adoptively transferred LAK cells (Loeffler *et al.* 1991), and produced 20-fold higher cytotoxicity than LAK (Yun *et al.* 1989). Further murine studies comparing anti-CD3 activated

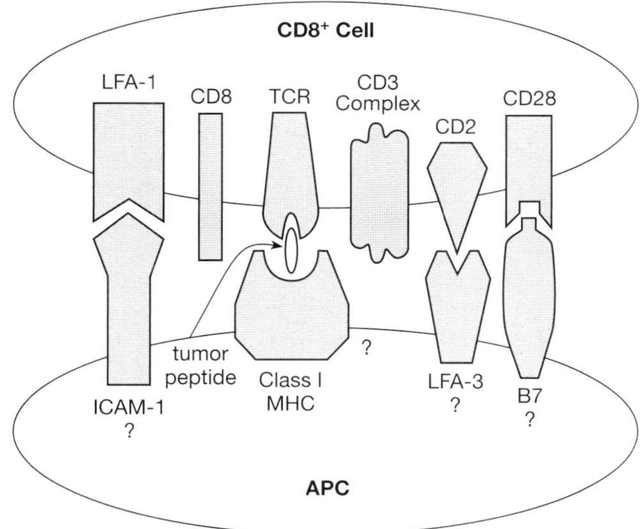

Fig. 43.1 Anti-CD3 anti-CD28 coactivation of T cells. Stimulation by both CD3 and CD28 receptors on the T cell leads to enhanced activation, proliferation, and cytokine production.

CD4+ versus CD8+ subsets and cyclophosphamide timing showed best results by the infusion of activated CD4+ cells with IL-2 given 4 days after cyclophosphamide (at greatest white blood cell nadir). This sequence produced the greatest antitumor effects and survival, and Th1 cytokine release in response to original but not unrelated syngeneic tumor (Saxton *et al.* 1997). Clinical trials in advanced cancer patients have been reported (Curti *et al.* 1993, 1998).

Anti-CD3/anti-CD28 coactivated T cells (COACTS)

While cross-linking of the TCR with anti-CD-3 may trigger a signaling cascade, other signals are probably needed for optimal immune activation and avoidance of anergy. These co-stimulatory signals are provided by interaction of CD28 or CTLA-4 receptor on T cells by anti-CD28 mAb or B7.1 and B7.2 (CD8O and CD 86) (Jenkins and Johnson 1993; Schwartz 1992) (Fig. 43.1). Co-stimulation of T cells leads to enhanced proliferation and stabilization of mRNA for a variety of Th1 cytokines, enhanced chemokine production (Thompson *et al.* 1989), and improved resistance to apoptosis due to induction of BCL-x (Boise *et al.* 1995). Preclinical murine models of COACTS demonstrated specific cytotoxicity against a B 16 tumor model (Harada *et al.* 1996). A phase 1 trial in patients with refractory cancers showed COACTS to be a feasible and safe approach, and induced immune modulation (Lum *et al.* 1998).

Monocyte-derived tumor-cytotoxic macrophages (MAC)

Peripheral blood monocytes obtained by pheresis can be cytokine activated *in vitro* with IFNγ to obtain monocyte-derived tumor-cytotoxic macrophages (MAC). These cells demonstrate cytotoxicity against malignant cells, and tumor-bearing animal studies have demonstrated the efficacy of the adoptive transfer of these cells (Fidler 1974). There have been small numbers of patients treated with MAC in clinical trials (Hennemann *et al.* 1997). The lack of efficacy in human trials of MAC will probably discourage further investigation of this cell population, and exploration of a related population of DC.

Dendritic cells (DC)

Tumor vaccine therapy has been explored for the treatment of metastatic RCC. However, tumor cells, by a variety of mechanisms, both evade immune surveillance and impair the host immune response. Many vaccine strategies attempt to make the tumor cell more immunogenic, or a more effective antigen-presenting cell (APC). RCC cell lines have been transfected with various cytokine genes in an attempt to make them more recognizable to the immune system. Phase I clinical trials have already applied vaccinations composed of GM-CSF-transduced autologous RCC (Simons *et al.* 1997) and allogeneic HLA-A2 + RCC lines transfected with the gene for IL-2 (Meyers *et al.* 1997). Other trials have used liposomal technology to deliver therapeutic genes to cells without the need for viral vectors. In RCC this has included the direct transfer *in vivo* of the liposomal IL-2 gene (Vical Inc San Diego CA) via intratumoral injection into a readily accessible metastatic lesion (Hoffman and Figlin 2000). A separate trial has assessed the intratumoral injection of DNA encoding both the class I MHC antigen HLA-B7 and beta 2 microglobulin (Genetic Therapy mc, Pasadena CA) (Rini *et al.* 1999). Ultimately, however, tumor cells are not efficient APC and for the most fail to elicit an adequate immune response in the tumor-bearing host.

Many ongoing vaccine trials in RCC and other cancers are now centered on the use of DC. DC are often referred to as 'the most potent APC'. The key feature of a vaccine-induced immune response should be effective antigen presentation by APC. In order for a cell to be an efficient APC, it must take up soluble antigen and process and present antigen in a way that is stimulatory to T cells. APC must express antigen in the context of MHC molecules, express co-stimulatory factors, and produce immunostimulatory cytokines in order to engage and activate T cells (Table 43.4).

DC are bone-marrow-derived leukocytes that lack cell surface markers typical for B, T, NK, or monocyte/macrophage cells. DC

Table 43.4 Features that make the DC the most potent APC

The form and distribution of DC fit their function of capturing antigens and selecting antigen-specific T cells

Immature DC are equipped with receptors to capture antigens by endocytosis

Mature DC are equipped with the components to stimulate antigen-specific T cells by expressing high levels of:
  MHC class I and II
  Costimulatory molecules (CD86)
  Adhesion molecules (LFA-3, ICAM-1)
  Immunostimulatory cytokines (IL-12)

are naturally found in trace numbers throughout the body, but mainly at sites of antigen encounter such as skin, gastrointestinal tract, and lung. They are expert at capturing and, processing antigen and then migrating to lymphoid organs where they present antigens to lymphocytes.

Dendritic cells can be pulsed with various forms of antigen including peptide-specific antigens (Nestle *et al.* 1998; Murphy *et al.* 1996), whole proteins in the form of lysates (Holtl *et al.* 1999; Gitlitz *et al.* 1999), and RNA encoding for antigens (Nair *et al.* 1999). DC-based phase I human trials have already shown promising results in patients with RCC (Holtl *et al.* 1999; Gitlitz *et al.* 1999; Kugler *et al.* 2000), melanoma (Nestle *et al.* 1998), prostate cancer (Murphy *et al.* 1996), B-cell lymphoma (Hsu *et al.* 1996), and multiple myeloma (Wen *et al.* 1998).

DC arise from at least two precursor populations including CD34+ stem cells originating from bone marrow and circulating CD 14+ monocytes. CD34+ stem cells mature into DC in response to GM-CSF and TNFα, an effect that is enhanced by other factors including IL-4, flt3-ligand, and CD4O-ligand (Banchereau and Steinman 1998). CD 14+ monocytes mature into DC primarily in response to the combination of GM-CSF and IL-4 (Kiertcher and Roth 1996), although similar effects have been reported when GM-CSF is combined with IFNα or CD40-ligand (Paquette *et al.* 1998; Brossart *et al.* 1998) (Fig. 43.2). These *in vitro* cultured DC exhibit all of the important morphologic, phenotypic, and functional features of APC that are crucial for the stimulation of both CD4 and CD8 T-cell subsets. Specifically, they express high levels of MHC class I and II, adhesion molecules (ICAM-l, LFA-3), and other important co-stimulatory molecules (CD40, CD8O, CD86) that are essential to the process of proper antigen presentation to T cells.

Primary renal cell cancers contain DC

The population of cells comprising human RCC include numerous lymphocyte populations (T and B cell), NK cells, and monocytes. Until recently, investigators have been primarily interested in the TIL populations for therapeutic application. For DC to be active in the process of antitumor immunity, they may be expected to migrate from blood or normal tissue into tumor via response to some chemotactic factor such as TNFα (Sallusto and Lanzavecchia 1994), 'take up' TAA, migrate to draining lymph

nodes, or interact with TIL to initiate immune response via T-cell activation. To date, however, there is a paucity of information about the process of DC migration into tumors, their activation state, and their interaction with TIL.

Using a culture system to capture cells emigrating from human RCC tumor explants, Thurnher *et al.* (1996) characterized DC populations from 17 tumors. Histologically, 'numerous' DC were identified by their pathognomonic cytoplasmic projections, or veils. These cells displayed the characteristics of mature DC including: expression of high levels of MHC and co-stimulatory molecules (CD88, B7-2), ability to stimulate naïve T cells in a mixed leukocyte reaction, and a reduced potential to capture soluble antigen. Up to 9 per cent of these emigrating leukocytes expressed CD83, a specific mature DC marker. These CD83+ cells were 40-fold enriched in tumor as compared to PBL. In Thurnher *et al.*'s (1996)conclusion, the failure of an antitumor response to RCC despite the presence of these tumor-derived DC suggests that these cells are suppressed by tumor-associated factors.

In a separate study, Troy *et al.* (1998) analyzed 14 nephrectomy specimens using both immunohistochemical and activation markers for both the detection of tumor-infiltrating DC and assessment of their functional/activation state. They found DCs accounting for less than 10 per cent of the leukocytes present in the tumors. More importantly, activated DC expressing the CD83 marker accounted for only 0.15 per cent of the total leukocyte population, and no specific tumor localization of DC was found over adjacent necrotic or inflammatory areas. Troy *et al.*'s (1998) findings suggest a lack of recruitment of DC into RCC tumors. Likewise, the tumor environment did not initiate the expected activation of DC.

A third study has also described DC infiltrating RCC (Schwaab *et al.* 1999). Similarly, however, their data also supports impaired antigen-presenting capability of these DC. Taken together these studies support the use of DC differentiated from PBL populations for clinical applications.

DC generation from PBL in RCC patients

Our UCLA Kidney Cancer Program has performed *in vitro* studies characterizing DC obtained specifically from patients with RCC (Mulders *et al.* 1999). Using common cytokine-based culture techniques (GM-CSF, IL-4 plus 10 per cent autologous serum), DC can be consistently isolated and expanded from the PBL of patients with metastatic RCC. When loaded with autologous RCC TuLy and co-cultured with autologous TIL, these DC induce: (1) lymphocyte growth expansion; (2) upregulation of CD3+, CD56– cell populations; (3) enhancement of autologous tumor lysis; and (4) upregulation of TIL, Th1 cytokine profile. Other studies confirm the finding of the ability to consistently generate functional DC from patients with RCC (Radmayr *et al.* 1995).

These *in vitro* DC culture methods require considerable resources when considering clinical/therapeutic applications including: large blood draws or leukopheresis; isolation of PBL; culture/differentiation in sterile conditions; loading with antigen; and patient vaccination. At UCLA, we have also demonstrated, via a novel phase I dose escalation trial, that DC can be generated *in vivo* by administering GM-CSF plus IL-4 subcutaneously to

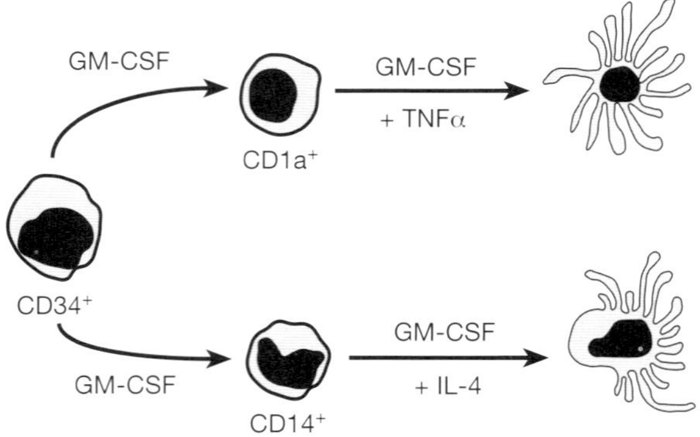

Fig. 43.2 Major dendritic cell differentiation pathways.

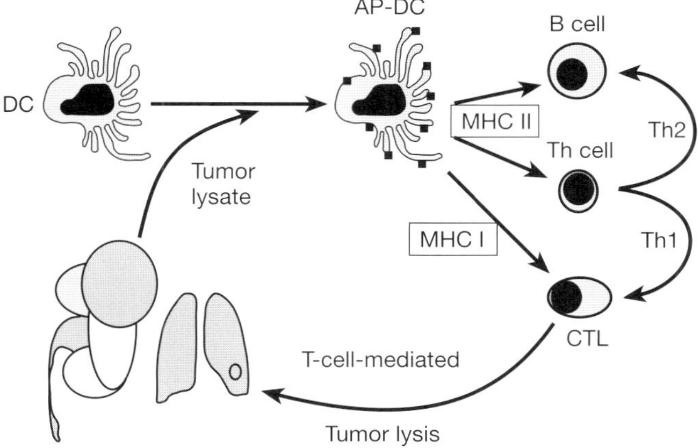

Fig. 43.3 Dendritic cell-based treatment of metastatic RCC.

patients with advanced cancers (including subjects with RCC) (Roth *et al.* 2000). These patients show minimally detectable DC at baseline, and have a marked increase in functional circulating DC after days 7–14 days of combined cytokine administration. These observations will underlie future DC-based clinical trials without the need for *ex vivo* processing of patient PBL to generate DC.

Dendritic-cell based clinical trials in renal cell carcinoma

At UCLA, we have an ongoing phase I clinical trial for patients with metatastic RCC, using TuLy obtained from primary RCC to produce an autologous TuLy-loaded DC vaccination (Gitlitz *et al.* 1999) (Figure 43.3). Using cytokine-derived DC obtained from peripheral blood precursors cultured in GM-CSF-, IL-4-, and 10 per cent autologous serum-containing media we have obtained an average of 4.9×10^6 DC range ($1.9–7.5 \times 10^6$) from ~ 90 cm^3 of blood. We have consistently cultured these DC for three consecutive weekly intradermal vaccine applications and we have not observed any dose-limiting toxicities. One subject showed *in vitro* evidence of enhanced antitumor immunity with upregulation of Th1 cytokine production from PBL and enhanced cytotoxicity against autologous tumor. This subject sustained a short-lived partial response but then developed brain metastases. In a mouse model it was found that IL-2 could augment the efficacy of a TuLy-pulsed DC vaccine (Shimizu *et al.* 1999). Future cohorts receiving our TuLy-loaded DC vaccine for the treatment of their metastatic RCC will receive this vaccine plus adjuvant systemic IL-2.

A similar study from Austria used cytokine-generated DC loaded with TuLy plus Keyhole-Limpet Hemocyanin (KLH) for intravenous application (Holtl *et al.* 1999). Again the vaccine was well tolerated with evidence of *in vitro* immune response to KLH and lysate. One of five subjects showed evidence of a partial clinical response.

More recently, a tumor cell–DC hybrid vaccination has demonstrated remarkable clinical response in patients with RCC (Kugler *et al.* 2000). To prepare this vaccine, allogeneic cytokino-derived DC plus autologous tumor cells are hybridized using an 'electrofusion' process. Allogeneic DCs are used to recruit allo-reactive

helper T cells. Seventeen subjects were vaccinated subcutaneously with a booster vaccine given after 6 weeks. All subjects without disease progression received further boosters every 3 months. Interestingly, a different allogeneic DC donor was used to prepare each vaccine. There were four complete and two partial responses observed (mean follow-up time, 13 months) with mild to moderate toxicity (fevers, tumor pain) and no evidence of autoimmune reaction. All subjects with objective response demonstrated a positive, delayed-type hypersensitivity (DTH) reaction to autologous tumor.

Conclusions

Since RCC is mostly resistant to conventional oncologic therapies, it has become a model to assess novel strategies. Although promising in both concept and early clinical trials, adoptive cellular immunotherapy with ALT, LAK, and TIL is not yet of proven benefit in patients with metastatic RCC. In the case of ALT, measurable tumor response has not correlated with survival advantage. The possible benefit of ALT awaits confirmation in a phase III trial using an appropriate control arm. Randomized phase III trials comparing LAK plus IL-2 versus IL-2 alone have failed to show a statistically significant improvement in response rate and survival with the addition of LAK. Adoptive therapy with TIL appears promising, although the results a phase III trial failed to show the feasibility of this therapy in a multi-institutional setting. In addition, the factors determining patient response are still poorly understood. The search for effector cells with antitumor activity has continued, yielding exciting preliminary results using DC-based therapies, TDLN, and COACTS. Dendritic cell vaccines are a relatively new type of therapy leaving many clinical questions to be answered with respect to the optimal number of DC to administer, the optimal antigen source and best route of vaccine administration (intravenous, subcutaneous, intramuscular) and how best to demonstrate *in vitro* immune response to these vaccines. In small, single-institution trials, there have already been promising results using DC-based vaccines for RCC. We look to the future to determine whether adoptive immunotherapy and DC-based vaccine strategies will continue to evolve into effective therapies that overcome cancer-related immunosuppression and produce durable remissions.

References

Aruga, A., Shu, S., and Chang, A.E. (1995). Tumor-specific granulocyte/macrophage colony-stimulating factor and interferon gamma secretion is associated with *in vivo* therapeutic efficacy of activated tumor-draining lymph node cells. *Cancer Immunol. Immunother.* **41** (5), 317–24.

Asher, A.L., Mule, J.J., Reichert, C.M., *et al.* (1987). Studies of the anti-tumor efficacy of systemically administered recombinant tumor necrosis factor against several murine tumors *in vivo. J. Immunol.* **138**, 963.

Bajorin, D., Sell, K.W., Richards, J.M., *et al.* (1990). A randomized trial of interleukin 2 plus lymphokine-activated killer cells versus interleukin 2 alone in renal cell carcinoma [abstract 1106]. *Proc. Am. Assoc. Cancer Res.* **31**, A1106.

Banchereau, J. and Steinman, R. (1998). Dendritic cells and the control of immunity. *Nature* **392**, 245–52.

Belldegrun, A., Pierce, W.C., Kaboo, R., *et al.* (1993). Interferon alpha-primed tumor-infiltrating lymphocytes combined with interleukin 2 and interferon alpha as a therapy for metastatic renal cell carcinoma. *J. Urol.* **150**, 1384.

Belldegrun, A., Tso, C.L., Kaboo, R., *et al.* (1996). Natural immune reactivity-associated therapeutic response in patients with metastatic renal cell carcinoma receiving tumor-infiltrating lymphocytes and IL-2 based therapy. *J. Immunother.* **19** (2), 149–61.

Bjorkman, P.J. and Parham, P. (1990). Structure, function and diversity of class I major histocompatibility complex molecules. *Ann. Rev. Biochem.* **59**, 253.

Bjorkman, P.J., Saper, M.A., Samraoui, B., *et al.* (1987). The foreign antigen binding site and T-cell recognition regions of class I histocompatibility antigens. *Nature* **329**, 512.

Boise, L.H., Noel, P.J., and Thompson, C.S. (1995). CD28 and apoptosis. *Curr. Opin. Immunol.* **7**, 620–5.

Boon, T., Coulie, P., Marchand, M., Weynants, P., Wolfel, P., and Brichard, V. (1994). Genes coding for tumor rejection agents: perspectives for specific immunotherapy. In *Biologic therapy of cancer updates* (ed. V.T. DeVita, S. Hellman, and S.A. Rosenberg), Vol. 14, p. 2. J.B. Lippincott, Philadelphia.

Brossart, P., Grunebach, F., Stuhler, G., *et al.* (1998). Generation of functional human dendritic cells from adherent peripheral blood monocytes by CD40 ligation in the absence of GM-CSF. *Blood* **92**, 4238–47.

Bukowski, R.M., Goodman, P., Crawford, E.D., *et al.* (1990). Phase II trial of high-dose intermittent interleukin 2 in metastatic renal cell carcinoma: a Southwest Oncology Group study. *J. Natl Cancer Inst.* **82**, 143.

Bukowski, R.M., Sharfman, W., Murthy, S., *et al.* (1991). Clinical results and characterization of tumor-infiltrating lymphocytes with or without recombinant interleukin 2 in human metastatic renal cell carcinoma. *Cancer Res.* **51**, 4199.

Cammarota, G., Scheirle, A., Takacs, B., *et al.* (1992). Identification of a CD4 binding site on the beta-2 domain of HLA-DR molecules. *Nature* **356**, 799.

Cantrell, D.A. and Smith, K.A. (1984). The interleukin 2 T-cell system: a new cell growth model. *Science* **224**, 1312.

Cardi, G., Heaney, J.A., Schned, A.R., *et al.* (1998). Expression of Fas (APO-1/CD95) in tumor-infiltrating and peripheral blood lymphocytes in patients with renal cell carcinoma. *Cancer Res.* **58** (10), 2078–80.

Chang, A.E., Aruga, A., Cameron, M.J., *et al.* (1997). Adoptive immunotherapy with vaccine-primed lymph node cells secondarily activated with anti-CD3 and IL-2. *J. Clin. Oncol.* **15** (2), 796–807.

Cheever, M.A., Greenberg, P.D., Fefer, A., *et al.* (1982). Augmentation of the anti-tumor therapeutic efficacy of long-term cultured lymphocytes by *in vivo* administration of purified interleukin 2. *J. Exp. Med.* **155**, 968.

Cheever, M.A., Greenberg, P.D., Irle, C., *et al.* (1984). Interleukin 2 administered *in vivo* induces the growth of cultured T cells *in vivo*. *J. Immunol.* **132**, 2259.

Clark, J.W., Smith, J.W., Steis, R.G., *et al.* (1990). Interleukin 2 and lymphokine-activated killer cell therapy: analysis of a bolus interleukin 2 and a continuous infusion interleukin 2 regimen. *Cancer Res.* **50**, 7343.

Curti, B.C., Longo, D.J., Ochoa, A.C., *et al.* (1993). Treatment of cancer patients with *ex vivo* anti-CD-3 activated killer cells and interleukin-2. *J. Clin. Oncol.* **11**, 653–60.

Curti, B.C., Ochoa, A.C., Powers, C.G., *et al.* (1998). Phase I trial of anti-CD-3 stimulated CD4⁺ T-cells, infusional interleukin-2 and cyclophosphamide in patients with advanced cancer. *J. Clin. Oncol.* **16**, 2752–60.

Dillman, R.O., Church, C., Oldham, R.K., *et al.* (1993). A randomized phase II trial of continuous infusion interleukin 2 in 788 patients with cancer. The National Biotherapy Study Group experience. *Cancer* **71**, 2358.

Donohue, J.H., Rosenstein, M., Chang, A.E., *et al.* (1984). The systemic administration of purified interleukin 2 enhances the ability of sensitized murine lymphocytes to cure a disseminated syngeneic lymphoma. *J. Immunol.* **132**, 2123.

Economou, J.S., Belldegrun, A.S., Glaspy, J., *et al.* (1996). *In vivo* trafficking of adoptively transferred interleukin-2 expanded tumor-infiltrating lympho-cytes and peripheral blood lymphocytes. Results of a double gene marking trial. *J. Clin. Invest.* **97**, 515–21.

Elsasser-Beile, U., Grussenmeyer, T., Gierschner, D., *et al.* (1999). Semiquantitative analysis of Th1 and Th2 cytokine expression in CD3+, CD4+, and CD8+ renal-cell-carcinoma-infiltrating lymphocytes. *Cancer Immunol. Immunother.* **48** (4), 204–8.

Elson, P.J., Witte, R.S., and Trump, D.L. (1988). Prognostic factors for survival in patients with recurrent or metastatic renal cell carcinoma. *Cancer Res.* **48**, 7310–13.

Ettinghausen, S.E., Lipford, E.H., Mule, J.J., *et al.* (1985). Recombinant interleukin 2 stimulates *in vivo* proliferation of adoptively transferred lymphokine-activated killer cells. *J. Immunol.* **135**, 3623.

Fallick, M.L., McDermott, D.F., LaRock, D., *et al.* (1997). Nephrectomy before interleukin-2 therapy for patients with metastatic renal cell carcinoma. *J. Urol.* **158** (5), 1691–5.

Ferrini, S., Biassoni, R., Moretta, A., Bruzzone, M., Nicolin, A., and Moretta, L. (1985). Clonal analysis of T lymphocytes isolated from ovarian carcinoma ascites fluid: phenotypic and functional characterization of T cell clones capable of lysing. *Int. J. Cancer* **36**, 337.

Fidler, I.J. (1974). Inhibition of pulmonary metastasis by intravenous injection of specifically activated macrophages. *Cancer Res.* **34**, 1074–8.

Figlin, R.A., Belldegrun, A., Moldawer, N., *et al.* (1992). Concomitant administration of recombinant human interleukin 2 and recombinant interferon alpha-2A: an active outpatient regimen in metastatic renal cell carcinoma. *J. Clin. Oncol.* **10**, 414.

Figlin, R.A., Pierce, W.C., Kaboo, R., *et al.* (1997). Treatment of metastatic renal cell carcinoma with nephrectomy, interleukin-2 and cytokine-primed or CD8(+) selected tumor infiltrating lymphocytes from primary tumor. *J. Urol.* **158**, 740–5.

Figlin, R.A., Thompson, J.A., Bukowski, M.D., *et al.* (1999). A multi-center, randomized, phase III trial of CD8⁺ tumor-infiltrating lymphocytes in combination with recombinant interleukin-2 in metastatic renal cell carcinoma. *J. Clin. Oncol.* **17** (8), 251–9.

Finke, J.H., Zea, A.H., Stanley, J., *et al.* (1993). Loss of T cell receptor zeta chain and p56lck in T-cells infiltrating human renal cell carcinoma. *Cancer Res.* **53**, 5613–16.

Finke, J.H., Rayman, P., Hart, L., *et al.* (1994). Characterization of tumor infiltrating lymphocyte subsets from human renal cell carcinoma: specific reactivity defined by cytotoxicity, interferon gamma secretion, and proliferation. *J. Immunother.* **15**, 91.

Flanigan, R.C. (1996). Role of surgery in patients with metastatic renal cell carcinoma. *Sem. Urol. Oncol.* **14** (4), 227–9.

Foon, K.A., Walther, P.J., Bernstein, Z.P., *et al.* (1992). Renal cell carcinoma treated with continuous-infusion interleukin 2 with *ex vivo*-activated killer cells. *J. Immunother.* **11**, 184.

Franklin, J.R., Figlin, R.A., Rauch, J., *et al.* (1996). Cytoreductive surgery in the management of metastatic renal cell carcinoma: the UCLA experience. *Sem. Urol. Oncol.* **14** (4), 230–6.

Gitlitz, B.J., Hinkel, A., Mulders, P., *et al.* (1999). Multi-antigen loaded dendritic cell vaccine for the treatment of metastatic renal cell carcinoma *in vitro* correlates. *Proc. Am. Urol. Assoc.* **161** (4), 137.

Goedegubuure, P.S., Douville, L.M., Li, H., *et al.* (1995). Adoptive immunotherapy with tumor-infiltrating lymphocytes and interleukin-2 in patients with metastatic malignant melanoma and renal cell carcinoma: a pilot study. *J. Clin. Oncol.* **13**, 1939–49.

Gold, J.E. and Osband, M.E. (1994). Autolymphocyte therapy. 1. *In vivo* tumour-specific adoptive cellular therapy of murine melanoma and carcinoma using *ex vivo* activated memory T lymphocytes. *Eur. J. Cancer* **30A**, 1871–82 [retracted *Eur. J. Cancer* (1998) **34** (6), 946].

Gold, J.E., Masters, T.R., and Osband, M.E. (1995). Autolymphocyte therapy III. Effective adjuvant adoptive cell therapy using *ex vivo* activated memory T-lymphocytes. *J. Surg. Res.* **59** (2), 279–86 [retracted *J. Surg. Res.* (1998) **74** (2), 196].

Grabmaier, K., Vissers, J.L.M., De Weigert, M.C.A., *et al.* (2000). Molecular cloning and immunogenicity of renal cell carcinoma-associated antigen G250. *Int. J. Cancer* **85** (6), 865–70.

Graham, S., Babayan, R.K., Lamm, D.L., *et al.* (1993). The use of *ex vivo* activated memory T cells (autolymphocyte therapy) in the treatment of metastatic renall cell carcinoma: final results from a randomized controlled multisite study. *Sem. Urol.* **11**, 27–34.

Gramata, J.W., Schmitz, P.I.M., Goey, S.H., *et al.* (1996). Modulation of immune parameter in patients with metastatic renal-cell cancer receiving combination immunotherapy (IL-2, IFNa and autologous IL-2-activated lymphocytes). *Int. J. Cancer* **65**, 152–60.

Grimm, E.A., Mazumder, A., Zhang, H.Z., and Rosenberg, S.A. (1982). Lymphokine-activated killer cell phenomenon. Lysis of natural killer-resistant fresh solid tumor cells by interleukin 2-activated autologous human peripheral blood lymphocytes. *J. Exp. Med.* **155**, 1823.

Grimm, E.A., Robb, J., Roth, J.A., *et al.* (1983). Lymphokine-activated killer cell phenomenon III. Evidence that IL-2 is sufficient for direct activation of peripheral blood lymphocytes into lymphokine-activated killer cells. *J. Exp. Med.* **158**, 1356.

Halapi, E., Yamamoto, Y., Juhlin, C., *et al.* (1993). Restricted T cell receptor V-beta usage in T cells from interleukin 2 cultured lymphocytes of ovarian and renal carcinomas. *Cancer Immunol. Immunother.* **36**, 191.

Harada, M., Okamoto, T., Omoto, K., *et al.* (1996). Specific immunotherapy with tumour-draining lymph node cells cultured with both anti-CD3 and anti-CD28 monoclonal antibodies. *Immunology* **87**, 446–53.

Hennemann, B., Rehm, A., Kottke, A., *et al.* (1997). Adoptive immunotherapy with tumor-cytotoxic macrophages derived from recombinant human granulocyte–macrophage colony-stimulating factor (rhuGM-CSF) mobilized peripheral blood monocytes. *J. Immunother.* **20** (5), 365–71.

Herberman, R.B., Hiserodt, J.C., Vujanovic, N.K., *et al.* (1987). Lymphokine-activated killer cell activity: characteristics of effector cells and progenitor cells in blood and spleen. *Immunol. Today* **8**, 178.

Herzberg, V.L. and Smith, K.A. (1987). T cell growth without serum. *J. Immunol.* **139**, 998.

Hiserodt, J.C. (1991). Some thoughts on the cytolytic activity of natural killer lymphocytes. *Cancer Cells* **3**, 530.

Hiserodt, J.C. (1993). Lymphokine-activated killer cells: biology and relevance to disease. *Cancer Invest.* **11**, 420.

Hoffman, D. and Figlin, R.A. (2000). Intratumoral IL-2 for renal cell carcinoma by direct gene transfer of a plasmid DNA/DMRIE/DOPE lipid complex. *World J. Urol.* **18** (2), 152–6.

Holtl, L., Rieser, C., Papesh, C., *et al.* (1999). Cellular and humoral immune responses in patients with metastatic renal cell carcinoma after vaccination with antigen pulsed dendritic cells. *J. Urol.* **161**, 777–82.

Hsu, F.J., Benike, C., Fagnoni, F., *et al.* (1996). Vaccination of patients with B-cell lymphoma using autologous antigen-pulsed dendritic cells. *Nature Med.* **2**, 52.

Itoh, K., Platisoucas, C.D., and Balch, C.M. (1988). Autologous tumor-specific cytotoxic T lymphocytes in the infiltrate of human metastatic melanomas: activation of interleukin 2 and autologous tumor cells, and involvement of the T cell receptor. *J. Exp. Med.* **168**, 1419.

Jenkins, M.K. and Johnson, J.G. (1993). Molecules involved in T-cell costimulation. *Curr. Opin. Immunol.* **5**, 361–7.

Kantoff, P.W., Kohn, D.B., Mitsuia, H., *et al.* (1986). Correction of adenosine deaminase deficiency in cultured human T and B cells by retrovirus-mediated gene transfer. *Proc. Natl Acad. Sci., USA* **83**, 6563.

Khan, M.M., Sansone, P., Englemen, E.G., *et al.* (1985). Pharmacologic effects of autacoids on subsets of T cells: regulation of expression function of histamine 2 receptors by a subset of suppressor cells. *J. Clin. Invest.* **75**, 1578.

Kiertcher, S. and Roth, M. (1996). Human CD14+ leukocytes acquire the phenotype and function of antigen-presenting dendritic cells when cultured in GM-CSF and IL-4. *J. Leuk. Biol.* **59**, 208–18.

Koo, A.S., Tso, C.L., Peyret, C., deKernion, J.B., and Belldegrun, A. (1991). Autologous tumor-specific cytotoxicity of tumor infiltrating lymphocytes derived from human renal cell carcinoma. *J. Immunother.* **10**, 347.

Kradin, R.L., Lazarus, D.S., Dubinett, S.M., *et al.* (1989). Tumour-infiltrating lymphocytes and interleukin 2 in treatment of advanced cancer. *Lancet* **1**, 577.

Kugler, A., Gernot, S., Walden, P., *et al.* (2000). Regression of human metastatic renal cell carcinoma after vaccination with tumor cell–dendritic cell hybrids. *Nature Med.* **6** (3), 332–6.

Lafreniere, R. and Rosenberg, S.A. (1985). Adoptive immunotherapy of murine hepatic metastases with lymphokine-activated killer cells and recombinant interleukin 2 can mediate the regression of both immunogenic and nonimmunogenic sarcomas and an adenocarcinoma. *J. Immunol.* **135**, 4273.

Lavin, P.T., Maar, R., Franklin, M., *et al.* (1992). Autolymphocyte therapy for metastatic renal cell carcinoma: initial clinical results from 335 patients treated in a multisite clinical practice. *Transplant. Proc.* **24**, 3057–62.

Loeffler, C.M., Platt, J.L., Anderson, P.M., *et al.* (1991). Antitumor effects of interleukin-2, liposomes and anti-CD3-stimulated T-cells against murine MCA 38 hepatic metastasis. *Cancer Res.* **51**, 2127–32.

Lum, L.G., LeFever, A.V., Treisman, J., *et al.* (1998). Phase I study of antiCD3/anti CD28 coactivated T cells (COACTS) in cancer patients: enhanced TH1 responses *in vivo* [abstract]. *Exp. Hematol.* **26**, 772.

Mazumdar, A., Eberlein, T.J., Grimm, E.A., *et al.* (1984). Phase I study of the adoptive immunotherapy of human cancer with lectin-activated autologous mononuclear cells. *Cancer* **53**, 896.

McCabe, M., Stablein, D., and Hawkins, M.J. (1991). The Modified Group C experience—phase III randomized trials of IL-2 versus IL-2/LAK in advanced renal cell cancer and advanced melanoma [abstract 714]. *Proc. Am. Soc. Oncol.* **10**, 213.

McGuire, K.L., Yang, J.A., and Rothenberg, E.V. (1988). Influence of activating stimulus on functional phenotype: interleukin 2 mRNA accumulation differentially induced by ionophore and receptor ligands in subsets of murine T cells. *Proc. Natl Acad. Sci., USA* **85**, 6503.

Merrouche, Y., Negrier, S., Bain, C., *et al.* (1995). Clinical application of retroviral gene transfer in oncology: results of a French study with tumor-infiltrating lymphocytes transduced with the gene of resistance to neomycin. *J. Clin. Oncol.* **13**, 410–18.

Meuer, S.C., Hodgdon, J.C., Hussey, R.E., *et al.* (1983). Antigen-like effects of monoclonal antibodies directed at receptors on human T cell clones. *J. Exp. Med.* **158**, 988–93.

Meyers, M.L., Minasian, L., Motzer, R.J., *et al.* (1997). Immunization with HLA-A2 matched allogeneic tumor cells that secrete interleukin-2 in patients with metastatic melanoma or metastatic renal cell carcinoma. *Proc. Am. Soc. Clin. Oncol.* **16**, 441a.

Morris, D.G. and Pross, H.F. (1989). Studies on lymphokine-activated killer cells. Evidence using novel monoclonal antibodies that most human LAK precursor cells share a common surface marker. *J. Exp. Med.* **169**, 717.

Mulders, P., Tso, C.L., Pang, S., *et al.* (1998). Adenovirus-mediated interleukin-2 production by tumors induces growth of cytotoxic tumor-infiltrating lymphocytes against human renal cell carcinoma. *J. Immunother.* **21**, 170–80.

Mulders, P., Tso, C.L., Gitlitz, B., *et al.* (1999). Presentation of renal tumor antigens by human dendritic cells activates tumor infiltrating lymphocytes against autologous tumor: implications for live kidney cancer vaccines. *Clin. Cancer Res.* **5**, 445–54.

Mule, J.J., Shu, S., and Rosenberg, S.A. (1985). The anti-tumor efficacy of lymphokine-activated killer cells and recombinant interleukin 2 *in vivo*. *J. Immunol.* **135**, 646.

Murphy, G., Tjoa, B., Ragde, H., *et al.* (1996). A phase I clinical trial: T-cell therapy for prostate cancer using autologous dendritic cells pulsed with HLA-A0201-specific peptides from prostate-specific membrane antigen. *Prostate* **26**, 371.

Nair, S.K., Hull, S., Coleman, D., *et al.* (1999). Induction of carcinoembryonic antigen (CEA)-specific cytotoxic T-lymphocyte responses in patients with metastatic malignancies expressing CEA. *Int. J. Cancer* **82** (1), 121.

Nestle, F.O., Alijagic, S., Gilliet, M., *et al.* (1998). Vaccination of melanoma patients with peptide- or tumor lysate-pulsed dendritic cells. *Nature Med.* **4**, 328.

Olencki, T., Finke, J., Lorenzi, V., *et al.* (1994). Adoptive immunotherapy (AIT) for renal cell carcinoma (RCC) tumor infiltrating lymphocytes (TILs) cultured *in vitro* with rIL-2, rhIL-4, and autologous tumor: a phase II trial [abstract 762]. *Proc. Am. Soc. Clin. Oncol.* **13**, 244.

Ortaldo, J.R. and Hiserodt, J.E. (1989). Mechanisms of cytotoxicity by natural killer cells. *Curr. Opin. Immunol.* **2**, 39.

Osband, M.E., Lavin, P.T., Babayan, R.K., *et al.* (1990). Effect of auto-lymphocyte therapy on survival and quality of life in patients with metastatic renal cell carcinoma. *Lancet* **335**, 994–8.

Palmer, P.A., Vinke, J., Evers, P., *et al.* (1992). Continuous infusion of recombinant interleukin 2 with or without autologous lymphokine-activated killer cells for the treatment of advanced renal cell carcinoma. *Eur. J. Cancer* **28A**, 1038.

Papa, M.Z., Mule, J.J., and Rosenberg, S.A. (1986). Antitumor efficacy of lymphokine-activated killer cells and recombinant interleukin 2 *in vivo*: successful immunotherapy of established pulmonary metastases from weakly immunogenic and nonimmunogenic tumors of three distinct histological types. *Cancer Res.* **46**, 4973.

Paquette, R.L., Hsu, N.C., Kiertscher, S.M., *et al.* (1998). Interferon alpha and GM-CSF differentiate peripheral blood monocytes into potent antigen presenting cells. *J. Leuk. Biol.* **64**, 358–67.

Parkinson, D.R., Fisher, R.I., Rayner, A.A., *et al.* (1990). Therapy of renal cell carcinoma with interleukin 2 and lymphokine-activated killer cells: phase II experience with a hybrid bolus and continuous infusion interleukin 2 regimen. *J. Clin. Oncol.* **8**, 1630.

Radmayr, C., Boch, G., Hobisch, A., *et al.* (1995). Dendritic antigen-presenting cells from the peripheral blood of renal-cell carcinoma patients. *Int. J. Cancer* **63**, 627–32.

Reichert, T.E., Rabinowich, H., Johnson, J.Y., and Whiteside, T.L. (1998). Mechanisms responsible for signaling and functional defects. *J. Immunother.* **21**, 295–306.

Ridolfi, R., Flamini, E., Riccobon, A., *et al.* (1998). Adjuvant adoptive immunotherapy with tumour-infiltrating lymphocytes and modulated doses of interleukin-2 in 22 patients with melanoma, colorectal and renal cancer, after radical metastasectomy, and in 12 advanced patients. *Cancer Immunol. Immunother.* **46**, 185–93.

Rini, B.I., Selk, L.M., Vogelzang, N.J., *et al.* (1999). Phase I study of direct intralesional gene transfer of HLA-B7 into metastatic renal cell carcinoma lesions. *Clin. Cancer Res.* **5** (10), 2766–72.

Rosenberg, S.A. (1984). Immunotherapy of cancer by systemic administration of lymphoid cells plus interleukin 2. *J. Biol. Response Mod.* **3**, 501.

Rosenberg, S.A. (1992). Karnofsky Memorial Lecture: the immunotherapy and gene therapy of cancer. *J. Clin. Oncol.* **10**, 180.

Rosenberg, S.A., Lotze, M.T., Muul, L.M., *et al.* (1985). Observations on the systemic administration of autologous lymphokine-activated killer cells and recombinant interleukin 2 to patients with metastatic cancer. *New Engl. J. Med.* **313**, 1485.

Rosenberg, S.A., Speiss, P.J., and Lafreniere, R. (1986). A new approach to the adoptive immunotherapy of cancer with tumor-infiltrating lymphocytes. *Science* **233**, 1318.

Rosenberg, S.A., Lotze, M.T., Yang, J.D., *et al.* (1989). Experience with the use of high-dose interleukin 2 in the treatment of 652 cancer patients. *Ann. Surg.* **210**, 474.

Rosenberg, S.A., Lotze, M.T., Yang, J.D., *et al.* (1993). Prospective randomized trial of high dose interleukin 2 alone or in conjunction with lymphokine-activated killer cells for the treatment of patients with advanced cancers. *J. Natl Cancer Inst.* **85**, 622.

Roth, M.D., Gitlitz, B.J., Kiertscher, S.M., *et al.* (2000). GM-CSF and interleukin-4 enhance the number and antigen presenting activity of circulating CD14+ and CD83+ cells in cancer patients. *Cancer Res.* **60** (7), 1934–41.

Sallusto, F. and Lanzavecchia, A. (1994). Efficient presentation of soluble antigen by cultured human dendritic cells is maintained by GM-CSF plus IL-4 and downregulated by TNF-a. *J. Exp. Med.* **179**, 1109–18.

Salter, R.D., Benjamin, R.J., Wesly, P.K., *et al.* (1990). A binding site for the T-cell co-receptor CD8 on the alpha-3 domain of HLA-A2. *Nature* **345**, 41.

Sawczuk, I.S. (1993). Autolymphocyte therapy in the treatment of metastatic renal cell carcinoma. *Urol. Clin. N. Am.* **20**, 297–301.

Sawczuk, I.S., Graham, S.D. Jr, Miesowicz, F., and the ALT Adjuvant Study Group, Cellcor Inc, Newton MA, Emory Clinic, Atlanta, GA, and Columbia University, New York NY (1997). Randomized, controlled trial of adjuvant therapy with *ex vivo* activated T cells (ALT) in $T_{1-3a,b,c}$ or $T_4N_+M_0$ renal cell carcinoma. *Proc. Am. Soc. Clin. Oncol.* **16**, 326a.

Saxton, M.L., Longo, D.L., Wetzel, H.E., *et al.* (1997). Adoptive transfer of anti-CD3-activated CD4+ T cells plus cyclophosphamide and liposome encapsulated interleukin-2 cure murine MC-38 and 3LL tumors and establish tumor specific immunity. *Blood* **89**, 2529–36.

Schendel, D.J. Gansbacher, B., Oberneder, R., *et al.* (1993). Tumor-specific lysis of human renal cell carcinoma by tumor-infiltrating lymphocytes I. HLA-A2 restricted recognition of autologous and allogeneic tumor lines. *J. Immunol.* **151**, 4209.

Schoof, D.D., Gramolini, B.A., Davidson, D.L., *et al.* (1988). Adoptive immunotherapy of human cancer using low dose recombinant interleukin 2 and lymphokine-activated killer cells. *Cancer Res.* **48**, 5007.

Schwaab, T., Schned, A.R., Heaney, J.A., *et al.* (1999). *In vivo* description of dendritic cells in human renal cell carcinoma. *J. Urol.* **162** (2), 567–73.

Schwartz, R.H. (1992). Costimulation of T lymphocytes: the role of CD28, CTLA-4, and B7/BB1 in interleukin-2 production and immunotherapy. *Cell* **71**, 1065–8.

Schwartzentruber, D.J., Topalian, S.L., Mancini, M.J., *et al.* (1991). Specific release of granulocyte–macrophage colony-stimulating factor, tumor necrosis factor-alpha, and interferon gamma by tumor-infiltrating lymphocytes after autologous tumor stimulation. *J. Immunol.* **146**, 3674.

Shimizu, K., Fields, R.C., Giedlin, M., *et al.* (1999). Systemic administration of interleukin-2 enhances the therapeutic efficacy of dendritic cell-based tumor vaccines. *Proc. Natl Acad. Sci., USA* **96** (5), 2268-73.

Simons, J.W., Jaffee, E.M., Weber, C.E., *et al.* (1997). Bioactivity of autologous irradiated renal cell carcinoma vaccines generated by *ex vivo* GM-CSF gene transfer. *Cancer Res.* **57**, 1537.

Sosman, J.A., Oettle, K.R., Hank, J.A., *et al.* (1989). Specific recognition of human leukemic cells by allogeneic T cell lines. *Transplantation* **48**, 486–95.

Speiss, P.J., Yang, J.C., and Rosenberg, S.A. (1987). *In vivo* antitumor activity of tumor infiltrating lymphocytes expanded in recombinant interleukin 2. *J. Natl Cancer Inst.* **79**, 1067.

Steffens, M.G., Boerman, O.C., Oosterwijk-Wakka, J.C., *et al.* (1997). Targeting of renal cell carcinoma with iodine-131-labeled chimeric monoclonal antibody G250. *J. Clin. Oncol.* **15**, 1529–37.

Steiner, T., Junker, U., Wunderlich, H., *et al.* (1999). Are renal cell carcinoma cells able to modulate the cytotoxic effect of tumor infiltrating lymphocytes by secretion of interleukin-6? *Anticancer Res.* **19** (2C), 1533–6.

Sznol, M., Clark, J.W., Smith, J.W., *et al.* (1992). Pilot study of interleukin 2 and lymphokine-activated killer cells combined with immunomodulatory doses of chemotherapy and sequenced with interferon alpha-2A in patients with metastatic melanoma and renal cell carcinoma. *J. Natl Cancer Inst.* **84**, 929.

Thompson, C.B., Lindsten, T., Ledbetter, J.A., *et al.* (1989). CD 28 activation pathway regulates the production of multiple T-cells derived lymphokines/cytokines. *Proc. Natl Acad. Sci., USA* **86**, 1333–7.

Thompson, J.A., Shulman, K.L., Benyunes, M.C., *et al.* (1992). Prolonged continuous intravenous infusion interleukin 2 and lymphokine-activated killer cell therapy for metastatic renal cell carcinoma. *J. Clin. Oncol.* **10**, 960.

Thurnher, M., Radmayr, C., Ramoner, R., *et al.* (1996). Human renal cell carcinoma tissue contains dendritic cells. *Int. J. Cancer* **67**, 1–7.

Topalian, S.L., Solomon, D., Frederick, P., *et al.* (1988). Immunotherapy of patients with advanced cancer using tumor-infiltrating lymphocytes and recombinant interleukin 2: a pilot study. *J. Clin. Oncol.* **6**, 839.

Treisman, J., Hwu, P., Yannelli, J.Y., *et al.* (1994). Upregulation of tumor necrosis factor-alpha production by retrovirally transduced human tumor-infiltrating lymphocytes using trans-retinoic acid. *Cell. Immunol.* **156** (2), 448–57.

Treisman, J., Hwu, P., Minamoto, S., *et al.* (1995). Interleukin-2 transduced lymphocytes grow in an autocrine fashion and remain responsive to antigen. *Blood* **85** (1), 139–45.

Troy, A., Summers, K.L., Davidson, P.J.T., *et al.* (1998). Minimal recruitment and activation of dendritic cells within renal cell carcinoma. *Clin. Cancer Res.* **4**, 585–93.

Vissers, J.L.M., DeVries, J.M., Schreurs, M.W.J., *et al.* (1999). The renal cell carcinoma-associated antigen G250 encodes a human leukocyte antigen (HLA)-A2.1-restricted epitope recognized by cytotoxic T lymphocytes. *Cancer Res.* **59** (21), 5554–9.

Walther, M.M., Alexander, R.B., Weiss, G.H., *et al.* (1993). Cytoreductive surgery prior to interleukin-2-based therapy in patients with metastatic renal cell carcinoma. *Urology* **42**, 250–8.

Wasserman, J., Petrini, B., and Blomgren, H. (1982). Radiosensitivity of T lymphocyte subpopulations. *J. Clin. Lab. Immunol.* **7**, 139.

Waymack, J.P., Guzman, R.F., Burleson, D.G., *et al.* (1989). Effect of prostaglandin E in multiple experimental models. *Prostaglandins* **38**, 345.

Weiss, G.R., Margolin, K.A., Aronson, F.R., *et al.* (1992). A randomized phase II trial of continuous infusion interleukin 2 or bolus injection interleukin 2 plus lymphokine-activated killer cells for advanced renal cell carcinoma. *J. Clin. Oncol.* **10**, 275.

Wen, Y.J., Ling, M., Bailey-Wood, R., *et al.* (1998). Idiotypic protein-pulsed adherent peripheral blood mononuclear cell-derived dendritic cells prime immune system in multiple myeloma. *Clin. Cancer Res.* **4**, 957–62.

Wolf, J.S. Jr, Aronson, F.R., Small, E.J., and Carroll, P.R. (1994). Nephrectomy for metastatic renal cell carcinoma: a component of systemic treatment regimens. *J. Surg. Oncol.* **55** (1), 7–13.

Yannelli, J.R., Hyatt, C., McConnell, S., *et al.* (1996). Growth of tumor-infiltrating lymphocytes from human solid cancers: summary of a 5-year experience. *Int. J. Cancer* **65**, 413–21.

Yoshizawa, H., Chang, A.E., and Shu, S. (1991). Specific adoptive immuno-therapy mediated by tumor-draining lymph node cells sequentially activated with anti-CD3 and IL-1. *J. Immunol.* **147**, 729–37.

Yron, I., Wood, T.A., Speiss, P., and Rosenberg, S.A. (1980). *In vitro* growth of murine T cells V. The isolation and growth of lymphoid cells infiltrating syngeneic solid tumors. *J. Immunol.* **125**, 238.

Yun, Y.S., Hargrove, M.E., and Tng, C.C. (1989). *In vivo* anti tumor activity of anti-CD3 induced activated killer cells. *Cancer Res.* **49**, 4770–4.

44. Role of nephrectomy in metastatic disease

Robert C. Flanigan and Paul Matthew Yonover

Introduction

When a patient presents with a diagnosis of renal cell carcinoma (RCC), a work-up for metastatic spread will be positive approximately one-third of the time. Common sites of metastatic spread include the lung, liver, bone, brain, and adrenal gland, with case reports detailing this cancer's capacity to appear almost anywhere in the body, including the thyroid, pancreas, labia, retina, etc. Of patients with clinically localized disease at time of diagnosis, another 20 to 50 per cent eventually will develop metastatic disease following nephrectomy (Flanigan 1996; Motzer and Russo 2000). Despite major advances in genitourinary oncology, those patients with metastatic RCC still face a dismal prognosis, with a median survival of only 6 to 10 months and a 2-year survival of 10 to 20 per cent (Figlin *et al.* 1997) (see Table 44.1).

The advent of systemic immunotherapy has brought renewed hope for this group of patients, although responses to date have been modest. These advances have also brought renewed interest in cytoreductive nephrectomy, whose role is currently being evaluated in the treatment of advanced RCC in conjunction with immune-based therapies.

In the past, nephrectomy in the face of known cancer spread was only thought to be indicated for palliative therapy. This logic has been revisited and is the center of an increasingly intense debate about the proper timing, if any, of removing the primary tumor in conjunction with biologic response modifier (BRM) therapy.

Epidemiology

In 2000, it is estimated that nearly 31 200 new cases of RCC will be discovered, with almost 11 900 deaths attributable to this disease each year in the USA alone (Greenlee *et al.* 2000). While RCC is only the seventh leading cause of cancer, it still remains a focal point for both the urologist and oncologist who seek to impart durable responses to therapies directed against advanced disease.

With fewer than 10 per cent of patients presenting with the classic triad of flank pain, hematuria, and a palpable mass, RCC is often referred to as the 'internist's tumor' because of its protean array of presenting signs and symptoms. Older studies show that hematuria is the most common presenting symptom of RCC, but certainly today's advanced imaging capabilities have made the 'incidental' finding of a renal tumor a much more common entity (Skinner *et al.* 1971).

Prognostic factors

The overall prognosis for advanced RCC is very poor. Identifying prognostic factors that correlate with survival has been the focus of investigators for many years. Pathologic stage, nuclear grade and cell type, tumor size, age, race, sex, and associated paraneoplastic syndromes have all been examined for discernible patterns that can distinguish subsets of patients who may benefit from aggressive therapies.

Pathologic stage

The consensus in the literature is that the prognosis of patients with RCC is inversely proportional to pathologic stage. Using the older Robson classification schema, several large studies reported the 5-year overall survival in patients with stage IV disease to be between 2 and 20 per cent (Thrasher and Paulson 1993). The Robson system is limited because it includes nodal involvement into stage III tumors, making it difficult to compare older studies with those that utilize the updated TNM (tumor–node–metastasis) system now in use. However, regardless of the system used, patho-

Table 44.1 Survival of patients with metastatic RCC*

		Survival (%)	
Reference	Number of patients	I year	5 years
Riches *et al.* 1951	409	33	0.5
Middleton 1967	141	10	0
Skinner *et al.* 1971	77	–	0
Johnson *et al.* 1975	93	26	–
Thompson *et al.* 1975	65	22	0
Klugo *et al.* 1977	64	12	3
Montie *et al.* 1977	78	18	–
deKernion *et al.* 1978	86	43	10
McNichols *et al.* 1981	56	–	14
Bassil *et al.* 1985	53	–	18
Golimbu *et al.* 1986	88	–	2
Giuiliani *et al.* 1990	50	–	7

* Adapted from Kavolius *et al.* (1998).

logic stage is the most powerful single prognostic factor identified to date. Those patients with any type of extrarenal extension display a much poorer prognosis (Thrasher and Paulson 1993).

Lymph node involvement has an adverse impact on survival comparable to that found in patients with distant metastases. For example, when comparing patients with nodal involvement versus distant metastatic disease, Libertino (1987) found no difference in overall 5-year survival between the two groups. Similarly, in a report from Bassil *et al.* (1985), the survival rate for patients with positive nodes ranged from 0 to 5 per cent over 10 years, suggesting that the grim outlook for metastatic disease is also seen in node-positive disease. Although data exist suggesting that a regional lymphadenectomy may confer some benefit to a subset of patients whose disease is limited in its spread, these studies are fraught with problems, including their small numbers and retrospective nature. Until good prospective studies show otherwise, one must equate nodal metastasis to systemic disease.

Nuclear grade and cell type

On the basis of characteristics of tumor nuclei, Fuhrman *et al.* (1982) developed a standard for grading RCC. In a study outlining this classification system, significant survival differences appeared in three distinct groups. Grade 1 tumors carried a favorable prognosis, Grade 4 had a very poor prognosis, and Grades 2 and 3 were intermediate.

RCC has several well described cell types, namely, clear cell, papillary, chromophobe, oncocytic, and collecting duct; sarcomatoid changes have been described with all of these histologic subtypes. It is unclear from the literature exactly how important these cell types are when evaluating prognosis but it would appear that pure clear cell or granular cell tumors are less aggressive than sarcomatoid cell-type RCC (Ro *et al.* 1987). Selli *et al.* (1983) concluded that survival in metastatic RCC was not related to the local extent of the primary tumor nor to the site of metastases but was dependent on cell type. However, since grade and stage correlate closely to cell type, it is impossible to look at cell type alone as an independent factor. For example, Skinner *et al.* reported that spindle (sarcomatoid) cancers were more malignant in nature, but the tumors in this cohort were all high nuclear grade (grade 3 or 4) tumors.

Other factors

Some authors have suggested that hypercalcemia related to metastatic RCC adversely affects survival compared to patients who are normocalcemic, although others have failed to confirm this observation. Weight loss, performance status, and the number and sites of metastases have also been noted as prognostic indicators (Johnson *et al.* 1975; Elson *et al.* 1988; Negrier *et al.* 1998; Motzer and Russo 2000).

Role of palliative nephrectomy

Patients with metastatic RCC usually do not present with severe symptomatology directly related to their primary tumor. Intractable hemorrhage, unrelenting flank pain, and the various paraneoplastic syndromes have, however, been associated with this cancer. RCC are known to be markedly vascular. This vascularity may be linked to vascular endothelial growth factor (VEGF), which is thought to be regulated by the von Hippel–Lindau (VHL) protein. Furthermore, loss of VEGF suppression may play an important role in the formation of tumor-associated angiogenesis (Figlin 1999). As a result, large arteriovenous fistulas have been associated with RCC. This, in turn, can lead to hypertension, cardiomegaly, and high-output heart failure. Nephrectomy has been advocated to relieve these symptoms (Freed 1977). Such dramatic tumors are unusual today, primarily because most cancers are discovered at an earlier stage.

Although most urologists agree that palliative nephrectomy may benefit the unusual patient presenting with these problems, up to 50 per cent of these patients are going to die within 4 to 12 months after palliative nephrectomy alone (Flanigan 1996). Given the poor prognosis these patients face, as outlined earlier, it is difficult to justify the morbidity associated with open surgery when less invasive techniques, such as angioinfarction, may satisfactorily control local symptoms.

Montie *et al.* (1977) cautioned that the systemic effects attributed to RCC may be produced by the metastases and not necessarily by the primary tumor itself; thus palliative nephrectomy may not bring relief for the problem it is meant to alleviate. For instance, in a study examining the effects of nephrectomy on hypercalcemia associated with RCC, Walther *et al.* (1997*a*) concluded that surgical extirpation of the primary tumor helped reduce calcium levels in 7 of 12 patients. However, four patients actually suffered an increase in their serum calcium and one patient had no change. Overall, patients benefiting from surgery, that is, those experiencing a decrease in calcium levels, did no better than those who failed to respond, both groups having a median survival time of approximately 6 months.

In a retrospective review of survival data of 93 patients with metastatic RCC, Johnson *et al.* (1975) observed that palliative nephrectomy alone increased survival in a small subset of patients. In this series, of the 27 patients with metastases limited to bone, median survival for those who underwent nephrectomy was 16.1 months compared to 10.6 months for those not undergoing surgery. The paper, however, did not comment on whether these differences were statistically significant. Interestingly, a subsequent published review by Montie *et al.* (1977) also noted that, of those patients undergoing adjunctive nephrectomy, patients with osseous metastases alone fared better than those who had metastases to other sites, based on 1-year survival data.

Fuselier and associates (1983) reported their experience at the Ochsner Clinic between 1945 and 1978. Of their patients who underwent nephrectomy, nearly 24 per cent had recognized distant metastases at the time of operation. These patients underwent palliative nephrectomy followed by adjuvant therapy by various modalities, including radiation, hormones, and chemotherapy. Fifty per cent of these patients died within 1 year, and no patient who had distant metastases at the time of operation experienced a regression of disease. Middleton (1967) reported a series of 141 patients at New York Hospital with metastatic RCC. For the 33 patients with documented multiple distant metastases who underwent palliative nephrectomy, survival was no different than for those who did not undergo surgery.

Another argument against liberal use of nephrectomy alone to treat these patients is the high operative mortality that has been observed. deKernion and Lindner (1982) noted a 6 per cent mortality rate even after excluding debilitated patients, while other studies have reported that up to 17 per cent of these patients die within 30 days of nephrectomy from surgery-related complications (see Table 44.6).

Overall, nephrectomy alone in the face of metastatic disease is not generally felt to offer any real survival benefit. Palliative nephrectomy not followed by other adjunctive therapy is not warranted except in patients with significant symptomatology from these primary tumors, which will only be required in very rare cases (Flanigan 1996).

Spontaneous regression

One of the most troubling aspects of this cancer is its unpredictable nature. Primary tumors have been observed to remain stable for years without growing or metastasizing and some metastatic lesions have displayed long periods of growth arrest or lengthened tumor doubling time. Anecdotal reports of spontaneous regression of distant metastases exist and it has been estimated to occur in approximately 0.4 to 0.8 per cent of patients (see Table 44.2). The mechanism by which this rare phenomenon occurs is unclear and there is as yet no established association between it and the removal of the primary tumor. More importantly, investigators have failed to demonstrate an improved survival in these patients. As deKernion and Lindner (1982) observed, most spontaneous regressions that do seem to occur are of short duration.

The idea that RCC can truly undergo spontaneous regression is not universally accepted, with several large series failing to exhibit this in any of their patients (Johnson *et al.* 1975; Montie *et al.* 1977; Fuselier *et al.* 1983).

Many of the reported cases of spontaneous regression have involved metastases to the lung. Of 51 cases of regression reviewed by Freed *et al.* (1977), 45 were examples involving pulmonary metastases. Given this trend, some speculate that suspicious lesions on chest radiographs are actually some other, more benign

Table 44.2 Spontaneous regression after nephrectomy*

Reference	Number of patients	
	Total	With regression
Rafla	14	0
Wagle and Scal	80	2
Bottinger 1970	100	0
Mims *et al.*	57	1
Middleton 1967	33	0
Johnson *et al.* 1975	43	0
Skinner *et al.* 197?	77	1
Lokich and Harrison 1975	45	0
Montie *et al.* 1977	25	0
Total	474	4 (0.8%)

* Adapted from Couillard *et al.* (1993).

condition such as old granulomatous lesions or fungal disease. Indeed, few of the cases reported have biopsy-proven histologic proof of being truly RCC. Of the four patients who Walther *et al.* (1993) claimed experienced regression of pulmonary nodules after surgery, only one was confirmed by biopsy. Non-neoplastic lung lesions are known to regress spontaneously at times, thus perhaps misleading the clinician into thinking a true regression of metastasis has occurred.

Angioinfarction plus nephrectomy

A large single-institution series from M.D. Anderson Cancer Center retrospectively reviewed an experience with angioinfarction followed by nephrectomy and postoperative hormonal therapy (medroxyprogesterone 400 mg intramuscularly twice weekly) for metastatic RCC (Swanson *et al.* 1983). The theory behind this approach was that tumor antigens released from the infarcted tissue would provide a powerful stimulus for the host immune system to fight the offending tumor cells. In 100 patients followed for at least 12 months, the overall response rate was 28 per cent (with complete responses in 7 patients, partial responses in 8 patients). The median survival for both of these groups was 19 months. It is of note that those patients most likely to benefit from this form of therapy demonstrated limited pulmonary parenchymal metastases, showing a 64 per cent 1- year survival rate. This study left many questions unanswered, including the effect of patient selection, the effect of postoperative progesterone therapy, and whether the patients in the stable disease category would have done as well without nephrectomy or with nephrectomy and no infarction.

Subsequent to this report, Kurth *et al.* (1986) reported an experience with 25 patients treated with embolization and delayed nephrectomy. One complete response of metastases was seen (lasting greater than 36 months) and stable disease was apparent in six patients (duration of 14 to 31 months), but 72 per cent of patients died after a median of 5.7 months.

A multi-institutional study by the Southwestern Oncology Group (SWOG) failed to document any significant efficacy for renal angioinfarction followed by nephrectomy (Gottesman 1985). Thirty patients with metastatic RCC were treated by renal infarction followed by delayed nephrectomy with a minimal follow-up of 1 year. There were no complete responses and only one partial remission, which lasted 21 months before progression of disease. Three patients displayed stable disease for at least 6 months, but eventually all patients showed evidence of progression. Furthermore, only 3 of 11 patients with metastases limited to the lung lived 1 year. An overall 21 per cent 1-year survival and a 7-month median survival were reported.

The significant side-effects of angioinfarction should not be overlooked. The postinfarction syndrome, which includes abdominal pain, nausea, vomiting, diarrhea, fevers, and ileus, has been well described (deKernion and Lindner 1982). Another potential complication of this therapy is the inadvertent embolization of peripheral vessels. In sum, angioinfarction, like palliative nephrectomy, should be reserved for controlling severe symptoms

Table 44.3 Five-year survival of patients with metastatic RCC after metastectomy

Reference	Number of patients	5-year survival (%)
Middleton 1967	59	34
Skinner et al. 1971	41	29
Tolia and Whitmore 1975	17	35
Klugo et al. 1977	10	50
O'Dea et al. 1978	44	16
deKernion et al. 1978	20	25
McNichols et al. 1981	13	69
Jett et al. 1983	44	27
Dernevik et al. 1985	33	21
Kierney et al. 1994	36	31
Kavolius et al. 1998	141	44

* Adapted from Kavolius et al. (1998).

or reducing the size of large tumors preoperatively and not as an attempt at prolonging survival and cure.

Nephrectomy with resection of metastases

Several series have demonstrated the efficacy of complete surgical resection of all tumor burden, including the removal of both the primary renal mass as well as metastatic deposits in patients with minimal volume metastatic RCC (see Table 44.3).

Kierney *et al.* (1994) described 41 patients in whom complete excision of all metastatic deposits and the primary tumor was possible in 88 per cent of cases. In 64 per cent, the metastatic process was in a single site. These investigators reported a 59 per cent 3-year and a 31 per cent 5-year survival in their patients, suggesting that long-term benefit for many patients with resectable metastatic disease may be realized by complete surgical excision.

One subset of patients who may benefit most from removal of the primary renal tumor and metastases are those with solitary pulmonary lesions amenable to resection. Tolia and Whitmore (1975) reported a 35 per cent 5-year survival period when solitary pulmonary metastases were excised along with the primary lesion. deKernion and Lindner (1982) also reported on a series of 12 patients who underwent excision of single or multiple pulmonary metastases with a 42 per cent 3-year and a 25 per cent 5-year survival. One of their patients was reported to be alive without evidence of disease more than 6 years after excision of pulmonary metastases. A similar retrospective study has shown overall 5-year overall survival rates of 44 per cent for patients undergoing a curative metastectomy (Kavolius *et al.* 1998). Among 94 patients with solitary metastases who underwent resection, lung metastases were more favorable than metastases to brain, with 5-year survival rates of 54 versus 18 per cent, respectively.

Although it is clear that the majority of such patients will manifest other signs of metastases over a period of time and die of metastatic RCC, nephrectomy and excision of minimal metastatic disease, particularly when confined to the lungs, may benefit a small number of patients.

Adjuvant therapies

Chemotherapy

Largely refractory to chemotherapy, RCC has long been recognized as a chemoresistant tumor. Little benefit has been derived from either single or combination regimens. Despite the advent of novel chemotherapeutic agents, responses have been poor at best. When Yagoda reviewed phase II trials of the mid-1980s involving 39 different agents, he found that an objective response was seen in less than 9 per cent of 2100 patients. In an update of this review, covering over 70 agents, this response rate became a mere 6.8 per cent with responses typically being of short duration (Yagoda 1990; Yagoda *et al.* 1995).

Similarly, deKernion and Lindner (1982) reviewed several studies looking at both single-agent and combined-agent therapies. The most optimistic was a retrospective review by Hrushesky and Murphy (1977) citing a 25 per cent overall objective response rate following therapy with vinblastine. deKernion and Lindner (1982) concluded that, overall, complete responses were rare and lacked durability.

In seven other studies cited in deKernion and Lindner's (1982) review, a total of 207 patients were treated with vinblastine-containing combination chemotherapies. With an overall response rate of 16 per cent, only 2 per cent were complete responders. deKernion and Lindner (1982) further warned that the significant toxicity weighed heavily against these questionable response rates and that these studies were small and failed to meet the rigors of a well-structured prospective trial.

The source of RCC's well-recognized resistance to chemotherapy is speculative, but two strong theories exist. The multidrug resistance (*MDR-1*) gene has been found in a high percentage of renal tumors and is thought to be linked to cell surface p170 glycoproteins. This abnormality may facilitate the active efflux of cytotoxic drugs out of the tumor cells, effectively neutralizing these agents. Unfortunately, the investigational use of MDR-inhibitors, particularly in combination with cytotoxic agents, has produced little success to date (Figlin 1999; Gitlitz *et al.* 1996; Bukowski 1997).

Secondly, given the slow or variable growth rate of some of these tumors, it is felt that long doubling times may also offer some protection for the cancer against drugs that poison rapidly dividing cells. To counter this, prolonged drug infusion techniques have been utilized in recent trials, using antimetabolites such as 5-fluorouracil (5-FU) and floxuridine. With various time-modified schedules, it is hoped that these drugs may produce improved responses when combined with biologic response modifiers (Bukowski 1997).

To date, combination chemotherapy/immunotherapy trials (interleukin 2 (IL-2), interferon alpha (IFNα), 5-FU) have had mixed results, as shown in Table 44.4 (Motzer and Russo 2000).

Table 44.4 Results with IFNα, IL-2, and 5-FU combinations

Reference	Number of patients	Number of responses		Overall response, number (%)	Median duration of response (months)
		CR	**PR**		
Kirchner et al.	246	26	54	80 (33)	—
Hofmockel et al.	34	9	10	13 (38)	12
Ellerhorst et al.	52	4	12	16 (31)	17
Joffe et al.	38	0	9	9 (24)	—
Dutcher et al.	50	1	7	8 (16)	9
Gitlitz et al. 1996	23	0	6	6 (26)	7
Olencki et al.	18	0	0	—	
Tourani et al.	62	1	11	12 (19)	13
Ravaud et al.	111	0	5	5 (2)	4

* Adapted from Motzer and Russo (2000).

Hormonal therapy

In the early 1970s, it was observed that the growth of diethylstilbe-strol (DES)-induced kidney tumors in the Syrian hamster was at least partially inhibited by progestational agents, sparking a flurry of clinical activity. Despite initially encouraging results, these agents are clearly of little value against these tumors. Although retrospective data were promising, subsequent prospective randomized trials failed to substantiate claims of durable responses and improved survival. Objective responses to medroxy-progesterone acetate (MPA), testosterone, tamoxifen, and other hormonal agents have been lackluster at best, with overall response rates reported as less than 5 per cent (deKernion and Lindner 1982; Harris 1983; Bukowski 1997). Currently, MPA has been relegated to providing symptomatic relief rather than achieving cure (*Lancet* 1999).

Immunotherapy

It has long been thought that the immune system holds the key to this devastating disease. The behavior of these tumors, at times dormant, perhaps even regressing, has driven speculation that the host immune system may affect its natural course.

Detailing the history and current status of immunotherapy for RCC is beyond the scope of this chapter. It is important to briefly touch on this area of research, however, because much of today's approach to cytoreductive nephrectomy is inexorably tied to adjuvant immune-based therapies. Furthermore, whether to deliver these biologic response modifiers *before* or *after* removal of the primary tumor is subject to intense debate.

The link between the immune system and RCC has been recog-nized for many years. As noted by Freed (1977), most examples of spontaneous regression are noted in lung metastases. He argued that lung tissue, with its rich supply of macrophages and lympho-cytes, may be able to contain the disease via host immune mechan-isms. He put forth a theory of 'proliferative suicide', speculating that the large antigen load presented by the tumor may be driving the lymphocytes to their 'end stage', thus paralysing the immune system. In further support of this hypothesis, he cited animal data that showed that cell-mediated cytotoxicity was diminished with the continuing growth of the tumor. Other authors have described

the primary tumor as an 'immunologic sink', essentially monopo-lizing the efforts of circulating lymphocytes and preventing any effective response against distant metastases (Spencer *et al.* 1992).

Serotherapy was a novel undertaking in the early 1970s to exploit these host immune responses, whereby the plasma from a patient previously cured of RCC was transfused into a family member suffering from metastatic disease. Success was limited, but demonstrated an early attempt to harness the natural immune system (deKernion and Lindner 1982).

Interferon therapy represented one of the first breakthroughs in immunotherapy for this disease. Once bound to the cell mem-brane, interferons initiate a complex sequence of intracellular events that include the induction of certain enzymes. This process is thought to be responsible for inhibition of virus replication in infected cells, suppression of cell proliferation, and immunomod-ulatory activities such as the enhancement of cytotoxicity of lym-phocytes for target cells. Increased natural killer (NK) cell activity and the induction of specific antigen expression have also been cited as potential antineoplastic effects of IFNα. Investigators have sought to capitalize on these properties, and early nonrandomized trials of interferon-based biologic therapy produced a small number of responses. Monotherapy trials have yielded response rates anywhere between 0 and 33 per cent (Flanigan 1996). The dosage schedule employed in these trials varied considerably.

An important pattern has been recognized among responders to IFNα therapy. Several studies have noted longer survival associ-ated with prior nephrectomy as well as a high performance status and predominantly lung metastases, leading some investigators to believe that removal of the primary tumor is an important part of IFNα therapy (Motzer and Russo 2000).

Cytokine therapy, particularly IL-2, forms an integral part of the modern immunotherapy armamentarium. IL-2 can support the generation and proliferation of cytotoxic T cells with non-specific antitumor cytotoxic activity (lymphokine-activated killer (LAK) cells) as well as specific antitumor cytotoxic T lymphocytes (tumor-infiltrating lymphocyte (TIL) cells).

Early trials utilizing IL-2 high-dose bolus monotherapy formed the basis of US Food and Drugs Administration (FDA) approval of this therapy. An overall response rate of 14 per cent (5 per cent complete response (CR) and 9 per cent partial response (PR)) was noted (Fyfe *et al.* 1995). More importantly, the mean duration of this small number of responses was considerable, lasting almost 2 years, with even longer durable responses seen in the complete responder group (Gitlitz *et al.* 1996).

Significant toxicity associated with this therapy has led investigators to alter the schedule of administration of IL-2 alone, as well as to evaluate the use of combination IL-2/ IFNα regimens, and triple therapy (for example, IL-2, IFNα, and 5-FU) (Flanigan 1997).

Cytoreductive nephrectomy

Given the advent of biologic response modifier therapy (BRM), removal of the primary tumor in the face of metastatic spread has been the focus of much renewed interest. As outlined above, nephrectomy alone is no longer felt to be of much benefit to the patient with systemic disease. When performed as part of a multimodality approach, however, cytoreductive surgery may have an expanded role.

There is some evidence that patients who undergo removal of their primary tumor followed by systemic immunotherapy have improved response rates when compared to those treated with biologic response modifiers with the tumor in place. The approach of performing nephrectomy initially also provides immunoreactive cells for certain treatment protocols. Theoretically, removing the primary tumor may prevent further seeding of metastases and may eliminate a potential source of pain and hemorrhage (Fallick *et al.* 1997; Walther *et al.* 1993).

On the other hand, some investigators cite a growing body of evidence that supports treating these patients initially with systemic immunotherapy. They propose that nephrectomy should be offered only to those that demonstrate an objective response to immunotherapy. This would select out those who would most be likely to benefit from surgery, thus preventing an unnecessary morbid and costly procedure for many patients. Trials continue to identify the benefits of these two pathways.

Tumor debulking theory

In an extensive review of cancer immunotherapy, Morton postulated that the surgical removal of tumor bulk would benefit the patient because the small volume of cancer cells left behind would be easier to control with immunotherapy. Other investigators have echoed this view, citing animal studies that suggest that adoptive immunotherapy is more effective with less tumor bulk (Robertson *et al.* 1990). This forms the core rationale for performing nephrectomy first, followed by BRM therapy.

There is increasing evidence to suggest that removing the tumor may enhance the host response to systemic immunotherapy, although convincing objective data are still lacking. Tumor-related host immune defects have been recognized, such as a decreased delayed-type hypersensitivity reaction, decreased lymphocyte cytolytic function, and a decreased lymphocyte proliferation response (Rackley *et al.* 1994). Researchers have yet to fully elucidate the mechanism behind this phenomenon. Tumor debulking may remove certain soluble factors, such as transforming growth factor-beta (TGFβ), secreted by the tumor itself which act as potent immunosuppressors, inhibiting the effects of IL-2 on T lymphocytes (Eggermont *et al.* 1987; Figlin *et al.* 1999). This is of only theoretical benefit, however, and no clinical data currently exist to support these contentions (Robertson *et al.* 1990).

Initial nephrectomy followed by systemic immunotherapy

The use of recombinant (r) IFNα alone has resulted in approximately a 15 per cent objective response rate in patients with metastatic RCC (Flanigan 1996). Several retrospective studies analyzing interferon trials have suggested that prior nephrectomy was an independent variable in determining patient response to interferon. Muss *et al.* (1987), for example, found a 23 per cent response rate in patients with prior nephrectomy, no prior non-surgical treatment, and a lack of bone metastases as compared with an 8 per cent response rate in the entire patient population. In a large multicenter study of 371 patients in Japan, Umeda and Niijma (1986) also showed a significantly higher response rate for patients who had undergone radical or palliative nephrectomy.

Similarly, patients with metastatic RCC treated with IL-2 and LAK cells have shown a poorer response rate when the primary tumor was intact. Fisher *et al.* (1988) reported only one objective response in 14 patients with an intact renal primary (7 per cent response rate) as compared to a 26 per cent response rate for all patients.

Rackley *et al.* (1994) examined their experience of 62 patients with metastatic RCC who presented for treatment at the Cleveland Clinic (see Table 44.7). They separated this cohort into two groups in a nonrandomized fashion. The first group contained 37 patients who were scheduled for nephrectomy first, followed by BRM therapy. A second group of 25 patients were identified who underwent initial BRM therapy, with nephrectomy reserved for those who demonstrated an objective response to immunotherapy. Of the 37 patients who underwent initial nephrectomy, 22 per cent were unable to go on to receive immunotherapy. Of those who did complete systemic treatment, a partial response was seen in 8 per cent with a median survival of 12 months (range of 1–57 months). No complete responders were seen. Performance status was evaluated using the Eastern Cooperative Oncology Group (ECOG) scale, in which '0' represents patients with normal activity level, '1' represents symptomatic but ambulatory patients, '2' represents patients who are bedridden less than 50 per cent of the time, '3' represents patients who are bedridden more than 50 per cent of the time, and '4' represents completely bedridden patients. This initial nephrectomy group all had an ECOG performance status of either 0 or 1. All the patients had a tumor burden and distribution of metastatic lesions typical for the disease, although none had brain metastasis. Four patients of the 37 (11 per cent) failed to go on to BRM because of rapid tumor progression.

In those patients receiving BRM therapy first, tumor burden and distribution of metastatic disease were similar to those in the initial nephrectomy group, though the performance status was slightly worse overall and two patients had central nervous system lesions. Five patients had received radiation treatment to metastatic lesions and one patient had been treated with hormonal therapy prior to immunotherapy. A 12 per cent objective response was demonstrated in the initial BRM arm (2 CR, 1 PR) with a median survival of 14 months (range 1–48 months). The three patients who enjoyed an objective response did so within 1 month of initiating therapy and all received at least four courses of systemic therapy before undergoing nephrectomy. One patient died of cardiopulmonary complications while receiving combination rIL-2/IFNα therapy. The paucity of responders in both groups makes it difficult to form any conclusions about patient factors that may favor a response with either approach. As a retrospective review of a nonrandomized trial, it has a significant selection bias. Therefore, no meaningful comparisons can be made between the two treatment strategies.

Other such studies can be found in the literature, although they too suffer from the same drawbacks, that is, they represent single-institution, retrospective, nonrandomized reviews, also making it difficult to properly interpret the results.

Bennett *et al.* (1995) examined their experience with 30 patients in order to determine the effect of cytoreductive surgery in preparation for immunotherapy. They concluded that nephrectomy prior to systemic therapy was ill-advised and should not be performed based on several observations. Ten of the 30 patients experienced rapid tumor progression after the primary tumor was removed. Furthermore, their series yielded a sobering 17 per cent mortality rate, with an additional 20 per cent experiencing non-fatal myocardial infarctions. Overall, 77 per cent of their patients could not go on to receive immunotherapy after surgery. This series did not represent a well-selected group of patients, a fact that certainly impacted on the results. Only five of the patients were screened preoperatively by a physician who would have subsequently provided immunotherapy to determine if they were eligible for postoperative immunotherapy. In addition, several patients in this group were undergoing 'palliative' nephrectomy, two for pain and three for gross hematuria. Overall, these patients had a poorer performance status than most: only two patients were ECOG 0, whereas 24 were ECOG 1 and four patients were ECOG 2. Almost one-third of the patients had brain metastasis, while 43 per cent had bone lesions and 37 per cent had evidence of hepatic metastases. However, for those seven patients who were able to undergo postoperative immunotherapy, the responses were better than most. Three achieved a complete response and one had a partial response, showing an overall response rate of greater than 50 per cent.

The value of good performance status in the selection of these patients has been emphasized by other studies. In an attempt to identify the characteristics associated with prolonged survival and to evaluate the value of nephrectomy, Naito *et al.* (1991) examined 57 cases of stage IV RCC. Improved survival was correlated to metastasis limited to a single organ site and the removal of the primary tumor. They also saw that the median survival for patients with good performance status (defined as greater than 80 per cent on the Karnofsky scale) was 13 months compared to only 4 months with patients with poor performance profiles, a difference that was highly significant.

With this in mind, Fallick *et al.* (1997) used very strict criteria in selecting patients who would qualify for nephrectomy prior to immunotherapy. Patients were excluded if they had evidence of central nervous system (CNS), liver, or bone metastasis, if they lacked adequate pulmonary and cardiac function, and if they had an ECOG score greater than 1. Also, patients who had biopsies that demonstrated histology that was not predominantly clear cell type were similarly excluded. Fallick *et al.*'s (1997) series of 28 patients who underwent initial nephrectomy with delayed adjuvant systemic immunotherapy had an overall response rate of 39 per cent, with 18 per cent CR and 21 per cent PR. Actuarial median survival of all 28 patients was 20.5 months from the initiation of treatment. The median duration of the responses was 10+ months, with eight of the responders remaining progression-free at intervals of 5 to 66 months after initiation of treatment. They had no episodes of rapid tumor progression and only one of the 28 patients (3.6 per cent) died in the postoperative period. Overall, only 7 per cent failed to go on to biologic therapy after surgery.

Examining the rates of receiving biological therapy after cytoreductive nephrectomy, Levy *et al.* (1998) reported that 18 per cent of patients were unable to receive systemic therapy after surgery. In this series of 66 patients, 82 per cent received therapy beginning a median of 40 days after nephrectomy, while 3 per cent died in the perioperative period. Again, their study reflects an emphasis on patient selection. They reported that, of the 79 patients who originally presented at their institution, 13 were not deemed fit for initial surgery and were referred for systemic biological therapy. The group who underwent initial surgery did have a much better ECOG performance profile. Unfortunately, they failed to establish and maintain formal selection criteria. An important point made by this study is that initial surgery, for those who qualify, avoids the pitfall of clinically overstaging the disease. For example, they report that one patient was found to have a pathologically proven primary lung tumor originally thought to be a metastatic renal lesion. Another patient had no metastatic spread despite hilar lymphadenopathy on computerized tomography (CT) that was presumed to represent localized spread. They contend that suspected lymph node involvement as the only site of metastatic spread deserves a confirmatory biopsy before referring that patient for initial systemic therapy to avoid such a problem. Other studies have shown that up to 10 per cent of patients with a presumptive diagnosis of RCC will actually harbor histology other than RCC, reinforcing the need for histologic proof of the disease before initiating systemic therapy (Figlin *et al.* 1999).

Perhaps the largest published retrospective series looking at the outcome of patients treated with cytoreductive surgery prior to immunotherapy is a review by Walther *et al.* (1997*b*) from the US National Cancer Institute (NCI). This paper, which updated previous reports, included 195 patients over an 11-year period who underwent initial nephrectomy in preparation for IL-2 therapy. Surgery consisted of removal of the primary tumor as well as contiguous or adjacent metastases.

Although this study concluded that surgery in selected patients could be performed safely before immunotherapy, only 62 per cent of patients were eligible for high-dose IL-2 therapy after surgery. Factors that prevented administration of adjuvant IL-2 included rapid tumor progression, refractory hypercalcemia, pulmonary emboli, regression of presumed metastatic disease, renal

Table 44.5 Survival in subgroups defined according to stratification factors

Category	Median survival		1-yr survival		P value*
	Interferon alone	Nephrectomy plus interferon	Interferon alone	Nephrectomy plus interferon	
	mo		%		
Not stratified	8.1	11.1	36.8	49.7	0.012
Stratification factor					
Measurable disease					0.010
Yes	7.8	10.3	34.7	46.6	
No	11.2	16.4	43.1	63.6	
Performance status†					0.080
0	11.7	17.4	49.2	63.6	
1	4.8	6.9	28.2	32.5	
Type of metastases					0.008
Lung only	10.3	14.3	41.5	58.5	
Other	6.3	10.2	34.6	45.1	

* P values for the comparison of median survival between groups were derived with the log-rank test.
† Performance was scored as 0 or 1, with 1 indicating decreased activity.

insufficiency, death, and refusal of treatment. In a previous report, they had noted that the only factor associated with a statistically significant risk of not receiving treatment after nephrectomy was an ECOG score greater than or equal to 2. They reported that 9 per cent of patients had surgical complications that prevented them from going on to receive BRM therapy. More concerning, however, was the 22 per cent of the 195 patients who experienced rapid progression of metastatic disease between time of surgery and scheduled time of immunotherapy, with disease progression seen in lung, bone, CNS, and liver. In this study, overall objective responses to therapy were a modest 18 per cent (19 of 107 patients). This included 3.7 per cent (4 patients) who demonstrated a complete response and 14 per cent (15 patients) with a partial response. The majority of responses were in patients receiving high-dose IL-2 alone, high-dose IL-2 plus IFNα, and IL-2 plus LAK cells. Interestingly, they also reported that four patients had spontaneous postoperative regression of pulmonary nodules.

Initial reports detailing the UCLA experience with IL-2 with TIL cell therapy trials have also shown promising results. Figlin *et al.* (1997) showed an overall response rate of 34.6 per cent (9 per cent CR and 25.5 per cent PR) with a median duration of response of 14 months. In this study of 55 patients, 32 patients underwent 'cytokine priming' with biologically active doses of cytokines (IL-2, IL-6, TNFα-a, IFNγ, or IFN-α-2a) administered subcutaneously before radical nephrectomy. The other 23 patients who did not receive presurgery priming were treated with CD8(+) enriched TIL harvested from nephrectomy specimens. The authors reported no perioperative deaths for the entire cohort, with 11 per cent of all patients not being able to go on from surgery to immunotherapy. Although the survival was not different between the two groups, the results were encouraging, prompting a phase III, multicenter, randomized trial (Figlin *et al.* 1999). This study prospectively evaluated outcomes in patients with metastatic RCC after receiving either rIL-2 monotherapy or combination CD8 (+) TIL with rIL-2 after nephrectomy. Neither

objective response rates nor 1-year survival rates were significantly different between the two groups (9.9 versus 11.4 per cent and 55 versus 47 per cent, respectively), and overall patients did not fare as well as in the original pilot study; hence this trial was closed early.

A recently reported SWOG trial (Flanigan *et al.* 2000) demonstrated that cytoreductive nephrectomy statistically significantly enhanced survival in patients with metastatic RCC randomized to IFNα-2b (Intron-A) or nephrectomy followed by interferon therapy. The overall survival advantage for the nephrectomy arm in the study of 246 patients was 50 per cent (8.1 versus 12.5 months) (see Table 44.5). The survival advantage persisted across all of the prestudy stratifications including performance status (0 or 1), site of metastases (lung only versus other), and measurable disease (present or absent). This study also demonstrated remarkably minimal surgical toxicity (5 per cent class IV toxicity), 1 per cent operative and perioperative mortality, and the ability of nearly all patients (98 per cent) to proceed from nephrectomy to interferon therapy. This study is the best current argument in favor of the concept of cytoreductive nephrectomy in patients with metastatic RCC to date.

Note on how response rates should be calculated

Fleischman's editorial comments to a 1993 report by Walther *et al.* point out an important caveat when evaluating studies that claim initial nephrectomy is a superior strategy when comparing it to initial systemic therapy strategies. He notes that the convention in assessing efficacy has been to calculate response rates based on the patients who actually *receive* immunotherapy as the denominator. He argues that this method would artificially inflate the response rate figures because they fail to include the *total* number of therapy candidates, that is, all those who undergo surgery with the intention of receiving adjuvant immunotherapy. Rather, reported response rates should include all those who enter a protocol, not simply those who actually go on to systemic therapy. As seen

Table 44.6 Cytoreductive nephrectomy in preparation for immunotherapy

Institution (year)	Number of patients	Mortality (%)	Unable to receive postoperative BMR therapy (%)	Rapid tumor progression (%)
Cleveland Clinic (1994)	37	3	22	11
UCSF (1994)	35	0	26	13
Albert Einstein (1995)	30	17	77	33
Tufts (1997)	28	4	7	0
NCI (1997)	195	1	38	23
UCLA (1997)	55	0	11	0
M.D. Anderson Clinic (1998)	66	3	17	—

in several reviews, this often leaves a significant portion of the population out of these response rate calculations.

Arguments against immediate cytoreductive surgery

Some investigators believe that performing surgery followed by immunotherapy is a suboptimal approach. Instead, they argue that patients with metastatic RCC should first receive BRM therapy. Only then should those who demonstrate objective response to systemic therapy go on to adjuvant nephrectomy and resection of remaining metastatic lesions. This argument is based on several key ideas, which we will discuss in the following subsections.

A substantial subset of patients fail to go on from surgery to BRM therapy
A review of the current literature reveals that, indeed, a certain fraction of patients will not be able to continue after surgery with systemic therapy (see Table 44.6). This may be the result of mortality or serious surgical morbidity, tumor progression, or a marked decline in performance status. Only very rarely will a patient not receive immunotherapy because they were deemed free of metastatic disease from overstaging or because of misdiagnosis (Figlin *et al.* 1999).

Failure to go on to BRM therapy depends on the expected toxicity associated with the planned BRM therapy and has been noted in recent series to range from 7 to as high as 77 per cent. In the NCI series of 195 patients, 38 per cent could not go on from surgery to IL-2 immunotherapy (see Table 44.6). In the SWOG trial, only 2 patients (2 per cent) who received nephrectomy could not go on receive IFNα-2b therapy.

Surgery has significant morbidity, mortality, and cost and should therefore be reserved for only those who demonstrate benefit from biologic therapy
Recent series examining the role of cytoreductive surgery in preparation for immunotherapy report a mortality rate anywhere between 0 and 17 per cent in this population. The argument follows that putting patients at risk for these complications is only indicated for those who have already shown that their disease is responsive to immunotherapy, which is much better tolerated and therefore better suited as a first-line therapy.

In an effort to reduce the prolonged recovery often seen with open nephrectomy, Walther *et al.* (1999) investigated the use of a laparoscopic modality of cytoreductive nephrectomy. Their study looked at three groups: open nephrectomy; laparoscopic surgery with tumor removal through a small incision ('laparoscopic-assisted'); or laparoscopic surgery with tumor morcellation. Time to IL-2 therapy was compared in all three groups. For open surgery, a median of 67 days elapsed before IL-2 could be administered after surgery (range 50–151 days), whereas laparoscopic-assisted patients took a median of 60 days (range 47–63 days). The group who appeared to benefit the most were those who had undergone laparoscopic morcellation of their renal tumors. This group was able to go on to systemic therapy a median of 37 days (range 37–57 days) after surgery.

The minimally invasive surgery was performed with morbidity and complication rates similar to those of the traditional open procedures. Tumor morcellation, at least in their hands, was feasible even with large tumors. The authors concluded that laparoscopy offered a reasonable method of performing cytoreductive nephrectomy in preparation for systemic therapy. In the SWOG trial there was only one operative death (1 per cent, including 30 days postoperatively). In addition, only 5 per cent of patients experienced class IV toxicity from surgery and 79 per cent of patients had no operative complications.

Immunosuppressive effects of surgery
Studies have demonstrated that the host immune system becomes impaired—at least temporarily—in the postoperative state, thereby hampering adjuvant immunotherapy efforts. In an elegant animal study examining the effects of laparotomy on intraperitoneal tumor growth, Eggermont *et al.* (1987) demonstrated how surgical trauma could reduce the effects of IL-2 and LAK cells on the tumor cells and thus enhance tumor propagation. Their data suggested that the inflamed peritoneal surfaces played a role in tumor promotion. They speculated that the peptide growth factors that are released during the inflammatory response cascade and the process of tissue repair, such as transforming growth factors TGFα and TGFβ and platelet-derived growth factor (PDGF), all may enhance tumor growth. By promoting the growth of natural tissues, these factors may be augmenting tumor cells as well while at the same time suppressing the immune system, hindering the host's natural antitumor responses.

Rapid tumor progression as a result of surgery
Although some series failed to document any cases of rapid tumor progression following removal of the primary tumor, it has been reported to occur in up to 22 per cent of cases (NCI) (Walther *et al.* 1997*b*). O'Reilly *et al.* (1994) observed a similar tumor

Table 44.7 Response rates for adjuvant immunotherapy

Institution	Number of patients	Response (%)		
		Overall	Complete	Partial
Cleveland Clinic (1994)	37	8	0	8
UCSF (1994)	35	9	4	4
Tufts (1997)	28	39	18	21
NCI (1997)	195	18	4	14
UCLA (1997)	55	35	9	26

progression after removal of the primary lesion in the Lewis lung carcinoma model. The authors thought that this phenomenon was related specifically to the loss of the angiogenesis inhibitor angiostatin, a substance secreted by the primary tumor, which may have been partially suppressing the growth of metastases. This may help explain the rapid disease progression reported after cytoreductive surgery.

The Groupe Franc[,]ais d'Immunothérapie reported on a large randomized trial of rIL-2, rIFNα, or a combination therapy for metastatic RCC (Negrier *et al.* 1998). They noted that several factors were associated with rapid tumor progression. They found that patients with multiple organs involved with metastases, metastasis to the liver, and the discovery of metastases less than 1 year after diagnosis of the primary tumor had a 70 per cent probability of experiencing rapid tumor progression despite cytokine therapy.

A retrospective analysis was undertaken at the M.D. Anderson Clinic in 1993 looking at the value of surgery after interferon therapy was given to patients with metastatic RCC (Sella *et al.* 1993). Seventeen patients with a mean age of 57 years who had demonstrated either a partial or minimal response to IFNα therapy underwent resection of residual masses presumed to represent residual tumor in order to render these patients tumor-free. A subset of eight patients presented with metastatic disease without prior nephrectomy. Sixty-five per cent of the 17 patients remained disease-free at a median of 12 months postoperatively with a median survival of 12 months. Of those 8 patients who presented with metastases with the primary tumor still in place, 6 had complete response of metastases and 2 had partial response of metastases. The authors concluded that surgery is indicated for patients who demonstrate a response to immunotherapy but that a randomized study is still needed to fully assess the role and timing of cytoreductive surgery in this disease process.

In 51 patients with metastatic RCC treated at the NCI with various immunotherapy regimens, including IL-2 and IFNα, a complete response was seen in one and partial responses were seen in two at extrarenal sites, yielding an overall response rate of 6 per cent (Wagner *et al.* 1999). No responses, however, were seen in the primary tumor. These three patients who did demonstrate a response in their metastatic lesions then underwent nephrectomy. After nephrectomy, two patients had a continued partial response for 4 and 11 months each before progression, while one patient had enjoyed a complete response for more than 88 months. The median survival for the entire cohort was 13 months.

Conclusion

When is nephrectomy justified in the face of metastatic disease? There is no simple answer. Our SWOG trial suggests that, in the era of BRM therapy, cytoreductive surgery may well prolong survival in patients with metastatic disease by 50 per cent for those receiving IFNα-2b monotherapy. We in SWOG therefore believe that, in suitable patients (especially those with good performance status), nephrectomy followed by BRM therapy using IFNα-2b ± other cytokine therapy should be the control arm for future phase III trials.

Adjuvant nephrectomy can also be advocated for control of a patient's current symptoms related to the primary disease process, that is, flank pain, hematuria, anemia, erythrocytosis, and hypercalcemia, and refractory to nonsurgical modalities and for patients with respectable (that is, minimal volume) metastases that may also be surgically removed.

References

Bassil, B., Dosoretz, D.E., Pruot, G.R., J.R. (1985). Validation of the tumor, nodes, and metastasis classification of renal cell carcinoma, *J. Urol.* **134**, 450.

Bennett, R.T., Lerner, S.E., and Taub, H.C. (1995). Cytoreductive surgery for stage IV renal cell carcinoma. *J. Urol.* **154** (1), 32.

Bottinger, L.E. (1970). Prognosis in renal carcinoma. *Cancer* **26**, 780.

Bukowski, R.M. (1997). Natural history and therapy of metastatic renal cell carcinoma. *Cancer* **80** (7), 1198.

Couillard, D.R. and de Vere White, R.W. (1993). Surgery of renal cell carcinoma. *Urol. Clin. N. Am.* **20** (2), 263–75.

de Kernion, J.B. and Lindner, A. (1982). Treatment of advanced renal cell carcinoma. In *Proceedings of the First International Symposium on Kidney Tumors* (ed. R. Kuss, G. Murphy, S. Khoury, and J. Karr), p. 641. Alan R. Liss, New York.

deKernion, J.B., Ramming, K.D., and Smith, R.B. (1978). The natural history of metastatic renal cell carcinoma: a computer analysis. *J. Urol.* **120**, 148.

Dernevik, L., Berggren, H., Larsson, S., *et al.* (1985). Surgical removal of pulmonary metastases from renal cell carcinoma. *Scand. J. Urol. Nephrol.* **19**, 133–7.

Dutcher, J., Atkins, M., Fisher, R., *et al.* (1997). IL-2-based therapy in metastatic renal cell carcinoma: Cytokine Working Group experience. *Proc. Am. Soc. Clin. Oncol.* **16**, 327.

Eggermont, A.M., Steller, E.P., and Sugarbaker, P.H. (1987). Laparotomy enhances intraperitoneal tumor growth and abrogates the antitumor effects of interleukin-2 and lymphokine-activated killer cells. *Surgery* **102** (1), 71.

Ellerhorst, J.A., Sella, A., Amato, R.J., *et al.* (1997). Phase II trial of 5-fluorouracil, interferon-alpha, and continuous infusion interleukin-2 for patients with metastatic renal cell carcinoma. *Cancer* **80**, 2128.

Elson, P.J., Witte, R.S., and Trump, D.L. (1988). Prognostic factors for survival in patients with recurrent or metastatic renal cell carcinoma. *Cancer Res.* **48**, 7310–13.

Fahn, H., Lee, Y., Chen, M., *et al.* (1991). The incidence and prognostic significance of humoral hypercalcemia in renal cell carcinoma. *J. Urol.* **145**, 248.

Fallick, M.L., McDermott, D.F., LaRock, D., *et al.* (1997). Nephrectomy before interleukin-2 therapy for patients with metastatic renal cell carcinoma. *J. Urol.* **158** (5), 1691–5.

Figlin, R.A. (1999). Renal cell carcinoma: management of advanced disease. *J. Urol.* **161** (2), 381.

Figlin, R.A., Pierce, W.C., Kaboo, R., *et al.* (1997). Treatment of metastatic renal cell carcinoma with nephrectomy, interleukin-2 and cytokine-primed or CD8(+) selected tumor infiltrating lymphocytes from primary tumor. *J. Urol.* **158** (3), 740–5.

Figlin, R.A., Thompson, J.A., Bukowski, M.D., *et al.* (1999). A multi-center, randomized, phase III trial of CD8$^+$ tumor-infiltrating lymphocytes in combination with recombinant interleukin-2 in metastatic renal cell carcinoma. *J. Clin. Oncol.* **17** (8), 2521–9.

Fisher, R.I., Coltman, C.A., Doroshaw, J.H., *et al.* (1988). Metastatic renal cancer treated with interleukin-2 and lymphokine-activated killer cells. *Ann. Intern. Med.* **108**, 518–23.

Flanigan, R.C. (1987*b*). The failure of infarction and/or nephrectomy in stage IV renal cell cancer to influence survival or metastatic regression. *Urol. Clin. N. Am.* **14** (4), 757–62.

Flanigan, R.C. (1996). Role of surgery in patients with metastatic renal cell carcinoma. *Sem. Urol. Oncol.* **14** (4), 227–9.

Flanigan, R.C. (1997). Advances in immunotherapy and chemotherapy for renal cell carcinoma. In *Urology annual* (ed. S. Rous), Chapter 7, pp. 95–105. Blackwell Sciences, Oxford.

Flanigan, R.C., Salmon, S., Blumenstein, B.A., *et al.* (2001). Nephrectomy followed by interferon alfa-2b compared with interferon alfa-2b alone for metastatic renal cell cancer. *New England Journal of Medicine*, **345** (23), 1655–9.

Freed, S. (1977). Nephrectomy for renal cell carcinoma with metastases. *Urology* **9** (6), 613.

Freed, S., Halperin, J., and Gordon, M. (1977). Idiopathic regression of metastases from renal cell carcinoma. *J. Urol.* **118**, 538.

Fuhrman, S., Lasky, C., and Limas, C. (1982). Prognostic significance of morphologic parameters in renal cell carcinoma. *Am. J. Surg. Pathol.* **6**, 655–63.

Fuselier, H.A., Guice, S.L., Brannan, W., *et al.* (1983). Renal cell carcinoma: the Ochsner Medical Institution experience (1945–78). *J. Urol.* **130**, 445.

Fyfe, G., Fisher, R.I., and Rosenberg, S.A. (1995). Results of treatment of 255 patients with metastatic renal cell carcinoma who received high-dose recombinant interleukin-2 therapy. *J. Clin. Oncol.* **13** (3), 688.

Gitlitz, B.J., Belldegrun, A., and Figlin, R. (1996). Immunotherapy and gene therapy. *Sem. Urol. Oncol.* **14** (4), 237.

Gitlitz, B.K., Dolan, N., Pierce, W., *et al.* (1996). Fluoropyrimidines plus interleukin-2 and interferon-alpha in the treatment of metastatic renal cell carcinoma: the UCLA Kidney Cancer Program. *Proc. Am. Soc. Clin. Oncol.* **15**, 248.

Giuliani, L., Gilberti, C., Martorana, G., *et al.* (1990). Radical extensive surgery for renal cell carcinoma: long-term results and prognostic factors. *J. Urol.* **143**, 468–73.

Golimbu, M., Al-Askari, S., Tessler, A., *et al.* (1986). Aggressive treatment of metastatic renal cancer. *J. Urol.* **136**, 805–7.

Golimbu, M., Joshi, P., Sperber, A., *et al.* (1989). Renal cell carcinoma: survival and prognostic factors. *Urology* **34**, 310.

Goltesman, J.E., Crawford, E.D., Grossman, H.S., *et al.* (1985). Infarction—nephrectomy for metastatic renal cell carcinoma. *Urology*, **25**, 248.

Greenlee, R.A., Murray, T., Bolden, S., *et al.* (2000). Cancer statistics, 2000. *CA Cancer J. Clin.* **50**, 7–33.

Harris, D.T. (1983). Hormonal therapy and chemotherapy for RCC. *Sem. Oncol.* **10**, 422–30.

Hofmockel, G., Langer, W., Theiss, M., *et al.* (1996). Immunocheotherapy for metastatic renal cell carcinoma using a regimen of interkeukin-2, interferon-alpha, and 5 flurouracil. *J. Urol.* **156**, 18.

Hrushesky, L.J. and Murphy, G.P. (1977). Current status of the therapy of advanced renal carcinoma. *J. Surg. Oncol.* **9**, 277.

Jett, J.R., Hollinger, C.G., Zinsmesiter, A.R., *et al.* (1983). Pulmonary resection of metastatic renal cell carcinoma. *Chest* **84**, 422–42.

Joffe, J.K., Banks, R.E., Forbes, M.A., *et al.* (1996). Phase II study of interferon-alpha, interleukin and 5-fluorouracil in advanced renal cell carcinoma. Clinical data and laboratory evidence of protease action. *Br. J. Urol.* **77**, 638.

Johnson, D.E., Kaesler, K.E., and Samuels, M.L. (1975). Is nephrectomy justified in patients with metastatic renal carcinoma? *J. Urol.* **114**, 27.

Kavolius, D.P., Mastorakos, C., Pavlovich, P., *et al.* (1998). Resection of metastatic renal cell carcinoma. *J. Clin. Oncol.* **16** (6), 2261–6.

Kierney, P.C., van Heerden, J.A., Segura, J.W., *et al.* (1994). Surgeon's role in the management of solitary renal cell carcinoma metastases occurring subsequent to initial curative nephrectomy: an institutional review. *Ann. Surg. Oncol.* **1**, 345–52.

Kirchner, H., Ber, J., Probst-Kepper, M., *et al.* (1998). Risk and longterm outcome in metastatic renal cell carcinoma patients receiving SC interleukin-2, SC interferon-alfa2a and IV 5 flurouracil. *Proc. Am. Soc. Clin. Oncol.* **17**, 310.

Kurth, K.H., Cinqualbre, J., Oliver, R.T.D., *et al.* (1986). Embolization and subsequent nephrectomy in metastatic renal cell carcinoma. *World J. Urol.* **2**, 122–6.

Levy, D.A., Swanson, D.A., and Slaton, J.W. (1998). Timely delivery of biological therapy after cytoreductive nephrectomy in carefully selected patients with metastatic renal cell carcinoma. *J. Urol.* **159** (4), 1168.

Libertino, J. (1987). Long term results of resection of renal cell cancer with extension into inferior vena cava. *J. Urol.* **137**, 21.

Lokick, J.J. and Harrison, J.H. (1975). Renal cell carcinoma: natural history and chemotherapeutic experience. *J. Urol.* **114**, 371.

McNichols, D.W., Segura, J.W., and DeWeerd, J.H. (1981). Renal cell carcinoma: long term survival and late recurrence. *J. Urol.* **126**, 17–23.

Medical Research Council Renal Cancer. Collaborator: Interferon-alpha and survival in metastatic renal cancer: results of a randomized controlled trial. (1999). *Lancet*, **353** (9146), 14–17.

Middleton, R.G. (1967). Surgery for renal cell carcinoma. *J. Urol.* **97**, 973.

Mims, M.M., Christenson, B., Schlumberger, F.C., *et al.* (1966). A ten year evaluation of nephrectomy for extensive renal cell carcinoma. *J. Urol.* **95**, 10.

Montie, J.E., Stewart, B.H., and Straffon, R.A. (1977). The role of adjunctive nephrectomy in patients with metastatic renal cell carcinoma. *J. Urol.* **117**, 272.

Morton, D.C. Cancer immunotherapy: an overview (1974). *Seminars in Oncology*, **1**(4), 297–310.

Motzer, R. and Russo, P. (2000). Systemic therapy for renal cell carcinoma. *J. Urol.* **163**, 408–17.

Muss, H., Constanzi, J.J., *et al.* (1987). Recombinant alpha interferon in renal cell carcinoma: randomized trial of two routes of administration. *J. Clin. Oncol.* **5**, 286–91.

Naito, S., Kimiya, K., and Sakamoto, N. (1991). Prognostic factors and value of adjunctive nephrectomy in patients with stage IV renal cell carcinoma. *Urology* **37** (2), 95.

Negrier, S., Escudier, B., and Lasset, C. (1998). Recombinant human interleukin-2, recombinant human interferon alfa-2a, or both in metastatic renal-cell carcinoma. *New Engl. J. Med.* **338**, 1272.

O'Dea, M.J., Zincke, H., Utz, D.C., *et al.* (1978). The treatment of renal cell carcinoma with solitary metastasis. *J. Urol.* **120**, 540–2.

Olencki, T., Bukowski, R.M., Budd, G.T., *et al.* (1996). Phase I/II trial of simultaneously administered rIL-2/rHuIFN and 5-FU in patients with metastatic renal cell carcinoma. *Proc. Am. Soc. Clin. Oncol.* **15**, 263.

O'Reilly, M.S., Holmgren, L., and Shing, Y. (1994). Angiostatin: a novel angiogenesis inhibitor that mediates the suppression of metastases by a Lewis lung carcinoma. *Cell* **2**, 315.

Rackley, R., Novick, A., and Klein, E. (1994). The impact of adjuvant nephrectomy on multimodality treatment of metastatic renal cell carcinoma. *J. Urol.* **152**, 1399.

Rafla, S. (1970). Renal cell carcinoma: Natural history and results of treatment. *Cancer* **25**, 26–40.

Ravaud, A., Audhuy, B., Gomez, F., *et al.* (1998). Subcutaneous interleukin-2, interferon alfa-2a, and continuous infusion of fluorouracil in metastatic renal cell carcinoma: a multicenter phase trial: Groupe Francois d'Immunotherapie. *J. Clin. Oncol.* **16**, 2728.

Riches, E.W., Griffiths, I.H., and Thackray, A.C. (1951). New growths of the kidney and ureter. *Br. J. Urol.* **23**, 297–356.

Ro, J.Y., Ayala, A.G., Sella, A., *et al.* (1987). Sarcomatoid renal cell carcinoma: a clinicopathologic study of 42 cases. *Cancer* **59**, 516.

Robertson, C.N., Linehan, W.M., and Pass, H.I. (1990). Preparative cytoreductive surgery in patients with metastatic renal cell carcinoma treated with adoptive immunotherapy with interleukin-2 or interleukin-2 plus lymphokine activated killer cells. *J. Urol.* **144**, 614.

Sella, A., Swanson, D.A., and Ro, J.Y. (1993). Surgery following response to interferon-based therapy for residual renal cell carcinoma. *J. Urol.* **149**, 19.

Selli, C., Hinshaw, W.M., Woodard, B.H., *et al.* (1983). Stratification of risk factors in renal cell carcinoma. *Cancer* **52**, 899–903.

Skinner, D.G., Colvin, R.V., Vermillion, C.D., *et al.* (1971). Diagnosis and management of renal cell carcinoma: a clinical and pathological study of 309 cases. *Cancer* **28**, 1165–77.

Skinner, D.G., Vermillion, C.D., and Colvin, R.B. (1972). The surgical management of renal cell carcinoma. *J. Urol.* **107**, 711.

Spencer, W.F., Linehan, W.M., and McClellan, M.W. (1992). Immunotherapy with interleukin-2 and interferon in patients with metastatic renal cell cancer *in situ* primary cancers: a pilot study. *J. Urol.* **147**, 24.

Swanson, D., Johnson, D., and von Eschenbach, A.C. (1983). Angioinfarction plus nephrectomy for metastatic renal cell carcinoma—an update. *J. Urol.* **130**, 449.

Thompson, I.M., Shannon, H., Ross, G. Jr, *et al.* (1975). An analysis of factors affecting survival in 150 patients with renal carcinoma. *J. Urol.* **117**, 272–5.

Thrasher, J.B. and Paulson, D.F. (1993). Prognostic factors in renal cancer. *Urol. Clin. N. Am.* **20** (2), 247.

Tolia, B.M. and Whitmore, W.F. Jr (1975). Solitary metastasis from renal cell carcinoma. *J. Urol.* **114**, 836–8.

Tourani, J.M., Pfister, C., Berdah, J.F., *et al.* (1998). Outpatient treatment with subcutaneous interleukin-2 and interferon alfa administration in combination with fluorouracil in patients with metastatic renal cell carcinoma: results of a sequential nonrandomized phase II study. Subcutaneous Administration Propeukin Program Cooperative Group. *J. Clin. Oncol.* **16**, 2505.

Umeda, T. and Niijima, T. (1986). Phase II study of alpha interferon on renal cell carcinoma. *Cancer* **58**, 1231–5.

Wagle, D.G., and Scal, D.R. (1970). Renal cell carcinoma. A review of 256 cases. *J. Surg. Oncol.* **2**, 23.

Wagner, J.R., McClellan, M., and Linehan, W.M. (1999). Interleukin-2 based immunotherapy for metastatic renal cell carcinoma with the kidney in place. *J. Urol.* **162** (1), 43.

Walther, M.M., Alexander, R.B., and Weiss, G.H. (1993). Cytoreductive surgery prior to interleukin-2-based therapy in patients with metastatic renal cell carcinoma. *Urology* **42** (3), 250.

Walther, M.M., Patel, B., and Choyke, P.L. (1997*a*). Hypercalcemia in patients with metastatic renal cell carcinoma: effect of nephrectomy and metabolic evaluation. *J. Urol.* **158** (3), 733.

Walther, M.M., Yang, J.C., and Pass, H.I. (1997*b*). Cytoreductive surgery before high dose interleukin-2 based therapy in patients with metastatic renal cell carcinoma. *J. Urol.* **158**, 158.

Walther, M.M., Lyne, J.C., Libutti, S.K., *et al.* (1999). Laparoscopic cytoreductive nephrectomy as preparation for administration of systemic interleukin-2 in the treatment of metastatic renal cell carcinoma: a pilot study. *Urology* **53** (3), 496–500.

Wolf, J.S. Jr, Aronson, F.R., Small, E.J., and Carroll, P.R. (1994). Nephrectomy for metastatic renal cell carcinoma: a component of systemic treatment regimens. *J. Surg. Oncol.* **55** (1), 7–13.

Yagoda, A. (1990). Phase II cytotoxic chemotherapy trials in RCC: 1983–1988. *Prog. Clin. Biol. Res.* **350**, 227–41.

Yagoda, A., Abi Rached, B., and Petrylak, D. (1995). Chemotherapy for advanced renal cell carcinoma, 1983–1993. *Sem. Oncol.* **22**, 42.

45. Surgical resection of metastases

Joel W. Slaton and David A. Swanson

Introduction

Renal cell carcinoma (RCC) is an aggressive tumor with a high propensity to metastasize. Historically, in fact, 25 to 48 per cent of patients already had metastases at the time of initial presentation (Skinner *et al.* 1971; deKernion *et al.* 1978), although this proportion has almost certainly decreased as ever-increasing numbers of tumors are being found incidentally (Bretheau *et al.* 1995*b*; Rodriguez *et al.* 1995). Additionally, between 8 and 43 per cent of patients will manifest metastasis after resection of apparently localized disease with the incidence dependent on the stage of the tumor (Levy *et al.* 1998). Patients who present with synchronous metastases have an average survival time of about 4 months with only 10 per cent surviving 1 year, whereas patients with metachronous metastases have a median survival time of 11 months (deKernion *et al.* 1978; Maldazys and deKernion 1986).

Metastatic RCC is relatively unresponsive to chemotherapy and radiotherapy. The current standard treatment of metastatic disease is immunotherapy, which produces objective responses in only 20 to 40 per cent of patients. Fewer than one-third of patients obtained complete regression of all metastases (Rosenberg *et al.* 1994; Taneja *et al.* 1994; Ellerhorst *et al.* 1997). Because of such poor response rates and the reasonable survival rates seen in patients who undergo resection of a solitary metastasis, metastasectomy has been offered to selected patients for more than 60 years. Herein, we review the published experience as well as our own data in an attempt to define the contemporary role of metastasectomy.

Selection of patients for metastasectomy: general considerations

In large series of patients with metastatic disease, approximately 2 to 4 per cent of patients have a solitary metastasis (deKernion *et al.* 1978; Maldazys and deKernion 1986; Rosenberg *et al.* 1994; Taneja *et al.* 1994; Ellerhorst *et al.* 1997). Thus, only a small number of patients with metastatic disease will be eligible for surgical resection of the metastasis as an attempt at definitive therapy. Furthermore, in patients with metastatic disease, a number of factors related to both the patient and the tumor have

been identified that predict for a shorter disease-free interval and survival: (1) poor performance status; (2) high nuclear grade; (3) sarcomatoid histology; (4) synchronous presentation of metastatic disease; (5) short interval between nephrectomy and appearance of metastasis; (6) metastatic sites other than lung, particularly liver; and (7) multiple organ sites of metastatic involvement (Skinner *et al.* 1971; deKernion *et al.* 1978; Fuhrman *et al.* 1982; Saitoh *et al.* 1982; Golimbu *et al.* 1986*b*; Neves *et al.* 1988; Landonio *et al.* 1994; Bretheau *et al.* 1995*a*; Guinan *et al.* 1997). The presence of one or more of these adverse prognostic indicators may make aggressive surgical resection of metastases less rational.

Different organs present different surgical challenges that may influence the surgeon's decision about proceeding with metastasectomy. The organ most amenable to resection of metastases is the lung because of the relative ease and safety of thoracotomy. In fact, some lesions can be removed by thoracoscopy. Some series that report the results of pulmonary metastasectomy for many different primary tumors (not just RCC) consider the number and size of lung metastases resected to be important predictors for survival with the best survival rates seen in patients with fewer than four metastases (Roth *et al.* 1985; Maeda *et al.* 1989; Pastorino *et al.* 1989, 1997). Others report that surgical resectability rather than the number of metastases is important; if all lesions can be surgically removed, the number of lesions resected does not matter (van Dongen *et al.* 1986). A long disease-free interval between diagnosis of the primary tumor and appearance of the first lung metastasis correlates with good survival after thoracotomy in many series (Kelm *et al.* 1988; Jablons *et al.* 1989; Pastorino *et al.* 1997). However, in other series across a variety of histological types, the disease-free interval was not found to be of prognostic importance (Roth *et al.* 1985).

Surgical resection of osseous metastases, which are present in 25 to 50 per cent of patients with metastatic RCC (Saitoh 1981), may pose special problems, particularly when there are axial skeletal lesions. Even appendicular lesions can be very vascular, although preoperative embolization may facilitate surgery. Osseous lesions frequently have a large soft tissue mass associated with them, particularly in the pelvis. Using contemporary techniques, however, even vertebral metastases can now be resected. Althausen *et al.* (1997) reported that patients undergoing resection of axial metastases, especially pelvic metastases, have a poorer survival rate than patients undergoing resection of an appendicular (extremity) metastasis ($p < 0.008$). They also noted that presentation initially without metastasis, long disease-free interval between nephrectomy and first metastasis, and solitary metastasis all correlated with longer survival.

About 50 per cent of patients with brain metastases secondary to various primary tumors have a solitary intracranial tumor and, of these, about 50 per cent will have resectable tumors by virtue of surgical accessibility and the performance status of the patients (Barr *et al.* 1992). Patients with minimal or no neurologic deficit at the time of craniotomy and infratentorial lesions showed a trend towards improved survival (Badalament *et al.* 1990). Some investigators have found that patients with metachronous metastases secondary to many different types of primary tumors have a trend towards improved survival (Torre *et al.* 1988), although others have not found a significant difference (Demange *et al.* 1989).

Although liver metastases are rarely resected in patients with RCC, they are frequently resected in patients with colorectal carcinoma. Most authors agree that the extent of liver involvement is an important predictor of outcome following surgical resection, regardless of the primary tumor type. Some have found that the total number of metastases is important (Fortner *et al.* 1984; Doci *et al.* 1991), while others report that the percentage of involvement of liver parenchyma is more predictive of outcome (Stief *et al.* 1997). Unilobar versus bilobar tumor, surgical resectability, and the absence of positive margins are the factors reported to be important for a good outcome (Bakalakos *et al.* 1998). Most investigators have not found a difference in survival rates between patients with synchronous metastases and those with metachronous metastases (Fortner *et al.* 1984; Stief *et al.* 1997).

Results after solitary metastasectomy

In 1939, Barney and Churchill reported what is believed to be the first excision of a clinically solitary pulmonary metastasis in a patient who had undergone prior nephrectomy. The patient survived for 23 years after resection and died of coronary artery disease. Metastasectomy for solitary metastasis was firmly established as potentially effective by the mid-1970s after several groups reported 5-year overall survival rates of 29 to 35 per cent (Middleton 1967; Skinner *et al.* 1971; Tolia and Whitmore 1975; O'Dea *et al.* 1978). Since then, additional reports have confirmed this initial experience (Klugo *et al.* 1977; Montie *et al.* 1977; McNichols *et al.* 1981; Jett *et al.* 1983; Dernevik *et al.* 1985; Golimbu *et al.* 1986*a*; Dineen *et al.* 1988; Tongaonkar *et al.* 1992; Kierney *et al.* 1994; Dreicer *et al.* 1997; Kavolius *et al.* 1998; van der Poel *et al.* 1999), and the cumulative 5-year survival rate in more than 450 patients is estimated to be about 35 per cent (Table 45.1).

Kavolius *et al.* (1998) reported on the largest single series of patients undergoing resection of a solitary metastasis as first recurrence of disease ($n = 94$). The sites resected were lung ($n = 50$), gland (including pancreas, adrenal, thyroid, and salivary; $n = 15$), brain ($n = 11$), bone ($n = 5$), and soft tissue ($n = 5$). Patients with completely resected solitary metastasis fared better than those who underwent complete resection of multiple meta-

Table 45.1 Survival after resection of solitary metastasis

Study	Number of patients	5-year survival rate (%)
Middleton 1967	59	34*
Skinner *et al.* 1971	41	29
Tolia and Whitmore 1975	17	35
Montie *et al.* 1977	5	20
Klugo *et al.* 1977	10	6
O'Dea *et al.* 1978	44	23
deKernion *et al.* 1978	20	≈25[†]
McNichols *et al.* 1981	13	69
Jett *et al.* 1983	16	≈25◊
Dernevik *et al.* 1985	15	27
Golimbu *et al.* 1986*a*	4	50
Dineen *et al.* 1988	29	13
Tongaonkar *et al.* 1992	19	16
Kierney *et al.* 1994	23	31[§]
Dreicer *et al.* 1997	18	39
Kavolius *et al.* 1998	94	44
van der Poel *et al.* 1999	40	29
Total	467	35‖

* Eight personal cases; 51 from review of prior literature.
[†] Estimated from survival curve; includes solitary metastasis and multiple metastases in single organ.
◊ Estimated from survival curves.
[§] Survival rate includes 13 patients with multiple metastases.
‖ Estimated overall survival.

stases ($n = 47$), with a 5-year overall survival rate of 52 compared with 29 per cent ($p < 0.005$). Disease-free survival rates by site were 44 per cent for patients with a solitary metastasis in the lung, 42 per cent gland, 20 per cent brain, 40 per cent bone, and 50 per cent for soft tissue metastases. Overall, survival rates for these patients by site were 54 per cent for patients with lung metastases, 63 per cent gland, 18 per cent brain, 40 per cent bone, and 75 per cent soft tissue metastases.

We recently reviewed The University of Texas M.D. Anderson Cancer Center's experience with resection of solitary metastasis. Among 2100 patients who were known to have metastatic RCC between 1984 and 1997, 179 (8.5 per cent) underwent resection for an apparently solitary metastatic lesion. Sites resected included lung ($n = 50$), axial bone ($n = 29$), appendicular bone ($n = 27$), visceral organ ($n = 23$), brain ($n = 23$), locoregional location, including renal fossa or regional lymph nodes ($n = 17$), and skin ($n = 10$). The overall 5-year survival rate was 29 per cent (Fig. 45.1(a)). The disease-specific 5-year survival rate for all sites was 19 per cent (Fig. 45.1(b)), but survival rates were dependent upon the location of the metastasis: 56 per cent for patients with a solitary metastasis in the lung, 49 per cent locoregional location, 28 per cent skin, 20 per cent visceral organs, 18 per cent appendicular bone, 13 per cent brain, and 9 per cent for axial bones. Rates for morbidity and operative mortality were acceptable at 11 and 3.7 per cent, respectively. Patients who developed a metachronous solitary metastasis fared better than those with a synchronous solitary metastasis (5-year survival rates of 39 and 22 per cent, respectively) regardless of the site of metastasis. Among the 40 patients with recurrent disease after resection of a lung meta-

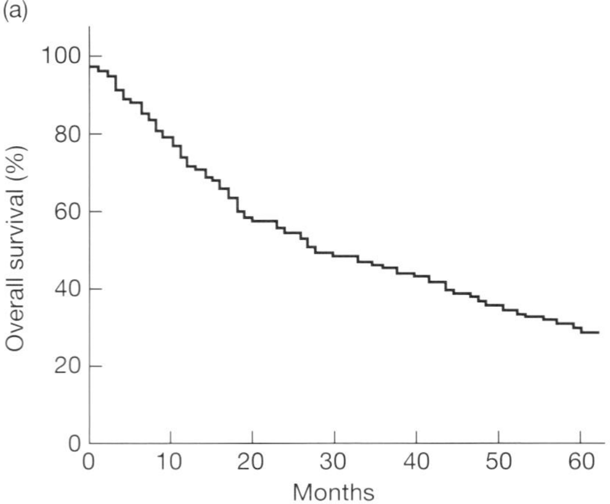

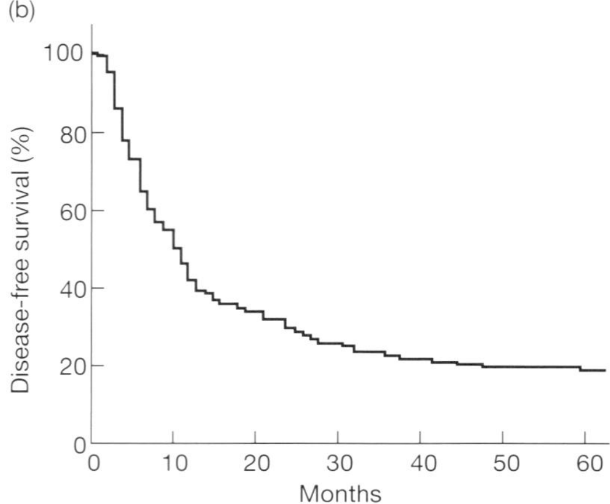

Fig. 45.1 (a) Overall and (b) disease-free survival for 179 patients after resection of an apparently solitary metastasis at the University of Texas M.D. Anderson Cancer Center.

stasis, 24 (60 per cent) were able to undergo a subsequent resection compared with only 14 (25 per cent) of the 56 patients with recurrent bone metastasis.

Overall, patients with solitary lung and locoregional metastases had the most favorable outcome in our series. The results support treating these patients initially with surgical resection. However, patients with a solitary metastasis in other organ sites may benefit from an approach that integrates surgery and biological therapy, similar to what we would recommend for patients with multiple metastases. Nonetheless, in the absence of a clinical trial that addresses the question of using biological therapy as initial treatment before resection or biological therapy as adjuvant therapy following resection of a solitary metastasis, we recommend resection as initial treatment for a solitary metastasis and biological therapy only if there is a recurrence.

The case of patient J.E.S. illustrates why adjuvant biological therapy should be given only when dictated by protocol. In September 1980, at age 56 years, 2 years after right radical nephrectomy for RCC, he underwent resection of a solitary metastasis in the contralateral left adrenal gland (Fig. 45.2(a), (b)). He did not receive adjuvant therapy postoperatively. The patient

did very well until 1996, when he began to complain of fatigue and left upper-quadrant pain. Computerized tomography (CT) scan showed an 8 cm × 10 cm × 11 cm poorly defined mass in the region of the celiac artery (Fig. 45.2(c)). Resection of this mass along with the spleen and tail of the pancreas in September 1996 again revealed metastatic RCC (Fig. 45.2(d)). Surgical margins were negative for tumor. The patient is currently alive without clinical evidence of disease almost 20 years after initial resection of a solitary adrenal metastasis.

Site-specific results of metastasectomy

Many of the reports in the literature on resection of metastases are organized by specific organ sites and often include malignancies other than RCC in the review. Although RCC may have unique features in terms of natural history and response to treatment, we cannot be sure that what we are seeing is disease-specific and not site-specific. For this reason, it seems appropriate to include the results of metastasectomy for other diseases.

Lung

As mentioned earlier, the lung is a favorable site for resecting metastasis or metastases for a number of reasons: (1) the ease of detection by chest radiography often results in earlier detection than in other organs; (2) the presence of a solitary metastasis, or even limited lung metastases, has minimal effect on organ physiologic function; and (3) the lung may have a microenvironment favorable for slow tumor growth (Barr *et al.* 1992). Nonetheless, the patients who tend to do best after lung metastasectomy are those who have tumors responsive to systemic therapy. Resection of solitary pulmonary metastases secondary to a number of different neoplasms has been reported, including metastases of melanoma (Kelm *et al.* 1988; Coit 1993; Sharpless and Das Gupta 1998), colon cancer (Sauter *et al.* 1990; De Giacomo *et al.* 1999; Kobayashi *et al.* 1999), breast cancer (Livartowski *et al.* 1998), transitional cell carcinoma (Cowles *et al.* 1982), osteogenic sarcoma (Belli *et al.* 1989; Skinner *et al.* 1992), and RCC (Jett *et al.* 1983; Dernevik *et al.* 1985; Thrasher *et al.* 1990; Cerfolio *et al.* 1994; Cozzoli *et al.* 1995; Tanguay *et al.* 1996*b*; Fourquier *et al.* 1997; Kavolius *et al.*1998). Patients with melanoma generally fare poorly, and those with carcinoma or sarcoma have intermediate results. Patients with resected metastases from osteogenic sarcoma have better survival rates than do those with adult soft-tissue sarcoma (Maeda *et al.* 1989).

The morbidity of the operation is usually low, and the operative mortality rates are 0–2 per cent. Although surgeons should strive to preserve enough parenchyma for adequate pulmonary function when treating these patients surgically, the goal should be to resect all known metastases (Barr *et al.* 1992). Pastorino *et al.* (1997) reported on 4572 patients who underwent complete surgical resection. The actuarial survival rates after complete metastasectomy were 36 per cent at 5 years, 26 per cent at 10 years, and 22 per cent at 15 years compared with 13 per cent at 5 years and 7 per cent at 10 years for patients who had incomplete resections.

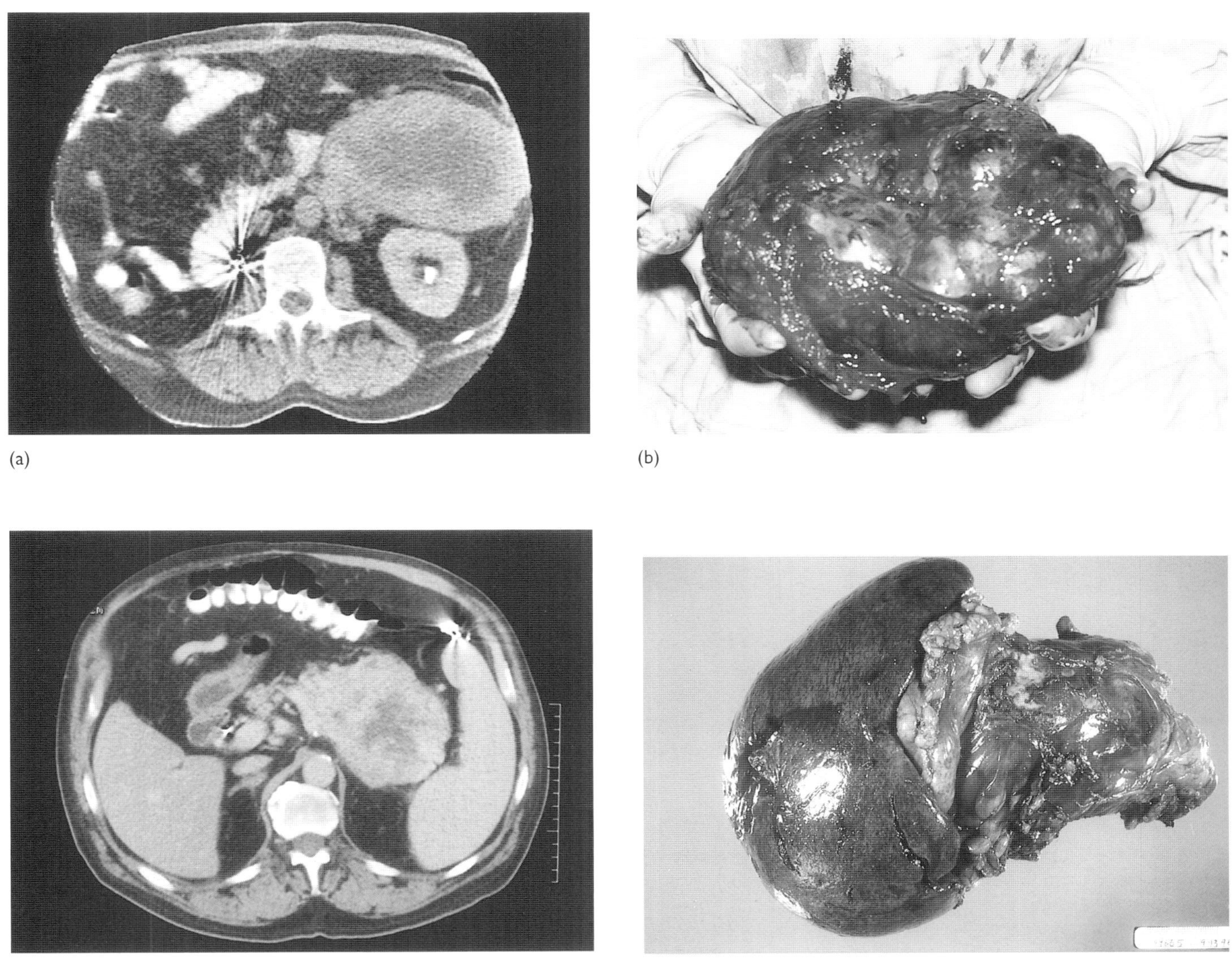

Fig. 45.2 Patient J.E.S. (a) CT scan of solitary left adrenal metastasis.(b) Surgical specimen weighing 895 g. (c) CT scan of recurrent tumor in adrenal bed. (d) Resected tumor, including spleen and tail of pancreas.

The 5-year survival rates were 33 per cent for patients with a disease-free interval of 0–11 months and 45 per cent for those with a disease-free interval of more than 36 months; the rates were 43 per cent for patients with single lesions and 27 per cent for those with four or more lesions.

The lungs are the most frequently involved organs for both solitary and multiple metastases secondary to RCC. Among patients with RCC, 3-year survival rates for patients undergoing resection of a solitary metastasis range from 42 to 60 per cent compared with 27–42 per cent for those undergoing resection of multiple metastases (Table 45.2) (Jett *et al.* 1983; Dernevik *et al.* 1985; Thrasher *et al.* 1990; Cerfolio *et al.* 1994; Cozzoli *et al.* 1995; Tanguay *et al.* 1996*b*; Fourquier *et al.* 1997; Kavolius *et al.* 1998). One report addressed the benefit of aggressive surgical resection in patients with recurrent disease in solitary or multiple sites or in

patients who had undergone prior metastasectomy (Kavolius *et al.* 1998). Among 50 patients with a solitary lung metastasis, including patients with multiple, unilateral metastases, the 5-year overall survival rate was 54 per cent. Survival rates after resection with curative intent of second and third metastases were not different from rates after initial metastasectomy (46 and 44 per cent, respectively).

Brain

The brain is another common site of metastasis for solid tumors. Brain metastases tend to be well-circumscribed tumors with a surrounding pseudocapsule, and they can often be removed with generally low morbidity and mortality (Barr 1989). The metastases are typically small, but they present with neurologic

Table 45.2 Overall survival after resection of RCC lung metastasis

Study	Number of patients	Follow-up (years)	Survival rate (%) for metastasis(es)		
			Solitary	Multiple	Mixed
Jett et al.1983	44	3	43*	46*	
Dernevik et al.1985	33	3	42	29	
Thrasher et al.1990	14	3	50		
Cerfolio et al.1994	96	3	46	27	
Cozzoli et al.1995	19	3	60		
Tanguay et al.1996b	22	5			55
Fourquier et al.1997	50	5			44
Kavolius et al.1998	50	5	54		

* Estimated from survival curve.

symptoms. A high percentage of patients undergoing resection of a solitary brain metastasis achieve immediate and prolonged improvement in neurological symptoms regardless of the primary histological type. For comparable tumors, the palliative benefit of surgical resection of brain metastases appears to be considerably greater than what can be achieved using radiotherapy or dexamethasone alone (Patchell *et al.* 1986; Wroński *et al.* 1997). This finding has been verified by a randomized trial of surgery with postoperative irradiation versus irradiation alone for solitary brain metastases in which a highly significant difference in performance status was found in favor of surgery (Patchell *et al.* 1990). The median time that patients undergoing surgery remained functionally independent was 38 weeks compared with 8 weeks for those receiving radiation alone.

Wroński *et al.* (1996) evaluated 50 consecutive patients with RCC brain metastases among 709 patients with brain metastases who underwent surgical resection at Memorial Sloan–Kettering Cancer Center. Ten patients had synchronous metastases and 40 had a metachronous metastasis, with a median interval between diagnosis of RCC and brain metastasis of 17 months. Overall, survival from time of diagnosis of RCC was 31.4 months; survival time from craniotomy was 12.6 months, with a postoperative mortality rate of 10 per cent. The 1-, 2-, 3-, and 5-year survival rates were 51, 24, 22, and 8.5 per cent, respectively. Similar results have been noted by other investigators (Decker *et al.* 1984; Badalament *et al.* 1990). Although patients with multiple metastases may be cured by complete surgical resection, the majority of patients with multiple metastases have unresectable disease and should be considered for brain irradiation (Badalament *et al.* 1990). In summary, there is good evidence that metastasectomy is superior to irradiation for solitary brain metastases. About 25 per cent of patients with such metastases have surgically resectable lesions and, therefore, surgical resection should be recommended (Barr *et al.* 1992).

Liver

Liver resection is commonly performed for metastases of such neoplasms as colorectal cancer (Ekberg *et al.* 1986; Sauter *et al.* 1990; Wanebo *et al.* 1996; Stief *et al.* 1997; Curley and Vecchio 1998; De Giacomo *et al.* 1999; Fong *et al.* 1999; Kobayashi *et al.* 1999) and breast cancer (Seifert *et al.* 1999). Operative mortality

rates are low, and survival rates of 10–32 per cent at 5 years appear promising compared with the overall outlook for patients with liver metastases (Ekberg *et al.* 1986; Barr *et al.* 1992; Wanebo *et al.* 1996; Fujisaki *et al.* 1997; Bakalakos *et al.* 1998; Curley and Vecchio 1998; Fong *et al.* 1999; Seifert *et al.* 1999).

However, the experience with liver metastasectomy in patients with RCC is more limited, in part because deKernion *et al.* (1978) reported that the presence of a liver metastasis in a patient correlated with a very poor overall outcome. Fujisaki *et al.* (1997) reported on three patients who had one, three, and six metastases resected. The patients with one and three lesions survived without tumor recurrence for 12 and 21 months, respectively, while the patient with six hepatic metastases had a tumor-free interval of only 2 months and died 10 months later. Stief *et al.* (1997) reported on 17 patients who underwent surgical exploration for metachronous liver metastases secondary to RCC. Resection was feasible in 13 patients and complete resection was accomplished in 11 patients. Mean survival time was 4 months in patients with unresectable disease and 16 months in the 13 patients who underwent resection. However, the mortality rate was 31 per cent (4 of 13) with significant morbidity in another two. In general, only a minority of patients with hepatic metastases will have resectable disease. Furthermore, the majority of patients who undergo successful liver resection for RCC develop recurrent disease either in the liver or other sites.

Osseous

Among patients with multiorgan metastases from RCC, 50 per cent will have osseous metastasis, 15 to 30 per cent of which will be solitary (Swanson *et al.* 1981; Kozlowski 1994). Eighty per cent of osseous metastases occur in the axial skeleton, thoracolumbar spine, and pelvis (all marrow-producing sites). When long bones are involved, only the proximal portions are likely to be the site of metastatic disease, and the involvement is typically lytic in nature (Swanson *et al.* 1981). RCC accounts for 10 per cent of all pathologic fractures in patients with osseous metastases and 5 per cent of all cases of spinal cord compression (Kozlowski 1994). We reported a number of years ago that the median survival time for patients with metachronous multiple osseous metastases was 1 year, and the 1-, 3-, and 5-year survival rates were 50, 20, and 0 per cent, respectively (Swanson *et al.* 1981). In contrast, the corresponding survival rates were 86, 70, and 45 per cent for patients with a metachronous solitary osseous metastasis from RCC. If the solitary metastasis was synchronous and the patient underwent radical nephrectomy, the survival rates were 74, 52, and 15 per cent, respectively. Several small series report similar results (Pongracz *et al.* 1988; Smith *et al.*1992; Althausen *et al.* 1997).

The goals of treating bone metastases are to: (1) relieve pain; (2) prevent pathologic fractures; (3) improve function; (4) reduce neurological symptoms in patients with spinal lesions; and (5) prolong survival (Nielsen *et al.* 1991). Resection of an osseous metastasis should be considered when an impending fracture appears imminent. If a lesion greater than 2–3 cm is present in a weight-bearing bone and the anticipated survival is greater than 6 weeks, the bone can and should be stabilized.

Spinal metastases present a unique challenge for treatment. Sioutos *et al.* (1995) studied 109 spinal metastases from a wide variety of neoplasms. All patients had cord compression and received adjuvant radiotherapy after surgical resection. The overall median survival was 10 months. Patients with RCC survived the longest, followed by those with breast, prostate, lung, and colon cancer. In patients with vertebral column involvement, poor leg strength and multiple vertebral body involvement were adverse prognostic factors. King *et al.* (1991) reported similar findings in 33 patients with RCC who underwent decompression. Of these 33 patients, 88 per cent had partial or complete relief of pain and 64 per cent who were bedridden before decompression were able to walk after it. Overall, survival was 8 months.

Because of its efficacy and safety, selective arterial embolization is advocated by some investigators as a preoperative adjunct to help with hemostasis in patients with bone metastases (Roscoe *et al.* 1989; Sun and Lang 1998). Although technically difficult, preoperative embolization of spinal metastases has also been effective in devascularizing these lesions and can be performed without serious neurologic complications (Sundaresan *et al.* 1990).

Local recurrence

Local recurrence in or near the renal fossa is a unique variant of advanced RCC that may, in fact, not truly represent metastatic disease. It may result from incomplete resection of the primary tumor or persistence of tumor in the regional lymph nodes, but it is generally associated with a poor prognosis, and usually surgical resection must be considered (deKernion *et al.* 1978). Renal fossa recurrences may not produce symptoms until adjacent structures are invaded, particularly the posterior abdominal wall, which contributes to its seeming to be unresectable. Thus, only a few programs have taken an aggressive surgical approach toward the resection of local recurrences (Fig. 45.2). Esrig *et al.* (1992) reported on 11 patients with renal fossa recurrences who underwent resection a median of 31 months after nephrectomy. There were two postoperative deaths, two patients died of disseminated disease (at 8 and 22 months), and three died of unrelated causes. Four patients had no clinical evidence of disease 47 months (median) after surgery. Tanguay *et al.* (1996*a*) resected 16 renal fossa recurrences; eight of these patients received preoperative immunotherapy. Complete resection was possible in 15 patients,

12 of whom also had negative surgical margins. Among the eight patients who did not receive immunotherapy, five of eight patients were alive 16 months (median) after surgery. These reports suggest that resection of a solitary local recurrence in a patient with no other sites of metastases, especially if a negative margin can be obtained, can be associated with long-term survival.

Miscellaneous sites

Analysis of radical nephrectomy specimens in a number of studies revealed ipsilateral adrenal involvement in 3.2–5.8 per cent of cases, with the majority found in association with upper pole tumors (Sagalowsky *et al.* 1994; Shalev *et al.* 1995; Sandock *et al.* 1997; Kessler *et al.* 1998; Wunderlich *et al.* 1999). The frequency of contralateral adrenal recurrence is less than 1 per cent. Factors predisposing to adrenal involvement include left-sided tumors, large tumors, upper pole tumors, and advanced tumor stage (Sagalowsky *et al.* 1994).

For patients with either bilateral adrenal metastases or a metachronous contralateral adrenal metastasis of many different neoplasms, surgical resection has provided long-term disease control. Authors have reported survival periods of 25.7 months in patients with metastatic melanoma (Haigh *et al.* 1999) and 24 months in those with metastatic lung cancer (Lo *et al.* 1996; Beitler *et al.* 1998; Porte *et al.* 1998). Nonetheless, protracted survival time depends on the secondary tumor being an isolated adrenal metastasis, which is not very common in RCC. Sagalowsky *et al.* (1994) reported that 30 per cent of 695 patients who underwent nephrectomy for RCC had evidence of metastases in other organs. Twenty-one of these patients underwent adrenalectomy, although 81 per cent died of disease by 27 months. Sagalowsky *et al.* (1994) estimated that resection of the adrenal metastasis accounted for a cure in only 0.43 per cent of the patients in this series.

Although patients with renal metastases in multiple organs will have a pancreatic metastasis in 15 per cent of cases, a patient with a solitary metastasis rarely presents with a lesion in the pancreas (Saitoh *et al.* 1982). Metachronous pancreatic metastases may appear more than 20 years after the nephrectomy. Fabre *et al.* (1995) reviewed 33 cases of solitary pancreatic metastases (nine synchronous and 24 metachronous). Over 50 per cent of the metachronous metastases were identified more than 10 years after nephrectomy. Median survival after resection was 13 months for patients with synchronous metastases and 14 months for metachronous metastases. Once widespread metastases have been ruled out, the authors recommend partial pancreatectomy.

RCC accounts for 6 per cent of head and neck metastases (Flocks and Boatman 1973; Kozlowski 1994). Nasal obstruction, discharge, and epistaxis are the most common presenting symptoms. In 50 per cent of cases the lesions are solitary (Eneroth *et al.* 1961; Flocks and Boatman 1973; Kozlowski 1994). Radical maxillectomy, radiation, and a combination of both are the primary modes of therapy (Matsumoto and Yanagihara 1982; Kozlowski 1994; Sesenna *et al.* 1995; Gottlieb and Roland 1998). Average survival times associated with surgery alone, radiation alone, and combined modality treatment are 32.3, 19.7, and 20 months, respectively (Kent and Majumdar 1985). RCC also accounts for up

Table 45.3 Overall survival after resection of residual disease following cytokine therapy

Study	Number of patients	Follow-up (months)	Overall survival (%)
Sella *et al.* 1993	17	12	65
Sherry *et al.* 1992	16	20	68
Kim and Louie 1992	11	21	100
Tanguay *et al.* 1996*a*	8	19	88
Tanguay *et al.* 1996*b*	29	48	66
Krishnamurthi *et al.* 1998	14	41	71

to 25 per cent of all metastases to the thyroid gland (Kim and Louie 1992; Kozlowski 1994; Chen *et al.* 1999). Surgical resection should be performed if possible.

Resection of metastatic disease after cytokine therapy

Resection of solitary metastasis is widely practised and is supported by the current literature with very good survival rates. However, patients with a solitary metastasis are relatively rare when compared with the number of patients with multiple metastases. For these latter patients, primary surgical resection is rarely employed unless the volume of disease is truly limited or unless one goal of the surgery is palliation. Instead, biological therapy alone or in combination with chemotherapeutic agents is generally used; these treatments will produce objective responses in up to 40 per cent of patients, although less than one-third of responding patients will have complete regression of all disease (Rosenberg *et al.* 1994; Taneja *et al.* 1994; Ellerhorst *et al.* 1997). For patients who respond but not completely, the residual mass creates a dilemma for the surgeon. Should this mass be surgically resected? The rationale for resecting a residual mass includes: (1) histologic confirmation of the response to systemic therapy, which may confirm unrecognized complete regressions; (2) the potential to remove all malignant tissue; (3) the opportunity to promote long-term survival in some patients. The role of surgery in this setting is not yet defined, but the reported experience of several groups helps us address this issue. Table 45.3 summarizes results of studies in which patients underwent resection of residual disease following cytokine therapy. Most surgeons reported resection of a residual mass after partial regression of metastatic disease following therapy with interleukin 2 (IL-2), although surgery was sometimes performed for stable disease after an interval without progression and occasionally after clinical relapse following a prior complete response.

Kim and Louie (1992) were among the first to address the issue of whether patients would benefit from surgical resection of residual tumor after partial response to IL-2 therapy. They reviewed the records of 399 patients with metastatic RCC enrolled in 14 clinical trials from multiple institutions who received IL-2 with or without lymphokine-activated killer (LAK) cell immunotherapy. Sixty-two patients demonstrated an objective response

(15.5 per cent), 18 (4.5 per cent) having a complete response and 44 (11.0 per cent) a partial response. Eleven patients (10 of whom had achieved a partial response and one who progressed following an initial complete response) underwent resection of residual tumor in the lung, kidney, retroperitoneum, or pelvis. At the time of publication, all 11 patients who had been rendered surgically free of disease after immunotherapy remained alive without clinical evidence of disease after a median follow-up of 21 months. In contrast, among patients who did not undergo surgery after immunotherapy, only 14 (78 per cent) of 18 patients who had had a complete response, and 15 (34 per cent) of 44 patients who had partial responses maintained their disease-free status.

Sherry *et al.* (1992) reported that seven of 16 patients with RCC who had undergone surgery for disease progression after prior complete response (5 patients), or partial response (11 patients), were free of tumor progression 4 to 44 months after surgery, and three of 12 patients rendered disease-free by surgery remained disease-free after 2 years. The same group later reported on 23 patients with only lung metastases, 18 of whom had previously received IL-2. They noted that patients who underwent complete resection of metastatic disease ($n = 15$) had a significantly longer survival (mean, 49 months) than did patients with incomplete resection (median, 16 months, $p = 0.02$) (Pogrebniak *et al.* 1992).

Sella *et al.* (1993) reported their experience with 17 patients with RCC who underwent surgical resection after prior interferon alpha (IFNα) therapy. They noted that 65 per cent of their patients were disease-free at 12 months despite a finding of viable cancer in the surgical specimen in 88 per cent. The 12-month disease-free rate was increased to 77 per cent for patients who were able to receive biological therapy after surgical resection in addition to the preoperative therapy. Subsequent reports from the same institution looked at patients with RCC who had pulmonary metastases or local recurrences. Tanguay *et al.* (1996*b*) reported on 51 patients with only lung metastases, 22 of whom were treated with surgical resection alone and 29 of whom were treated with biologic therapy followed by surgery. It should be emphasized that this was not a randomized study. In the initial surgery group, only two patients had more than two nodules, and the average number of nodules resected was two; in the initial biologic therapy group, 23 patients had more than two nodules, and the average number resected was 4.5. Of the 22 patients treated with surgery without prior biologic therapy, 12 (55 per cent) were alive after a median follow-up of 57 months, and 19 of the 29 (66 per cent) treated with surgical resection after prior biologic therapy were alive after a median follow-up of 48 months. Only eight of 46 patients in whom lung metastases were completely resected had no relapse, including five who had prior biologic therapy and three treated with surgery alone. Median time to relapse was 8.5 months in patients treated with combination therapy and 6 months in those treated with initial surgical resection. At the time of evaluation, 31 (61 per cent) of the 51 patients were alive, including 15 who were disease-free; a total of 19 (37 per cent) patients died of progressive disease.

As previously mentioned, Tanguay *et al.* (1996*a*) also reported on 16 patients undergoing resection of renal fossa recurrence. Eight of these patients had received biologic therapy before surgical resection. Of the eight patients treated with combination therapy, 50 per cent had no evidence of disease compared with 25 per cent of those treated with surgery alone. Complete resection with negative surgical margins was found to be very important for long-term success.

Krishnamurthi *et al.* (1998) reported on 14 patients with metastatic RCC who were treated at the Cleveland Clinic with initial biologic therapy followed by surgery to resect residual primary or metastatic RCC lesions. Nine patients had an objective response to systemic therapy and five had stable disease. All patients were then rendered disease-free by surgical excision of residual or recurrent metastatic lesions and the primary tumor (if not previously resected). The cancer-specific survival rate at 3 years was 81.5 per cent. Seven patients were alive and disease-free after a mean follow-up of 41 months, three patients were alive with recurrent disease (mean survival, 48 months), three patients had died of metastatic disease (mean survival, 28 months), and one patient had died of an unrelated cause 54 months after therapy.

We recently updated our experience with metastasectomy and retrospectively analyzed results for 81 patients who underwent resection of residual or stable disease after cytokine therapy. Forty-four patients underwent 52 resections of lung metastases after a median of 8 months of immunotherapy (range, 2–19 months). The median time to recurrence in these patients was 9 months, and the median survival was 47 months (range, 8–160 months). Eighteen patients underwent resection of locoregional recurrences after a median of 7 months of immunotherapy (range, 3–11 months), nine of whom had recurrent disease (3 locally) a median of 14 months (range, 11–32 months) after resection. Median survival was 23 months (range, 6–68 months), with symptomatic patients having a more dire prognosis. Twenty patients with lung metastases and 11 patients with local recurrence also received postoperative immunotherapy for 4 months. Patients who received postoperative immunotherapy had a trend towards improved survival of approximately 5 months compared with those not receiving immunotherapy after resection, although this difference was not statistically significant (Fig. 45.3). The remaining 19 of the 81 metastasectomy patients

underwent resections of supradiaphragmatic lymph nodes ($n = 5$), spine ($n = 5$), brain ($n = 3$), liver ($n = 2$), pancreas ($n = 2$), and appendicular bone ($n = 2$) with a median survival of 15 months (range, 1–62 months) for all presentations.

Patient G.P.L. illustrates the remarkable clinical course that is possible in some patients with metastatic RCC who undergo aggressive surgical resection of disease in combination with biological therapy. In October 1980, at age 43 years, he presented with a right renal mass and two pulmonary nodules. He underwent arterial embolization of the right kidney followed by radical nephrectomy and was started on medroxyprogesterone acetate. The pulmonary nodules remained stable until August 1987 when they were excised because of growth. A second wedge resection of the lung was performed in September 1989. In December 1990, he presented with jaundice, and a CT scan showed a liver metastasis plus several lesions in the pancreas (Fig. 45.4(a)). The patient was treated with IFNα and floxuridine. His serum bilirubin level returned to normal, and the masses regressed more than 50 per cent. In January 1992, resection of 95 per cent of the pancreas, wedge resection of the liver, and resection of the gall bladder and

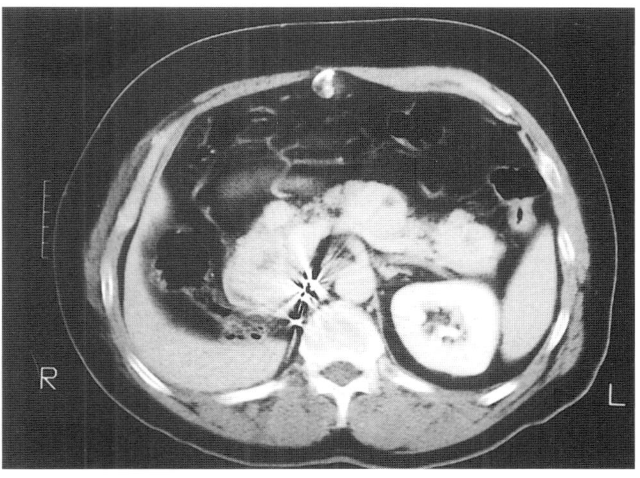

(a)

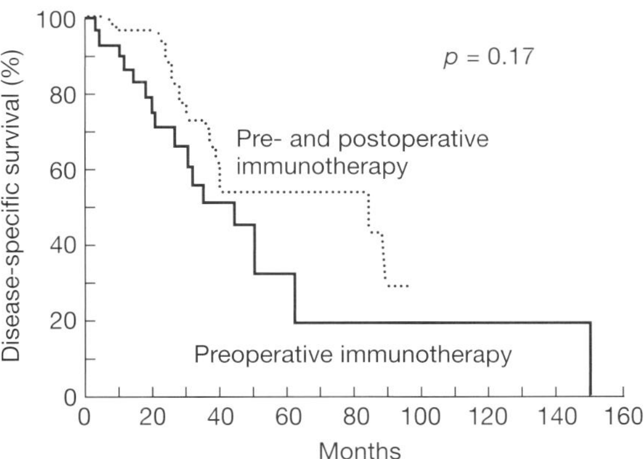

Fig. 45.3 Disease-specific survival of 44 patients who underwent resection of residual or stable disease in the lungs after biological therapy, some of whom received adjuvant therapy following resection.

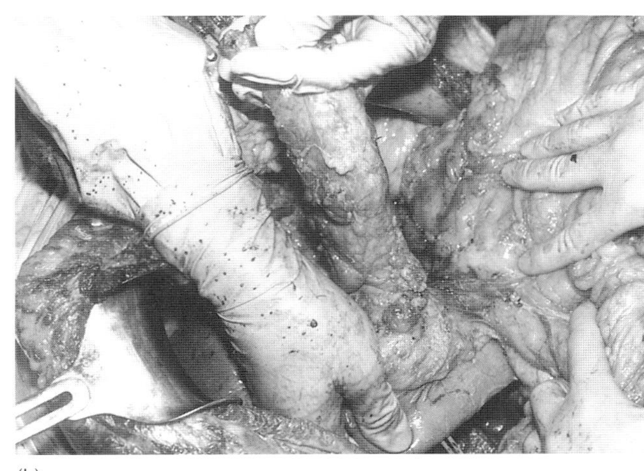

(b)

Fig. 45.4 Patient G.P.L. (a) CT scan showing metastatic lesions in pancreas. (b) Intraoperative photograph showing subtotal pancreatectomy.

the first and second portions of the duodenum revealed eight metastatic RCC nodules up to 3.8 cm in diameter; all soft tissue margins were negative for tumor (Fig. 45.4(b)). The patient did not receive additional biologic therapy postoperatively and did well until late 1999, when he was noted to have a palpable nodule in his parotid gland. A left parotidectomy performed in February 2000 revealed two RCC metastases; the patient is clinically-free of disease at this time.

Our retrospective analysis of patients subjected to aggressive surgical management after biologic therapy reinforces the need to find better therapeutic modalities in order to achieve complete eradication of disease in metastatic sites. In truth, most patients treated with biologic therapy will never achieve a response sufficient to make them candidates for surgical resection of residual disease. Although it is tempting to say that a partial or stable response to biologic therapy, particularly in combination with surgery, is beneficial, it is not possible to do so with any authority, in part at least because the results in patients treated with combination therapy are so strongly influenced by patient selection.

Summary

The role of metastasectomy for RCC in the era of biologic therapy is not yet defined except, perhaps, for solitary metastasis. We would encourage aggressive surgical resection of the clinically apparent solitary metastasis, whether synchronous or metachronous. For patients with multiple metastases, however, initial systemic therapy followed by resection of any residual disease seems to be supported by our results. We have observed apparently prolonged survival times after systemic therapy followed by surgery in highly selected patients, as have some other investigators, despite finding viable cancer in the overwhelming majority of specimens. One must be mindful of the morbidity of treatment, however, and try to assess preoperatively the potential complications associated with an attempt to remove all known disease. If the morbidity of the surgical procedure is likely to be high, then we must be relatively certain that surgery is, in fact, directly benefiting the patient. If the morbidity is likely to be low, then even simple palliation would be a sufficient reason for the patient to undergo surgery. Only a prospective, randomized trial will ever confirm the value of an aggressive surgical approach to metastatic RCC. In the meantime, however, metastasectomy at the very least offers the opportunity to confirm the histologic response to systemic therapy, render some patients disease-free, and possibly promote long-term survival in selected patients.

References

Althausen, P., Althausen, A., Jennings, L.C., and Mankin, H.J. (1997). Prognostic factors and surgical treatment of osseous metastases secondary to renal cell carcinoma. *Cancer* **80**, 1103–9.

Badalament, R.A., Gluck, R.W., Wong, G.Y., Gnecco, C., Kreutzer, E., Herr, H.W., *et al.* (1990). Surgical treatment of brain metastases from renal cell carcinoma. *Urology* **36**, 112–15.

Bakalakos, E.A., Kim, J.A., Young, D.C., and Martin, E.W. Jr (1998). Determinants of survival following hepatic resection for metastatic colorectal cancer. *World J. Surg.* **22**, 399–404.

Barney, J.D. and Churchill, E.J. (1939). Adenocarcinoma of the kidney with metastasis to the lung: cured by nephrectomy and lobectomy. *J. Urol.* **42**, 269–76.

Barr, L.C. (1989). Review: the encapsulation of tumours. *Clin. Exp. Metastas.* **7**, 277–82.

Barr, L.C., Skene, A.I., and Thomas, J.M. (1992). Metastasectomy. *Br. J. Surg.* **79**, 1268–74.

Beitler, A.L., Urschel, J.D., Velagapudi, S.R.C., and Takita, H. (1998). Review article: surgical management of adrenal metastases from lung cancer. *J. Surg. Oncol.* **69**, 54–7.

Belli, L., Scholl, S., Livartowski, A., Ashby, M., Palangié, T., Levasseur, P., *et al.* (1989). Resection of pulmonary metastases in osteosarcoma: a retrospective analysis of 44 patients. *Cancer* **63**, 2546–50.

Bretheau, D., Lechevallier E., de Fromont, M., Sault, M. C., Rampal, M., and Coulange, C. (1995a). Prognostic value of nuclear grade of renal cell carcinoma. *Cancer* **76**, 2543–9.

Bretheau, D., Lechevallier, E., Eghazarian, C., Grisoni, V., and Coulange, C. (1995b). Prognostic significance of incidental renal cell carcinoma. *Eur. Urol.* **27**, 319–23.

Cerfolio, R.J., Allen, M.S., Deschamps, C., Daly, R.C., Wallrichs, S.L., Trastek, V.F., *et al.* (1994). Pulmonary resection of metastatic renal cell carcinoma. *Ann. Thorac. Surg.* **57**, 339–44.

Chen, H., Nicol, T.L., and Udelsman, R. (1999). Clinically significant, isolated metastatic disease to the thyroid gland. *World J. Surg.* **23**, 177–81.

Coit, D.G. (1993). Role of surgery for metastatic malignant melanoma: a review. *Sem. Surg. Oncol.* **9**, 239–45.

Cowles, R.S., Johnson, D.E., and McMurtrey, M.J. (1982). Long-term results following thoracotomy for metastatic bladder cancer. *Urology* **20**, 390–2.

Cozzoli, A., Milano, S., Cancarini, G., Zanotelli, T., and Cunico, C. (1995). Surgery of lung metastases in renal cell carcinoma. *Br. J. Urol.* **75**, 445–7.

Curley, S.A. and Vecchio, R. (1998). New trends in the surgical treatment of colorectal cancer liver metastases. *Tumori* **84**, 281–8.

Decker, D.A., Decker, V.L., Herskovic, A., and Cummings, G.D. (1984). Brain metastases in patients with renal cell carcinoma: prognosis and treatment. *J. Clin. Oncol.* **2**, 169–73.

De Giacomo, T., Rendina, E.A., Venuta, F., Ciccone, A.M., and Coloni, G.F. (1999). Thoracoscopic resection of solitary lung metastases from colorectal cancer is a viable therapeutic option. *Chest* **115**, 1441–3.

DeKernion, J.B., Ramming, K.P., and Smith R.B. (1978). The natural history of metastatic renal cell carcinoma: a computer analysis. *J. Urol.* **120**, 148–52.

Demange, L., Tack, L., Morel, M., Dubois de Montreynaud, J.M., Pauchet, P., Froissart, D., *et al.* (1989). Single brain metastasis of non-small cell lung carcinoma. Study of survival among 54 patients. *Br. J. Neurosurg.* **3**, 81–8.

Dernevik, L., Berggren, H., Larsson, S., and Roberts, D. (1985). Surgical removal of pulmonary metastases from renal cell carcinoma. *Scand. J. Urol. Nephrol.* **19**, 133–7.

Dineen, M.K., Pastore, R.D., Emrich, L.J., and Huben, R.P. (1988). Results of surgical treatment of renal cell carcinoma with solitary metastasis. *J. Urol.* **140**, 277–9.

Doci, R., Gennari, L., Bignami, P., Montalto, F., Morabito, A., and Bozzetti, F. (1991). One hundred patients with hepatic metastases from colorectal cancer treated by resection: analysis of prognostic determinants. *Br. J. Surg.* **78**, 797–801.

Dreicer, R., Galbraith, S.S., Davis, C.S., and See, W.A. (1997). Surgical resection of metastatic renal cell carcinoma: the University of Iowa experience. *Urol. Oncol.*, **3**, 99–101.

Ekberg, H., Tranberg, K.G., Andersson, R., Lundstedt, C., Hägerstrand, I., Ranstam, J., *et al.* (1986). Determinants of survival in liver resection for colorectal secondaries. *Br. J. Surg.* **73**, 727–31.

Ellerhorst, J.A., Sella, A., Amato, R.J., Tu, S.M., Millikan, R.E., Finn, L.D., *et al.* (1997). Phase II trial of 5-fluorouracil, interferon-α and continuous infusion interleukin-2 for patients with metastatic renal cell carcinoma. *Cancer* **80**, 2128–32.

Eneroth, C.M., Mårtensson, G., and Thulin, A. (1961). Profuse epistaxis in hypernephroma metastases. *Acta Oto-Laryngol.* **53**, 546–50.

Esrig, D., Ahlering, T.E., Lieskovsky, G., and Skinner, D.G. (1992). Experience with fossa recurrence of renal cell carcinoma. *J. Urol.* **147**, 1491–4.

Fabre, J.M., Rouanet, P., Dagues, F., Blanc, F., Baumel, H., and Domergue, J. (1995). Various features and surgical approach of solitary pancreatic metastasis from renal cell carcinoma. *Eur. J. Surg. Oncol.* **21**, 683–92.

Flocks, R.H. and Boatman, D.L. (1973). Incidence of head and neck metastases from genito-urinary neoplasms. *Laryngoscope* **83**, 1527–39.

Fong, Y., Fortner, J., Sun, R.L., Brennan, M.F., and Blumgart, L.H. (1999). Clinical score for predicting recurrence after hepatic resection for metastatic colorectal cancer: analysis of 1001 consecutive cases. *Ann. Surg.* **230**, 309–21.

Fortner, J.G., Silva, J.S., Golbey, R.B., Cox, E.B., and Maclean, B.J. (1984). Multivariate analysis of a personal series of 247 consecutive patients with liver metastases from colorectal cancer. 1. Treatment by hepatic resection. *Ann. Surg.* **199**, 306–16.

Fourquier, P., Regnard, J.F., Rea, S., Levi, J.F., and Levasseur, P. (1997). Lung metastases of renal cell carcinoma: results of surgical resection. *Eur. J. Cardiothorac. Surg.* **11**, 17–21.

Fuhrman, S.A., Lasky, L.C., and Limas, C. (1982). Prognostic significance of morphologic parameters in renal cell carcinoma. *Am. J. Surg. Pathol.* **6**, 655–63.

Fujisaki, S., Takayama, T., Shimada, K., Yamamoto, J., Kosuge, T., Yamasaki, S., et al. (1997). Hepatectomy for metastatic renal cell carcinoma. *Hepatogastroenterology* **44**, 817–19.

Golimbu, M., Al-Askari, S., Tessler, A., and Morales, P. (1986a). Aggressive treatment of metastatic renal cancer. *J. Urol.* **136**, 805–7.

Golimbu, M., Joshi, P., Sperber, A., Tessler, A., Al-Askari, S., and Morales, P. (1986b). Renal cell carcinoma: survival and prognostic factors. *Urology* **27**, 291–301.

Gottlieb, M.D. and Roland, J.T. Jr (1998). Paradoxical spread of renal cell carcinoma to the head and neck. *Laryngoscope* **108**, 1301–05.

Guinan, P., Stuhldreher, D., Frank, W., and Rubenstein, M. (1997). Report of 337 patients with renal cell carcinoma emphasizing 110 with stage IV disease and review of the literature. *J. Surg. Oncol.* **64**, 295–8.

Haigh, P.I., Essner, R., Wardlaw, J.C., Stern, S.L., and Morton, D.L. (1999). Long-term survival after complete resection of melanoma metastatic to the adrenal gland. *Ann. Surg. Oncol.* **6**, 633–9.

Jablons, D., Steinberg, S.M., Roth, J., Pittaluga, S., Rosenberg, S.A., and Pass, H. I. (1989). Metastasectomy for soft tissue sarcoma: further evidence for efficacy and prognostic indicators. *J. Thorac. Cardiovasc. Surg.* **97**, 695–705.

Jett, J.R., Hollinger, C.G., Zinsmeister, A.R., and Pairolero, P.C. (1983). Pulmonary resection of metastatic renal cell carcinoma. *Chest* **84**, 442–5.

Kavolius, J.P., Mastorakos, D.P., Pavlovich, C., Russo, P., Burt, M.E., and Brady, M.S. (1998). Resection of metastatic renal cell carcinoma. *J. Clin. Oncol.* **16**, 2261–6.

Kelm, C., Achatzy, R., Ritscher, R., Wahlers, B., Wörn, H., and Kunze, W. P. (1988). Chirurgie von Lungenmetastasen. *Thorac. Cardiovasc. Surgeon* **36**, 118–21.

Kent, S.E. and Majumdar, B. (1985). Metastatic tumours in the maxillary sinus: a report of two cases and a review of the literature. *J. Laryngol. Otol.* **99**, 459–62.

Kessler, O.J., Mukamel, E., Weinstein, R., Gayer, E., Konichezky, M., and Servadio, C. (1998). Metachronous renal cell carcinoma metastasis to the contralateral adrenal gland. *Urology* **51**, 539–43.

Kierney, P.C., van Heerden, J.A., Segura, J.W., and Weaver, A.L. (1994). Surgeon's role in the management of solitary renal cell carcinoma metastases occurring subsequent to initial curative nephrectomy: an institutional review. *Ann. Surg. Oncol.* **1**, 345–52.

Kim, B. and Louie, A. C. (1992). Surgical resection following interleukin 2 therapy for metastatic renal cell carcinoma prolongs remission. *Arch. Surg.* **127**, 1343–9.

King, G. J., Kostuik, J. P., McBroom, R. J., and Richardson, W. (1991). Surgical management of metastatic renal carcinoma of the spine. *Spine* **16**, 265–71.

Klugo, R.C., Detmers, M., Stiles, R.E., Talley, R.W., and Cerny, J.C. (1977). Aggressive versus conservative management of stage IV renal cell carcinoma. *J. Urol.* **118**, 244–6.

Kobayashi, K., Kawamura, M., and Ishihara, T. (1999). Surgical treatment for both pulmonary and hepatic metastases from colorectal cancer. *J. Thorac. Cardiovasc. Surg.* **118**, 1090–6.

Kozlowski, J.M. (1994). Management of distant solitary recurrence in the patient with renal cancer. Contralateral kidney and other sites. *Urol. Clin. N. Am.* **21**, 601–24.

Krishnamurthi, V., Novick, A.C., and Bukowski, R.M. (1998). Efficacy of multimodality therapy in advanced renal cell carcinoma. *Urology* **51**, 933–7.

Landonio, G., Baiocchi, C., Cattaneo, D., Ferrari, M., Gottardi, O., Majno, M., et al. (1994). Retrospective analysis of 156 cases of metastatic renal cell carcinoma: evaluation of prognostic factors and response to different treatments. *Tumori* **80**, 468–72.

Levy, D.A., Slaton, J.W., Swanson, D.A., and Dinney, C.P.N. (1998). Stage specific guidelines for surveillance after radical nephrectomy for local renal cell carcinoma. *J. Urol.* **159**, 1163–7.

Livartowski, A., Chapelier, A., Beuzeboc, P., Dierick, A., Asselain, B., Dartevelle, P., et al. (1998). Exérèse chirurgicale de métastases pulmonaires de cancer du sein: à propos de 40 patientes. *Bull. Cancer* **85**, 799–802.

Lo, C.Y., van Heerden, J.A., Soreide, J.A., Grant, C.S., Thompson, G.B., Lloyd, R.V., et al. (1996). Adrenalectomy for metastatic disease to the adrenal glands. *Br. J. Surg.* **83**, 528–31.

Maeda, H., Nakahara, K., Ohno, K., Fujii, Y., Hashimoto, J., Miyoshi, S., et al. (1989). Surgical treatment of pulmonary metastases from osteogenic sarcoma—significance of aggressive resection of bilateral multiple metastases and tumors invading adjacent organs. *Nippon Kyobu Geka Gakkai Zasshi* **37**, 344–9.

Maldazys, J.D. and deKernion, J.B. (1986). Prognostic factors in metastatic renal carcinoma. *J. Urol.* **136**, 376–9.

Matsumoto, Y. and Yanagihara, N. (1982). Renal clear cell carcinoma metastatic to the nose and paranasal sinuses. *Laryngoscope* **92**, 1190–3.

McNichols, D.W., Segura, J.W., and DeWeerd, B.H. (1981). Renal cell carcinoma: long-term survival and late recurrence. *J. Urol.* **126**, 17–22.

Middleton, R.G. (1967). Surgery for metastatic renal cell carcinoma. *J. Urol.* **97**, 973–7.

Montie, J.E., Stewart, B.H., Straffon, R.A., Banowsky, L.H.W., Hewitt, C.B., and Montague, D.K. (1977). The role of adjunctive nephrectomy in patients with metastatic renal cell carcinoma. *J. Urol.* **117**, 272–5.

Neves, R.J., Zincke, H., and Taylor, W.F. (1988). Metastatic renal cell cancer and radical nephrectomy: identification of prognostic factors and patient survival. *J. Urol.* **139**, 1173–6.

Nielsen, O.S., Munro, A.J., and Tannock, I.F. (1991). Bone metastases: pathophysiology and management policy. *J. Clin. Oncol.* **9**, 509–24.

O'Dea, M.J., Zincke, H., Utz, D.C., and Bernatz, P.E. (1978). The treatment of renal cell carcinoma with solitary metastasis. *J. Urol.* **120**, 540–2.

Pastorino, U., Valente, M., Gasparini, M., Azzarelli, A., Santoro, A., Alloisio, M., et al. (1989). Lung resection for metastatic sarcomas: total survival from primary treatment. *J. Surg. Oncol.* **40**, 275–80.

Pastorino, U., Buyse, M., Friedel, G., Ginsberg, R.J., Girard, P., Goldstraw, P., et al., and the International Registry of Lung Metastases (1997). Long-term results of lung metastasectomy: prognostic analyses based on 5206 cases. *J. Thorac. Cardiovasc. Surg.* **113**, 37–49.

Patchell, R.A., Cirrincione, C., Thaler, H.T., Galicich, J.H., Kim, J.H., and Posner, J.B. (1986). Single brain metastases: surgery plus radiation or radiation alone. *Neurology* **36**, 447–53.

Patchell, R.A., Tibbs, P.A., Walsh, J.W., Dempsey, R.J., Maruyama, Y., Kryscio, R.J., et al. (1990). A randomized trial of surgery in the treatment of single metastases to the brain. *New Engl. J. Med.* **322**, 494–500.

Pogrebniak, H.W., Haas, G., Linehan, W.M., Rosenberg, S.A., and Pass, H.I. (1992). Renal cell carcinoma: resection of solitary and multiple metastases. *Ann. Thorac. Surg.* **54**, 33–8.

Pongracz, N., Zimmerman, R., and Kotz, R. (1988). Orthopaedic management of bony metastases of renal cancer. *Sem. Surg. Oncol.* **4**, 139–42.

Porte, H.L., Roumilhac, D., Graziana, J.P., Eraldi, L., Cordonier, C., Puech, P., et al. (1998). Adrenalectomy for a solitary adrenal metastasis from lung cancer. *Ann. Thorac. Surg.* **65**, 331–5.

Rodriguez, R., Fishman, E.K., and Marshall, F.F. (1995). Differential diagnosis and evaluation of the incidentally discovered renal mass. *Seminars in Urol. Oncol.* **13**, 246–53.

Roscoe, M.W., McBroom, R.J., Louis, E.S., Grossman, H., and Perrin, R. (1989). Preoperative embolization in the treatment of osseous metastases from renal cell carcinoma. *Clin. Orthopaed. Rel. Res.* **238**, 302–7.

Rosenberg, S.A., Yang, J.C., Topalian, S.L., Schwartzentruber, D.J., Weber, J.S., Parkinson, D.R., *et al.* (1994). Treatment of 283 consecutive patients with metastatic melanoma or renal cell cancer using high-dose bolus interleukin 2. *J. Am. Med. Assoc.* **271**, 907–13.

Roth, J.A., Putnam, J.B. Jr, Wesley, M.N., and Rosenberg, S.A. (1985). Differing determinants of prognosis following resection of pulmonary metastases from osteogenic and soft tissue sarcoma patients. *Cancer* **55**, 1361–6.

Sagalowsky, A.I., Kadesky, K.T., Ewalt, D.M., and Kennedy, T.J. (1994). Factors influencing adrenal metastasis in renal cell carcinoma. *J. Urol.* **151**, 1181–4.

Saitoh, H. (1981). Distant metastasis of renal adenocarcinoma. *Cancer* **48**, 1487–91.

Saitoh, H., Hida, M., Nakamura, K., Shimbo, T., Shiramizu, T., and Satoh, T. (1982). Metastatic processes and a potential indication of treatment for metastatic lesions of renal adenocarcinoma. *J. Urol.* **128**, 916–18.

Sandock, D.S., Seftel, A.D., and Resnick, M.I. (1997). Adrenal metastases from renal cell carcinoma: role of ipsilateral adrenalectomy and definition of stage. *Urology* **49**, 28–31.

Sauter, E.R., Bolton, J.S., Willis, G.W., Farr, G.H., and Sardi, A. (1990). Improved survival after pulmonary resection of metastatic colorectal carcinoma. *J. Surg. Oncol.* **43**, 135–8.

Seifert, J.K., Weigel, T.B., Gonner, U., Bottger, T.C., and Junginger, T. (1999). Liver resection for breast metastases. *Hepatogastroenterology* **46**, 2935–40.

Sella, A., Swanson, D.A., Ro, J.Y., Putnam, J.B. Jr, Amato, R.J., Markowitz, A.B., *et al.* (1993). Surgery following response to interferon-α-based therapy for residual renal cell carcinoma. *J. Urol.* **149**, 19–22.

Sesenna, E., Tullio, A., and Piazza, P. (1995). Treatment of craniofacial metastasis of a renal adenocarcinoma: report of case and review of literature. *J. Oral Maxillofac. Surg.* **53**, 187–93.

Shalev, M., Cipolla, B., Guille, F., Staerman, F., and Lobel, B. (1995). Is ipsilateral adrenalectomy a necessary component of radical nephrectomy? *J. Urol.* **153**, 1415–17.

Sharpless, S.M. and Das Gupta, T.K. (1998). Surgery for metastatic melanoma. *Sem. Surg. Oncol.* **14**, 311–18.

Sherry, R.M., Pass, H.I., Rosenberg, S.A., and Yang, J.C. (1992). Surgical resection of metastatic renal cell carcinoma and melanoma after response to interleukin-2-based immunotherapy. *Cancer* **69**, 1850–5.

Sioutos, P.J., Arbit, E., Meshulam, C.F., and Galicich, J.H. (1995). Spinal metastases from solid tumors: analysis of factors affecting survival. *Cancer* **76**, 1453–9.

Skinner, D.G., Colvin, R.B., Vermillion, C.D., Pfister, R.C., and Leadbetter, W.F. (1971). Diagnosis and management of renal cell carcinoma: a clinical and pathologic study of 309 cases. *Cancer* **28**, 1165–77.

Skinner, K.A., Eilber, F.R., Holmes, E.C., Eckardt, J., and Rosen, G. (1992). Surgical treatment and chemotherapy for pulmonary metastases from osteosarcoma. *Arch. Surg.* **127**, 1065–71.

Smith, E.M., Kursh, E.D., Makley, J., and Resnick, M.I. (1992). Treatment of osseous metastases secondary to renal cell carcinoma. *J. Urol.* **148**, 784–7.

Stief, C.G., Jähne, J., Hagemann, J.H., Kuczyk, M., and Jonas, U. (1997). Surgery for metachronous solitary liver metastases of renal cell carcinoma. *J. Urol.* **158**, 375–7.

Sun, S. and Lang, E.V. (1998). Bone metastases from renal cell carcinoma: preoperative embolization. *J. Vasc. Intervent. Radiol.* **9**, 263–9.

Sundaresan, N., Choi, I.S., Hughes, J.E.O., Sachdev, V.P., and Berenstein, A. (1990). Treatment of spinal metastases from kidney cancer by presurgical embolization and resection. *J. Neurosurg.* **73**, 548–54.

Swanson, D.A., Orovan, W.L., Johnson, D.E., and Giacco, G. (1981). Osseous metastases secondary to renal cell carcinoma. *Urology* **18**, 556–61.

Taneja, S.S., Pierce, W., Figlin, R., and Belldegrun, A. (1994). Management of disseminated kidney cancer. *Urol. Clin. N. Am.* **21**, 625–37.

Tanguay, S., Pisters, L.L., Lawrence, D.D., and Dinney, C.P.N. (1996a). Therapy of locally recurrent renal cell carcinoma after nephrectomy. *J. Urol.* **155**, 26–9.

Tanguay, S., Swanson, D.A., and Putnam, J.B. Jr (1996b). Renal cell carcinoma metastatic to the lung: potential benefit in the combination of biological therapy and surgery. *J. Urol.* **156**, 1586–9.

Thrasher, J.B., Clark, J.R., and Cleland, B.P. (1990). Surgery for pulmonary metastases from renal cell carcinoma: army experience from 1977–1987. *Urology* **35**, 487–91.

Tolia, B.M. and Whitmore W.F. Jr (1975). Solitary metastasis from renal cell carcinoma. *J. Urol.* **114**, 836–8.

Tongaonkar, H.B., Kulkarni, J.N., and Kamat, M.R. (1992). Solitary metastases from renal cell carcinoma: a review. *J. Surg. Oncol.* **49**, 45–8.

Torre, M., Barbieri, B., Bera, E., Locicero, S., Pieri Nerli, F., and Belloni, P.A. (1988). Surgical therapy in lung cancer with single brain metastasis. *Eur. J. Cardiothorac. Surg.* **2**, 336–9.

van der Poel, H.G., Roukema, J.A., Horenblas, S., van Geel, A.N., and Debruyne, F.M.J. (1999). Metastasectomy in renal cell carcinoma: a multicenter retrospective analysis. *Eur. Urol.* **35**, 197–203.

van Dongen, J.A., Hart, A.M., Jonk, A., Postuma, H.S., Vos, A., and van Zandwijk, N. (1986). Resection of pulmonary metastases: results, prognostic factors, reappraisal of selection criteria. *Thorac. Cardiovasc. Surgeon* **34**, 140–2.

Wanebo, H.J., Chu, Q.D., Vezeridis, M.P., and Soderberg, C. (1996). Patient selection for hepatic resection of colorectal metastases. *Arch. Surg.* **131**, 322–9.

Wroński, M., Arbit, E., Russo, P., and Galicich, J. H. (1996). Surgical resection of brain metastases from renal cell carcinoma in 50 patients. *Urology* **47**, 187–93.

Wroński, M., Maor, M.H., Davis, B.J., Sawaya, R., and Levin, V.A. (1997). External radiation of brain metastases from renal carcinoma: a retrospective study of 119 patients from the M.D. Anderson Cancer experience. *Int. J. Rad. Oncol. Biol. Phys.* **37**, 753–9.

Wunderlich, H., Schlichter, A., Reichelt, O., Zermann, D. H., Janitzky, V., Kosmehl, H., *et al.* (1999). Real indications for adrenalectomy in renal cell carcinoma. *Eur. Urol.* **35**, 272–6.

46. Gene therapy for metastatic kidney cancer

Nejd F. Alsikafi and Mitchell H. Sokoloff

Introduction

In the year 2000, kidney tumors (of which renal cell carcinoma (RCC) predominates) were diagnosed in more than 31 200 people and resulted in nearly 12 000 deaths (Greenlee *et al.* 2000). While localized lesions are amenable to cure with surgery, metastatic disease continues to be a major source of morbidity and mortality. Approximately one-third of patients with RCC present with evidence of disseminated disease. Moreover metastasis will subsequently develop in an additional 30 to 40 per cent of patients with localized or locally advanced disease (Figlin 1999; Vogelzang and Stadler 1998). While the 5-year survival of patients with localized disease treated surgically is greater than 90 per cent, 5-year survival of patients with metastatic RCC remains less than 30 per cent despite recent advances in systemic therapies (Figlin 1999; Vogelzang and Stadler 1998).

Metastatic RCC is immunologically sensitive and can be treated with cytokines. Interleukin 2 (IL-2) has emerged as the single most effective immune modulator against kidney cancer. Among 1712 patients treated with IL-2 alone, a 15.4 per cent overall response rate was achieved including a complete response rate of 3.8 per cent (Figlin 1999; Figlin and Raghavan 1999; Vogelzang and Stadler 1998; Belldegrun 2000). When combined with interferon α (IFNα), the overall response rate increased to 20.6 per cent (Vogelzang and Stadler 1998). Cytokine therapy is accompanied by significant clinical side-effects, however, which limit its application (Smith 1997). In an attempt to overcome this toxicity, other immunotherapeutic approaches, such as tumor-infiltrating lymphocyte (TIL) and dendritic cell (DC) therapies have been developed. These have demonstrated success, albeit limited, against metastatic RCC (Gitlitz *et al.* 1996; Hoffman *et al.* 2000).

In contrast to immunotherapy, chemotherapy has been remarkably ineffective in treating metastatic RCC. A review of more than 70 agents used in phase II trials in more than 4500 patients between 1983 and 1993 demonstrated an objective response in 6.8 per cent of patients, all with a short duration of response (Yagoda *et al.* 1995). Chemotherapy's poor efficacy is hypothesized to result from a high multidrug resistance (MDR)-1 gene product and p-glycoprotein that work to actively transport the chemotherapeutic metabolites out of the tumor cells.

Because of the limitations of systemic cytokine administration and the established cellular therapies for RCC, novel treatments are being developed that capitalize on RCC's hallmark therapeutic characteristic, its immunosensitivity. Gene therapy is one such approach. On the basis of successes in using gene therapy techniques to enhance the efficacy of TIL therapy (Rosenberg *et al.* 1990, 1993; Cao *et al.* 1998), researchers have examined the potential of expanding the role of gene therapy in kidney cancer (Galanis *et al.* 1999; Schmidt-Wolf *et al.* 1999). Such studies are still in the early phases of development and several paramount issues remain unresolved, including the identification of optimal kidney cancer-killing genes, developing efficient methods of gene delivery, and refining the role of gene transfer in adoptive (that is, TIL) and active (that is, vaccine) therapies. In fact, at the time of publication, gene therapy for RCC is truly experimental and little clinical data regarding its efficacy exist. Nonetheless, it holds promise for becoming a powerful component of our anti-RCC armamentarium and warrants discussion. As such, this chapter will review the methodology of gene therapy and the identification of important cytokine and non-cytokine therapeutic agents. The principal investigative strategies employing gene therapy strategies against RCC and current US federally funded protocols utilizing gene therapy regimens against RCC will be summarized.

Principles and practice of gene therapy

Gene therapy involves the introduction of genetic material into a cell with the intent of replacing (or reconstituting) the original DNA or adding additional sequences capable of enhancing or suppressing normal cellular function (Hwu and Rosenberg 1999; Morgan and Anderson 1993; Mulligan 1993). To be effective, the methodology of gene therapy must include the selection of an effective and selective gene transfer vector, efficient incorporation of the gene of interest into the target cell, and activation of the genetic material to induce a therapeutic effect. With regard to anticancer gene therapy, the intended result may involve the direct destruction of tumor cells or, alternatively, the enhancement of a host antitumor immune response (Fig. 46.1). To illustrate the latter approach, Fig. 46.2 demonstrates how a gene encoding granulocyte–macrophage colony-stimulating factor (GM-CSF) may be utilized to help a patient mount an anticancer immune response.

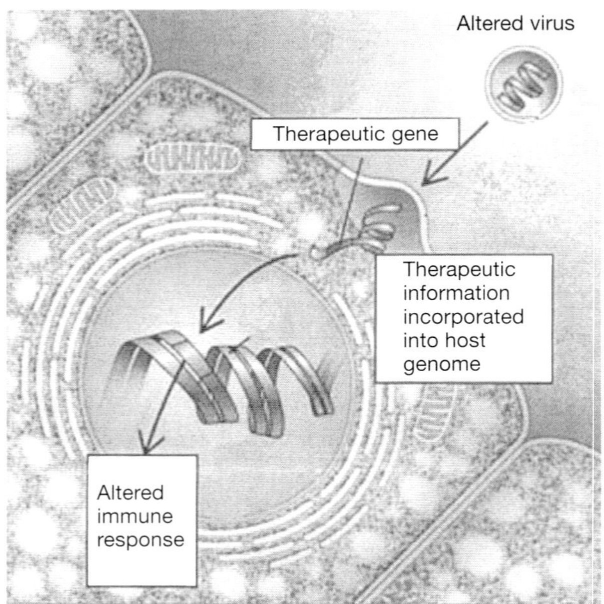

Fig. 46.1 Illustration of how gene therapy can be utilized to enhance the host antitumor immune response and/or directly eradicate tumor cells *in vivo*.

Fundamentals of gene therapy

Gene therapy can be defined as the transfer of new genetic material into the cells of an individual with a resulting therapeutic benefit to that individual (Hwu and Rosenberg 1999; Morgan and Anderson 1993; Mulligan 1993). Contemporary strategies to treat various forms of cancer must include that of gene therapy, as malignancies appear to be the result of a number of genetic lesions, often the activation of dominant-acting oncogenes or the inactivation of tumor suppressor genes (Israel 1993). Gene therapy can be used to restore the activity of the normal allelic make-up of these cells by directly introducing functional homologs or by inhibiting oncogene activity. Gene therapy can also be used to enhance the cytotoxic and immunostimulatory effects of natural host defence mechanisms. Finally, gene therapy offers the ability to deliver toxic products to tumor cells or to confer sensitivity to toxic drugs.

Therapeutic genes

Neoplastic development involves a complex interplay between endogenous and external factors (Weinberg 1989). The conversion of a normal cell to a malignant tumor cell involves genetic alterations such as mutations, rearrangements, amplifications, or deletions. The events that occur depend upon the genetic susceptibility of the host, numerous growth factors and hormones that regulate cellular differentiation, and, often, the expression of oncogenes and suppressor genes. Any of these can be targets for gene therapy.

Oncogenes and suppressor genes

Cellular growth and proliferation are regulated by a balance between growth-promoting oncogenes and growth-constraining suppressor genes (Weinberg 1989, 1991; Peehl 1993). Activation of an oncogene is believed to involve the loss of associated negative regulatory (tumor suppressor) genes. Loss of suppressor gene activity removes a constraint on oncogene expression and allows cell proliferation and tumorigenesis. Gene therapy affords a mechanism by which these negative regulatory sequences can be reinstated, thus preventing neoplastic development. By inserting wild-type suppressor genes into tumor cells, the resemblance of orderly growth control can be restored and tumor cells can revert to a more normal growth pattern.

Cytokines

Cytokines are soluble factors that are responsible for communication between cells of the immune system. They are important elements in the antitumor immune response: in addition to direct

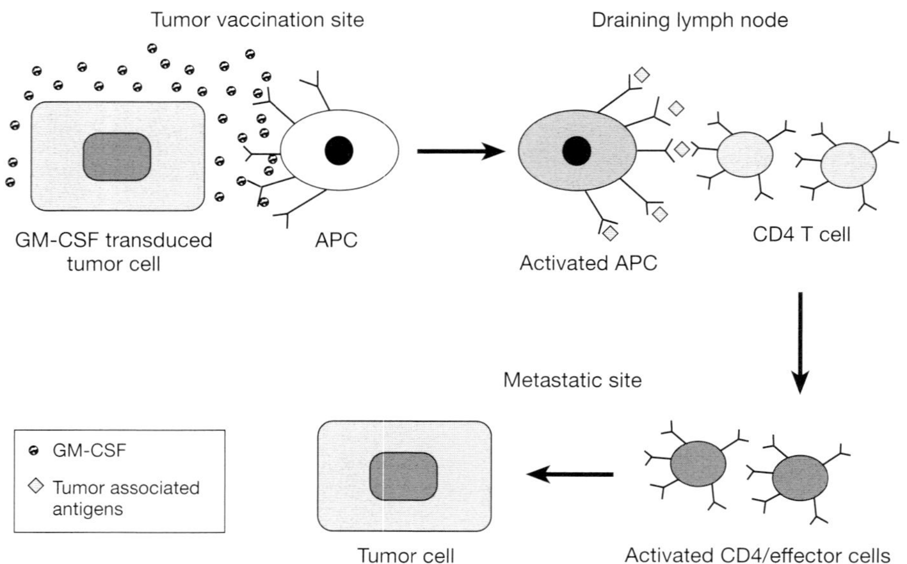

Fig. 46.2 Specific schematic of a GM-CSF-secreting tumor vaccine.

tumoricidal effects, they also activate effector components of the immune system (Knuth *et al.* 2000; Wolf *et al.* 2000). The introduction of cytokine genes into tumor cells has been proven to enhance antitumor immune responses in both *in vitro* and *in vivo* studies.

Suicide and toxic genes

Another strategy to combat cancer involves the targeted delivery to tumor cells of genes that either encode a toxic product or confer sensitivity to a toxic drug (Hwu and Rosenberg 1999; Shalev *et al.* 2000). One such example is the use of the herpes simplex virus-thymidine kinase (HSV-tk) 'suicide' gene. Cells transfected with, and thus expressing, the thymidine kinase gene show enhanced ability to incorporate acyclovir and gancyclovir into newly synthesized DNA. When these drugs are given systemically after cellular incorporation of the tk gene, DNA strand breaks occur, which ultimately prevents cellular proliferation and causes apoptosis (programmed cell death) (Shirakawa *et al.* 1999). The gene encoding for cytosine deaminase can also be used to prime cell death. Cells expressing this gene are able to synthesize 5-fluorouracil (5-FU) from 5-fluorocytosine (a nontoxic drug delivered systemically), causing cell lysis in only those cells transfected with the cytosine deaminase gene (Shirakawa *et al.* 1999). In theory, a deadly cytotoxic agent, such as the diphtheria toxin gene, can be selectively delivered to a tumor cell, causing cell death (Vallera *et al.* 2000).

An important concept germane to gene therapy is that of the 'bystander effect'. This describes the process by which an entire tumor mass is successfully destroyed despite subtotal transfection of the tumor cells with the target gene. Complete tumorilysis can occur when expression of gene products on the transfected subset of tumor cells attracts enough immune effector cells to destroy the entire lesion, or when endogenous cytotoxic substances are released from successfully transfected cells, which then lyse surrounding cells.

Gene transfer vectors: introducing DNA into cells

The critical first step in gene therapy is transduction, the process of transferring DNA into appropriate target cells (Hwu and Rosenberg 1999; Mulligan 1993). Different methods for delivering genetic material in a highly efficient manner have been developed, each suitable for different forms of therapy. Transfers can be accomplished either *ex vivo* (removing the target cells from the individual, transducing the cells *in vitro*, followed by reintroducing the modified cells back to the patient) or *in vivo* (in which genetic material is directly transferred into cells and tissues of the patient).

The choice of a particular gene transfer technique will depend on the biologic requirements of the specific therapeutic strategy. Gene transfers are performed by vectors, the term given to biologic constructs that transfer the engineered DNA or RNA sequences that encode therapeutic information (Hwu and Rosenberg 1999; Mulligan 1993). Vectors are categorized into two main classes: viral and nonviral. The viral vectors are attenuated viruses in which the therapeutic gene is introduced. These include retroviruses, adeno- and adeno-associated viruses (AAV), pox viruses, and lentiviruses (Wivel and Wilson 1998; Nayak *et al.* 1996; Yei *et al.* 1994; Lipkowitz *et al.* 1999; Wild *et al.* 1990; Lever *et al.* 1999). Examples of nonviral vectors include cationic lipids, calcium phosphate transfection, microinjection, and the 'gene-gun' gene transfer (Dass *et al.* 2000; Seigne *et al.* 1999; Mendriatta

et al. 1999; Coleman *et al.* 1998). While transfection rates with nonviral vectors are much less than with viral vectors, they are convenient and have obvious safety advantages over viral methods. Currently, no single vector has been identified or designed with all the desirable features of every therapeutic application of cancer gene therapy (Simons and Marshall 1998; Steiner and Gingrich 2000). An analysis of each of the viral and nonviral vectors is beyond the scope of this chapter. An overview schematic of the different characteristics of the vectors are catalogued in Table 46.1.

Gene therapy for renal cell carcinoma

Rationale for anti-RCC gene therapy and putative applications

Early observations of spontaneous regression of human RCC tumors suggested a role for immunotherapy in treating metastatic disease. Subsequently, over the past two decades, various applications of immunotherapy for RCC have been advanced (Figlin 1999; Figlin and Raghavan 1999; Vogelzang and Stadler 1998; Belldegrun 2000). These immunotherapeutic approaches offer a golden opportunity to apply the principles and practice of gene therapy.

We have already referred to three mechanisms by which gene therapy can be applied to treat human cancers. Because of RCC's inherent immunogenicity, two such approaches hold the most promise for treating metastatic RCC. In the first, cytokine or other immunogenic genes (such as major histocompatibility (MHC) B7-1) can be inserted into RCC tumor cells to enhance the tumor's inherent immunogenicity. This produces a 'tumor vaccine' that is intended to stimulate a cellular immune response against the tumor cells (Parmiani *et al.* 2000; Belldegrun *et al.* 1993*a*). This can be accomplished by introducing cytokine genes into tumor cells *ex vivo*, followed by the reintroduction of the genetically altered tumor cells back into the patient, resulting in active immunization against the tumor. Alternatively, the immune-enhancing genes can be given systemically, with a vector engineered to selectively target tumor cells. In either case, the resulting immune response would, hopefully, involve acute cytotoxic activity (T-cell mediated) as well as memory against subsequent corruption with the tumor (T- and B-cell mediated).

Gene therapy can also be used to directly augment the antitumor activity of immune system effector cells. The introduction of cytokines into RCC TIL cells has been shown to increase their antitumor activity, enhance their survival in circulation, and enable the delivery of large quantities of cytokines directly to a tumor site without many of the adverse side-effects seen with systemic immunotherapy (Schmidt-Wolf *et al.* 1999; Belldegrun *et al.* 1993*a*; Hathorn *et al.* 1994).

In addition to immunotherapeutic applications, gene therapy has been touted as a promising anticancer therapy because of the fundamental doctrine that oncogenesis results from mutations or deletions of cellular DNA. The third application of anticancer gene therapy is, therefore, to introduce genetic material into tumor cells *in vivo* (such as tumor suppressor genes, anti-sense and ribozyme genes, suicide genes, and toxic genes (for example, diphtheria toxin)), with the intent of inducing tumor cell death.

RCC is particularly apropos to such an approach, as specific genetic aberrations have been implicated in the development of kidney cancer (Zisman *et al.* 2000; Chen *et al.* 1995). These include von Hippel–Lindau (VHL) gene mutations and overexpression of c-myc (a DNA regulatory protein involved with DNA repair and cellular proliferation) and Pax-2 (an embryonic transcriptional factor suspected in the development of the metanephric blastoma). In addition, G250, a cellular surface antigen of unknown function that is found almost exclusively on neoplastic kidney cells, affords a potential target for selective delivery of genetic material to kidney cancer cells (Durrbach *et al.* 1999).

Immunotherapy: the foundation of anti-RCC gene therapy

The immune system contributes to the surveillance and destruction of tumor cells (Knuth *et al.* 2000; Wolf *et al.* 2000; Hrounda *et al.* 1997). Multiple cellular and humoral immune effectors inhibit tumor proliferation. Cellular mediators with antitumor activity include MHC-restricted cytotoxic T cells (Tc) and natural killer (NK) cells. The goal of immunotherapy is to sensitize these immune effector cells to tumor antigen(s) and induce a tumori-lytic response directed against the tumor with minimal systemic toxicity. Gene therapy offers the ability to deliver immunogenic elements directly to tumor cells.

Adoptive immunotherapy

Adoptive immunotherapy involves the *ex vivo* manipulation and modification of immune effector cells before reintroduction into the host (Gitlitz *et al.* 1996; Hoffman *et al.* 2000). Immune cells with antitumor reactivity are expanded before being transferred back to the tumor-bearing host to attack sites of cancerous cells. One such example is TIL cells, which have been shown to cause regression in RCC (Hoffman *et al.* 2000). TIL are isolated from solid tumors and are grown by preparing a single-cell suspension of tumor tissue and then culturing these cells with IL-2. After expansion of these cells in culture, they are given back to the patient in the hope that they will destroy tumor sites within the body as well as help stimulate the host immune system to recognize tumor cells. Transfection of the TIL cells with IL-2 increases HLA antigen presentation and enhances activation of the cellular immune system *in vivo*.

Table 46.1 Characteristics of viral and nonviral vectors

Vector	Insert size (kb)	Potential advantages	Potential disadvantages
Viral vectors			
Retrovirus	4–5	Integration into genome Requirement of cell division for transduction	Low transduction efficiency Packaging cell line required No tissue-specific targeting Replication competent
Adenovirus	30–40	High transduction efficiency Infection of many cell types Transduction does not require cell division Large insert size Immunogenic	No integration into genome Packaging cell line required Immunogenic No tissue-specific targeting Replication competence
Adeno-associated virus	5	Integration Infection does not require cell division Immunogenic	No tissue-specific targeting Packaging cell line required Immunogenic
Vaccinia	25	Large insert size Immunogenic	No tissue-specific targeting Moderate to high toxicity Low transduction efficiency Immunogenic
Avipox	5–10	Transduction does not require cell division Large insert size Immunogenic	No tissue-specific targeting Low transduction efficiency Moderate to high toxicity Immunogenic
Herpes simplex	40–50	Neuronal tropism Large insert size Latency	No tissue-specific targeting Packaging cell line required Moderate to high toxicity
Nonviral vectors			

Mechanical	N/A	No limitation on size of
		  nucleic acid
			No tissue-specific targeting
			Possible requirement for surgical
			  procedure
			Low transduction efficiency

Cationic lipid complexes	N/A	Completely synthetic No limitation on size and type of nucleic acid	No tissue-specific targeting Inefficient

Active immunotherapy

Tumor vaccine protocols also utilize the ability of cytokines to increase tumor cell immunogenicity, thereby increasing the ability of the host immune system to recognize and destroy cancer foci. Autologous tumor cells are transfected *ex vivo* with cytokine-producing genes. These transfected cells, now producing cytokines and expressing increased MHC class I antigens, are implanted into the host where they stimulate a tumor-specific immune response (Parmiani *et al.* 2000; Zisman *et al.* 2000). Dendritic cell therapy is also a form of active immunotherapy. In this case, host antigen-presenting cells (APC) are harvested and exposed ('pulsed') by tumor antigens, whereby they become activated. They are then infused back into the host, where they stimulate a tumor-specific immune response (Schreurs *et al.* 2000). Both tumor vaccine and dendritic cell protocols have been applied to RCC. Active immunotherapy can also utilize the systemic infusion of immune, toxic, suppressor, and/or suicide genes conjoined to a tumor-specific vector, with the intent that the vector will selectively target tumor cells deposits and induce tumor cell death. At this time, such a systemic approach has not been widely applied to RCC.

Cytokines: potential therapeutic genes for anti-RCC-directed gene therapy

Cytokines have a prominent function in the stimulation of the immune response and the enhancement of tumor immuno-genicity (Knuth *et al.* 2000; Wolf *et al.* 2000). Systemic cytokine therapy has been used with some success to treat RCC and is, in a pure sense, the most simplistic application of anti-RCC active immunotherapy (Figlin 1999; Figlin and Raghavan 1999; Vogelzang and Stadler 1998; Belldegrun 2000; Gitlitz *et al.* 1996). Cytokines can also be effective when introduced into either immune-effector or kidney tumor cells (Cao *et al.* 1998; Galanis *et al.* 1999; Schmidt-Wolf *et al.* 1999). A major advantage of genetically introducing cytokines into tumor cells is the production of very high levels of cytokines in the tumor microenvironment. This results in the recruitment and attachment of immune effector cells directly to sites of cancer cell deposition. The immune cells can then stimulate a systemic anticancer host response. In contrast, systemic administration of cytokines results in low concentrations *in vivo*, is associated with more severe side-effects, and less accurately mimics the paracrine nature by which cytokines normally interact to regulate immune responses. Cytokine therapy has shown success in the treatment of metastatic RCC and promises to maintain a principal role in anti-RCC gene therapy. In fact, at this time, genes that encode cytokine production are the most promising type of genetic material to be used in anti-RCC gene therapy.

Interleukin 2

IL-2 is produced by activated T cells (Belldegrun 2000; Smith 1997). It enhances NK- and T-cell proliferation, survival, and effector function, namely, cytolysis of tumor cells. IL-2 is the most commonly used cytokine to treat metastatic RCC. The combination of IL-2 with other cytokines, including IFNα, IFNγ, IL-10, IL-12, and IL-18 may improve its efficacy (Zisman *et al.* 2000). Low-dose IL-2 may have counterproductive effects, inducing significant immunosuppression as a result of T-cell apoptosis in the absence of effective T-cell receptor cross-linking or the provision of co-stimulatory signals necessary for an effective immune response (Lenardo 1991; Boehme and Lenardo 1993). In the light of this, the use of low-dose IL-2 therapy may need to be re-evaluated.

Interleukin 4

Preclinical and clinical studies have indicated that IL-4 also has potent antitumor activity (Vokes *et al.* 1998; Obiri *et al.* 1993). Although a precise mechanism of action has yet to be defined, it is hypothesized that broad activation of eosinophils, macrophages, CD8+ T cells, and dendritic cells plays a role. IL-4 acts synergistically with IL-2 in the generation of tumor-specific killer cells. It increases humoral cell production and differentiation and recruits antigen-presenting macrophages to tumor sites, which then enhance the T-cell response. In addition, an increase in endothelial cell intercellular adhesion molecule expression, which facilitates targeting and migration of eosinophils, may contribute.

IFNα and IFNγ

In cancers that are traditionally considered to be immunosensitive, interferon therapy is advocated because of its ability to stimulate subsets of immune effector cells capable of attacking established systemic disease (Belldegrun *et al.* 1993*b*; Tomita *et al.* 1992; Ogasawar and Rosenberg 1993). IFNα has direct antitumor activity, induces a marked increase in the surface expression of class I MHC antigens, and upregulates adhesion molecule expression on the surface of tumor cells, aiding the immune response. IFNγ augments and enhances the cytotoxic activity of both T and NK cells. In addition, IFNγ can upregulate the cellular expression of MHC class I and class II antigens, thereby improving the presentation of antigenic peptides to T helper cells. Although initial results were promising, the current role of interferon therapy in RCC is controversial (Zisman *et al.* 2000; Naitoh and Belldegrun 1998).

Tumor necrosis factor

Tumor necrosis factor (TNF) augments the antitumor activity of cytotoxic T and NK cells, enhances the expression of HLA class I and intercellular adhesion molecule (ICAM)-1 molecules on the tumor cell surface, and lymphokine-activated killer cells (LAK) cell activity (Goldman 1997; Griffith *et al.* 2000). TNF has been used in several clinical trials for a variety of solid organ malignancies with moderate partial and complete response rates (Braczkowski *et al.* 1998).

Granulocyte–macrophage colony-stimulating factor

GM-CSF stimulates the differentiation of hematopoietic progenitor cells into dendritic cells, the most potent antigen-presenting cell, which can induce an immune response (Zisman *et al.* 2000; Schreurs *et al.* 2000; Bubenick 1999). GM-CSF increases the presentation of tumor antigens on dendritic cells, thereby stimulating both CD4+ and CD8+ T-cell-mediated tumor immunity. The use of GM-CSF has been shown to generate an antineoplastic immune response in poorly immunogenic tumor models, and its efficacy has been shown in preclinical models of RCC and prostate carcinoma, as well as others (Nelson *et al.* 2000; Simons *et al.* 1997). Clinical trials using GM-CSF-transfected RCC tumor vaccines have had minimal therapeutic effect (Simons *et al.* 1997).

Noncytokine genes used to treat RCC

HLA-B7

HLA-B7 is an adhesion molecule that binds to the CD28 receptor of T cells and is classified as a co-stimulator of the cellular immune response (Jung *et al.* 1998; Antonia and Seigne 2000). T cells need two signals before they can mount a cytotoxic response. The first is the binding of the T-cell receptor (TCR) to an antigenic tumor peptide presented in conjunction with the MHC molecule. The second is the binding of CD28 on the T cell to B7-1 on the 'foreign' cell. RCC cells do not normally express B7-1. Therefore, the expression induced by transfection of RCC cells by an exogenous B7-1 gene might increase the immunogenicity of the tumor cells. This has been demonstrated in mice, in which the injection of tumor cells transfected with B7-1 resulted in the T-cell-mediated rejection of tumor cells (Antonia and Seigne 2000).

Tumor-specific delivery

The use of suicide and toxic genes has yet to be explored in clinical trials for RCC. As with any gene therapy trial using such an approach, tissue-specific delivery is paramount. The therapeutic genes must be delivered selectively to the tumor deposits without infecting (and injuring) normal, healthy tissue. As such, the gene or the vector can be engineered so as to include a tissue- or tumor-specific promoter so that expression is limited to the cancer cells (Steiner and Gingrich 2000). This approach has received much attention in prostate cancer, where prostate-specific antigen (PSA) and prostate membrane antigen (PSMA) have tissue-specific expression (Steiner and Gingrich 2000; Latham *et al.* 2000).

A tissue-specific antigen, known as G250, has been characterized in RCC. Approximately 90 per cent of primary and 50–80 per cent of metastatic RCC lesions express G250 (Vissers *et al.* 1999; Oosterwijk *et al.* 1995). G250 is absent in normal tissue. The toxicity, pharmacokinetics, and localization capabilities of radiolabeled G250 have been assessed in patients with RCC (Oosterwijk *et al.* 1993). More than 90 per cent of primary and metastatic RCC sites were visualized in this manner, including some tumor deposits that were later confirmed by surgery despite being absent on computerized tomography (CT) and magnetic resonance imaging (MRI) scans. Subsequently, two phase I/II trials using ^{131}I-labeled G250 were undertaken. In the first, 33 patients were given escalating doses of ^{131}I-labeled murine anti-G250 monoclonal antibody (mAb) (Divgi *et al.* 1998). All tumors > 2 cm were successfully targeted by the radioactively labeled antibodies. Although there were no major responses, 17 of the 33 patients had stable disease. The treatment was generally well-tolerated, with minimal toxicity. In the second study, 12 patients received a chimeric ^{131}I-labeled anti-G250 mAb (Steffens *et al.* 1999). One patient had stable disease while a second experienced a partial response. Two patients experienced grade 4 toxicity. These studies demonstrate that G250 affords a target by which a gene therapy cassette or a liposome-coated vector can be directed specifically to RCC cells.

Anti-RCC clinical trials in gene therapy

Tumor vaccines: modification of tumor cells with genes that enhance immunogenicity

In the first human clinical trial of genetically engineered cancer cell vaccines for RCC, 18 patients with kidney cancer were treated with a GM-CSF-transfected RCC vaccine (Nelson *et al.* 2000; Simons *et al.* 1997). Kidney cancer cells were removed at surgery, propagated *ex vivo*, and then genetically modified to secrete high levels of GM-CSF via transduction with a GM-CSF-containing retrovirus. After being irradiated, the kidney tumor cells were administered subcutaneously as vaccines to 18 patients with advanced kidney cancer. The vaccine treatment was well tolerated, with only minor toxicities. Anticancer immune responses were triggerred, as manifest by conversion of delayed-type hypersensitivity (DTH) skin responses against irradiated autologous cancer cells after vaccination. In addition, biopsies of vaccine sites yielded evidence of vaccine cell recruitment of dendritic cells, T cells, and eosinophils. One patient with measurable kidney cancer metastases treated at the highest vaccine dose level experienced a partial treatment response. Correlative studies were also performed (Baccala *et al.* 1998).

The HLA-B7 gene, encoding allogeneic MHC class I antigen, has also been introduced into RCC cells in the hope of restoring the expression of surface antigens required for appropriate cytotoxic T lymphocyte (CTL) stimulation (Jung *et al.* 1998). Recently, at our institution, 15 patients were treated with escalating amounts of a lipid-formulated plasmid DNA encoding for the MHC HLA-B7 gene product, Allovectin-7 (Rini *et al.* 1999). Allovectin-7 was injected directly into tumor deposits. The treatment was safe and asociated with minimal toxicity. Although there were no significant clinical responses, three patients had evidence of TIL infiltrates at their tumor sites. In a second clinical trial, patients with metastatic RCC were treated with an autologous gene modified tumor cell vaccine expressing HLA-B7.1 in combination with systemic IL-2 (Antonia and Seigne 2000; Seigne *et al.* 2000). Toxicity was minimal and several patients experienced increased DTH responses with a large perivascular T-cell infiltration. In one patient there was a 90 per cent reduction in lung metastases. A second patient experienced stable disease. Current trials of HLA-B7 are ongoing at several academic centers (Zisman *et al.* 2000).

Genetic modification of immune effector cells

Since 1990, when the first human clinical gene transfer trial into TIL cells was approved for patients with metastatic melanoma (Rosenberg *et al.* 1990), researchers have expanded the potential of TIL transduction to include the introduction of cytokine and other immune-modulating genes. TNF has been transduced into TIL cells after murine studies demonstrated potent antitumor activity (Rosenberg 1992). In clinical trials, however, TNF toxicity was high. IL-2 has also been introduced into TIL, under the hypothesis that, with increased expression of IL-2, the TIL cells would become able to stimulate themselves in an autocrine fashion, proliferating in an IL-2-independent fashion while still maintaining antigen specificity (Galanis *et al.* 1999; Schmidt-Wolf *et al.* 1999; Yamada *et al.* 1987; Karsuyama *et al.* 1989; Treisman *et al.* 1995). This is precisely what happened, and prolonged cell survival was demonstrated. Investigators at UCLA transfected an

Table 46.2 NIH-funded clinical trials for renal cell cancer

Title of clinical trial	Institution
Phase I pilot study of immunization with allogeneic HLA-A2-matched RCC cells transduced with a gene for IL-2 in patients with advanced RCC	MSKCC
Phase I pilot study of IFNγ-transduced autologous tumor cell vaccine for metastatic RCC	NCI
Phase I study of B7-1 gene modified autologous tumor cell vaccine plus IL-2 in patients with stage IV RCC	MSKCC
Phase I study of gene therapy with intralesional allovectin-7, an HLA-B7 plasmid DNA–lipid complex, plus concurrent low-dose IL-2 for metastatic RCC	NCI
	UCLA
Phase I study of vaccination with nonviable autologous tumor cells with or without transduction with a GM-CSF-secreting gene for metastatic RCC	Johns-Hopkins
Phase I/II trial of leuvectin as an immunotherapeutic agent by direct gene transfer in patients with metastatic melanoma, RCC, and sarcoma	Mayo Clinic
	UCLA
Phase II study of gene therapy with intralesional allovectin-7, an HLA-B7 plasmid DNA–lipid complex, for metastatic cancer	NCI

* MSKCC, Memorial Sloan–Kettering Cancer Center; NCI, US National Cancer Institute.

autologous RCC tumor line with the IL-2 gene as a potent immune stimulant for propagating TIL (Mulders *et al.* 1998). TIL grown in this manner had enhanced CD4+ and CD8+ populations, cytokine production, and HLA-restricted tumor-specific cytotoxicity. Additional efforts are focusing on identifying promotor-enhancer regions that result in higher levels of gene expression in order to optimize this treatment strategy.

Current trials

A list of US National Institutes of Health (NIH)-funded clinical trials for RCC is presented in Table 46.2.

Conclusions

Disappointing clinical outcomes and recent scrutinization by government and regulatory agencies have exposed a number of practical and technical weaknesses in the principles and practice of anticancer gene therapy. As a result, its future is unclear. Certainly, at the present time, systemic gene therapy is not the 'magic bullet' that will eradicate human cancer as it was once hailed. Improvements in tumor-specific targeting and the development of more effective therapeutic genes are needed. Nonetheless, gene therapy as a technique is a powerful resource with which other anticancer treatments can be augmented and enhanced.

Moreover, as a result of compelling preclinical studies, gene therapy continues to hold promise that it some day might evolve into an effective anticancer therapeutic modality. In particular, successful utilization of gene therapy techniques to improve upon immunotherapeutic approaches for cancer has established a role for it. This is especially pertinent to renal cell cancer, in which gene therapy has been used to enhance the propogation and potency of anti-RCC immune effector cells. It is impossible to speculate whether tumor vaccines or the systemic delivery of cytotoxic genetic material will ever prove effective against RCC. However, as long as the excitement over results from preclinical studies is maintained, research efforts will continue to focus on optimizing the role of gene therapy in the treatment of cancer.

References

Antonia, S.J. and Seigne, J.D. (2000). B7-1 gene-modified autologous tumor-cell vaccines for renal-cell carcinoma. *World J. Urol.* **18** (2), 157.

Baccala, A.A., Zhong, H., Clift, S.M., *et al.* (1998). Serum vascular endothelial growth factor is a candidate biomarker of metastatic tumor response to *ex vivo* gene therapy of renal cell carcinoma. *Urology* **51** (2), 327.

Belldegrun, A. (2000). Expanding the indications for surgery and adjuvant interleukin-2-based immunotherapy in patients with advanced renal cell carcinoma. *Cancer J. Sci. Am.* **6** (1), 88.

Belldegrun, A.S., Tso, C.L., Sakata, T., *et al.* (1993*a*). Human renal carcinoma line transfected with interleukin-2 and/or interferon-alpha genes: implications for live cancer vaccines. *J. Natl Cancer Inst.* **85** (3), 207.

Belldegrun, A., *et al.* (1993*b*). Interferon-alpha primed tumor infiltrating lymphocytes combine with IL-2 and interferon-alpha as therapy for metastatic renal cell cancer. *J. Urol.* **150** (5), 1384.

Boehme, S.A. and Lenardo, M.J. (1993). Propriocidal apoptosis of mature T lymphocytes occurs at S phase of the cell cycle. *Eur. J. Immunol.* **23**, 1552.

Braczkowski, R., Zubelewicz, B., Romanowski, W., *et al.* (1998). Possible biological indicators of the response to recombinant tumour necrosis factor alpha in patients with advanced neoplasms. *J. Exp. Cancer Res.* **17** (3), 349.

Bubenick, J. (1999). Granulocyte–macrophage colony-stimulating factor gene-modified vaccines for immunotherapy of cancer. *Folia Biol.* **45** (4), 115.

Cao, L., Kulmburg, P., Veelken, H., *et al.* (1998). Cytokine gene transfer in cancer therapy. *Stem Cells* **16** (suppl. 1), 251.

Chen, F., Kishida, T., Duh, F.M., *et al.* (1995). Suppression of growth of renal carcinoma cells by von Hippel–Lindau tumor supressor gene. *Cancer Res.* **55** (21), 4804.

Coleman, M., Muller, S., Quezada, A., *et al.* (1998). Nonviral interferon-alpha gene therapy inhibits growth of established tumors by eliciating a systemic immune response. *Hum. Gene Ther.* **9** (15), 2223.

Dass, C.R., Walker, T.L., Kalle, W.H., and Burton, M.A. (2000). A microsphere-liposome vector for targeted gene therapy of cancer. *Drug Deliv.: J. Deliv. Target. Ther. Agents* **7** (1), 15.

Divgi, C.R., Bander, N.H., Scott, A.M., *et al.* (1998). Phase I/II radio-immunotherapy trial with iodine-131-labeled monoclonal antibody G250 in metastatic renal cell carcinoma. *Clin. Cancer Res.* **4** (11), 2729.

Durrbach, A., Angevin, E., Poncet, P., *et al.* (1999). Antibody-mediated endo-cytoloysis of G250 tumor associated antigen allows targeted gene transfer to human renal cell carcinoma *in vitro*. *Cancer Gene Ther.* **6** (6), 564.

Figlin, R.A. (1999). Renal cell carcinoma: management of advanced disease. *J. Urol.* **161** (2), 381.

Galanis, E., Hersh, E.M., Stopeck, A.T., *et al.* (1999). Immunotherapy of advanced malignancy by direct gene transfer of an interleukin-2 DNA/DMRIE/DOPE lipid complex: phase I/II experience. *J. Clin. Oncol.* **17** (10), 3313.

Gitlitz, B.J., Belldegrun, A.S., and Figlin, R.A. (1996). Immunotherapy and gene therapy. *Sem. Urol. Oncol.* **14** (4), 237.

Goldman, M. (1997). Advances in immunotherapy. Cellular and molecular basis of modern immunotherapy. *Acta Clin. Belg.* **52** (4), 193.

Greenlee, R.T., Murray, T., Bolden, S., and Wingo, P.A. (2000). Cancer statistics, 2000. *CA Cancer J. Clin.* **50** (1), 7.

Griffith, T.S., Anderson, R.D., Davidson, B.L., *et al.* (2000). Adenoviral-mediated transfer of the TNF-related apoptosis-inducing ligand/Apo-2 ligand gene induces tumor cell apoptosis. *J. Immunol.* **165** (5), 2886.

Hathorn, R.W., Tso, C.L., Kaboo, R., *et al.* (1994). *In vitro* modulation of the invasive and metastatic potentials of human renal cell carcinoma by interleukin-2 and/or interferon-alpha gene transfer. *Cancer* **74** (7), 1904.

Hoffman, D.M., Belldegrun, A.S., and Figlin, R.A. (2000). Adoptive cellular therapy. *Sem. Oncol.* **27** (2), 221.

Hrounda, D., Muir, G.H., and Dalgleish, A.G. (1997). The role of immunotherapy for urological tumours. *Br. J. Urol.* **79** (3), 307.

Hwu, P. and Rosenberg, S.A. (1999). Gene therapy of cancer. In *Cancer: principles and practice of oncology* (ed. V.T. DeVita, *et al.*). Lippincott Williams and Wilkins, Philadelphia, 3005–19.

Israel, M.A. (1993). Molecular approaches to cancer therapy. *Advan. Cancer Res.* **61**, 57.

Jung, D., Jaeger, E., Cayeux, S., *et al.* (1998). Strong immunogenic potential of a B7 retroviral expression vector: generation of HLA-B7-restricted CTL response against selectable marker genes. *Hum. Gene Ther.* **9** (1), 53.

Karsuyama, H., Tohyama, N., and Tada, T. (1989). Autrocrine growth and tumorigenicity of interleukin 2-dependent helper T cells transfected with IL-2 gene. *J. Exp. Med.* **169**, 13.

Knuth, A., Jager, D., and Jager, E. (2000). Cancer immunotherapy in clinical oncology. *Cancer Chemother. Pharmacol.* **46** (suppl.), 46.

Latham, J.P., Searle, P.F., Mautner, V., and James, N.D. (2000). Prostate-specific antigen promoter-enhancer driven gene therapy for prostate cancer: construction and testing of a tissue-specific adenovirus vector. *Cancer Res.* **60** (2), 334.

Lenardo, M. (1991). Interleukin-2 programs mouse alpha beta T lymphocytes for apoptosis. *Nature* **353**, 858.

Lever, A.M., Kaye, J.F., McCann, E., *et al.* (1999). Lentivirus vectors for gene therapy. *Biochem. Soc. Trans.* **27** (6), 841.

Lipkowitz, M.S., Hanss, B., Tulchin, N., *et al.* (1999). Transduction of renal cells *in vitro* and *in vivo* by adeno-associated virus gene therapy vectors. *J. Am. Soc. Nephrol.* **10** (9), 1908.

Mendriatta, S.K., Quezada, A., Matar, M., *et al.* (1999). Intratumoral delivery of IL-12 gene by polyvinyl polymeric vector system to murine renal and colon carcinoma results in potent antitumor immunity. *Gene Ther.* **6** (5), 833.

Morgan, R.A. and Anderson, W.F. (1993). Human gene therapy. *Ann. Rev. Biochem.* **62**, 191.

Mulders, P.H., Tso, C.L., Pang, S., *et al.* (1998). Adenovirus-mediated interleukin-2 production by tumors induces growth of cytotoxic tumor-infiltrating lymphocytes against human renal cell carcinoma. *J. Immunother.* **21** (2), 170.

Mulligan, R.C. (1993). The basic science of gene therapy. *Science* **260** (5110), 926.

Naitoh, J. and Belldegrun, A. (1998). Interferon and kidney cancer: a promise unfulfilled? *Cancer J. Sci. Am.* **4** (3), 155.

Nayak, S.K., McCallister, T., Han, L.J., *et al.* (1996). Transduction of human renal carcinoma cells with human gamma-interferon via retroviral vector. *Cancer Gene Ther.* **3** (3), 143.

Nelson, W.G, Simons, J.W., Mikhak, B., *et al.* (2000). Cancer cells engineered to secrete granulocyte–macrophage colony-stimulating factor using *ex vivo* gene transfer as vaccines for the treatment of genitourinary malignancies. *Cancer Chemother. Pharmacol.* **46** (suppl.), 67.

Obiri, N.I., Hillman, G.G., Haas, G.P., *et al.* (1993). Expression of high-affinity interleukin-4 receptors on human renal cell carcinoma cells and inhibition of tumor cell growth *in vitro* by interleukin-4. *J. Clin. Invest.* **91** (1), 88.

Ogasawar, M. and Rosenberg, S.A. (1993). Enhanced expression of HLA molecules and stimulation of autologous human tumor infiltrating lymphocytes following transduction of melanoma cells with gamma-interferon genes. *Cancer Res.* **35**, 3561–8.

Oosterwijk, E., Bander, N.H., Divgi, C.R., *et al.* (1993). Antibody localization in human renal cell carcinoma. *J. Clin. Oncol.* **11**, 738.

Oosterwijk, E., Debruyne, F.M.J., and Schalken, J.A. (1995). The use of monoclonal antibody G250 in the therapy of renal cell carcinoma. *Sem. Oncol.* **22** (1), 34.

Parmiani, G., Rodolfo, M., and Melani, C. (2000). Immunological gene therapy with *ex vivo* gene-modified tumor cells: a critique and a reappraisal. *Hum. Gene Ther.* **11** (9), 1269.

Peehl, D.M. (1993). Oncogenes in prostate cancer. *Cancer Suppl.* **71** (3), 1159.

Rini, B.I., Selk, L.M., and Vogelzang, N.J. (1999). Phase I study of direct intralesional gene transfer of HLA-B7 into metastatic renal cell carcinoma lesions. *Clin. Cancer Res.* **5** (10), 2766.

Rosenberg, S.A. (1992). The immunotherapy and gene therapy of cancer. *J. Clin. Oncol.* **10** (1), 180.

Rosenberg, S.A., Aebersold, P., Cornetta, K., *et al.* (1990). Gene transfer into humans: immunotherapy of patients with advanced melanoma, using tumor-infiltrating lymphocytes modified by retroviral gene transduction. *New Engl. J. Med.* **323**, 570.

Rosenberg, S.A., Anderson, W.F., Blaese, M., *et al.* (1993).The development of gene therapy for the treatment of cancer. *Ann. Surg.* **218**, 455.

Schmidt-Wolf, I.G., Finke, S., Trojaneck, B., *et al.* (1999). Phase I clinical study applying autologous immunological effector cells transfected with the interleukin-2 gene in patients with metastatic renal cancer, colorectal cancer, and lymphoma. *Br. J. Cancer* **81** (6), 1009.

Schreurs, M.W., Eggert, A.A., Punt, C.J., *et al.* (2000). Dendritic cell-based vaccines: from mouse models to clinical cancer immunotherapy. *Crit. Rev. Oncogen.* **11** (1), 1.

Seigne, J., Turner, J., Diaz, J., *et al.* (1999). A feasibility study of gene gun mediated immunotherapy for renal cell carcinoma. *J. Urol.* **162** (4), 1259.

Seigne, J.D., Diaz, J.I., Muro-Cacho, C., *et al.* (2000). Preliminary results of a phase I trial of an autologous gene modified tumor cell vaccine expressing B7.1 in combination with systemic interleukin-2 in metastatic renal cell carcinoma. *J. Urol.* **163** (4, suppl.), 179.

Shalev, M., Kadmon, D., The, B.S., *et al.* (2000). Suicide gene therapy toxicity after multiple and repeat injections in patients with localized prostate cancer. *J. Urol.* **163** (6), 1747.

Shirakawa, T., Gardner, T.A., Ko, S.C., *et al.* (1999). Cytotoxicity of adenoviral-mediated cytosine deaminase plus 5-fluorocytosine gene therapy is superior to thymidine kinase plus acyclocir in a human renal cell carcinoma model. *J. Urol.* **162** (3, part 1), 949.

Simons, J.W. and Marshall, F.F. (1998). The future of gene therapy in the treatment of urologic malignancies. *Urol. Clin. N. Am.* **25** (1), 23.

Simons, J.W., Jaffee, E.M., Weber, C.E., *et al.* (1997). Bioactivity of autologous irradiated renal cell carcinoma vaccines generated by *ex vivo* granulocyte– macrophage colony-stimulating factor gene transfer. *Cancer Res.* **57** (8), 1537.

Smith, K.A. (1997). Rational interleukin-2 therapy. *Cancer J. Sci. Am.* **3**, 137.

Steffens, M.G., Boerman, O.C., Mulder, P.H., *et al.* (1999). Phase I radioimmotherapy of metastatic renal cell carcinoma with 131I-labeled chimeric monoclonal antibody G250. *Clin. Cancer Res.* **5** (10, suppl.), 3268.

Steiner, M.S. and Gingrich, J.R. (2000). Gene therapy for prostate cancer: where are we now? *J. Urol.* **164** (4), 1121.

Tomita, Y., *et al.* (1992). Interferon-gamma but not tumor necrosis factor alpha decreases susceptibility of human renal cancer cell lines to lymphokine-activated killer cells. *Cancer Immunol. Immunother.* **35**, 381.

Treisman, J., Hwu, P., Minamoto, S., *et al.* (1995). Interleukin-2-transduced lymphocytes grow in an autocrine fashion and remain responsive to antigen. *Blood* **85**, 139.

Vallera, D.A., Jin, N., Baldrica, J.M., *et al.* (2000). Retroviral immunotoxin gene therapy of acute myelogenous leukemia in mice using cytotoxic T cells transduced with an interleukin-4/diphtheria toxin gene. *Cancer Res.* **60** (4), 976.

Vissers, J.L., De Vries, I.J., Schreurs, M.W., *et al.* (1999). The renal cell carcinoma-associated antigen G250 encodes a human leukocyte antigen (HLA)-A2.1-restricted epitope recognized by cytotoxic T lymphocytes. *Cancer Res.* **59** (21), 5554.

Vogelzang, N.J. and Stadler, W.M. (1998). Kidney cancer. *Lancet* **352** (9141), 1691.

Vokes, E.E., Figlin, R., Hochster, H., *et al.* (1998). A phase II study of recombinant human interleukin-4 for advanced or recurrent non-small cell lung cancer. *Cancer J. Sci. Am.* **4** (1), 46.

Weinberg, R.A. (1989). Oncogenes, antioncogenes, and the molecular bases of multistep carcinogenesis. *Cancer Res.* **49**, 3713.

Weinberg, R.A. (1991). Tumor suppressor genes. *Science* **254**, 1138.

Wild, F., Giraudon, P., Spehner, D., *et al.* (1990). Fowlpox virus recombinant encoding the measles virus fusion protein: protection of mice against fatal measles encephalitis. *Vaccine* **8**, 441.

Wivel, N.A. and Wilson, J.M. (1998). Methods of gene delivery. *Hematol. Oncol. Clin. N. Am.* **12** (3), 483.

Wolf, S.F., Lee, K., Swiniarski, H., *et al.* (2000). Cytokines and cancer immunotherapy. *Immunol. Invest.* **29** (2), 143.

Yagoda, A., Abi-Rached, B., and Petrylak, D. (1995). Chemotherapy for advanced renal cell carcinoma, 1983–1993. *Sem. Urol. Oncol.* **22** (1), 42.

Yamada, G., Kitamura, Y., Sonada, H., *et al.* (1987). Retroviral expression of the human IL-2 gene in a murine T cell line results in cell growth autonomy and tumorigenicity. *EMBO J.* **6**, 2705.

Yei, S., Mittereder, N., Tank, K., O'Sullivan, C., and Trapnell, B.C. (1994). Adenovirus-mediated gene transfer for cystic fibrosis: quantitative evaluation of repeated *in vivo* vector administration to the lung. *Gene Ther.* **1**, 192.

Zisman, A., Pantuck, A.J., and Belldegrun, A.S. (2000). Immune and genetic therapies for advanced renal cell carcinoma. *Rev. Urol.* **2** (1), 54.

47. Brain metastases

Gregory J. Rubino

For patients with renal cell carcinoma (RCC), one of their most frightening moments occurs when they learn that their disease has spread to the central nervous system (CNS). Most physicians hold the perception that patients with RCC metastatic to the brain have a poor prognosis (Halperin and Harisiadis 1983; Decker *et al.* 1984). While brain metastases generally occur during the later stages of cancer, many modern treatment options are highly effective in controlling intracranial disease. This chapter reviews the incidence of CNS metastasis, the symptoms, patient prognostic factors, and historical and current treatment options.

Incidence

The yearly incidence of brain metastases is rising. Recent estimates of all brain metastases exceed 150 000 new cases each year (Young 1998). Factors contributing to this rise include improved neurologic imaging, which is capable of detecting smaller intracranial tumors, and increased imaging use for staging. With advances in systemic treatments, patients who live longer are more likely to develop distant metastases, including brain metastases. One-third of patients with RCC will already have metastatic disease at initial presentation (Kavolius *et al.* 1998; Kozlowski 1994; Ritchie and deKernion 1987; Giuliani *et al.* 1990). The most common sites for renal cell cancer metastasis are the lung (57 per cent), bone (19 per cent), lymph nodes (11 per cent), and brain (8 per cent) (Kavolius *et al.* 1998). Others have reported incidence of brain metastases from 4 to 13 per cent (Marshall *et al.* 1990; Gay *et al.* 1987; Mori *et al.* 1998). Autopsy series demonstrate a 10 per cent incidence of brain metastases (Becker *et al.* 1999; Saitoh *et al.* 1982). More than half of patients with RCC brain metastases have multiple brain metastases (Mori *et al.* 1998).

Brain metastases are hematogenously spread, arising at the gray–white junction where circulating tumor emboli lodge and grow (O'Neill *et al.* 1994; Delattre *et al.* 1988). The valveless vertebral epidural venous system (Batson's plexus) has been implicated in disseminating intrapelvic tumors (Batson 1942). The distribution of RCC brain metastases parallels brain weight and blood flow, with approximately 80 per cent found in the cerebral hemispheres and 20 per cent found in the posterior fossa (Delattre *et al.* 1988).

Symptoms

Patients suffering from brain metastases present with a myriad of symptoms. Largely due to the increasing frequency of obtaining brain magnetic resonance imaging (MRI) scans in asymptomatic patients, a significant number of asymptomatic brain metastases have been reported (Seaman *et al.* 1995). RCC brain metastases often induce a large amount of peritumoral edema that may cause CNS symptoms. Either a large intracranial tumor volume or large amount of peritumoral edema may cause nonlocalizing symptoms from increased intracranial pressure, including headache, nausea, and vomiting. Headache is the most common presenting symptom, seen in 24–34 per cent of patients with brain metastases. Focal symptoms are observed when the tumor's mass or edema disrupts eloquent cortical areas, subcortical pathways, or brainstem nuclei, or compresses cranial nerves. Focal weakness is the presenting symptom in 16–32 per cent of patients. Other presenting symptoms include sensory deficits (2–4 per cent), ataxia (9–12 per cent), cranial nerve dysfunction (7–22 per cent), aphasia (9–12 per cent), or behavioral changes (14–24 per cent) (Nussbaum *et al.* 1996; Culine *et al.* 1998; Wronski *et al.* 1997). Between 10 and 16 per cent of patients present with seizure.

Factors contributing to prognosis

Many studies describe factors that portend improved survival, thereby attempting to provide guidance to physicians about which patient groups would most benefit from aggressive treatment. These studies often contradict each other. The most consistent favorable prognostic factor for patients with RCC brain metastases is long (> 1 year) disease-free interval, defined as the time from diagnosis of the primary tumor to the diagnosis of metastatic disease (Kavolius *et al.* 1998; Culine *et al.* 1998; Maldazys and deKernion 1986; deKernion *et al.* 1978; Buatti *et al.* 1995). Other studies place importance upon number of metastatic foci (Neves *et al.* 1988), completeness of resection of the primary tumor and the metastases (deKernion *et al.* 1978), and patient performance status (Decker *et al.* 1984; Maldazys and deKernion 1986; Nieder *et al.* 2000).

Diagnosis

Brain MRI is the diagnostic study of choice. While computer-assisted tomography (CT) may demonstrate larger intracranial tumors, a contrast-enhanced MRI is the most sensitive study available to show numbers of brain metastases and size of tumors. Due to its superior definition of neural structures and triplanar imaging, MRI best defines the tumors' relationship to intracranial structures. Brain MRI is also capable of demonstrating sub-arachnoid spread of disease. For patients with symptoms localizable to the spine, the cervical, thoracic, and lumbar spine may be surveyed with MRI for intradural disease. CT provides superior bone imaging for spine metastases when assessing structural stability. Because extent of systemic disease factors into choosing the best treatment option, the oncologist may re-assess the extent of systemic disease with CT scans of the chest, abdomen, and pelvis and with a bone scan.

Treatment options

Without treatment, 1-month median survival is reported for patients who present with neurologic symptoms (Mehta *et al.* 1992; Posner 1974). The short duration from presentation to death does not necessarily reflect rapid tumor growth. Our experience from observing the growth of untreated brain metastases on serial MRI indicates that many smaller tumors grow relatively slowly. Tumors measuring less than 2 mm in diameter often take 3–6 months to grow to greater than 1 cm in diameter. The short survival typically reported is the result of selection bias toward symptomatic patients. These patient present with neurologic symptoms because their metastases are either great in number or in size. Patients with large brain tumor burden or large lesions have short survivals.

Patients with neurologic symptoms should receive corticosteroids. The exact mechanism of action is unknown. Corticosteroids enhance extracellular fluid absorption and decrease capillary permeability. Corticosteroids decrease brain edema and often relieve the patient's symptoms. Prolonged use may cause diabetes, gastrointestinal bleeding, myopathy, and immune and adrenal suppression. After treatment and upon resolution or stabilization of neurologic deficits, corticosteroids should be tapered to limit their potentially damaging side-effects.

Most patients found to have intracranial metastases should be treated with prophylactic anti-epileptic medication. The presence of the tumor, the surrounding edema, and the subsequent treatments all contribute to lowering the patient's seizure threshold. While usually causing no permanent neurologic injury, most generalized seizures frighten both patients and families and can be avoided with medical prophylaxis.

Radiotherapy: whole-brain

Whole-brain radiotherapy has been used to treat brain metastases for over four decades (Black 1993; Cairncross *et al.* 1980; Berk 1995; Coia 1992). It has become the community standard for patients who suffer from brain metastases. Because the prognosis for this patient population has been considered grim, radiation oncologists have tailored this palliative treatment to achieve the best results with the least number of treatments.

Many fractionation schemes have been examined with the goal of optimizing tumor control in the shortest time and with the lowest morbidity. There is a trade-off between convenience and efficacy of large fractions delivered in short periods and the safety of smaller fractions delivered over longer periods. Hendrickson (1977) compared several fractionation schemes (10 Gy single dose, 20 Gy/1 week, 30 Gy/2 weeks, 30 Gy/3 weeks, 40 Gy/3 weeks, 40 Gy/4 weeks), finding that higher doses in shorter schedules provided more prompt and durable symptomatic improvement

Table 47.1 Whole-brain radiotherapy

Reference	Number of subjects	Histology	Median survival (months)	Radiation dose (Gy)
Culine *et al.* 1998	68	Renal cell	7	
Wronski *et al.* 1997	19	Renal cell	4.4	30
Rodriguez *et al.* 1992	13	Ovarian	7	
Noordjik *et al.* 1994	31	Mixed	6	40
Boogerd *et al.* 1993	29	Breast	2.5	
Sundstrom *et al.* 1998	75	Mixed	4	25
Cairncross *et al.* 1980	183	Mixed	3	
Epstein *et al.* 1993	30	Mixed	4.9	48
	53	Mixed	5.4	54
	44	Mixed	7.2	64
	26	Mixed	8.2	70
Ryan *et al.* 1995	283	Lung	3.2	< 30
	63	Lung	4.8	> 30
Wong *et al.* 1996	86	Mixed	4	20*

* Re-irradiated after failure at 30 Gy.

but no change in the survival of 4.8 months. Cairncross *et al.* (1980) used a higher whole-brain dosing regimen of three fractions of 5 Gy/fraction, followed 4 days later with eight additional fractions of 3 Gy/fraction. His analysis revealed that patients treated with whole-brain radiotherapy lived longer and with fewer neurologic symptoms than untreated patients. Median survival was only 3 months because most patients treated with whole-brain radiotherapy died of systemic disease prior to succumbing to their intracranial disease.

The most common current fractionation schedule is 10 fractions of 3 Gy/fraction delivered over 2 weeks. However, higher fractionation schemes are still being evaluated. Epstein *et al.* (1993) reported superior survival times and improved neurologic function in patients with solitary brain metastases with whole-brain doses of 32 Gy administered in 1.6 Gy fractions twice daily (also called 'hyperfractionation'), followed by boost doses to 48, 54, 64, and 70 Gy. Survivals increased with increasing dose, from 4.9 months with 48 Gy to 8.2 months with 70 Gy. The survivals achieved with whole-brain radiotherapy treatments, summarized in Table 47.1, range from 2.5 to 8 months.

RCC is widely considered to be radioresistant (Onufrey and Mohiuddin 1985). Perhaps because of its biologic radioresistance and the limited efficacy of whole-brain radiotherapy, studies focusing on patients with renal cell metastases report poor survivals with whole-brain radiotherapy similar to those of the general studies discussed above (Culine *et al.* 1998; Maor *et al.* 1988). Wronski *et al.* (1997) reported a median survival of 4.4 months for 119 patients with renal cell brain metastases treated with whole-brain radiotherapy only. He found improved survival in subgroups of patients with one brain metastasis (versus multiple lesions), with the absence of extracranial metastases, and with small (< 2 cm) tumors.

Side-effects of whole-brain radiotherapy include fatigue, hair loss, nausea, and serous otitis media. Fatigue affects the majority of patients undergoing treatment, beginning 12–14 days after the start of treatment and lasting 2–6 weeks after treatment. About 5 per cent of patients will experience a resurgence of somnolence 2 months after treatment. Hair thinning and loss may be expected in all patients receiving greater than 10 Gy. Hair often grows back 2–6 months after treatment. Nausea and serous otitis media affect 10 per cent of patients and may last for 2–4 weeks after treatment completion.

Complications from whole-brain radiotherapy are minimized because survival is poor. Similarly to Cairncross *et al.*'s (1980) findings, patients with metastatic disease often succumb to systemic disease before developing neurocognitive decline from the cranial radiotherapy. Many patients surviving more than 1 year after whole-brain radiotherapy develop some degree of cognitive impairment. In 20 patients who survived 2.4–10.6yrs after whole-brain radiotherapy, Johnson *et al.* (1985) report that 60 per cent suffered abnormal mental status examinations and 65 per cent had abnormal neuropsychological testing. DeAngelis *et al.* (1989) report that 2–5 per cent of long-term survivors suffered radiation-induced dementia, and advocate delivery of smaller fractions (1.8–2 Gy/fraction daily to 40–45 Gy) for patients with controlled systemic disease.

Due to its toxic effects to normal brain parenchyma, many believe that whole-brain radiotherapy may be used once to treat patients with intracranial metastases. New brain metastases are common after whole-brain radiotherapy. Treatment options for recurrence after whole-brain radiotherapy include additional palliative re-irradiation with whole-brain radiotherapy (Wong *et al.* 1996), radiosurgery, or surgical excision.

Radiotherapy: stereotactic radiosurgery

Over the past several decades, stereotactic radiosurgery has been used to successfully treat patients with brain metastases from RCC. By focusing a single lethal dose of radiation to a limited target volume, stereotactic radiosurgery is far more effective at treating RCC brain metastases than whole-brain radiotherapy, with reduced neurotoxicity. There are two methods by which focused radiation may be delivered: linear accelerator (LINAC)-based radiosurgery and 'gamma-knife' radiosurgery. LINAC utilizes converging arcs or shaped-beams and gamma-knife uses 201 converging beams to focus the radiation. Both LINAC and gamma-knife systems utilize the convergence of multiple radiation beams to accomplish high central doses and sharp 'drop-off' of radiation dose. By focusing the radiation upon a small target volume, lethal doses of radiation may be delivered to the tumor while the surrounding brain parenchyma receives a minimal radiation dose. This limits the potential injury to the brain or neural structures adjacent to the brain metastasis. The treatment volumes generated by converging beams are spherical, which conveniently matches the spherical shape of most brain metastases. Treatment volumes are generally small so that dose drop-off is rapid and does not damage surrounding neural structures.

Lars Leksell (1989) developed the gamma-knife system in Stockholm during the 1950s. Current gamma-knife units contain 201 cobalt sources, radially distributed over the convexity segment of the skull (Lunsford *et al.* 1990). The circular beams are collimated towards a common point located in the center of a collimator helmet. To deliver the focused radiation to the brain metastasis, the tumor must be placed at the center where the beams converge. Changing collimator helmets that have beam diameters of 4 to 18 mm varies the treatment volume. Single isocenter treatment volumes may range in size from 3 to 17 mm. Larger and nonspherical tumors may be treated with multiple isocenters. However, the dose distribution of a multiple isocenter plan is inhomogeneous, meaning that different parts of the tumor receive different radiation dosages. The gamma-knife system focusing accuracy is reported to be 0.3 mm (Wu *et al.* 1990). Radiosensitive structures may be shielded by obstructing single beam channels.

The alternative system to the gamma-knife, the linear accelerator (LINAC, Fig. 47.1), was adapted to deliver focused radiation by many groups from around the world during the 1980s. Betti *et al.* (1983, 1989, 1991) first coupled a commercial LINAC unit with the Talairach stereotactic system to precisely focus radiation with multiple radiation arcs. Columbo, Benedetti, and colleagues (1985, 1986) built a stereotactic frame to fix the intracranial target to the rotational isocenter of a LINAC. The Heidelberg group

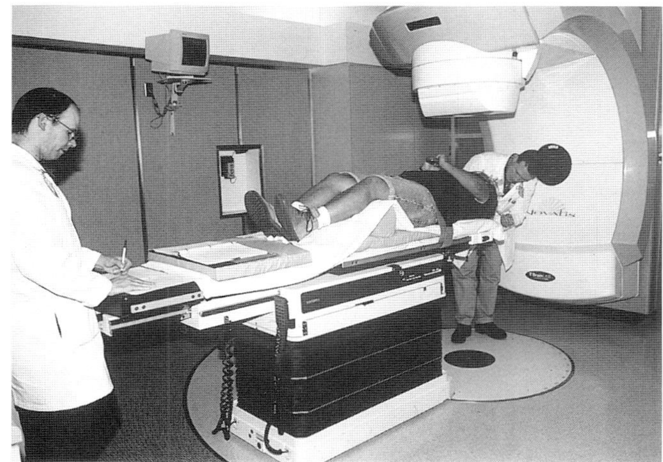

Fig. 47.1 Linear accelerator dedicated to stereotactic radiosurgical use.

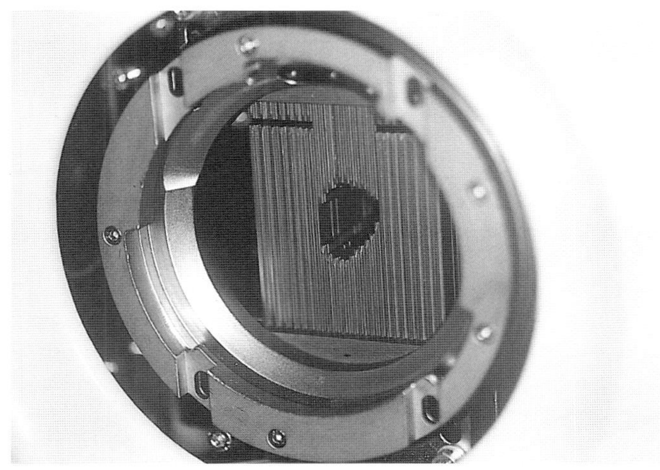

Fig. 47.2 Mini-multileaf collimator made up of 26 paired leaves that are computer-controlled to match the tumor shape.

(Hartmann *et al.* 1985; Sturm *et al.* 1987) utilized collimated narrow beams, a localizing system, and a special computer program to concentrate dose into small, precise volumes. The Montreal group (Podgorsak *et al.* 1988) describes dynamic radiosurgery whereby both the couch and gantry move simultaneously. Kooy and the Boston group (Kooy *et al.* 1991) improved upon targeting accuracy by separating the stereotactic head fixation from the patient couch and rigidly fixing it to the floor over the couch rotation bearings. The University of Florida group (Friedman and Bova 1989; Friedman *et al.* 1992) further refined the accuracy with a mechanical system of precision bearings that control patient and linear accelerator movements. Winston and Lutz (Lutz *et al.* 1988) developed accuracy tests that are still commonly used by radiosurgical centers for quality control.

All LINAC-based systems utilize a moving beam that is focused upon a single stereotactic target, thus generating an 'arc' of radiation. Multiple arcs are often used to generate near-spherical treatment volumes. Collimators vary in size from 5 to 40 mm and produce treatment volume diameters of 4 to 35mm. LINAC-based radiosurgical systems can accommodate larger lesions with single isocenter plans than can Gamma-knife systems. The treatment volume is shaped to accommodate nonspherical lesions by manipulating the length, orientation, and number of radiation arcs. Radiosensitive structures are excluded from the radiation arcs. Current LINAC systems use sophisticated image processing and fusion of multiple imaging modalities (CT, MRI, angiography) to improve targeting accuracy. The accuracy for LINAC-based radiosurgery systems ranges from 1 to 2 mm. However, centers equipped with linear accelerators dedicated to radiosurgical treatment may achieve system accuracy as low as 0.4 mm.

The refinement of LINAC-based radiosurgery continues. At UCLA, we currently utilize both arc-based radiosurgery, described above, and beam-based radiosurgery. The radiation beams are shaped by a 10 cm square collimator into which 26 paired computer-controlled leaves may be interposed (Fig. 47.2). This collimator is referred to as the mini-multileaf collimator. Using sophisticated image processing, the leaves within the collimator are moved to reflect the two-dimensional shadow of the tumor shape. Between 10 and 20 beams, each shaped to match the two-dimensional shadow of the tumor visualized from a 'beam's eye view', are focused upon the target from multiple angles (Fig. 47.3). These 'shaped' radiation beams converge upon a target volume, thereby delivering a homogeneous radiation dose to large and irregularly shaped lesions.

Whether gamma-knife or LINAC systems are utilized, stereotactic radiosurgery is a single-day, outpatient procedure. The patient undergoes application of a stereotactic frame followed by a series of magnetic resonance and CT scan images during the morning of treatment. The radiation oncologist, physicist, and neurosurgeon outline targets and develop a treatment plan. The

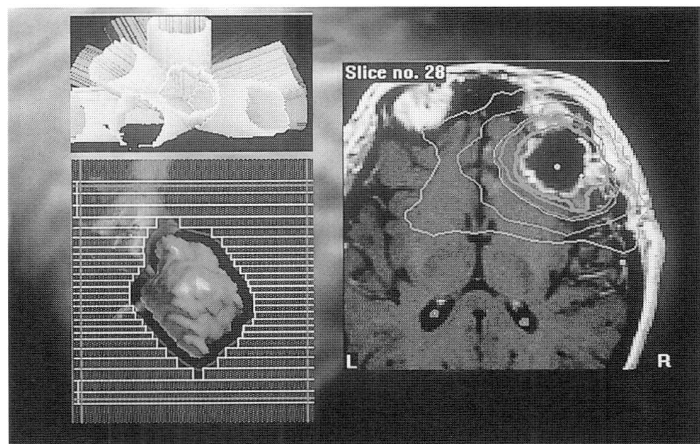

Fig. 47.3 Computer planning of stereotactic radiosurgery case using shaped beams and mini-multileaf collimator. Upper left diagram shows the converging 'shaped beams'. Lower left diagram shows the computer representation of the collimator after adding a treatment margin to the tumor volume. The right diagram shows the rapid drop-off of radiation dose. The high-isodose lines (70, 80, and 90 per cent) tightly surround the target volume while the low-isodose lines (30 and 10 per cent) spread small radiation dose.

patient undergoes the radiotherapy and is allowed to return home the same day. Patient satisfaction is high because the procedure requires only one day and is non-invasive.

Because radiosurgery is non-invasive, it may be used to treat any patient with brain metastases irrespective of their degree of disability or extent of systemic illness. Even patients with advanced systemic disease, who cannot tolerate more aggressive surgical interventions, can often tolerate radiosurgery. However, it is usually reserved for patients whose systemic disease does not limit life expectancy to less than 3 months. Radiosurgery may generate local tumor and brain edema. Therefore, patients who present with significant debilitating neurologic deficits due to large tumor size or large areas of peritumoral edema may suffer an exacerbation of their pretreatment symptoms.

Patients with up to five brain metastases may be treated with single-fraction radiosurgery. While this number is not an absolute limit to treatment, total brain radiation dose, and hence risk of toxicity, increases when treating large numbers of metastases. In addition, treatment plans become unusually complex when treating more than five lesions.

Radiosurgery is most effective when used to treat small tumors. Mehta *et al.* (1992) report that the highest tumor control rates are reported for tumors smaller than 2 cm^3. Large tumor volumes must be treated with lower total radiation doses to prevent brain injury. Radiation doses below 15 Gy undertreat the tumor, leading to ineffectual treatment and rapid recurrence. Shiau *et al.* (1997) report that doses over 18 Gy are needed for good tumor control. In general, we find that RCC brain metastases with maximal diameters under 2 cm can be effectively treated with radiosurgery. Success in treating tumors larger than 2 cm with radiosurgery is limited, probably due to RCC's biologic radioresistance.

Because the radiation is delivered with stereotactic precision and submillimeter accuracy, brain tumors located nearly any-where within the skull can be treated. The lethal radiation dosage at the center of the convergent radiation beams or arcs drops rapidly outside the intended treatment volume. Therefore, tumors located within the deep subcortical nuclei, eloquent cortical areas, and the brainstem can be treated with radiosurgery with minimal risk to the surrounding critical neural structures.

For patients who have undergone whole-brain radiotherapy, new brain metastases and tumors that continue to grow despite the whole-brain radiation treatment may be retreated focally with radiosurgery. These patients are at risk for radiation-induced cognitive decline if they receive additional whole-brain radiotherapy. Because radiosurgery focuses the radiotherapy and delivers only small additional radiation doses to the brain tissue outside the treatment volume, it is ideally suited for patients who have had whole-brain radiotherapy and suffer intracranial recurrence.

Radiosurgery is highly effective in treating brain metastases. Series from the last three decades demonstrate consistently that this treatment rivals the efficacy of surgical excision. Table 47.2 summarizes the success of gamma-knife and LINAC-based radiosurgical treatment of brain metastases. Local control rates range from 60 to 97 per cent and survival ranges from 6 to 13 months. Even for radiation-resistant brain metastases such as those associated with RCC (Fertil and Malaise 1985; Nieder *et al.* 1996), multiple studies have demonstrated local control rates between 85 and 95 per cent and survivals of 6 to 12 months using single-fraction radiosurgery (Becker *et al.* 1999).

Side-effects of radiosurgery may be immediate or delayed. Immediate side-effects include the increased risk of seizure, which usually lasts for 2–4 days after treatment. A temporary boost of prophylactic anti-epileptic medication often reduces this immediate risk. Increase in peritumoral edema may be observed within a few days of treatment, and may be treated with corticosteroids if

Table 47.2 Radiosurgery

Reference	Number of subjects/tumors	Histology	Tumor control rate (%)	Median survival (months)
Gamma-knife				
Mori *et al.* 1998	35/52	Renal cell	90	11
Somaza *et al.* 1993	23/32	Melanoma	97	9
Flickinger *et al.* 1994	116/116	Mixed	85 at 1 year 67 at 2 years	11
Mehta *et al.* 1992	40/58	Mixed	82	6.5
Jokura *et al.* 1994	25/77	Mixed		8.5
Schoeggl *et al.* 1999	97/266	Mixed	94	6
Kihlstrom *et al.* 1993	160/235	Mixed	94	7
Peterson *et al.* 1999	48/78	Mixed	90 at 1 year 61 at 2 years	12
LINAC				
Hawighorst *et al.* 1997	25/35	Mixed	88	10.5
Alexander *et al.* 1995	248/421	Mixed	85 at 1 year 65 at 2 years	9.4
Joseph *et al.* 1996	120/189	Mixed	94	8
Engenhart *et al.* 1993	69/102	Mixed	95	6
Auchter *et al.* 1996	122/122	Mixed	86	13
Fuller *et al.* 1992	27/47	Mixed	88	8.3
Adler *et al.* 1992	33/52	Mixed	91	10.5

symptomatic. Intratumoral hemorrhage may occur 1–2 months after radiosurgery. Metastatic RCC is particularly susceptible to intratumoral hemorrhage due to the vascular nature of the tumor (Bitoh *et al.* 1984; Kaiser *et al.* 1983; Bucci *et al.* 1986). It is believed that the friable tumor vessels are left without tissue support as the tumor decays and involutes, leading to vessel rupture and hemorrhage. Small and asymptomatic hemorrhages may be observed and usually resolve without intervention. Larger and clinically symptomatic hemorrhages should be surgically removed. Hemorrhage may spread viable tumor cells into the surrounding brain parenchyma, leading to diffuse recurrence.

Radiation necrosis is a late complication that may be observed from 4 months to years after treatment. While the goal of radiosurgical treatment is to induce tumor necrosis, the process occasionally extends beyond the tumor borders into the brain parenchyma. Radiation necrosis induces brain edema. When symptomatic, brain edema may be treated with corticosteroids. However, there is currently no effective medical therapy to stop the progression of radiation necrosis. Surgical resection of the necrotic brain is sometimes required for larger necrotic areas or when neurologic symptoms do not improve with steroids. Interestingly, histologic examination of radiation necrotic brain tissue often reveals nests of viable tumor cells, which may explain late recurrence.

Because radiosurgery is a focused treatment and intentionally does not deliver therapeutic radiation dose to the entire brain, small and radiographically occult tumors are not treated by radiosurgery. These tumors may grow and lead to recurrence of intracranial disease, necessitating additional radiosurgical sessions or whole-brain radiotherapy. As with whole-brain radiotherapy, new seeding of the brain with new crops of brain metastases may occur after radiosurgery. Unlike whole-brain radiotherapy, radiosurgical treatments may be repeated multiple times to effectively treat new 'crops' of tumors.

Should patients who undergo radiosurgical treatment of their brain metastases also undergo whole-brain radiotherapy? Fuller *et al.* (1992) report a higher local control rate and lower incidence of new metastases with adjuvant whole-brain radiotherapy. Additional studies, however, indicate that additional metastases may be treated effectively with additional radiosurgical sessions rather than whole-brain radiotherapy without changing survival.

Chemotherapy

While remarkable advances have been made in the systemic treatment of RCC and other cancers, the brain remains a privileged site in the body, which usually resists the beneficial effects of systemic chemical and immunologic therapies. The blood–brain barrier, while obviously imperfect for intracranial tumor vessels, appears to limit the effective treatment of brain metastases by chemotherapy. Elson *et al.* (1988) found a median survival of 4 months in 43 patients with brain metastases treated with chemotherapy. Over the past decade, wafers impregnated with chemotherapeutic drugs have been placed in the tumor resection beds of patients with high-grade gliomas. This treatment has demonstrated limited success in this patient population. If a highly effective chemotherapeutic treatment were discovered for

RCC, these wafers might prove an effective delivery vehicle because they bypass the blood–brain barrier. These wafers must be surgically implanted, and may prove to be a useful adjuvant to surgical resection.

Surgery

Surgical excision is the 'gold' standard of therapy for metastatic renal cell cancer to the brain. Neurosurgical extirpation of renal cell brain metastases offers patients the longest survival with the best quality of life (O'Dea *et al.* 1978; Salvati *et al.* 1992; Badalament *et al.* 1990; Wronski *et al.* 1996). Over the past 30 years, neurosurgical techniques and technology have improved dramatically, allowing surgical resection of lesions that were once considered unresectable with lower surgical morbidity.

Both patient and tumor factors are considered when considering surgical excision of brain metastases. The patient must be medically able to tolerate the surgical intervention. The patient's systemic disease should either be stable or slowly advancing. The patient ought to have an expected lifespan greater than 6 months to fully enjoy the benefits of surgical excision. The number of intracranial metastases is important. When surgery was first being evaluated as a treatment option, only patients with single brain metastases were considered surgical candidates (Patchell *et al.* 1990). The literature now supports surgical resection of up to three brain metastases (Bindal *et al.* 1993; Sawaya *et al.* 1996) through three separate craniotomies. The metastasis must be considered surgically accessible, with careful consideration of the expected morbidity associated with tumor access. Surgical excision is not limited by tumor size, as is radiosurgery. In fact, surgery is the preferred treatment for large tumors because it is the only treatment that will immediately relieve the tumors' mass effect and deliver symptomatic relief from neurologic symptoms.

The morbidity associated with surgery has decreased as neurosurgical access and equipment have improved. Utilization of the operating microscope facilitates extremely delicate tissue manipu-

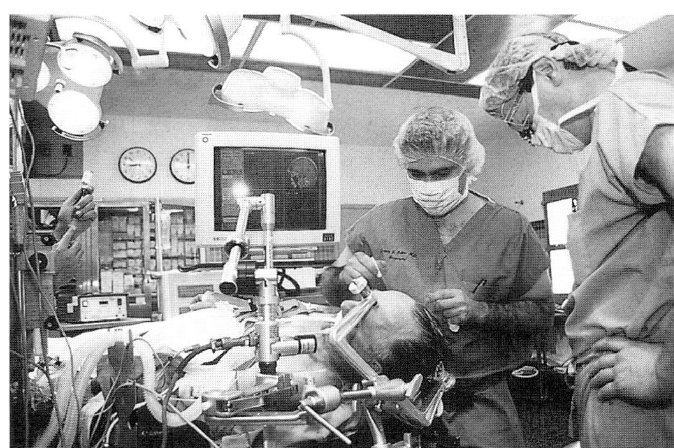

Fig. 47.4 The ISG Wand, an arm-based navigation system seen in the foreground, is rigidly fixed to the head clamp. The monitor screen is seen in the background, above the patient. The surgeon is using the system to plan a small craniotomy (see Fig. 47.5(a), (b)).

lation, thereby decreasing morbidity. Even tumors in 'eloquent' cortex, such as primary motor and speech cortex, can be removed safely, with resolution or improvements in neurologic deficits caused by the tumor (Tobler and Stanley 1994; Sawaya *et al.* 1998).

Neuronavigation

Neuronavigation instruments have contributed to the decline in surgical morbidity. Neuronavigation systems may be wand-based, or arm-based as depicted in Fig. 47.4. A typical wand-based neuronavigation system is composed of: passive reflective markers attached rigidly to the patient's head frame and to any surgical instrument or pointing 'wand' to be tracked; 2–3 infrared cameras that emit infrared light and track location of the patient's head and the surgical equipment; a computer system that both stores the preoperative MR images and drives the 'real-time' navigation system; a monitor to display images in three planes.

To use neuronavigation, the patient with metastatic tumors must undergo a volumetric, T1-weighted imaging sequence with contrast administration to highlight the tumor prior to surgery. After anesthetic induction, the patient's head is immobilized in a rigid head holder, such as the Mayfield head holder, and a reference post with reflective markers is attached to the head holder. The camera array must have direct line of sight of the reference post and the surgical area for the navigation system to work. A registration process is then performed that aligns the preoperative volumetric MR images to the patient's current head position using a surface-matching program. After calibration, the cameras may track any tool with reflective markers attached, including the pointing 'wand'. The monitor displays the location of the tool or wand in the three planes of the brain MRI. The 'wand' tool can be used before the opening to precisely map where that tumor lies beneath the skin. For deeper tumors, the neuronavigation system identifies the location of the wand's tip on the preoperative MRI (seen on the monitor), thus allowing the surgeon to precisely identify current location and 'navigate' through the patient's brain.

Arm-based systems differ from the wand-based system described above by replacing the camera system with a multi-jointed arm that is rigidly fixed to the patient's head holder. Each joint has precision sensors so that the tip of the pointer is determined by summing the position of each joint. After a similar registration process based upon surface landmarks, as detailed above, this wand can be used in a similar way to 'point' to extracranial and intracranial structures on the preoperative MRIs. The camera system is not needed in this system because the pointing arm is always rigidly connected to the patient's head. The mechanical arm can sometimes obstruct or interfere with surgical access. Other neuronavigation instruments have been developed that utilize sound or magnetic fields to track pointers. After a decade of experimentation, the camera-based system has become the commercial favorite due to its accuracy and ease of use and is most widely used.

Neuronavigation allows the surgeon to 'see' below the skin and plan surgical entry prior to starting the surgery. Figure 47.5(a) and (b) illustrates how small and directed the opening may be with neuronavigation. The craniotomy size need be only as large as the tumor, because the craniotomy can be directly placed over the

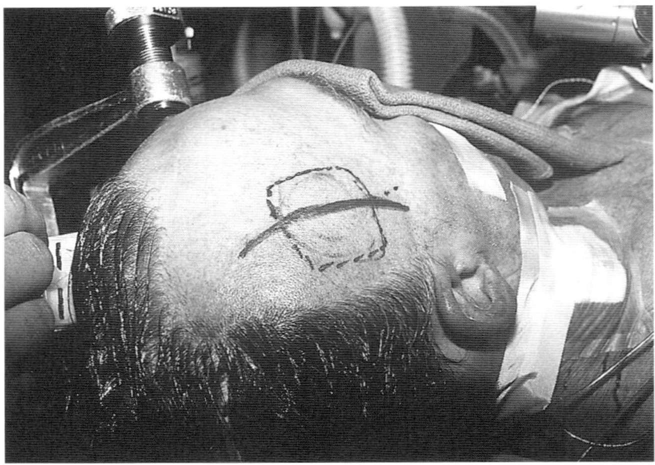

(a)

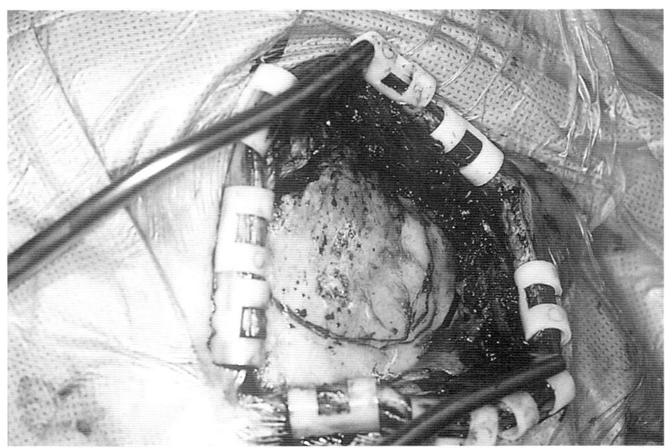

(b)

Fig. 47.5 (a) The ISG Wand was used prior to opening to outline the tumor (circle) and plan a small craniotomy (square) and skin incision. (b) The second photograph shows the small skin incision and craniotomy.

surgical access route. The small craniotomy minimizes surgically induced trauma to the scalp, muscle, and dura, limiting postoperative discomfort and speeding recovery. Because only enough brain tissue to allow surgical access is uncovered, surgical risk to the brain is also reduced. Neuronavigation may be used after opening to direct the surgeon through the brain tissue to deep-seated and smaller tumors. This guidance also limits trauma to the brain and reduces the risk of postoperative deficits.

Manufacturers of camera-based neuronavigation systems claim hardware accuracy of less than 0.5 mm and clinical accuracy of 1–2 mm, which is adequate to find and remove brain metastases. Wirtz *et al.* (1998) report the accuracy for wand-based systems as 3.3 mm for camera-based systems and for arm-based systems as 2.9 mm. Because of their high accuracy, these systems can also be used to perform frameless' stereotactic brain biopsies.

One flaw inherent to all neuronavigation systems is that their accuracy relies upon preoperatively acquired MRI. Many factors associated with surgery, including hypocarbia, mannitol diuretics, and release of cerebrospinal fluid after dural opening, and removal of mass lesions, contribute to changes in brain conformation. These brain shifts cannot be accommodated by the current neuronavigation systems. Newer systems are attempting to incorporate ultrasound guidance to update the preoperative images to reflect brain shift. While useful for leading the surgeon to the tumor, the neuronavigation system cannot demonstrate tumor removal.

iMR-guidance

The current state-of-the-art procedure for removing brain metastases is interventional MRI (iMR)-guidance. iMR allows surgeons to navigate towards the tumor, visualize the resection process, confirm complete tumor removal, and assess for intraoperative complications. The concept of intraoperative MRI and the introduction of MRI scanning equipment into the surgical suite originated in Boston during the early 1990s. The original device utilized a double-donut design: two magnets shaped like donuts are vertically positioned. The patient lies on a table and can slide through the 'donut holes', while the surgeon operates in the gap between the two donuts (Black *et al.* 1997). Because the patient's head remains within the imaging space of the magnet, new images may be acquired at any time during the surgery. The disadvantages of this concept include a small and restricted surgical space and the requirement that all surgical instrumentation and equipment must be non-ferrous and 'MRI-compatible'.

A competing concept developed in Heidelberg (Tronnier *et al.* 1997) and Erlangen (Steinmeier *et al.* 1998) wherein a twin operating room was built, one containing standard surgical equipment and the adjacent room, magnetically shielded from the first room, containing the MRI scanner. The patient is transported via a specially designed surgical table from one room to the other. The obvious advantage is that the surgeon may use all standard equipment and is not encumbered by the confines of the magnet. However, the steps necessary to acquire imaging add to the surgical time and effectively limit the number of intraoperative scans that may be obtained for each case. Practically speaking, this concept allows for one 'postresection' imaging session to check for residual tumor and complications, but is not practical for use as a neuronavigation tool.

At UCLA, we developed a third concept, termed the 'fringe-field' approach to iMR-guidance (Rubino *et al.* 2000). This concept attempts to minimize the flaws inherent in the two earlier concepts while maintaining the advantages. The UCLA concept capitalizes upon the rapid fall-off of magnetic fields around some MRI scanners. The surgery and the imaging are performed in the same room, which is divided into zones on the basis of the magnetic field strength. The surgical zone is outside the strong magnetic field. Standard surgical equipment and ferrous instruments may be used to perform surgery in this weak magnetic 'fringe-field'. Figure 47.6 shows a typical surgical set-up where all standard equipment is being used to perform a craniotomy. A rotating surgical table moves the patient's head from the surgical zone to the imaging zone when imaging is needed. Because the

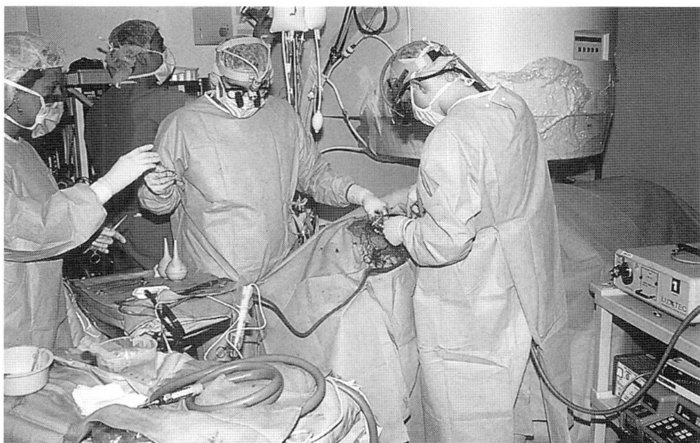

Fig. 47.6 All standard surgical instruments and equipment may be used in the weak fringe fields of the UCLA 0.2 T iMR suite. To acquire intraoperative imaging, the patient's head is moved from 'operating position' (current position) to 'imaging position', in the MRI's isocenter, seen in the background.

transition from surgical position to imaging position is relatively simple and can be accomplished in less than 1 minute, multiple imaging sessions do not unduly slow the operation. The UCLA 'fringe-field' approach is also being developed at Case Western and in Minnesota. The Minnesota group (Hall *et al.* 1999) has incorporated a 1.5 T magnet into the operating suite that permits high-resolution anatomic imaging, MR spectroscopy, diffusion-weighted imaging, and functional (BOLD) imaging.

The usual procedure for iMR-guided resection of brain metastases starts with a 'presurgical planning' imaging session. After anesthetic induction and positioning, MR markers are placed over the planned skin incision. This first set of images demonstrates whether these markers are accurately placed over the tumor. The markers may be adjusted and re-imaged until the ideal incision is identified directly over the surgical access route. The patient's head is then rotated out of the magnetic isocenter (imaging position) and into the surgical position. Figure 47.7's schematic demonstrates the movement from operating to imaging positions. The craniotomy is then opened in standard fashion using all standard surgical equipment, including electrical cautery and mechanical drills. After opening the dura, the head is rotated back into imaging position, and a contrast-enhanced set of images is acquired. An access route is planned based upon these images that minimizes risk of injury to the normal brain parenchyma adjacent to the brain metastasis. For cystic tumors, the cyst is often drained and additional images are taken, revealing the extent of solid tumor present. Only iMR can yield this type of intraoperatively acquired information. For tumors located deep within the brain, a ventricular catheter may be placed using 'MR fluoroscopy' to guide the catheter from the cortical surface to the tumor surface. This catheter leads the surgeon from the cortical surface to the tumor surface. As tumor is removed, additional imaging is acquired as is clinically dictated. Through this iterative process of partial tumor resection and imaging, the surgeon can visualize the progress made in removing the tumor and the effect that tumor removal has had upon both the adjacent brain and the

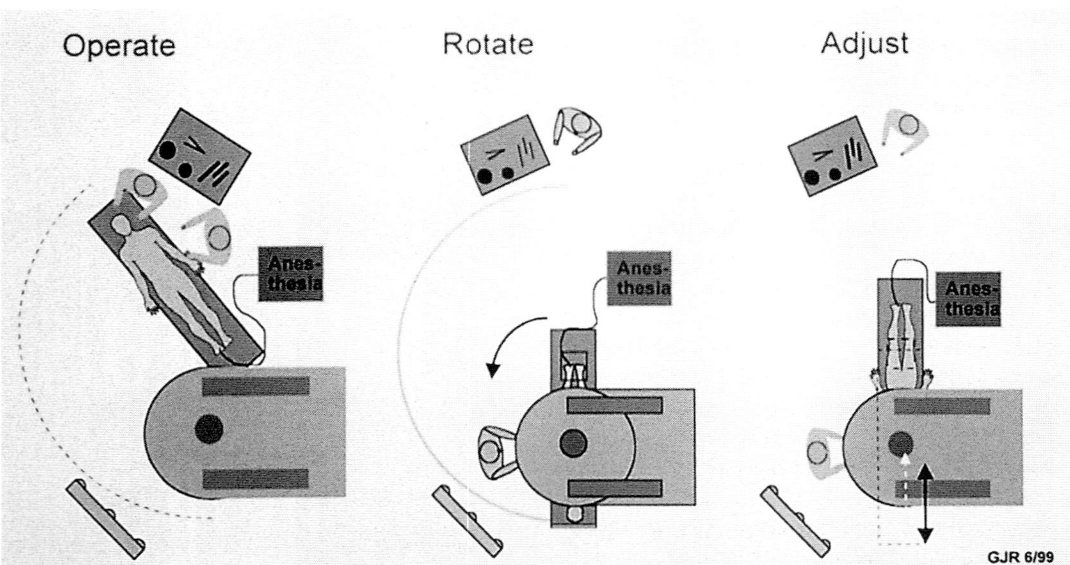

Fig. 47.7 The MRI schematic diagram demonstrates that rotation of the surgical table transitions the patient's head from 'operating' position (left) to 'imaging' position (right)

global brain. The surgeon can be confident that the entire tumor has been removed before closing using iMR-guidance. After closing the craniotomy, a final set of images is obtained to ensure that no hematoma has collected in the tumor resection cavity, the subdural, or epidural space during the closure.

iMR-guidance for tumor resection appears to offer several advantages over conventional neuronavigation systems. When used for removing cystic tumors, the intraoperative images often yield unanticipated information. After cyst decompression, cyst walls that appear on all preoperative imaging to have no significant tumor bulk expand to reveal additional tumor tissue on the intraoperative images. Intraoperative imaging facilitates the diagnosis and treatment of many causes of intraoperative brain swelling, including hematoma formation, subarachnoid hemorrhage, trapped irrigation fluid, and acute obstructive hydrocephalus. These problems can be addressed immediately, thereby limiting their potential to cause permanent injury.

iMR-guidance can visualize and allow the surgeon to compensate for brain shift. When removing tumors near functional cortex such as those in primary motor areas, mapping the cortical surface using somatosensory evoked potentials and cortical stimulation identifies the location and margins of eloquent cortex. These margins may be marked with MR markers so that the relationship between the functional brain and underlying tumor can be appreciated with intraoperative imaging. As surgery progresses, the cortex shifts up to several centimeters in response to removal of the mass lesion. By leaving the cortical markers in place and repeating the imaging during the tumor removal process, the changing relationship between eloquent cortex and surgical resection cavity can be followed, thereby avoiding injury to cortical function. Conventional neuronavigation cannot demonstrate brain shift, leaving the surgeon to judge extent of brain shift and the location of eloquent cortex without the benefit of imaging.

Surgical removal of multiple brain metastases is also made safer using iMR-guidance. To perform multiple craniotomies during the same surgical procedure requires that the surgeon make every effort to minimize each opening so as to reduce blood loss and superficial trauma. After performing the first craniotomy, brain shift makes conventional neuronavigation an inaccurate tool for guiding the second or later craniotomies. In addition, changes in head position would require re-calibration of 'wand-based' systems. iMR-guidance visualizes the brain shift caused by the first craniotomy and accurately directs the surgeon during the second and subsequent craniotomies, so that all intracranial disease can be removed with the highest level of safety. In addition, the global images from iMR allow the surgeon to continue to monitor the resection beds from earlier craniotomies for hematoma accumulation, further reducing the risk of multiple craniotomies.

RCC brain metastases are vascular tumors. When removing larger lesions, it would be helpful to know where the dominant feeding vessels to the tumor are located so that they can be coagulated early in the tumor removal and blood loss may be reduced. The field strength of our current 0.2 T iMR suite scanner is too low to perform angiographic studies. After completion of our second iMR suite equipped with a 1.5 T MRI, we will be capable of performing an intraoperative MR angiogram, which may prove useful in demonstrating where the larger feeding vessels are located when removing RCC brain metastases.

The continued utilization of iMR-guidance during surgical excision may allow craniotomy size to further shrink. If direct visualization of the surgical sight is no longer needed, because intraoperative imaging can allow the surgeon to 'see' below the surface, craniotomies may be reduced to burr holes large enough to fit instruments through. Endoscopic, minimally invasive surgery becomes safely feasible with iMR-guidance. This would further minimize surgical trauma and increase speed of recovery.

Treatment indications

RCC brain metastases often cause focal neurologic symptoms, such as weakness or aphasia, either by direct compression of functional neurologic tissue or functional disruption by peritumoral edema. Tumors may also cause general symptoms of increased intracranial pressure, such as headache, nausea, vomiting, or diplopia. Large tumor size may contribute to the neurologic symptoms. Peritumoral edema is often severe for RCC brain metastases and is often out of proportion to tumor size compared to other cancers metastatic to the brain. Tumor hemorrhage, also common for RCC metastases, may contribute to neurologic symptoms. Surgical removal immediately decompresses neighboring cortex and removes the tumor tissue that is inducing the edema. Therefore, patients with preoperative neurologic symptoms or focal deficits often enjoy rapid relief from these symptoms and recovery of function. Surgical removal is the only treatment that offers immediate benefits. The tumor size does not change the safety or efficacy of surgical intervention. Large tumors are particularly well suited for surgical excision because whole-brain radiotherapy and stereotactic radiosurgery are largely ineffective in treating larger masses.

Surgical excision is also the default treatment when other treatments have failed. RCC brain metastases may continue to grow after whole-brain or stereotactic radiosurgery. Even additional treatments of stereotactic radiosurgery sometimes fail to halt the tumor growth. For these patients, surgical removal provides the definitive, effective therapy. For patients who have undergone radiosurgery and have developed symptomatic necrosis, surgical excision of the necrotic tissue often relieves symptoms. After surgical excision, if tumor recurs either locally or at another intracranial location, re-resection has been proven to offer patients meaningful survival (Bindal *et al.* 1995; Arbit *et al.* 1995).

Surgery is the most direct and aggressive approach for patients with brain metastases, offering patients the longest disease-free intervals, the longest survivals, and the greatest opportunity to recover from a tumor-induced neurologic deficit or symptom. Table 47.3 summarizes the reported survivals achieved with surgery. The refinements in surgical technique described above decrease the likelihood of new neurologic deficits, foster a rapid recovery, and lead to short hospital stays. On average, patients who undergo craniotomy for resection of brain metastases spend 1 postoperative night in the intensive care unit and an additional 1–3 inpatient hospital days. With additional minimization of craniotomy size, hospital stay may shorten to a point where a single overnight observation period is required. Patients typically complain of moderate headaches that resolve within 1–2 weeks. Incisional pain is minimal and treated with oral analgesics. If patients are not already on prophylactic anti-epileptic medication, an anti-epileptic may be administered during surgery and for at least one postoperative week to minimize perioperative seizure risk.

Surgical treatment, which offers the greatest benefit, also carries the most risk of any brain metastasis treatment, even with the recent refinements in surgery. Unlike radiotherapy, where the risks of peritumoral edema, intratumoral hemorrhage, and radiation necrosis exist for months to years after treatment, all the surgical

Table 47.3 Surgery

Reference	Number of Subjects	Tumors	Histology*	Median survival (months)
Badalament *et al.* 1990	22		Renal	20.9
Wronski *et al.* 1996	47		Renal	12
Bindal *et al.* 1993	30	40	Mixed	6
	52	81	Mixed	14
Bindal *et al.* 1994	21	24	Sarcoma	11.8
Bindal *et al.* 1995	48		Mixed	11.5
Bindal *et al.* 1996	62		Mixed	16.4
Wronski *et al.* 1995	231	295	NSC lung	11
Arbit *et al.* 1995	32[†]		NSC lung	10
White *et al.* 1981	122	122	Mixed	7
Salvati *et al.* 1995	100	100	Mixed	10.8
Nakagawa *et al.* 1994	89		Lung	11.6
Noordijk *et al.* 1994	32		Mixed	10
Sundaresan and Galicich 1985	125	125	Mixed	12
Ryan *et al.* 1995	32		Lung	6.5
Andrews *et al.* 1996	25	28	NSC lung	13.1
Hazuka *et al.* 1993	46		Mixed	11

* NSC, Non-small-cell.
[†] Recurrent.

risks are immediate and associated with the time during and immediately after the procedure. During surgery, the direct mechanical or thermal trauma to neural structures near the area of resection may result in temporary or permanent neurologic deficits. Injury to cortical blood vessels around a tumor may cause a stroke and resulting neurologic sequelae. After surgery, hemorrhage may occur into the tumor resection bed or in the subdural or epidural space. Risk of hemorrhage is greatest during the first 24 hours after surgery, and diminishes rapidly over the 2 postoperative weeks. Small hemorrhages may be observed, but larger hemorrhages, especially those that cause neurologic deficit or mass effect, should be removed during an additional surgical procedure. Infection may develop during the 2 weeks after craniotomy. Seeding of a resection cavity or surgical site due to later bacteremia is possible but uncommon. The risk of significant complication associated with a craniotomy is less than 5 per cent at major medical centers.

Carcinomatous meningitis is a risk specifically associated with surgical removal of posterior fossa tumors. Carcinomatous meningitis is the subarachnoid spread of metastatic tumor along the skull base and cranial nerves, resulting in headaches, cranial neuropathy, and rapid demise. Van der Ree *et al.* (1999) report a 33 per cent risk of developing carcinomatous meningitis after surgical removal of posterior fossa masses. If posterior fossa masses are small, stereotactic radiosurgery may be the preferred method of treating these tumors so as to avoid this devastating risk. For larger tumors, preoperative radiotherapy may reduce this risk.

It has become the standard of care to follow surgical excision of brain metastases with adjuvant whole-brain radiotherapy, delivered in 10 fractions of 3 Gy/fraction. The goal of adjuvant radiotherapy is threefold: to kill any tumor cells remaining in the surgical bed; to kill tumor cells released into the subarachnoid space during surgery; to kill any 'microscopic' tumors that are too small to be visualized on the perioperative imaging. Most of the surgical series listed in Table 47.3 follow surgical excision with adjuvant whole-brain radiotherapy. Studies have demonstrated that postsurgical adjuvant radiotherapy decreases the local recurrence rate (Smalley *et al.* 1987, 1992). DeAngelis *et al.* (1998) report that adjuvant radiotherapy delays both local and distant intracranial recurrence, but does not improve survival. Armstrong *et al.* (1994) report that adjuvant radiotherapy reduces the rate of tumor recurrence in the resection bed but does not reduce recurrence of distant intracranial disease. Armstrong's finding refutes the popular notion that whole-brain radiotherapy 'sterilizes' the brain of micrometastases.

Recently, surgeons have questioned the need for adjuvant radiotherapy. Why expose the entire brain to the risk of radiation injury when only a portion of the brain may require this adjuvant therapy? Two alternative treatments are available to decrease the risk of radiation-induced dementia. First, a longer radiotherapy course using smaller fractions (1.8 Gy/fraction × 28 fractions) both reduces the risk of neurocognitive decline and may enhance the therapeutic value of radiation. For patients with favorable long-term prognosis, this fractionation scheme may be preferable to the standard one. Second, the radiation may be focused to only the tumor bed using stereotactic targeting. Single-fraction radiosurgical treatment of the tumor bed has been used to sterilize the surgical resection bed. This treatment nearly guarantees radiation injury to any normal cortex within the treatment volume and will miss any tumor cells within the subarachnoid space outside the radiosurgical treatment volume. Another approach to limiting radiation injury is fractionation. The subject of an ongoing clinical trial at UCLA examines whether adjuvant fractionated stereotactic radiotherapy can provide the therapeutic effects of whole-brain radiotherapy while limiting the risk of radiation injury. In this experimental protocol, we treat a 1 cm tissue rim of normal brain surrounding the resection cavity with five daily fractions of 5 Gy, using a Gill Thomas Cosman relocatable frame (Kooy *et al.* 1994) and a LINAC stereotactic system.

Factors influencing treatment decision

How does the clinician decide which of the three treatment modalities described above, whole-brain radiotherapy, radiosurgery, or surgical excision, is best for his or her patient? Multiple factors contribute to the decision-making process. Tumor number, tumor size, tumor location, patient symptoms, and the status of the patient's systemic disease are all important to consider.

The number of tumors is critical in deciding which treatment option to offer patients. If the patient presents with more than five intracranial metastases, whole-brain radiotherapy is indicated. While radiosurgery may be technically feasible for many small tumors, their presence may indicate that there are additional tumor seeds below the limits of the MRI's resolution. These 'micrometastases' will be treated by whole-brain radiation but missed by the focused radiation of stereotactic radiosurgery. These patients must be followed with serial imaging. Treatment failures and recurrences may be treated with radiosurgery or surgery when clinically indicated. Additional factors need to be considered in deciding whether surgery or radiosurgery is preferable for treating patients with fewer than five tumors.

Tumor size also bears upon the treatment decision issue. Small tumors are more radiosensitive and hence more sensitive to radiotherapy. Tumors smaller than 3 mm may be adequately treated by whole-brain radiotherapy. RCC tumors between 3 mm and 2 cm can usually be destroyed with radiosurgical treatment. Tumors between 2 and 4 cm may be treated with radiosurgery. However, for the reasons previously described in the dose–volume discussion above, these larger tumors will probably fail radiosurgical treatment and require surgery. For tumors larger than 2 cm, surgical excision is the treatment of choice, offering patients the greatest opportunity for long-term survival. In addition, larger tumors usually cause neurologic symptoms that will resolve most rapidly with surgical removal.

Tumor location is important when choosing treatment options. For tumors located in non-eloquent brain areas, such as the nondominant temporal lobe, the premotor frontal lobes, and the cerebellum, surgical excision is not likely to cause any new deficits and is the preferred treatment option. Tumor size is critical when considering how location impacts upon choosing the optimal treatment for tumors located in eloquent cortex. Eloquent cortex is defined as motor, speech, and visual cortex, the deep gray matter, and brainstem. Small tumors are often found incidentally in asymptomatic patients. While small tumors may be surgically 'accessible', surgery in eloquent cortex incurs a significant and unnecessary risk of temporary or permanent neurologic damage. For small, asymptomatic tumors in eloquent brain, radiosurgery is highly effective and less likely than surgical resection to cause neurologic deficits in the asymptomatic patient. Therefore, stereotactic radiosurgery is the preferred treatment for small asymptomatic tumors in eloquent brain. As tumors in eloquent cortex become larger, they often produce deficits or symptoms. For larger tumors in eloquent brain, surgical excision will remove the mass causing the deficit and provide the most rapid resolution of the neurologic deficit. Therefore, surgery is the preferred treatment for larger tumors in eloquent brain areas.

Treatment choice is influenced by the effect the tumor has upon the patient. If the tumor causes clinically significant neurologic deficits or symptoms due to size or a large amount of peritumoral edema, surgery will most rapidly reverse these symptoms. Whole-brain radiotherapy may also ameliorate the symptoms, but will do so only over the course of weeks. Radiosurgery may exacerbate the symptoms caused by larger tumors and tumors causing edema and is not an appropriate treatment.

The patient's overall prognosis and current medical condition bear upon treatment decisions. Severely debilitated patients and those with extensive, uncontrolled disease who are not expected to live long enough to derive benefit from aggressive treatment are often palliated with whole-brain radiotherapy. Because the risk of radiation-induced cognitive decline often takes more than a year to develop, this patient population with life expectancy below 1 year is not at risk. For patients who have medical conditions that prohibit surgery, radiosurgery is the next best treatment option. Surgery should be considered for all patients who are expected to survive their systemic disease for longer than 6 months and can tolerate general anesthesia.

The UCLA approach is to limit the use of whole-brain radiotherapy and treat focal intracranial disease focally. Patients who present with fewer than six brain metastases are considered for radiosurgery if all lesions are smaller than 3 cm in diameter and not causing significant neurologic symptoms. Patients with larger tumors, or symptomatic lesions, are offered surgical resection of the larger lesion(s) or all lesions (< three tumors). The goal of this approach is to deliver the most effective treatment while minimizing the number and risk of treatments. Whole-brain radiotherapy is reserved for patients who present with more than five intracranial metastases.

Applying this approach aggressively, we have achieved some remarkable long-term survivors (> 5 years) who enjoy high quality of life. Some patients return every 6–12 months for radiosurgical treatment of their new crop of brain metastases while enjoying active lives. When focused radiotherapy fails, surgical resection with iMR-guidance is used to remove recalcitrant tumors. Whole-brain radiotherapy is reserved for if and when patients develop multiple small tumors. If patients present with many small recurrent tumors after whole-brain radiotherapy, radiosurgery is used to treat the five largest tumors or any tumors

in critical neurologic areas. We believe that this aggressive approach offers patients the best quality of life and opportunity for long-term survival. This approach challenges our oncology colleagues to offer equally aggressive and effective systemic therapies.

References

Adler, J.R., Cox, R.S., Kaplan, I., and Martin, D.P. (1992). Stereotactic radiosurgical treatment of brain metastases. *J. Neurosurg.* **76** (3), 444–9.

Alexander, E. 3rd, Moriarty, T.M., Davis, R.B., Wen, P.Y., Fine, H.A., Black, P.M., Kooy, H.M., and Loeffler, J.S. (1995). Stereotactic radiosurgery for the definitive, noninvasive treatment of brain metastases. *J. Natl Cancer Inst.* **87** (1), 34–40.

Andrews, R.J., Gluck, D.S., and Konchingeri, R.H. (1996). Surgical resection of brain metastases from lung cancer. *Acta Neurochir.* **138** (4), 382–9.

Arbit, E., Wronski, M., Burt, M., and Galicich, J.H. (1995). The treatment of patients with recurrent brain metastases. A retrospective analysis of 109 patients with nonsmall cell lung cancer. *Cancer* **76** (5), 765–73.

Armstrong, J.G., Wronski, M., Galicich, J., Arbit, E., Leibel, S.A., and Burt. M. (1994). Postoperative radiation of lung cancer metastatic to the brain. *J. Clin. Oncol.* **12** (11), 2340–4.

Auchter, R.M., Lamond, J.P., Alexander, E., Buatti, J.M., Chappell, R., Friedman, W.A., Kinsella, T.J., Levin, A.B., Noyes, W.R., Schultz, C.J., Loeffler, J.S., and Mehta, M.P. (1996). A multi-institutional outcome and prognostic factor analysis of radiosurgery for resectable single brain metastasis [see comments]. *Int. J. Rad. Oncol. Biol. Phys.* **35** (1), 27–35.

Badalament, R.A., Gluck, R.W., Wong, G.Y., Gnecco, C., Kreutzer, E., Herr, H.W., Fair, W.R., and Galicich, J.H. (1990). Surgical treatment of brain metastases from renal cell carcinoma. *Urology* **36** (2), 112–17.

Batson, O.V. (1942). Role of vertebral veins metastatic processes. *Ann. Intern. Med.* **16**, 38–45.

Becker, G., Duffner, F., Kortman, R., Weinmann, M., Heinrich Grote, E., and Bamberg, M. (1999). Radiosurgery for the treatment of brain metastases in renal cell carcinoma. *Anticancer Res.* **19**, 1611–18.

Berk, L. (1995). An overview of radiotherapy trials for the treatment of brain metastases. *Oncology* **9** (11), 1205–12; discussion 1212–16.

Betti, O. and Derechinsky, V. (1983). Multiple-beam stereotaxic irradiation. *Neuro-Chirurgie* **29** (4), 295–8.

Betti, O., Munari, C., and Rosler, R. (1989). Stereotactic radiosurgery with the linear accelerator: treatment of arteriovenous malformations. *Neurosurgery* **24**, 311–21.

Betti, O., Galamarini, D., and Derechinsky, V. (1991). Radiosurgery with a linear accelerator: methodical aspects. *Stereotac. Funct. Neurosurg.* **27** (1–2), 87–98.

Bindal, R.K., Sawaya, R., Leavens, M.E., and Lee, J.J. (1993). Surgical treatment of multiple brain metastases. *J. Neurosurg.* **79** (2), 210–16.

Bindal, R.K., Sawaya, R.E., Leavens, M.E., Taylor, S.H., and Guinee, V.F. (1994). Sarcoma metastatic to the brain: results of surgical treatment. *Neurosurgery* **35** (2), 185–90; discussion 190–1.

Bindal, R.K., Sawaya, R., Leavens, M.E., Hess, K.R., and Taylor, S.H. (1995). Reoperation for recurrent metastatic brain tumors. *J. Neurosurg.* **83** (4), 600–4.

Bindal, A.K., Bindal, R.K., Hess, K.R., Shiu, A., Hassenbusch, S.J., Shi, W.M., and Sawaya, R. (1996). Surgery versus radiosurgery in the treatment of brain metastasis. *J. Neurosurg.* **84** (5), 748–54.

Bitoh, S., Hasegawa, H., Ohtsuki, H., Obashi, J., Fujiwara, M., and Sakurai, M. (1984). Cerebral neoplasms initially presenting with massive intracerebral hemorrhage. *Surg. Neurol.* **22** (1), 57–62.

Black, P. (1993). Solitary brain metastases: radiation, resection, or radiosurgery? *Chest* **103**, 367S–9S.

Black, P.M., Moriarty, T., Alexander, E., Stieg, P., Woodard, E.J., Gleason, L., Martin, C.H., Kikinis, R., Schwartz, R.B., and Jolesz, F.A. (1997).

Development and implementation of intraoperative magnetic resonance imaging and its neurosurgical applications. *Neurosurgery* **41**, 831–45.

Boogerd, W., Vos, V.W., Hart, A.A., and Baris, G. (1993). Brain metastases in breast cancer; natural history, prognostic factors and outcome. *J. Neurooncol.* **15** (2), 165–74.

Buatti, J.M., Freidman, W.A., Bova, F.J., and Mendenhall, W.M. (1995). Treatment selection factors for stereotactic radiosurgery of intracranial metastases. *Int. J. Rad. Oncol. Biol. Phys.* **32**, 1161–6.

Bucci, L., Giannini, A., Bellotti, R., Castellano, A.E., and Carillo, C. (1986). [Role of hypernephroma in a case of intracerebral hemorrhage as a first sign of metastasis. Case report.] *Riv. Neurol.* **56** (5), 325–35.

Cairncross, J.G., Kim, J.H., and Posner, J.B. (1980). Radiation therapy for brain metastases. *Ann. Neurol.* **7** (6), 529–41.

Coia, L.R. (1992). The role of radiation therapy in the treatment of brain metastases. *Int. J. Rad. Oncol. Biol. Phys.* **23** (1), 229–38.

Colombo, F., Benedetti, A., Pozza, F., Avanzo, R.C., Marchetti, C., Chierego, C., and Zanardo, A. (1985). External stereotactic irradiation by linear accelerator. *Neurosurgery* **16**, 154–60.

Colombo, F., Benedetti, A., Pozza, F., Avanzo, R., Chierego, G., Marchetti, C., Bernardi, P., and Pinna, L. (1986). Radiosurgery using a 4 MV linear accelerator. Technique and radiobiologic implications. *Acta Radiol.* **369**, 603–7.

Culine, S., Bekradda, M., Kramar, A., Rey, A., Escudier, B., and Droz, J.P. (1998). Prognostic factors for survival in patients with brain metastases from renal cell carcinoma. *Cancer* **83** (12), 2548–53.

DeAngelis, L.M., Dellatre, J.Y., and Posner, J.B. (1989). Radiation-induced dementia in patients cured of brain metastases. *Neurology* **39**, 789–96.

DeAngelis, L.M., Mandell, L.R., Thaler, T., Kimmel, D.W., Galicich, J.H., Fuks, Z., and Posner, J.B. (1998). The role of postoperative radiotherapy after resection of single brain metastases. *Neurosurgery* **24** (6), 798–805.

Decker, D.A., Decker, V.L., Herskovic, A., and Cummings, G.D. (1984). Brain metastases in patients with renal cell carcinoma: prognosis and treatment. *J. Clin. Oncol.* **2**, 169–73.

deKernion, J.B., Ramming, K.P., and Smith, R.B. (1978). The natural history of metastatic renal cell carcinoma: a computer analysis. *J. Urol.* **120** (2), 148–52.

Delattre, J.Y., Krol, G., Thaler, H.T., and Posner, J.B. (1988). Distribution of brain metastases. *Arch. Neurol.* **45**, 741–4.

Elson, P.J., Witte, R.S., and Trump, D.L. (1988). Prognostic factors for survival in patients with recurrent or metastatic renal cell carcinoma. *Cancer Res.* **48** (24, Pt. 1), 7310–13.

Engenhart, R., Kimmig, B.N., Heover, K.H., Wowra, B., Romahn, J., Lorenz, W.J., vanKaick, G., and Wannenmacher, M. (1993). Long-term follow-up for brain metastases treated by percutaneous stereotactic single high-dose irradiation. *Cancer* **71** (4), 1353–61.

Epstein, B.E., Scott, C.B., Sause, W.T., Rotman, M., *et al.* (1993). Improved survival duration in patients with unresected solitary brain metastasis using accelerated hyperfractionated radiation therapy total doses of 54.4 gray and greater. *Cancer* **71**, 1362–7.

Fertil, B. and Malaise, E.P. (1985). Intrinsic radiosensitivity of human cell lines is correlated with radioresponsiveness of human tumors: analysis of 101 published survival curves. *Int. J. Rad. Oncol. Biol. Phys.* **11** (9), 1699–707.

Flickinger, J.C., Kondziolka, D. Lunsford, L.D., Coffey, R.J., Goodman, M.L., Shaw, E.G., Hudgins, W.R., Weiner, R., Harsh, G.R. 4th, Sneed, P.K., *et al.* (1994). A multi-institutional experience with stereotactic radiosurgery for solitary brain metastasis. *Int. J. Rad. Oncol. Biol. Phys.* **28** (4), 797–802.

Friedman, W.A. and Bova, F.J. (1989). The University of Florida radiosurgery system. *Surg. Neurol.* **32** (5), 334–42.

Friedman, W.A., Bova, F.J., and Spiegelmann, R. (1992). Linear accelerator radiosurgery at the University of Florida. *Neurosurg. Clin. N. Am.* **3** (1), 141–66.

Fuller, B.G., Kaplan, I.D., Adler, J., Cox, R.S., and Bagshaw, M.A. (1992). Stereotaxic radiosurgery for brain metastases: the importance of adjuvant whole brain irradiation. *Int. J. Rad. Oncol. Biol. Phys.* **23**, 413–18.

Gay, P.C., Litchy, W.J., and Cascino, T.L. (1987). Brain metastasis in hypernephroma. *J. Neurooncol.* **5** (1), 51–6.

Giuliani, L., Giberti, C., Martorana, G., and Rovida, S. (1990). Radical extensive surgery for renal cell carcinoma: long-term results and prognostic factors. *J. Urol.* **143** (3), 468–73; discussion 473–4.

Hall, W.A., Martin, A.J., Liu, H., Nussbaum, E.S., Maxwell, R.E., and Truwit, C.L. (1999). Brain biopsy using a high-field strength interventional magnetic resonance imaging. *Neurosurgery* **44**, 807–14.

Halperin, E.C. and Harisiadis, L. (1983). The role of radiation therapy in the management of metastatic renal cell carcinoma. *Cancer* **51**, 614–17.

Hartmann, G.H., Schlegel, W., Sturm, V., Kober, V., Pastyr, O., and Lorenz, W.J. (1985). Radiation surgery using moving field irradiation at a linear accelerator. *Int. J. Rad. Oncol. Biol. Phys.* **11**, 1185–92.

Hawighorst, H., Essig, M., Debus, J., Knopp, M.V., Engenhart-Cabilic, R., Scheonberg, S.O., Brix, G., Zuna, I., and van Kaick, G. (1997). Serial MR imaging of intracranial metastases after radiosurgery. *Mag. Res. Imag.* **15** (10), 1121–32.

Hazuka, M.B., Burleson, W.D., Stroud, D.N., Leonard, C.E., Lillehei, K.O., and Kinzie, J.J. (1993). Multiple brain metastases are associated with poor survival in patients treated with surgery and radiotherapy. *J. Clin. Oncol.* **11** (2), 369–73.

Hendrickson, F.R. (1977). The optimum schedule for palliative radiotherapy for metastatic brain cancer. *Int. J. Rad. Oncol. Biol. Phys.* **2**, 165–8.

Johnson, B.E., Becker, B., Goff, W.B., Petronas, N., Krehbiel, M.A., Makuch, R.W., McKenna, G., Glatstein, E., and Ihde, D.C. (1985). Neurologic, neuropsychologic, and computed cranial tomography scan abnomalies in 2- to 10-year survivors of small-cell lung cancer. *J. Clin. Oncol.* **3**, 1659–67.

Jokura, H., Takahashi, K., Kayama, T., and Yoshimoto, T. (1994). Gamma knife radiosurgery of a series of only minimally selected metastatic brain tumours. *Acta Neurochir. Suppl.* **62**, 77–82.

Joseph, J., Adler, J.R., Cox, R.S., and Hancock, S.L. (1996). Linear accelerator-based stereotaxic radiosurgery for brain metastases: the influence of number of lesions on survival. *J. Clin. Oncol.* **14** (4), 1085–92.

Kaiser, M.C., Rodesch, G., and Capesius, P. (1983). Blood-fluid levels in multiloculated cystic brain metastasis of a hypernephroma. A case report. *Neuroradiology* **25** (5), 339–41.

Kavolius, J.P., Mastorakos, D.P., Pavlovich, C., Russo, P., Burt, M.E., and Brady, M.S. (1998). Resection of metastatic renal cell carcinoma. *J. Clin. Oncol.* **16** (6), 2261–6.

Kihlstrom, L., Karlsson, B., and Lindquist, C. (1993). Gamma knife surgery for cerebral metastases. Implications for survival based on 16 years experience. *Stereotact. Funct. Neurosurg.* **61**, 45–50.

Kooy, H.M., Nedzi, L.A., Loeffler, J.S., Alexander, E., Cheng, C.W., Mannari, C., Holupka, E.J., and Siddan, R.L. (1991). Treatment planning for stereotactic radiosurgery for intracranial lesions. *Int. J. Rad. Oncol. Biol. Phys.* **21** (3), 683–93.

Kooy, H.M., Dunbar, S.F., Tarbell, N.J., Mannarino, E., Ferarro, N., Shusterman, S., Bellerive, M., Finn, L., McDonough, C.V., and Loeffler, J.S. (1994). Adaptation and verification of the relocatable Gill–Thomas–Cosman frame in stereotactic radiotherapy. *Int. J. Rad. Oncol. Biol. Phys.* **30** (3), 685–91.

Kozlowski, J.M. (1994). Management of distant solitary recurrence in the patient with renal cancer. Contralateral kidney and other sites. *Urol. Clin. N. Am.* **21**, 601–24.

Leksell, D. (1989). Radiosurgery, *Neurosurgery*, **24**, 297–8.

Lunsford, L.D., Flickinger, J., Coffey, R.J., *et al.* (1990). Stereotactic gamma knife radiosurgery: initial North American experience in 207 patients. *Arch. Neurol.* **24**, 151–75.

Lutz, W., Winston, K.R., and Maleki, N. (1988). A system for stereotactic radiosurgery with a linear accelerator. *Int. J. Rad. Oncol. Biol. Phys.* **14** (2), 373–81.

Maldazys, J.D. and deKernion, J.B. (1986). Prognostic factors in metastatic renal carcinoma. *J. Urol.* **136** (2), 376–9.

Maor, M.H., Frias, A.E., and Oswald, M.J. (1988). Palliative radiotherapy for brain metastases in renal carcinoma. *Cancer* **62** (9), 1912–17.

Marshall, M.E., Pearson, T., Simpson, W., Butler, K., and McRoberts, W. (1990). Low incidence of asymptomatic brain metastases in patients with renal cell carcinoma. *Urology* **36** (4), 300–2.

Mehta, M.P., Rozenthal, J.M., Levin, A.B., Mackie, T.R., *et al.* (1992). Defining the role of radiosurgery in the management of brain metastases. *Int. J. Rad. Oncol. Biol. Phys.* **24**, 619–25.

Mori, Y., Kondziolka, D., Flickinger, J., Logan, T., and Lunsford, L.D. (1998). Stereotactic radiosurgery for brain metastasis from renal cell carcinoma. *Cancer* **83**, 344–52.

Nakagawa, H., Miyawaki, Y., Fujita, T., Kubo, S., Tokiyoshi, K., Tsuruzono, K., Kodama, K., Higashiyama, M., Doi, O., and Hayakawa, T. (1994). Surgical treatment of brain metastases of lung cancer: retrospective analysis of 89 cases. *J. Neurol. Neurosurg. Psychiat.* **57** (8), 950–6.

Neves, R.J., Zincke, H., and Taylor, W.F. (1988). Metastatic renal cell cancer and radical nephrectomy: identification of prognostic factors and patient survival. *J. Urol.* **139** (6), 1173–6.

Nieder, C., Niewald, M., and Schnabel, K. (1996). Treatment of brain metastases from hypernephroma. *Urologia Int.* **57** (1), 17–20.

Nieder, C., Nestle, U., Motaref, B., Walter, K., Niewald, M., and Schnabel, K. (2000). Prognostic factors in brain metastases: should patients be selected for aggressive treatment according to recursive partitioning analysis (RPA) classes? *Int. J. Rad. Oncol. Biol. Phys.* **46** (2), 297–302.

Noordijk, E.M., Vecht, C.J., Haaxma-Reiche, H., Padberg, G.W., Voormolen, J.H., Hoekstra, F.H., Tans, J.T., Lambooij, N., Metsaars, J.A., Wattendorff, A.R., *et al.* (1994). The choice of treatment of single brain metastasis should be based on extracranial tumor activity and age [see comments]. *Int. J. Rad. Oncol. Biol. Phys.* **29** (4), 711–17.

Nussbaum, E.S., Djalilian, H.R., Cho, K.H., and Hall, W.A. (1996). Brain metastases: histology, multiplicity, surgery, and survival. *Cancer* **78** (8), 1781–8.

O'Dea, M.J., Zincke, H., Utz, D.C., and Bernatz, P.E. (1978). The treatment of renal cell carcinoma with solitary metastasis. *J. Urol.* **120** (5), 540–2.

O'Neill, B.P., Buckner, J.C., Coffey, R.J., Dinapoli, R.P., and Shaw, E.G. (1994). Brain metastatic lesions. *Mayo Clin. Proc.* **69**, 1062–8.

Onufrey, V. and Mohiuddin, M. (1985). Radiation therapy in the treatment of metastatic renal cell carcinoma. *Int. J. Rad. Oncol. Biol. Phys.* **11** (11), 2007–9.

Patchell, R.A., Tibbs, P.A., Walsh, J.W., Dempsey, R.J., Maruyama, Y., Kryscio, R.J., Markesbery, W.R., Macdonald, J.S., and Young, B. (1990). A randomized trial of surgery in the treatment of single metastases to the brain. *New Engl. J. Med.* **322** (8), 494–500.

Peterson, A.M., Meltzer, C.C., Evanson, E.J., Flickinger, J.C., and Kondziolka, D. (1999). MR imaging response of brain metastases after gamma knife stereotactic radiosurgery. *Radiology* **211** (3), 807–14.

Podgorsak, E.B., Olivier, A., Pla, M., Lefebvre, P.Y., and Hazel, J. (1988). Dynamic stereotactic radiosurgery. *Int. J. Rad. Oncol. Biol. Phys.* **14** (1), 115–26.

Posner, J. (1974). Diagnosis and treatment of metastases to the brain. *Clin. Bull.* **4**, 47–57.

Ritchie, A.W. and deKernion, J.B. (1987). The natural history and clinical features of renal carcinoma. *Sem. Nephrol.* **7**, 131–9.

Rodriguez, G.C., Soper, J.T., Berchuck, A., Oleson, J., Dodge, R., Montana, G., and Clarke-Pearson, D.L. (1992). Improved palliation of cerebral metastases in epithelial ovarian cancer using a combined modality approach including radiation therapy, chemotherapy, and surgery. *J. Clin. Oncol.* **10** (10), 1553–60.

Rubino, G.J., Farahani, K., McGill, D., Van de Wiele, B., Villablanca, J.P., and Wang-Mathieson, A. (2000). Magnetic resonance imaging-guided neurosurgery in the magnetic fringe fields: the next step in neuronavigation. *Neurosurgery* **46**, 643–54.

Ryan, G.F., Ball, D.L., and Smith, J.G. (1995). Treatment of brain metastases from primary lung cancer. *Int. J. Rad. Oncol. Biol. Phys.* **31** (2), 273–8.

Saitoh, H., Shimbo, T., Tasaka, T., Iida, T., and Hara, K. (1982). Brain metastasis of renal adenocarcinoma. *Tokai J. Exp. Clin. Med.* **7** (3), 337–43.

Salvati, M., Scarpinati, M., Orlando, E.R., Celli, P., and Gagliardi, F.M. (1992). Single brain metastases from kidney tumors. Clinico-pathologic considerations on a series of 29 cases. *Tumori* **78** (6), 392–4.

Salvati, M., Cervoni, L., and Raco, A. (1995). Single brain metastases from unknown primary malignancies in CT-era. *J. Neurooncol.* **23** (1), 75–80.

Sawaya, R., Ligon, B.L., Bindal, A.K., Bindal, R.K., and Hess, K.R. (1996). Surgical treatment of metastatic brain tumors. *J. Neurooncol.* **27**, 269–77.

Sawaya, R., Hammound, M., Schoppa, D., Hess, K.R., Wu, S.Z., Shi, W.M., and Wild, D.M. (1998). Neurosurgical outcomes in a modern series of 400 craniotomies for the treatment of parenchymal tumors. *Neurosurgery* **42** (5), 1044–55.

Schoeggl, A., Klitz, K., Ertl, A., Reddy, M., Bavinzski, G., and Schneider, B. (1999). Prognostic factor analysis for multiple brain metastases after gamma knife radiosurgery: results in 97 patients. *J. Neurooncol.* **42**, 169–75.

Seaman, E.K., Ross, S., and Sawczuk, I.S. (1995). High incidence of asymptomatic brain lesions in metastatic renal cell carcinoma. *J. Neurooncol.* **23** (3), 253–6.

Shiau, C.Y., Sneed, P.K., Shu, H.K., Lamborn, K.R., McDermott, M.W., *et al.* (1997). Radiosurgery for brain metastases: relationship of dose and pattern of enhancement to local control. *Int. J. Rad. Oncol. Biol. Phys.* **37** (2), 375–83.

Smalley, S.R., Schray, M.F., Laws, E.R., and O'Fallon, J.R. Adjuvant radiation therapy after surgical resection of solitary brain metastasis: association with pattern of failure and survival. *Int. J. Rad. Oncol. Biol. Phys.* **13**, 1611–16

Smalley, S.R., Laws, E.R. Jr, O'Fallon, J.R., Shaw, E.G., and Schray, M.F. (1992). Resection for solitary brain metastasis. Role of adjuvant radiation and prognostic variables in 229 patients. *J. Neurosurg.* **77** (4), 531–40.

Somaza, S., Kondziolka, D., Lunsford, L.D., Kirkwood, J.M., and Flickinger, J.C. (1993). Stereotactic radiosurgery for cerebral metastatic melanoma. *J. Neurosurg.* **79** (5), 661–6.

Steinmeier, R., Fahlbusch, R., Ganslandt, O., Nimsky, C., Buchfelder, M., Kaus, M., Heigl, T., Lenz, G., Kuth, R., and Huk, W. (1998). Intraoperative magnetic resonance imaging with the Magnetom Open scanner: concepts, neurosurgical indications and procedures: a preliminary report. *Neurosurgery* **43**, 739–48.

Sturm, V., Kober, B., Hover, K.H., Schlegel, W., Boesecke, R., Pastyr, O., Hart, G.H., Schabbert, S., Zum Zinkel, K., Kunze, S., *et al.* (1987). Stereotactic percutaneous single dose irradiation of brain metastases with a linear accelerator. *Int. J. Rad. Oncol. Biol. Phys.* **13** (2), 279–82.

Sundaresan, N. and Galicich, J.H. (1985). Surgical treatment of brain metastases. Clinical and computerized tomography evaluation of the results of treatment. *Cancer* **55** (6), 1382–8.

Sundstrom, J.T., Minn, H., Lertola, K.K., and Nordman, E. (1998). Prognosis of patients treated for intracranial metastases with whole-brain irradiation. *Ann. Med.* **30** (3), 296–9.

Tobler, W.D. and Stanley, M. (1994). Stereotactic resection of brain metastases in eloquent brain. *Stereotact. Funct. Radiosurg.* **63**, 38–44.

Tronnier, V.M., Wirtz, C.R., Knauth, M., Lenz, G., Pastyr, O., Bonsanto, M.M., Albert, F.K., Kuth, R., Staubert, A., Schlegel, W., Sartor, K., and Kunze, S. (1997). Intraoperative diagnostic and interventional magnetic resonance imaging in neurosurgery. *Neurosurgery* **40**, 891–902.

Van der Ree, T.C., Dippel, D.W., Avezaat, C.J., Sillevis Smitt, P.A., Vecht, C.J., and Bent, M.J. (1999). Leptomeningeal metastasis after surgical resection of brain metastases. *J. Neurol. Neurosurg. Psychiat.* **66** (2), 225–7.

White, K.T., Fleming, T.R., and Laws, E.R. Jr (1981). Single metastasis to the brain. Surgical treatment in 122 consecutive patients. *Mayo Clin. Proc.* **56** (7), 424–8.

Wirtz, C.R., Knauth, M., Hassfeld, S., Tronnier, V.M., Albert, F.K., Bonsanto, M.M., and Kunze, S. (1998). Neuronavigation—first experiences with three different commercially available systems. *Zentralbl. Neurochir.* **59** (1), 14–22.

Wong, W.W., Schild, S.E., Sawyer, T.E., and Shaw, E.G. (1996). Analysis of outcome in patients reirradiated for brain metastases. *Int. J. Rad. Oncol. Biol. Phys.* **34**, 585–90.

Wronski, M., Arbit, E., Burt, M., and Galicich, J.H. (1995). Survival after surgical treatment of brain metastases from lung cancer: a follow-up study of 231 patients treated between 1976 and 1991. *J. Neurosurg.* **83** (4), 605–16.

Wronski, M., Arbit, E., Russo, P., and Galicich, J.H. (1996). Surgical resection of brain metastases from renal cell carcinoma in 50 patients. *Urology* **47** (2), 187–93.

Wronski, M., Maor, M.H., Davis, B.J., Sawaya, R., and Levin, V.A. (1997). External radiation of brain metastases from renal carcinoma: a retrospective study of 119 patients from M.D. Anderson Cancer Center. *Int. J. Rad. Oncol. Biol. Phys.* **37** (4), 753–9.

Wu, A., Lindner, G., Maitz, A.H., Kalend, A.M., Lunsford, L.D., Flickinger, J.C., and Bloomer, W.D. (1990). Physics of gamma knife approach on convergent beams in stereotactic radiosurgery. *Int. J. Rad. Oncol. Biol. Phys.* **18** (4), 941–9.

Young, R.F. (1998). Radiosurgery for the treatment of brain metastases. *Sem. Surg. Oncol.* **14** (1), 70–8.

48. Palliative therapy of advanced renal cell carcinoma

Sophie D. Fosså and the MRC Renal Cell Cancer Group

Introduction

The primary goal of palliative cancer therapy in advanced (metastatic) renal cell carcinoma (RCC) is to relieve existing symptoms. Secondary aims are prevention of symptoms and prolongation of life. Adequate palliative treatment of a cancer patient requires that the physician, the patient, and the patient's relatives know and accept that cure is no longer the aim of therapy, but rather symptom relief and, eventually, prolongation of life. The achievement of the above goals does not necessarily require the use of any specific anticancer treatment, though radiotherapy, surgery, chemotherapy, and/or immunotherapy may represent

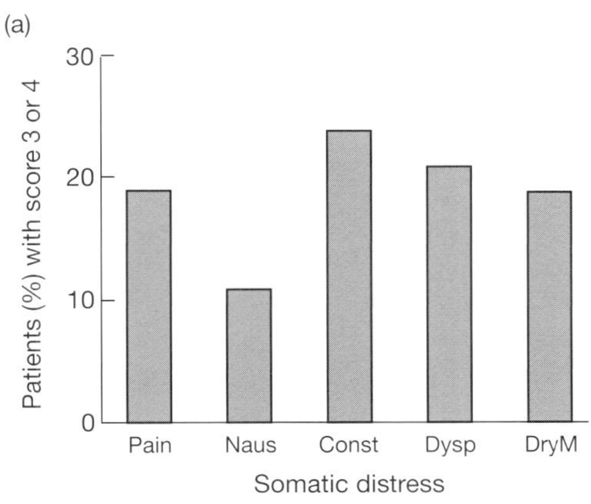

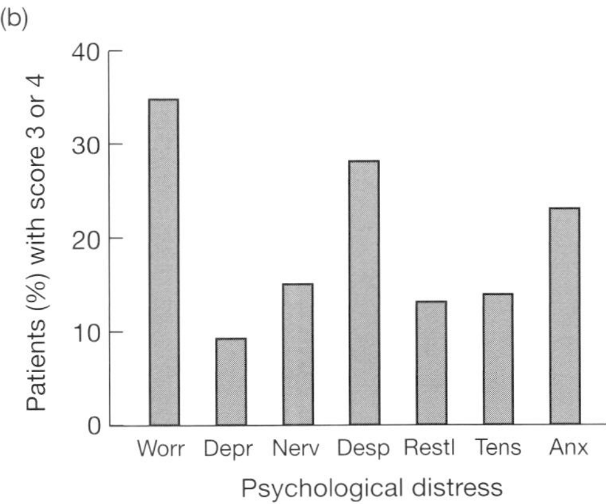

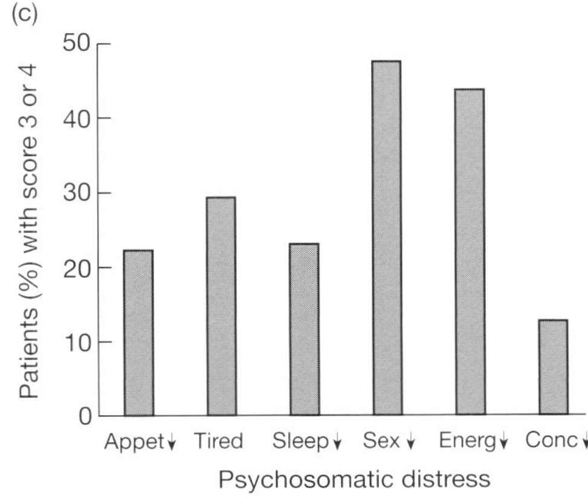

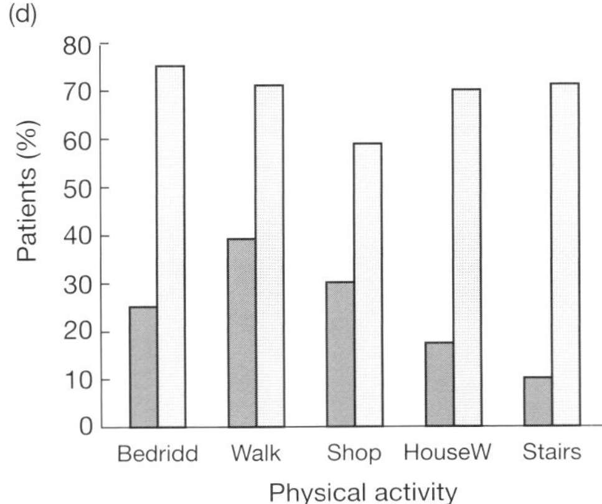

Fig. 48.1 Quality of life parameters (Rotterdam Symptom Check List (de-Haes *et al.* 1990; Medical Research Council Renal Cancer Collaborators, 1999)) in 278 patients with metastatic RCC before start of systemic treatment with IFNα or medroxyprogesterone acetate (1). (a) Somatic distress: pain, nausea (Naus), constipation (Const), dyspnea (Dysp), dry mouth (Dry M). (b) Psychological distress: worrying (Worn), depressed (Depr), nervous (Nerv), despondent or other (Desp), restless (Restl), tense (Tens), anxious (Anx). (c) Psychosomatic distress: reduced appetite (Appet↓), tiredness, disturbed sleep (Sleep↓), reduced sexual interest (Sex↓), lack of energy (Energy↓), difficulty with concentration (Conc↓). (d) Physical activity: bedridden (Bedridd), outdoor walk (Walk), shopping (Shop), light house work (HouseW), stairs. Black bar: score 3-4, great difficulty or unable; hatched bar: score 1-2, no or only limited difficulty/able.

effective means to reduce physical symptoms such as pain or dyspnea. However, good palliative care also requires the medical team to be aware of the patient's psychosocial suffering and other aspects of health-related quality of life (QL). The pretreatment QL data from the UK Medical Research Council's (MRC) trial on interferon (Medical Research Council Renal Cancer Collaborators 1999; de-Haes *et al.* 1990) indicate lack of energy, tiredness, and reduced everyday physical activity in 25–45 per cent of patients with metastatic RCC (scored as 3 or 4 on the 4-point scale of the Rotterdam symptom checklist) (Fig. 48.1). Ten to 35 per cent of the 278 patients recorded psychological distress. Significant somatic distress was reported by only 11–25 per cent of the patients. In other words, the patient's healthcare team should take into account the different psychological and psychosomatic dimensions of QL, and not only consider the patient's somatic disease and treatment-related symptoms.

Though metastatic RCC does not differ essentially from other advanced malignancies as to the needs of palliation some more specific characteristics have to be considered during the treatment of a patient with advanced RCC. This chapter aims to review some of the most frequently encountered clinical scenarios and principles of their management.

Specific anticancer treatment

In contrast to the situation in many other malignancies the patient with metastatic RCC has to recognize at an early phase of the disease that no standard anticancer treatment exists for the condition. Therefore, whenever possible, inclusion of patients in a trial evaluating new drugs and new therapeutic modalities should be considered. At present, immunotherapy is the best systemic anticancer treatment one can offer to a patient with advanced

RCC, if he/she accepts the unavoidable side-effects (fever, flu-like symptoms) (Fossa 2000; Atzpodien *et al.* 1990). Prolongation of life and occasionally long-lasting complete remission can be observed after treatment with interferon α (IFNα) with or without interleukin 2 (IL-2) (Fig. 48.2). However, modern immunomodulatory therapy has a chance of being effective only in selected patients, for example, those with good performance status, no prior weight loss, and with a sedimentation rate < 30–50 mm.

Palliative surgery

Palliative surgery is an important tool in the care of patients with advanced RCC, even though a patient's survival is considered to be limited. Solitary metastases (pulmonal, skeletal) are sometimes resected with an attempted cure, though the life-prolonging or curative significance of such an approach has not been documented. Surgery of symptomatic metastases may, however, represent effective palliation in patients with an expected lifetime of several months or even years. Resection of large ulcerating hemorrhagic and infected tumor masses reduces general symp-

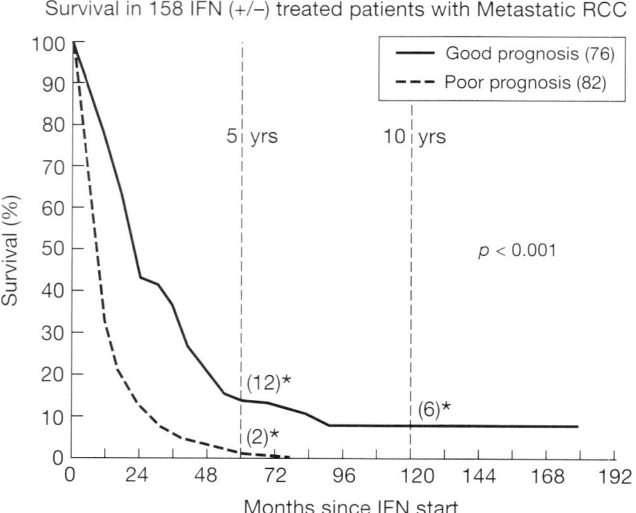

Fig. 48.2 Overall survival of patients with metastatic RCC treated with IFNα based immunotherapy (without IL-2) according to risk groups, based on performance status, weight loss, and sedimentation rate. (Five patients survived without evidence of disease for 10 years; a sixth is alive with metastases.) *Numbers in brackets represent number of patients at risk.

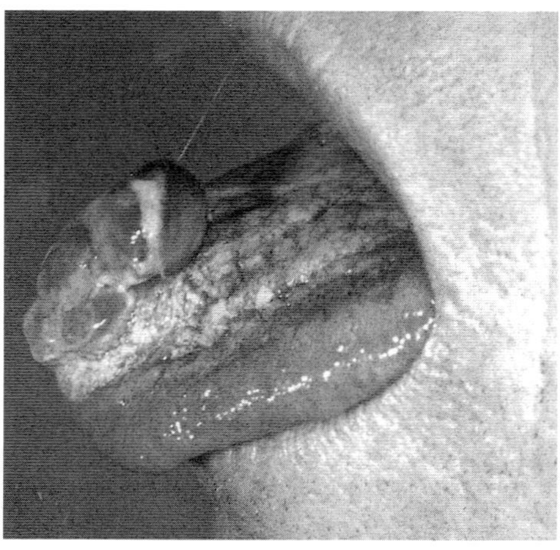
(a)

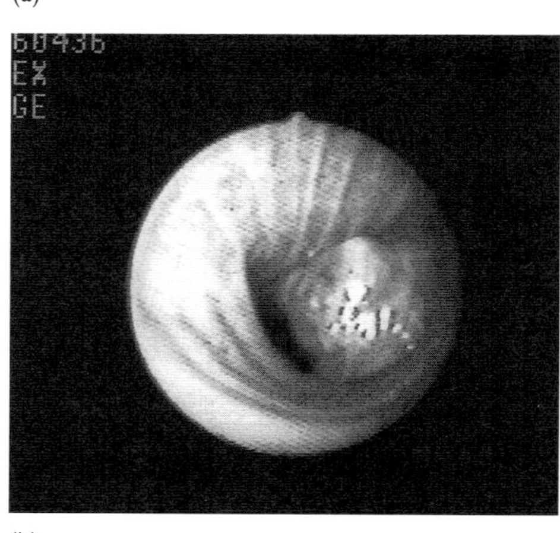
(b)

Fig. 48.3 Metastasis from RCC (a) to the tongue and (b) to the trachea

toms such as fever and malaise and lowers the risk of hypercalcemia. It is not rare for patients with advanced RCC to display metastases with unusual localization: vagina, gall bladder, upper airways, gastrointestinal tract (Fig. 48.3), thyroid. Excellent palliation can be achieved by resection of even small metastases to the aerodigestive tract, causing stenosis and hemorrhage, or by extirpation of symptomatic cerebral metastases. On the basis of the limited radiosensitivity of RCC surgical intervention should always be considered first in cases of spinal cord compression due to metastases (laminectomy). Of particular value is stabilizing orthopedic surgery in the case of osteolytic metastases in weight-bearing parts of the skeleton (columna, lower extremities). For the patients and their relatives it makes a significant difference to their daily life activity if the patient's walking ability is preserved for as long as possible.

Palliative radiotherapy

In most patients with metastatic RCC referred to radiotherapy units, the median survival is only 6–10 months. Long-term survivors may occasionally be observed, even after treatment for brain metastases (Fig. 48.4).

RCC is a relatively radioresistant tumor. Usually, high target doses are required for radiotherapy of osteolytic bone metastases (3 Gy × 10–12 or 2 Gy × 20–23). When defining the target field, radiotherapists should have in mind that large soft-tissue tumors may surround the skeletal metastasis, without being sufficiently visualized by routine skeletal X-rays (Fig. 48.5). Objective response to radiotherapy is observed in about 30 per cent of the patients; subjective response is recorded by about 60–80 per cent (Fossa *et al.* 1982). Though not well documented in the medical literature, postoperative radiotherapy may be considered in cases of incompletely resected metastases in a patient with expected long-term survival, in order to delay or prevent re-growth of residual malignant cells.

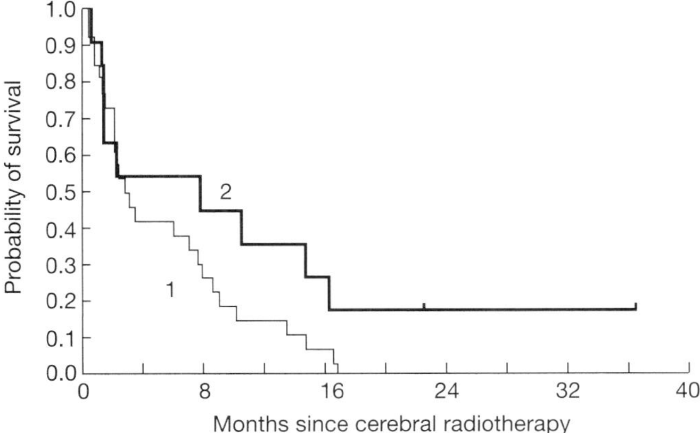

Fig. 48.4 Overall survival in 37 patients with brain metastases from RCC. (1) Cerebral metastases and other metastatic lesions (11 patients). (2) Cerebral lesion(s) as the only metastatic site (26 patients).

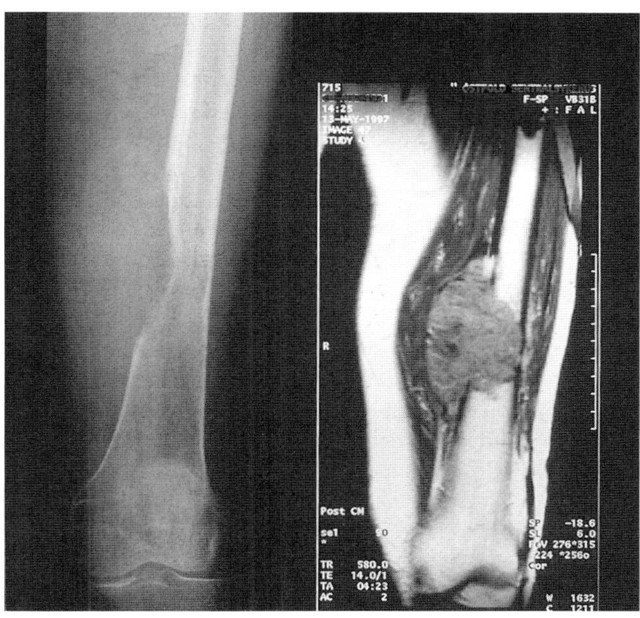

Fig. 48.5 Skeletal X-ray of an osteolytic metastasis to the femur (left) with large surrounding magnetic resonance (MR)-visualized soft-tissue component (right).

Treatment of symptoms

Pain

Pain in patients with advanced RCC is caused by tissue damage of an organ (nociceptive pain) or by direct nerve affection (neuropathic pain), both of which may develop separately (Portenoy 1992). Furthermore, pain may occur secondarily due to pathological fractures or stenosis of hollow organs (ureter, bowel, biliary tract). Concomitant psychological distress will increase the patient's perception of pain.

Rapidly increasing back pain extending to the legs, with increasing sensory and/or motor symptoms must raise the suspicion of imminent paraplegia, an emergency condition for oncological or neurosurgical units. If this development can be excluded, pain relief can be attempted to increasing doses of analgesics, to be used without restriction as to the type and amount of analgesics. Physicians and patients should, however, have realistic aims with pain treatment. Complete pain relief is not obtained in all patients, but all patients can reach an acceptable level through the combined attempts of their family doctors, oncologists, and, if necessary, a 'pain team'.

The first step in the management of pain is to evaluate its cause and contributing factors. The solution to local problems should be attempted using palliative surgery or radiotherapy. In the case of psychological distress psychopharmaceuticals (tricyclic antidepressives) can contribute to achieve an acceptable pain level.

Drug treatment of pain should start with non-opiates. The combination of paracetamol (4–6 g daily in patients with normal liver function) combined with nonsteroidal anti-inflammatory drugs represents the first step on the WHO pain ladder. It is important that the patient is told to use the medication regularly even if he/she is pain-free, in order to prevent pain exacerbation. A few patients may have increased pain relief if paracetamol is combined with dextropropoxyphen.

If non-opiates do not relieve pain sufficiently, opiates should be prescribed, usually on a regular basis. At that stage non-opiates should be discontinued, and an anti-inflammatory preparation, eventually low-dose cortisone, is recommended if no major dyspepsia develops. There is no upper limit of the doses of opiates in order to achieve pain relief in a cancer patient. Morphine is available for oral, rectal, and parenteral use. One should start with a morphine formulation that has a short half-life (to be given every 4 hours) increasing the daily dose until sufficient pain relief is obtained. Thereafter slow-release medications can be used (half-life 10–12 hours, to be given twice daily). In cases where the intermittent pain worsens, morphine tablets (10 mg) should be made available for the patient.

During the use of high-dose analgesics health-care providers should be aware of the problem of constipation and prescribe laxatives on a regular basis. Anti-emetics may be required during the treatment with opiates.

Hypercalcemia

The development of hypercalcemia should always be considered in patients with advanced RCC. Hypercalcemia is most often associated with skeletal metastases, but may develop in non-metastatic patients with large primary tumors. The clinical symptoms are fatigue, nausea, dehydration, and confusion. In such cases the tumor cells may produce parathyroid-related peptides, which activate osteoclast activity and increase calcitonin reabsorption in the renal tubuli. Such endocrine hypercalcemia may be more therapy-resistant than hypercalcemia associated with skeletal metastases and may by itself require reductive palliative surgery of a large tumor mass.

Seventy-five per cent of serum calcium is bound to serum albumin, whereas it is the free or ionized calcium that is responsible for the clinical symptoms of hypercalcemia. In the case of low serum albumin, total calcium may be measured within the normal range despite the increase in free calcium. If possible, laboratories should therefore measure ionized calcium directly. If this is not possible, the measured value of total calcium has to be corrected according to the following 'rule of the thumb':

$$\text{Corrected calcium} = \text{measured calcium} + (40 - \text{albumin level} \ (g/l)) \times 0.02.$$

Treatment of hypercalcemia starts with excessive hydration (4–6 l NaCl 0.9 per cent) with furosemide, which leads to increased excretion of calcium. Biphosphanates reduce the osteoclast activity thus decreasing serum calcium. Two to four hours intravenous (IV) infusions of pamidronate 60–90 mg or clodronate 300–600 mg are applied daily for 3–4 days, and should be repeated with 3–4 week intervals. Maintenance treatment with clodronate can also be given orally.

Severe symptomatic hypercalcemia combined with reduced kidney function is initially treated with IV infusions of calcitonin or mitramycin. The role of glucocorticoids in the treatment of hypercalcemia in patients with metastatic RCC is not clear, but is probably minimal.

Fever

Tumor-induced fever (38–39°C) is a quite frequent symptoms in patients with advanced RCC. Its cause has to be discriminated from an ongoing infection. Tumor-induced fever is controlled by paracetamol (500 mg × 4 orally daily) or, if necessary, by corticosteroids such as prednisone (10 mg × 2–3 orally daily). If given for long periods the risk of steroid-induced peptic ulcer should, however, not be overlooked.

Dyspnea

Lung and mediastinal metastases, and/or pleural effusions are frequent tumor manifestations in advanced RCC and may cause considerable somatic distress and anxiety during the terminal phase, both for the patient and his/her relatives. Intraluminal metastases may cause stenosis of the trachea or larger bronchi (Fig. 48.3). These can be treated by (repeated) endoscopic reactions and/or intraluminar laser beam irradiation or brachytherapy.

Only if hypoxemia is documented by blood gas analysis is the use of oxygen indicated. In all other cases morphine, applied subcutaneously, or intravenously, is the treatment of choice in patients suffering from severe terminal dyspnea.

Hematuria

Severe macroscopic hematuria may be the cause of anemia. Blood clots may lead to obstruction of the urinary tract resulting in pain and micturition problems. Not least, patients are alarmed and psychologically distressed by repeated hematuria.

These local problems can be avoided by early nephrectomy even in metastatic patients, in particular in patients with a large primary tumor, low metastatic tumor burden, and expected long survival time. If nephrectomy is not possible an interventional radiologist should be consulted for selective embolization of the tumor's main arteries (Roy *et al.* 1999). Microscopic or minor macroscopic hematuria does not usually require any treatment except for psychological support of the distressed patient.

Fatigue/cachexia

During recent years the impact of fatigue on QL in a cancer patient has been repeatedly emphasized. It is, however, unclear to what degree fatigue is related to the psychological and/or somatic concerns of the patient. Some investigators, but not all, have found a correlation with depression. Fatigue is a frequent palliation-demanding dimension in patients with metastatic RCC. Fatigue may or may not be associated with cachexia (reduced appetite, weight loss). If this is the case, high-dose medroxy-progesterone (500 mg × 2 orally daily), megestrol (160 mg orally daily), or prednisone (10 mg × 2–3 orally daily) may be helpful.

Fatigue and cachexia may or may not be associated with anemia. If so, blood transfusions and treatment with recombinant erythropoietin may transiently be beneficial (Leitgeb *et al.* 1994).

Quality of life and psychological distress

A patient's health-related QL is usually assessed by valid and reliable multidimensional instruments evaluating symptoms (pain, fatigue, dyspnea, nausea, vomiting) and functional status (physical, social, emotional) (de Haes *et al.* 1990; Aaronson *et al.* 1993). Though most of the available questionnaires cover the above domains, an individual patient's QL may additionally be affected by generally unaddressed domains such as financial issues or spiritual problems. Such 'paramedical' problems should be identified and solutions should be sought.

The information that cure can no longer be expected and the experience of gradual disease progression (increasing pain, reduced performance status, and the development of new metastases) are often accompanied by increasing anxiety and depression. In many situations medication with modern antidepressive drugs can control the situation, together with the repeated confirmation of the availability of supportive and palliative therapy, whenever necessary. Counseling by a psychologist, psychiatrist, or by a spiritual counselor should be considered in individual cases.

Not unexpectedly, many patients with metastatic RCC and their relatives will explore and try unconventional 'therapeutic' approach such as homeopathy, acupuncture, healing, etc., often without daring to inform the responsible physician about their attempts. Representatives of academic medicine have to understand and have to accept these attempts of their patients as an expression of psychological distress in a life-threatening situation. It is important that the health-care providers within conventional medicine continue an open dialogue with the patient and offer him/her support based on scientifically proven methods, though the patient may also follow less documented advice.

In summary, due to the multitude and variability of the problems, palliative care of a patient with metastatic RCC represents a considerable scientific and personal challenge for the responsible specialist and family doctor.

References

Aaronson, N.K., Ahmedzai, S., Bergman, B., Bullinger, M., Cull, A., Duez, N.J., Filiberti, A., Flechtner, H., Fleishman, S.B., de Haes, J.C., *et al.* (1993). The European Organization for Research and Treatment of Cancer QLQ–C30: a quality-of-life instrument for use in international clinical trials in oncology. *J. Natl Cancer Inst.* **85**, 365–76.

Atzpodien, J., Korfer, A., Franks, C.R., Poliwoda, H., and Kirchner, H. (1990). Home therapy with recombinant interleukin-2 and interferon-alpha 2b in advanced human malignancies. *Lancet* **335**, 1509–12.

de Haes, J.C., van-Knippenberg, F.C., and Neijt, J.P. (1990). Measuring psychological and physical distress in cancer patients: structure and application of the Rotterdam Symptom Checklist. *Br J Cancer* **62**, 1034–8.

Fosså, S.D. (2000). Interferon in metastatic renal cell carcinoma. *Sem. Oncol.* **27**, 187–93.

Fossa, S.D., Kjolseth, I., and Lund, G. (1982). Radiotherapy of metastases from renal cancer. *Eur Urol* **8**, 340–2.

Leitgeb, C., Pecherstorfer, M., Fritz, E., and Ludwig, H. (1994). Quality of life in chronic anemia of cancer during treatment with recombinant human erythropoietin. *Cancer* **73**, 2535–42.

Medical Research Council Renal Cancer Collaborators (1999). Interferon-alpha and survival in metastatic renal carcinoma: early results of a randomised controlled trial. *Lancet* **353**, 14–17.

Portenoy, R.K. (1992). Cancer pain: pathophysiology and syndromes. *Lancet* **339**, 1026–31.

Roy, C., Tuchmann, C., Morel, M., Saussine, C., Jacqmin, D., and Tongio, J. (1999). Is there still a place for angiography in the management of renal mass lesions? *Eur Radiol* **9**, 329–35.

Part 2, Adrenal tumors

49.   Imaging of adrenal masses

Susan Teeger, Nicholas Papanicolaou, and E Darracott Vaughan, Jr

Introduction

Adrenal masses are relatively common, and have been reported to occur in about 9 per cent of post mortem examinations (Hedeland *et al.* 1968). Detection of adrenal masses has increased substantially since the advent of cross-sectional imaging techniques and especially computerized tomography (CT). One of the most common problems that one faces in daily practice is the discovery of an incidental adrenal mass. Most incidentally detected adrenal masses are nonfunctioning adenomas; however, they need to be distinguished from primary or secondary malignant lesions (Reed Dunnick *et al.* 1996). Even in patients with a documented malignancy elsewhere, only approximately 50 per cent (Katz and Shirkhoda 1985) or fewer (Oliver *et al.* 1984) of adrenal lesions are proved to represent metastases at pathology. Thus, the approach to the evaluation of these incidentally detected masses is dependent on whether or not the patient has a known underlying malignancy, as the work-up is different in these two clinical scenarios.

In the non-oncologic patient, the differentiation is between a primary adrenal neoplasm and an incidentally detected, nonfunctioning adrenal adenoma, which is the most common benign cause of an incidentally detected adrenal mass. (Other benign causes of an incidentally detected adrenal mass are cyst, hemorrhage, or myelolipoma; however, these have imaging features that are often sufficiently characteristic that one can make a relatively confident diagnosis.) In most institutions in the USA, adrenal masses larger than 5 cm in size are resected. Lesions ranging in size between 3 and 5 cm are more problematic as in some centers additional imaging is performed to exclude a malignant neoplasm. Smaller lesions can be presumed to represent adenomas as it is rare for metastases to present first in the absence of a known primary tumor; however, detection of an incidental small adrenal mass often necessitates follow-up imaging at yearly intervals to ensure stability in size, further characterization with CT or magnetic resonance imaging (MRI), or, rarely, biopsy.

In patients with a known underlying malignancy, in whom an adrenal mass is potentially the only evidence of metastatic disease, differentiation is between nonfunctioning adenoma and metastases. It is essential to distinguish the two in this subgroup of patients as tumor staging and treatment strategies are affected. The two imaging modalities currently employed to help in the differentiation between an adrenal adenoma and a malignant neoplasm are CT and MRI.

Adrenal adenomas

Adrenal adenomas are either hyperfunctioning (secrete an unregulated amount of hormone) or non-hyperfunctioning (behave like normal adrenal cortex) (Reed Dunnick *et al.* 1996). Functioning adenomas may present with hypersecretion of cortisol (Cushing's syndrome), aldosterone (Conn's syndrome), or androgens (adrenal virilization). Adenomas causing Cushing's syndrome measure on average 4 cm or more in diameter, whereas aldosteronomas tend to be much smaller (Reed Dunnick *et al.* 1996). Detection of an adrenal mass in a patient in the appropriate clinical setting with biochemical documentation of the suspected disease process implies a hyperfunctioning adenoma and these lesions should be removed.

CT features of an adenoma include a smooth contour, sharp margination, homogeneous density, and diameter less than 4 cm (Fig. 49.1(a), (b)). Occasionally, adenomas may be heterogeneous because of the presence of cystic degeneration or hemorrhage. Most adenomas are unilateral, although bilateral lesions occur. With MR, non-complicated adenomas are usually isointense with liver on both T1- and T2-weighted sequences, or may be slightly hyperintense to liver on T2-weighted images. Enhancement of adenomas occurs with intravenous (IV) gadolinium and iodinated contrast administration.

Adrenal carcinoma

CT features typical of adrenal carcinoma are size larger than 5 cm, central areas of low attenuation due to tumor necrosis, tumoral calcification, inhomogeneous enhancement with intravenous (IV) contrast, and evidence of extraadrenal spread (Fig. 49.2). Uncomplicated adrenal carcinomas are hypointense to liver on T1-weighted images and hyperintense to liver on T2-weighted images. MRI with vascular techniques is useful in defining intravascular extension. Coronal and sagittal MR images are better for revealing the most cephalad extent of tumor invasion into the inferior vena cava, than are the axial images.

In general, metastases can be larger than adrenal adenomas, have heterogeneous attenuation, are less well defined, and have thick, irregular enhancing walls (Fig. 49.3). They can be unilateral or bilateral. The MRI findings of adrenal metastases include an

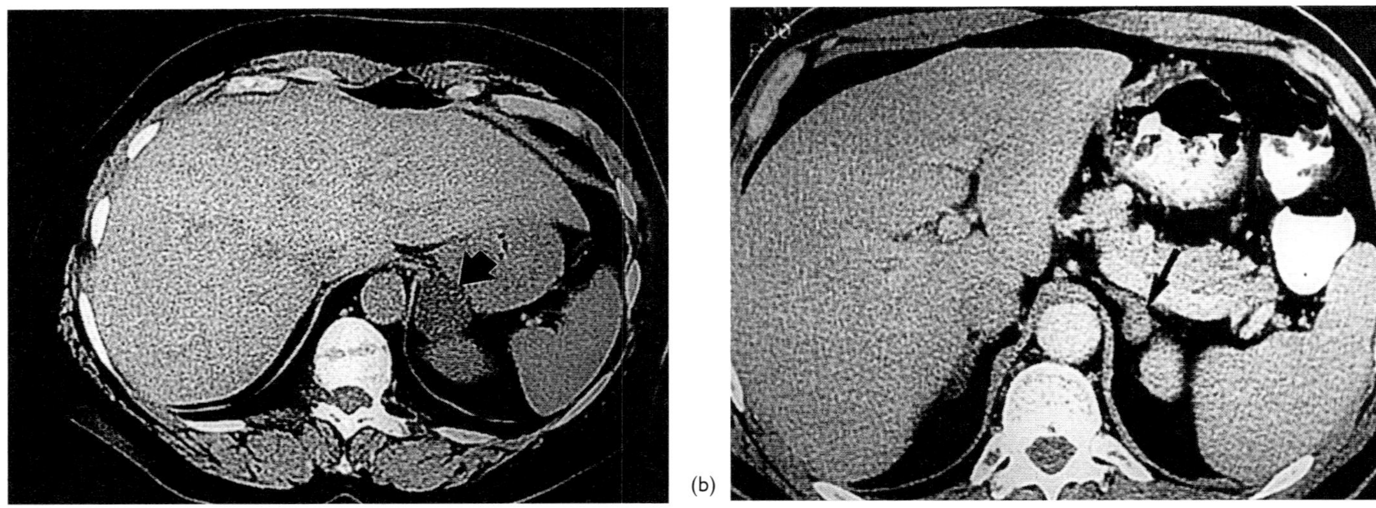

(a)

(b)

Fig. 49.1 (a) Non-hyperfunctioning adenoma of the left adrenal gland seen on nonenhanced CT (arrow). (b) Aldosteronoma of the left adrenal gland on contrast-enhanced CT (arrow). The lesion is typically small.

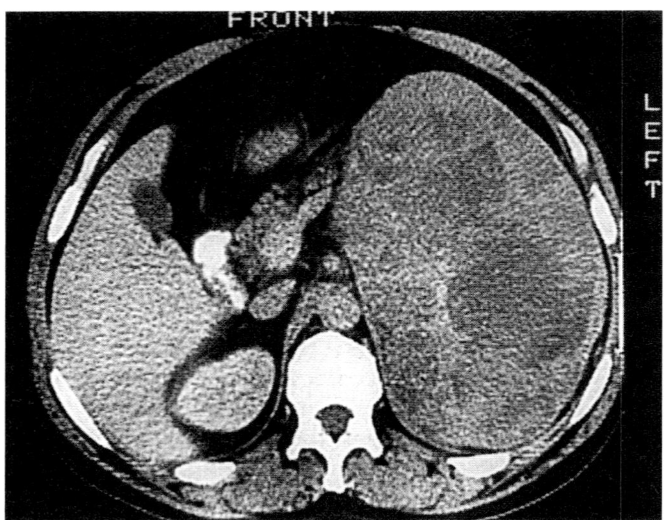

Fig. 49.2 Large, heterogeneous mass in left upper quadrant represents an adrenocortical carcinoma.

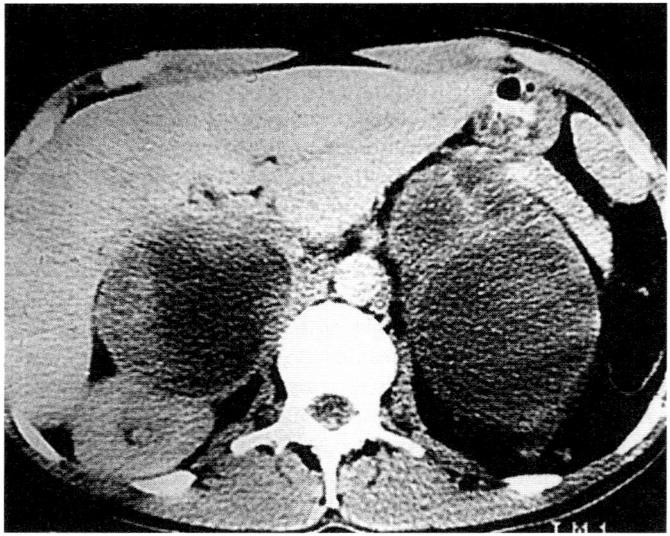

Fig. 49.3 Bilateral, large heterogeneous adrenal masses on CT represent adrenal metastases. The primary was melanoma.

adrenal mass of varying size, which is often isointense or slightly less intense than the liver or spleen on T1-weighted sequences and considerably increased in signal intensity on T2-weighted images, possibly representing an increased water content. They may, however, be atypical and may be isointense or hypointense relative to the liver on T2-weighted images. Unfortunately, CT and MRI features alone do not usually allow differentiation of adrenal adenoma from metastasis. One approach to this problem is to biopsy all these masses; however, recently, methods to characterize the tissue in the lesion have been devised, which often obviates the need for biopsy. These methods are described below.

Differentiating adrenal adenoma from metastasis

CT scans

Benign non-hyperfunctioning adrenal adenomas consist of lipid-laden cells. Metastases to the adrenal glands reflect the histology of the primary neoplasm, and few contain cytoplasmic lipid. Although lipid within adenomas contributes to their often low attenuation on CT scans, confident detection of lipid requires documentation of negative Hounsfield units at unenhanced CT.

Lee and his colleagues (1991) were the first to demonstrate the use of unenhanced CT attenuation values in distinguishing between adrenal adenomas and malignant adrenal masses. Subsequently, several other studies (van Erkel *et al.* 1994; Korobkin *et al.* 1996*a, b*) have corroborated the value of unenhanced CT densitometry in making this important distinction. Unfortunately, CT cannot reliably distinguish between adenomas and metastases with 100 per cent sensitivity and specificity; however, if the mass measures 0 Hounsfield units (HU) or less on unenhanced CT, the likelihood of this being a benign mass is almost 100 per cent. In fact, a relatively high specificity (> 90 per cent) can be achieved even if one uses a density of 10 HU on unenhanced CT. In many centers, including our own, a threshold of 10 HU is used as the cut-off to distinguish between adenomas and metastases. Some centers use a threshold of 18 HU. Unfortunately, as most staging and routine CT scans are obtained after the IV infusion of contrast material, the patient often has to return on another day for an unenhanced scan to obtain reliable CT values. Recently, several studies have shown that delayed scans obtained as early as 5–15 minutes after enhancement may differentiate between adenomas and metastases with high specificity and reasonable sensitivity (Szolar and Kammerhuber 1997; Korobkin *et al.* 1997; Boland *et al.* 1997). Adrenal adenomas have shown a rapid washout of contrast enhancement compared to non-adenomatous lesions. The need to return for a repeat unenhanced CT examination may, thus, be avoided if delayed imaging can be performed.

MRI

MRI has also been used to differentiate between adenomas and metastases, with a high degree of specificity and an acceptable sensitivity (Mitchell *et al.* 1992; Outwater and Mitchell 1994; Outwater *et al.* 1995). Many different techniques were previously utilized; however, currently, chemical shift MRI is the imaging technique most commonly utilized to distinguish between adenomas and metastases (Mitchell *et al.* 1992; Outwater and Mitchell 1994; Outwater *et al.* 1995). The premise with this technique, as with unenhanced CT, is that adenomas contain lipid, while in general malignant lesions do not. This technique takes advantage of the different resonant frequency peaks for the hydrogen atom in water and triglyceride (lipid) molecules and, if appropriate imaging parameters are chosen, water and lipid magnetic dipoles will be out of phase and their signals will cancel, resulting in a decrease in signal intensity of tissue containing both lipid and water, compared to tissue containing no lipid on what are termed 'opposed phase' images. Using this lipid-sensitive imaging sequence, adrenal adenomas, unlike malignant lesions, will show lower signal intensity on opposed-phase than on what are termed conventional in-phase MR images, where they exhibit a signal intensity that is similar or greater compared to the spleen or liver (Fig. 49.4 (a), (b)).

Because CT and MRI both depend on the presence of lipid in the adrenal adenoma for a specific diagnosis, it is unclear whether CT or MRI is more accurate for discriminating adrenal adenomas from metastasis. Furthermore, for lesions that do not adhere to the above-mentioned criteria, needle biopsy or surgery is warranted.

Adrenal scintigraphy

One other imaging technique that has been developed at the University of Michigan is adrenal scintigraphy (Francis *et al.* 1992; Gross *et al.* 1994). Adenomas larger than 2 cm, because they contain functioning adrenal cortical cells, accumulate a cortical-labeling radionuclide tracer known as I-131 NP-59, an analog of 19-iodocholesterol, whereas metastases do not (Fig. 49.5). When an area of uptake on an NP-59 scan is concordant with a mass seen on CT, the mass represents an adenoma. If the mass does not take up tracer, the mass is not an adenoma, but could represent a metastasis or another benign lesion such as a cyst or hemorrhage. Unfortunately, I-131 NP-59 is currently not widely available and it may result in false-negative examinations; therefore, this technique is not often utilized.

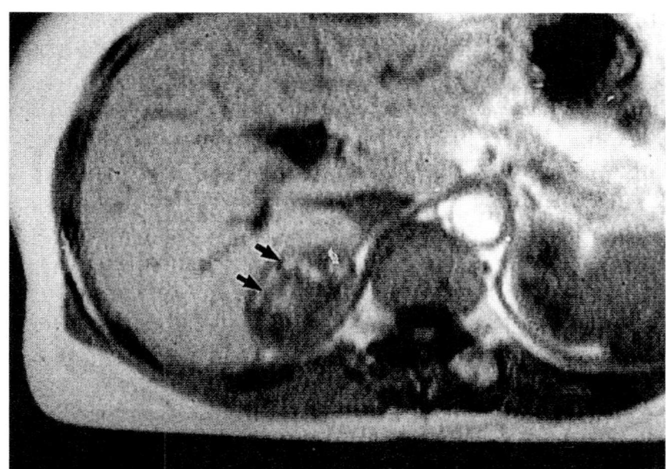

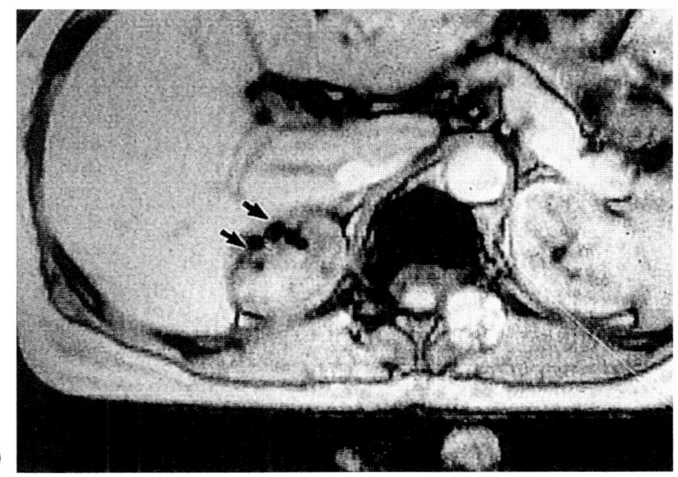

Fig. 49.4 Chemical-shift MRI of adrenal adenoma. (a) In-phase image shows foci of increased signal intensity within a right adrenal mass (arrows). (b) Out-of-phase imaging shows a drop-off in signal intensity confirming the presence of lipid within the adenoma (arrows).

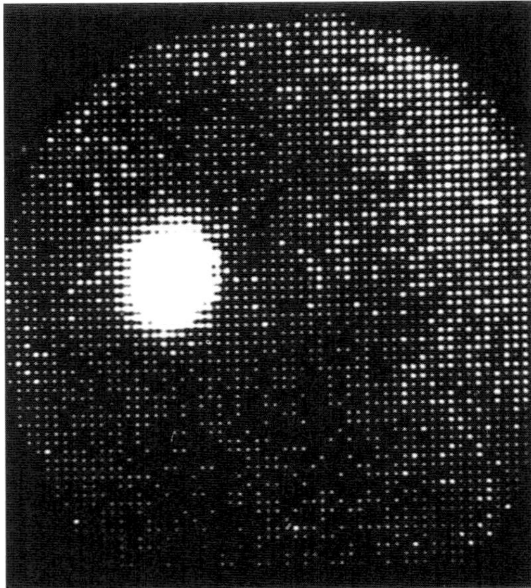

Fig. 49.5 Scintigraphic image of left adrenal adenoma using I-131 NP-59. There is intense focal uptake by the lesion.

The role of percutaneous biopsy

Although the above-mentioned imaging techniques can characterize most adrenal masses as benign adenomas, masses suspected to be metastases still require percutaneous biopsy for confirmation in patients with a known primary neoplasm and either no other evidence of metastatic disease or no other lesion more amenable to biopsy (Korobkin *et al.* 1996*c*). A patient who has a positive biopsy will usually not undergo resection of the primary neoplasm, whereas a negative biopsy may allow for potentially curative resection of the primary malignancy (Korobkin *et al.* 1996*c*). The overall accuracy of percutaneous biopsy is approximately 90 per cent (Welch *et al.* 1994). If neither malignant cells nor benign adrenal tissue are seen on the biopsy specimen, the result is considered non-diagnostic (Reed Dunnick *et al.* 1996). These patients may often be successfully diagnosed with a repeat biopsy but, if not, a surgical biopsy should be considered (Reed Dunnick *et al.* 1996). Histologic distinction between benign adenoma and well differentiated primary adrenal carcinoma may be difficult, and there is a small risk of tumor seeding. Percutaneous biopsy is therefore not recommended to differentiate between an adrenal adenoma and adrenocortical carcinoma (Korobkin *et al.* 1996*c*). Percutaneous biopsy is also not advised to confirm a pheochromocytoma as it can precipitate a hypertensive crisis and even death (Korobkin *et al.* 1996*c*).

Other adrenal pathologies

Other adrenal pathologies include adrenal hyperplasia, medullary tumors such as pheochromocytoma and ganglioneuroma, adrenal cysts, hemorrhage, extramedullary hematopoiesis, lymphoma, and myelolipoma.

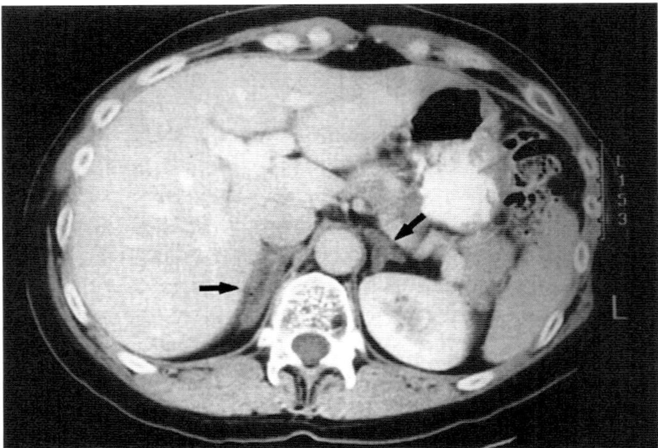

Fig. 49.6 Bilateral adrenal hyperplasia is demonstrated on CT (arrows).

Adrenal hyperplasia causes diffuse enlargement of the adrenal gland (Fig. 49.6). A variant of adrenal hyperplasia, macronodular hyperplasia, is characterized by nodular thickening of the adrenal glands. MRI has little to offer over CT in the evaluation of adrenal hyperplasia.

Pheochromocytomas are usually located in the adrenal glands, but can occur elsewhere in the retroperitoneum, thorax, or pelvis. They usually occur sporadically, but can be seen in association with MEN syndromes, neurofibromatosis, von Hippel–Lindau disease, Sturge–Weber syndrome, and Carney's syndrome. Sporadic tumors are usually large and intraadrenal, and can undergo necrosis and hemorrhage. Because a hypertensive crisis may be precipitated with the use of IV contrast, patients suspected of having a pheochromocytoma are often examined with unenhanced CT or MRI. Suggestive MRI findings are very high signal intensity on T2-weighted images, a pseudocapsule around the adrenal mass, and, frequently, the presence of internal hemorrhage (Fig. 49.7). Even the high signal inten-

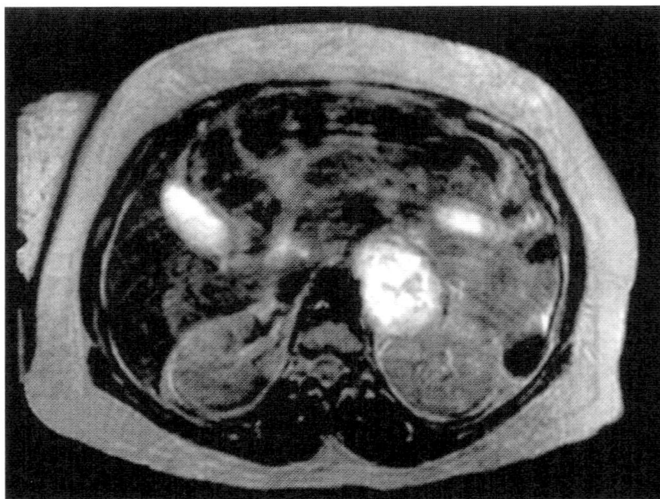

Fig. 49.7 T2-weighted MRI of the left adrenal gland demonstrates a large, heterogeneous, mostly hyperintense mass with a pseudocapsule consistent with pheochromocytoma.

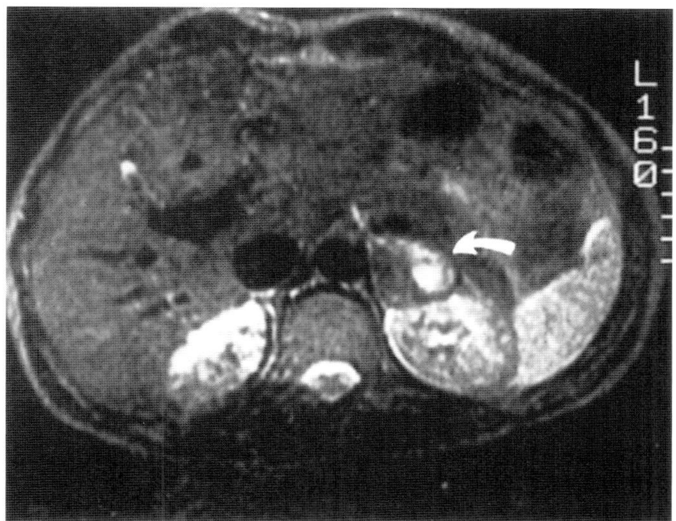

Fig. 49.8 T2-weighted MRI shows a heterogeneous mass with foci of high signal intensity in the left adrenal gland (curved arrow). The lesion was a ganglioneuroma.

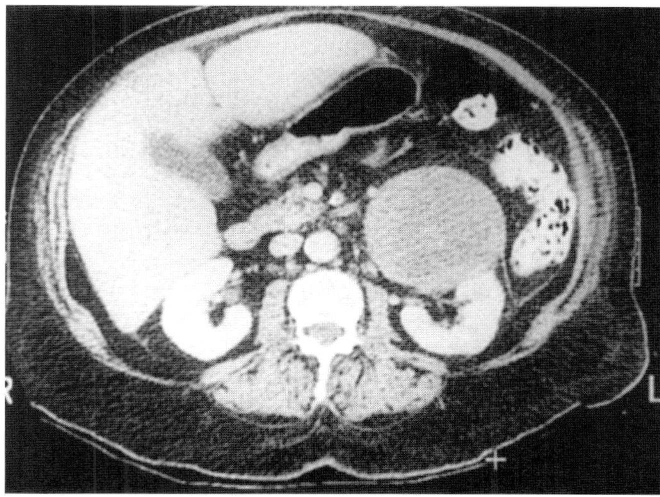

Fig. 49.9 Large, nonenhancing mass in the left renal, suprarenal region on CT, representing an adrenal pseudocyst.

sity on T2-weighted images, however, is not specific enough for the accurate diagnosis of a pheochromocytoma. Imaging features sometimes overlap between pheochromocytomas and other adrenal lesions. Furthermore, pheochromocytomas may present as relatively low signal intensity lesions on T2-weighted images (Varghese *et al.* 1997). In addition, they do not demonstrate chemical shift evidence of lipid. The clinical situation is, however, often helpful, as a patient with biochemical evidence of a pheochromocytoma and an adrenal mass is highly likely to have a pheochromocytoma. Coronal MRI images are often helpful to demonstrate the relationship between the pheochromocytoma and the adjacent vessels. Pheochromocytomas can also be detected with I-131 metaiodobenzyl-guanidine (MIBG) scintigraphy, with an accuracy of approximately 90 per cent. Since I-131 metaiodobenzyl-guanidine (MIBG) scintigraphy is capable of whole-body imaging, it is useful for the detection of metastatic disease in patients with pheochromocytoma, as well as in the detection of extraadrenal tumors.

Adrenal ganglioneuromas typically show heterogeneous high signal intensity on T2-weighted images (Fig.49.8) and may have areas of internal calcifications.

Benign adrenal cysts are usually homogeneous, nonenhancing round masses with a thick, often calcified wall, and water density (Fig. 49.9). They will be dark on T1-weighted MR images and homogeneously bright on T2-weighted-images. The diagnosis is usually reliably made with CT and only rarely is MRI necessary.

Adrenal hemorrhage usually appears as an oval or round mass on CT scans (Fig. 49.10). Acute hemorrhage has high density measurements (50–90 HU) and can be easily characterized, if necessary, with MRI. Follow-up studies reveal a diminution in size of the mass and a gradual decrease in attenuation value. As the hematoma resolves, calcification may occur (Fig. 49.10).

Extramedullary hematopoiesis may arise in the hematopoietic marrow in the adrenal gland, and it may appear as a large inhomogeneous mass in the adrenal gland.

Adrenal lymphoma is usually secondary lymphoma and most commonly appears as a solid homogeneous soft-tissue density mass in the adrenal gland.

Myelolipoma is an uncommon, benign tumor composed of mature adipose and hematopoietic tissue, which will be of fat density on CT (Fig. 49.11), of high signal intensity on T1-weighted MR images, and of low signal intensity on fat-suppressed T1-weighted MR images. The diagnosis is usually reliably made with CT and only rarely is MRI necessary.

Infections occurring in the adrenal glands include granulomatous infections such as tuberculosis and histoplasmosis, and pneumocystis carinii. Tuberculosis is the most common infec-

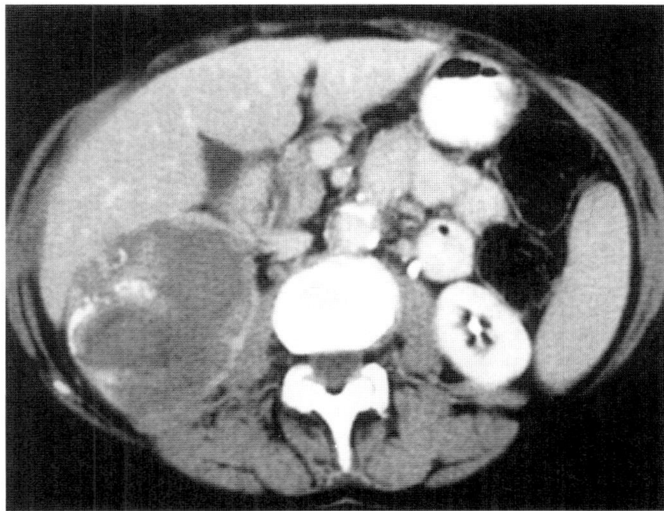

Fig. 49.10 Right adrenal hemorrhage on CT. The lesion is heterogeneous with thick walls and wall calcifications.

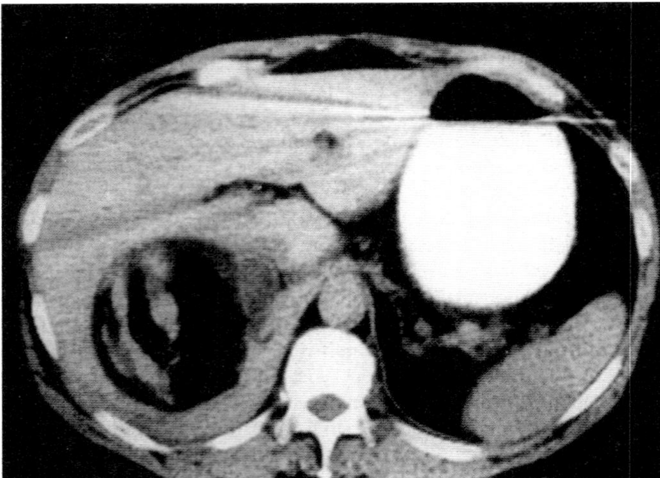

Fig. 49.11 Fat-containing mass in the right adrenal gland is diagnostic of a myelolipoma. The soft tissue density surrounding the lesion represents hemorrhage.

tious cause of Addison's disease. Disseminated histoplasmosis usually occurs in endemic areas and usually occurs in immuno-compromised patients. CT findings in granulomatous infection include bilateral enlargement of the adrenal glands with a central area of hypodensity, and a peripheral rim of enhancement. In the healing phase of infection, the adrenal glands may contain variable amounts of calcification (Fig. 49.12) and often become atrophic. Patients with disseminated pneumocystis carinii infection may have punctate or coarse calcifications in the adrenal glands, as well as the spleen, liver, kidneys, and lymph nodes. Adrenal abscesses are rare, and most are found in neonates with pre-existing adrenal hemorrhage.

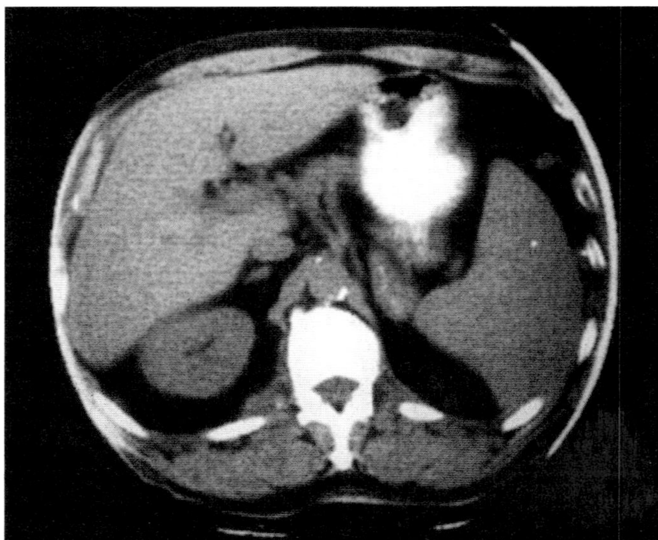

Fig. 49.12 Mild adrenal enlargement with calcifications in a patient with tuberculosis and Addison's disease. Also note splenic granuloma.

Conclusion

In conclusion, although the optimal algorithm for non-invasive imaging assessment of adrenal masses has not yet been conclusively established, one or more of the imaging techniques described above can often clearly characterize many adrenal masses. Adrenal cysts, adrenal hemorrhage, and myelolipoma are usually easily characterized because of their distinctive imaging characteristics. Using unenhanced CT with densitometry, delayed enhanced CT with densitometry, chemical shift MRI, or NP-59 scintigraphy, most benign adrenal adenomas can be distinguished from a malignant neoplasm. For adrenal lesions that cannot be characterized as benign using the available imaging techniques described above, in an oncology patient who has no other evidence of metastatic disease, or to confirm suspected adrenal lymphoma, percutaneous biopsy is still necessary. Surgical resection is recommended when non-invasive imaging techniques suggest the possibility of adrenocortical carcinoma or pheochromocytoma.

References

Boland, G., Hahn, P.F., Pena, C., and Mueller, P.R. (1997). Adrenal masses: characterization with delayed contrast-enhanced CT. *Radiology* **202**, 693–6.

Francis, I.R., Gross, M.D., Shapiro, B., *et al.* (1992). Integrated imaging of adrenal disease. *Radiology* **184**, 1–13.

Gross, M.D., Shapiro, B., Francis, I.R., *et al.* (1994). Scintigraphic evaluation of clinically silent adrenal masses. *J. Nucl. Med.* **35**, 1145–52.

Hedeland, H., Ostberg, G., and Hokfeld, B. (1968). The prevalence of adrenocortical adenomas in autopsy material in relation to hypertension and diabetes. *Acta Med. Scand.* **184**, 211–14.

Katz, R.L. and Shirkhoda, A. (1985). Diagnostic approach to incidental adrenal nodules in the cancer patient. *Cancer* **55**, 1995–2000.

Korobkin, M.T., Brodeur, F.J., Yutzy, G.G., *et al.* (1996*a*). Differentiation of adrenal adenomas from non adenomas by using CT attenuation values. *Am. J. Roentgenol.* **166**, 531–6.

Korobkin, M.T., Giordano, T.J., Brodeur, F.J., *et al.* (1996*b*). Adrenal adenomas: relationship between histologic lipid and CT and MR findings. *Radiology* **200**, 743–7.

Korobkin, M., Francis, I.R., Kloos, R.T., and Reed Dunnick, N. (1996*c*). The incidental adrenal mass. *Radiol. Clin. N. Am.* **34**, 1037–54.

Korobkin, M.T., Brodeur, F.J., Francis, I.R., *et al.* (1997). CT time-attenuation washout curves of adrenal nonadenomas. *Am. J. Roentgenol.* **170**, 747–52.

Lee, M.J., Hahn, P.F., Papanicolaou, N., Egglin, T.K., Saini, S., Mueller, P.R., and Simeone, J.F. (1991). Benign and malignant adrenal masses: CT distinction with attenuation coefficients, size and observer analysis. *Radiology* **179**, 415–18.

Mitchell, D.G., Crovello, M., Matteuci, T., Petersen, R.O., *et al.* (1992). Benign adrenocortical masses: diagnosis with chemical shift MR imaging. *Radiology* **185**, 345–51.

Oliver, T.W. Jr, Bernardino, M.E., Miller, J.I., Mansour, K., Greene, D., and Davis, W.A. (1984). Isolated adrenal masses in nonsmall-cell bronchogenic carcinoma. *Radiology* **153**, 217–18.

Outwater, E.K. and Mitchell, D.G. (1994). Differentiation of adrenal masses with chemical shift imaging. *Radiology* **193** (3), 877–8.

Outwater, E.K., Siegelman, E.S., Radecki, P.D. *et al.* (1995). Distinction between benign and malignant adrenal masses: value of T1-weighted chemical shift MR imaging *Am. J. Roentgenol.* **165**, 579–83.

Reed Dunnick, N., Korobkin, M.T., and Francis, I.R. (1996). Adrenal radiology: distinguishing benign from malignant adrenal masses. *Am. J. Roentgenol.* **167**, 861–7.

Szolar, D.H. and Kammerhuber, F. (1997). Quantitative CT evaluation of adrenal gland masses: a step forward in the differentiation between adenomas and nonadenomas. *Radiology* **202**, 517–21.

van Erkel, A.R., van Gillis, A.P.G., Lequin, M., *et al.* (1994). CT and MR distinction of adenomas and non adenomas of the adrenal gland. *J. Comput. Assist. Tomogr.* **18**, 432–8.

Varghese, J.C., Hahn, P.F., Papanicolaou, N., *et al.* (1997). MR differentiation of pheochromocytoma from other adrenal lesions based on qualitative analysis of T2 relaxation times. *Clin. Radiol.* **57**, 603–6.

Welch, T.J., Sheedy, P.F., Stephens, D.H., Johnson, C.M., and Swensen, S.J. (1994). Percutaneous adrenal biopsy: review of a 10-year experience. *Radiology* **193**, 341–4.

50.   Diagnostic tests of adrenal cortical and medullary function

Zhenqi Liu, Helmy M. Siragy, and Robert M. Carey

Introduction

The adrenal glands are paired retroperitoneal organs situated above the upper pole of each kidney and lying lateral to the twelfth thoracic and first lumbar vertebrae. The glands are composed of two distinct structural units. The cortex composes the outer layer and completely surrounds the centrally located medulla. The average weight of the gland in the adult is 4 g irrespective of sex (Studzinski *et al.* 1963).

The blood supply to the gland arises from three main groups of arteries: a superior group from the distal portion of the terminal branches of the inferior phrenic artery; a middle group—the superior, middle, and inferior adrenal arteries—directly from the aorta; and an inferior group from the renal artery. The numerous arteries and their branches ramify over the surface of the gland to form a thin subcapsular plexus from which the sinusoidal circulation of the cortex is formed. Large capillaries traverse the cortex and reunite to form the plexus reticularis at the corticomedullary junction. The medulla has both arterial and venous blood supply. A few arterioles pass through the subcapsular plexus, the cortex, and the plexus reticularis to feed the medulla directly. The venous supply is via the plexus reticularis. This plexus and the venous sinuses that drain the medulla form a portal system that allows blood from the cortex to bathe the cells of the medulla. The venous sinuses anastomose, establishing the adrenal vein that drains into the inferior vena cava on the right and the renal vein of the left. The numerous arterial channels protect the gland from infarction (Dobbie and Symington 1966; Netter 1965).

Embryology and postnatal development

The gland develops from two separate germ cell lines. The cortex evolves from primordial mesoderm just medial to the urogenital ridge and can be identified by the fourth week of gestation. The medulla, which arises from the neural crest cells and is of ectodermal origin, invades the primordium of the cortex during the fourth week of gestation. By the fifth week the relative positions of the cortex and the medulla are established (Crowder 1957; Buster 1980; Artal 1980). The fetal cortex attains its maximum size during the fourth fetal month and then slowly begins to decrease in size. At birth the adrenal gland consists of three distinct, concentric tissue layers: the true cortex lying immediately beneath the connective tissue capsule; the fetal cortex, a middle layer of tissue;

and a thin central zone, the medulla, surrounding the venous sinuses (Keene and Hewer 1926). The fetal cortex, comprising 80 per cent of the adrenal gland at birth, rapidly undergoes involution during the first 3 weeks of life. This process continues such that by the third month of life only a remnant of the fetal cortex composed mostly of connective tissue encapsulates the medulla (Tahka 1951). From the first month of life, the true cortex dominates the gland. The adrenal medulla does not become distinct and compact until the atrophy of the fetal cortex. In the adult the cortex comprises 90 per cent and the medulla 10 per cent of the adrenal gland by weight (Fig. 50.1) (Weiss and Greep 1977).

Histology

Histologically, the cortex can be divided into three concentric sections—the zona glomerulosa (directly beneath the tissue capsule), the zona fasciculata, and the zona reticularis (the section immediately surrounding the medulla) (Fig. 50.2). They comprise 15, 75, and 7 per cent of the adult cortex by volume, respectively (Neville and Mackay 1972).

The zona glomerulosa and the zona fasciculata can be delineated at birth, while the time of appearance of the zona reticularis has been controversial, with estimates ranging from the first postnatal week to the third month of life (Keene and Hewer 1926; Blackman 1946). The major change in the true cortex in the first year of life is the increase in the size of the fascicular zona (Keene and Hewer 1926). The zona reticularis remains very thin until the third year of life, at which time it gradually thickens (Blackman 1946).

The medulla occupies approximately 10 per cent of the adrenal gland throughout life. The major change that takes place in the medulla is the relative production of norepinephrine (also called noradrenaline) and epinephrine (also called adrenaline) (West *et al.* 1951). This change will be discussed later in the chapter.

Steroid synthesis

Through a series of biochemical alterations of a common precursor—cholesterol—the zones of the adrenal cortex produce steroid hormones for salt retention, metabolic homeostasis, and the development of adrenarche (Fig. 50.3). The zona glomerulosa is the only source of the mineralocorticoid aldosterone. This

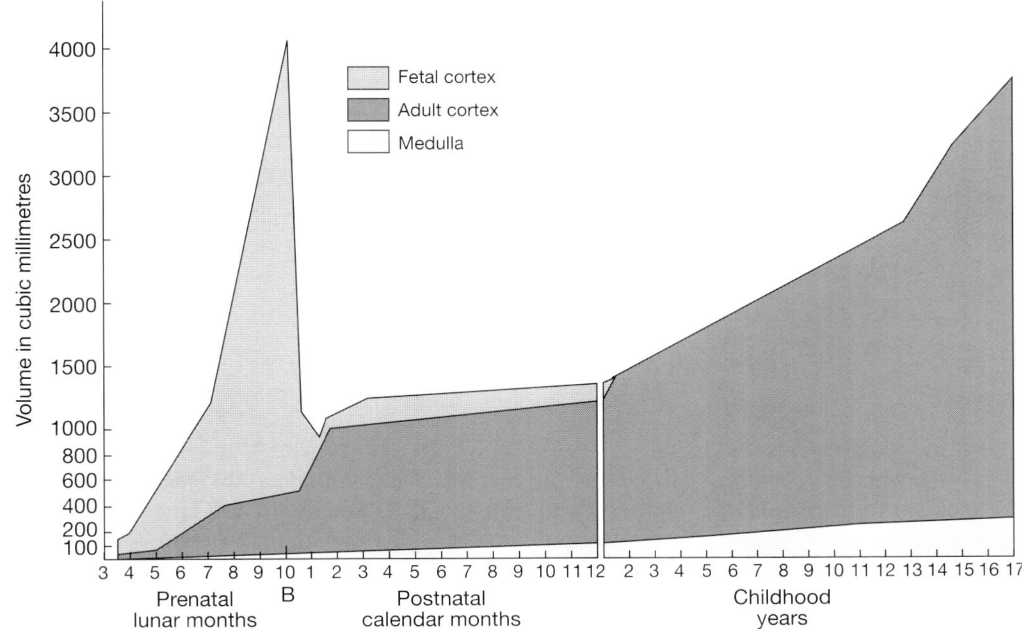

Fig. 50.1 Growth of the human adrenal gland. (Adapted from Swinyard C.A., Anat Rec 87: 146, 1943.)

hormone regulates sodium retention in the kidney, the gut, and the salivary and sweat glands. The zona fasciculata and the zona reticularis produce and secrete cortisol (the major glucocorticoid hormone with slight mineralocorticoid activity), the androgens, and the estrogens. The principal androgens produced are dehydroepiandrosterone (DHEA), dehydroepiandrosterone sulfate (DHEA-S), and androstenedione. The rate-limiting step in the formation of all of these hormones is the conversion of cholesterol to pregnenolone (Nelson 1980*a*). For the major pathways, products, and urinary metabolites, see Fig. 50.4.

The adrenal has three sources from which to obtain the foundation for steroid hormone synthesis: (1) uptake of cholesterol from low-density and high-density lipoproteins; (2) endogenous synthesis of cholesterol in the gland; (3) hydrolysis of stored cholesterol esters (Brown *et al.* 1979; Kovanen *et al.* 1979). Once the process of transforming cholesterol has begun, the enzymes present in the different zones of the adrenal dictate the ultimate product.

In the zona glomerulosa cholesterol is converted to aldosterone with the intermediate by-products of pregnenolone, progesterone, deoxycorticosterone, and corticosterone. The final step in the formation of aldosterone requires the conversion of the 18-methyl group of corticosterone to an aldehyde. This process is catalyzed by CYP11B2 (aldosterone synthase, 18-hydrosteroid dehydrogenase). This enzyme is only found in the zona glomerulosa and thus aldosterone is solely produced there (Stachenko and Giroud 1959; Tait *et al.* 1970). The lack of CYP17 (17α-hydroxylase) prevents the cells of the zona glomerulosa from synthesizing cortisol, estrogen, and the androgens (Tait *et al.* 1970; Finkelstein and Shaefer 1979).

The presence of CYP17 (17α-hydroxylase) in the zona fasciculata and the zona reticularis allows pregnenolone and progesterone to enter the glucocorticoid and androgen pathways. 17-Hydroxypregnenolone undergoes isomerase and dehydro-

genase reactions. The OH group at the 3 position is converted to a ketone, and the 5–6 double bond in the B ring is converted to a 4–5 double bond in the A ring. The product, 17-OH-progesterone, undergoes hydroxylation at the 21 and 11 positions, and thus cortisol is formed.

The major androgen formed in the adrenal is DHEA. The action of CYP17 (17,20-desmolase) on 17-hydroxypregnenolone removes the C20–C21 side chain from the 17 position and converts the 17-OH group to a ketone, forming DHEA. Androstenedione can be synthesized from either 17-OH-progesterone or DHEA. Androstenedione is the immediate precursor of testosterone and estrone. Despite the fact that DHEA can be converted to androstenedione, most of the androstenedione is formed from the conversion of 17-OH-progesterone (Samuels and Nelson 1975). DHEA may also undergo sulfation by a sulfokinase to form DHEA-S.

Glucocorticoids

Glucocorticoid metabolism

Glucocorticoid secretion

Adrenocorticotropin (ACTH) is a 39 amino acid polypeptide (molecular weight 4.5 k) that exerts a major influence on the function of the adrenal cortex (Hoffman 1974). This polypeptide is produced by cleavage of a large protein of 290 amino acids (13 k), termed proopiomelanocortin (POMC). This protein is also a common precursor for other polypeptide hormones, for example, β-LPH, α-MSH, β-MSH, β-endorphin (Fig. 50.5), and methionine enkephalin (Mains and Eipper 1980).

The biologic activity of ACTH is dictated by its amino acid sequence. Experiments altering the length of the parent compound have revealed that $ACTH_{1-24}$ is equipotent to $ACTH_{1-39}$. Further shortening of the amino acid sequence to $ACTH_{1-18}$

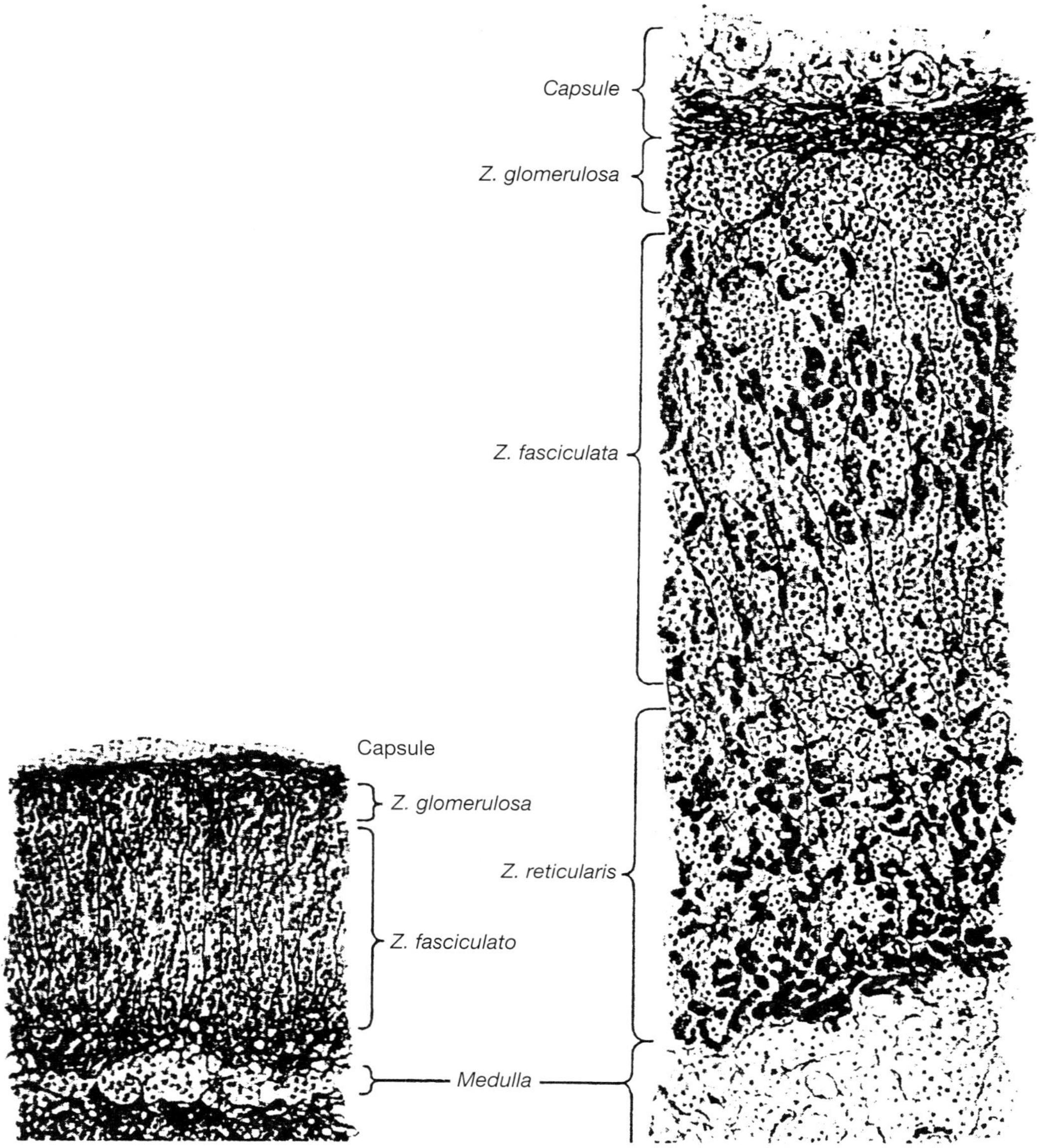

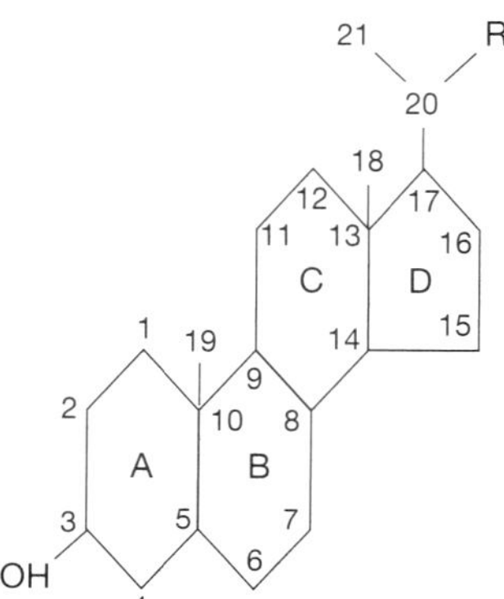

Fig. 50.2   Histology of the human adrenal gland at 6 months of age (left) and in the adult (right). (Adapted from Bloom and Fawett, 'A Textbook of a histology,' p 361, 1992.

Fig. 50.3   Basic structure of the common cholesterol precursor.

decreases the biologic effect of the compound (Seelig and Sayers 1973; Hofmann *et al.* 1970; Li *et al.* 1961; Sayers and Portanova 1975). The minimum sequence needed for any biologic activity is $ACTH_{1-10}$. The biological half-life of $ACTH_{1-39}$ is less than 10 min (Krieger and Allen 1975).

Catabolism of ACTH takes place primarily in the liver. ACTH maintains immunologic reactivity long after biologic activity has ceased. The catabolic event that alters the bioeffect but not the immunologic effect of the molecule is not known (Krieger and Allen 1975; Nicholson *et al.* 1978).

ACTH secretion is controlled by three components: (1) an inherent diurnal rhythm; (2) 'stress' (physical and emotional); and (3) circulating cortisol levels (Frohman 1981). The influence of stress overrides the other controlling factors.

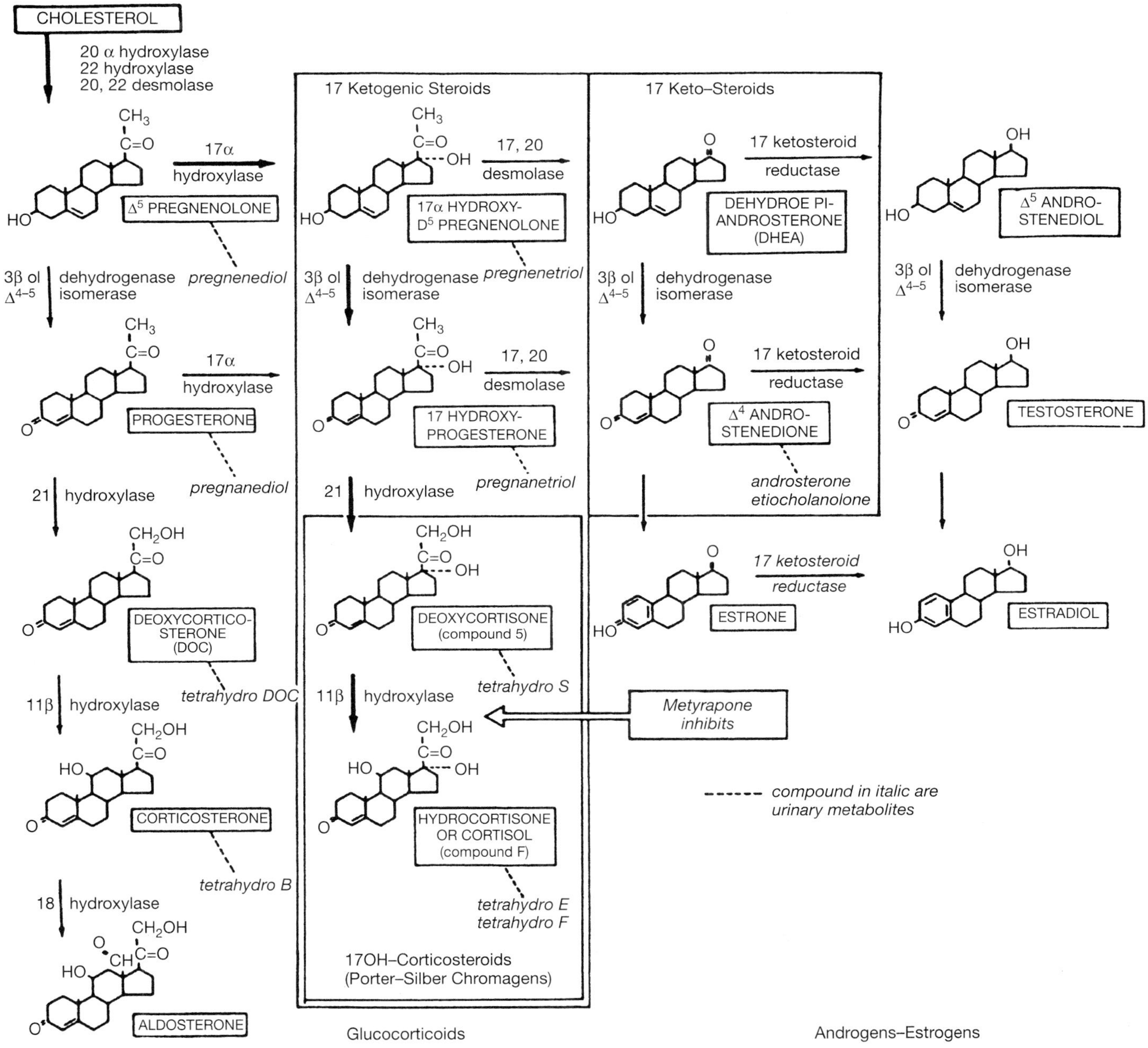

Fig. 50.4 Major steroid pathways in the adrenal including urinary metabolites. Although estrone is 17-ketosteroid, it is not a significant contributor to the 17-ketosteroid level in the urine and therefore not included in the brackets. (Adapted from Urology (Suppl) 7:4, 1976.)

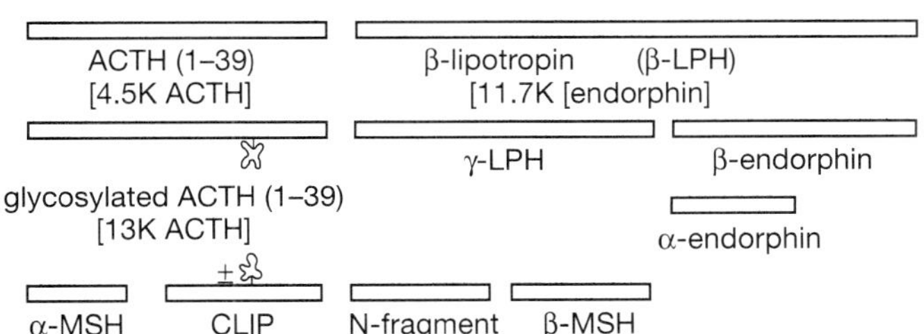

Fig. 50.5 Structural relationships of peptides whose parental compound is proopiomelanocortin. (Adapted from Eipper, B.A., Mains, R.E., Endocr Rev 1:2, 1980.)

ACTH appears to have three effects on the adrenal cortex: (1) a possible trophic effect; (2) the ability to increase the production of cortisol and its precursors; and (3) the ability to stimulate the release of cortisol (Frohman 1981).

Early experiments in animals first drew attention to the possible trophic properties of ACTH. Cortical atrophy was observed a short time after total hypophysectomy (Schumacker and Firor 1934). Adrenal cortical hypertrophy was induced in both intact and hypophysectomized animals by treatment with corticotropic hormone (Emery and Atwell 1933; Reese and Moon 1938). The removal of one adrenal in the intact animal was promptly followed by a compensatory increase in the size of the cortex of the remaining gland. This process did not occur in the hypophysectomized animal but did occur if adrenocorticotropic hormone was administered to such an animal (Soffer *et al.* 1961).

More recent information has called this concept into question. Antiserum to ACTH has been shown to inhibit steroid synthesis but not to decrease the size of the adrenal cortex. Antiserum given to intact, unilaterally adrenalectomized animals did not prevent hypertrophy of the remaining gland (Ajagannadha *et al.* 1978). These data suggest that a non-ACTH pituitary factor may be responsible for the size of the adrenal cortex and that the early experiments utilized adrenocorticotropin contaminated with this pituitary factor or factors. ACTH has also been shown to inhibit rather than stimulate the growth of isolated adrenal cells (Gill *et al.* 1979). Further work is required to confirm the trophic capabilities of ACTH or the existence of an adrenal cortical weight-maintaining factor of pituitary origin.

The role of ACTH in the synthesis and secretion of cortisol appears to be that of a modulator rather than an initiator. This concept is supported by the fact that low levels of cortisol have been detected in the plasma of individuals who have undergone total hypophysectomy (Nelson 1980*a*). Also, a gland that has been exposed chronically to low levels of ACTH may require 24–72 h of priming with ACTH before a normal increase in cortisol is observed after the acute administration of corticotropin (Cope 1972).

The mechanism whereby ACTH stimulates the secretion of cortisol appears to be intimately tied to hormone production. There is little storage of cortisol by the adrenal (Holzbauer 1957), yet plasma cortisol rises within 3 min of the administration of ACTH (Blair-West *et al.* 1970; Espiner *et al.* 1972; Sayers *et al.* 1973). Therefore, it is believed that the response of the cortex to corticotropin is primarily due to increased hormone production (Holzbauer 1957). How ACTH stimulates cortisol synthesis is not clear but roles for cyclic AMP, calcium ion, and phospholipase A_2 have been suggested.

ACTH appears to act at several fronts to alter the rate-limiting step, the conversion of cholesterol to pregnenolone, and thus increase steroidogenesis. It decreases the activity of cholesterol ester synthetase, increases the activity of cholesterol esterase, and stimulates intrinsic cholesterol production by activating 3-hydroxy-3-methyglutaryl CoA reductase (HMG CoA reductase). Each of these actions works to increase the level of free cholesterol in cortical cells (Gill 1979; Brown *et al.* 1979). ACTH has also been implicated in the increased uptake of low-density lipoproteins by adrenal cells, making available more free cholesterol (Kovanen *et al.* 1979). Despite all these efforts to increase substrate, no significant intracellular rise in free cholesterol has been described after exposure to ACTH (Brown *et al.* 1979). These data offer indirect evidence for an effect of ACTH on the enzyme complex that converts cholesterol to pregnenolone. Data suggesting a direct action on this enzyme complex are lacking.

Other substances have been reported to stimulate steroid secretion in the hypophysectomized animal. Pitressin, serotonin, histamine, prostaglandins, splanchnic nerve stimulation, acetylcholine, thyroxine, and the catecholamines are among those substances (Nelson 1980*a*).

Circulating concentrations

In the circulation under physiologic conditions, 80 per cent of cortisol is bound to corticosteroid-binding globulin (CBG, transcortin), 10–15 per cent is bound to albumin and α_1 acid glycoprotein, and 7–10 per cent is free. All binding proteins are synthesized in the liver. Certain states raise CBG levels (estrogen therapy, pregnancy, hyperthyroidism, diabetes mellitus), and other processes lower CBG levels (liver disease, multiple myeloma, nephrotic syndrome, obesity). Variations in binding proteins influence the total plasma cortisol value but not the free cortisol level. It appears that only the free fraction of cortisol is metabolically active (Baxter and Tyrrell 1981).

Cortisol catabolism

The half-life of plasma cortisol varies from 60 to 120 min in adults (Weitzman *et al.* 1971; Peterson 1959; Brown *et al.* 1957) and from 175 to 255 min in the newborn. The longer half-life in newborns is secondary to decreased hepatic enzyme activity (Reynolds *et al.* 1962; Bongiovanni *et al.* 1958). By 1 year of age, the half-life of cortisol is equal to that in the adult (Bongiovanni *et al.* 1958).

The liver is the primary site for cortisol catabolism (Nelson and Harding 1952). The major reaction is a reduction of the double bond of the A ring of cortisol and cortisone to form dihydrocortisol (dihydrocortisone). This transformation inactivates the glucocorticoid. Dihydrocortisol is then converted rapidly to tetrahydrocortisol (tetrahydrocortisone) by 3-hydroxysteroid dehydrogenase (Peterson 1971). The tetrahydrocompounds can undergo reduction of the 20-ketone to form cortols and cortolones (Rosenfield *et al.* 1967). Sixty to 70 per cent of the metabolites of cortisol are conjugated to glucuronides with a small fraction of the metabolites bound to sulfate. The addition of glucuronide or sulfate makes the substances more water-soluble and therefore more easily excreted by the kidney (Fig. 50.6) (Rosenfeld *et al.* 1967; Pasqualini and Jayle 1961).

Assays

Plasma ACTH

The plasma level of ACTH can be assessed by three different methods—bioassay, radioimmunoassay, and immunoradiometric assay.

The bioassay technique measures the ability of an individual's plasma to increase steroidogenesis. Its major pitfall is measurement of the steroidogenic activity of substances other than $ACTH_{1-39}$. The offending fragments are usually shortened ACTH molecules. Liotta and Krieger (1975) developed a bioassay system using dispersed rat adrenal cells. Prior to exposure of the adrenal cells to the patient's plasma, an extraction is performed that removes the major interfering substances. The steroidogenic potential of the individual serum is then assessed. The assay is now only used as a research tool.

Radioimmunoassay (RIA) of ACTH is a tool that is accessible to the clinician. This process involves development of an antibody that recognizes a portion of the ACTH molecule. Numerous antibodies to different portions of the ACTH molecule are available. Thus the antibody interacts with any molecule containing the

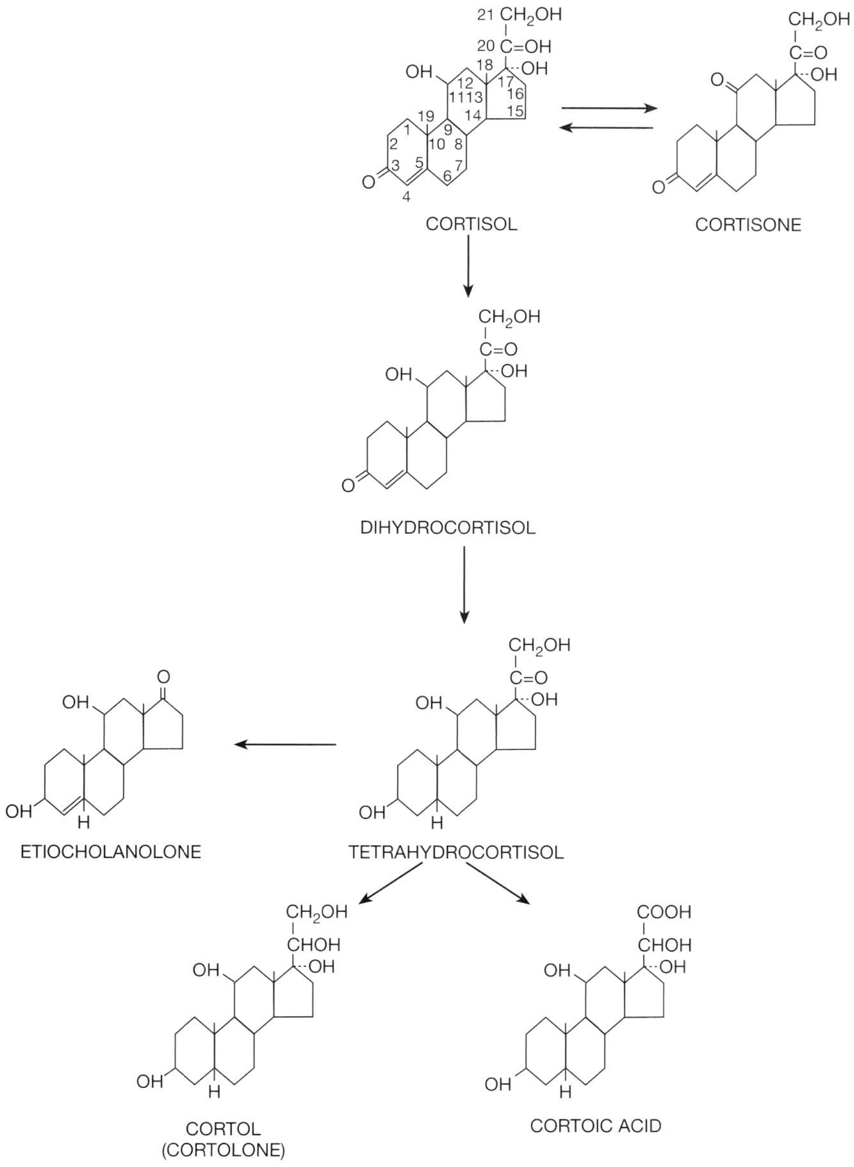

Fig. 50.6 Cortisol catabolism. (Adapted from Nelson, D., 'The Adrenal Cortex: Major Problems in Internal Medicine,' W.B. Saunders, Philadelphia, p 80, 1980.)

given amino acid sequence it has been programmed to recognize. The substance with which the antibody reacts may not be $ACTH_{1-39}$. The antibody may recognize fragments of $ACTH_{1-39}$ or substances sharing common amino acid sequence such as β-LPH, α-MSH, α-LPH, and big ACTH (Mains and Eipper 1980). These substances may not be biologically active. Thus, one must be aware of the cross-reactivity of the antibody that is used in the radioimmunoassay before the assay can be interpreted accurately.

Immunoradiometric assay (IRMA) is now the method of choice for measuring ACTH in clinical laboratories. Unlike RIA, IRMA uses saturating concentrations of two antisera that recognize noncompeting epitopes present in the ACTH molecule. An anti-ACTH antibody-coated bead captures ACTH in the sample and then the amount of captured ACTH is determined by a ^{125}I radiolabelled anti-ACTH antibody, which attaches to the bead-bound ACTH. There is no or very weak cross-reactivity with ACTH fragments and IRMA is 5- to 100-fold more sensitive in basal range than RIA (Segre and Brown 1998; Kertesz *et al.* 1998; Rosano *et al.* 1995).

Plasma cortisol
Assessment of plasma cortisol values has been developed using the competitive binding protein assay (CBPA), the fluorometric assay (FA), and radioimmunoassay (RIA). CBPA and FA played a major role in validating the dynamic studies of the hypothalamic–pituitary–adrenal axis. Therefore, these assays are reviewed. RIA is the present method of choice.

CBPA utilizes the competition between radiolabeled cortisol and endogenous substances in the patient's plasma competing for binding sites available on a known concentration of corticosteroid-binding globulin (CBG). The level of naturally occurring elements is assessed by the degree of inhibition of binding of radiolabeled cortisol to CBG (Murphy 1975). Substances other than cortisol that can bind to CBG are cortisone, corticosterone, 17-OH-progesterone, progesterone, 11-deoxycortisol, 11-deoxycorticosterone, and 21-deoxycortisol (Murphy 1967, 1975). In normal conditions these substances are present in negligible amounts. Pregnancy and disease states involving enzyme deficiency or abnormality can increase cortisol precursors that compete for CBG. Synthetic steroids—prednisolone and 6-methylprednisolone—can interfere with measurement of endogenous cortisol. Extraction techniques have been developed to eliminate cross-reactivity (Murphy 1967; Newsome *et al.* 1972; Sheridan and Mattingly 1975). The clinician must be cognizant of the potential interaction of endogenous substances to obtain an accurate measure of plasma cortisol.

The FA exploits the fluorescent property of steroids containing 21- and 11-hydroxyl groups and ketones at the 3 and 20 positions. Thus, cortisol, corticosterone, 20-hydroxycortisol (a metabolite of cortisol), and 21-deoxycortisol (a precursor of cortisol) are measured with this technique (Nielson and Asfeldt 1967). Except in errors of biosynthesis, these compounds are not found in significant amounts. Investigators have measured a nonspecific background fluorescence in plasma that may lead to an overestimation of plasma cortisol by 2–3 mg/dl compared with other techniques. Certain drugs can also interfere with this assay—spironolactone, quinacrine, fusidic acid, niacin, quinidine, and heparin preparations that contain benzyl alcohol (Baxter and Tyrrell 1980).

Radioimmunoassay (RIA) is the assay method of choice. Polyclonal or monoclonal antibodies are raised to a steroid analog that has been conjugated to a protein carrier. The accuracy of RIA in defining cortisol levels is directly related to the specificity of the antibody. Cross-reaction has been documented with all precursors in the glucocorticoid pathway, all substances in the mineralocorticoid pathway, and DHEA, estradiol, testosterone, prednisone, dexamethasone, spironolactone, and 21-deoxycortisol (Krieger 1979). The specificity and potential for cross-reaction differs among antisera. The clinician must be aware of the possible cross-reaction in the assay utilized.

High-performance liquid chromatography (HPLC) has been used to separate cortisol from other steroids and steroid metabolites and cortisol can then be measured fluorometrically or spectrophotometrically (Gotelli *et al.* 1981). The radioreceptor assay uses the type II glucocorticoid receptor as cortisol-binding agent (Ballard *et al.* 1975). Both assays are very specific, but not widely used due to tedious procedural processes and/or availability (Orth and Kovacs 1998).

Plasma-free cortisol

The unbound or free fraction of cortisol found in the plasma gives a measure of the physiologically active portion of total plasma cortisol. The laboratory can define this fraction by using gel filtration, equilibrium dialysis, and competition between radiolabeled dexamethasone and plasma cortisol for glucocorticoid receptors in intact cells (Ballard *et al.* 1975; Robin *et al.* 1977). This test can aid the clinician in defining states of cortisol excess and deficiency.

Urinary 17-ketosteroids

Urinary extracts with a 17-ketone group react with M-dinitrobenzene to form a pink substance (Fig. 50.7). This colorimetric reaction

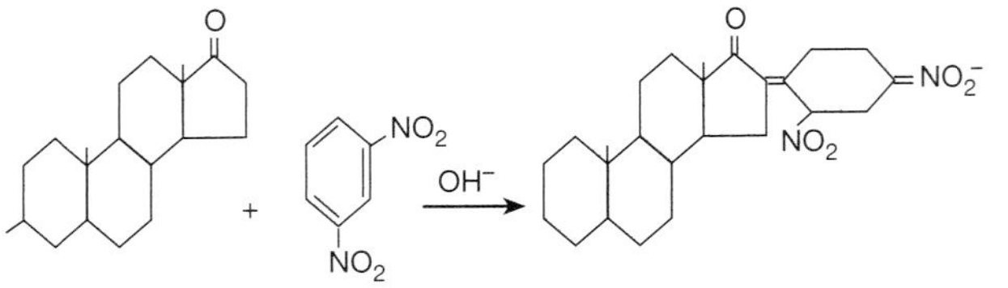

Fig. 50.7 The 17-ketosteroid reaction. Conjugates of 17-KS are cleaved by mild acid hydrolysis to yield free 17-KS. The free 17-KS are extracted by ether to remove interfering compounds. The extracted 17-KS react with m-dinitrobenzene in an alkaline solution to form a reddish-purple complex. (Adapted from 'Pioneering in Diagnostic Reagents,' Am J Med, Wycell Inc., 1974).

is used to assess the concentration of 17-ketosteroids present in the urine (Ryan *et al.* 1964; Drekter *et al.* 1952). The steroids that undergo this reaction are androstenedione, androsterone, etiocholanolone, dehydroepiandrosterone, 11-ketoandrosterone, 11-ketoetiocholanolone, 11-β-hydroxyandrosterone, and 11-β-hydroxyetiochiolanolone.

Urinary 17-ketogenic steroids

When C_{21} steroids with a hydroxyl group at the C17 position are treated with sodium periodate, the C20–C21 side chain is removed, generating a 17-ketosteroid (Fig. 50.8). The concentration of the newly formed ketosteroid can be measured by the colorimetric reaction depicted in Fig. 50.7. All compounds that can be converted to 17-ketosteroids by sodium periodate are 17-ketogenic steroids. These compounds are cortisol, 11-deoxycortisol, cortisone, 17-OH-progesterone, 17-OH-pregnenolone, tetrahydrocortisol, tetrahydrocortisone, tetrahydrodeoxycortisone, pregnanediol, and pregnentriol (Fig. 50.4). Penicillin G in large doses can elevate 17-ketogenic steroid levels. Meprobamate, glucose duographin, and conray can reduce the levels.

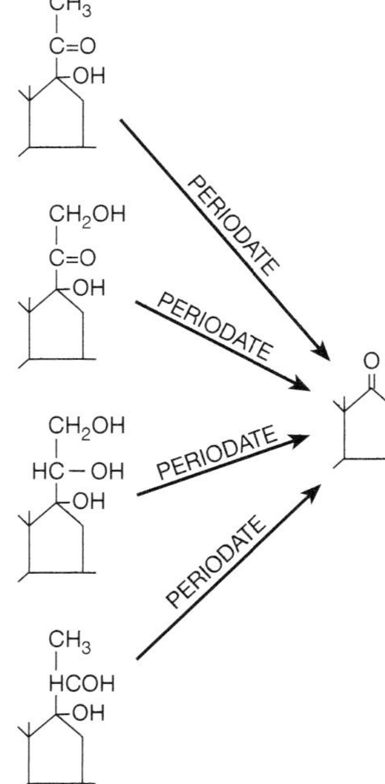

Fig. 50.8 Oxidation of 17-KGS to 17-KS. Prior to the oxidation, naturally occurring 17-KS are extracted and measured (Fig. 50.7). After oxidation the newly formed 17-KS are measured by the m-dinitrobenzene reaction. (Adapted from 'Bioscience Handbook,' 11ᵗʰ E.D., Bioscience Laboratory, Van Nuys, 1975.)

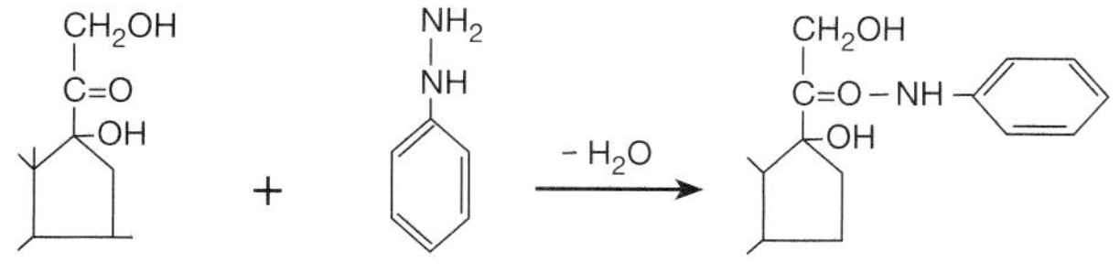

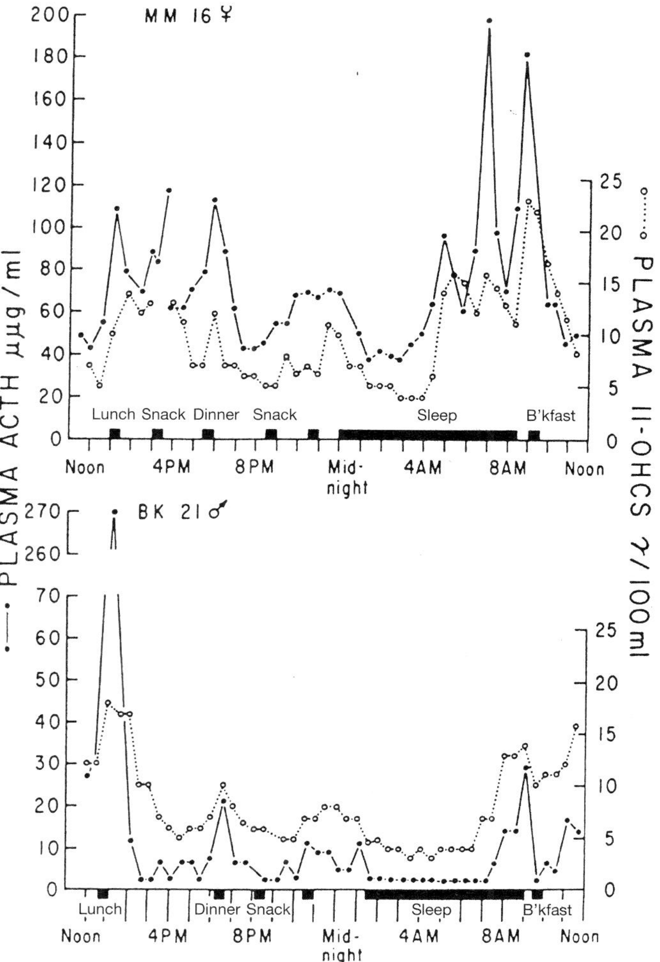

Fig. 50.9 17-OHCS reaction (Porter-Silber). (Adapted from 'Bioscience Handbook,' 11th Ed, Bioscience Laboratory, Van Nuys, 1975.)

Urinary 17-hydroxycorticosteroids (17-OHCS)

17-OHCS are C_{21} steroid hormones containing 17,21-dihydroxy, 20-ketone configuration in the side chain. This side chain reacts in an acid medium with phenylhydrazine to form a yellow derivative, phenylhydrazone (Fig. 50.9). Colorimetric assessment of this reaction allows measurement of the concentration of 17-OHCS. Compounds that undergo this reaction are cortisol, deoxycortisone, cortisone, and their tetrahydro derivatives. These compounds are also referred to as Porter–Silber chromagens. Drugs that directly interfere with this assay are spironolactone, chlordiazepoxide, hydroxyzine, meprobamate, phenothiazines, quinine, and triacetyloleandomycine.

Basal function of the hypothalamic–pituitary–glucocorticoid axis

Circadian rhythm of ACTH and cortisol

ACTH stimulates the release of cortisol. Studies measuring plasma levels of ACTH and cortisol reveal that the pulsatile secretion of ACTH is followed very closely by a parallel change in the concentration of cortisol (Krieger 1975; Krieger *et al.* 1971; Gallagher *et al.* 1973) (Fig. 50.10). Observations over a 24-hour period showed the highest levels of ACTH and cortisol in the early morning, 2–4 hours prior to awakening. Levels of both substances gradually fall during the course of the day, with the lowest levels seen in the evening (Weitzman *et al.* 1971; Krieger *et al.* 1971). This circadian rhythm for cortisol and ACTH has been closely linked to the sleep/wake cycle in man. When the cycle was changed to 12-, 19-, or 33-hour periods, a new rhythm developed within several days that was synchronous with the new sleep/wake cycle (Orth *et al.* 1967).

Corticotropin-releasing hormone (CRH) has been implicated in the development and maintenance of the circadian rhythm. Experiments utilizing a bioassay for CRH demonstrated a circadian variation in the concentration of hypothalamic corticotropin-releasing activity (CRA) and changes in the CRA preceded parallel alterations in steroidogenesis in normal rats (Hiroshige and Sakakura 1971; Hiroshige *et al.* 1969). These data suggest a rise in the hypothalamic CRH prior to a rise in plasma steroids. This process maintains a regular 24-hour rhythm. A temporal relationship has also been described in rats between the earliest detection of CRA and the establishment of the circadian rhythm (Hiroshige and Sato 1970). The feeding schedules also greatly influenced the circadian rhythm in the rat (Miyabo *et al.* 1980; Kato *et al.* 1980).

By measuring the variation of plasma 17-OHCS from 8 a.m. to 8 p.m. in different age groups, it has been established that the

Fig. 50.10 Circadian rhythm of plasma 11-OHCS and ACTH. Characterization of the normal temporal pattern of plasma corticosteroid levels. (Adapted from Kreiger *et al.*, J Clin Endocrinol Metab. 32:269, 1971.)

circadian rhythm of cortisol is present by 3 years of age and probably can be found in some individuals as early as 1 year of age (Franks 1967) (Fig. 50.11). In the adult, it has been shown that the circadian rhythm of ACTH dictates the rhythm of cortisol (Krieger 1975; Krieger *et al.* 1971; Gallagher *et al.* 1973) (Fig. 50.10).

Plasma ACTH concentration

A single random plasma ACTH level offers limited useful information concerning the hypothalamic–pituitary–adrenal axis. The pulsatile manner of secretion imposed on the circadian rhythm limits interpretation of an isolated ACTH level except in two circumstances—ectopic ACTH production and the assessment of adequacy of exogenous glucocorticoid therapy.

The production of ACTH by an extrapituitary source is found in certain neoplasms. A majority of these tumors are found in the thorax—carcinoma of the lung and thymomas. Pancreatic cell tumors, medullary carcinoma of the thyroid, and adrenal cortical and medullary tumors have also been found to secrete an ACTH-like substance (Gewirtz and Yallow 1974; Salyer *et al.* 1976; Keusch *et al.* 1977). Analysis of this compound revealed immunoreactive

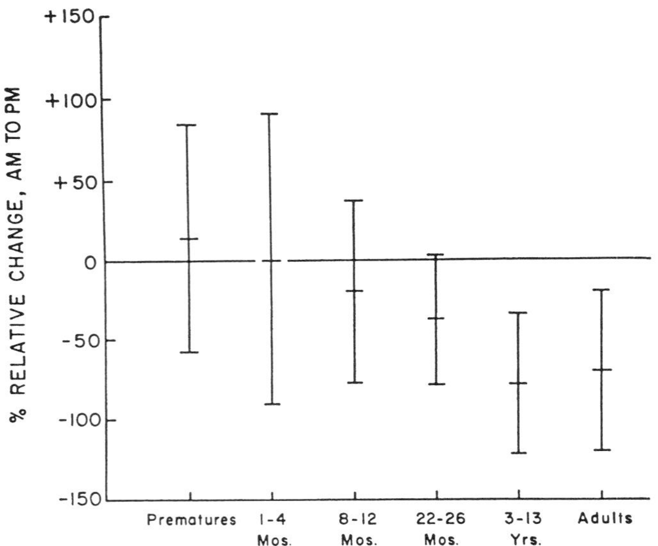

Fig. 50.11 Mean percent relative change in plasma 17-OHCS by age. (Adapted from Franks R.C. *et al.*, *J Clin Endocrinol Metab* 27:78, 1967.)

ACTH with a higher molecular weight than $ACTH_{1-39}$ (Hofmann *et al.* 1970). This fraction is called 'big ACTH'. It has varied biological potency.

Normal values for plasma ACTH vary with each assay. Tables 50.1 and 50.2 state examples of normal values from literature that may assist in the interpretation of reported plasma values. A high evening ACTH level or a lack of diurnal rhythm suggests a state of hypersecretion of ACTH or lack of adequate exogenous glucocorticoid replacement.

Plasma cortisol concentration

Episodic secretion and the circadian rhythm also prevent the use of a random cortisol level in assessing the hypothalamic–pituitary–adrenal axis. The use of morning and evening cortisol levels can allow the clinician to draw limited conclusions. Morning cortisol levels should vary between 10 and 25 μg/dl, and evening levels should be at least 50 per cent less than the 8 a.m. level. This rhythm should be present by 1–3 years of age.

Some guidelines for different ages are presented in Tables 50.3–50.5. Please note the type of assay utilized. Normal values for different laboratories and assays may differ.

Table 50.2 Plasma ACTH concentration as a function of time

Patient and time	Plasma ACTH
Normal adult (8–10 a.m.)	10–80 pg/ml
Normal adult (8–10 p.m.)	Minimum 50% ↓ from morning level

Adapted from Besser G.M., *Clin Endocrinol* 2; 175–186, 1973; Ratcliffe J.G., *Clin Endocrinol* 1:37, 1972; and Besser G.M. *et al.*, *Br Med J* 4:552–554, 1968.

Table 50.3 Plasma cortisol concentrations in the postnatal period

Group	Plasma cortisol by protein-binding assay (μg/dl)[a]	
	Cord blood	Femoral vein blood[b]
Term infant–vaginal delivery	13.1 ± 1.1 (20)[c]	12.3 ± 1.1 (22)
Term infant–vaginal delivery with distressed labor	13.2 ± 0.5 (6)	22.2 ± 5.3 (7)
Postmature infant–vaginal delivery with distressed labor	13.3 ± 4.1 (6)	7.5 ± 1.8 (8)
Postmature infant–cesarean	10.6 ± 1.6 (3)	4.6 ± 1.5 (6)

[a] Mean ± SEM.
[b] 8 a.m. values obtained with 24 h of birth.
[c] Numbers in parentheses.
Adapted from Nwosu U.C. *et al.*, *Am J Obstet Gynecol* 122:969–974, 1975.

Table 50.4 Plasma cortisol concentrations in infancy through adolescence

Group	Source	Plasma cortisol by fluorescence (μg/dl)[a]	
		8 a.m.	8 p.m.
1–4 months (13)[b]	Antecubital vein	6.3 ± 1.0	6.8 ± 1.1
22–26 months (6)	Antecubital vein	15.3 ± 1.8	11.2 ± 2.1
3–13 years (13)	Antecubital vein	17.3 ± 2.0	7.3 ± 1.3

[a] Mean ± SEM.
[b] Numbers in parentheses.
Adapted from Franks R.C. *et al.*, *J Clin Endocrinol Metab* 27:75–78, 1967.

When evaluating plasma cortisol levels, one also must assess the relationship of cortisol to plasma ACTH. An inappropriate relationship between cortisol and ACTH helps differentiate primary from secondary disease.

Table 50.1 Plasma ACTH concentrations as a function of age

Group	No. of subjects	Source of blood	Plasma ACTH[a] (pg/ml)
12–19 weeks gestation	7	Umbilical cord	249 ± 65.7
20–34 weeks gestation	8	Umbilical cord	234 ± 29.0
35–42 weeks gestation	376	Umbilical cord	143 ± 7.0
1–7 days postnatal (time drawn not recorded)	46	Heel stick	120 ± 8.3
Normal adult (1–4 p.m.)	22	Antecubital vein	43 ± 3.7

[a] Mean ± SEM for ACTH.
Adapted from Winters A.J. *et al.*, *J Clin Endocrinol Metab* 39:269–273, 1974.

Table 50.5 Plasma cortisol concentrations in adults

Group	Source	Plasma cortisol by fluorescence (μg/dl)[a]	
18–53 years[c] (12)[b]	Antecubital vein	14.6 ± 1.2 (8 a.m.)	5.7 ± 1.1 (10 p.m.)
72–95 years[d] (16)	Antecubital vein	19.6 ± 1.6 (8 a.m.)	10.0 ± 1.0 (8 p.m.)

[a] Mean ± SEM.
[b] Numbers in parentheses.
Adapted from [c]Migeon *et al.*, *J Clin Endocrinol Metab* 16:622–633, 1956, and
[d]Silverberg *et al.*, *J Clin Endocrinol Metab* 28:1661–1663, 1968.

Table 50.6 Urinary 17-ketosteroids as a function of age

Age	17-Ketosteroids (range in mg/24 h)
< 2 years	0.2–1.2
2–8 years	0.2–1.8
9 years to puberty	0.6–6.2
Adolescent	
Male	

Urinary 17-ketosteroids

17-Ketosteroid levels in the urine reflect the excretion of androgens and their metabolites (Fig. 50.4). Prior to puberty, the adrenal is the major contributor to the level of urinary ketosteroids. The increase in 17-ketosteroids in the urine at 8–9 years of age reflects the onset of adrenarche with subsequent increases hailing the onset of puberty. In normal adult males, two-thirds of 17-ketosteroids are derived from the adrenal. In adult females, the ovary makes a minimal contribution to 17-ketosteroid concentration. Normal values are listed in Table 50.6. Isolated 17-ketosteroid values offer the clinician no specific diagnostic tool.

Urinary 17-ketogenic steroids

Normal levels for17-ketogenic steroids are 2.0–3.0 times higher than expected 17-OHCS levels for children of the same age. The normal ranges for adults are listed in Table 50.7 (Ernest 1966).

17-Ketogenic steroids have been used to assess baseline secretion of the glucocorticoid pathway.(Fig. 50.4) Very high levels strongly suggest a diagnosis of cortisol hypersecretion. Difficulties arise in defining the presence or absence of disease when values in the urine fall within the upper limit of normal to slightly above the highest acceptable level of the control population. In these situations, distinguishing between a hypersecretory state and the normal is impossible. One must resort to other tests to make the distinction.

Another difficulty in interpreting 17-ketogenic steroid levels is that they are usually elevated in the CYP21A2 (21-hydroxylase) or

Table 50.7 Urinary 17-ketogenic steroids in adults

	17-Ketogenic steroid (mg/24 h)	
	Mean ± SD	Range
Normal adults	13.4 ± 3.6	7.6–22.7
Normal females[a]	—	3.5–13
Normal males[a]	—	5–17

[a] From Eddy R.L. *et al.*, *Am J Med* 55:621–630, 1973.

the CYP11B1 (11β-hydroxylase) varieties of congenital adrenal hyperplasia, but the clinical situation is a deficiency of cortisol and aldosterone.

Today the 17-ketogenic steroid assay has little value in clinical practice due to availability of the 17-OHCS and free cortisol assays.

Urinary 17-OHCS

A 24-hour urine collection for 17-OHCS can be a valuable tool in evaluating the functional state of a patient's adrenal cortex. When the raw values obtained are below normal, a pathological process involved with the steroid production is suggested. Classically, in congenital adrenal hyperplasia of CYP21A2 (21-hydroxylase), 3β-hydroxysteroid dehydrogenase (3β-HSD), CYP11A1 (cholesterol side-chain cleavage enzyme, desmolase), and CYP17 (17α-hydroxylase) varieties, 17-OHCS levels are decreased. In adrenal insufficiency, 17-hydroxysteroids are also low. In congenital adrenal hyperplasia of the CYP11B1 (11β-hydroxylase) type, 17-OHCS levels are high, as they also are in situations with excess cortisol secretion.

Difficulty can arise in discriminating the obese but normal individual from the patient with hypersecretion of glucocorticoids. The obese individual secretes and excretes a greater amount of 17-OHCS than the normal individual. The excretion rate for normal individuals with range of age from 2 to 76 years is 3.1 ± 1.1 mg/m^2/24 h (mean ± SD). Obese adolescents and adults excrete 4.35 ± 1.87 mg/m^2/24 h (Migeon *et al.* 1963). Clearly, obese individuals have raw 17-OHCS excretion values higher than normal individuals. An additional problem is that some individuals with hypersecretion of cortisol can fall into the normal range for age.

When 17-OHCS excretion in the urine is expressed as a function of grams of creatinine excreted in the same urine collection, one can separate all normal individuals more than 3 years of age as well as obese adolescents and adults from individuals with hypersecretion of cortisol (Fig. 50.12). The range for normal and obese individuals was 2.0–6.5 mg/24 h/g creatinine. Those individuals with an excess secretion of cortisol had higher levels. Please note that the youngest individual in the normal age range was more than 3 years of age, the youngest obese individual was 4 years of age, and the youngest patient with hypersecretion was 8 years old (Streeten *et al.* 1969; Franks 1973). The creatinine correction may not prove to be helpful at a younger age. In the range of ages studied, however, separation of the normal population from those with cortisol excess was accomplished effectively by this maneuver.

Urine free cortisol

Numerous attempts have been made to correlate basal urine free cortisol values with excess and deficient cortisol secretion. Twenty-four-hour urine collections for free cortisol have proved valuable in screening for the hypersecretory state but are of no value in defining the deficient situation (Streeten *et al.* 1969; Ross 1960). Combined data from 15 studies revealed that 3.3 per cent of lean, obese, or chronically ill individuals had elevated 24-hour urine free cortisol values and that 5.6 per cent of patients with Cushing's syndrome had normal urine free cortisol. Normal ranges varied with each laboratory, and different laboratory

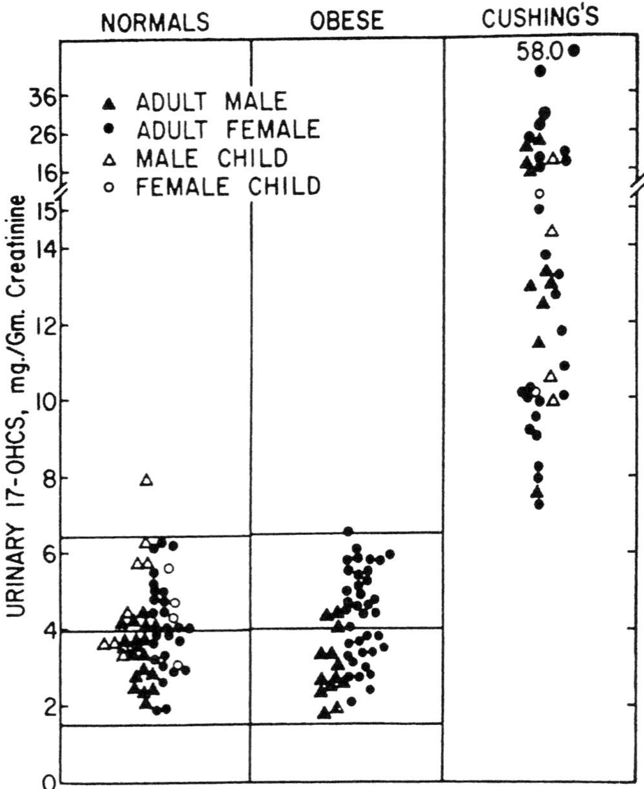

Fig. 50.12 Urinary 17-OHCS excretion per gram creatinine in normal individuals, obese subjects, and patients with Cushing's syndrome. Diagnosis of hypercortisolism. Biochemical criteria differentiate patients of lean from obese normal and from females on oral contraceptives. (Adapted from Streeten D.N. et al., J Clin Endocrinol Metab 29:1200, 1969.)

Table 50.8 Urinary free cortisol in different age groups

	Adults (11)[a]	Children (30)
Urinary free cortisol (μg/24 h)	96 ± 35	41 ± 23
Urinary free cortisol (μg/g creatinine /24 h)	68 ± 15	75 ± 18

All values are mean ± SD
[a] Numbers in parentheses.
Adapted from Franks R.C., J Clin Endocrinol Metab 36:702–705, 1973.

predictor of the pathologic state can be established for this age group. Whether correcting free cortisol values by gram creatinine improves the accuracy of the test needs to be defined. Free cortisol in the urine does not separate normal from deficient states.

High fluid intake (5 liters/day) has been shown to increase urine free cortisol excretion without an increase in urine 17-OHCS (Mericq and Cutler 1998). Therefore, mild to moderate increases in urine free cortisol excretion may not indicate hypercortisolism in such individuals.

Salivary cortisol

The salivary cortisol concentration accurately reflects plasma free cortisol concentration since plasma free cortisol diffuses freely into saliva and it is independent of salivary flow rate (Vining *et al.* 1983). Saliva can be obtained easily by the patient, either by unstimulated flow or after chewing a cotton tube. Cortisol in the saliva is very stable and can be stored at room temperature for many days (Chen *et al.* 1992) or frozen for extended periods. Salivary cortisol concentrations can be determined using either CBPA or RIA. Normal reference range varies in different laboratories depending on the methods of assay used and the time saliva was collected. Both the CBPA and RIA cross-react with other steroids, such as 17-hydroxyprogesterone and 11-deoxycortisol. RIA are more specific. Cortisol can be chromatographically separated from other steroids before assay to reduce the interference (Laudat *et al.* 1988).

Morning salivary cortisol concentrations are decreased in adrenal insufficiency, while late evening salivary cortisol concentrations are increased in Cushing's syndrome. Studies have shown that there was significant overlap in salivary cortisol between patients with Cushing's syndrome and normal subjects at 8 a.m. but no overlap at 8 or 11 p.m. (Laudat *et al.* 1988; Raff *et al.* 1998; Findling and Raff 1999). The data suggest that measuring a late evening salivary cortisol level can distinguish most patients with Cushing's syndrome from those with the pseudo-Cushing's status (Raff *et al.* 1998). The ability to sample saliva in the evening over several days or weeks makes this test particularly useful in the evaluation of patients with cyclical Cushing's syndrome (Mosnier-Pudar *et al.* 1995; Hermus *et al.* 1993).

Combination of the low-dose dexamethasone suppression test and salivary cortisol determination may improve the diagnostic sensitivity and specificity (Barrou *et al.* 1996).

Dynamic function of the hypothalamic–pituitary–glucocorticoid axis: stimulation tests

Metyrapone

Metyrapone inhibits the enzyme CYP11B1 (11β-hydroxylase), thus decreasing the amount of cortisol produced by the adrenal

methods were utilized. In the two studies utilizing the rapid CBPA to assess free cortisol values, 108 mg/24 h was the upper limit of normal and clearly separated normals from those with Cushing's syndrome (Crapo 1979).

There is a paucity of information concerning urine free cortisol values in children. Franks (1973) studied 30 normal children (4–12 years of age) and 11 normal adults utilizing the CBPA (Table 50.8). In the study he also examined the urine free cortisol levels of a child with bilateral adrenocortical hyperplasia and an adult with metastatic adrenocortical carcinoma. The child's free urine cortisol levels were not consistently above the values of the normal population, but the adult's urine cortisol levels were above those of the normal population. When Franks depicted the absolute values per gram creatinine, the pathologic state was separable from that of the normal individuals. Table 50.8 describes the normal values per gram creatinine in Franks' control population.

Thus, 24-hour urine collections for urine free cortisol by CBPA offer a reliable screening tool for hypersecretion of cortisol in the adult population when normal values are clearly defined for a given laboratory. With the development of high-affinity antisera that react specifically with the D-ring of cortisol, most laboratories switched to RIA for urine free cortisol measurement, with higher sensitivity and less interference by other steroids than in CBPA. More data from a pediatric population with hypersecretion are needed before the value of free cortisol in the urine as a

glands (Fig. 50.4). The subsequent decrease in circulating cortisol stimulates the hypothalamic–pituitary axis to increase ACTH secretion. Corticotropin activates the production of glucocorticoids and increases the precursors of cortisol in the glucocorticoid pathway. In the individual with a normal hypothalamic–pituitary–adrenal axis, there is a fall in plasma cortisol, an increase in plasma 11-deoxycortisol, and an increase in urinary 17-OHCS.

Overnight single-dose metyrapone test (Spiger et al. 1975; Limal et al. 1976; Fiad et al. 1994)

Test. At 24.00 h, 30 mg/kg up to 2 g for individuals less than 70 kg, 2.5 g for individuals 70–90 kg, and 3 g for patients over 90 kg of metyrapone is given by mouth. A snack is taken with the metyrapone. At 08.00 h, plasma 11-deoxycortisol and cortisol levels are obtained.

Normal response. A plasma 11-deoxycortisol level of 7–20 μg/dl and a plasma cortisol level < 10 μg/dl.

This test is a safe, simple, and reliable index of the hypothalamic–pituitary axis integrity and gives information similar to that given by the insulin tolerance test (Fiad et al. 1994). Patients with a normal response of 11-deoxycortisol and cortisol have a normal hypothalamic–pituitary–adrenal axis. Individuals with a low 11-deoxycortisol and a low plasma cortisol response may have adrenal insufficiency. Four per cent of normal individuals will have subnormal 11-deoxycortisol and cortisol responses.

A low response of 11-deoxycortisol and a cortisol level above 10 μg/dl suggest that either not enough metyrapone was given, there was a lack of absorption of the metyrapone, or metyrapone failed to inhibit the CYP11B1 enzyme adequately.

A high level of 11-deoxycortisol with a cortisol level above 10 μg/dl suggests rapid absorption/metabolism of metyrapone with insufficient block of cortisol production at the time the blood sample was obtained.

Patients with congestive heart failure, obesity, or hypothyroidism and those taking oral contraceptives may not have as great an increase in 11-deoxycortisol. Patients taking phenytoin may also respond with a subnormal increase in 11-deoxycortisol secondary to hypermetabolism of metyrapone (Spiger et al. 1975; Limal et al. 1976; Meikle et al. 1969).

Three-day metyrapone test (Avgerinos et al. 1996; Steiker et al. 1961; Liddle et al. 1959; Richmond et al. 1964; Bacon et al. 1975)

Test. Day 1, 24-h urine collection for 17-OHCS. Day 2, 300 mg/m^2 to a maximum dose of 750 mg metyrapone every 4 hours by mouth for six doses; 24-hour urine collection for 17-OHCS. Day 3, 24-hour urine collection for 17-OHCS; a blood sample obtained for 11-deoxycortisol.

Normal response. An increase of urinary 17-OHCS of two- to threefold above the baseline on either the day of metyrapone administration or the day after.

A subnormal response of 17-OHCS suggests adrenal insufficiency, hypermetabolism of metyrapone, or a pathological state with decreased excretion of 17-OHCS. Patients taking anticonvulsants may hypermetabolize metyrapone, not permitting the expected block of CYP11B1 and not allowing an increase in 17-OHCS in the urine (Meikle et al. 1969). Patients on estrogen therapy may excrete subnormal amounts of steroids in the urine, lowering the expected 17-OHCS levels. Subnormal urinary response to metyrapone also can be observed in hypothyroidism, cirrhosis of the liver, renal failure, and malnutrition. By measuring changes in plasma cortisol and 11-deoxycortisol after the administration of metyrapone, one can define a normal response to metyrapone in individuals in whom an excretion of 17-OHCS is unreliable.

The metyrapone test may precipitate an adrenal crisis in patients with primary adrenal insufficiency or inadequate ACTH reserve. Such patients must be monitored closely while they receive metyrapone.

The test can also be used to confirm the etiology of Cushing's syndrome. In Cushing's disease of pituitary origin, urinary 17-OHCS excretion increases with metyrapone, whereas in the presence of an adrenal tumor the levels of urinary 17-OHCS usually do not rise.

The six-dose standard metyrapone test has a sensitivity and specificity for the differential diagnosis of ACTH-dependent Cushing's syndrome nearly identical to that of the overnight metyrapone test (Avgerinos et al. 1996) and that of the standard high-dose dexamethasone suppression test (Avgerinos et al. 1994).

Intravenous metyrapone test (Bacon et al. 1975)

Test. 70 mg/kg metyrapone to a maximum dose of 1 g is infused over 4 hours in a subject who has fasted overnight. Blood samples are obtained for 11-deoxycortisol and cortisol at 0, 240, and 480 min.

Normal response. Plasma cortisol decreases to < 8 μg/dl, and the maximum plasma 11-deoxycortisol exceeds 6 μg/dl.

Other than the presence of an IV line, there are no significant drawbacks to this test.

In summary, the metyrapone test is the most sensitive test of pituitary ACTH secretory reserve. An individual who responds normally to any of the metyrapone tests has an intact hypothalamic–pituitary–adrenal axis and requires no further investigation. The metyrapone test can establish the diagnosis of adrenal insufficiency but does not define whether the disease is primary or secondary in nature. When interpreting the results of the metyrapone test, remember that: (1) anticonvulsant therapy alters the metabolism of metyrapone; (2) exogenous estrogen therapy and other diseases can affect the excretion of steroids; and (3) certain exogenous steroid preparations can be measured by some of the assays for plasma cortisol.

ACTH

ACTH increases steroid production and release within 3 min of administration (see previous section on glucocorticoid metabolism). Investigators have utilized this property to develop tests to define the ability of the fasciculata and reticularis to produce cortisol. The response to ACTH varies with the underlying disorder. In patients with secondary adrenal insufficiency, the intrinsically normal adrenal gland should respond to exogenous ACTH if given for a long enough time. The response may be sluggish initially due to adrenal atrophy. In patients with primary adrenal insufficiency, there should be little or no adrenal response to exogenous ACTH.

Rapid standard-dose ACTH stimulation test (Grieg et al. 1967; Speckart et al. 1971; May and Carey 1985; Dickstein et al. 1991; Parker et al. 2000; Oelkers 1996)

Test. Test may be done at any time of the day without fasting the patient. Cosyntropin (synthetic ACTH$_{1-24}$) 250 μg is administered by rapid IV injection. Blood samples are drawn for plasma cortisol levels at 0, 30, and 60 min.

Normal response. Using RIA to determine plasma cortisol, a normal response is a rise in plasma cortisol concentration after 30 or 60 minutes to a peak of 18 to 20 μg/dl or more. A subnormal response confirms the diagnosis of adrenal insufficiency, but further studies are necessary to establish its type and cause.

A normal response to the cosyntropin stimulation tests effectively excludes the diagnosis of primary adrenal insufficiency (Fig. 50.13). A subnormal response to cosyntropin does not always establish the diagnosis of adrenal insufficiency. Normal individuals have been described who do not respond to the rapid test but do respond to more prolonged ACTH stimulation. Pre- and post-menopausal women respond to ACTH stimulation similarly (Parker *et al.* 2000).

In a patient with adrenal insufficiency and a subnormal response to cosyntropin, this 'rapid test' does not separate those patients with primary adrenal insufficiency from those with secondary adrenal insufficiency. High plasma ACTH suggests adrenal cortical failure. Conversely, low circulating ACTH suggests adrenal failure based on a central lesion. Patients with secondary adrenal insufficiency usually respond to more prolonged ACTH exposure.

A patient who has adrenal insufficiency because of a relative or absolute lack of ACTH may respond normally to cosyntropin but may fail to respond with as great an increase in plasma cortisol as the normal individual to stress of surgery. Thus, a normal rapid ACTH test does not guarantee the clinician that his patient will be 'covered' for stress by endogenous cortisol as adequately as the normal individual.

In patients with secondary adrenal insufficiency, a subnormal cosyntropin response predicts a subnormal rise in plasma cortisol in response to the stress of insulin hypoglycemia, metyrapone, and surgery (Nelson and Tindall 1978; Lindholm *et al.* 1978). It is recommended that steroid coverage be initiated for individuals with secondary adrenal insufficiency who fail to respond normally to cosyntropin. Whether the individuals who respond normally to cosyntropin should be covered by exogenous glucocorticoid is controversial. The clinician must remember that an inadequate hypothalamic–pituitary response to surgical stress may be observed despite a normal screening cosyntropin test.

In a patient with suspected adrenal insufficiency whose clinical situation dictates immediate glucocorticoid therapy, the cosyntropin test can be performed while one treats the patient with the synthetic steroid dexamethasone (Sheridan and Mattingly 1975).

Rapid low-dose ACTH stimulation test (Dickstein et al. 1991, 1997; Tordjman et al. 1995, 2000; Mayenknecht et al. 1998; Ambrosi et al. 1998; Zarkovic et al. 1999; Darmon et al. 1999; Oelkers 1998; Thaler and Blevins 1998; Park et al. 1999)

Test. Test may be done at any time of the day without fasting the patient. Cosyntropin (synthetic ACTH$_{1-24}$) 1 μg is administered by rapid IV injection. Blood samples are obtained for plasma cortisol levels at 0 and 30 min.

Normal response. Using RIA to determine plasma cortisol, a normal response is a rise in plasma cortisol concentration to a peak of 18 μg/dl or more. A subnormal response confirms the diagnosis of adrenal insufficiency, but further studies are necessary to establish its type and cause.

Though the rapid standard-dose ACTH stimulation test using 250 μg of synthetic ACTH$_{1-24}$ has been widely used for an initial assessment of adrenal function, many investigators believe that the dose of 250 μg ACTH is supraphysiological and a maximal adrenal response can be obtained with much smaller doses of ACTH. A normal cortisol response to 250 μg of ACTH may misleadingly imply that adrenal function is normal in some patients with adrenal insufficiency and may subject these patients to life-threatening complications. Numerous studies in the past several years have provided substantial evidence that the low-dose ACTH stimulation test involves more physiological plasma concentrations of ACTH and provides a similar or more sensitive index of adrenocortical responsiveness. Currently, there is no 1-μg cosyntropin vial available commercially and one needs to prepare the low-dose solution by diluting the standard 250 μg vial using normal saline as diluent.

Eight-hour ACTH stimulation test (Orth and Kovacs 1998)

Test. Cosyntropin (250 μg) is infused intravenously over 8 hours in 500 ml of normal saline. A 24-hour urine specimen is collected the day before

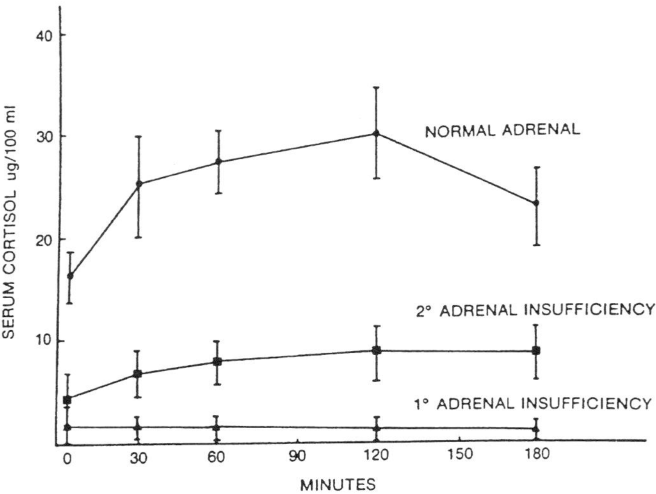

Fig. 50.13 Response of cortisol (CBG assay) to acute ACTH infusion. Mean ± SD. (Adapted from Speckart, P.F. *et al.*, Arch Intern Med 128:761–763, 1971.)

and the day of the infusion for 17-OHCS and creatinine measurement. Plasma cortisol is determined at the end of the infusion.

Normal response. Urinary 17-OHCS should increase three- to fivefold over baseline on the day of ACTH infusion. Plasma cortisol should reach 20 μg/dl 30 to 60 minutes after the infusion is begun and exceed 25 μg/dl after 6 to 8 hours.

The infusion solution must contain isotonic saline (154 mEq/l NaCl) because patients with adrenal insufficiency can become severely hyponatremic if given hypotonic solutions since they may already be hyponatremic and lack aldosterone prior to the test. This test is rarely performed today.

Two-day ACTH infusion test (Orth and Kovacs 1998; Rose *et al.* 1970)

Test. Similar to the 8-hour infusion test, except that the same dose of ACTH is infused for 8 hours on 2 consecutive days. Alternatively, 250 μg of a depot formulation of purified bovine ACTH in gelatin is injected intramuscularly every 12 hours for 48 hours.

Normal response. Urinary 17-OHCS should exceed 27 mg during the first 24 hours of infusion and 47 mg during the second 24 hours. Plasma cortisol should reach 20 μg/dl 30 to 60 minutes after the ACTH infusion is begun and exceed 25 μg/dl after 6 to 8 hours. Both plasma and urinary steroid values increase progressively thereafter, but the ranges of normal are not well defined.

This test is the most widely used prolonged ACTH stimulation test and it may be helpful in distinguishing secondary from tertiary adrenal insufficiency. The 1-day 8-hour test might be too short for this purpose, while longer tests add little further useful information.

Insulin

Insulin tolerance test (Orth and Kovacs 1998; Erturk *et al.* 1998; Leisti *et al.* 1978; Zurburgg and Joss 1970; Landon *et al.* 1963; Greenwood *et al.* 1966)

Test. Test is begun at 08.00 h after an overnight fast. Plasma cortisol and glucose values are obtained at time 0. A dose of 0.15 U/kg regular insulin is administered by rapid IV injection. The dose should be decreased to 0.05–0.1 U/kg if growth hormone deficiency is suspected. The standard dose may be increased by 0.1 U/kg in cases of insulin resistance (for example, obesity, acromegaly, or Cushing's syndrome). At 30, 45, 60, and 90 min, plasma cortisol and glucose levels are obtained.

Normal response. Plasma glucose must decrease to 50 per cent of baseline or < 40 mg/dl to ensure an adequate stimulus. Plasma cortisol concentration is measured by RIA and should reach 18–20 μg/dl at some point during the test. Failure to reach this level is indicative of an inadequate response only if the plasma glucose fell to 35 mg/dl or less. If this was not achieved, the stimulus was inadequate and the test must be repeated.

The nadir of plasma glucose is usually seen 30–45 min after the injection of insulin. The peak response of plasma cortisol is seen 45–90 min after insulin administration.

As a result of the inherent risks associated with hypoglycemia, a physician must be in attendance, and a 25 or 50 per cent dextrose solution suitable for intravenous use must be at the bedside. If the patient becomes unarousable, the concentrated glucose solution should be given immediately. After the glucose is administered, one should continue to obtain plasma cortisol levels at the designated times. The test is contraindicated in patients with epilepsy, cardiac disease, or cerebrovascular disease.

The insulin tolerance test is an effective tool in defining the stress response of the pituitary–adrenal axis. It does not differentiate between primary or secondary adrenal insufficiency. Patients with decreased ACTH secretory reserve may have a subnormal ACTH but normal cortisol response because the normal increment of plasma ACTH during the test is greater than necessary for stimulating serum cortisol to levels > 18 μg/dl and it is unlikely that they are at increased risk of developing an adrenal crisis in stressful situations unless their pituitary function deteriorates (Tuchelt *et al.* 2000).

Corticotropin-releasing hormone (CRH) stimulation test (Orth and Kovacs 1998; Nieman *et al.* 1989, 1993)

Test. After 4-hour fasting, synthetic ovine CRH (1 μg/kg body weight) is injected intravenously. Blood samples are collected for ACTH and cortisol measurement at 15 and 0 min before and 5, 10, 15, 30, 45, 60, 90, and 120 min after CRH injection.

Normal response. In patients with Cushing's syndrome, an increase of 35 per cent or more above basal plasma ACTH or 20 per cent or more above basal plasma cortisol concentration distinguishes those with Cushing's disease from those with ectopic ACTH syndrome. The responses are quite variable among individuals and in the same individual (Chrousos *et al.* 1984; DeCherney *et al.* 1985).

This test can be used to assess the ACTH response to the exogenous CRH to distinguish Cushing's disease from ectopic ACTH secretion: those with pituitary Cushing's disease respond while those with ectopic ACTH secretion do not. It has also been used in the differential diagnosis between secondary and tertiary adrenal insufficiency.

Patients may experience mild, brief facial flushing immediately after injection. There are no other side-effects at the dose used. In normal subjects, the peak ACTH value is greater in the morning than in the afternoon and the peak cortisol value is similar at both times of day. In patients with Cushing's syndrome, results are similar at any time of day due to lack of circadian rhythm.

Dexamethasone–CRH test (Yanovski *et al.* 1993, 1998)

Test. The CRH test is performed 2 hours after a standard low-dose dexamethasone suppression test. Dexamethasone 0.5 mg is given orally every 6 hours for eight doses, starting at noon 2 days prior to CRH test (that is, at 12.00, 18.00, 24.00, 06.00, 12.00, 18.00, 24.00, and 06.00 hours). CRH is then given intravenously at the dose of 1 μg/kg of body weight at 08.00 hours. Plasma cortisol levels are obtained at −15, −10, −5, and 0 min and then at 5, 15, 30, 45, and 60 min.

Normal values. A plasma cortisol concentration greater than 1.4 μg/dl measured 15 min after the administration of CRH correctly identified all cases of Cushing's syndrome while the level is found to be less than 1.4 μg/dl in all patients with pseudo-Cushing's syndrome and normal subjects.

This combined test is more sensitive than both the low-dose dexamethasone suppression test and the CRH test alone in differentiating pseudo-Cushing's syndrome from true Cushing's syndrome. It is useful in patients with suspected pseudo-Cushing's syndrome who have equivocal diagnostic test results. However, single midnight plasma cortisol concentration measurement may provide similar sensitivity and specificity (Newell-Price *et al.* 1995; Papanicolaou *et al.* 1998). There is no head-to-head comparison between these two tests.

CRH plus arginine vasopressin or desmopressin test (Dickstein *et al.* 1996; Newell-Price *et al.* 1997)

The CRH, arginine vasopressin, and desmopressin tests all yield a significant number of false-negative results in Cushing's disease patients. Both arginine vasopressin and desmopressin are known ACTH secretagogues and preliminary studies have shown that CRH plus arginine vasopressin or desmopressin improved the false-negative responses associated with each test alone. More studies are needed to further validate the usefulness of these combined tests in clinical practice.

Dynamic function tests of the hypothalamic–pituitary–glucocorticoid axis: suppression tests

Low-dose overnight dexamethasone test (Crapo 1979; Cronin *et al.* 1990; Montwill *et al.* 1994; Hindmarsh and Brook 1985)

Test. Patient ingests 1 mg of dexamethasone by mouth at 23.00 h, and a plasma cortisol value is obtained at 08.00 h the next morning. A dose of 0.3 mg/m^2 surface area can be used in children (Hindmarsh and Brook 1985). ACTH and dexamethasone levels are also obtained by some clinicians.

Normal response. Normal individuals have an 08.00 h plasma cortisol level of < 5 μg/dl. Plasma ACTH should be less than 10 pg/ml, and plasma dexamethasone from about 2 to 6.5 ng/ml (Meikle et al. 1975).

It should be noted that normal values for this test have not yet been defined in all pediatric ages. It is likely that similar criteria apply after 3 years of age in that: (1) the diurnal rhythm of cortisol is established at 3 years of age (Franks 1967); and (2) dexamethasone given once daily in a dose of 1.25 mg/100 lb decreases the excretion of urinary 17-OHCS within 48 hours of the initial dose (Migeon *et al.* 1963). The clinician is forewarned that urinary excretion and plasma levels are not equivalent, so interpretation of the overnight suppression test in the pediatric population may present some difficulties.

High estrogen states (pregnancy and patients on oral contraceptives) often have elevated plasma cortisol levels that can be equal to those of patients with Cushing's syndrome. Patients with elevated estrogens maintain a diurnal rhythm of cortisol, but cortisol levels are higher (Aron *et al.* 1981). As a result they may suppress with dexamethasone, but not below the goal of 5 μg/dl. Some investigators demonstrated normal plasma cortisol suppression when the dose of estrogen was less than 1.25 mg of equine estrogen per day (Treece *et al.* 1977). Other investigators found lack of normal suppression with various types and doses of estrogen (Eddy *et al.* 1973). A 24-hour urine collection for free cortisol is normal in patients with high estrogens (Grant *et al.* 1965). A 2-day dexamethasone test results in suppression of urinary 17-OHCS to normal levels (Streeten *et al.* 1969).

Patients on phenytoin (Dilantin) may fail to suppress their plasma cortisol level adequately with dexamethasone. This phenomenon results from increased dexamethasone degradation in the liver, lower blood levels, and less biologic effect of a given dose (Haque *et al.* 1972). This has also been described with other hepatic microsomal enzyme inducers, such as phenobarbital (Brooks *et al.* 1972). Although such patients have accelerated degradation of dexamethasone, they do not have increased catabolism of hydrocortisone. To eliminate the diagnosis of hypercortisolism in these patients, the overnight hydrocortisone test has been devised.

Overnight hydrocortisone test (Meikle *et al.* 1974)

Test. At 08.00 h, plasma corticosterone levels are obtained. At midnight that evening, 50 mg of hydrocortisone is given by mouth. The following morning at 08.00 h, another plasma corticosterone level is obtained.

Normal response. In individuals not receiving anticonvulsants, the 08.00 h plasma corticosterone level is less than 120 ng/dl and less than 50 per cent of baseline. In individuals on anticonvulsants, the 08.00 h plasma corticosterone level is < 270 ng/dl or < 50 per cent of baseline.

Obese patients, although they usually have normal plasma cortisol levels and normal diurnal rhythm, occasionally will not suppress with the overnight dexamethasone test (Eddy *et al.* 1973). These patients will have normal urine free cortisol values and will suppress with longer-term dexamethasone administration.

Low-dose 2-day dexamethasone suppression test (Orth and Kovacs 1998; Streeten *et al.* 1969; Orth 1995; Liddle 1960)

Test. Baseline 24-h urine collections for 17-OHCS, free cortisol, and creatinine are obtained on days 1 and 2. At 08.00 h on day 3, the patient begins taking dexamethasone 1.25 mg/100 lb up to 2 mg/day. One-quarter of the daily dose is given every 6 hours by mouth. Dexamethasone is administered for a total of 48 hours. Urine collections continue on days 3 and 4 for same measurements. Blood samples can be drawn at the end of urine collection for assay of cortisol, ACTH, and dexamethasone.

Normal response. Normal individuals will have suppression of 17-OHCS to < 2.5 mg/day, urinary free cortisol to < 10 μg/day by day 4, and plasma cortisol < 5 μg/dl.

In most instances, the low-dose 2-day dexamethasone suppression test is able to separate normal or obese individuals from those with Cushing's syndrome (Streeten *et al.* 1969; Crapo 1979). Unfortunately most patients with Cushing's disease also demonstrate a significant reduction in urinary free cortisol and

17-OHCS excretion and the test has relatively low sensitivity (69 per cent), specificity (74 per cent), and diagnostic accuracy (71 per cent) when used alone (Yanovski *et al.* 1993). Many patients with mild Cushing's disease may suppress urinary steroid secretion to undetectable ranges with low doses of dexamethasone. In addition, as many as 15 to 25 per cent of patients with pseudo-Cushing's states may have false-positive tests. Clinicians must be very careful in interpreting the test results. Because of the expense and cumbersome nature of consecutive urine collections and the frequent need for dexamethasone administration, this test is now used infrequently in clinical practice.

High-dose overnight dexamethasone test (Orth and Kovacs 1998; Orth 1995; Tyrrell *et al.* 1986)

Test. Patient ingests 8 mg of dexamethasone by mouth at 23.00 h, and a plasma cortisol value is obtained at 08.00 h the next morning. ACTH and dexamethasone levels are also obtained by some clinicians.

Normal response. Normal individuals have an 08.00 h plasma cortisol level of < 5 μg/dl and it is usually undetectable. Most patients with Cushing's disease have an 08.00 h plasma cortisol level of < 5 μg/dl. Plasma ACTH is low and usually undetectable.

This test is used in differentiating patients with Cushing's disease from patients with Cushing's syndrome caused by ectopic ACTH syndrome or adrenal adenoma. If plasma cortisol values suppress to at least 50 per cent of baseline, the presumptive diagnosis of Cushing's disease is made. Patients with either ectopic ACTH syndrome or adrenal tumor do not demonstrate a 50 per cent decrease in plasma cortisol.

High-dose 2-day dexamethasone suppression test (Orth and Kovacs 1998; Crapo 1979; Orth 1995; Liddle 1960; Flack *et al.* 1992; Dichek *et al.* 1994)

Test. Days 1–4: four 24-hour urine collections accomplished and 17-OHCS, free cortisol, and creatinine measured. On days 3 and 4, 3.7 mg/100 lb/day up to 8 mg/day of dexamethasone is administered by mouth in four equal doses. Blood samples can be drawn at the end of the study for assay of cortisol, ACTH, and dexamethasone.

Normal response. In normal individuals, urinary 17-OHCS excretion is suppressed to less than 2.5 mg per 24 hours and urinary free cortisol excretion is less than 5 μg per 24 hours. Plasma cortisol and ACTH concentrations are low and usually undetectable. Patients with Cushing's disease (pituitary adenoma) suppress their 17-OHCS and free cortisol in the urine to 50 per cent of the baseline values. Patients with adrenal tumors or ectopic ACTH syndrome do not suppress to > 50 per cent from baseline values.

The high-dose dexamethasone test is based on the fact that patients with pituitary Cushing's syndrome have a higher set point for glucocorticoid-induced suppression than normals. Thus, patients with hypothalamic–pituitary Cushing's syndrome respond to high-dose glucocorticoids, and individuals with ectopic ACTH syndrome or an adrenal tumor do not suppress urinary 17-OHCS or free cortisol excretion when exposed to higher-dose dexamethasone. Therapeutic intervention can be implemented rationally on the basis of this test.

Unfortunately, some individuals with Cushing's disease do not have adequate suppression. In such cases, very-high-dose dexamethasone suppression test (32 mg/day given in four divided doses for 1 day or 36 mg/day given in six divided doses for 2 days) may reveal hypothalamic–pituitary pathology (al-Saadi *et al.* 1998; West and Meikle 1979).

Other methods for defining the pathology of Cushing's syndrome include measurement of plasma ACTH concentration, the 2-day metyrapone test, and the 48-h ACTH infusion test. In patients with Cushing's syndrome because of an adrenal tumor, plasma ACTH levels are very low (< 20 pg/ml) (Besser and Edwards 1972). In patients with Cushing's disease of hypothalamic–pituitary origin, the plasma ACTH concentration may be in the 'normal range' but is inappropriately high for the degree of hypercortisolism. Most ACTH levels are < 100 pg/ml, and virtually all are < 200 pg/ml (Besser and Edwards 1972). In ectopic ACTH syndrome, the ACTH values are rarely < 100 pg/ml and usually > 200 pg/ml (Besser and Edwards 1972).

The 2-day metyrapone test and the 48-hour ACTH infusion test have been discussed. In pituitary Cushing's disease, patients respond with an elevation of urinary 17-OHCS to metyrapone and an elevation of plasma cortisol to ACTH. Such response reflects the altered set point of ACTH secretion observed in hypothalamic–pituitary Cushing's disease versus the autonomy of adrenocortical function with tumors.

Mineralocorticoids

Mineralocorticoid pathway

The work of numerous investigators has helped to define the factors responsible for aldosterone secretion. See Fig. 50.14 for a detailed description of the mineralocorticoid pathway. Major elements controlling aldosterone secretion are the renin–angiotensin system and circulating potassium concentration with lesser contributions by ACTH and plasma sodium concentration.

Regulators of aldosterone secretion

Renin–angiotensin system

The major elements of the renin–angiotensin system are depicted in Fig. 50.15. Renin is a proteolytic enzyme synthesized, stored, and secreted into the circulation mainly by the juxtaglomerular apparatus of the kidney. Renin circulates until it undergoes inactivation by the liver, by plasma proteolytic enzymes, or is excreted into urine or bile. The half-life of renin in a normal subject is 10–20 min. Renin release is stimulated by a reduction of systemic arterial pressure, change from supine to upright posture, sympathetic neuronal discharge, a decrease in plasma sodium level, a decrease in the plasma potassium level, salt depletion, or an increase in catecholamine levels. Increased systemic blood pressure, changing from an erect to a supine posture, salt loading, increased angiotensin II levels, antidiuretic hormone (ADH), and increased plasma potassium levels all suppress renin release (Freeman and Davis 1977).

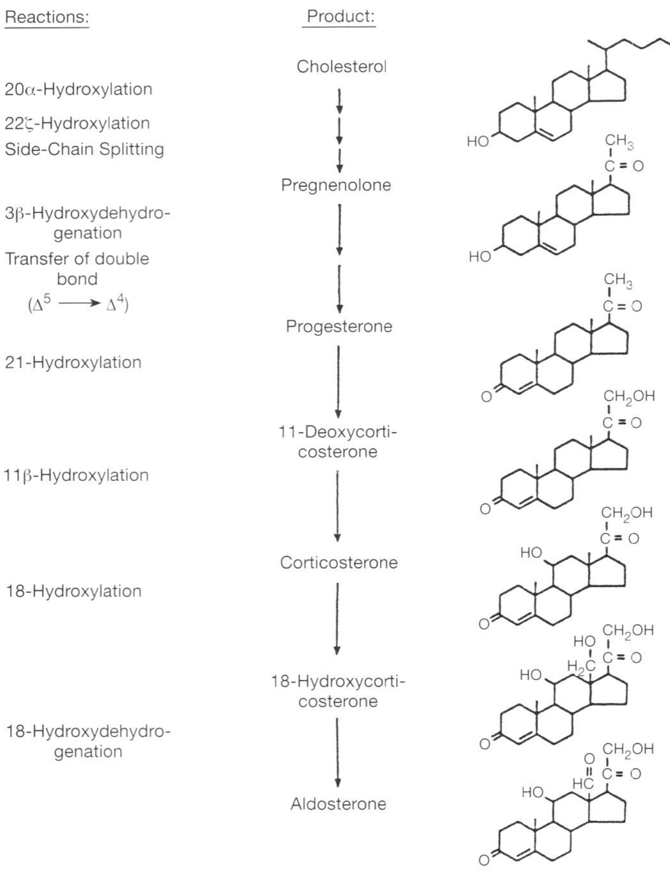

Fig. 50.14   Mineralocorticoid pathway. (Adapted from Genest, J. (ed), 'Hypertension,' McGraw-Hill, New York, p 267, 1977.)

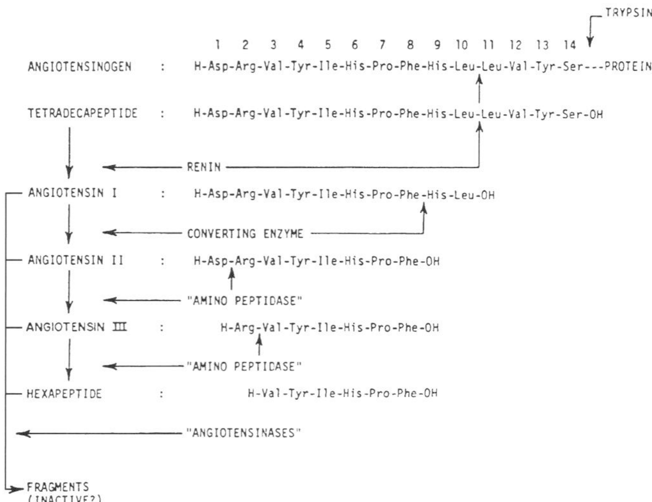

Fig. 50.15   The renin-angiotensin system. (Adapted from Genest, J. (ed), 'Hypertension,' McGraw-Hill, New York, p 141, 1977.)

Renin acts on a α_2-globulin, renin substrate (angiotensinogen), synthesized by the liver to produce the decapeptide angiotensin I. Angiotensin I stimulates catecholamine secretion by the adrenal medulla, raises systemic blood pressure via a central mechanism, and induces thirst. It has no known direct influence on mineralocorticoid function (Peach 1971; Solomon *et al.* 1974; Fitzsimmons 1971).

Angiotensin I is converted to angiotensin II by converting enzyme. This process is accomplished by the cleavage of two amino acids (His, Leu) from the carboxyterminus of angiotensin I. Converting enzyme activity has been found in the lung, the kidney, the liver, and the systemic vascular bed.

Angiotensin II has two major functions. First, angiotensin II is the most potent vasoconstrictor found in mammals. The rise in blood pressure is a result of the direct action of angiotensin II on the arterioles. Second, angiotensin II stimulates the production and the secretion of aldosterone by the cells of the zona glomerulosa of mammals including man. It increases the conversion of cholesterol to pregnenolone as well as that of corticosterone to aldosterone in laboratory animals (Kramer *et al.* 1980; Laragh *et al.* 1960; Aquilera and Catt 1980). The point(s) of action in the mineralocorticoid pathway in man have not yet been defined.

Angiotensin II and angiotensin III are inactivated by cleavage of these compounds to smaller peptides. A family of aminopeptidases, endopeptidases, and carboxypeptidases, collectively known as angiotensinases, attack the peptide chains of angiotensin II and angiotensin III. The resulting peptide fragments have no known biologic activity. Angiotensinases are found in the vascular bed, plasma, kidney, liver, and lung. The vascular bed is believed to be the major site of angiotensin II and III inactivation. Fifty per cent of these angiotensins are removed in one pass through the capillary bed.

Plasma potassium concentration

Plasma potassium levels play an intimate role in the regulation of aldosterone production and secretion. Alterations as small as 0.1 mEq/l can affect aldosterone (Himathongkam *et al.* 1975). An increased plasma potassium level stimulates aldosterone and, conversely, a decrease in plasma potassium inhibits aldosterone. The influence of changing potassium concentration is zone-specific. Dexamethasone-suppressed and metyrapone-blocked human subjects demonstrated alterations of steroidogenesis only in the mineralocorticoid pathway with potassium administration (Brown *et al.* 1972). *In vitro* studies on rat and canine adrenals have revealed that changes in potassium concentration can act on three different steps in the aldosterone pathway: (1) the conversion of cholesterol to pregnenolone (Muller 1971); (2) the conversion of deoxycorticosterone to corticosterone (Burwell *et al.* 1969); and (3) the conversion of corticosterone to aldosterone (Baumann and Muller 1972). Specific sites of action in man have not been determined.

ACTH

Increases in aldosterone production are seen after an acute infusion of ACTH in normal human subjects (Nichols *et al.* 1975; Kem *et al.* 1975). The response of aldosterone to continuous

ACTH administration is transient. Aldosterone secretion will return to normal in 72–96 h despite continued administration of ACTH (Laragh *et al.* 1975). It has been postulated that ACTH may mediate the rise in aldosterone secretion observed during stress, evidenced by the observation that normal humans had higher urinary 17-OHCS, lower urinary sodium/potassium ratios, and a higher level of aldosterone in the initial 24 h after surgery (Llaurado 1955; Venning *et al.* 1958) than patients who had just undergone surgical hypophysectomy (Llaurado 1957) and that hypophysectomy or creation of a lesion of the median eminence in canines significantly inhibited the increase in urinary 17-OHCS and aldosterone in response to surgical stress (Ganong *et al.* 1965). Such experiments suggest that a pituitary factor, possibly ACTH, could mediate the rise in aldosterone seen with surgery, but these studies did not control for other stimuli of aldosterone secretion (potassium, sodium).

Experiments in sheep also add to the pool of data. After autotransplant of the left adrenal into a carotid jugular skin loop, ewes underwent the stress of placement of an external jugular line without anesthesia. Serial measurements of cortisol, aldosterone, potassium, and angiotensin II were accomplished after line placement in animals with and without dexamethasone suppression. Dexamethasone treatment prevented the rise in cortisol and aldosterone observed in untreated animals. Circulating potassium and angiotensin II concentrations did not change in either set of animals (Espiner *et al.* 1978).

Plasma sodium concentration

Changes in plasma sodium concentration in the dog *in vivo* have been linked to changes in aldosterone levels. A decrease in plasma sodium of 12 mEq/l below normal values of 140–146 mEq/l by direct infusion of 5 per cent dextrose solution into the adrenal artery was associated with an increase in aldosterone secretion (Davis *et al.* 1963).

In vitro experiments utilizing canine adrenal cortical slices bathed with fluid in which the sodium level varied from 120 to 160 mEq/l demonstrated changes in aldosterone secretion with each 10 mEq/l change in the extracellular fluid sodium concentration. There was an inverse relationship between extracellular sodium concentration and aldosterone secretion. The osmolality and the extracellular potassium level were held constant (Lobo *et al.* 1978).

Experiments in man have been difficult to interpret because of the inability to control the influence of the other regulating elements of aldosterone secretion when manipulating the plasma sodium concentration.

Aldosterone metabolism

Circulating aldosterone

Aldosterone is poorly bound to albumin and plasma proteins. The half-life of aldosterone is 20–30 min. Virtually 100 per cent of the aldosterone is metabolized on a single pass through a normal liver.

Aldosterone catabolism

The major metabolite of aldosterone is tetrahydroaldosterone (THA). THA results from a reduction of a double bond in the A ring. THA comprises 30–40 per cent of the excreted aldosterone.

The other significant metabolic by-product is the 18-glucuronide. It comprises 15–20 per cent of the aldosterone excreted in the urine. The 18-glucuronide metabolite is also known as the 'acid-labile' conjugate, because reduction of the urinary pH to 1 liberates free aldosterone. The 'acid-labile' form is the usual substance measured when assessing the excretion of aldosterone in the urine (Horton 1973).

Mineralocorticoid function tests

Plasma renin activity

A satisfactory system to measure plasma renin directly is currently not available. Most laboratories utilize the plasma renin activity (PRA) as the indicator of normal or pathologic levels of renin. PRA assesses the amount of angiotensin I produced under specific laboratory conditions by a sample of plasma drawn from a patient. The angiotensin I level is measured by RIA.

The numerical value generated by this assay is meaningless unless rigid criteria are followed when processing the sample. The blood should be drawn as rapidly as possible into tubes that have been immersed in ice and that contain inhibitors of angiotensinases. As soon as possible after collection, the sample should be placed in ice and centrifuged in the cold. If the plasma is not immediately processed, the sample should be frozen.

When measuring the angiotensin I generated by the sample, time, pH, and temperature must be carefully controlled. Alterations in any of these factors will lead to erroneous PRA values.

The PRA is usually normal in secondary adrenal insufficiency, elevated in primary adrenal insufficiency, and normal or suppressed in Cushing's syndrome. Interpretation of reported PRA is fraught with many difficulties. Numerous physiologic conditions such as posture, sodium balance, adrenergic nerve activity, and age can alter PRA levels. A diurnal rhythm has been described in the supine adult (Gordon *et al.* 1966) but not in the upright individual (Lightman *et al.* 1981). Thus, time of day also may influence PRA levels. All of these physiologic variables make it difficult if not impossible to interpret a random PRA. The renin profile has been developed to attempt to control these variables and intelligently interpret the PRA value.

The 'renin profile' entails a comparison of PRA obtained at noon after 4 hours of upright posture with a 24-hour urine excretion of sodium completed the morning the sample for PRA is obtained (Fig. 50.16). This protocol has been used to standardize the influence of sodium balance, diurnal rhythm, and posture on a patient's PRA. This PRA–sodium index gives the clinician a tool with which to evaluate outpatients on an *ad libitum* sodium intake (Laragh *et al.* 1972; Wood *et al.* 1976).

Attempts to define normal PRA in the pediatric population have been less successful. Numerous authors report normal values for infants and children, but time of day, sodium balance, and posture were not adequately controlled. Despite these difficulties, such studies have demonstrated that PRA is highest in infants and gradually decreases with age to levels seen in adults (Pipkin *et al.* 1981; Dillion and Ryness 1975; Sassard *et al.* 1975).

Several attempts have been made to standardize diet, posture, and time of day when assessing PRA in children. In these studies, Berenson *et al.* (1979) were unable to demonstrate an age-related

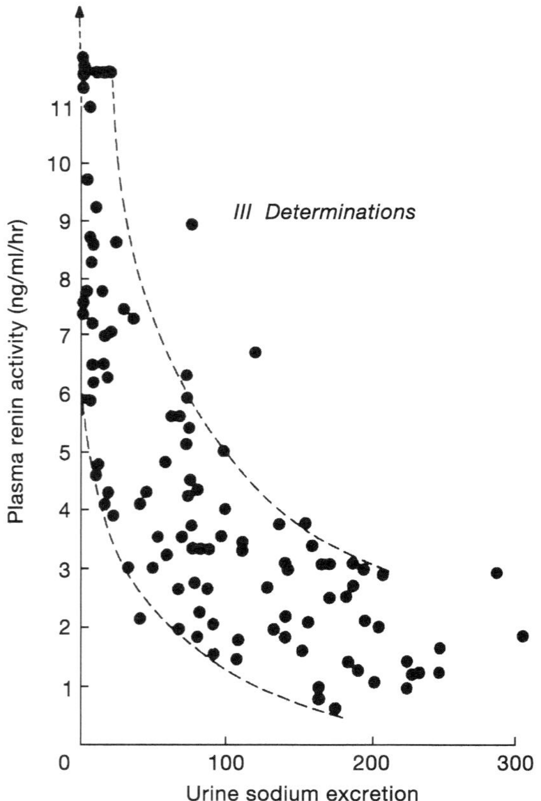

Fig. 50.16 Relation of noon plasma renin activity to the concurrent daily sodium excretion in 52 normal adults. (Adapted from Brunner *et al.*, N Eng J Med 286:443, 1972.)

difference of PRA in individuals 5–15 years of age. Hiner *et al.* (1976) documented a decrease in PRA with age in patients taking a normal diet (2–17 years) but found no relationship with excretion of sodium when sodium excretion was corrected per 1.73 m². Giovannelli *et al.* (1981) found an inverse correlation between PRA measured in either the supine or upright position in children (2 months to 14 years) and sodium excreted in the urine per 24 hours (range of sodium intake, 10–160 mEq/m²/24 h) whether or not the sodium excretion was corrected for differences in the surface areas of the individuals (Figs 50.17 and 50.18). These two nomograms are the closest estimations of a 'renin profile' available in pediatrics.

Peripheral renin activity

Furosemide stimulation test (outpatient procedure) (Carey et al. 1972)

Test. PRA is drawn after 3 hours of upright posture following overnight administration of 40 mg of Lasix at 18.00, 23.00, and 06.00 h.

Normal response. Normal individuals will have PRA 1.7 ng/ml/h.

Saline suppression test and dietary sodium depletion (inpatient procedure) (Grim *et al.* 1977)

Test. Day 1, Patient admitted to hospital and placed on an intake of 150 mEq/day sodium and 70 mEq/day potassium. Day 3, Patient is awakened at 06.00 h and assumes an upright posture for 2 h. At 08.00 h blood is drawn for PRA and plasma aldosterone. Patient then assumes supine position and 2 l of normal saline is infused over 4 h. At 12.00 h a PRA and plasma aldosterone are drawn. Patient may then eat. Total sodium intake for day 3 must approximate 458 mEq. Day 4, Patient is awakened at 06.00 h and assumes an upright posture for 2 h. At 08.00 h a PRA is drawn. After blood drawing the diet is changed to 10 mEq sodium, 60 mEq potassium, and 25 ml/kg free water. Lasix (40 mg) is administered at 09.00, 13.00, and 17.00 h. Day 5: At 08.00 h, after 2 h of upright posture, a PRA is drawn.

Normal response. See Table 15.9.

All medications that affect PRA (antihypertensive drugs, diuretics, etc.) must be discontinued for at least 2 weeks prior to testing.

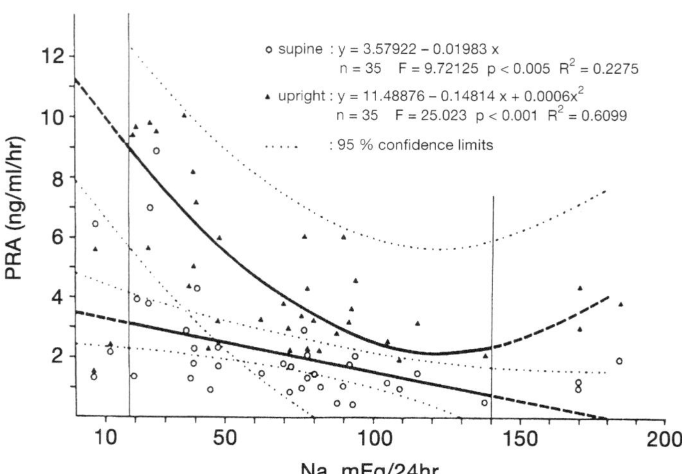

Fig. 50.17 Plasma renin activity level vs. urinary sodium excretion at equilibrium of sodium balance in the supine and upright positions in 38 normal children. (Adapted from Giovannelli, G. (ed), 'Hypertension in Childhood and Adolescents,' Raven Press, New York, p 131, 1981.)

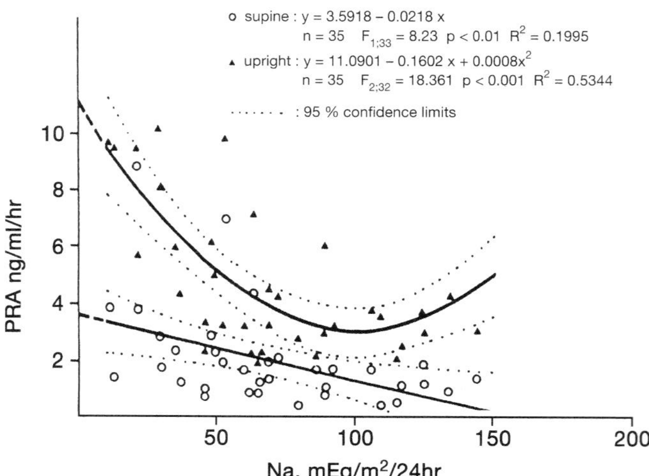

Fig. 50.18 Plasma renin activity level vs. urinary sodium excretion (mEq/m²/24 h) at equilibrium of sodium balance in supine and upright positions in 35 normal children. (Adapted from Giovannelli, G. (ed), 'Hypertension in Childhood and Adolescents,' Raven Press, New York, p 133, 1981.)

Table 50.9 Plasma renin activity and aldosterone response to saline suppression test and dietary sodium depletion

	Age (years)	PRA (ng/ml/3 h)			PA (ng/100ml)		
		Before saline	After saline	Before furosemide	After furosemide	Before saline	After saline
Normal subjects (114)[a]							
Mean	33	5.2	0.9	3.2	22.8	34	4.8
±SD	14	3.4	0.6	2.5	14.4	20	2.7
Renovascular hypertension (38)							
Mean	45	21.0	4.9	12.4	42.0	82	7.2
±SD	13	15.0	4.6	11.1	37.0	59	3.8
Primary aldosteronism (28)							
Mean	48	0.8	0.6	0.8	1.1	54	30.0
±SD	11	0.8	1.0	0.8	0.8	50	18.0
Essential hypertension (170)							
Mean	42	9.3	2.5	5.3	20.0	45	6.4
±SD	13	12.0	3.6	5.3	22.0	35	9.0
Low renin (27)							
Mean	49	1.6	0.6	1.0	1.9	32	5.8
±SD	10	1.2	0.5	0.7	0.9	21	2.3
Normal renin (92)							
Mean	41	7.3	1.2	4.3	21.6	44	5.5
±SD	13	7.5	0.7	4.5	23.2	34	3.0
High renin (51)							
Mean	40	17.2	5.7	9.7	27.7	58	8.9
±SD	13	17.0	5.2	5.2	19.0	40	15.6

[a] Numbers in parentheses.
Adapted from Grim C.E. *et al.*, *JAMA* 237:1334, 1997.

Spironolactone and exogenous estrogen must be stopped 4 weeks and 3 months before testing, respectively.

Some authors prefer to use the stimulation test at the initial PRA screen rather than use the random profile. Although there are some quantitative differences, a general correlation exists between the PRA profile and the stimulation test. Most of the controversy lies in identifying the border between low-renin and normal-renin essential hypertension.

The response of PRA to these tests does not differentiate entities within the high- or low-PRA groups. The stimulation tests can help to identify patients with renal vascular hypertension. Such patients have an excessive response of PRA to sodium restriction. The lack of suppression of plasma aldosterone can aid in the identification of patients with primary aldosteronism (Grim *et al.* 1977).

Renal vein renin activity

Renal vascular hypertension test (Gunnels *et al.* 1969; Stone *et al.* 1977; Stockigt *et al.* 1972; Bourgoignie *et al.* 1970; Vaughan *et al.* 1981)

Test. Patient is admitted the night before the study and maintained on a regular diet. Patient remains supine throughout the night and is transported to the radiology suite without a change in posture. Blood for peripheral PRA is obtained, and a catheter is introduced through the femoral vein. The catheter is positioned by fluoroscopy in the renal vein. Blood samples are obtained from each renal vein and the inferior vena cava for PRA.

Normal response. Individuals with surgically remediable renovascular hypertension have a renal venous PRA (R) ÷ contralateral renal venous PRA (Rc) of > 1.5. The contralateral renal venous PRA should be equal to the inferior vena cava PRA. Also, in patients who respond to surgery, the renal vein PRA on the same side of the lesion, minus the inferior vena cava PRA, divided by inferior vena cava renin is ≥ 0.5.

Patients should discontinue as many antihypertensive medications as possible prior to testing. Some authors use a low-sodium diet to attempt to enhance PRA (Genest 1977). The R/Rc of 1.5 is valid whether a low or normal sodium diet is utilized.

Selective renal vein PRA measurement is an effective method of defining individuals with renal artery stenosis who have a high likelihood of responding to surgical correction of the lesion. Results in individual series vary, but two reviews quote a 95 per cent accuracy in predicting individuals with renal artery stenosis who will respond to surgery when the renal venous renin ratio R/Rc is > 1.5.

Patients whose lesion occludes at least 80 per cent of the renal arterial lumen and does not fulfil the R/Rc ratio requirement should be treated with antihypertensive medication and restudied in 1 year (Genest 1977).

Unfortunately, the renal venous PRA tests alone do not select from the hypertensive population those individuals who would benefit from surgery. Two studies, investigating the renal vein renin test in patients with essential hypertension and either normal renal arteriograms (Stone *et al.* 1977; Genest 1977) or normal excretory urograms and renal scans (Maxwell *et al.* 1975), documented 14 and 20 per cent of the individuals, respectively, as having an R/Rc ratio > 1.5. Thus, the renal renin test does not exclude the need for renal angiography.

One study (Stone *et al.* 1977) addressed the effect of contrast material on renal vein PRA. As a group, renal PRA samples drawn 1, 5, and 15 min after selective angiography were not statistically different from preangiographic renal PRA, but there were major differences in some of the values.

Plasma aldosterone concentration

Plasma aldosterone concentration can be measured by RIA. An isolated value reflects only the physiologic response of the individual at that specific moment as influenced by posture, salt balance, time of day, ACTH, and plasma potassium concentration. When plasma aldosterone is measured in a standardized situation, limited inferences can be made with respect to a single value. Correlation with simultaneous PRA can expose pathologic states.

Table 50.10 depicts plasma aldosterone levels in normal individuals of various ages on a salt diet > 100 mEq/1.73 m^2 obtained between 09.00 and 10.00 h with the patients in a supine position, after an overnight fast, and not on any medications (Stark *et al.* 1975). Aldosterone values for adults are similar to those of children and adolescents (Kowarski *et al.* 1974) in a similar clinical setting. In adults on a normal sodium intake and not taking drugs that affect aldosterone, a plasma aldosterone level > 30 ng/dl is highly suggestive of an aldosterone excess (Biglieri *et al.* 1974; Ganguly *et al.* 1973).

Upright morning plasma aldosterone levels (Kowarski *et al.* 1974) and 24-hour integrated plasma aldosterone values (Zadik and Kowarski 1980) in normal individuals on a normal diet at different ages have been reported (Figs 50.19 and 50.20). Although these values have not been compared to those of patients with known adrenal cortical pathology, they may be helpful in defining patients with abnormalities of aldosterone production.

In the normal supine individual, plasma aldosterone exhibits a circadian rhythm with its zenith in the early morning hours (06.00–10.00 h) and its nadir in the late evening (22.00–24.00 h) (Armbuster *et al.* 1975; Katz *et al.* 1975; Cain *et al.* 1972). This rhythm can be exaggerated if the patient is placed on a low sodium diet (Armbuster *et al.* 1975; Katz *et al.* 1975).

The circadian rhythm of plasma aldosterone in normal individuals assuming upright posture from 08.00 to 22.00 h and then remaining supine until the following morning exhibits two peaks. The first peak is in the early morning hours, and the second is between 08.00 and 12.00 h. These individuals continue to have the

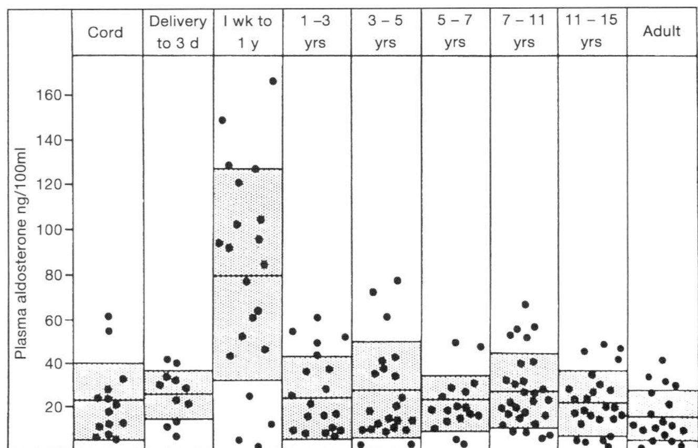

Fig. 50.19 Plasma alsosterone concentrations measured in the upright position in the morning on a normal diet in normal individuals by age. (Adapted from Kowarski, A. *et al.*, J Clin Endocrinol Metab 38:490, 1974.)

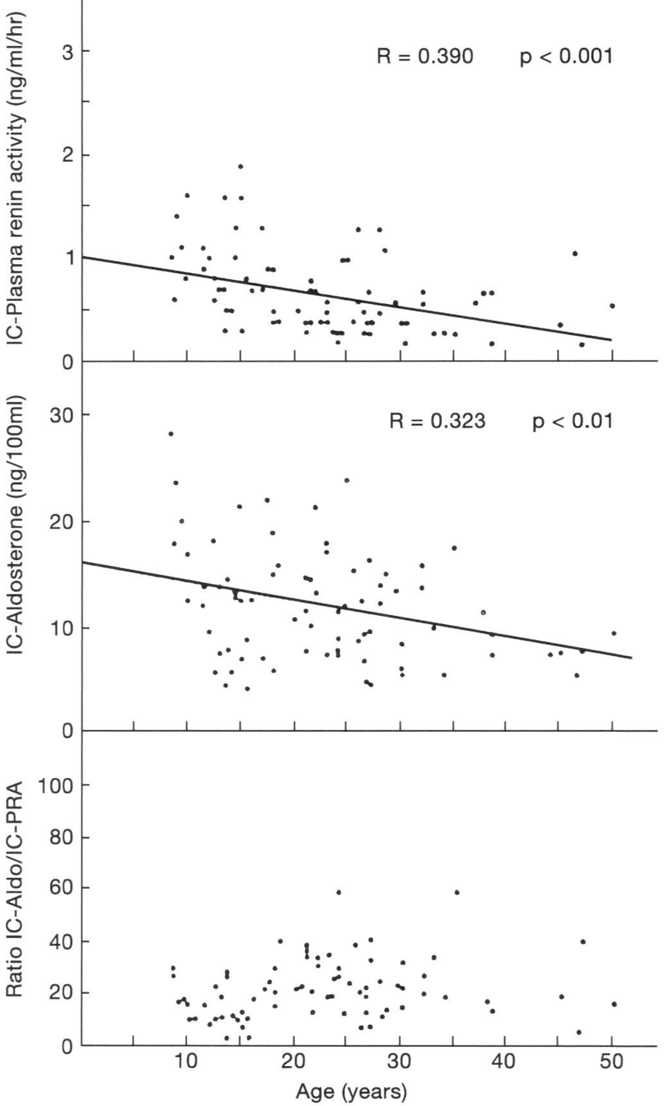

Fig. 50.20 Integrated concentration of aldosterone and plasma renin activity by age. (Adapted from Zadik, Z. *et al.*, J Clin Endocrino Metab 50:868, 1980.)

Table 50.10 Plasma aldosterone concentration by age

Group	Age (years)	N	Plasma aldosterone (ng/100ml) X	Range
I	0–1	13	43.3	4.8–132.0
II	1–4	8	25.9	4.6–60.00
III	4–8	11	19.2	3.6–76.0
IV	8–12	21	9.5	2.8–28.0
V	12–16	9	8.5	0.6–17.6
VI	Adults	10	5.9	2.5–7.8

Value at 0800h. No dietary control.
Adapted from Stark *et al.*, *Helv Paediatr Acta* 30:353, 1975.
Mean and range of morning plasma aldosterone in healthy individuals of various ages. Groups I, II, IV were significantly higher than group VI (p<.025).

nadir in the cycle in the late evening (Biglieri *et al.* 1974; Grim *et al.* 1974). The factors governing this rhythm have not been fully defined. The principal participants appear to be ACTH, renin as altered by sodium intake, posture, and renal nerve activity (Armbuster *et al.* 1974, 1975).

Plasma aldosterone to renin ratio (Gordon 1995; Ganguly 1998; Weinberger and Fineberg 1993; Blumenfeld and Vaughan 1999; Blumenfeld *et al.* 1994; Vallotton 1996)

Plasma aldosterone (PA) to plasma renin activity (PRA) ratio has emerged as an effective screening test for primary hyperaldosteronism due to the presence of high PA and low PRA in these patients. Most patients have a value of 30 or more, compared with 4 to 5 in normal individuals or patients with essential hypertension. The combination of a plasma aldosterone concentration above 20 ng/dl and a PA/PRA ratio above 30 has a 90 per cent sensitivity and specificity (Weinberger and Fineberg 1993).

It is important to remember that it is essential to eliminate other factors that can affect renin and aldosterone prior to the test, including correction of hypokalemia with potassium chloride supplements and discontinuing medications such as diuretics, angiotensin-converting enzyme (ACE) inhibitors, and beta blockers.

Test for response of aldosterone to change in posture (Biglieri *et al.* 1974)

Diet. 120 mEq sodium per day.

Test. Plasma aldosterone is obtained at 08.00 h after overnight recumbancy. Patient assumes an upright posture, and at 12.00 h a second plasma aldosterone value is obtained.

Normal response. See Fig. 50.21. 08.00 h recumbent < 14 ng/dl; 12.00 h upright = an increase by a minimum of 100 per cent from baseline.

Adrenal adenoma response. 08.00 h recumbent > 19.5 ng/dl; 12.00 h upright decreases from recumbent value or rises less than 25 per cent.

Adrenal hyperplasia response. 08.00 h recumbent ~ 19.5 ng/dl; 12.00 h upright increases above recumbent by minimum of 72 per cent.

This test has been useful in distinguishing between the surgically responsive (aldosterone-producing adenoma) and the surgically resistant (idiopathic adrenal hyperplasia) as causes of primary aldosteronism. The lack of rise of plasma aldosterone with aldosterone-producing adenoma is the result of an expanded plasma volume that eliminates the renin-stimulated response of aldosterone to upright posture.

Urinary aldosterone excretion

Twenty-four-hour urine collection for aldosterone gives the clinician the advantage of documenting a patient's mineralocorticoid status over an extended period of time rather than just at a particular instant. The urinary aldosterone sodium excretion index constitutes an accurate assessment of excess or deficient aldosterone excretion (Figs 50.22 and 50.23). The procedure can be accomplished in outpatients.

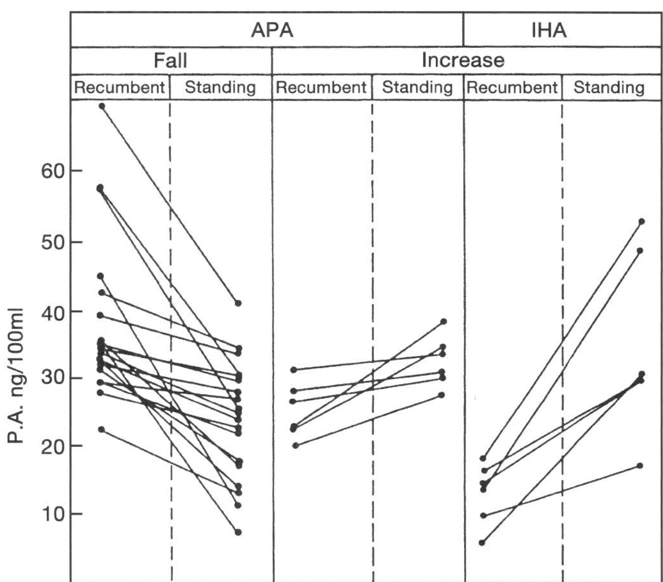

Fig. 50.21 Response of plasma aldosterone (P.A.) concentration to postural change in surgically proven cases of aldosterone-producing adenoma (APA) and idiopathic hyperaldosteronism (IHA). (Adapted from Biglieri, E.G. *et al.*, Circ Res (Suppl) 34/35:1–186, 1974.)

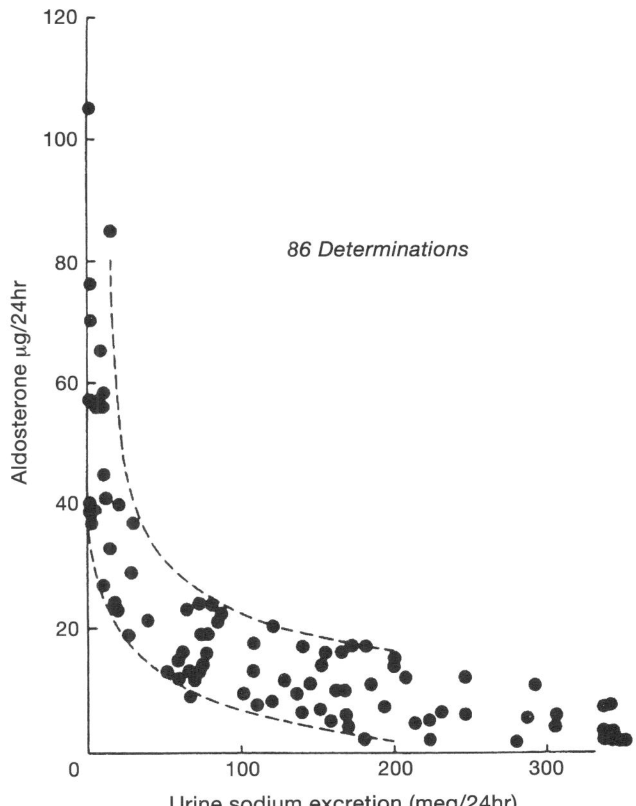

Fig. 50.22 Excretion of aldosterone per 24 h with concurrent sodium excretion in normal adults. (Adapted from Brunner, H.R. *et al.*, N Engl J Med 286: 1443, 1972.)

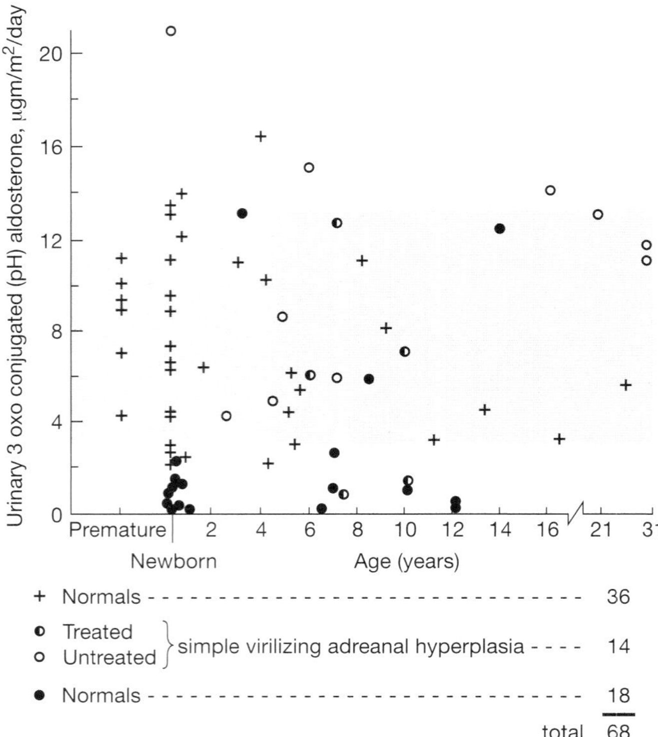

Fig. 50.23 Twenty-four-hour excretion of the 3-oxoconjugate of aldosterone per square meter by age. Shaded area represents normal adult values. (Adapted from New, M.I. et al., J Clin Invest 45:420, 1966.)

Figure 50.22 depicts aldosterone excretion in adults on various amounts of dietary sodium. Figure 50.23 shows aldosterone production per square meter in the pediatric population on an 'unrestricted' sodium intake (New *et al.* 1966). When the values are adjusted for surface area, normal children and adults have similar excretion rates. It is not known whether this relationship would hold if the children were placed on sodium restriction. The fraction of aldosterone measured in the urine was the C18 glucuronide (3-oxo-conjugate, acid-labile conjugate) fraction of aldosterone.

The lack of suppressibility of urinary aldosterone to changes in dietary sodium with a constant potassium intake has been used to identify patients with primary aldosteronism.

Dietary sodium and urinary aldosterone test (Cain *et al.* 1972)

Test. 3-day equilibration period on a diet of 10 mEq of sodium and 100 mEq potassium is accomplished. On the fourth day a 24-hour urine collection for aldosterone is completed. The diet is changed to 200 mEq Na and 100 mEq K per day. Another 3-day equilibration period is completed. The next day a 24-hour urine collection for aldosterone is accomplished.

Normal response. See Table 50.11.

When dietary criteria are rigidly upheld, this is an effective test for identifying the adult patient with primary aldosteronism. Control values are not available for the pediatric population.

Aldosterone suppression tests

Deoxycorticosterone suppression test (Biglieri et al. 1967, 1972)

*Test.*Patient is placed on 120 mEq/day sodium diet. After 3 days of equilibration, a 24-hour urine collection for sodium is accomplished. On day 5 the patient receives 10 mg of deoxycorticosterone acetate intramuscularly (IM) every 12 hours for a total of six doses. Another 24-hour urine collection is made during the last 24 hours of the deoxycorticosterone administration.

Normal response. See Fig. 50.24.

Figure 50.24 depicts the responses of normal individuals and patients with an aldosterone-producing adenoma, idiopathic hyperplasia, and indeterminate hyperplasia. Although not shown, there is also marked suppression of aldosterone in patients with essential hypertension. As can be seen by the graph, this test differentiates only the indeterminate type of adrenal hyperplasia from the other forms of primary aldosteronism. With appropriate aldosterone suppression and the clinical picture of hypertension, hypokalemia, normal cortisol production, and suppressed PRA, a diagnosis of primary aldosteronism—indeterminate type—can be made.

Fluorohydrocortisone test

The fluorohydrocortisone test relies on the ability of an exogenously administered mineralocorticoid to expand plasma volume and suppress aldosterone secretion. The test can be used to sepa-

Table 50.11 Influence of dietary sodium in normals and patients with primary aldosteronism[a]

Determination	Normal subjects		Patients with primary aldosteronism	
	10 mEq	200 mEq	10 mEq	200 mEq
Serum sodium (mEq/L)	141 ±1	142 ± 1	144 ± 1	145 ± 1
Serum potassium (mEq/L)	4.5 ± 0.1	4.4 ± 0.1	4.0 ± 0.1	3.3 ± 0.2
Upright plasma aldosterone (ng/100 ml)	96 ± 9	22 ± 3	93 ± 18	53 ± 11
Upright PRA (ng/ml/3 h)	17.6 ± 0.9	3.2 ± 0.5	1.8 ± 0.2	1.3 ± 0.2
Urine sodium (mEq/day)	5 ± 2	195 ± 20	16 ± 2	186 ± 16
Urine potassium (mEq/day)	85 ± 5	86 ± 7	73 ± 4	104 ± 10
Aldosterone secretion rate (μg/day)	755 ± 30	150 ± 60	830 ± 104	488 ± 47

[a] All subjects on a 100 mEq potassium intake.
Adopted from Cain et al., AM J Med 53:630, 1972.

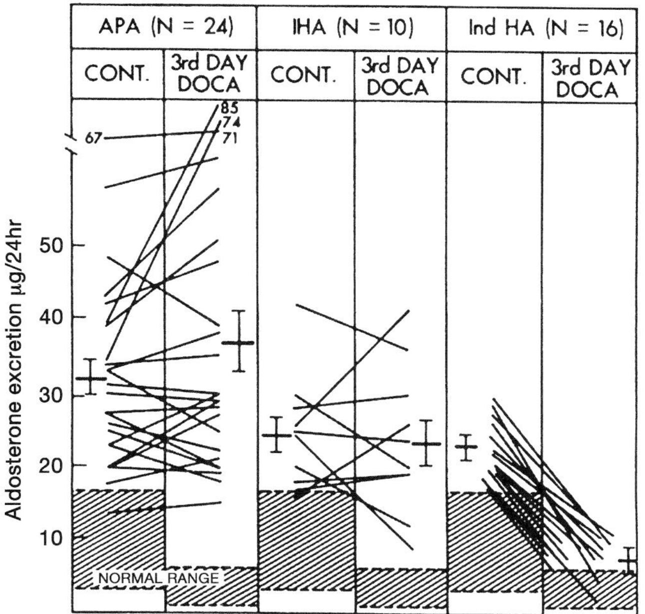

Fig. 50.24 Aldosterone excretion in patients with aldosterone-producing adenoma (APA), idiopathic hyperplasia (IHA), and indeterminate hyperaldosteronism (Ind HA) on 120 mEq of sodium intake and after 3 days of treatment with deoxycorticosterone acetate (DOCA). (Adapted from Felig, P. (ed), 'Endocrinology and Metabolism,' McGraw-Hill, New York, p 573, 1981.)

rate patients with primary aldosteronism from normal individuals and from those with essential hypertension. The test does not discriminate between causes of primary aldosteronism. False-positive and false-negative results occur with this test. Interpretation of this test is not always straightforward. The test does not usually add to the clinician's knowledge but may be used as an adjunct in defining the presence or absence of primary aldosteronism. References are given for those who desire to use this test (Padfield *et al.* 1975; Biglieri *et al.* 1970; Ferris *et al.* 1978).

Saline suppression test (Kem *et al.* 1971)

Test. Patient arises at 06.00 h and remains in the upright position for 2 hours. At 08.00 h a plasma aldosterone is obtained. Patient is placed in the supine position, and 2 l of isotonic saline is administered intravenously at an even rate over 4 hours. At 12.00 h, with the patient still in the supine position, a plasma aldosterone is obtained. Diet is not controlled for this test.

Normal response. Normal adults and patients with essential hypertension all suppress plasma aldosterone to < 5 ng/dl after saline infusion. Patients with primary aldosteronism fail to reduce their plasma aldosterone level to 5 ng/dl.

This test is a rapid means for assessing the suppressibility of aldosterone and failure to suppress the aldosterone is very suggestive of primary aldosteronism.

Dexamethasone suppression test (Litchfield *et al.* 1997)

Glucocorticoid-remediable aldosteronism is a subset of patients with primary aldosteronism who have been described as respond-

ing to glucocorticoids. It is caused by a chimeric gene in which the ACTH-responsive 5 -promoter of the 11β-hydroxylase gene is fused to coding sequences of the aldosterone synthase gene (Litchfield *et al.* 1995; Lifton 1992; Dluhy and Lifton 1995, 1999; Williams and Dluhy 1995). This results in ectopic expression of aldosterone synthase activity in zona fasciculata cells of the adrenal cortex under the regulation of ACTH, with resultant production of aldosterone and the novel steroids such as 18-oxocortisol and 18-hydroxycortisol. Clinical manifestations are related to hyperaldosteronism and respond to treatment with glucocorticoids. Direct genetic testing is 100 per cent sensitive and specific in making the diagnosis. The Dexamethasone suppression test can probably be used as a screening test and needs further validation.

Aldosterone stimulation tests

ACTH stimulation test (Dluhy *et al.* 1974)

Test. At time 0, plasma aldosterone is obtained and 0.25 mg of cosyntropin is administered IM or IV. At 30 and 60 min after cosyntropin administration, additional samples are obtained for plasma aldosterone.

Normal response. A minimum rise of aldosterone of 4 ng/dl from the baseline value is seen in normal individuals. The mean increase is 14 ng/dl, with a range of 4–29 ng/dl in the normal population.

ACTH stimulates rapid short-term release of aldosterone (Biglieri *et al.* 1969). This fact can aid the clinician in assessing the patient suspected of adrenal insufficiency. Individuals with secondary adrenal insufficiency as a result of panhypopituitarism or exogenous steroid administration usually have normal aldosterone responses to acute ACTH stimulation. In patients with primary adrenal insufficiency the disease generally compromises all layers of the adrenal cortex, and there is no response of cortisol or aldosterone to exogenously administered ACTH (Dluhy *et al.* 1974).

Adrenal vein aldosterone test (Gordon 1995; Horton and Finck 1972; Nichols *et al.* 1972; Doppman and Gill 1996; Young *et al.* 1996; Sheaves *et al.* 1996)

Test. After an overnight fast the patient is brought to the radiology suite in the recumbent position. A venous catheter is passed through the femoral vein, and samples are taken from the right and left adrenal veins and peripheral vein for plasma aldosterone and cortisol concentrations before and 15 min after IV injection of 0.25 mg synthetic ACTH.

Normal response. In patients with a unilateral tumor producing aldosterone, the plasma aldosterone level from the adrenal vein on the side of the adenoma far exceeds the contralateral adrenal vein plasma aldosterone level (usually greater than 10-fold). Minimum ratios reported from different sources are 26:1 (Nichols *et al.* 1972), 12:1 (Melby 1972), and 10:1 (Horton and Finck 1972).

ACTH acutely stimulates aldosterone release and increases the difference between the two sides with an adrenal adenoma. The cortisol concentration should be the same in both adrenal veins, but much higher than that in a peripheral vein.

Adrenal vein aldosterone levels can be very helpful in distinguishing between an adrenal adenoma and hyperplasia. Patients with bilateral adrenal hyperplasia characteristically have left adrenal vein aldosterone levels 25 per cent greater than the right adrenal vein aldosterone level. This difference has been related to differences in tissue mass, with the left characteristically greater than the right (Melby 1972). If catheterization of one of the veins is not possible, a comparison between the peripheral level and the side obtained will suggest where the pathology lies in a patient whose other tests *strongly* point to an adenoma. If the tumor is on the same side as the sample obtained, the plasma aldosterone value will far exceed the peripheral value. If the tumor is on the opposite side, the sample drawn from the adrenal vein will approximate the peripheral value. In the latter situation, if the patient has adrenal hyperplasia, a comparison of one adrenal vein aldosterone value with a peripheral aldosterone concentration might suggest a tumor on the sampled side. Thus, accurate identification of the position of a tumor when only one adrenal vein is sampled can only be accomplished when other tests strongly support the presence of an adenoma.

Androgens

Androgen pathway

The androgens secreted in the greatest quantities by the adrenal cortex are dehydroepiandrosterone (DHEA), dehydroepiandrosterone sulfate (DHEA-S), and androstenedione. The production and release of these compounds is not well understood. It is known that ACTH can stimulate the release of androgens, but other mechanisms also influence androgen secretion. Peripheral tissues convert DHEA to DHEA-S, thus contributing to plasma DHEA-S levels (Dluhy and Lifton 1999).

Acute IV administration of ACTH results in a rise in DHEA without a simultaneous change in the level of DHEA-S. More prolonged administration of ACTH (IM gel every 4 hours for 48 hours) elicits a rise in both compounds. The slow peripheral conversion of DHEA to DHEA-S is believed to be responsible for the lack of rise in DHEA-S during short-term exposure to ACTH (Vaitukaitis *et al.* 1969).

The diurnal variation of DHEA mimics the rhythm of cortisol. In contrast, a patient with an adrenal adenoma and elevated cortisol levels had an extremely low level of DHEA and no diurnal rhythm (Rosenfield *et al.* 1975). These observations suggest that ACTH plays a role in the production and secretion of androgens. Although the androgen pathway has not been extensively studied, the enzymatic steps at which ACTH acts in the androgen pathway are believed to be identical to those in the glucocorticoid channel.

ACTH is not the only regulator of androgen secretion. It has long been known that urinary metabolites of the androgens (17-ketosteroids) begin to increase in both sexes at 6–8 years of age with a continued rise until after the completion of puberty (Nathanson *et al.* 1941; Talbot *et al.* 1943). Urinary metabolites of cortisol (17-OHCS) demonstrate a steady rate of excretion

(3.1 ± 1.1 mg/m²/24 h) from infancy to adulthood. There is no incremental increase between ages 6 and 8 years (Migeon *et al.* 1963). In children 2–12 years of age, no significant change in plasma cortisol occurs despite a progressive increase in DHEA and DHEA-S with advancing age. These data suggest dissociation of the androgen and the glucocorticoid pathways as the individual progresses through adrenarche. Evidence has also been presented to suggest that adrenarche may be regulated by physiologic processes other than puberty (Parker *et al.* 1978; Sklar *et al.* 1980).

Authors have suggested three possible mechanisms to explain non-ACTH-stimulated androgen secretion: (1) maturational shift in the pathway of adrenal steroid biosynthesis; (2) secretion at the age of adrenarche of an extrapituitary adrenal androgen-stimulating hormone (AASH); and (3) secretion of AASH by the pituitary (Grumbach 1980). The meager amount of data available concerning adrenarche dictates further investigation of this process in normal maturation.

Androgen binding and catabolism

Circulating DHEA, DHEA-S, and androstenedione are weakly but significantly bound to albumin (Plager 1965; Forest *et al.* 1968). After sulfation, excretion of these compounds is primarily in the urine.

DHEA has several metabolic fates (Fig. 50.25). DHEA can be secreted by the adrenal as a free compound with sulfation taking place in the liver or the kidney, or it can be secreted by the adrenal as a sulfate conjugate. DHEA can then be converted to either DHEA-diol, androsterone, etiocholanolone, androdiol, or etiodiol. Androstenedione suffers a similar metabolic fate. The liver is the major site of these conversions. All compounds must undergo conjugation with sulfate or glucuronide before excretion in the urine (Migeon 1972).

Androgen function tests

Plasma DHEA

A unique characteristic of DHEA is that it is the only androgen that is not produced in significant quantities by a tissue other than

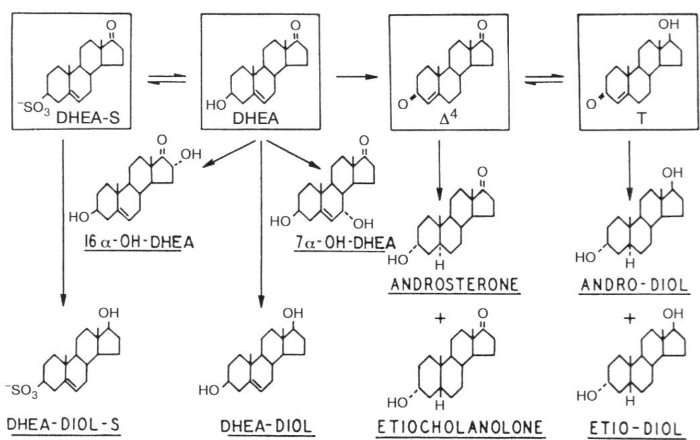

Fig. 50.25 Androgen catabolism. (Adapted from Migeon, C.J., AM J Med 53:611, 1972.)

Table 50.12 Plasma DHEA concentration (ng/dl) by age

	Age (years)					
	<6	6–8	8–10	10–12	12–14	>14
Females						
n	10	9	8	9	6	6
X	28.6	109.3	116.4	351.7	370.1	465.9
CL	19.4–42.1	72.6–164.5	74.4–179.6	233.7–529.4	224.3–610.6	282–770
p		<.0001		<.0005		
Males						
n	6	9	7	11	10	6
X	43.4	43.8	84.7	264.8	352.9	505.9
CL	26.3–71.7	29.1–66.0	53.3–134.6	183.0–383.3	239.5–520.3	306.7–834.6
p			<.05	<.0005		

Values obtained between 0900 and 1100 h. Key: n, number of observations; X, mean; CL, 95% confidence limit; p, probability.

the adrenal gland in the healthy individual. Thus, the reported laboratory value gives the clinician a picture of adrenal androgen metabolism that is usually not clouded by ovarian, testicular, or peripheral tissue contributions.

In the adult, plasma DHEA has been shown to have a circadian rhythm that parallels that of plasma cortisol (Rosenfield *et al.* 1975). The increment between the zenith and nadir can be as much as 600 ng/dl. Studies in children have not been performed to document or refute a similar finding, but it is reasonable to expect a circadian variation of DHEA. Thus, it is important to consider the time of day a sample for DHEA is obtained before interpreting the results.

Table 50.12 describes plasma DHEA measured between 09.00 and 11.00 h in normal children. Significant increases in plasma levels are seen at a younger age in females than males (Vaitukaitis *et al.* 1969). Afternoon DHEA values have been documented for both sexes from 8 years to adulthood (Hopper and Yen 1975). Other authors have described morning plasma DHEA levels of 6- to 14-year-old females and afternoon plasma DHEA levels in males of the same age (Sizonenko and Paunier 1975). Figure 50.26 shows normal values in infancy; the time of day that the samples were obtained was not standardized.

Low plasma DHEA values are found in late adrenarche (Sklar *et al.* 1980). Elevated DHEA levels are found in idiopathic hirsutism (Nelson 1980*b*) and in adrenal androgen-producing tumor (AAPT) (Osborn and Yannone 1971; Mahesh *et al.* 1968). High DHEA levels can sometimes be found in disorders of the gonad—polycystic ovary syndrome (Osborn and Yannone 1971) and gonadal androgen-producing tumor (GAPT) (Nelson 1980*b*).

Differentiation between polycystic ovary syndrome, GAPT, idiopathic hirsutism, and AAPT in the laboratory can be difficult. Comparison of the plasma levels of the different androgens is the initial step. In virilizing syndromes of gonadal origin, testosterone dominates the plasma androgen profile, whereas in diseases of adrenal origin, DHEA predominates. The second step is the measurement of 17-ketosteroids in a 24 hour urine collection. Patients with high DHEA levels have high urinary 17-ketosteroids. Those with a primary elevation of testosterone do not have elevated 17-ketosteroids. These two steps usually differentiate pathology of gonadal and adrenal origin.

To separate autonomously functioning adrenal tissue (adenoma) from other adrenal pathology, the response of DHEA and 17-ketosteroids to dexamethasone is assessed. A response to 2 mg of dexamethasone administered every 6 hours is seen within 72–96 hours (Mahesh *et al.* 1968). Lack of suppression of DHEA and 17-ketosteroids suggests an autonomous adrenal source of the plasma androgens. Thus, the dominant androgen and suppressibility to dexamethasone should differentiate most clinical entities that present with increased plasma DHEA (Nelson 1980*b*).

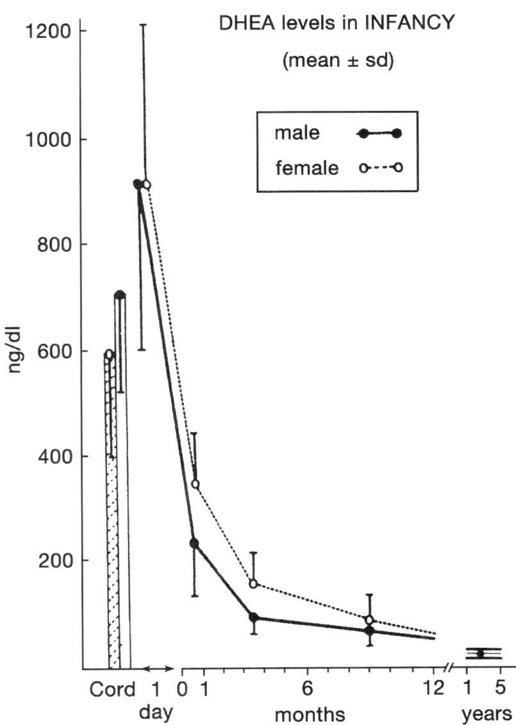

Fig. 50.26 Plasma dehydroepiandrosterone (DHEA) by age. (Adapted from James, V.H.T. (ed), 'The Endocrine Function of the Human Adrenal Cortex,' Academic Press, New York, p 574, 1978.)

It should be noted that AAPT suppressed by dexamethasone administration has been reported (Mahesh *et al.* 1968).

DHEA levels may be elevated or normal in untreated patients with congenital adrenal hyperplasia (Reiter *et al.* 1977). DHEA levels routinely decrease in treated patients with congenital adrenal hyperplasia but do not reflect the degree of control attained with a given dose of glucocorticoid or mineralocorticoid. As a result, DHEA cannot be used for accurate diagnosis or assessment of the adequacy of management of congenital adrenal hyperplasia (Korth-Schutz *et al.* 1978; Guisti *et al.* 1978).

Plasma DHEA-S

Plasma DHEA-S has two sources. It is secreted directly by the adrenal cortex, and it is produced by peripheral tissue sulfokinase, converting DHEA to DHEA-S. When monitored at frequent intervals over a 24 hour period, little fluctuation and minimal synchrony with cortisol are noted. Thus, it is believed that DHEA-S does not have a circadian rhythm (Rosenfeld *et al.* 1975).

Levels of DHEA-S have been described for normal individuals (Hopper and Yen 1975; Reiter *et al.* 1977) (see Figs 50.27 and 50.28). With minimal daily fluctuations, DHEA-S is considered to be reflective of day-to-day rather than moment-to-moment adrenal androgen production. For this reason DHEA-S is more commonly used than DHEA to assess androgen secretion by the adrenal cortex. A less than normal plasma DHEA-S is found in delayed adrenarche (Sklar *et al.* 1980). DHEA-S is increased in idiopathic hirsutism, adrenal androgen-producing adenoma, polycystic ovary syndrome, and gonadal androgen-producing tumors (Nelson 1980*b*; Osborn and Yannone 1971; Mahesh *et al.*

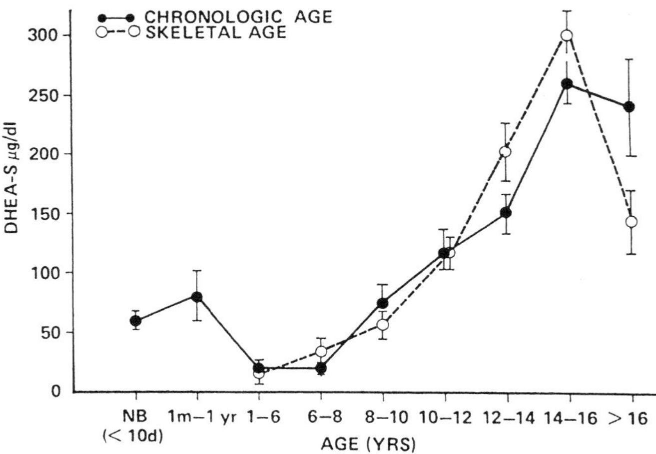

Fig. 50.28   Serum dehydroepiandrosterone-sulfate related to chronologic and skeletal age. (Adapted from Reites E.O. *et al.*, J Pediatr 90: 767, 1977.)

1968). Laboratory differentiation of the above entities has been discussed in the section on plasma DHEA.

DHEA-S can be elevated or normal in untreated congenital adrenal hyperplasia. If the initial DHEA-S level is elevated, a continued elevated level is evidence of poor control, but a normal level does not necessarily reflect good control (Guisti *et al.* 1978; Golden *et al.* 1978).

Plasma androstenedione

Androstenedione has a circadian rhythm that parallels that of cortisol (James *et al.* 1978). As much as a 50 per cent change in plasma concentration has been documented in a 24-hour period (Givens 1976). The age of onset of this pattern has not been established.

Androstenedione levels also have a cyclic relationship with the menstrual period. The highest androstenedione levels are found on the day of ovulation, and the lowest in the first few days prior to menses (Abraham 1974).

Normal values are shown in Fig. 50.29 and Table 50.13. The values presented in Table 50.13 were obtained between 09.00 and 11.00 h; the values in Fig. 50.29 are not standardized for time of day. Menstruating women reach a mean of 210 ng/dl on the day of luteinizing hormone (LH) peak and 110 ng/dl in the final days of the luteal phase (Abraham 1974).

The clinical use of plasma androstenedione is limited. Androstenedione can aid the clinician in assessing androgen excess but cannot be used to define specific pathologic states. Elevated plasma androstenedione levels have been found in untreated congenitalhyperplasia, adrenal androgen-producing tumors, idiopathic hirsutism, polycystic ovary syndrome, and androgen-producing gonadal tumors (Osborn and Yannone 1971; Mahesh *et al.* 1968; Cavollo *et al.* 1979; Keenam *et al.* 1979). Because androstenedione is produced by both the adrenal cortex and the gonad, it is difficult if not impossible to define the source of excess androgen by using plasma levels of androstenedione or the response of androstenedione to dexamethasone.

Some authors have advocated the use of plasma androstenedione in assessing treatment of patients with congenital adrenal

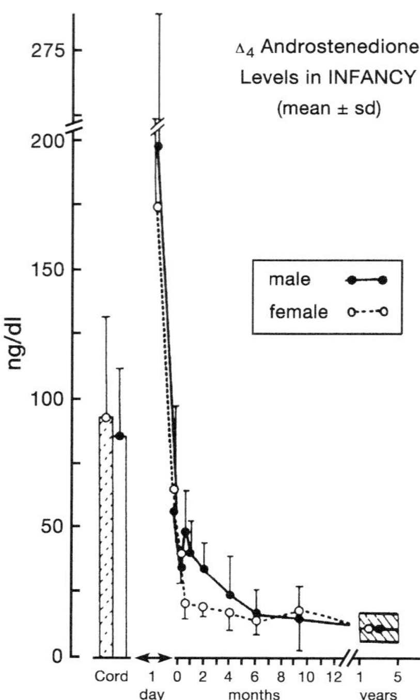

Fig. 50.27   Plasma dehydroepiandrosterone-sulfate (DHEA-S) by age. (Adapted from James, V.H.T. (ed), "The Endocrine Functions of the Human Adrenal Cortex," Academic Press, New York, p 575, 1978.)

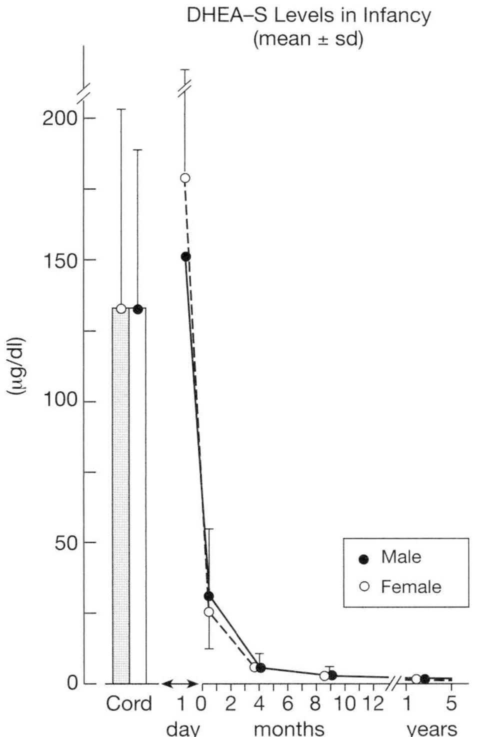

Fig. 50.29 Plasma androstenedione by age. (Adapted from James, V.H.T. (ed), 'The Endocrine Function of the Human Adrenal Cortex,' Academic Press, New York, p 572, 1978.)

hyperplasia (Cavollo *et al.* 1979; Keenam *et al.* 1979), but it has not been validated unequivocally.

Serum 17-hydroxyprogesterone

17-hydroxyprogesterone is the normal substrate for CYP21A2 (21-hydroxylase) and is measured by RIA. Its concentration is significantly increased (usually several hundredfold) in patients with typical CYP21A2 deficiency. These patients also display an exaggerated serum 17-hydroxyprogesterone response to ACTH stimulation (White *et al.* 1987*a*; Witchel *et al.* 1997). In patients with late-onset CYP21A2 deficiency, basal serum concentrations may be only slightly elevated during follicular phase, but the

response to ACTH is also exaggerated (Azziz *et al.* 1994). Heterozygotes have smaller responses to ACTH, which may overlap with those of normal subjects (Gutai *et al.* 1977).

Serum 11-deoxycortisol and 11-deoxycorticosterone

Both 11-deoxycortisol and 11-deoxycorticosterone are the normal substrates for CYP11B1 (11β-hydroxylase) and are measured by RIA. Patients with CYP11B1 deficiency have high basal and ACTH-stimulated serum concentrations of 11-deoxycortisol and 11-deoxycorticosterone (White *et al.* 1987*a*, *b*, 1994; Lashansky *et al.* 1991, 1992). 11-Deoxycorticosterone, but not 11-deoxycortisol is increased in patients with CPY17 (17α-hydroxylase) deficiency.

Rapid standard-dose ACTH stimulation test (New 1998)

Test. Cosyntropin (synthetic ACTH$_{1-24}$) 0.25 mg is administered by rapid IV injection and blood samples are drawn at 0, 30, and 60 min for measurements of serum 17-hydroxyprogesterone, 11-deoxycortisol, and/or 11-deoxycorticosterone.

Normal response. As described above. Each laboratory has its own reference range and special attention has to be paid to the value of 17-hydroxyprogesterone, which varies significantly during the menstrual cycle.

Urinary 17-ketosteroids

The assay and normal values of urinary 17-ketosteroids have been discussed in the section on glucocorticoids. The diagnostic capabilities of this laboratory test are limited. A 24-hour urine collection for 17-ketosteroids can be used to confirm excess or reduced androgen production for age by the adrenal cortex. Suppressibility to dexamethasone has been discussed in the section on plasma DHEA.

Adrenal medulla

Histology

The adrenal medulla is composed of large epithelioid cells, a supporting connective tissue matrix, and scattered ganglion cells. The epithelioid cells compose the endocrine parenchyma and are arranged in small clusters and short cords in intimate association

Table 50.13 Plasma androstenedione concentration (ng/dl) by age

	Age (years)					
	<6	6–8	8–10	10–12	12–14	>14
Females						
n	9	9	11	9	9	6
X	14.8	17.7	32.1	64.5	123.2	131.4
CL	9.6–22.9	11.5–27.4	21.6–47.4	41.7–99.6	79.8–190.4	77.2–223.9
P		<.05		<.05	<.05	
Males						
n	7	9	9	12	11	6
X	11.6	16.1	20.2	44.7	66.6	82.0
CL	7.1–19.0	10.4–24.8	13.1–31.3	30.7–65.2	44.9–98.7	48.2–139.7
P			<.01			

Values drawn between 0900 and 1100 h. Key: n, number of observations; X, means; CL, 95% confidence limit; p, probability. Adapted from Ducharme J.R. *et al.*, *J Clin Endocrinol Metab* 42:472, 1976.

with the capillaries and venules. Fine granules in the cells stain brown when exposed to chromium salts. This reaction is the result of oxidation and polymerization of epinephrine and norepinephrine and is referred to as the chromaffin reaction. Thus, the cells are called chromaffin cells. Other histochemical reactions can also separate the chromaffin cells into norepinephrine cells (those that autofluoresce with argentaffin and potassium iodide) and epinephrine-containing cells (those that have a high affinity for azocarmine and a positive acid phosphatase reaction).

Pre- and postnatal development

During gestation and extrauterine existence, the medulla does not undergo significant anatomic change. It occupies 10 per cent of the adrenal gland by weight. The cells do undergo a significant change in the ratio of norepinephrine/epinephrine production. This alteration is believed to be linked to the intimate association of the medulla with the cortex and the two-pronged blood supply to the chromaffin cells (see 'Introduction' for details).

Investigators have long noted a change in the ratio of norepinephrine to epinephrine with advancing age. Experiments in cats, rabbits, guinea pigs, rats, and dogs measuring total epinephrine and norepinephrine in chromaffin cells have shown a predominance of norepinephrine *in utero*, a progressive decrease in the total amount of norepinephrine with growth, and an increase in the amount of epinephrine with advancing age. These changes result in dramatic fall in the norepinephrine/epinephrine ratio (Shepherd and West 1951; Hokfelt 1951) (Fig. 50.30). Analysis of catecholamine fractions from the medulla in the fetus, the child, and the adult reveals a similar pattern in man (West *et al.* 1951; Shepherd and West 1951; Hokfelt 1951; Niemineva and

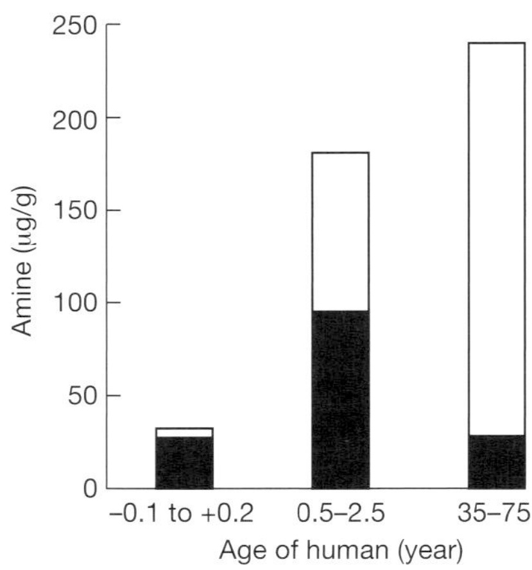

Fig. 50.31 Amine content (fresh tissue) by age in the adrenal gland of the human. Shaded area is norepinephrine; plain area is epinephrine. (Adapted from Shepherd, D.M. *et al.*, Br J Pharmacol Chemother 6:668, 1951.)

Pekkarinen 1953; Axelrod 1962; Fuller and Hunt 1967; Wurtman 1966; Wurtman and Axelrod 1965) (Fig. 50.31).

Phenylethanolamine-*N*-methyl transferase (PNMT) is the enzyme that catalyzes the final steps in epinephrine formation—the methylation of norepinephrine to form epinephrine—and it is localized almost exclusively in the adrenal medulla (Axelrod 1962). Experiments in the rat have demonstrated parallel increases in PNMT activity, the volume of medulla, and the amount of epinephrine in the medulla with advancing age (Fuller and Hunt 1967). Hypophysectomy reduced the weight of the adrenal gland, the amount of PNMT activity, and the concentration of epinephrine in the medulla when compared to weight- and age-matched

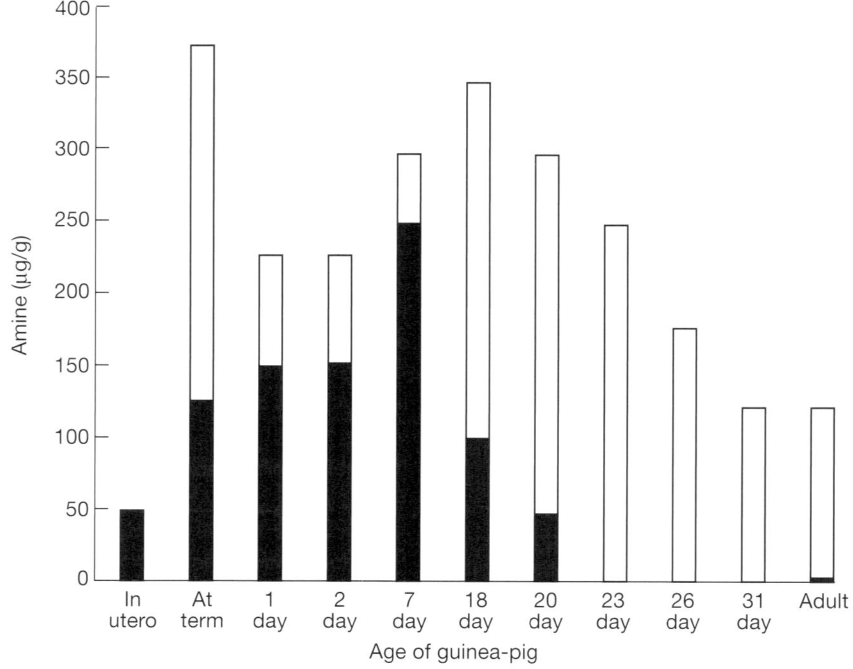

Fig. 50.30 Amine content (fresh tissue) by age in the adrenal gland of the guinea pig. Shaded area is norepinephrine; plain area is epinephrine. (Adapted from Shepherd, D.M. *et al.*, Br J Pharmacol Chemother 6:671, 1951.)

control animals. Treatment of the hypophysectomized rat with ACTH resulted in the return of PNMT activity to normal. There was also an increase in the weight of the gland and adrenaline production with ACTH therapy, but these levels did not return to normal. Dexamethasone treatment of normal rats produced a decrease in the weight of the adrenal gland (cortical atrophy), but there was a slight increase in PNMT activity over the control animals. Hypophysectomized rats treated with dexamethasone had a reduction in the weight of the adrenal gland, elevated PNMT levels, and slightly decreased epinephrine concentrations when compared to the control group (Wurtman and Axelrod 1965). These experiments suggest that glucocorticoids alter the activity of PNMT and the pituitary–adrenal cortical unit may significantly influence the production of epinephrine.

In a separate experiment a dose–response relationship was constructed between different doses of ACTH, various doses of glucocorticoid, and epinephrine synthesis in hypophysectomized rats. The experiments demonstrated that the dose of ACTH required to restore epinephrine biosynthesis to normal was the same as that needed to maintain the adrenal gland at its normal weight and the dose of exogenous steroid needed to maintain a normal medullary concentration of adrenaline was 100 times greater than the normal replacement dose of glucocorticoid (Wurtman 1966). These data suggest that, in adrenal cortex of normal weight (implying cortical cells secreting normal amounts of cortisol), high levels of glucocorticoids may be required to regulate PNMT activity and therefore epinephrine production. This possible prerequisite for epinephrine production may explain why the medullary cells are bathed in the venous effluent of the cortex. Such blood would have a very high concentration of glucocorticoids.

Catecholamine synthesis

Catecholamines are naturally occurring compounds containing a catechol nucleus (3,4-dihydroxyphenyl) linked to an amine (Fig. 50.32). Three such compounds occur in man. They are dopamine, norepinephrine, and epinephrine.

The sequential order of the reactions required for the synthesis of catecholamines was constructed from work done by numerous authors on tissue slices, homogenates, and subcellular fractions of the medulla utilizing radiolabeled substrates (Kishner 1975). Such studies delineated the pathway shown in Fig. 50.33.

Catecholamine synthesis has been demonstrated in three different locations—the adrenal medulla, the adrenergic nerve terminals, and the central nervous system. The amount and type of the end products are dictated by the enzymes present. The relatively exclusive presence and activity of PNMT in the medulla

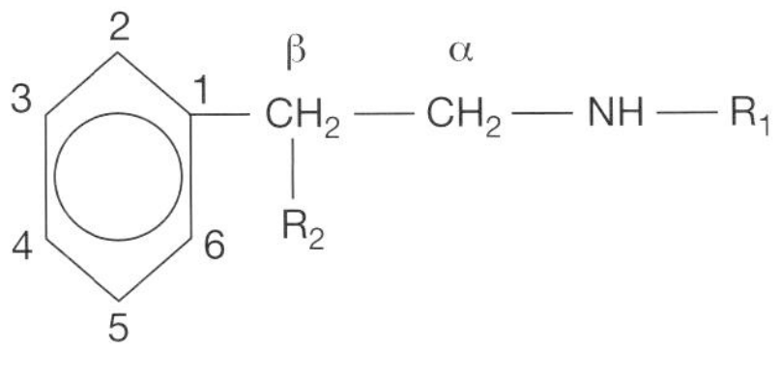

Fig. 50.32 Nomenclature of the catecholamines. (Adapted from Goodman, A.G., Goodman, L.S., Gillman, A. (eds), 'The Pharmacologic Basis of Therapeutics,' 6th Ed, Macmillan, New York, p 142, 1980.)

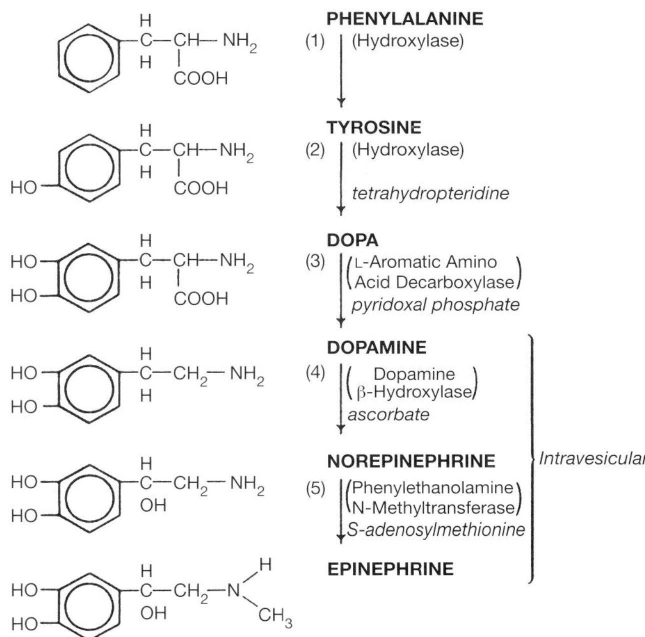

Fig. 50.33 Enzymatic pathway for dopamine, norepinephrine, and epinephrine synthesis. Enzymes are in parentheses; cofactors are in italics. (Adapted from Goodman, A.G., Goodman, L.S., Gillman, A. (eds), 'The Pharmacologic Basis of Therapeutics,' 6th Ed, Macmillan, New York, p 72, 1980.)

are reflected by the dominance of epinephrine in the mature animal (Kishner 1975). Dopamine and norepinephrine are found in the central nervous system, and norepinephrine is mainly present in the axons of the postganglionic adrenergic nervous system.

Dietary tyrosine and phenylalanine converted by phenylalanine hydroxylase to tyrosine are the sources of substrate for catecholamine synthesis. After uptake into the cytoplasm of the cell, tyrosine is converted to dihydroxyphenylalanine (dopa) by the addition of a hydroxyl group in the 3 position. The removal of the carboxyl group from the alpha carbon by the cytoplasmic enzyme dopa carboxylase leads to the formation of dopamine. In epinephrine- and norepinephrine-producing cells, dopamine diffuses into cytoplasmic storage vesicles. There, the placement of a hydroxyl group of the beta carbon produces norepinephrine. Norepinephrine either remains in these vesicles until it is secreted or, in the medullary cells, diffuses into the cytoplasm, where the addition of a methyl group by PNMT forms epinephrine. Epinephrine then re-enters a different group of storage vesicles. Norepinephrine and epinephrine remain in their storage vesicles until secreted.

Activation and suppression of tyrosine hydroxylase activity (THA) appear to be a major regulator of catecholamine biosynthesis (Levitt et al. 1965). Chronic stimulation (24 hours) of the sympathetic nervous system increases catecholamine production with a parallel increase in THA (Kishner 1975). The metabolic intermediate dopa and the catecholamines, dopamine, norepinephrine, and epinephrine, all directly inhibit THA (DeQuattro et al. 1979; Nagatsu et al. 1964).

Other factors can also influence catecholamine production. Acute stimulation of the sympathetic nervous system increases catecholamine production. No change in THA levels has been noted. The mechanism of the sympathetic nervous system's influence remains obscure (Kishner 1975).

The adrenal cortex also appears to play a role in the regulation of THA activity. Hypophysectomy in rats decreased THA activity and administration of ACTH raised the levels of THA in those animals. The administration of glucocorticoids to the hypophysectomized rats failed to raise THA (Mueller *et al.* 1970). These experiments have led to speculation that either ACTH or another adrenal cortical product induced by ACTH might alter THA. Subsequent experiments revealed that one possible cortical product, cyclic AMP, increases THA (Gewirtz *et al.* 1971). The adrenal cortex also influences the production of catecholamines at a later step. This influence of glucocorticoids on PNMT has previously been described.

Catecholamine release

Norepinephrine and epinephrine are stored in separate vesicles in the chromaffin cells. The vesicles contain a high concentration of the catecholamines and adenosine triphosphate (ATP) as well as specific proteins (chromogranins) and the enzyme dopamine β-hydroxylase (DHB). Under the appropriate stimuli, the catecholamines and the other contents of the vesicles are released by exocytosis.

The preganglionic sympathetic nerve release of acetylcholine is a major stimulus for catecholamine release (Feldberg *et al.* 1934; Lee and Trendelenburg 1967; DelCastillo and Katz 1955; Douglas and Rubin 1961). This action is believed to involve the influx of calcium ions, which results in release of the contents of the chromaffin granules (Douglas and Rubin 1961; Schober *et al.* 1977).

Studies have revealed a variety of physiologic stimuli that activate the release of catecholamines by increasing sympathetic activity. Stress (emotional and physical), upright posture, cold, heat, asphyxia, hypotension, hypoglycemia, and sodium depletion have all been found to increase catecholamine release by activation of the sympathetic nervous system (Lewis 1975). Other substances have been shown to release catecholamines without intervention by the sympathetic nervous system. Acetylcholine, histamine, bradykinins, angiotensin II, angiotensin III, and related compounds directly stimulate the medullary cells to release catecholamines (Peach 1971; Douglas and Rubin 1961; Boadle-Biber *et al.* 1974). These substances do not appear to act on the same receptor. Their role in non-emergency states has yet to be established.

Catecholamine catabolism

The levels of circulating catecholamines depend on the secretion rate, the cellular uptake rate, and the rate of catabolism of norepinephrine and epinephrine.

Norepinephrine enters the circulation from two major sources. The principal source of norepinephrine is secretion by the postganglionic sympathetic axons. A lesser but still significant contributor is the adrenal medulla. In contrast, epinephrine originates almost exclusively from the medulla. Secretion rates of the catecholamines depend on the relative input of factors governing the activity of the sympathetic nervous system and the adrenal medulla. Both substances are rapidly removed from the circulation, with each having a plasma half-life under 20 seconds (Ferrerira and Vane 1967). The rapid half-life is a result of rapid uptake of the catecholamines by tissues, inactivation in the circulation, and inactivation by the liver.

Catecholamines are metabolized to inactive compounds by catechol-O-methyltransferase (COMT) and by monoamine oxidase (MAO) (Fig. 50.34). COMT aids in the replacement of the hydrogen in the 3 position of the phenol ring with a methyl group (Axelrod *et al.* 1958). MAO removes the amine group from the beta carbon. Either COMT or MAO can act initially on the catecholamine to begin the degradative process. The primary metabolite in the urine is vanillylmandelic acid (VMA) with

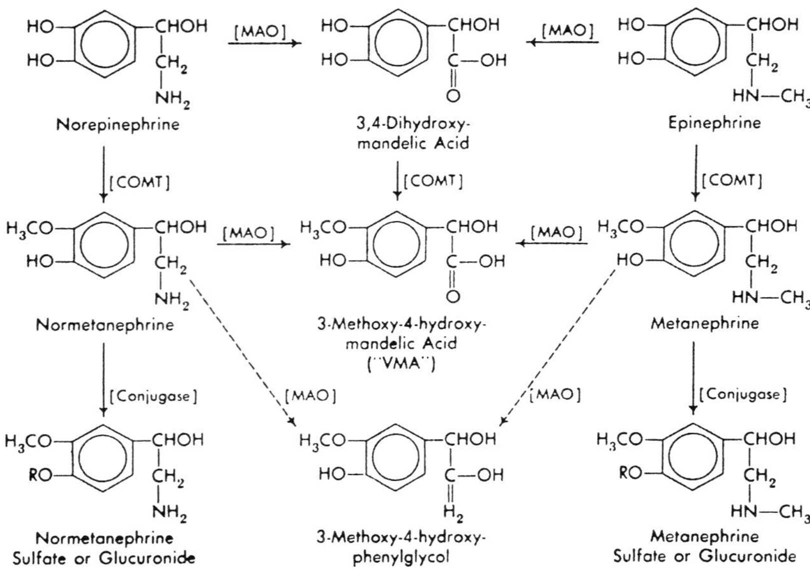

Fig. 50.34 Metabolic fate of the catecholamines. Enzymes are in brackets; COMT is catechol-O-methyltransferase, and MAO is monoamine oxidase. VMA is also known as vanillylmandelic acid. (Adapted from Goodman, A.G., Goodman, L.S., Gillman, A. (eds), 'The Pharmacologic Basis of Therapeutics,' 6th Ed, Macmillan, New York, p 77, 1980.)

metanephrine, normetanephrine, and their sulfates and glucuronide derivatives also contributing. COMT is widely distributed in mammalian tissues—blood vessels, intestine, kidney, liver, spleen, skin, skeletal muscle, adipose tissue, red blood cells, and the nervous system. COMT is largely confined to the cytoplasm of these cells. The fraction found in the liver is important in the catabolism of the catechols (Assicot and Bohuon 1966; Axelrod and Cohen 1971; Axelrod and Tomchick 1958; Bamshad *et al.* 1964; Traiger and Calvert 1969; Mayes 1980).

MAO is also found in many locations. Rich sources are present in the liver, nervous system, and salivary glands; lesser amounts in smooth muscle, cardiac muscle, and the gonads; and low concentrations in skeletal muscle, plasma, and red blood cells (Blaschko 1952; Collins and Sandler 1971; Robinson *et al.* 1968). The enzyme is found chiefly in the mitochondria of these cells.

The administration of the inhibitors of COMT, MAO, or both has little effect on the action of norepinephrine or epinephrine. Thus, COMT and MAO are not believed to play a major role in the rapid elimination of the catecholamines (Celander and Mellander 1955; Crout 1961; Corne and Graham 1957; Kamijo *et al.* 1955).

Investigators have found that the uptake of catecholamines by tissues is the major reason for the brief half-lives of epinephrine and norepinephrine. This process of uptake by the tissues has been divided into two categories. Uptake$_1$ refers to the ability of the postganglionic sympathetic neurons to remove catecholamines from the circulation. Uptake$_2$ is the term used to describe the phenomenon of nonneuronal tissue-accumulating catecholamines (Iverson 1975).

Studies on the removal of catecholamines from the circulation by uptake$_1$ have shown that norepinephrine avidly accumulates in neurons, is sequestered in storage vesicles and in the axons of these neurons, and is secreted from these storage vesicles when the sympathetic nervous system is activated (Iverson 1967; Iverson and Whitby 1963; Potter 1967; Mussachio *et al.* 1965). This process is believed to be accomplished by an active transport system in the membrane of the sympathetic axons. These neurons have a higher affinity for norepinephrine than for epinephrine (Iverson 1975).

Certain properties of uptake$_2$ have also been described. First, uptake$_2$ is characterized by greater affinity for epinephrine than for norepinephrine (Iverson 1967, 1975). Second, epinephrine and norepinephrine uptake by extraneuronal tissue can be inhibited by the catecholamine metabolites metanephrine and normetanephrine (Iverson 1975; Burgen and Iverson 1965). This suggests that, after accumulation of the catecholamines in extraneuronal tissue, norepinephrine and epinephrine undergo degradation.

Thus, the evidence suggests that catecholamines are rapidly removed from the circulation by tissue uptake. Norepinephrine is principally removed from the circulation by uptake$_1$ and becomes a part of the intraneuronal catecholamine stores. A lesser portion of norepinephrine is removed by uptake$_2$ and undergoes catabolism. Epinephrine is sequestered from the bloodstream by extraneuronal tissue and undergoes rapid degradation. A small amount of epinephrine accumulates in the nervous system. The catabolic metabolites of the catecholamines are eliminated in the urine.

Catecholamine function tests

Establishing accurate and reproducible laboratory tests for the measurement of catecholamines and their metabolites has been and continues to be a difficult process. The following is a summary of the methods that are available for assessing the concentration of catecholamines in plasma and urine.

Fluorometric assay (FA)

The FA is used to document free (unconjugated) norepinephrine, epinephrine, or dopamine levels in the urine or plasma (Nagatsu 1973). The method is based on the conversion of catecholamines to highly fluorescent substances. The process requires two major steps. The first is oxidation of the sample by potassium ferricyanide, iodine, or manganese dioxide. The product then undergoes molecular rearrangement with either trihydroindole or ethylenediamine to form the fluorescent compound. The concentration of the parent substance is calculated from the degree of fluorescence of the final product. By manipulating the pH of the oxidation reaction or by fractionation of the products, one can identify epinephrine, norepinephrine, and dopamine. Routinely, there is no hydrolysis step in the assay. Only free catecholamines are measured. If hydrolysis is a part of the assay, total (free and conjugated) catecholamines are defined.

Spectrophotometric assay

The spectrophotometric assay (SA) is used to measure the concentration of total metanephrines (metanephrine and normetanephrine) and vanillylmandelic acid in the urine (Nagatsu 1973). The process is established on the basis of the emission of ultraviolet (UV) light by the common end product, vanillin. The initial step in the assay is the separation of the metanephrines from VMA by the use of a cation exchange column. Once these two substances have been fractionated, they are oxidized by periodate to vanillin. The emission of UV light is measured by the spectrophotometer, and the level of the original substances is calculated. The vast majority of the metanephrines but not VMA are conjugated prior to excretion. A hydrolysis step in the assay liberates the metanephrines from sulfate and glucuronide. Thus, the SA measures all metanephrines and VMA in the urine.

Double isotope derivative technique

The double isotope derivative technique (DIT) is used for measuring low levels of epinephrine and norepinephrine (Nagatsu 1973). The process is based on the controlled enzymatic conversion of epinephrine and norepinephrine to radiolabeled products in the presence of ^{14}C-methyl group or ^{3}H-acetic anhydride. The products are separated by extraction procedures, and their concentrations measured. The appropriate end products reflect the initial level of epinephrine or norepinephrine. This assay is effective in measuring catecholamine level below the limit of the spectrophotometric and fluorometric assays.

Radioenzymatic method

The radioenzymatic method (REM) is the most widely used assay for assessing norepinephrine, epinephrine, and dopamine

(Sole and Hussain 1977; Vlachakis and Mendlowitz 1980). This test exposes the catecholamines to COMT. The parent substances are converted to their *O*-methylated ^{3}H derivatives: [^{3}H]normetanephrine, [^{3}H]metanephrine, and [^{3}H]methoxytyramine. These derivatives are purified by solvent extraction and isolated by one-dimensional silica gel thin-layer chromatography. The isolates are counted by liquid scintillation, thus giving an assessment of the parent catecholamine concentration.

Electron capture technique

The electron capture technique (ECT) is another method available to measure catecholamine levels (Riggin and Kissinger. 1977). This technique extracts the catecholamines on a cation exchange column and separates them by chromatography. Actual catecholamine levels are calculated by comparing the peaks of the specimen with samples of known catecholamine concentrations.

High-performance liquid chromatography (HPLC) (Hjemdahl 1984)

The development of sensitive detectors has allowed the use of HPLC for measurements of catecholamines in extracts of plasma, urine, and tissue samples. Separation of the catecholamines may be effected by reversed phase chromatography or cation-exchange chromatography and quantitation can be done by electrochemical detection (EC) or by fluorimetry coupled with postcolumn derivatization according to the trihydroxyindole (THI) method. EC has a somewhat lower sensitivity than the THI method for norepinephrine and epinephrine. The THI method is insensitive to dopamine.

Plasma norepinephrine

Plasma norepinephrine levels can vary dramatically over the course of the day (Levin *et al.* 1979). Upright posture (Cryer *et al.* 1974), exercise (Ziegler *et al.* 1976), and severe sodium depletion (Cryer 1976) can elevate plasma norepinephrine levels compared to supine baseline levels. As a result, it is important when measuring plasma norepinephrine to standardize as many of these factors as possible.

Baseline samples should be drawn at least 30 min after placement of a venous catheter with the patient supine and resting quietly during the interval. After the initial blood sample is obtained, the patient assumes the upright position, and samples are obtained at 2, 5, and 10 min. Table 50.14 documents normal levels in the laboratory using the double isotope derivative method. The clinician must be aware of normal values for the technique used by the specific laboratory. It should be noted that some authors have documented an increase in plasma norepinephrine with age (10 years to adulthood) in the supine position, in the upright position, and after exercise (Ziegler *et al.* 1976; Aedersen and Christensen 1975). Other authors have not found a rise in norepinephrine with advancing age (Cryer 1976).

Normal and adrenalectomized patients have the same rise in norepinephrine in response to change in posture (Cryer 1981). Thus, it is felt that the sympathetic nervous system is the major source of norepinephrine.

Baseline norepinephrine and the response to change in posture have been used as indices of sympathetic neuronal activity. Individuals with autonomic dysfunction have low baseline norepinephrine and poor responses to upright posture (Fig. 50.35). Impaired sympathetic neuronal function results from an abnormality in the reflex arc. The disease process could involve any or all of the components of the arc: the afferent nerves, the integrating centers of the central nervous system, or the efferent nerves. Some of the disease states that influence the arc are listed in Table 50.15.

High plasma catecholamine levels are found in sodium depletion (Cryer 1976) and pheochromocytoma (Louis *et al.* 1975) and in some patients with essential hypertension (Aedersen and Christensen 1975; Louis *et al.* 1975; De Quattro *et al.* 1976; Lake *et*

Table 50.14 Normal plasma norepinephrine and epinephrine concentrations

Reference	Sex	N	Position	NE (pg/ml)	E (pg/ml)
Engelman *et al.*	Both	22	Supine	200 ± 80[a] (100–370)	50 ± 30[a] (0–110)
	F	12	Supine	210 ± 90	40 ± 30
	M	10	Supine	200 ± 80	50 ± 40
Pederson and Christensen	Both	32	Supine	254 (80–750)	48 (0–190)
	F	6	Supine	238	58
	M	26	Supine	258	45
Cryer *et al.*	Both	50	Supine	234 ± 81[a] (102–406)	35 ± 18[a] (8–103)
	F	20	Supine	234 ± 82	32 ± 21
	M	30	Supine	234 ± 81	37 ± 16
	Both	35	Supine	226 ± 14[b]	32 ± 3[b]
			2 min standing	364 ± 24	43 ± 5
			5 min standing	513 ± 28	55 ± 6
			10 min standing	535 ± 35	57 ± 5

[a] Standing deviation.
[b] Standard error.
Adapted from Cryer P.E., *Diabetes* 25:1072,1976.

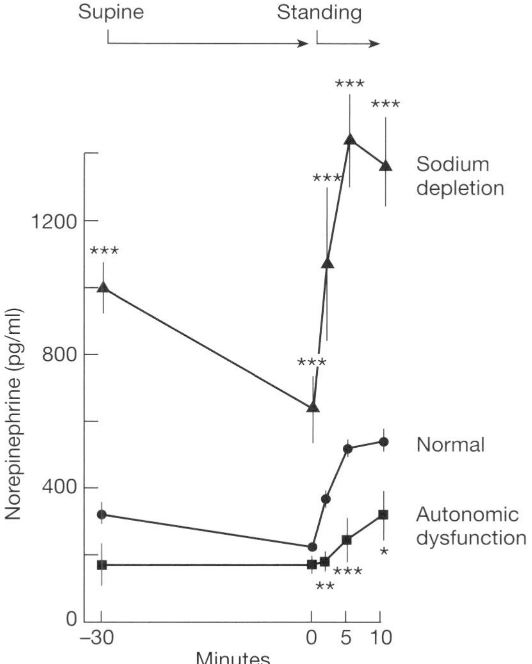

Fig. 50.35 Response of norepinephrine to postural change in normal individuals (n=35), sodium-depleted subjects (n=3), and patents with primary autonomic dysfunction (n=6). The asterisks denote p values (vs. normals) of .05*, .01**, and .001***. (Adapted from Cryer, P.E., Diabetes 25: 1075, 1976.)

Table 50.16 Plasma catecholamine responses to graded levels of exercise

Exercise level	Norepinephrine (ng/ml)	Epinephrine (ng/ml)
Rest	0.40 ± 0.06	0.07 ± 0.01
Mild	0.44 ± 0.09	0.07 ± 0.01
Moderate	1.30 ± 0.30	0.12 ± 0.02
Heavy	2.20 ± 0.39	0.42 ± 0.13

Means ± SE.
Taken from Galbo H. *et al. J Appl Physiol* **38**:72, 70–76, 1975.

that many factors other than neuronal release of norepinephrine can influence the plasma norepinephrine level.

Plasma epinephrine
Plasma epinephrine levels are also a function of posture, exercise, and sodium depletion (Cryer 1976) (Tables 50.14 and 50.16). Along with its role in blood pressure homeostasis, epinephrine acts as a counterregulatory hormone to maintain plasma glucose (Cryer 1981).

There are no standardized function tests involving plasma epinephrine, but measurement of plasma levels can be useful in some situations. Some patients with pheochromocytoma have elevated plasma epinephrine levels. Plasma levels will be decreased in some patients with autonomic dysfunction. The lack of rise of epinephrine with hyperglycemia documents adrenal medullary dysfunction (Cryer 1981).

Plasma free metanephrine
Plasma free metanephrines (metanephrine plus normetanephrine) can be measured using the HPLC method and their measurement may represent a more accurate and sensitive diagnostic test for pheochromocytoma compared with plasma and urinary catecholamines (Lenders *et al.* 1995; Eisenhofer *et al.* 2000; Raber *et al.* 2000). Plasma metanephrine concentrations are largely unsusceptible to external influences such as change of posture or the mechanical stress imposed by either endoscopic or open surgery (Raber *et al.* 2000). Their levels are also insensitive to short-term increase of plasma catecholamine levels (Eisenhofer *et al.* 1998).

Levels of urine catecholamines and their metabolites
Concentrations of epinephrine, norepinephrine, and their metabolites—normetanephrine, metanephrine, homovanillic acid, and vanillylmandelic acid—have been used effectively to

al. 1977). Authors have attempted to subdivide the patients with essential hypertension and elevated plasma norepinephrine by virtue of their renin values (De Quattro *et al.* 1976; Mitchell *et al.* 1977). No clear-cut subgroup has been universally accepted.

The plasma norepinephrine baseline value and response to change in posture have been presented as indices of the activity of the sympathetic nervous system. They are at best a crude measurement of such activity. Norepinephrine level is the function of exocytosis at the efferent sympathetic nerve terminal, exocytosis from the adrenal medulla, plasma inactivation, neuronal uptake, and excretion in the urine. Alterations in one or simultaneous changes in more than one of these areas will influence the numerical report of the laboratory. Even though we have used the norepinephrine level to assess sympathetic neural activity, the clinician must remember

Table 50.15 Disease states of the autonomic reflex arc

Central nervous system	*Spinal cord*	*Peripheral autonomic nerve*
Familial dysautonomia	Trauma	Diabetes mellitus
Encephalopathy	Cervical transection	Amyloidosis
Toxic	Tabes dorsalis	Prophyria
Nutritional	Pernicious anemia	Alchoholism
Cerebrovascular disease	Syringomyelia	
Neoplasms		
Trauma		
Infections		
Degenerative diseases of the white matter		

Adapted from Cryer P.E., Diseases of the adrenal medullac and sympathetic nervous system, in 'Endocrinology and Metabolism.' McGraw-Hill, New York, pp 535–6, 1981.

diagnose disorders involving the adrenal medulla and other tissues that develop from neural crest cells. The standard procedure is to collect a 24-hour urine or an accurately timed urine specimen. The sample is analyzed for the previously mentioned compounds and creatinine. A timed specimen is extrapolated to represent a 24-hour collection. The concentration of creatinine is analyzed to determine if the urine specimen approximates the collection time interval reported by the patient. The calculated catecholamine level and the level of catecholamine metabolites are compared with normal standards. Tables 50.17 and 50.18 represent the normal values for the parent compounds and their metabolic products. The values differ between laboratories and depend on the assay used. Please note that the values in Table 50.18 have been adjusted for creatinine excretion.

Currently the 24-hour urinary excretion rates of catecholamines and their metabolites are the tests of choice to screen for catecholamine-secreting tumors (Young 1997). Single-voided urine for metanephrine and normetanephrine assay has been reported to have high sensitivity and specificity in diagnosing pheochromocytoma (Ito *et al.* 1998).

Pediatric patients have a wide normal range for the excretion of these products. Such variability has been reduced by correcting the specimen per milligram creatinine (Gitlow *et al.* 1968). Other laboratories adjust the pediatric values by the child's weight (Hakulinen 1971). This maneuver also reduces the variability seen in the pediatric group (Table 50.19). Both methods have their proponents.

The presence of biogenic amines, vanilla, vanillin, and phenolic acids in the diet was previously thought to factitiously increase catecholamine degradation products in the urine. Studies in children and adults have documented that dietary restriction is not necessary (Weetman *et al.* 1976; Rayfield *et al.* 1977).

Table 50.19 Urinary catecholamines adjusted for weight

	Adult (μg)	Infant and child (μg/kg) range
Norepinephrine	<80	0.4–1.6
Epinephrine	<25	0.02–0.7
VMA	<8	83 ± 26
Normetanephrine	<450	4.9–20.8
Metanephrine	<300	3.1–15.6

Catecholamine values for 24-h urine collection.
Adapted from University of Virginia Catecholamine Laboratory, February 1982.

Studies of urine excretion in pheochromocytoma revealed elevated urinary catecholamines, total metanephrines, and VMA. Cases have been reported in which VMA and total metanephrines have not been elevated (Voochess 1966). Neuroblastoma patients excrete increased amounts of homovanillic acid (HVA) and VMA. Urine catecholamine levels are not always elevated (Jaffee 1976).

Patients with familial dysautonomia excrete decreased amounts of VMA and increased amounts of HVA (Smith *et al.* 1963). Patients with phenylketonuria characteristically have low levels of urinary catecholamines and their metabolites (Hung *et al.* 1978).

Factitious alterations in the catecholamine profile
Stress and exercise are the most common physiologic factors that raise plasma and urinary catecholamine levels. Diagnostic evaluation should attempt to minimize if not eliminate these factors.

Urine and plasma catecholamine profiles can also be influenced by many drugs. Catecholamines or drugs that increase

Table 50.17 Normal range for urinary catecholamines and metabolites by age (μg/24 h)

Age (years)	Norepinephrine	Epinephrine	Dopamine	VMA
0–1	5–16	0.6–5	17–99	169–1,350
1–5	8–31	0.8–9	48–217	465–2,200
6–15	19–71	1–11	79–365	1,050–3,740
>15	34–87	3–13	179–377	2.050–4,250

Adapted from Hung W., 'Pediatric Endocrinology,' Medical Examination Publishing, p. 226, 1978.

Table 50.18 Normal values for VMA, HVA, and metanephrine-normetanephrine by age (μg/mg Creatinine)

No. of subjects	Age (years)	VMA Mean	VMA SD	VMA Range	HVA Mean	HVA SD	HVA Range	M–N Mean	M–N SD	M–N Range
43	0–1	6.9	3.2	1.4–15.0	12.9	9.6	1.2–35.0	1.6	1.3	0.0–4.6
15	1–2	4.6	2.2	1.3– 8.0	12.6	6.3	4.0–23.0	1.7	1.1	0.3–5.4
21	2–5	3.9	1.7	1.5– 7.5	7.6	3.6	0.5–13.5	1.3	0.7	0.4–2.9
23	5–10	3.3	1.4	0.5– 6.0	4.7	2.7	0.5– 9.0	1.1	0.8	0.4–2.7
24	10–15	1.9	0.8	0.3– 3.3	2.5	2.4	0.3–12.0	0.6	0.5	0.0–1.9
14	15–18	1.3	0.6	0.1– 2.8	1.0	0.7	0.5– 2.0	0.3	0.2	0.0–0.7

Adapted from Gitlow S.E. *et al. J Lab Clin Med* 72:614,1968.

catecholamines taken while testing is being done will increase the measured products. Amphetamines, methylxanthines, ephedrine, α-adrenergic blocking agents, and vasodilating agents are the common offenders. Another common offender is α-methyldopa. During catabolism, α-methyldopa is converted to α-methylnorepinephrine and α-methylnormetanephrine. The alpha group on the alpha carbon prevents monoamine oxidase from converting α-methylnormetanephrine to VMA. The alphamethyl compounds are measured by the fluorimetric assay but not by the spectrophotometric assay. Thus, a fluorimetric profile would reveal elevations in 'dopamine' and 'norepinephrine', whereas spectrophotometric analysis would show no elevation of catecholamines or degradation products.

Drugs can be measured directly by the laboratory method used, thus producing factitiously elevated levels. Some drugs measured in the fluorimetric assay are tetracycline, erythromycin, quinidine, quinine, chloral hydrate, bromosulfophthalein, phenolsulfophthalein, nicotinic acid, riboflavin, mandelamine, methenamine, bretylium, and methocarbomal. Nalidixic acid falsely elevates the spectrophotometric assay for VMA, because this compound is extracted from the urine with VMA. P-aminosalicylic acid, bromosulfophthalein, and phenolsulfophthalein also artificially increase VMA.

Hypertensive drugs that suppress sympathetic function decrease urine and plasma catecholamines—for example, clonidine. MAO inhibitors prevent the formation of VMA, falsely lowering VMA. Clofibrate and mandelamine can also artificially lower VMA.

It is evident that a drug history is vital to the selection and interpretation of catecholamine assays.

Glucagon stimulation test (Lawrence 1967; Bravo 1991; Grossman et al. 1991)

Test. A constant infusion of 10 per cent glucose at 2 ml/min is administered throughout the test. Twenty minutes after the initiation of the infusion, baseline blood pressure is measured four times at 5-min intervals. The patient is then given 1 ml of normal saline by IV push. Blood pressure is recorded every 15 s for 5 min. If the blood pressure remains stable, the patient is given a 0.5 mg glucagon IV push. Blood pressure measurement continues every 15 s. If there is no response within 5 min, an additional dose of 1.0 mg glucagon is given. Plasma catecholamines are measured at baseline and 2 min after the infusion.

Normal response. Patients with pheochromocytoma will have rapid, dramatic increase in blood pressure within 2–5 min after glucagon administration and either a threefold increase in plasma catecholamine concentrations or an absolute value above 2000 pg/ml.

It is important to note that both false-positive and false-negative data can be generated from the glucagon test. Thus a positive test is suggestive but not diagnostic of a pheochromocytoma. Patients can be pretreated with an α-blocker (prazosin or phenoxybenzamine) or a calcium channel blocker (nifedipine) if the clinician is very concerned about the acute hypertensive response. If the hypertensive response is excessive or prolonged, phentolamine (5.0 mg) should be readily available to alleviate such a response.

Phentolamine test (Spergel et al. 1970; De Quattro and Campese 1979)

Test. A constant infusion of 10 per cent glucose at a rate of 2 ml/min is administered into an antecubital vein throughout the test. A scalp vein is inserted distal to the site of the glucose infusion, and subsequent samples are drawn from this cannula. Twenty minutes after the start of the glucose infusion, four samples are collected at 5 min intervals for plasma glucose. At the end of the control period, 1 ml normal saline is rapidly injected intravenously. Blood pressure measurement and blood samples are obtained at 30s intervals for 3 min. Test doses of 0.5 and 1.0 mg phentolamine are given. If there is no hypotensive response, 5.0 mg of phentolamine is administered. Blood pressure measurements and blood samples are obtained as described previously. If there is a pressure response, it is monitored closely until it returns to baseline.

Normal response. Patients with a pheochromocytoma will have a decrease in blood pressure of at least 35–50/35 mm Hg (systolic/diastolic) and a decrease in blood glucose of at least 50 mg/dl.

As a result of simultaneous measurement of blood pressure and plasma glucose, changes after phentolamine have been employed to eliminate false-positive tests. Phentolamine offsets the α-adrenergic suppression of insulin release by high circulating catecholamine levels. Thus, blood sugar falls in patients with excess circulating catecholamines. The glucose response to phentolamine helps the clinician differentiate the true decrease in pressure seen in catechol excess from the false-positive response.

False-positive changes in blood pressure can occur in many settings. Simultaneous administration of barbiturates, an elevated blood urea nitrogen (BUN), and antiadrenergic drugs taken within 2 weeks of the test can result in a decrease in blood pressure to phentolamine. Some individuals may have a decline in pressure to phentolamine for no apparent reason.

Clonidine suppression test (Bravo 1991; Bravo et al. 1981; Grossman et al. 1991; Lenz et al. 1998)

Test. The subject is fasted for 10 hours overnight and remains supine throughout the study period. An IV catheter is placed in the forearm vein and kept patent with a 0.9 per cent NaCl solution containing 2 units of heparin/ml. After 30 min of rest in the supine position, a blood sample is obtained for plasma norepinephrine. The patient receives oral clonidine (300 μg as the hydrochloride) with 250 ml of water. A blood sample is obtained 180 min after the administration of clonidine for measurement of plasma norepinephrine.

Normal response. Patients without a pheochromocytoma have a decrease in their plasma norepinephrine level to the normal range or below. Subjects with documented pheochromocytoma do not have suppression of their plasma norepinephrine to the normal range.

The clonidine should be given at least 12 hours after antihypertensive medications have been discontinued except for α-adrenergic blockers, which do not interfere with the test. This test has been shown in a small number of adults to be an effective test for identifying individuals with a pheochromocytoma. Clonidine acts by inhibition of centrally mediated adrenergic systems. Such inhibition decreases the release of norepinephrine from sympathetic nerve terminals, resulting in a decrease of circulating norepinephrine. An autonomously functioning pheochromocytoma does not respond to a centrally acting drug. Thus, plasma norepinephrine levels do not fall to the normal range. Although the initial report appears impressive, the efficacy of this test in a large number of patients with pheochromocytoma and in the pediatric population must be established.

References

Abraham, G. (1974). Ovarian and adrenal contribution to peripheral androgens during the menstrual cycle. *J. Clin. Endocrinol. Metab.* **39**, 340–6.

Aedersen, E.B. and Christensen, N.J. (1975). Catecholamines in plasma and urine in patients with essential hypertension determined by double isotope derivative method. *Acta Med. Scand.* **198**, 373–7.

Ajagannadha, R.J., Long, J.A., and Ramachandran, J. (1978). Effects of antiserum to adrenocorticotropin on adrenal growth and function. *Endocrinology* **102**, 371–8.

al-Saadi, N., Diederich, S., and Oelkers, W. (1998). A very high dose dexamethasone suppression test for differential diagnosis of Cushing's syndrome. *Clin. Endocrinol.* **48**, 45–51.

Ambrosi, B., Barbetta, L., Re, T., Passini, E., and Faglia, G. (1998). The one microgram adrenocorticotropin test in the assessment of hypothalamic–pituitary–adrenal function. *Eur. J. Endocrinol.* **139**, 575–9.

Aquilera, G. and Catt, K.J. (1980). Loci of action of regulators of aldosterone biosynthesis in isolated glomerulosa cells. *Endocrinology* **104**, 1046–52.

Armbuster, H., Vetter, W., Uhlschmid, G., Zaruba, K., Beckerhoff, B., Nussberger, J., Vetter, H., and Siegenthaler, W. (1974). Circadian rhythm of plasma renin activity and plasma, aldosterone in normal man and in renal allograft recipients. *Proc. Eur. Dialysis Transplant. Assoc.* **11**, 268–76.

Armbuster, H., Vetter, W., Beckeroff, R., Nussberger, J., Vetter, H., and Siegenthaler, W. (1975). Diurnal variations of plasma aldosterone in supine man: relationship to plasma renin activity and plasma cortisol. *Acta Endocrinol.* **80**, 95–103.

Aron, D.C., Tyrrell, J.B., Fitzgerald, P.A., Findling, J.W., and Forsham, P.H. (1981). Cushing's syndrome: problems in diagnosis. *Medicine* **60**, 25–33.

Artal, R. (1980). Fetal adrenal medulla. *Clin. Obstet. Gynecol.* **23**, 825–7.

Assicot, M. and Bohuon, C. (1966). Catechol-O-methyltransferase activity in skeletal muscle. *Nature* **212**, 861–2.

Avgerinos, P., Yanovski, J., Oldfield, E., Nieman, L., and Cutler, G.J. (1994). The metyrapone and dexamethasone suppression tests for the differential diagnosis of the adrenocorticotropin-dependent Cushing's syndrome: a comparison. *Ann. Intern. Med.* **121**, 318–27.

Avgerinos, P., Nieman, L., Oldfield, E., and Cutler, G.J. (1996). A comparison of the overnight and the standard metyrapone test for the differential diagnosis of adrenocorticotrophin-dependent Cushing's syndrome. *Clin. Endocrinol.* **45**, 483–91.

Axelrod, J. (1962). Purification and properties of phenylethanolamine-N-methyl transferase. *J. Biol. Chem.* **237**, 1657–60.

Axelrod, J. and Cohen, C.K. (1971). Methyltransferase enzymes in the red blood cells. *J. Pharmacol. Exp. Ther.* **176**, 650–4.

Axelrod, J. and Tomchick, R. (1958). Enzymatic O-methylation of epinephrine and other catechols. *J. Biol. Chem.* **233**, 710–15.

Axelrod, J., Senoh, S., and Witkop, B. (1958). O-methylation of catecholamines in-vivo. *J. Biol. Chem.* **233**, 697–701.

Azziz, R., Dewailly, D., and Owerbach, D. (1994). Clinical review 56: nonclassic adrenal hyperplasia: current concepts. *J. Clin. Endocrinol. Metab.* **78**, 810–15.

Bacon, G.E., Larson, R.M., Spencer, M.L., and Kelch, R.P. (1975). Intravenous metopyrone testing. *Am. J. Dis. Child.* **129**, 1042–4.

Ballard, P.L., Carter, J.P., Graham, B.S., and Baxter, J.D. (1975). A radioreceptor assay for evaluation of the plasma glucocorticoid activity of natural and synthetic steroids in man. *J. Clin. Endocrinol. Metab.* **41**, 290–304.

Bamshad, J., Lerner, A.P., and McGuire, J.S. (1964). Catechol-O-methyltransverase in skin. *J. Invest. Dermatol.* **43**, 111–13.

Barrou, Z., Guiban, D., Maroufi, A., Fournier, C., Dugue, M., Luton, J., and Thomopoulos, P. (1996). Overnight dexamethasone suppression test: comparison of plasma and salivary cortisol measurement for the screening of Cushing's syndrome. *Eur. J. Endocrinol.* **134**, 93–6.

Baumann, K. and Muller, J. (1972). Effect of potassium intake on the final step of aldosterone biosynthesis in the rat. I. 18-Hydroxylation and 18-hydroxydehydrogenation. *Acta Endocrinol.* **69**, 701–17.

Baxter, J.D. and Tyrrell, J.B. (1981). The adrenal cortex. In *Endocrinology and metabolism* (ed. P. Felig), pp. 385–510. McGraw-Hill, New York.

Berenson, G.S., Voors, A.W., Dablers, E.R., Webber, L.S., and Shuler, S.E. (1979). Creatinine clearance, electrolytes and plasma renin activity related to blood pressure of white and black children—the Bogalusa Heart Study. *J. Lab. Clin. Med.* **93**, 535–48.

Besser, G.M. and Edwards, C.R.W. (1972). Cushing's syndrome. *Clin. Endocrinol. Metab.* **1**, 451–90.

Biglieri, E.G., Slaton, P.E., Kronfield, S.J., and Schambelan, M. (1967). Diagnosis of an aldosterone-producing adenoma in primary aldosterone. *J. Am. Med. Assoc.* **201**, 510–18.

Biglieri, E.G., Shambelan, M., and Slaton, P.E. (1969). Effect of adrenocorticotropin on desoxycorticosterone, corticosterone and aldosterone excretion. *J. Clin. Endocrinol. Metab.* **29**, 1090–101.

Biglieri, E.G., Stockigt, J.M., and Schambelan, M. (1970). A preliminary evaluation for primary aldosterone. *Arch. Intern. Med.* **126**, 1004–7.

Biglieri, E.G., Stockigt, J.R., and Schambelan, M. (1972). Adrenal mineralocorticoids causing hypertension. *Am. J. Med.* **52**, 623–32.

Biglieri, E.G., Schambelam, M., Brust, N., Chang, B., and Hogan, M. (1974). Plasma aldosterone concentration. *Circ. Res.* (suppl.) **34/35**, I183–I189.

Blackman, S.S. (1946). Concerning the function and origin of the reticular zone of the adrenal cortex. *Bull. Johns Hopkins Hosp.* **78**, 180–208.

Blair-West, J.R., Coghlan, J.P., Denton, D.A., Scoggins, B.A., Wintour, E.M., and Wright, R.D. (1970). The onset of ACTH, angiotensin II and raised plasma potassium concentration on the adrenal cortex. *Steroids* **15**, 433–48.

Blaschko, H. (1952). Amine oxidase and amine metabolism. *Pharmacol. Rev.* **4**, 415–58.

Blumenfeld, J.D. and Vaughan, E.D. Jr (1999). Diagnosis and treatment of primary aldosteronism. *World J. Urol.* **17**, 15–21.

Blumenfeld, J., Sealey, J., Schlussel, Y., Vaughan, E.J., Sos, T., Atlas, S., Muller, F., Acevedo, R., Ulick, S., and Laragh, J. (1994). Diagnosis and treatment of primary hyperaldosteronism. *Ann. Intern. Med.* **121**, 877–85.

Boadle-Biber, M.C., Morgenroth, V.H., and Roth, R.H. (1974). Activation of tyrosine hydroxylase by angiotensin II and des (asp[1])-angiotensin II heptapeptide [abstract]. *Pharmacologist* **16**, 213.

Bongiovanni, A.M., Eberlein, W.R., Westphal, M., and Boggs, T. (1958). Prolonged turnover rate of hydrocortisone in the newborn infant. *J. Clin. Endocrinol. Metab.* **18**, 1127–30.

Bourgoignie, J., Kurz, S., Catanzaro, F.J., Serirat, P., and Perry, H.M. (1970). Renal venous renin in hypertension. *Am. J. Med.* **48**, 332–42.

Bravo, E. (1991). Pheochromocytoma: new concepts and future trends. *Kidney Int.* **40**, 544–56.

Bravo, E.L., Tarazi, R.C., Fouad, F.M., Vidt, D.G., and Gifford, R.W. (1981). Clonidine-suppression test. *New Engl. J. Med.* **305**, 623–6.

Brooks, S.M., Werk, E.E., Ackerman, S.T., Sullivan, I., and Thrasher, K. (1972). Adverse effects of phenobarbital on corticosteroid metabolism in patients with bronchial asthma. *New Engl. J. Med.* **286**, 1125–8.

Brown, H., Englert, E., Wallach, S., and Simons, E.L. (1957). Metabolism of free and conjugated 17-OHCSs in normal subjects. *J. Clin. Endocrinol. Metab.* **17**, 1191–201.

Brown, M.S., Kovanen, P.T., and Goldstein, J.L. (1979). Receptor-mediated uptake of lipoprotein-cholesterol and its utilization for steroid synthesis in the adrenal cortex. *Recent Prog. Horm. Res.* **35**, 215–57.

Brown, R.D., Strott, C.A., and Liddle, G.W. (1972). Site of stimulation of aldosterone biosynthesis by angiotensin and potassium. *J. Clin. Invest.* **51**, 1413–18.

Burgen, A.S. and Iverson, L.L. (1965). The inhibition of noradrenaline uptake by sympathomimetic amines in the isolated rat heart. *Br. J. Pharmacol. Chemother.* **25**, 34–49.

Burwell, L.R., Davis, W.W., and Bartter, F.C. (1969). Studies on the loci of action of stimuli to the biogenesis of aldosterone. *Proc. R. Soc. Med.* **62**, 1254–7.

Buster, J.E. (1980). Fetal adrenal cortex. *Clin. Obstet. Gynecol.* **23**, 803–6.

Cain, J.P., Tuck, M.L., Williams, G.H., Dluhy, R.G., and Rosenoff, S.H. (1972). The regulation of aldosterone secretion in primary aldosteronism. *Am. J. Med.* **53**, 627–37.

Carey, R.M., Douglas, J.G., Schweikert, J.R., and Liddle, G.W. (1972). The syndrome of essential hypertension and suppressed plasma renin activity. *Arch. Intern. Med.* **130**, 849–54.

Carey, R.M., Vaughan, E.D., Peach, M.J., and Ayers, C.R. (1978). Activity of [des-asparty1[1]] II and angiotensin II in man. *J. Clin. Invest.* **61**, 20–31.

Cavollo, A., Corn, C., Bryan, G.T., and Myer, W.J. (1979). The use of plasma androstenedione in monitoring therapy of patients with congenital adrenal hyperplasia. *J. Pediatr.* **95**, 33–7.

Celander, O. and Mellander, S. (1955). Elimination of adrenaline and noradrenaline from the circulating blood. *Nature* **176**, 973–4.

Chen, Y., Cintron, N., and Whitson, P. (1992). Long-term storage of salivary cortisol samples at room temperature. *Clin. Chem.* **38**, 304–5.

Chrousos, G., Schulte, H., Oldfield, E., Gold, P., Cutler, G.J., and Loriaux, D. (1984). The corticotropin-releasing factor stimulation test. An aid in the evaluation of patients with Cushing's syndrome. *New Engl. J. Med.* **310**, 622–6.

Collins, G.G. and Sandler, M. (1971). Human blood platelet monamine oxidase. *Biochem. Pharmacol.* **20**, 289–96.

Cope, C.L. (1972). *Adrenal steroids and disease.* J.B. Lippincott, Philadelphia.

Corne, S.J. and Graham, J.D. (1957). The effect of inhibition of amine oxidase *in vivo* on administered adrenaline, noradrenaline, tyramine and serotonin. *J. Physiol.* **135**, 339–49.

Crapo, L. (1979). Cushing's syndrome. A review of diagnostic tests. *Metabolism* **28**, 955–77.

Cronin, C., Igoe, D., Duffy, M., Cunningham, S., and McKenna, T. (1990). The overnight dexamethasone test is a worthwhile screening procedure. *Clin. Endocrinol.* **33**, 27–33.

Crout, J.R. (1961). Effect of inhibiting both catechol-O-methyl transferase and monamine oxidase on cardiovascular responses to norepinephrine. *Proc. Soc. Exp. Biol. Med.* **108**, 482–4.

Crowder, R.E. (1957). The development of the adrenal gland in man, with special reference to origin and ultimate location of cell types and evidence in favor of the "cell migration" theory. In *Contributions to embryology*, Vol XXXVI, No. 251, pp. 195–210. Carnegie Institute, Washington, DC.

Cryer, P.E. (1976). Isotope derivative measurements of plasma norepinephrine and epinephrine in man. *Diabetes* **25**, 1071–82.

Cryer, P. (1981). Diseases of the adrenal medulla and sympathetic nervous system. In *Endocrinology and metabolism* (ed. P. Felig), pp. 511–50. McGraw-Hill, New York.

Cryer, P.E., Santiago, J.V., and Shak, S.D. (1974). Measurement of norepinephrine and epinephrine in small volumes of human plasma by single isotope derivative method: response to upright posture. *J. Clin. Endocrinol. Metab.* **39**, 1025–9.

Darmon, P., Dadoun, F., Frachebois, C., Velut, J.-G., Boullu, S., Dutour, A., Oliver, C., and Grino, M. (1999). On the meaning of low-dose ACTH (1–24) tests to assess functionality of the hypothalamic–pituitary–adrenal axis. *Eur. J. Endocrinol.* **140**, 51–5.

Davis, J.O., Urquhart, J., and Higgins, J.T. (1963). The effects of alterations of plasma sodium and potassium concentration on aldosterone secretion. *J. Clin. Invest.* **42**, 597–609.

DeCherney, G., DeBold, C., Jackson, R., Sheldon, W.J., Island, D., and Orth, D. (1985). Diurnal variation in the response of plasma adrenocorticotropin and cortisol to intravenous ovine corticotropin-releasing hormone. *J. Clin. Endocrinol. Metab.* **61**, 273–9.

DelCastillo, J. and Katz, B. (1955). On the localization of acetylcholine receptors. *J. Physiol.* **128**, 157–81.

DeQuattro, V. and Campese, V.M. (1979) Pheochromocytoma: diagnosis and therapy. In *Endocrinology* (ed. L. DeGroot), Vol 2, pp. 1281–3. Grune and Stratton, New York.

De Quattro, V., Campese, V., Miura, Y., and Meijer, D. (1976). Increased plasma catecholamines in high renin hypertension. *Am. J. Cardiol.* **38**, 801–4.

DeQuattro, V., Meyers, M.R., and Campese, V.M. (1979). Anatomy and biochemistry of the sympathetic nervous system. In *Endocrinology* (ed. L. DeGroot), Vol. 2, p. 1249. Grune and Stratton, New York.

Dichek, H., Nieman, L., Oldfield, E., Pass, H., Malley, J., and Cutler, G.J. (1994). A comparison of the standard high dose dexamethasone suppression test and the overnight 8-mg dexamethasone suppression test for the differential diagnosis of adrenocorticotropin-dependent Cushing's syndrome. *J. Clin. Endocrinol. Metab.* **78**, 418–22.

Dickstein, G., Shechner, C., Nicholson, W., Rosner, I., Shen-Orr, Z., Adawi, F., and Lahav, M. (1991). Adrenocorticotropin stimulation test: effects of basal cortisol level, time to day, and suggested new sensitive low dose test. *J. Clin. Endocrinol. Metab.* **72**, 773–8.

Dickstein, G., DeBold, C., Gaitan, D., DeCherney, G., Jackson, R., Sheldon, W.J., Nicholson, W., and Orth, D. (1996). Plasma corticotropin and cortisol responses to ovine corticotropin-releasing hormone (CRH), arginine vasopressin (AVP), CRH plus AVP, and CRH plus metyrapone in patients with Cushing's disease. *J. Clin. Endocrinol. Metab.* **81**, 2934–41.

Dickstein, G., Spigel, D., Arad, E., and Shechner, C. (1997). One microgram is the lowest ACTH dose to cause a maximal cortisol response. There is no diurnal variation of cortisol response to submaximal ACTH stimulation. *Eur. J. Endocrinol.* **137**, 172–5.

Dillion, M.J. and Ryness, J.M. (1975). Plasma renin activity and aldosterone concentration in children. *Br. Med. J.* **4**, 316–19.

Dluhy, R. and Lifton, R. (1995). Glucocorticoid-remediable aldosteronism (GRA): diagnosis, variability of phenotype and regulation of potassium homeostasis. *Steroids* **60**, 48–51.

Dluhy, R. and Lifton, R. (1999). Glucocorticoid-remediable aldosteronism. *J. Clin. Endocrinol. Metab.* **84**, 4341–4.

Dluhy, R.G., Himathongkam, T., and Greenfield, M. (1974). Rapid ACTH test with plasma aldosterone levels. *Ann. Intern. Med.* **80**, 693–6.

Dobbie, J.W. and Symington, T. (1966). The human adrenal gland with special reference to the vasculature. *J. Endocrinol.* **34**, 479–90.

Doppman, J. and Gill, J.J. (1996). Hyperaldosteronism: sampling the adrenal veins. *Radiology* **198**, 309–12.

Douglas, W.W. and Rubin, R.P. (1961). The mode of action of acetylcholine on the adrenal medulla [abstract]. *Biochem. Pharmacol.* **8**, 20.

Drekter, I.J., Heisler, A., Scism, G.R., Stern, S., Pearson, S., and McGavack, T.H. (1952). The determination of urinary steroids. I. The preparation of pigment-free extracts and a simplified procedure for the estimation of total 17-ketosteroids. *J. Clin. Endocrinol. Metab.* **12**, 55–65.

Eddy, R.L., Jones, A.L., Gilliland, P.F., Ibarra, J.D., Thompson, J.Q., and McMurray, J.F. (1973). Cushing's syndrome, a prospective study of diagnostic methods. *Am. J. Med.* **55**, 621–30.

Eisenhofer, G., Keiser, H., Friberg, P., Mezey, E., Huynh, T., Hiremagalur, B., Ellingson, T., Duddempudi, S., Eijsbouts, A., and Lenders, J. (1998). Plasma metanephrines are markers of pheochromocytoma produced by catechol-O-methyltransferase within tumors. *J. Clin. Endocrinol. Metab.* **83**, 2175–85.

Eisenhofer, G., Walther, M., Keiser, H., Lenders, J., Friberg, P., and Pacak, K. (2000). Plasma metanephrines: a novel and cost-effective test for pheochromocytoma. *Braz. J. Med. Biol. Res.* **33**, 1157–69.

Emery, F.E. and Atwell, W.J. (1933). Hypertrophy of adrenal glands following administration of pituitary extracts. *Anat. Rec.* **58**, 17–24.

Ernest, I. (1966). Steroid excretion and plasma cortisol in 41 cases of Cushing's syndrome. *Acta Endocrinol.* **51**, 511–25.

Erturk, E., Jaffe, C., and Barkan, A. (1998). Evaluation of the integrity of the hypothalamic–pituitary–adrenal axis by insulin hypoglycemia test. *J. Clin. Endocrinol. Metab.* **83**, 2350–4.

Espiner, E.A., Jensen, C.A., and Hart, D.S. (1972). Dynamics of adrenal response to sustained local ACTH infusions in conscious sheep. *Am. J. Physiol.* **222**, 570–7.

Espiner, E.A., Lun, S., and Hart, D.S. (1978). The role of ACTH, angiotensin and potassium in stress-induced aldosterone secretion. *J. Steroid Biochem.* **9**, 109–13.

Feldberg, W., Minz, B., and Tsudzimura, H. (1934). The mechanism of nervous discharge of adrenaline. *J. Physiol.* **81**, 286–304.

Ferreira, S.H. and Vane, J.R. (1967). Half-lives of peptides and amines in the circulation. *Nature* **215**, 1237–40.

Ferris, J.B., Beevers, D.G., Brown, J.J., Fraser, R., Lever, A.F., Padfield, P.L., and Robertson, J.I.S. (1978). Low renin (primary) hyperaldosteronism. *Am. Heart J.* **95**, 641–58.

Fiad, T., Kirby, J., Cunningham, S., and McKenna, T. (1994). The overnight single-dose metyrapone test is a simple and reliable index of the hypothalamic–pituitary–adrenal axis. *Clin. Endocrinol.* **40**, 603–9.

Findling, J. and Raff, H. (1999). Newer diagnostic techniques and problems in Cushing's disease. *Endocrinol. Metab. Clin. N. Am.* **28**, 191–210.

Finkelstein, M. and Shaefer, J.M. (1979). Inborn errors of steroid biosynthesis. *Physiol. Rev.* **59**, 353–406.

Fitzsimmons, J.T. (1971). The effect on drinking of peptide processors and of shorter chain peptide fragments of angiotensin II injected into the rat's diencephalon. *J. Physiol.* **214**, 295–303.

Flack, M., Oldfield, E., Cutler, G.J., Zweig, M., Malley, J., Chrousos, G., Loriaux, D., and Nieman, L. (1992). Urine free cortisol in the high-dose dexamethasone suppression test for the differential diagnosis of the Cushing syndrome. *Ann. Intern. Med.* **116**, 211–17.

Forest, M.G., Rivarola, M.A., and Migeon, C.J. (1968). Percentage of binding of testosterone, androstenedione and dehydroisoandrosterone in human plasma. *Steroids* **12**, 323–43.

Franks, R.C. (1967). Diurnal variation of plasma 17-OHCSs in children. *J. Clin. Endocrinol. Metab.* **27**, 75–8.

Franks, R.C. (1973). Urinary 17-OHCS and cortisol excretion in childhood. *J. Clin. Endocrinol. Metab.* **36**, 702–5.

Freeman, R.H. and Davis, J.O. (1978). The control of renin secretion and metabolism. In *Hypertension* (ed. J. Genest, E. Koiw, and O., Kuchel), pp. 210–40. McGraw-Hill, New York.

Frohman, L.A. (1981). Diseases of the anterior pituitary. In *Endocrinology* and *metabolism* (ed. P. Felig), pp. 157–9. McGraw-Hill, New York.

Fuller, R.W. and Hunt, J.M. (1967). Activity of phenolethanolamine-N-methyl transferase in the adrenal glands of fetal and neonatal rats. *Nature* **214**, 190.

Gallagher, T.F., Yoshido, K., Reffworg, H.D., Fukushima, D.K., Weitzman, E.D., and Hellman, L. (1973). ACTH and cortisol secretory patterns in man. *J. Clin. Endocrinol. Metab.* **36**, 1058–68.

Ganguly, A. (1998). Primary aldosteronism. *New Engl. J. Med.* **339**, 1828–34.

Ganguly, A., Melada, G.A., Leutscher, J.A., and Dowdy, A.J. (1973). Control of plasma aldosterone in primary aldosteronism: distinction between adenoma and hyperplasia. *J. Clin. Endocrinol. Metab.* **37**, 765–75.

Ganong, W.F., Lieberman, A.H., Daily, W.J., Yuen, V.S., Mulrow, P.J., Leutscher, J.A., and Bailey, R.E. (1965). Aldosterone secretion in dogs with hypothalamic lesions. *Endocrinology* **65**, 18–28.

Genest, J. (1977). Renovascular hypertension. In *Hypertension* (ed. J. Genest), p. 828. McGraw Hill, New York.

Gewirtz, G. and Yallow, R.S. (1974). Ectopic ACTH production in carcinoma of the lung. *J. Clin. Invest.* **53**, 1022–32.

Gewirtz, G.P., Kvetnansky, R., Weise, V.K., and Kopin, I.J. (1971). Effect of ACTH and dibutyryl cyclic AMP on catecholamine synthesizing enzymes in the adrenals of hypophysectomized rats. *Nature* **230**, 462–4.

Gill, G.N. (1979). ACTH regulation of the adrenal cortex. In *Pharmacology of adrenal cortical hormones*, (Gill, G. N. eds) pp. 35–66. Pergamon, Oxford.

Gill, G.N., Hornsby, P.J., and Simonian, M.H. (1979). Regulation of growth and differentiated function of cultured bovine adrenocortical cells. In *Hormones and cell culture* (ed. G.H. Sato and R. Ross), pp. 701–15. Cold Spring Harbor Laboratory, Cold Spring Harbor, New York.

Giovannelli, G., Ammenti, A., Virdis, R., Bernasconi, S., Nori, G., and Rocca, M. (1981). Plasma renin activity in the pediatric age. In *Hypertension in children and adolescents* (ed. G. Giovannelli), pp. 129–46. Raven Press, New York.

Gitlow, S.E., Mendlowitz, M., Wilk, E.K., Wilk, S., Wolf, R.L., and Bertani, L.M. (1968). Excretion of catecholamine catabolites by normal children. *J. Lab. Clin. Med.* **72**, 612–20.

Givens, J.R. (1976). Hirsutism and hyperandrogenism. *Advan. Intern. Med.* **21**, 221–47.

Golden, M.P., Lippe, B.M., Kaplan, S.A., Lavin, N., and Slavin, J. (1978). Management of congenital adrenal hyperplasia using serum dehydroepiandrosterone sulfate and 17 hydroxyprogesterone concentrations. *Pediatrics* **61**, 867–71.

Gordon, R. (1995). Primary aldosteronism. *J. Endocrinol. Invest.* **18**, 495–511.

Gordon, R.D., Wolfle, L.K., Island, D.P., and Liddle, G.W. (1966). A diurnal rhythm in plasma renin activity in man. *J. Clin. Invest.* **45**, 1587–92.

Gotelli, G., Wall, J., Kabra, P., and Marton, L. (1981). Fluorometric liquid-chromatographic determination of serum cortisol. *Clin. Chem.* **27**, 441–3.

Grant, S.D., Pavlatos, F., and Forsham, P.H. (1965). The effects of estrogen therapy on cortisol metabolism. *J. Clin. Endocrinol. Metab.* **25**, 1057–66.

Greenwood, F.C., Landon, J., and Stamp, T.C.B. (1966). The plasma sugar, free fatty acid, cortisol and growth hormone response to insulin. I. In control subjects. *J. Clin. Invest.* **45**, 429–36.

Greig, W.R., Jasani, M.K., Boyle, J.A., and Maxwell, J.D. (1967). Corticotropin stimulation tests. *Mem. Soc. Endocrinol.* **17**, 175–92.

Grim, C., Winnacker, J., Peters, T., and Gilbert, G. (1974). Low renin "normal" aldosterone and hypertension: circadian rhythm of renin, aldosterone, cortisol, and growth hormone. *J. Clin. Endocrinol. Metab.* **39**, 247–56.

Grim, C.E., Weinberger, M.H., Higgins, J.T., and Kramer, N.J. (1977). Diagnosis of secondary forms of hypertension. *J. Am. Med. Assoc.* **237**, 1331–5.

Grossman, E., Goldstein, D., Hoffman, A., and Keiser, H. (1991). Glucagon and clonidine testing in the diagnosis of pheochromocytoma. *Hypertension* **17**, 733–41.

Grumbach, M.H. (1980). The neuroendocrinology of puberty. *Hosp. Pract.* **15**, 51–60.

Guisti, G., Mannelli, M., Forti, G., Fiorelli, G., Giannotti, P., Basi, F., Calabresi, E., Borsi, L., Bartolozze, G., Bernini, G., Mannelli, F., and Serio, M. (1978). Plasma steroid values in congenital adrenocortical hyperplasia. In *The endocrine function of the human adrenal cortex* (ed. V.H.T. James), pp. 271–87. Academic Press, New York.

Gunnels, J.C., McGuffin, W.L., Johnsrude, I., and Robinson, R.R. (1969). Peripheral and renal venous plasma renin activity in hypertension. *Ann. Intern. Med.* **71**, 555–75.

Gutai, J., Kowarski, A., and Migeon, C. (1977). The detection of the heterozygous carrier for congenital virilizing adrenal hyperplasia. *J. Pediatr.* **90**, 924–9.

Hakulinen, A. (1971). Urinary excretion of vanillylmandelic acid of children in normal and certain pathological conditions. *Acta Paediatr. Scand. Suppl.* 212.

Haque, N., Thrasher, K., Werk, E.E., Knowles, H.C., and Sholiton, L.J. (1972). Studies on dexamethasone metabolism in man: effect of diphenylhydantoin. *J. Clin. Endocrinol. Metab.* **34**, 44–50.

Hermus, A., Pieters, G., Borm, G., Verhofstad, A., Smals, A., Benraad, T., and Kloppenborg, P. (1993). Unpredictable hypersecretion of cortisol in Cushing's disease: detection by daily salivary cortisol measurements. *Acta Endocrinol.* **128**, 428–32.

Himathongkam, T., Dluhy, R.G., and Williams, G.H. (1975). Potassium–aldosterone–renin interrelationships. *J. Clin. Endocrinol. Metab.* **41**, 153–9.

Hindmarsh, P. and Brook, C. (1985). Single dose dexamethasone suppression test in children: dose relationship to body size. *Clin. Endocrinol.* **23**, 67–70.

Hiner, L.B., Gruskin, A.B., Baluarte, H.J., and Cote, M.L. (1976). Plasma renin activity in normal children. *J. Pediatr.* **89**, 258–60.

Hiroshige, T. and Sakakura, M. (1971). Circadian rhythm of corticotropin-releasing activity in the hypothalamus of normal and adrenalectomized rats. *Neuroendocrinology* **7**, 25–36.

Hiroshige, T. and Sato, T. (1970). Postnatal development of circadian rhythm of corticotropin releasing activity in the rat hypothalamus. *Endocrinol. Jpn* **17**, 1–6.

Hiroshige, T., Sakakura, M., and Itoh, S. (1969). Diurnal variation of corticotropin releasing activity in the rat hypothalamus. *Endocrinol. Jpn* **16**, 465–7.

Hjemdahl, P. (1984). Catecholamine measurements by high-performance liquid chromatography. *Am. J. Physiol.* **247**, 13–20.

Hofmann, K. (1974). Relations between chemical structure and function of adrenocorticotropin and melanocyte stimulating hormones. In *Handbook of physiology*, Section 7, Part 2 *Endocrinology*, Vol. IV: The pituitary and its neuroendocrine control, pp. 29–58. American Physiologic Society, Washington, DC.

Hofmann, K.R., Andreatta, R., Bohm, H., and Moroder, L. (1970). Studies on polypeptides. XLV. Structure–function studies in beta-corticotropin series. *J. Med. Chem.* **13**, 339–45.

Hokfelt, B. (1951). Noradrenaline and adrenaline in mammalian tissues. *Acta Physiol. Scand.* **92** (suppl.), 48–58.

Holzbauer, M. (1957). The corticosterone content of rat adrenals under different experimental conditions. *J. Physiol.* **139**, 294–305.

Hopper, B.R. and Yen, S.S. (1975). Circulating concentrations of dehydroepiandrosterone and dehydroepiandrosterone sulfate during puberty. *J. Clin. Endocrinol. Metab.* **40**, 458–61.

Horton, R. (1973). Aldosterone: review of its physiology and diagnostic aspects of primary aldosterone. *Metabolism* **22**, 1525–45.

Horton, R. and Finck, E. (1972). Diagnosis and localization in primary aldosteronism. *Ann. Intern. Med.* **76**, 885–90.

Hung, W., August, G.P., and Glasgow, A.M. (1978). *Pediatric endocrinology*. Medical Examination Publishing, New Hyde Park.

Ito, Y., Obara, T., Okamoto, T., Kanbe, M., Tanaka, R., Iihara, M., Okamoto, J., Yamazaki, K., and Jibiki, K. (1998). Efficacy of single-voided urine metanephrine and normetanephrine assay for diagnosing pheochromocytoma. *World J. Surg.* **22**, 684–8.

Iverson, L.L. (1967). *The uptake and storage of noradrenaline in sympathetic nerves*. Cambridge University Press, London.

Iverson, L.L. (1975). Uptake of circulating catecholamines. In *Handbook of physiology*, Section 7. *Endocrinology*, Vol. VI: Adrenal gland (ed. H. Blaschko, G. Sayers, and A.D. Smith), pp. 713–22. American Physiologic Society, Washington, DC.

Iverson, L.L. and Whitby, L.G. (1963). The subcellular distribution of catecholamines in normal and tyramine-depleted mouse hearts. *Biochem. Pharmacol.* **12**, 582–4.

Jaffee, N. (1976). Neuroblastoma: review of the literature and an examination of factors contributing to its enigmatic character. *Cancer Treat. Rep.* **3**, 61–82.

James, V.H.T., Tanbridge, R.D., Wilson, G.A., Hutton, J., Jacobs, H.S., and Rippon, A.E. (1978). Steroid profiling: a technique for exploring adrenocortical physiology. In *Endocrine function of the human adrenal cortex* (ed. V.H.T. James), pp.179–92. Academic Press, New York.

Kamijo, K., Koelle, B.G., and Wagner, H.H. (1955). Modification of the effects of sympathimimetic amines and of adrenergic nerve stimulation by 1-isonicotinyl-2-isopropylhydrazine and isonicotinic acid hydrozide. *J. Pharmacol. Exp. Ther.* **117**, 213–27.

Kato, H., Saito, M., and Suda, M. (1980). Effect of starvation on the circadian rhythm in rats. *Endocrinology* **106**, 918–21.

Katz, F., Romfh, P., and Smith, J.A. (1975). Diurnal variation of plasma aldosterone cortisol and renin activity in supine man. *J. Clin. Endocrinol. Metab.* **40**, 125–34.

Keenam, B.S., McNeel, R., Barrett, G.N., Holcombe, J.H., Kirkland, R.T., and Clayton, G.W. (1979). Plasma androgens in congenital adrenal hyperplasia. *J. Lab. Clin. Med.* **94**, 799–808.

Keene, M.F. and Hewer, E.E. (1926). Observations on the development of the suprarenal gland. *J. Anat.* **61**, 302–24.

Kem, D.C., Weinberger, M.H., Mayes, D.M., and Nugent, C.A. (1971). Saline suppression of plasma aldosterone in hypertension. *Arch. Intern. Med.* **128**, 380–6.

Kem, D.C., Gomez-Sanchez, C., Kramer, N.J., Holland, O.B., and Higgins, J.R. (1975). Plasma aldosterone and renin activity response to ACTH infusion in dexamethasone-suppressed normal and sodium replete man. *J. Clin. Endocrinol. Metab.* **40**, 116–24.

Kertesz, G., Bourcier, B., Cailla, H., and Jean, F. (1998). Immunoradiometric assay of succinylated corticotropin: an improved method for quantification of ACTH. *Clin. Chem.* **44**, 78–85.

Keusch, G., Binswanger, U., Dambacher, M.A., and Fischer, J.A. (1977). Ectopic ACTH syndrome and medullary thyroid carcinoma. *Acta Endocrinol.* **86**, 306–16.

Kishner, N. (1975). Biosynthesis of the catecholamines. In *Handbook of physiology*, Section 7. *Endocrinology*, Vol. VI: Adrenal gland (ed. H. Blaschko, G. Sayers, and A.D. Smith), pp. 341–55. American Physiologic Society, Washington, DC.

Korth-Schutz, S., Virdis, R., Saenger, P., Chow, D.M., Levine, L.S., and New, M.I. (1978). Serum androgens as a continuing index of adequacy of treatment of congenital adrenal hyperplasia. *J. Clin. Endocrinol. Metab.* **46**, 452–8.

Kovanen, P.T., Faust, J.R., Brown, M.S., and Goldstein, J.L. (1979). Low density lipoprotein receptors in bovine adrenal cortex. I. Receptor-mediated uptake of low density lipoprotein and utilization of its cholesterol for steroid synthesis in cultured adrenocortical cells. *Endocrinology* **104**, 599–609.

Kowarski, A., Katz, H., and Migeon, C. (1974). Plasma aldosterone concentration from infancy to adulthood. *J. Clin. Endocrinol. Metab.* **38**, 489–91.

Kramer, R.E., Gallant, S., and Brownie, A.C. (1980). Actions of angiotensin II on aldosterone synthesis in the rat adrenal cortex. *J. Biol. Chem.* **255**, 3442–7.

Krieger, D.T. (1975). Rhythms of ACTH and corticosteroid secretion in health and disease and their experimental modification. *J. Steroid Biochem.* **6**, 785–91.

Krieger, D.T. (1979). Plasma ACTH and corticosteroids. In *Endocrinology* (ed. L. DeGroot), p. 1145. Grune and Stratton, New York.

Krieger, D.T and Allen, W. (1975). Relationship of bioassayable and immunoassayable plasma ACTH and cortisol concentrations in normal subjects and in patient's with Cushing's disease. *J. Clin. Endocrinol. Metab.* **40**, 675–87.

Krieger, D.T., Allen, W., Rizzo, F., and Krieger, H.P. (1971). Characterization of the normal temporal pattern of plasma corticosteroid levels. *J. Clin. Endocrinol. Metab.* **32**, 266–84.

Lake, C.R., Ziegler, M.G., Coleman, M.D., and Kopin, I.J. (1977). Age-adjusted plasma norepinephrine levels are similar in normotensive and hypertensive subjects. *New Engl. J. Med.* **296**, 208–9.

Landon, J., Wynn, V., and James, V.H.T. (1963). The adrenocortical response to insulin-induced hypoglycemia. *J. Endocrinol.* **27**, 183–92.

Laragh, J.H., Angers, M., Kelly, W.G., and Lieberman, S. (1960). Hypotensive agents and presser substances. *J. Am. Med. Assoc.* **174**, 234–40.

Laragh, J.H., Buer, L., Brunner, H.R., Buhler, F.R., Sealey, J.E., and Vaughan, E.D. Jr (1972). Renin, angiotensin and aldosterone system in pathogenesis and management of hypertensive vascular disease. *Am. J. Med.* **52**, 633–52.

Laragh, J.H., Sealey, J.E., and Brunner, H.R. (1975). The control of aldosterone secretion in normal and hypertensive man: abnormal renin–aldosterone patterns in low renin hypertension. In *Manual of hypertension* (ed. J.H. Laragh), pp. 203–205. Yorke Medical Books, New York.

Lashansky, G., Saenger, P., Fishman, K., Gautier, T., Mayes, D., Berg, G., Di Martino-Nardi, J., and Reiter, E. (1991). Normative data for adrenal steroidogenesis in a healthy pediatric population: age- and sex-related changes after adrenocorticotropin stimulation. *J. Clin. Endocrinol. Metab.* **73**, 674–86.

Lashansky, G., Saenger, P., Dimartino-Nardi, J., Gautier, T., Mayes, D., Berg, G., and Reiter, E. (1992). Normative data for the steroidogenic response of mineralocorticoids and their precursors to adrenocorticotropin in a healthy pediatric population. *J. Clin. Endocrinol. Metab.* **75**, 1491–6.

Laudat, M., Cerdas, S., Fournier, C., Guiban, D., Guilhaume, B., and Luton, J. (1988). Salivary cortisol measurement: a practical approach to assess pituitary-adrenal function. *J. Clin. Endocrinol. Metab.* **66**, 343–8.

Lawrence, A. (1967). Glucagon provocative test for pheochromocytoma. *Ann. Intern. Med.* **66**, 1091–6.

Lee, F. and Trendelenburg, U. (1967). Muscarinic transmission of pre-ganglionic impulses to the adrenal medulla of the cat. *J. Pharmacol. Exp. Ther.* **158**, 73–9.

Leisti, S. and Perheentupa, J. (1978). Vasopressin test: diagnostic inaccuracy in evaluation of hypothalamic–pituitary–adrenocortical axis. *Acta Endocrinol.* **87**, 28–39.

Lenders, J., Keiser, H., Goldstein, D., Willemsen, J., Friberg, P., Jacobs, M.-C., Kloppenborg, P., Thien, T., and Eisenhofer, G. (1995). Plasma metanephrines in the diagnosis of pheochromocytoma. *Ann. Intern. Med.* **123**, 101–9.

Lenz, T., Ross, A., Schumm-Draeger, P., Schulte, K., and Geiger, H. (1998). Clonidine suppression test revisited. *Blood Pressure* **7**, 153–9.

Levin, B.E., Rappaport, M., and Natelson, B.H. (1979). Ultradian variations of plasma noradrenaline in humans. *Life Sci.* **25**, 621–8.

Levitt, M., Spector, S., Sjoredsma, A., and Udenfriend, S. (1965). Elucidation of the rate limiting step in norepinephrine biosynthesis in the perfused guinea-pig heart. *J. Pharmacol. Exp. Ther.* **148**, 1–8.

Lewis, G.P. (1975). Physiological mechanisms controlling secretory activity of adrenal medulla. In *Handbook of physiology*, Section 7. *Endocrinology*, Vol. VI: Adrenal gland (ed. H. Blaschko, G. Sayers, and A.D. Smith), pp. 309–19. American Physiologic Society, Washington, DC.

Li, C.H., Meienhofer, J., Schnabel, E., Chung, D., Lo, T.B., and Ramachandran, J. (1961). Synthesis of a biologically active nonadecapeptide corresponding to the first nineteen amino acid residues of adrenocorticotropins. *J. Am. Chem. Soc.* **83**, 4449–57.

Liddle, G.W. (1960). Tests of pituitary–adrenal suppressibility in the diagnosis of Cushing's syndrome. *J. Clin. Endocrinol. Metab.* **20**, 1539–60.

Liddle, G.W., Estep, H.L., Kendall, J.W., Williams, W.C., and Townes, A.W. (1959). Clinical application of a new test of pituitary reserve. *J. Clin. Endocrinol. Metab.* **19**, 875–94.

Lifton, R., Dluhy, R., Powers, M., Rich, G., Cook, S., Ulick, S., and Lalouel, J.M. (1992). A chimaeric 11β-hydroxylase/aldosterone synthase gene causes glucocorticoid-remediable aldosteronism and human hypertension. *Nature* **355**, 262–5.

Lightman, S.L., James, V.H.T., Linsell, C., Mullen, P.E., Peart, W.S., and Sever, P.S. (1981). Studies of diurnal changes in plasma renin activity and noradrenaline, aldosterone and cortisol concentrations in man. *Clin. Endocrinol.* **14**, 213–23.

Limal, J.M., Basmaciogullari, A., and Rappaport, R. (1976). Evaluation of single oral dose metyrapone tests in children with hypopituitarism. *Acta Pediatr. Scand.* **65**, 177–83.

Lindholm, J., Kehlet, H., Blichert-Toft, M., Dinesen, B., and Riishede, J. (1978). Reliability of the 30 minute ACTH test in assessing hypothalamic-pituitary-adrenal function. *J. Clin. Endocrinol. Metab.* **47**, 272–5.

Liotta, A.L. and Krieger, D.T. (1975). A sensitive bioassay for the determination of human plasma ACTH levels. *J. Clin. Endocrinol. Metab.* **40**, 268–77.

Litchfield, W., Dluhy, R., Lifton, R., and Rich, G. (1995). Glucocorticoid-remediable aldosteronism. *Comprehens. Ther.* **21**, 553–8.

Litchfield, W., New, M., Coolidge, C., Lifton, R., and Dluhy, R. (1997). Evaluation of the dexamethasone suppression test for the diagnosis of glucocorticoid-remediable aldosteronism. *J. Clin. Endocrinol. Metab.* **82**, 3570–3.

Llaurado, J.G. (1955). Increased excretion of aldosterone immediately after operation. *Lancet* **1**, 1295–8.

Llaurado, J.G. (1957 Aldosterone excretion following hypophysectomy in man: relation to urinary Na/K ratio. *Metabolism* **6**, 556–63.

Lobo, M.V., Marusic, E.T., and Aquilera, G. (1978). Further studies on the relationship between potassium and sodium levels and adrenocortical activity. *Endocrinology* **102**, 1061–8.

Louis, W.J., Doyle, A.E., and Anavekar, S.N. (1975). Plasma noradrenaline concentration and blood pressure in essential hypertension, phaeochromocytoma and depression. *Clin. Sci. Mol. Med.* **48**, 239S–242S.

Mahesh, V.B., Greenblatt, R.B., and Coniff, R.F. (1968). Urinary steroid excretion before and after dexamethasone administration and steroid content of adrenal tissue and venous blood in virilizing adrenal tumors. *Am. J. Obstet. Gynecol.* **100**, 1043–54.

Mains, R.E. and Eipper, B.A. (1980). Structure and biosynthesis of pro-adrenocorticotropin/endorphin and related peptides. *Endocr. Rev.* **1**, 1–27.

Maxwell, M.H., Marks, L.S., Varady, P.D., Lupu, A.N., and Kaufman, J.J. (1975). Renal vein renin in essential hypertension. *J. Lab. Clin. Med.* **86**, 901–9.

May, M. and Carey, R. (1985). Rapid adrenocorticotropic hormone test in practice. *Am. J. Med.* **79**, 679–84.

Mayenknecht, J., Diederich, S., Bahr, V., Plockinger, U., and Oelkers, W. (1998). Comparison of low and high dose corticotropin stimulation tests in patients with pituitary disease. *J. Clin. Endocrinol. Metab.* **83**, 1558–62.

Mayes, S. (1980). Neurohumoral transmission and the autonomic nervous system. In *Pharmacological basis of therapeutics* (ed. A.G. Goodman, L.S. Goodman, and A. Gilman), p. 76. Macmillan, New York.

Meikle, A.W., Jubig, W., Matsukura, S., West, C.D., and Tyler, F. (1969). Effect of diphenylhydantoin on the metabolism and release of ACTH in man. *J. Clin. Endocrinol. Metab.* **29**, 1553–8.

Meikle, A.W., Stanchfield, J.B., West, C.D., and Tyler, F.H. (1974). Hydrocortisone suppression test for Cushing's syndrome. *Arch. Intern. Med.* **134**, 1068–71.

Meikle, A., Lagerquist, L., and Tyler, F. (1975). Apparently normal pituitary–adrenal suppressibility in Cushing's syndrome: dexamethasone metabolism and plasma levels. *J. Lab. Clin. Med.* **86**, 472–8.

Melby, J.C. (1972). Identify the adrenal lesion in primary aldosteronism. *Ann. Intern. Med.* **76**, 1039–41.

Mericq, M. and Cutler, G.J. (1998). High fluid intake increases urine free cortisol excretion in normal subjects. *J. Clin. Endocrinol. Metab.* **83**, 682–4.

Migeon, C.J. (1972). Adrenal androgens in man. *Am. J. Med.* **53**, 606–26.

Migeon, C.J., Green, O.C., and Ernest, J.P. (1963). Study of adrenal function in obesity. *Metabolism* **12**, 718–39.

Mitchell, J.R., Taylor, A.A., Pool, J.L., Lake, C.R., Rollins, D.E., and Bartter, F.C. (1977). Renin–aldosterone profiling in hypertension. *Ann. Intern. Med.* **87**, 596–612.

Miyabo, S., Yanagisawa, K., Ooya, E., Hisada, T., and Kishida, S. (1980). Ontogeny of the circadian corticosteroid rhythm in female rats: effects of periodic matured deprivation and food restriction. *Endocrinology* **106**, 442–636.

Montwill, J., Igoe, D., and McKenna, T. (1994). The overnight dexamethasone test is the procedure of choice in screening for Cushing's syndrome. *Steroids* **59**, 296–8.

Mosnier-Pudar, H., Thomopoulos, P., Bertagna, X., Fournier, C., Guiban, D., and Luton, J. (1995). Long-distance and long-term follow-up of a patient with intermittent Cushing's disease by salivary cortisol measurements. *Eur. J. Endocrinol.* **133**, 313–16.

Mueller, R.A., Thoenen, H., and Axelrod, J. (1970). Effect of the pituitary and ACTH on the maintenance of basal tyrosine hydroxalase activity in the rat adrenal gland. *Endocrinology* **86**, 751–5.

Muller, J. (1971). *Regulation of aldosterone biosynthesis*. Springer-Verlag, New York.

Murphy, B.E. (1967). Some studies of the protein binding steroids and their application to the routine micro and ultramicro measurement of various steroids in body fluids by competitive-binding radioassay. *J. Clin. Endocrinol. Metab.* **27**, 973–90.

Murphy, B.E. (1975). Non-chromatographic radiotransinassay for cortisol. Application to human adult serum, umbilical cord and amniotic fluid. *J. Clin. Endocrinol. Metab.* **41**, 1050–7.

Mussachio, J.M., Kopin, I.J., and Weise, V.K. (1965). Subcellular distribution of some sympathomimetic amines and their B-hydroxylated derivatives in the rat heart. *J. Pharmacol. Exp. Ther.* **148**, 22–8.

Nagatsu, T. (1973). *Biochemistry of catecholamines*. University Park Press, Baltimore.

Nagatsu, T., Levitt, M., and Udenfriend, S. (1964). Tyrosine hydroxylase. *J. Biol. Chem.* **239**, 2910–17.

Nathanson, I.T., Towne, L.E., and Aub, J.C. (1941). Normal secretion of sex hormones in childhood. *Endocrinology* **28**, 851–65.

Nelson, D.H. (1980*a*). The adrenal cortex: physiological function and disease. *Major Prob. Intern. Med.* **18**, 1–281.

Nelson, D.H. (1980*b*). Adrenal hirsutism and virilization. The adrenal cortex. *Major Prob. Intern. Med.* **18**, 199–210.

Nelson, H.G. and Harding, B.W. (1952). Effect of liver on blood levels of 17-OHCSs in the dog. *Fed. Proc.* **11**, 379.

Nelson, J.C. and Tindall, D.J. (1978). A comparison of the adrenal responses to hypoglycemia, metapyrone and ACTH. *Am. J. Med. Sci.* **275**, 165–72.

Netter, F.H. (1965). *CIBA collection of medical illustrations*, Vol. 4. *Endocrine system and selected metabolic diseases*, pp. 77–8. CIBA Pharmaceutical, Summit, New Jersey.

Neville, A.M. and Mackay, A.M. (1972). The structure of the human adrenal cortex in health and disease. *Clin. Endocrinol. Metab.* **1**, 361–95.

New, M. (1998). Diagnosis and management of congenital adrenal hyperplasia. *Ann. Rev. Med.* **49**, 311–28.

New, M.I., Miller, B., and Peterson, R.E. (1966). Aldosterone excretion in normal children and in children with adrenal hyperplasia. *J. Clin. Invest.* **45**, 412–28.

Newell-Price, J., Trainer, P., Perry, L., Wass, J., Grossman, A., and Besser, M. (1995). A single sleeping midnight cortisol has 100 per cent sensitivity for the diagnosis of Cushing's syndrome. *Clin. Endocrinol.* **43**, 545–50.

Newell-Price, J., Perry, L., Medbak, S., Monson, J., Savage, M., Besser, M., and Grossman, A. (1997). A combined test using desmopressin and corticotropin-releasing hormone in the differential diagnosis of Cushing's syndrome. *J. Clin. Endocrinol. Metab.* **82**, 176–81.

Newsome, H.H., Clements, A.S., and Bourm, E.A. (1972). The simultaneous assay of cortisol, corticosterone, 11-deoxycortisol, and cortisone in human plasma. *J. Clin. Endocrinol. Metab.* **34**, 473–83.

Nichols, G.L., Mitty, H., Modlinger, R.S., and Gabrilove, J.L. (1972). Percutaneous adrenal venography. *Ann. Intern. Med.* **76**, 899–909.

Nichols, M.G., Espiner, E.A., and Donald, R.A. (1975). Plasma aldosterone response to low dose ACTH stimulation. *J. Clin. Endocrinol. Metab.* **41**, 186–8.

Nicholson, W.E., Liddle, R.A., Puett, D., and Liddle, G.W. (1978). Adrenocorticotropic hormone biotransformation, clearance and catabolism. *Endocrinology* **103**, 1344–51.

Nielson, E. and Asfeldt, V.H. (1967). Studies on the specificity of fluorimetric determination of plasma corticosteroids. *Scand. J. Clin. Lab. Invest.* **20**, 185–94.

Nieman, L., Cutler, G.J., Oldfield, E., Loriaux, D., and Chrousos, G. (1989). The ovine corticotropin-releasing hormone (CRH) stimulation test is superior to the human CRH stimulation test for the diagnosis of Cushing's disease. *J. Clin. Endocrinol. Metab.* **69**, 165–9.

Nieman, L., Oldfield, E., Wesley, R., Chrousos, G., Loriaux, D., and Cutler, G.J. (1993). A simplified morning ovine corticotropin-releasing hormone stimulation test for the differential diagnosis of adrenocorticotropin-dependent Cushing's syndrome. *J. Clin. Endocrinol. Metab.* **77**, 1308–12.

Niemineva, K. and Pekkarinen, A. (1953). Determination of adrenalin and noradrenalin in the human foetal adrenal and aortic bodies. *Nature* **171**, 436–7.

Oelkers, W. (1996). Current concepts: adrenal insufficiency. *New Engl. J. Med.* **335**, 1206–12.

Oelkers, W. (1998). The role of high- and low-dose corticotropin tests in the diagnosis of secondary adrenal insufficiency. *Eur. J. Endocrinol.* **139**, 567–70.

Orth, D. (1995). Medical progress: Cushing's syndrome. *New Engl. J. Med.* **332**, 791–803.

Orth, D. and Kovacs, W. (1998). The adrenal cortex. In *Williams textbook of endocrinology* (ed. J. Wilson, D. Foster, H. Kronenberg, and P. Larsen), pp. 517–664. W.B.Saunders, Philadelphia.

Orth, D.N., Island, D.P., and Liddle, G.W. (1967). Experimental alteration of the circadian rhythm in plasma cortisol concentration in man. *J. Clin. Endocrinol. Metab.* **27**, 549–55.

Osborn, R.H. and Yannone, M.E. (1971). Plasma androgens in the normal and androgenic female. *Obstet. Gynecol. Surv.* **26**, 195–228.

Padfield, P.L., Allison, E.M., Brown, J.J., Ferris, J.B., Fraser, R., Lever, A.F., Luke, R.G., and Robertson, J.I.S. (1975). Response of plasma aldosterone to fludrocortisone in primary hyperaldosteronism and other forms of hypertension. *Clin. Endocrinol.* **4**, 493–500.

Papanicolaou, D., Yanovski, J., Cutler, G., Chrousos, G., and Nieman, L. (1998). A single midnight serum cortisol measurement distinguishes Cushing's syndrome from pseudo-Cushing states. *J. Clin. Endocrinol. Metab.* **83**, 1163–7.

Park, Y., Park, K., Kim, J., Shin, C., Kim, S., and Lee, H. (1999). Reproducibility of the cortisol response to stimulation with the low dose (1 μg) of ACTH. *Clin. Endocrinol.* **51**, 153–8.

Parker, C.J., Slayden, S., Azziz, R., Crabbe, S., Hines, G., Boots, L., and Bae, S. (2000). Effects of aging on adrenal function in the human: responsiveness and sensitivity of adrenal androgens and cortisol to adrenocorticotropin in premenopausal and postmenopausal women. *J. Clin. Endocrinol. Metab.* **85**, 48–54.

Parker, L.N., Sack, J., Fisher, D., and O'Dell, W. (1978). The adrenarche: prolactin, gonadotropins, adrenal androgens and cortisol. *J. Clin. Endocrinol. Metab.* **46**, 396–401.

Pasqualini, J.R. and Jayle, M.F. (1961). Corticosteroid 21-sulphates in human urine. *Biochem. J.* **81**, 147–9.

Peach, M.J. (1971). Adrenal medullary stimulation induced by angiotensin I, angiotensin II, and analogues. *Circ. Res.* **28** (suppl. 2), II107–II117.

Peterson, R.E. (1959). The miscible pool and turnover rate of adrenocortical steroids in man. *Recent Prog. Horm. Res.* **15**, 231–74.

Peterson, R.E. (1971). Metabolism of adrenal steroids. In *The human adrenal cortex* (ed. N.P. Christy), pp. 87–189. Harper and Row, New York.

Pipkin, F.B., Somales, O.R., and O'Callaghan, M.J. (1981). Renin and angiotensin levels in children. *Arch. Dis. Child.* **56**, 298–302.

Plager, J.E. (1965). The binding of androsterone sulfate, etiocholanolone sulfate and dehydroepiandrosterone sulfate by human plasma protein. *J. Clin. Invest.* **44**, 1234–9.

Potter, L.T. (1967). Role of intraneuronal vesicles in the synthesis, storage and release of noradrenaline. *Circ. Res.* **20** (suppl. 3), III13–III24.

Raber, W., Raffesberg, W., Bischof, M., Scheuba, C., Niederle, B., Gasic, S., Waldhausl, W., and Roden, M. (2000). Diagnostic efficacy of unconjugated plasma metanephrines for the detection of pheochromocytoma. *Arch. Intern. Med.* **160**, 2957–63.

Raff, H., Raff, J., and Findling, J. (1998). Late-night salivary cortisol as a screening test for Cushing's syndrome. *J. Clin. Endocrinol. Metab.* **83**, 2681–6.

Rayfield, E.J., Cain, J.P., Carey, M.P., Williams, G.H., and Sullivan, J.M. (1977). Influence of diet on urinary VMA excretion. *J. Am. Med. Assoc.* **221**, 704–5.

Reese, J.D. and Moon, H.D. (1938). Golgi apparatus of cells of adrenal cortex after hypophysectomy and on administration of adrenocortocotropic hormone. *Anat. Rec.* **70**, 543–56.

Reiter, E.O., Fuldauer, V.G., and Root, A.W. (1977). Secretion of the adrenal androgen, dehydroepiandrosterone sulfate, during infancy childhood and adolescence in sick infants and in children with endocrinologic abnormalities. *J. Pediatr.* **90**, 766–70.

Reynolds, J.W., Colle, E., and Ulstrom, R.A. (1962). Adrenocortical steroid metabolism in newborn infants. V. Physiologic disposition of exogenous cortisol loads in early neonatal period. *J. Clin. Endocrinol. Metab.* **22**, 245–54.

Richmond, L., Chappell, J., and Cleveland, W. (1964). Response of children to metopirone. *J. Pediatr.* **64**, 381–6.

Riggin, R.M. and Kissinger, P.T. (1977). Determination of catecholamines in urine by reverse-phase liquid chromatography with electrochemical detection. *Anal. Chem.* **49**, 2109–11.

Robin, P., Predine, J., and Milgrom, E. (1977). Assay of unbound cortisol in plasma. *J. Clin. Endocrinol. Metab.* **46**, 277–83.

Robinson, D.S., Lovenberg, W., Keiser, H., and Sjoerdsma, A. (1968). Effect of drugs on human blood platelet and plasma amine oxidase activity *in-vitro* and *in-vivo*. *Biochem. Pharmacol.* **17**, 109–19.

Rosano, T., Demers, L., Hillam, R., Dybas, M., and Leinung, M. (1995). Clinical and analytical evaluation of an immunoradiometric assay for corticotropin. *Clin. Chem.* **41**, 1022–7.

Rose, L., Williams, G., Jagger, P., and Lauler, D. (1970). The 48-hour adrenocorticotropin infusion test for adrenocortical insufficiency. *Ann. Intern. Med.* **73**, 49–54.

Rosenfeld, R.S., Fukushima, D.K., and Gallagher, T.F. (1967). Metabolism of the adrenal cortical hormones. In *The human adrenal cortex* (ed. A.B. Eisenstein), pp. 103–31. Little, Brown, Boston.

Rosenfeld, R.S., Rosenberg, B.J., Fukushima, D.K., and Hellman, L. (1975). 24 Hour secretory pattern of dehydroisoandrosterone and dehydroisoandrosterone sulfate. *J. Clin. Endocrinol. Metab.* **40**, 850–5.

Ross, R.J. (1960). Urinary excretion of cortisol in Cushing's syndrome: effect of corticotropin. *J. Clin. Endocrinol. Metab.* **20**, 1360–5.

Ryan, W.T., Ferro, W.F., and Beyler, A.L. (1964). An improved method for the measurement of urinary 17 ketosteroids of small laboratory animals. *Clin. Chem.* **10**, 191–6.

Salyer, W.R., Salyer, D.C., and Eggleston, J.C. (1976). Carcinoid tumors of the thymus. *Cancer* **37**, 958–73.

Samuels, L.T. and Nelson, D.H. (1975). Biosynthesis of corticosteroids. In *Handbook of physiology*, Section 7. *Endocrinology*, Vol. VI: Adrenal gland (ed. H. Blaschko, G. Sayers, and A.D. Smith), pp. 57–60. American Physiologic Society, Washington, DC.

Sassard, J., Sann, L., Vincent, M., Francois, R., and Cier, J.F. (1975). Plasma renin activity in normal subjects from infancy to puberty. *J. Clin. Endocrinol. Metab.* **40**, 524–5.

Sayers, G.R. and Portanova, R. (1975). Regulation of the secretory activity of the adrenal cortex: cortisol and corticosterone. In *Handbook of physiology*, Section 7. *Endocrinology*, Vol. VI: Adrenal gland (ed. H. Blaschko, G. Sayers, and A.D. Smith), p. 43. American Physiologic Society, Washington, DC.

Sayers, G.R., Beall, R.J., Seelig, S. and Cummins, K. (1973). Assay of ACTH: isolated adrenal cortex cells. In *Brain–pituitary–adrenal interrelationships* (ed. A. Brodish and E.S. Redgate), pp. 16–35. Karger, Basel.

Schober, R., Nitsch, C., Rinne, U., and Morris, S.J. (1977). Calcium induced displacement of membrane-associated particles upon aggregation of chromaffin granules. *Science* **195**, 495–7.

Schumacker, H.B. and Firor, W.M. (1934). Interrelationship of adrenal cortex and anterior lobe of hypophysis. *Endocrinology* **18**, 676–92.

Seelig, S. and Sayers, G. (1973). Isolated adrenal cortex cells: ACTH agonists, partial agonists, antagonists: cyclic AMP and corticosterone production. *Arch. Biochem. Biophys.* **154**, 230–9.

Segre, G. and Brown, E. (1998). Measurement of hormones. In *Williams textbook of endocrinology* (ed. J. Wilson, D. Foster, H. Kronenberg, and P. Larsen), pp. 43–54. W.B. Saunders Company, Philadelphia.

Sheaves, R., Goldin, J., Reznek, R., Chew, S., Dacie, J., Lowe, D., Ross, R., Wass, J., Besser, G., and Grossman, A. (1996). Relative value of computed tomography scanning and venous sampling in establishing the cause of primary hyperaldosteronism. *Eur. J. Endocrinol.* **134**, 308–13.

Shepherd, D.M. and West, G.B. (1951). Noradrenaline and the suprarenal medulla. *Br. J. Pharmacol. Chemother.* **6**, 665–74.

Sheridan, P. and Mattingly, P. (1975). Simultaneous investigative treatment of suspected acute adrenal insufficiency. *Lancet* **2**, 676–8.

Sizonenko, P.C. and Paunier, L. (1975). Hormonal changes in puberty. III. Correlation of plasma dehydroepiandrosterone, testosterone, FSH and LH with stages of puberty and bone age in normal boys and girls in patients with Addison's disease or hypogonadism or premature or late adrenarche. *J. Clin. Endocrinol. Metab.* **41**, 894–904.

Sklar, C., Kaplan, S.L., and Grumbach, M.M. (1980). Evidence for dissociation between adrenarche and gonadarche: studies in patients with idiopathic precocious puberty, gonadal dysgenesis, isolated gonadotropin deficiency and constitutionally delayed growth and adolescence. *J. Clin. Endocrinol. Metab.* **51**, 548–56.

Smith, A.A., Taylor, T., and Wortis, S.B. (1963). Abnormal catecholamine metabolism in familial dysautonomia. *New Engl. J. Med.* **268**, 705–7.

Soffer, L.J., Dorfman, R.I., and Garilove, J.L. (1961). *The human adrenal cortex.* Lea and Febiger, Philadelphia.

Sole, M.J. and Hussain, M.N. (1977). A simple specific assay for the simultaneous measurement of picogram quantities of norepinephrine, epinephrine and dopamine in plasma and tissues. *Biochem. Med.* **18**, 301–7.

Solomon, T.A., Cavero, I., and Buckley, J.P. (1974). Inhibition of the arterial presser effect of angiotensin I and II. *J. Pharmaceut. Sci.* **63**, 511–15.

Speckart, P.F., Nicoloff, J.T., and Bethune, J.E. (1971). Screening for adrenocortical insufficiency with cosyntropin. *Arch. Intern. Med.* **128**, 761–3.

Spergel, G., Levy, L.J., Chowdhury, F.R., Rodman, H.M., Ertel, N.H., and Bleicher, S.J. (1970). A modified phentolamine test for the diagnosis of pheochromocytoma. *J. Am. Med. Assoc.* **211**, 266–9.

Spiger, M., Jubiz, W., Meikle, A.W., West, C.D., and Tylor, F.H. (1975). Single dose metapyrone test. *Arch. Intern. Med.* **135**, 698–700.

Stachenko, J. and Giroud, C.J. (1959). Functional zonation of the adrenal cortex: pathways of corticosteroid biogenesis. *Endocrinology* **64**, 730–42.

Stark, P., Beckerhoff, R., Leumann, E.P., Vetter, W., and Siegenthaler, W. (1975). Control of plasma aldosterone in infancy and childhood. *Helv. Paediatr. Acta* **30**, 349–56.

Steiker, D.O., Bongiovanni, A.M., Eberlein, W.R., and Leboeut, G. (1961). Adrenocortical and adrenocorticotropic function in children. *J. Pediatr.* **59**, 884–9.

Stockigt, J.R., Collins, R.D., Noakes, C.A., Schambelan, M., and Biglieri, E.G. (1972). Renal vein renin in various forms of renal hypertension. *Lancet* **1**, 1194–8.

Stone, R.A., Talner, L.B., and Coel, M.C. (1977). Renal vein activity in primary hypertension: variability and influence of contrast material. *Invest. Radiol.* **12**, 455–61.

Streeten, D.H., Stevenson, C.T., Dalakos, T.G., Nickolas, J.J., Denick, L.G., and Fellerman, H. (1969). The diagnosis of hypercortisolism. Biochemical criteria differentiating patient from lean and obese normal subjects and from females on oral contraceptives. *J. Clin. Endocrinol. Metab.* **29**, 1191–211.

Studzinski, G.P., Hay, D.C., and Symington, T. (1963). Observations on the weight of the human adrenal gland and the effect of preparation of corticotrophin of different purity on the weight and morphology of the human adrenal. *J. Clin. Endocrinol. Metab.* **23**, 248–54.

Tahka, H. (1951). On weight and structure of adrenal glands and the factors affecting them, in children of 0–2 years. *Acta Pediatr. Suppl.* **81**, 7–95.

Tait, S.A., Schulster, D., Okamoto, M., Flood, C., and Tait, J.F. (1970). Production of steroids by *in vitro* superfusion of endocrine tissue. II. Steroid output from bisected whole, capsular, and decapsulated adrenals of normal intact, hypophysectomized and hypophysectomized nephrectomized rats as a function of time superfusion. *Endocrinology* **86**, 360–82.

Talbot, N.B., Butler, A.M., Berman, R.A., Rodriguez, P.M., and MacLuchlan, E.A. (1943). Excretion of 17-ketosteroids by normal and abnormal children. *Am. J. Dis. Child.* **65**, 364–75.

Thaler, L. and Blevins, L.J. (1998). The low dose (1-μg) adrenocorticotropin stimulation test in the evaluation of patients with suspected central adrenal insufficiency. *J. Clin. Endocrinol. Metab.* **83**, 2726–9.

Tordjman, K., Jaffe, A., Grazas, N., Apter, C., and Stern, N. (1995). The role of the low dose (1 microgram) adrenocorticotropin test in the evaluation of patients with pituitary diseases. *J. Clin. Endocrinol. Metab.* **84**, 1301–5.

Tordjman, K., Jaffe, A., Trostanetsky, Y., Greenman, Y., Limor, R., and Stern, N. (2000). Low-dose (1 μg) adrenocorticotrophin (ACTH)stimulation as a screening test for impaired hypothalamo–pituitary–adrenal axis function: sensitivity, specificity and accuracy in comparison with the high-dose (250 μg) test. *Clin. Endocrinol.* **52**, 633–40.

Traiger, G.J. and Calvert, D.N. (1969). O-methylation of ^{3}H-norepinephrine by epididymal adipose tissue. *Biochem. Pharmacol.* **18**, 109–17.

Treece, G.L., Magelssen, D.J., and Fariss, B.L. (1977). Conjugated estrogens and the overnight dexamethasone suppression test. *Obstet. Gynecol.* **50**, 407–9.

Tuchelt, H., Dekker, K., Bahr, V., and Oelkers, W. (2000). Dose–response relationship between plasma ACTH and serum cortisol in the insulin-hypoglycaemia test in 25 healthy subjects and 109 patients with pituitary disease. *Clin. Endocrinol.* **53**, 301–7.

Tyrrell, J., Findling, J., Aron, D., Fitzgerald, P., and Forsham, P. (1986). An overnight high-dose dexamethasone suppression test for rapid differential diagnosis of Cushing's syndrome. *Ann. Intern. Med.* **104**, 180–6.

Vaitukaitis, J.L., Dale, S.L., and Melby, J.C. (1969). Role of ACTH in the secretion of free dehydroopiandrosterone and its sulfate ester in man. *J. Clin. Endocrinol. Metab.* **29**, 1443–7.

Vallotton, M. (1996). Primary aldosteronism. Part I Diagnosis of primary hyperaldosteronism. *Clin. Endocrinol.* **45**, 47–52.

Vaughan, E.D., Sos, T.A., Sniderman, K.W., Pickering, T.G., Case, D.B., Sealey, J.E., and Laragh, J.H. (1981). Renal venous renin secretory patterns before and after percutaneous transluminal angioplasty: verification of analytic data. In *Frontiers in hypertension research* (ed. J.H. Laragh), pp. 173–80. Springer-Verlag, New York.

Venning, E.H., McCorriston, J.R., Dyranfruth, I., and Beck, J.C. (1958). Aldosterone excretion following trauma. *Metabolism* **7**, 293–300.

Vining, R., McGinley, R., and Symons, R. (1983). Hormones in saliva: mode of entry and consequent implications for clinical interpretation. *Clin. Chem.* **29**, 1752–6.

Vlachakis, N.D. and Mendlowitz, M. (1980). Plasma catecholamines in primary hypertension. *Biochem. Med.* **23**, 35–46.

Voochess, M.L. (1966). Functioning neural tumors. *Pediatr. Clin. N. Am.* **1**, 1–18.

Weetman, R.M., Rider, P.S., Oei, T.O., Hempil, J.S., and Baehner. R.L. (1976). Effect of diet on urinary excretion of VMA, HVA, metanephrine, total free catecholamines in normal preschool children. *J. Pediatr.* **88**, 46–50.

Weinberger, M. and Fineberg, N. (1993). The diagnosis of primary aldosteronism and separation of two major subtypes. *Arch. Intern. Med.* **153**, 2125–9.

Weiss, L. and Greep, R.O. (1977). *Histology*, 4th edn. McGraw-Hill, New York.

Weitzman, E.D., Fukushima, D.K., Nogeire, C., Roffwarg, H., Gallagher, T.F., and Hellman, L. (1971). Twenty-four hour pattern of the episodic secretion of cortisol in normal subjects. *J. Clin. Endocrinol. Metab.* **33**, 14–22.

West, C.D. and Meikle, A.W. (1979). Laboratory tests for the diagnosis of Cushing's syndrome and adrenal insufficiency and factors affecting those tests. In *Endocrinology* (ed. L. DeGroot), p. 1171. Grune and Stratton, New York.

West, G.B., Shepherd, D.M., and Hunter, R.B. (1951). Adrenaline and noradrenaline concentrations in adrenal glands at different ages and in some diseases. *Lancet* **2**, 966–9.

White, P., New, M., and Dupont, B. (1987*a*). Congenital adrenal hyperplasia. (1). *New Engl. J. Med.* **316**, 1519–24.

White, P., New, M., and Dupont, B. (1987*b*). Congenital adrenal hyperplasia (2). *New Engl. J. Med.* **316**, 1580–6.

White, P., Curnow, K., and Pascoe, L. (1994). Disorders of steroid 11 beta-hydroxylase isozymes. *Endocr. Rev.* **15**, 421–38.

Williams, G. and Dluhy, R. (1995). Glucocorticoid-remediable aldosteronism. *J. Endocrinol. Invest.* **18**, 512–17.

Witchel, S., Nayak, S., Suda-Hartman, M., and Lee, P. (1997). Newborn screening for 21-hydroxylase deficiency: results of CYP21 molecular genetic analysis. *J. Pediatr.* **131**, 328–31.

Wood, J.W., Pittman, A.W., Pullman, C.C., Werk, E.E., Waider, W., and Allen, C.A. (1976). Renin profiling in hypertension and its use in treatment with propranolol and chlorthalidone. *New Engl. J. Med.* **294**, 1137–43.

Wurtman, R.J. (1966). Control of epinephrine synthesis in the adrenal medulla by the adrenal cortex: hormonal specificity and dose–response characteristics. *Endocrinology* **79**, 608–14.

Wurtman, R.J. and Axelrod, J. (1965). Adrenalin synthesis: control by the pituitary gland and adrenal glucocorticoids. *Science* **150**, 1464–5.

Yanovski, J., Cutler, G., Chrousos, G., and Nieman, L. (1993). Corticotropin-releasing hormone stimulation following low-dose dexamethasone administration—a new test to distinguish Cushing's syndrome from pseudo-Cushing's states. *J. Am. Med. Assoc.* **268**, 2232–8.

Yanovski, J., Cutler, G.J., Chrousos, G., and Nieman, L. (1998). The dexamethasone-suppressed corticotropin-releasing hormone stimulation test differentiates mild Cushing's disease from normal physiology. *J. Clin. Endocrinol. Metab.* **83**, 348–52.

Young, W.J. (1997). Pheochromocytoma and primary aldosteronism: diagnostic approaches. *Endocrinol. Metab. Clin. N. Am.* **26**, 801–27.

Young, W.J., Stanson, A., Grant, C., Thompson, G., and van Heerden, J. (1996). Primary aldosteronism: adrenal venous sampling. *Surgery* **120**, 913–20.

Zadik, Z. and Kowarksi, A.A. (1980). Normal integrated concentration of aldosterone and plasma renin activity: effect of age. *J. Clin. Endocrinol. Metab.* **50**, 867–9.

Zarkovic, M., Ciric, J., Stojanovic, M., Penezic, Z., Trbojevic, B., Drezgic, M., and Nesovic, M. (1999). Optimizing the diagnostic criteria for standard (250-μg) and low dose (1-μg) adrenocorticotropin tests in the assessment of adrenal function. *J. Clin. Endocrinol. Metab.* **84**, 3170–3.

Ziegler, M.G., Lake, C.R., and Kopin, I.J. (1976). Plasma noradrenaline increases with age. *Nature* **261**, 333–4.

Zurburgg, R.P. and Joss, E.E. (1970). Diagnostic procecures in hypopituitary dwarfism. II. Evaluation of ACTH deficiency: metopirone test: daily oscillation of plasma cortisol and its response to exogenous ACTH, lysin, vasopressin, insulin-induced hypoglycemia and general anesthesia. *Helv. Paediatr. Acta* **25**, 382–96.

51.   Selection of patients with incidentally discovered adrenal masses for operation

Masaru Murai and Ken Marumo

Introduction

Since the early 1980s, incidentally discovered adrenal masses have become a common clinical problem as a result of the more widespread use of computerized tomography (CT), magnetic resonance imaging (MRI), and ultrasonography (US). Although technical advances solve many clinical problems, they may also create new management dilemmas. In patients without a known extra-adrenal primary malignancy, the vast majority of these lesions are benign and non-hypersecretory. The challenge is to identify the rare hyperfunctioning or malignant adrenal tumor that should be removed while avoiding unnecessary testing and surgery in the majority of patients whose adrenal lesion is non-hyperfunctioning and benign.

The current clinical approach to incidentally discovered adrenal masses must balance diagnostic costs, discomfort, risks, consequences of false-positive results, and low disease prevalence against the value of making an expeditious diagnosis that may result in curative therapy in the minority of patients in whom intervention would be indicated. This article reviews the prevalence of incidentally discovered adrenal masses, their differential diagnosis, and currently used strategies for evaluation and treatment of adrenal masses.

There are various definitions and terminology seen in the literature. Incidentally discovered adrenal masses were defined as adrenal tumors that were detected incidentally primarily as lesions on occasions unrelated to tumor signs and symptoms. Under the definition, previously unsuspected adrenal masses found at a routine health examination, or during diagnostic or therapeutic procedures for unrelated diseases were considered to be incidental adrenal tumors even if the patient retrospectively proved to have had symptoms or signs attributable to an adrenal tumor.

The term 'hypersecretion' is applied to adrenal mass lesions that produce sufficient hormonal secretions so as to be recognizably abnormal on standard, global biomechanical screening procedures such as the 1 mg overnight dexamethasone suppression test for glucocorticoid autonomy, or catecholamine evaluation for the diagnosis of pheochromocytoma. Therefore the term 'function' or 'functioning' should not be used to describe hormonal biochemical status. The term 'function' refers to the ability of a mass lesion to accumulate adrenocortical tracers to permit scintigraphic visualization.

Incidence

Adrenal masses are found in approximately 0.29–1.30 per cent of patients imaged with CT for reasons other than suspected adrenal pathology (Abecassis *et al.* 1985; Belldegrun *et al.* 1986; Glazer *et al.* 1982; Lopez *et al.* 1990). However, the incidence of adrenal adenoma at autopsies was reported to be from 1.45 to 15.50 per cent, depending on the size of the tumor and the age of the patient (Abecassis *et al.* 1985; Spain and Weinsaft 1964). Hedeland *et al.* (1968) found 64 adrenocortical adenomas of 0.2 cm and over in diameter among 739 consecutive autopsied patients aged over 20 years.

It is clear that a further increase in the prevalence of incidentally discovered masses may occur if the spatial resolving capacity of abdominal imaging technology progresses and if abdominal imaging is used more frequently.

Pathology

The clinical importance of adrenal incidentalomas depends on their pathology. They may represent both malignant and hypersecretory tumors but also abnormalities that do not require resection. Simple adrenal cyst, myelolipoma, and adrenal hematoma can usually be identified by CT alone (Moulton 1988).

In our department over the past 30 years, 287 adrenalectomies were performed on primary adrenal lesions for various reasons. Most of them were hypersecretory adrenal tumors including 111 aldosterone-producing adenomas, one hyperplasia causing primary aldosteronism, 62 cortical adenomas causing Cushing's syndrome, 4 hyperplasias causing Cushing's syndrome, 4 nodular hyperplasias causing Cushing's syndrome, 2 cortical carcinomas causing Cushing's syndrome, two virilizing tumors, one feminizing tumor, and 40 pheochromocytomas. Of the 287 cases with surgical adrenal diseases, 61 cases were incidentally discovered adrenal masses (Table 51.1). Fifteen cases of the 61 incidentalomas were hypersecretory tumors, including 11 cases of pheochromocytoma, one case of Cushing's syndrome, one primary aldosteronism, one 11-deoxycorticosterone (DOC)-producing tumor, and one feminizing tumor. Of the 61 incidentalomas, four proved to be adrenocortical carcinoma.

According to Gajraj and Young (1993) who reviewed 171 adrenal incidentalomas in 8 series, only eight (4.7 per cent) were

Table 51.1 Surgical pathology of incidentally discovered adrenal masses in 61 patients

Type	Number
Non-hypersecretory	
Cortical adenoma	26
Cortical carcinoma	2
Ganglioneuroma	5
Myelolipoma	5
Cyst	6
Hematoma	1
Hypersecretory	
Cortical adenoma	
Cushing's syndrome	1
Aldosteronism	1
DOC-producing tumor*	1
Cortical carcinoma	
Feminizing tumor	1
Virilizing tumor	1
Pheochromocytoma	11
Total	61

*DOC, 11-deoxycorticosterone.

primary carcinomas. Of 171 incidental adrenal masses, seven (4.1 per cent) were metastases with no obvious primary malignant condition. Metastatic adrenal carcinoma is extremely uncommon in the absence of an obvious primary lesion. Among patients known to have a malignancy, metastasis is the most common cause of an incidental adrenal mass. Belldegrun *et al.* (1986) described 33 patients with a known malignancy in association with an adrenal mass, of whom 24 were found to have an adrenal metastasie. In contrast, of 988 autopsy reports describing the adrenal gland, 73 glands were found to have a pathologic abnormality of which 50 (68 per cent) were metastases although most of the patients were already known to be suffering from malignant disease. Of the remaining 23 adrenal glands with a pathologic abnormality, 19 were cortical adenomas, two myelolipomas, one a hematoma, and one a pheochromocytoma. However, excluding metastatic malignant disease, most adrenal masses at autopsy proved to be benign cortical adenomas. This is also true of adrenal incidentaloma. Of 171 inci-

dentalomas described, 44 (2.5 per cent) proved to be cortical adenoma, only one of which was a hypersecretory tumor causing Cushing's syndrome. One adrenal incidentaloma was found to be a pheochromocytoma and was associated with firm biochemical evidence of catecholamine excess. Aso and Homma (1992) reported 210 cases of adrenal incidentaloma in a nationwide Japanese survey. The most common diagnosis was 69 nonfunctioning cortical adenomas, followed by 49 pheochromocytomas, 18 cysts, and 15 myelolipomas. A total of 14 malignant tumors (6.7 per cent) and 16 hypersecretory benign cortical lesions was also found.

Differential diagnosis of adrenal incidentaloma

Finding an 'incidentaloma' should alert the referring physician to re-examine the patients, looking for symptoms and signs of adrenocortical or adrenomedullary disease, or of a malignancy. Management of adrenal incidentaloma depends first on whether there is an excess of adrenal hormone and second on distinguishing between benign and malignant adrenal masses. The following is our diagnostic approach to incidentally discover adrenal masses (Table 51.2).

Diagnosis of hypersecretory masses

Hypersecretory masses require specific therapy, which is most often surgical extirpation. Evidence of excess secretion of cortisol, androgens, estrogens, mineralocorticoids, and catecholamines should be considered in the patient's history and physical examination. Clues obtained from this evaluation should obviously be pursued. However, the need for initial adequate biochemical screening of all adrenal masses without an obvious radiological diagnosis, regardless of a nonsuggestive history and examination, cannot be overemphasized.

Primary aldosteronism

Blood pressure and serum potassium should be measured in all patients to exclude mineralocorticoid excess. Sodium restriction

Table 51.2 Recommended biochemical screening tests and imaging studies for incidentally discovered adrenal masses in all patients unless specified*

Hypersecretory state	Screening test	Imaging study
Mineralocorticoid excess	Blood pressure	
	Serum potassium	
	Upright PRA and PAC	
Cushing's or pre-Cushing's syndrome	1 mg oral dexamethasone overnight suppression test	
Virilizing tumor	Serum DHES	
Feminizing tumor	Serum estradiol	
Pheochyromocytoma	Serum catecholamines	[^{123}I]- or [^{131}I]-MIBG scintigraphy
	24 hour urinary catecholamines	T2-weighted MRI
	24 hour urinary metanephrines	
Adrenocortical carcinoma	24 hour urinary steroid profiles	

*PRA, plasma renin activity; PAC, plasma aldosterone concentrations; DHES, dehydroepiandrosterone sulfate; MIBG, metaiodobenzylguanidine.

leads to potassium retention and minimizes hypokalemia. The amount of daily dietary sodium intake should be adequate when serum potassium is determined in these patients. In patients with hypertension, upright plasma renin activity (PRA) and plasma aldosterone concentration (PAC) should be determined. The presence of an elevated PAC along with suppressed PRA suggests the diagnosis of primary aldosteronism regardless of the patient's medications.

Patients taking β blockers and antisympathetic agents may have falsely reduced PRA values; however, these agents do not cause elevation of PAC. Meanwhile, calcium channel blockers may rarely increase PRA and reduce PAC to normal in patients with primary aldosteronism (Carpene *et al.* 1989). The presence of suppressed PRA and PAC with hypokalemia suggests the presence of suppressed PRA and PAC with hypokalemia suggests the presence non-aldosterone-mediated mineralocorticoid hypertension, such as in DOC-producing tumors.

Cushing's and pre-Cushing's syndrome

A large amount of data indicates that a spectrum of cortisol excess exists and that clinically obvious manifestations may occur relatively late along this spectrum, while loss of diurnal variation and loss of cortisol suppressibility often occur before baseline steroid hormone excretion exceeds established normal limits (Kloos *et al.* 1994). We followed up for 10 years a patient with bilateral adrenal adenoma that was initially non-hypersecretory. Excess of cortisol secretion gradually developed 8 years after the initial discovery of the masses. Central obesity, osteoporosis, and diabetes mellitus became obvious, when she underwent right adrenalectomy and left partial adrenalectomy (Figs 51.1 and 51.2). This case may suggest the functional shift of the adrenal incidentaloma from non-hypersecretory tumor to hypersecretory tumor and the existence of preclinical Cushing's or pre-Cushing's syndrome which is a term used to refer to biochemical evidence of Cushing's syndrome without physical stigmata. Thus, we recommend that the cortisol secretory status of patients with incidentalomas be initially investigated with an overnight 1.0 mg dexamethasone suppression test. The determination of cortisol secretory rhythm is also considered to be useful. However, studies to support surgical intervention in the absence of diurnal variation of cortisol level with a normal overnight dexamethasone suppression test and absence of physical stigmata of Cushing's syndrome are not available (Osella *et al.* 1994). The diagnosis and management of so-called pre-Cushing's syndrome has been controversial. In 1998, the Japanese Study Group of Adrenal Diseases proposed diagnostic criteria for preclinical Cushing's syndrome (Table 51.3). Patients with pre-Cushing's syndrome who are not being operated upon certainly require a more careful follow-up than those with small non-hypersecretory adrenal tumors.

Virilizing or feminizing tumor

Dehydroepiandrosterone sulfate (DHES) as a marker of adrenal androgen excess (and thus as a marker of adrenal carcinoma) should be measured in all incidentalomas. As the incidence of benign adrenocortical adenomas secreting masculinizing or feminizing hormones is rare, the determinations of testosterone or estradiol level are not considered as routine screening tests in

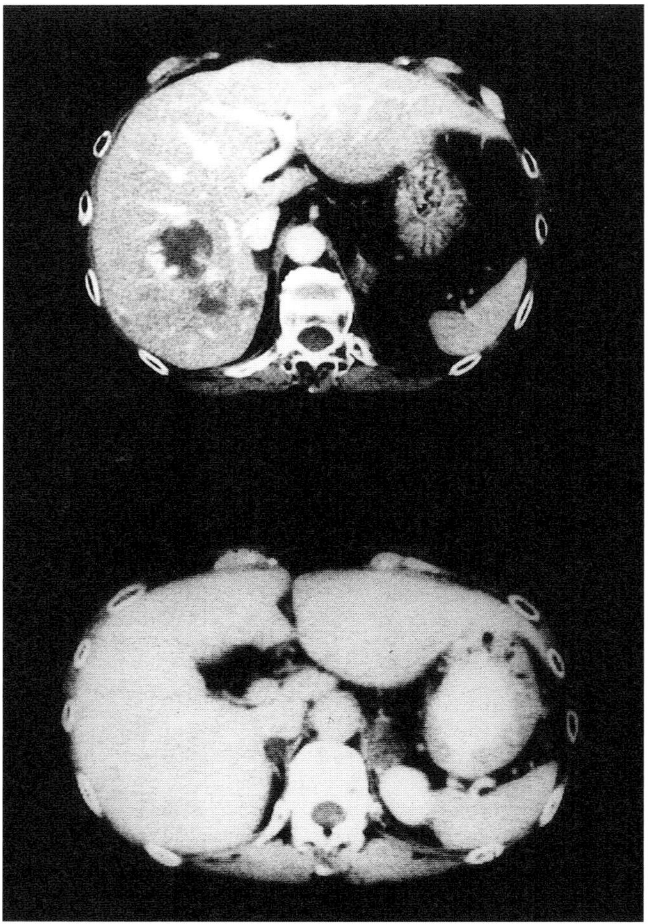

Fig. 51.1 A 62-year-old woman, who was initially found to have bilateral adrenal masses by CT scan, was followed up for 10 years until she developed Cushing's syndrome. Initial CT scan revealed bilateral adrenal mass (above). The masses were enlarged 10 years later (below).

asymptomatic patients. Congenital adrenal hyperplasia should always be considered in the differential diagnosis of androgen or mineralocorticoid excesses.

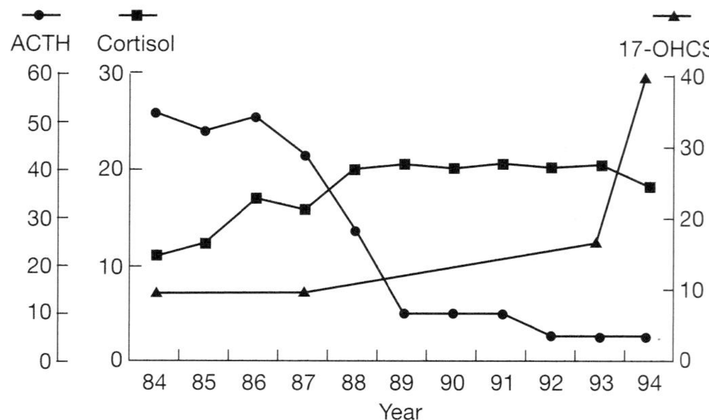

Fig. 51.2 Levels of serum cortisol, adrenocorticotropin (ACTH), and urinary 17-hydroxycorticosteroid (17-OHCS) of the patient with incidentally discovered bilateral adrenal masses in Fig. 51.1 as measured over a 10-year period.

Table 51.3 Diagnostic criteria for pre-clinical Cushing's syndrome

1	Adrenal tumor detected by imaging studies
2	Lack of clinical features of Cushing's syndrome
3	Laboratory findings*
	Normal level of serum cortisol
	Autonomous secretion of cortisol
	Suppression of ACTH level
	Accumulation of adrenocortical tracers in scintigraphy
	Lack of diurnal variation of cortisol level
	Low level of serum DHEA-S
	Adrenocortical malfunction after removal of the tumor

* One of the seven laboratory findings is necessary. ACTH, adrenocorticotropin; DHES, dehydroepiandrosterone sulfate.

Pheochromocytoma

Although a large percentage of pheochromocytomas are not diagnosed during lifetime, a tumor only discovered at autopsy may, in fact, have been the cause of death (Sutton *et al.* 1981). High mortality rates among patients with unsuspected pheochromocytoma who underwent surgery or anesthesia are well known. We, therefore, strongly advocate that a screening biochemical investigation should be done in all patients to exclude the possibility of pheochromocytoma. We reviewed 17 resected pheochromocytomas comprising 7 from symptomatic patients, and 10 unsuspected and incidentally discovered tumors (Miyajima *et al.* 1997). Although the clinical signs and findings in patients with incidental tumors were weaker than in those with symptomatic disease, they were correctly diagnosed by excess secretion of catecholamines.

MRI and [123]I- or ^{131}I-metaiodobenzylguanidine (MIBG) scintigraphy were also useful in diagnosing incidentally discovered pheochromocytoma (Figs 51.3 and 51.4). The utility of scintigraphy in patients with normal biochemistry and discordant adrenocortical scintigraphy is not yet determined.

Diagnosis of malignant tumor

Once an adrenal mass has been deemed hormonally non-hypersecretory, the possibility of primary or metastatic malignancy must be excluded. The mass, especially bilateral mass in patients known to have a malignancy, should be considered to be a metastasis. CT- or US-guided fine needle aspiration biopsy is occasionally indicated to diagnose metastatic malignancy. Primary adrenocortical carcinoma is rare. Ochiai *et al.* (1997) reported the usefulness of the US-guided needle biopsy for incidentally discovered adrenal tumors. Eighteen specimens of the 21 biopsies were pathologically adequate specimens and reported to be benign. Nakano (1988) reported that minotic activity is useful for diagnosis and vimentine-positive or cytokeration-positive findings are immunohistologically thought to be malignant. DNA histogram by flow cytometric analysis provides aneuploid patterns for malignant tumors but is not always reliable. Detection of telomerase activity seems an excellent method for the future (Hirano *et al.* 1998). However, it is not very easy to diagnose whether the tumor is malignant or not by biopsy specimen, and surgical treatment should not be determined by biopsy alone.

The determination of DHES level is valuable in differentiating primary adrenocortical carcinoma. We analyzed 24-hour urinary

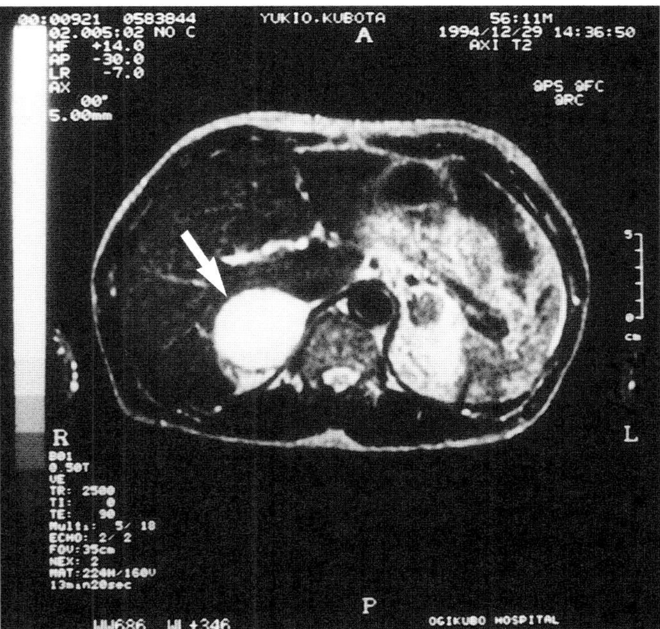

Fig. 51.3 A 57-year-old man who presented with epigastralgia was incidentally found to have bilateral adrenal mass on CT scan. The CT scan revealed a right adrenal mass measuring 5 cm in diameter with inhomogeneous enhancement of contrast (black arrow). A high-density mass measuring 2 cm in diameter was also visualized adjacent and anterior to the upper pole of the left kidney.

Fig. 51.4 T2-weighted MRI of the patient in Fig. 51.3 revealed high signal intensity of the right adrenal mass (white arrow) and relatively low intensity of the left adrenal mass. Pathologic study of the surgical specimen proved that it was pheochromocytoma of the right adrenal gland and cortical adenoma of the left adrenal gland.

steroids from patients with adrenocortical adenoma and carcinoma by gas chromatography/mass spectrometry (Kikuchi *et al.* 2000). Increased levels of metabolites of 11-deoxycortisol or 3-beta-hydroxy-5-ene steroids were observed in patients with adrenocortical carcinomas. By contrast, patients with adrenocortical adenomas from primary hyperaldosteronism had increased metabolites of 18-hydroxycorticosterone had increased metabolites of 18-hydroxycorticosterone and aldosterone, and those with Cushing's syndrome had elevated excretion of 11-deoxycortisol, cortisol, 18-hydroxycortisol, and cortisone metabolites.

Hormonally non-hypersecretory carcinomas tend to present in males and in older patients, with a larger size and at a more advanced clinical stage (Van Erkel *et al.* 1994). Attempts to separate benign from malignant lesions on the basis of anatomical imaging studies initially focused on size and subsequently on other characteristics. Belldegrun and co-workers (1986), reviewing six series, found that 105 of 114 adrenocortical carcinomas were more than 6 cm in size. Accordingly, solid adrenal lesions of more than 6 cm should be considered malignant until proven otherwise by exploration and adrenalectomy. The size of four adrenocortical carcinomas in our series ranged from 4.5 to 6.7 cm in diameter.

The masses less than 6 cm in diameter can be followed by serial CT scans at 6- to 12-month intervals. Enlargement of the masses is an indication for resection. Irregular margin of the mass or heterogeneous enhancement of the solid component with dynamic contrast enhancement may suggest the possibility of malignancy. The use of MRI to distinguish benign from malignant adrenal masses utilizing adrenal-to-liver signal intensity ratio on T2-weighted spin-echo images has been advocated (Fishman *et al.* 1987). On ^{131}I-6β-iodomethyl-norcholesterol adrenocortical scintigraphy, nonfunctioning primary and secondary malignancies of the adrenal gland demonstrate an imaging pattern of decreased or absent radiocholesterol uptake by the affected adrenal gland (Gross *et al.* 1987).

Management of incidentally discovered adrenal masses

Recently, laparoscopic or retroperitoneoscopic adrenalectomy has been performed as a minimally invasive procedure (Baba *et al.* 1997) Until 1993, incidentally discovered adrenal masses over 3 cm in diameter were resected in our series. However, surgical intervention for incidentally discovered adrenal masses should be limited to malignant or hypersecretory tumors. Management of the incidentaloma must be guided by the high prevalence of benign and clinically unimportant adrenal adenomas compared with the rarity of occult nonfunctioning adrenocortical carcinomas or hypersecretory adenomas (Fig. 51.5). We have operated on only two patients with incidentally discovered adrenal masses while 33 patients have been followed without surgery since 1994. Although hormonal assessments to differentiate hypersecretory tumor are important, particularly in small lesions, the potential benefit of early removal of the rare primary adrenal carcinoma must be balanced against the morbidity and mortality associated

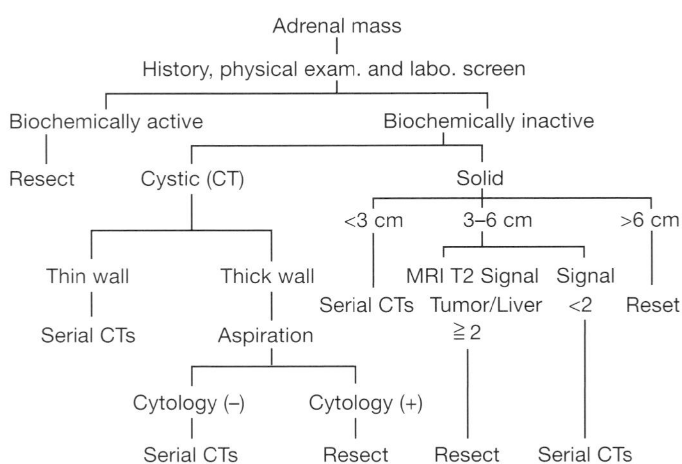

Fig. 51.5 Flow chart for management of incidentally discovered adrenal masses.

with surgery for the more common benign lesions. Serial CT and MRI can be applied in the follow-up of the masses less than 6 cm in diameter.

References

Abecassis, M.M., McLoughlin, M.J., Langer, B., and Kudlow, J.E. (1985). Serendipitous adrenal mass: prevalence, significance and management. *Am. Surg.* **149**, 783–8.

Aso, Y. and Homma, Y. (1992). A survey on incidental adrenal tumors in Japan. *J. Urol.* **147**, 1478–81.

Baba, S., Miyajima, A., Uchida, A., Asanuma, H., Miyakawa, A., and Murai, M. (1997). A posterior approach for retroperitoneoscopic adrenalectomy: assessment of surgical efficacy. *Urology* **50**, 19–24.

Belldegrun, A., Hussain, S., Selzer, S.E., Loughlin, K.R., Gittes, R.F., and Richie, J.P. (1986). Incidentally discovered mass of the adrenal gland. *Surg. Gynecol.* **163**, 203–8.

Carpene, G., Rocco, S., Opocher, G., and Mantero, F. (1989). Acute and chronic effect of nifedipine in primary aldosteronism. *Clin. Exp. Hypertens.* **11A**, 1263–72.

Fishman, E.K., Deutsch, B.M., Hartman, D.S., Goldman, S.M., Zerhouni, E.A., and Siegelman, S.S. (1987). Primary adrenocortical carcinoma: CT evaluation with clinical correlation. *Am. J. Roentgenol.* **148**, 531–5.

Gajraj, H. and Young, A.E. (1993). Adrenal incidentaloma. *Br. J. Surg.* **80**, 422–6.

Glazer, H.S., Weyman, P.J., Sagel, S.S., Levitt, R.G., and McClennan, B.L. (1982). Nonfunctioning adrenal masses: incidental discovery on computed tomography. *Am. J. Roentgenol.* **139**, 81–5.

Gross, M.D., Wilton, G.P., Shapiro, B., Cho, K., Samuels, B.I., Bouffard, J.A., Glazer, G., Grekin, R.J., and Brady, T. (1987). Functional and scintigraphic evaluation of the silent adrenal mass. *J. Nucl. Med.* **28**, 1401–7.

Hedeland, H., Ostberg, G., and Hokfelt, B. (1968). On the prevalence of adrenocortical adenomas in an autopsy material in relation to hypertension and diabetes. *Acta Med. Scand.* **184**, 211–14.

Hirano, Y., Fujita, K., Suzuki, K., Ushima, T., Ohtawara, Y., and Tsuda, F. (1998). Telomerase activity as an indicator of potentially malignant adrenal tumor. *Cancer* **83**, 772–6.

Kikuchi, E., Yanaihara, H., Nakashima, J., Homma, K., Ohigashi, T., Asakura, H., Tachibana, M., Shibana, H., Saruta, T., and Murai, M. (2000).

Urinary steroid profile in adrenocortical tumor. *Biomed. Pharmacother.* **54**, Suppl 1, 194–7.

Kloos, R.T., Gross, M.D., and Shapiro, B. (1994). Investigation of incidentally discovered, biochemically non-hypersecretory benign adrenal adenomas: a review of the current knowledge and areas for future investigation. *Intern. Med.* **2**, 9–15.

Lopez, J.M., Fardella, C., and Artega, E. (1990). Adrenal macrotumors diagnosed by computed tomography. *J. Endocrinol. Invest.* **13**, 581–5.

Miyajima, A., Nakashima, J., Baba, S., Tachibana, M., Nakamura, K., and Murai, M. (1997). Clinical experience with incidentally discovered pheochromocytoma. *J. Urol.* **157**, 1566–8.

Moulton, J.S. (1988). CT of the adrenal glands. *Sem. Roentgenol.* **33**, 288–303.

Nakano, M. (1988). Adrenocortical carcinoma. A clinicopathological and immunohistochemical study of 91 autopsy cases. *Acta Pathol. Jpn* **38**, 163–80.

Ochiai, A., Inui, E., Ukimura, O., Kojima, M., and Watanabe, H. (1997). Clinical evaluation of scintigraphy and tumor biopsy for incidentally detected adrenal masses. *Jpn J. Urol.* **88**, 807–17.

Osella, G., Terzolo, M., Borretta, G., Magro, G., Ali, A., Piovesan, A., Paccotti, P., and Angeli, A. (1994). Endocrine evaluation of incidentally disovered adrenal masses (incidentalomas). *J. Clin. Endocrinol. Metab.* **79**, 1532–9.

Spain, D.M. and Weinsaft, P. (1964). Solitary adrenal cortical adenomas in elderly females. *Arch. Pathol.* **78**, 231–3.

Sutton, M.G., Sheps, S.G., and Lie, J.T. (1981). Prevalence of clinically unsuspected pheochromocytoma. Review of a 50-year autopsy series. *Mayo Clin. Proc.* **56**, 354–60.

Van Erkel, A.R., van Gils, A.P., Lequin, M., Kruitwagen, C., Bloem, J.L., and Falke, T.H. (1994). CT and MR distinction of adenomas and non-adenomas of the adrenal gland. *J. Comput. Assist. Tomogr.* **18**, 432–8.

52. Diagnosis and treatment of primary aldosteronism

Jon D. Blumenfeld and E. Darracott Vaughan, Jr

Introduction

Primary aldosteronism is a syndrome characterized by hypertension, hypokalemia with renal potassium wasting, suppressed plasma renin activity (PRA), chloride-resistant metabolic alkalosis, and elevated levels of urinary and plasma aldosterone. The spectrum of adrenal disorders that now meet these diagnostic criteria extends beyond the functioning adrenal adenoma to include diagnostic subgroups with distinct physiologic and biochemical characteristics and with heterogeneous blood pressure responses to unilateral adrenalectomy (Biglieri *et al.* 1995). Although the prevalence of this disorder is thought to represent 0.5–2.0 per cent of all hypertension, this is probably an underestimate.

Diagnostic subsets (Table 52.1)

Aldosterone-producing adenoma (APA)

About two-thirds of all cases of primary aldosteronism are caused by an APA (Biglieri *et al.* 1995; Blumenfeld *et al.* 1994). Mineralocorticoid excess is more severe in APA than in idiopathic hyperaldosteronism (IHA), with higher systolic and diastolic pressures, lower serum potassium level, and more severe metabolic alkalosis. Aldosterone (ALDO) secretion by an APA is autonomous from renin–angiotensin, and is designated as angiotensin II unresponsive APA (AII-U APA). This feature provides a basis for preoperative diagnostic evaluation (see below) (Biglieri *et al.* 1995; Blumenfeld *et al.* 1994; Fontes *et al.* 1991; Gordon *et al.* 1987; Melby 1984). However, in fewer than 5 per cent of APA, ALDO production is stimulated by renin–angiotensin, as determined by the rise in aldosterone levels during exogenous angiotensin II (AII) infusion or postural stimulation (Gordon *et al.* 1987). This variant, referred to as AII-responsive aldosterone-producing adenoma (AII-R APA), has other unique biochemical and histological features. Unlike AII-U APA, in which 'hybrid' cortisol C18-oxygenated metabolites are overproduced (that is, 18-oxocortisol (18-oxo-F), 18-hydroxycortisol (18-OHF); see below), AII-R APA do *not* synthesize high levels of these steroids. In addition, plasma cortisol levels are suppressible in AII-U APA, but not in AII-R APA (Tunny *et al.* 1991). Although AII-R APA are much less common then AII-U APA, it appears that hypertension in both variants can be cured by unilateral adrenalectomy (Fontes *et al.* 1991).

Nonadenomatous adrenal hyperplasia

Bilateral adrenal hyperplasia associated with idiopathic hyperaldosteronism (IHA) occurs in about one-third of all cases of primary aldosteronism. Although the PRA level is low, ALDO production can be influenced by maneuvers that increase or decrease renin–angiotensin secretion and, therefore, this variant is not as autonomous as AII-U APA. Moreover, the magnitude of mineralocorticoid excess is less severe in IHA than in AII-U APA, with lower levels of 18-hydroxycorticosterone (18-OHB) and hybrid steroids (Biglieri *et al.* 1995; Irony *et al.* 1990).

A variant in which ALDO production is highly autonomous from renin–angiotensin, but in which an adenoma cannot be identified, has been referred to as primary adrenal hyperplasia (PAH) (Biglieri *et al.* 1995; Irony *et al.* 1990). The adrenals in this disorder are hyperplastic, frequently with a dominant nodule. As in patients with AII-U APA, metabolic abnormalities are corrected and hypertension is cured by unilateral adrenalectomy in PAH.

Adrenal carcinoma

This is a rare cause of primary aldosteronism (Arteaga *et al.* 1984; Vaughan and Blumenfeld 1998). Aldosterone production by the carcinoma is autonomous and markedly increased, causing severe hypokalemia. In contrast with APA, malignant tumors are quite large (> 5 cm), have internal calcification that is evident on computerized tomography (CT) scan, and may also produce excess amounts of androgens and cortisol. Metastasis often occurs prior to diagnosis and the prognosis is poor.

Table 52.1 Diagnostic subsets of primary aldosteronism

Aldosterone-producing adenoma (60–70%)
Angiotensin II unresponsive
Angiotensin II responsive
Nonadenomatous adrenal hyperplasia (25–35%)
Idiopathic hyperaldosteronsim (pseudoprimary)
Primary adrenal hyperplasia
Glucocorticoid-remediable aldosteronism (< 1%)

Monogenic forms of hypertension

Glucocorticoid-remediable aldosteronism (GRA)

This is an autosomal dominant form of mineralocorticoid hypertension in which ALDO biosynthesis is regulated by adrenocorticotropin (ACTH), rather than by the renin–angiotensin system (Lifton 1996; Lifton and Dluhy 1995). Clinical features include early onset hypertension, which may be complicated by cerebral hemorrhage or aortic dissection, and there is a strong family history of hypertension with target organ injury (Rich *et al.* 1992; Litchfield *et al.* 1998). The genetic defect is a chimeric $P\text{-}450_{11\beta}/P\text{-}450_{C18}$ gene that arises from unequal crossing over between the $5'$ regulatory region of $P\text{-}450_{11\beta}$ and the coding sequences of $P\text{-}450_{C18}$. This hybrid gene product can catalyze the terminal methyl oxidation reactions required for ALDO synthesis, but is regulated as the $P\text{-}450_{11\beta}$ by ACTH instead of by renin–angiotensin. The enzymatic product of this chimeric gene utilizes cortisol as a substrate for C18 oxidation to the cortisol–ALDO hybrid steroids (for example, 18-OHF). Affected family members may exhibit low renin hypertension and high urinary levels of hybrid steroids, but they may be overlooked because hypokalemia and other metabolic abnormalities (for example, hypokalemia) are often mild or absent (Rich *et al.* 1992; Litchfield *et al.* 1997). Therefore, genetic screening should be performed in all relatives of patient with GRA.

Treatment of this syndrome with low doses of exogenous glucocorticoid inhibits ACTH secretion, suppresses ALDO production, normalizes PRA, and corrects hypertension and other metabolic abnormalities. However, there is concern regarding the adverse effects associated with lifelong glucocorticoid administration (for example, osteoporosis). Alternative treatments include potassium-sparing diuretics, such as amiloride and spironolactone (Mantero *et al.* 1995).

Apparent mineralocorticoid excess

Normally, the mineralocorticoid receptor *in vitro* binds cortisol and aldosterone with equal affinity, whereas cortisone binding is less avid (Arriza *et al.* 1987). Although the serum concentration of cortisol is normally 1000-fold greater than that of aldosterone, cortisol is inactivated by conversion to cortisone at mineralocorticoid-responsive tissues by 11β-hydroxysteroid dehydrogenase (Funder 1995; Funder *et al.* 1988). This allows aldosterone, rather than cortisol, to gain access to the mineralocorticoid receptor. Thus, it is 11β-hydroxysteroid dehydrogenase rather than the mineralocorticoid receptor *per se* that confers tissue specificity for aldosterone.

Apparent mineralocorticoid excess (type 1) is characterized by hypertension, low PRA, low urinary aldosterone excretion rate, and increased urinary excretion of metabolites of cortisol rather than cortisone (an increased ratio of free cortisol:cortisone and terahydrocortisols:tetrahydrocortisone) (Stewart 1999). The disorder is caused by reduced conversion of cortisol to cortisone due to impaired activity of the type 1 isoenzyme of 11β-hydroxysteroid dehydrogenase (11β-HSD) (Ulick *et al.* 1979). The serum cortisol is normal and does not aid in the diagnosis. Homozygous inactivating mutations of this enzyme have been identified in patients with apparent mineralocorticoid excess (AME) (Dave-Sharma *et al.* 1998). Treatment options include (1) blockade of either the mineralocorticoid receptor (for example, spironolactone) or the renal apical sodium channel (for example, amiloride), or (2) suppression of endogenous cortisol production with dexamethasone, which has a low affinity for the mineralocorticoid receptor.

Licorice ingestion can cause hypertension with features that are similar to those of AME (Dave-Sharma *et al.* 1998). Glycerrhyzic acid, and its hydrolytic product (glycyrrhytenic acid), are the active ingredients of licorice that inhibit 11β-HSD and thereby allow cortisol to gain access to the mineralocorticoid receptor.

In patients with Cushing's syndrome, cortisol can become the active mineralocorticoid, especially in the ectopic ACTH syndrome where cortisol secretion is extremely high. In this disorder, mechanisms of cortisol inactivation are overwhelmed, allowing it to gain access to the mineralocorticoid receptor (Ulick *et al.* 1992*a*).

Liddle's syndrome

Liddle's syndrome is an autosomal dominant condition characterized by low renin hypertension, hypokalemia, renal potassium wasting, and low levels of aldosterone (Warnock 1998). The genetic defects responsible for this syndrome are deletion mutations in the C-terminus of the β/γ subunits of the renal epithelial sodium channel (ENaC) (Hansson *et al.* 1995; Schild *et al.* 1995). These gain of function mutations lead to constitutive activation of ENaC, resulting in electrogenic sodium reabsorption and kaliuresis. Amiloride, which blocks the apical sodium channel, is effective treatment. By contrast, mineralocorticoid receptor blockade (for example, spironolactone) is ineffective because renin, angiotensin II, and aldosterone levels are all suppressed by the sodium-dependent hypertension.

Diagnostic strategies

There are no clinical features that reliably distinguish primary aldosteronism from essential hypertension or other hypertensive disorders. Several laboratory tests are available to screen the hypertensive patient population for primary aldosteronism and thus identify patients with curable forms of this syndrome.

Serum potassium concentration

Spontaneous hypokalemia with urinary potassium wasting ($\geq$ 40 mEq/24 hours) is the hallmark of hyperaldosteronism. Hypokalemia attenuates aldosterone production and, therefore,

Table 52.2 Diagnostic tests

Plasma renin activity
24-hour urine aldosterone, cortisol, Na, K, creatinine
Plasma aldosterone-to-renin ratio
Serum 18-hydroxycorticosterone
24-hour urine 18-hydroxycortisol
Postural stimulation test
Sodium loading
Adrenal vein sampling during ACTH infusion
Adrenal CT scan

aldosterone excretion rates may be underestimated when serum K levels are very low. However, serum K levels between 3.5 and 4.0 mEq/l occur in about 20 per cent of untreated patients with primary aldosteronism and hypokalemia is less severe when dietary Na intake is restricted. Therefore, dietary loading of Na (daily intake ≥ 5 grams (> 200 mEq)) and K (≥ 80 mEq/day) is required during diagnostic evaluation (Blumenfeld *et al.* 1994).

In contrast to most patients with primary aldosteronism in whom serum K levels are low, GRA patients characteristically have normal serum K levels despite the moderate-to-severe hypertension and suppressed PRA level. This may be due to the blunted rise in aldosterone secretion during K loading in GRA patients, which, together with the diurnal fall in ACTH-mediated aldosterone secretion, produces a milder degree of hyperaldosteronism and potassium wasting (Litchfield *et al.* 1997).

Renin system profiling

An elevated 24-hour urine ALDO level indexed against urinary Na and K excretion, together with a corresponding low PRA, are the hallmark features of primary aldosteronism (Biglieri *et al.* 1995). However, this information does not distinguish APA from other diagnostic subsets and therefore does not predict the potential for surgical cure.

Aldosterone-to-renin ratio

The relative autonomy of ALDO secretion from renin–angiotensin can also be expressed as the ratio of plasma ALDO (PA; expressed as ng/dl) to PRA (expressed as ng/ml/h). Accordingly, the PA/PRA ratio ≥ 50 is a useful screening test for primary aldosteronism (Blumenfeld *et al.* 1994; Gordon *et al.* 1995; Gomez-Sanchez 1998). However, there is considerable overlap between APA and other variants of primary aldosteronism, so this index cannot differentiate diagnostic subsets or reliably predict surgical cure.

Sodium loading

In primary aldosteronism, renin secretion is chronically suppressed, so that additional volume expansion does not further reduce ALDO levels (Biglieri *et al.* 1995). Sodium loading can be achieved by increasing dietary Na intake (≥ 200 mEq/day for 3 days), or oral fludrocortisone (Florinef 0.4 mg/day for 5 days). On a high-Na diet, 24-hour urinary ALDO excretion is below 10 μg in normal individuals, but exceeds 14 μg in primary aldosteronism. After intravenous saline (1.25–2 liters over 90–120 minutes), a ratio of serum 18-OHB to cortisol > 3 identifies patients with AII-U APA, but is lower in idiopathic hyperaldosteronism. Alternatively, acute Na depletion by furosemide stimulates renin in essential hypertension but not in primary aldosteronism. However, this test does not discriminate surgically curable subsets of the syndrome.

Posture test

During the postural stimulation test, plasma levels of ALDO and cortisol are drawn at 8:00 a.m. while supine, after an overnight recumbence, and again while upright after 2 to 4 hours of ambulation (Fontes *et al.* 1991). In normal subjects and in essential hypertension, upright posture stimulates renin–angiotensin secretion and, consequently, plasma ALDO levels rise acutely. By contrast, in curable subsets of primary aldosteronism (that is, AII-U APA and PAH), during upright posture ALDO either falls or increases by less than 30 per cent above the supine level. This 'paradoxical' response reflects the diurnal fall in ACTH, which is normally a minor stimulus of ALDO secretion, but is unmasked by the complete suppression of renin secretion. In GRA, ALDO production also falls during the posture test because ALDO biosynthesis is stimulated by ACTH, potentially confounding the distinction between GRA and surgically curable forms of primary aldosteronism.

Response to spironolactone

Preoperative treatment with spironolactone at high doses (400 mg/day) for 3 to 5 weeks decreases blood pressure (BP) to normal in patients with an adenoma who are most likely to have their high BP cured by unilateral adrenalectomy (Celen *et al.* 1996). By contrast, in patients with idiopathic hyperaldosteronism, blood pressure often remains high during monotherapy with spironolactone. Therefore, this has been advocated as a screening test for identifying surgically curable forms of primary aldosteronism. However, patients with low renin essential hypertension may also become normotensive during treatment with spironolactone, so that the additional biochemical evaluation described herein is required to confirm the diagnosis of primary aldosteronism.

Steroid metabolites

Urinary excretion of C18 methyloxygenated metabolites of cortisol (that is, 18-OHF and 18-oxo-F) are elevated in patients with APA, but not in those with idiopathic hyperaldosteronism or AII-R-APA (Gordon *et al.* 1987; Ulick *et al.* 1992*b*). Although very high levels are also found in GRA, a comparable genetic mutation has not been reported in patients with APA.

Adrenal localization

Lateralization of ALDO secretion to one adrenal gland is a characteristic of patients who are most likely to have a significant reduction in BP after unilateral adrenalectomy. Successful catheterization can be confirmed by simultaneous measurements of cortisol and ALDO in adrenal vein samples obtained during exogenous ACTH infusion (cosyntropin 250 μg in 500 ml dextrose, infused at 50 ml/hour beginning 30 minutes prior to and during the sampling procedure). Lateralization is defined as an ALDO level greater than 10-fold higher in the ipsilateral adrenal vein or, alternatively, an ipsilateral ratio (adrenal (aldosterone/cortisol ratio))/(IVC (aldosterone/cortisol ratio)) > 1 and a ratio < 1 from the contralateral gland (Blumenfeld *et al.* 1994; Melby 1984; Celen *et al.* 1996).

Although contrast-enhanced CT scan could identify adenoma with a diameter of about 5–10 mm, radiographic evaluation may be misleading. For example, IHA with a dominant nodule may be incorrectly interpreted as an adenoma or, alternatively, the adrenal may appear normal or hyperplastic in surgically curable disease. Magnetic resonance imaging (MRI) currently has lower spatial resolution than CT scan and, therefore, is less useful for identifying APA. Adrenal scintigraphy with ^{131}I iodocholesterol is generally less sensitive than other localizing techniques and is not routinely used at our center. Therefore, contrast-enhanced CT scan and adrenal vein sampling of ALDO and cortisol during ACTH-stimulation are the preferred methods for visualizing the adrenals and determining whether ALDO secretion lateralizes.

It is important to recognize that incidental, nonfunctioning masses ('incidentalomas') occur in 0.6 per cent of all CT scans of the abdomen, and 2 to 9 per cent of adults have grossly visible adenomas at autopsy (Vaughan and Blumenfeld 1998). Therefore, to avoid unnecessary, expensive, and invasive procedures that may provide inconclusive or misleading results, radiographic imaging and adrenal venous sampling should be withheld until after biochemical confirmation of primary aldosteronism.

The sensitivity and specificity of the diagnostic maneuvers described above can be adversely influenced by concurrent use of antihypertensive medications. For example, β-adrenoceptor antagonists and clonidine both suppress PRA in essential hypertension and may confound the interpretation of these tests (Ulick *et al.* 1992*b*). Hypokalemia, when caused by thiazide or loop diuretics in essential hypertension, may be difficult to distinguish from primary aldosteronism, although the PRA level is usually elevated during diuretic use (Blumenfeld *et al.* 1994; Laragh and Sealey 1992; Vaughan *et al.* 1978; Weber *et al.* 1977). Angiotensin-converting enzyme (ACE) inhibitors reportedly reduce ALDO biosynthesis and improve hypokalemia in some patients with idiopathic hyperaldosteronism (Melby 1984). Therefore, antihypertensive medications should be discontinued for at least 2 weeks before diagnostic evaluation and potassium supplements provided to hypokalemic patients. Spironolactone and other diuretics should be discontinued for at least 1 month before these biochemical tests because of their prolonged effects on the renin system.

Figure 52.1 is a diagnostic algorithm for the evaluation of primary aldosteronism. Surgery may be recommended, without additional testing, in a patient with biochemical criteria for primary aldosteronism, if CT scan identifies a solitary unilateral adrenal mass in an otherwise normal gland. Although adrenal vein sampling is not essential in this case, lateralization of ALDO secretion confirms the diagnosis and indicates a high likelihood of surgical cure. Therefore, we recommend adrenal vein sampling in all patients with primary aldosteronism prior to unilateral adrenalectomy. In addition, we recommend a more comprehensive evaluation because of the limitations of radiographic imaging and the relatively high rate of persistent hypertension after unilateral adrenalectomy (see below). This preoperative evaluation is followed by several weeks of adequate control of hypertension and correction of hypokalemia and other metabolic abnormalities.

When biochemical criteria for primary aldosteronism are confirmed, but the patient's adrenal CT scan is normal or indicates hyperplasia, additional evaluation is required before

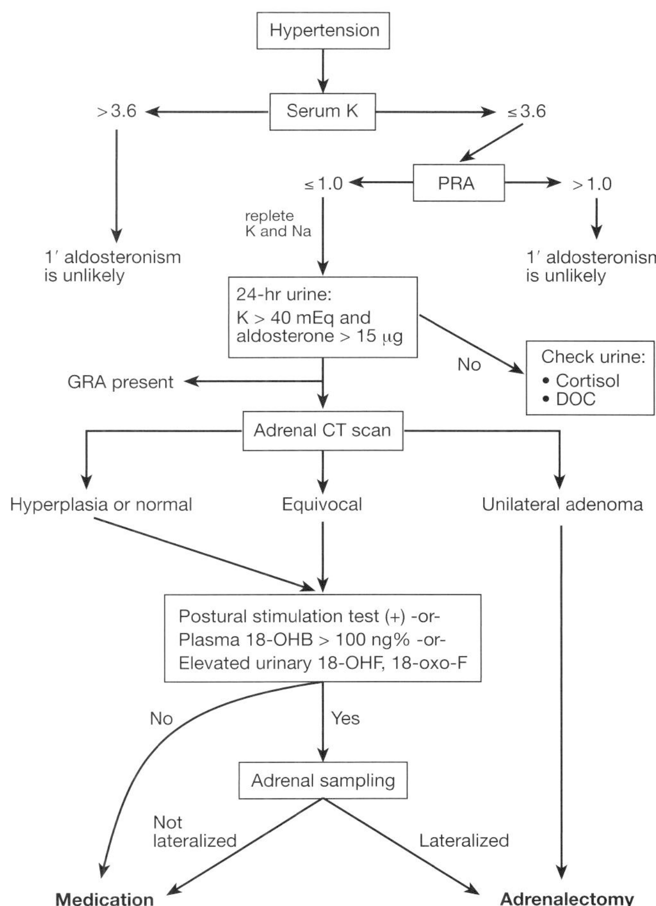

Fig. 52.1 Algorithm for evaluating and treating patients with primary aldosteronism. 18-OHB, 18 hydroxycorticosterone; 18-OHF, 18-hydroxycortisol; 18-oxo-F, 18-oxocortisol; CT, computerized tomography; DOC, deoxycorticosterone; PRA, plasma renin activity, GRA, glucocorticoid-remediable aldosteronism (adapted from Blumenfeld *et al.* (1994)).
ng% = ng/dl

resigning the patient to lifelong antihypertensive medication, because a subgroup can be cured by unilateral adrenalectomy (Biglieri *et al.* 1995; Blumenfeld *et al.* 1994). Additional diagnostic tests, which suggest the potential for surgical cure, include a positive postural stimulation test, lateralization of ALDO secretion, and elevated levels of plasma 18-OHB and urinary 18-OHF. Adrenalectomy is not indicated if the patient has bilateral ALDO secretion, a negative postural stimulation test, and low levels of these cortisol metabolites. If secretion is bilateral, or sampling is unsuccessful and the ancillary diagnostic tests described above indicate autonomous ALDO production, then the patient should be treated medically and re-evaluated in 6 to 12 months, including adrenal vein sampling.

When primary aldosteronism is confirmed by biochemical and hormonal measurements, all patients should undergo genetic screening for GRA because of the profound implications regarding treatment and clinical outcome for the patient and their family.

Table 52.3 Drug treatment for primary aldosteronism

Drug	Action	Indication	Advantage	Disadvantage
Spironolactone	Competitive antagonist of aldosterone for mineralcorticoid receptor	All patients	Effective control of hypertension and metabolic abnormalities	Gynecomastia, menstrual irregularity, nausea
Amiloride	Epithelial Na channel blocker	Intolerance to spironolactone	Few side-effects	Less effective in many patients
Triamterene	K-sparing diuretic	Intolerance to spironolactone and amiloride	Few side-effects	Less effective than amiloride or spironolactone; may form renal calculi
Hydrochlorothiazide	Kaliuretic diuretic	Potentiates diuretic action of K-sparing diuretics	If side-effects, can reduce dose of spironolactone	Provokes hypokalemia if used without K-sparing diuretic
Calcium channel blockers (verapamil, diltiazem, dihydropyridine)	Blockade calcium-mediated vasoconstriction and aldosterone production; natriuretic	Incomplete blood pressure response to spironolactone or other K-sparing diuretic	Effectively lowers blood pressure	Short-acting agents have been associated with cardiovascular complications and bleeding
ACE inhibitors	Inhibit angiotensin II formation and angiotensin-mediated aldosterone production	Selected patients with idiopathic hyperaldosteronism and AII-R adenoma	May reduce requirement for spironolactone	Not very effective in most patients

Medical treatment

Diuretics

Medical treatment is required initially for all patients to reduce BP and correct metabolic abnormalities, regardless of whether surgery is also planned. The cornerstone of medical therapy is spironolactone, an antagonist of aldosterone binding to the mineralocorticoid receptor (MR) (Fanestil 1988). Spironolactone also attenuates ALDO production in patients with APA, but not in those with IHA (Kater *et al.* 1983). This inhibitory effect does not occur when diuretics other than spironolactone are used (for example, amiloride).

The antihypertensive efficacy of spironolactone relates to the reduction in plasma volume (Bravo *et al.* 1973). Although a low dose (for example, ≤ 50 mg/day) will usually correct hypokalemia and metabolic alkalosis within a few days, higher doses are usually required for antihypertensive efficacy. Therefore, we begin with 50 mg twice a day and continue this dose for at least 2 to 4 weeks. Side-effects commonly occur when the daily dose exceeds 100 mg. If hypertension persists and there are no side-effects, then the dose is increased by 25 mg/day at 2 to 4 week intervals. If side-effects occur, the dose should be reduced and hydrochlorothiazide 25 mg/day added. A reactive rise in PRA occurs at doses that reduce extracellular volume and BP. However, this preoperative rise in renin does not hasten the postoperative recovery of ALDO production by the contralateral adrenal gland (Bravo *et al.* 1975). Although the antihypertensive response to spironolactone has been associated with improved chances of surgical cure, it does not reliably predict outcome for all diagnostic subgroups (Celen *et al.* 1996) (see above).

Side-effects of spironolactone include painful gynecomastia, erectile dysfunction, decreased libido, and menstrual irregularities that are caused by nonspecific binding to cellular receptors for progesterone and dihydrotesterone. In a study of 182 patients with essential hypertension treated with spironolactone, daily doses of 75–100 mg/day lowered blood pressure as effectively as 150–300 mg/day. Overall, gynecomastia developed in 13 per cent of patients and its occurrence was dose-related—6.9 per cent of patients taking 50 mg/day were symptomatic compared with 52 per cent of those taking a dose of 150 mg/day or more (de Gasparo *et al.* 1989). Compounds such as eplerenone that possess a high affinity for the MR but low affinity for the androgen and progesterone receptors have been synthesized and are promising substitutes for spironolactone (Delyani, 2000).

Other common side-effects associated with spironolactone include nausea and anorexia. Prerenal azotemia and hyper-kalemia can occur, especially at higher doses in patients with pre-existing renal insufficiency, so that serum electrolytes, creatinine, and blood urea nitrogen (BUN) should be measured at monthly intervals until a stable dose is achieved. Addition of a thiazide diuretic potentiates the antihypertensive effect of spironolactone but rarely causes hypokalemia (Bravo *et al.* 1973).

Amiloride inhibits Na reabsorption by directly blocking the apical Na channel of the principal cell in the collecting duct. This agent can effectively lower BP and correct hypokalemia. It is indicated for use in patients who are unable to tolerate side-effects related to spironolactone (Mantero *et al.* 1995). The effective daily dose of amiloride ranges from 10 to 30 mg/day.

Triamterene is a relatively weak potassium-sparing diuretic that inhibits Na reabsorption and potassium secretion at the distal nephron. The daily dose ranges from 50 to 300 mg. Although triamterene has been identified in renal calculi from treated patients, the pathogenic role of the diuretic in stone formation has not been established.

Calcium channel blockers

Dihydropyridine calcium channel antagonists can acutely decrease BP and ALDO secretion (Litchfield and Dluhy 1995). Studies of longer duration, however, failed to demonstrate these beneficial effects when nifedipine was used as monotherapy. However, when used in combination with potassium-sparing diuretics, in patients who remain hypertensive during diuretic monotherapy, calcium channel blockers effectively lower blood pressure. Based upon evidence of increased risks reported with short-acting calcium channel blockers (for example, nifedipine) in other hypertensive and cardiovascular disorders, these agents should be avoided in patients with primary aldosteronism (Grossman *et al.* 1996). Although longer-acting calcium blockers (diltiazem and verapamil) can also effectively lower blood pressure, they should used with caution.

Other treatments

ACE inhibitors have been reported to effectively control hypertension in IHA (Melby 1984). Presumably, AII receptor (AT1) antagonists will be as effective for these ACE-inhibitor-responsive patients. In our experience, ACE inhibitors and other anti-renin agents (that is, β-blockers) are ineffective as monotherapy for the treatment of primary aldosteronism. However, these agents may reduce blood pressure in patients who are resistant to diuretic monotherapy. As in essential hypertension, the reactive rise in the renin–angiotensin level that is stimulated by diuretic therapy promotes angiotensin-mediated vasoconstriction. In this circumstance, addition of a β-blocker, ACE inhibitor, or angiotensin II receptor antagonist can further reduce BP (Laragh and Sealey 1992; Vaughan *et al.* 1978).

Phentolamine reportedly did not acutely reduce BP in patients with primary aldosteronism, therefore, a role for α-adrenergic receptor blockade has not been established (Bravo *et al.* 1985). Nevertheless, long-term treatment with prazosin is effective in low-renin essential hypertension, suggesting that α-adrenergic receptor blockade may have an ancillary role in the treatment of primary aldosteronism.

Surgical outcomes

Patients with primary aldosteronism who demonstrate autonomous ALDO production should be managed with excision of the adrenal gland containing the adenoma or, when an adenoma cannot be identified, the gland from which ALDO secretion is predominant (Biglieri *et al.* 1995; Blumenfeld *et al.* 1994). Both the metabolic abnormalities and the hypertension are alleviated by unilateral adrenalectomy in most of these patients. By contrast, patients with IHA usually do not have significant improvement in hypertension after unilateral or bilateral adrenalectomy.

In the Cornell study, hypertension was cured postoperatively (BP $\leq$ 140/90 mm Hg, without concurrent antihypertensive medication) in about 35 per cent of patients with an APA (Blumenfeld *et al.* 1994). Hypertension improved after adrenalectomy in another 56 per cent of the APA group (BP < 140/90 mm Hg or lower with medication). Thus, hypertension was either cured or improved in more than 90 per cent of the patients with APA. Hypertension was more difficult to control in APA patients who were unable or unwilling to undergo adrenalectomy. Of the small group of patients with nonadenomatous hyperplasia who underwent adrenalectomy, 37 per cent were cured. When data were pooled from those adenoma and hyperplasia patients who were cured by adrenalectomy, they were found to be significantly younger than those who required antihypertensive medication postoperatively. In addition, preoperative PRA $\leq$ 0.2 was an important predictor of surgical cure.

There are a variety of surgical approaches to the adrenal gland, which are reviewed in detail in Chapter 57. The proper technique to use depends upon the underlying adrenal disorder, the size of the adrenal gland and associated lesion, the body habitus, and the experience and preference of the surgeon. This requires a collaborative effort between the internist, anesthesiologist, and surgeon.

Summary

Disorders of the adrenal cortex and medulla are often associated with hypertension, which, in many cases, can be cured surgically or which may require specific medical treatments. Therefore, knowledge of adrenal physiology, biochemistry, and molecular biology is essential so that an appropriate diagnostic evaluation can be conducted efficiently. The most common hypertensive disorder of the adrenal cortex is primary aldosteronism. Aldosterone-producing adenoma is the most common form of this syndrome and is most likely to be cured by unilateral adrenalectomy. Characteristics that increase the likelihood of surgical cure include aldosterone production that is highly autonomous from renin– angiotensin, that lateralizes to one adrenal gland, and that is associated with overproduction of 18-hydroxycorticosterone and C18-methyloxygenated metabolites of cortisol. Variants of adrenal hyperplasia that share these characteristics can also be cured by unilateral adrenalectomy. Variants of mineralocorticoid hypertension and of apparent mineralocorticoid excess syndromes with Mendelian patterns of inheritance should be considered in the differential diagnosis of primary aldosteronism.

References

Arriza, J.L., Weinberger, C., Cerelli, G., *et al.* (1987). Cloning of human mineralocorticoid receptor complementary DNA: structural and functional kinship with the glucocorticoid receptor. *Science* **237**, 268–75.

Arteaga, E., Biglieri, E.G., Kater, C.E., Lopez, J.M., and Schambelan, M. (1984). Aldosterone-producing adrenocortical carcinoma. Preoperative recognition and course in three cases. *Ann. Intern. Med.* **101**, 316–21.

Biglieri, E., Kater, C., and Mantero, F. (1995). Adrenocortical forms of human hypertension. In *Hypertension: pathophysiology, diagnosis and management*, Vol. 2 (ed. J. Laragh and B. Brenner), pp. 2145–62. Raven Press, New York.

Blumenfeld, J.D., Sealey, J.E., Schlussel, Y., *et al.* (1994). Diagnosis and treatment of primary hyperaldosteronism [see comments]. *Ann. Intern. Med.* **121**, 877–85.

Bravo, E., Dustan, H., and Tarazi, R. (1973). Spironolactone as a non-specific treatment for primary aldosteronism. *Circulation* **48**, 491–8.

Bravo, E., Dustan, H., and Tarazi, R. (1975). Selective hypoaldosteronism despite prolonged pre-and postoperative hyperreninema in primary aldosteronism. *J. Clin. Endocrinol. Metab.* **41**, 611–17.

Bravo, E., Tarazi, R., Dustan, H., and Fouad, F. (1985). The sympathetic nervous system and hypertension in primary aldosteronism. *Hypertension* **7**, 90–6.

Celen, O., O'Brien, M., Melby, J., and Beazeley, R. (1996). Factors influencing outcome of surgery for primary aldosteronism. *Arch. Surg.* **131**, 646–50.

Dave-Sharma, S., Wilson, R.C., Harbison, M.D., *et al.* (1998). Examination of genotype and phenotype relationships in 14 patients with apparent mineralocorticoid excess. *J. Clin. Endocrinol. Metab.* **83**, 2244–54.

de Gasparo, M., Whitebread, S.E., Preiswerk, G., Jeunemaitre, X., Corvol, P., and Menard, J. (1989). Antialdosterones: incidence and prevention of sexual side effects. *J. Steroid Biochem.* **32**, 223–7.

Delyani, J.A. (2000). Mineralcorticoid receptor antagonists: the evolution of utility and pharmacology. *Kidney Int.* **57**, 1408–11.

Fanestil, D. (1988). Mechanism of action of aldosterone blockers. *Sem. Nephrol.* **8**, 249–63.

Fontes, R., Kater, C., Biglieri, E., and Irony, I. (1991). Reassessment of the predictive value of the postural stimulation test in primary aldosteronism. *Am. J. Hypertens.* **4**, 786–91.

Funder, J.W. (1995). Apparent mineralocorticoid excess. *Endocrinol. Metab. Clin. N. Am.* **24**, 613–21.

Funder, J.W., Pearce, P.T., Smith, R., and Smith, A.I. (1988). Mineralocorticoid action: target tissue specificity is enzyme, not receptor, mediated. *Science* **242**, 583–5.

Gomez-Sanchez, C.E. (1998). Primary aldosteronism and its variants. *Cardiovasc. Res.* **37**, 8–13.

Gordon, R.D., Gomez-Sanchez, C.E., Hamlet, S.M., Tunny, T.J., and Klemm, S.A. (1987). Angiotensin-responsive aldosterone-producing adenoma masquerades as idiopathic hyperaldosteronism (IHA: adrenal hyperplasia) or low-renin essential hypertension. *J. Hypertens. Suppl.* **5**, S103–6.

Gordon, R.D., Stowasser, M., Klemm, S.A., and Tunny, T.J. (1995). Primary aldosteronism—some genetic, morphological, and biochemical aspects of subtypes. *Steroids* **60**, 35–41.

Grossman, E., Messerli, F.H., Grodzicki, T., and Kowey, P. (1996). Should a moratorium be placed on sublingual nifedipine capsules given for hypertensive emergencies and pseudoemergencies? [see comments]. *J. Am. Med. Assoc.* **276**, 1328–31.

Hansson, J.H., Nelson-Williams, C., Suzuki, H., *et al.* (1995). Hypertension caused by a truncated epithelial sodium channel gamma subunit: genetic heterogeneity of Liddle syndrome. *Nat. Genet.* **11**, 76–82.

Irony, I., Kater, C.E., Biglieri, E.G., and Shackleton, C.H. (1990). Correctable subsets of primary aldosteronism. Primary adrenal hyperplasia and renin responsive adenoma. *Am. J. Hypertens.* **3**, 576–82.

Kater, C., Biglieri, E., Schambelan, M., and Aretaga ,E. (1983). Studies of impaired aldosterone response to spironolactone-induced renin and

potassium elevations in adenomatous but not hyperplastic primary aldosteronism. *Hypertension* **5**, V115–V121.

Laragh, J.H. and Sealey, J.E. (1992). Renin–angiotensin–aldosterone system and the renal regulation of sodium, potassium, and blood pressure homeostasis. In *Handbook of physiology*, Vol. II. *Renal physiology* (ed. E.E. Windhager), pp. 1409–541. Oxford Press, New York.

Lifton, R. (1996). Molecular genetics of human blood pressure variation. *Science* **272**, 676–80.

Lifton, R. and Dluhy, R. (1995). Inherited forms of mineralocorticoid hypertension. In *Hypertension: pathophysiology, diagnosis and management*, Vol. 2 (ed. J. Laragh and B. Brenner), pp. 2163–6. Raven Press, New York.

Litchfield, W. and Dluhy, R. (1995). Primary aldosteronism. *Endocrinol. Metab. Clin. N. Am.* **24**, 593–612.

Litchfield, W.R., Coolidge, C., Silva, P., *et al.* (1997). Impaired potassium-stimulated aldosterone production: a possible explanation for normokalemic glucocorticoid-remediable aldosteronism [see comments]. *J. Clin. Endocrinol. Metab.* **82**, 1507–10.

Litchfield, W.R., Anderson, B.F., Weiss, R.J., Lifton, R.P., and Dluhy, R.G. (1998). Intracranial aneurysm and hemorrhagic stroke in glucocorticoid-remediable aldosteronism. *Hypertension* **31**, 445–50.

Mantero, F., Opocher, G., Rocco, S., and Armanini, D. (1995). Long-term treatment of mineralocorticoid excess syndromes. *Steroids* **60**, 81–6.

Melby, J. (1984). Primary aldosteronism. *Kidney Int.* **26**, 769–78.

Rich, G.M., Ulick, S., Cook, S., Wang, J.Z., Lifton, R.P., and Dluhy, R.G. (1992). Glucocorticoid-remediable aldosteronism in a large kindred: clinical spectrum and diagnosis using a characteristic biochemical phenotype. *Ann. Intern. Med.* **116**, 813–20.

Schild, L., Canessa, C.M., Shimkets, R.A., Gautschi, I., Lifton, R.P., and Rossier, B.C. (1995). A mutation in the epithelial sodium channel causing Liddle disease increases channel activity in the *Xenopus laevis* oocyte expression system. *Proc. Natl Acad. Sci., USA* **92**, 5699–703.

Stewart, P.M. (1999). Mineralocorticoid hypertension. *Lancet* **353**, 1341–7.

Tunny, T.J., Gordon, R.D., Klemm, S.A., and Cohn, D. (1991). Histological and biochemical distinctiveness of atypical aldosterone-producing adenomas responsive to upright posture and angiotensin. *Clin. Endocrinol. (Oxford)* **34**, 363–9.

Ulick, S., Levine, L.S., Gunczler, P., *et al.* (1979). A syndrome of apparent mineralocorticoid excess associated with defects in the peripheral metabolism of cortisol. *J. Clin. Endocrinol. Metab.* **49**, 757–64.

Ulick, S., Wang, J.Z., Blumenfeld, J.D., and Pickering, T.G. (1992*a*). Cortisol inactivation overload: a mechanism of mineralocorticoid hypertension in the ectopic adrenocorticotropin syndrome [see comments]. *J. Clin. Endocrinol. Metab.* **74**, 963–7.

Ulick, S., Blumenfeld, J., Atlas, S., Wang, J., and Vaughan, E.J. (1992*b*). The unique steroidogenesis of the aldosteronoma in the differential diagnosis of primary aldosteronism. *J. Clin. Endocrinol. Metab.* **76**, 873–8.

Vaughan, E.J. and Blumenfeld, J. (1998). The adrenals. In *Campbell's urology*, 7th edn, Vol. 3 (ed. P. Walsh, A. Retik, and E.J. Vaughan), pp. 2915–72. W.B. Saunders, Philadelphia.

Vaughan, E.D. Jr, Carey, R.M., Peach, M.J., Ackerly, J.A., and Ayers, C.R. (1978). The renin response to diuretic therapy. A limitation of antihypertensive potential. *Circ. Res.* **42**, 376–81.

Warnock, D.G. (1998). Liddle syndrome: an autosomal dominant form of human hypertension. *Kidney Int.* **53**, 18–24.

Weber, M.A., Drayer, J.I., Rev, A., and Laragh, J.H. (1977). Disparate patterns of aldosterone response during diuretic treatment of hypertension. *Ann. Intern. Med.* **87**, 558–63.

53. Adrenocortical carcinoma

Richard D. Schulick and Murray F. Brennan

Introduction

Adrenocortical carcinoma is rare, can occur at any age, and is slightly more common in women. Patients present with signs and symptoms of steroid excess and/or mass effect depending on whether the tumors are functional or nonfunctional. Functional tumors may produce corticosteroids, androgens, estrogens, or mineralocorticoids. Most patients with this disease present with a large mass and late-stage disease. Abdominal computerized tomography (CT) and magnetic resonance imaging (MRI) are useful for the evaluation of primary disease, local invasion, lymph node involvement, and metastatic disease to the liver and peritoneal cavity. The most effective treatment, and the only potentially curative treatment for adrenocortical carcinoma, is complete resection. Early stage and complete resection are the two clinical factors that predict long-term survival. Mitotane is the chemotherapeutic agent most often used to treat adrenocortical carcinoma. Its efficacy in prolonging survival is limited. Local recurrence and metastatic disease are common even for patients who undergo complete resection. Patients who develop local recurrence or metastatic disease should be evaluated for repeat resection. Long-term survival is possible in patients who can undergo complete repeat resection.

Incidence and demographics

Adrenocortical carcinoma is a rare tumor with an annual incidence of between 0.5 and 2 cases per million (Brennan 1987; National Cancer Institute 1975). This is in contrast to the incidence of adenomas of the adrenal gland yielding a relatively frequent finding of an 'incidentaloma' in patients having cross-sectional imaging of their abdominal cavities. As many as 2 per cent of all autopsies show adenomatous changes in the adrenal gland (Brennan 1987).

Most series find multiple peaks of occurrence by age, with one peak occurring at less than 5 years of age and a second peak, in the fourth to sixth decades of life (Norton 1997; Pommier and Brennan 1991). A series of 113 patients admitted to Memorial Sloan–Kettering Cancer Center for treatment of adrenocortical carcinoma had a small peak of occurrence at less than 5 years of age, a second broad peak from 20 to 60 years, and a third peak from 65 to 75 years (Schulick and Brennan 1999) (Fig. 53.1). Most

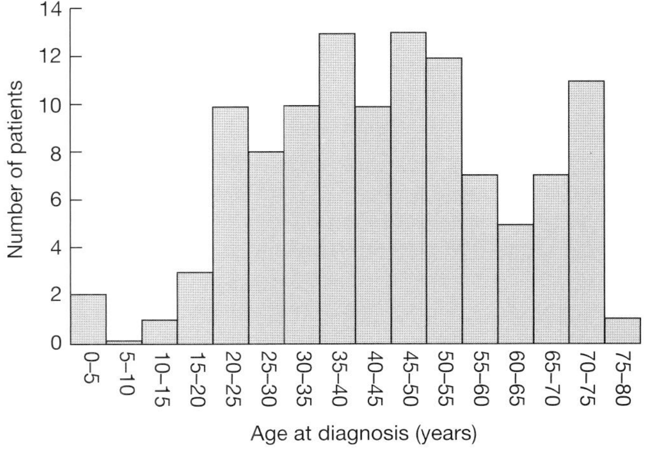

Fig. 53.1 Age distribution of 113 patients who presented to Memorial Sloan–Kettering Cancer Center with adrenocortical carcinoma (Schulick and Brennan 1999).

series find a slight preponderance of female over male patients but a few series find the opposite (Percapio and Knowlton 1976; Soreide *et al.* 1992). Wooten and King (1993) reviewed the English literature between 1952 and 1992 and found 87 series containing 1891 patients. They found a slight female predominance (4:3). The incidence of carcinoma on the left side was 52.8 per cent and in 2.4 per cent of the cases it was bilateral. The overall incidence of functional lesions was 59.3 per cent. More often than males, females with adrenocortical carcinoma manifest functional tumors. If tumors in males show signs and symptoms of hormonal function, they tend to occur before the age of 20 years, and most nonfunctional tumors tend to occur in men over the age of 40 years (Cohn *et al.* 1986).

Etiology

The etiology of adrenocortical carcinoma is as yet unknown. It has been argued that the carcinoma develops from a sequential progression of hyperplastic nodules that develop into adenomas that later develop into a malignant phenotype much like the adenoma–carcinoma sequence of colon cancer. In support of this hypothesis, some patients have abnormal adrenal steroid produc-

Table 53.1 Staging of adrenocortical carcinoma and stage at presentation of patients (*N* = 113) in Memorial Sloan–Kettering Cancer Center series (Schulick and Brennan 1999)

Stage	Characteristics	Number (%) of patients
I	< 5 cm, no local invasion, negative lymph nodes, no metastases	5 (4)
II	> 5 cm, no local invasion, negative lymph nodes, no metastases	52 (46)
III	Local invasion or positive lymph nodes	12 (11)
IV	Either local invasions and positive lymph nodes, or metastases	44 (39)

tion decades before the development of adrenocortical carcinoma (Hamwi *et al.* 1957; Plager 1984). Cytogenetic analysis suggests that loss of heterozygosity on chromosomes 11p, 13q, or 17p may be important in the pathogenesis (Henry *et al.* 1989; Yano *et al.* 1989). Several studies have implicated p53 in the pathogenesis of sporadic adrenocortical carcinoma (McNicol *et al.* 1997; Ohgaki *et al.* 1993; Reincke 1998). This is probably a late event, as mutations in the conserved regions of p53 are detected more frequently in carcinomas than in adenomas.

Classification and staging

Adrenocortical carcinomas are classified as either functional or nonfunctional. Patients develop symptoms due to excess amounts of steroidogenesis. Corticosteroid, androgen, and estrogen excesses are much more common than mineralocorticoid excess. Some patients express signs and symptoms of more than one type of hormone excess. Adrenocortical carcinomas can be inefficient in steroidogenesis and may not show obvious clinical syndromes of excess, even with large bulky disease. Care must be taken to assay for an abnormal presence of steroid in the blood and urine samples of these patients, if there is any clinical suspicion that the contralateral gland may be suppressed.

Adrenocortical carcinoma is staged on the basis of the TNM (tumor–node–metastasis) system (Norton 1997), which follows the original staging system first popularized by MacFarlane (1958) (Table 53.1). Stage I disease is tumor measuring less than or equal to 5 cm without local invasion and without nodal or distant metastases. Stage II disease is the same except that the tumor is greater than 5 cm. Stage III disease is associated with local invasion or positive lymph nodes. Stage IV disease is associated with local invasion and positive lymph nodes or distant metastases. In a recent report of patients with adrenocortical carcinoma treated at Memorial Sloan–Kettering Cancer Center, 4 per cent (4/113) presented with stage I disease, 46 per cent (52/113) with stage II disease, 11 per cent (12/113) with stage III disease, and 39 per cent (44/113) with stage IV disease (Schulick and Brennan 1999) (Table 53.1).

Presentation

Adrenocortical carcinoma presents either with the signs and symptoms of a functional tumor or secondary to mass effect. The functional lesions are broadly divided into four groups based on the type of hormone they produce (corticosteroid, virilizing sex hormone, feminizing sex hormone, or mineralocorticoid excess). Corticosteroid excess is the most common and more readily recognized presentation of the functional adrenocortical carcinomas. Lesions that produce corticosteroid excess can cause patients to have truncal obesity, rounded facies, buffalo hump, stria, hypertension, glucose intolerance, thinning of the skin, and osteoporosis (the classic stigmata of Cushing's syndrome). They sometimes present with renal calculi and even psychiatric conditions if the hormonal excess is high. Lesions that produce sex hormone excess can cause patients to present with excessive or early virilization or feminization. Lesions that produce mineralocorticoid excess are rare but cause patients to present with hypertension and hypokalemia. Patients with nonfunctional lesions usually present with a large mass and associated symptoms due to size, pressure, and invasion of contiguous structures.

In the Memorial Sloan–Kettering Cancer Center series, 55 per cent of patients presented with clinically evident functional tumors and 45 per cent presented with clinically nonfunctional tumors (Schulick and Brennan 1999). Nonfunctional tumors were defined as those tumors that did not produce signs or symptoms of excess adrenal hormone production, even if excess hormone production was subsequently shown by laboratory analysis of blood and urine. In the group that presented with functional tumors (62/113), 56 per cent had Cushing's syndrome, 21 per cent had virilization, 10 per cent had both, 8 per cent had feminization, and 5 per cent had hyperaldosteronism (Fig. 53.2). In the group that presented with nonfunctional tumors (51/113), 65 per cent had pain, 33 per cent

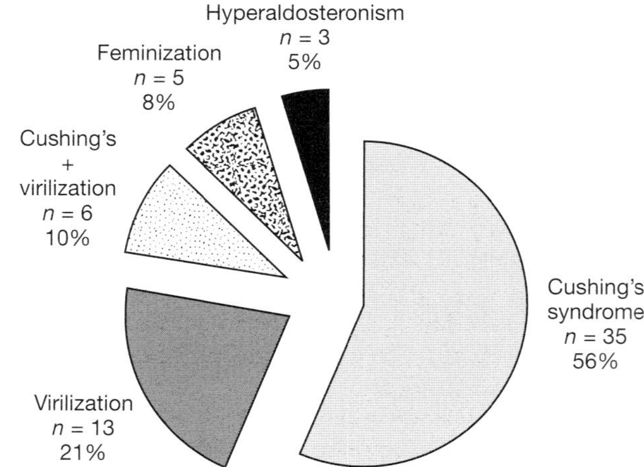

Fig. 53.2 Signs and symptoms in 62 patients with functional adrenocortical carcinomas out of 113 total patients who presented to Memorial Sloan–Kettering Cancer Center for treatment (Schulick and Brennan 1999).

Table 53.2 Signs and symptoms of nonfunctional lesions in Memorial Sloan–Kettering Cancer Center series (51 of 113 patients) (Schulick and Brennan 1999). (Some patients presented with more than one major sign/symptom.)

Sign/symptom	Number of patients (%)
Pain	33 (65)
Palpable mass	17 (33)
Weight loss	6 (12)
Hematuria	2 (4)
Varicocele	1 (2)
Dyspnea	1 (2)
Asymptomatic	6 (6)

had a palpable mass, 12 per cent had weight loss, 4 per cent had hematuria, 2 per cent had varicocele, 2 per cent had dyspnea, and 6 per cent were asymptomatic (Table 53.2).

Many patients with adrenocortical carcinoma present with large masses. This is especially true of patients with nonfunctional lesions who do not have signs and symptoms to indicate the presence of lesion before any mass effect occurs. In the Memorial Sloan–Kettering Cancer Center series, the median size at presentation of the lesions was 14 cm (range 4–25 cm) and the median weight at presentation was 750 g (range 4–2600 g) (Schulick and Brennan 1999). A series from France with 156 cases reported a mean size at presentation of 12 cm (range 3–30 cm) and mean weight at presentation of 714 g (range 12–4750 g) (Icard *et al.* 1992).

Diagnosis

Adrenocortical carcinomas are typically large, lobulated, inhomogeneous, and hemorrhagic, have central necrosis, and have calcifications on cross-sectional imaging. These characteristics are nonspecific and may be seen in conjunction with adenomas, metastatic disease, pheochromocytomas, or granulomatous infections. However, when seen in conjunction with the signs and symptoms detailed in the previous section, they are suggestive of adrenocortical carcinoma.

Adrenal incidentaloma refers to any adrenal mass discovered incidentally during an abdominal imaging evaluation. Multiple radiology series have shown the prevalence of incidentalomas of the adrenal gland to be in the range of 1–2 per cent (Ross and Aron 1990; Tutuncu and Gedik 1999). In the evaluation of an incidentaloma, the possibility of metastatic disease must be considered and excluded. Patients should then be evaluated for potential adrenal function based on history and physical examination as well as serum and urine chemistries. The presence of a functional lesion is a clear indication for surgical removal. Lesions larger than 5 cm should be removed in an otherwise healthy patient because of the higher incidence of adrenocortical carcinoma in this group.

Extent of disease

Metastatic disease is common in adrenocortical carcinoma. In the Memorial Sloan–Kettering Cancer Center series (Schulick and Brennan 1999), 39 per cent of the patients presented with

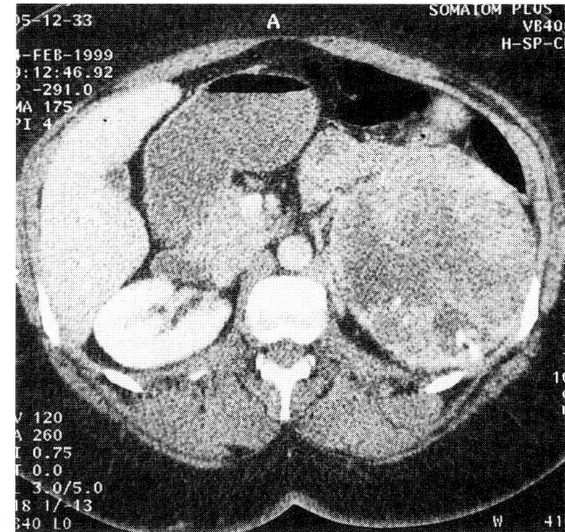
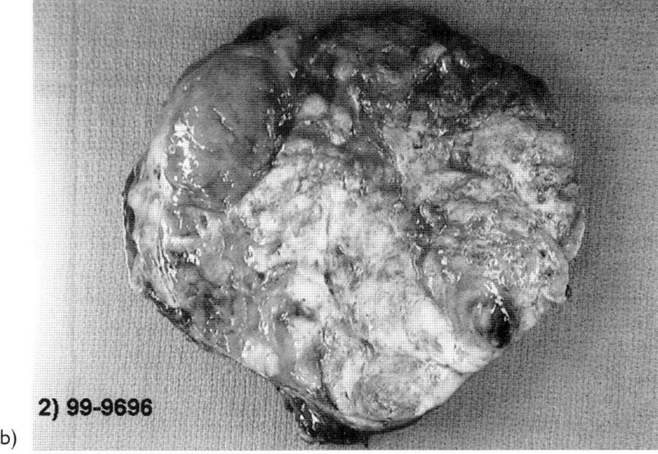

Fig. 53.3 CT image and gross specimen photo of a left sided adrenocortical carcinoma.

metastatic disease. The sites of metastatic disease were liver (64 per cent), lung (39 per cent), omentum/peritoneum (18 per cent), bone (7 per cent), distal lymph nodes (7 per cent), and soft palate (2 per cent).

CT scan of the abdomen is the radiology study of choice once an adrenocortical carcinoma is suspected (Fig. 53.3). Abdominal CT provides information about general resectability, presence of bilateral renal function, and presence of metastatic disease to the liver, lymph nodes, and other sites. CT does not reliably predict invasion of the tumor into the liver, kidney, or inferior vena cava. Approximation and adherence of the tumor to the liver and kidney are common but actual invasion occurs less frequently (Brennan 1987). MRI can sometimes better delineate planes between the tumor and adjacent organs. Additionally, MRI may discriminate between the different types of adrenal tumors on the basis of T1- and T2-weighted signal intensities (Egglin *et al.* 1988; Peppercorn and Reznek 1997). Adrenocortical carcinomas characteristically have signal intensities that are similar to liver on T1-weighted images and hyperintense to liver on T2-weighted images. These characteristics, however, do not absolutely allow discrimination between certain adrenocortical carcinomas, adrenal metastases, and benign adrenal cortical adenomas. MRI better

Table 53.3 Presentation with stage IV disease (44 of 113 patients) in Memorial Sloan–Kettering Cancer Center series (Schulick and Brennan 1999). (Some patients presented with more than one site of metastasis.)

Organ/site	Number of patients (%)
Liver	28 (64)
Lung	17 (39)
Omentum/peritoneum	8 (18)
Bone	3 (7)
Distal lymph node	3 (7)
Palate	1 (2)

defines inferior vena cava or renal vein involvement. Lesions that involve the inferior vena cava tend to arise from the right side (83 per cent) and tend to be large (Hedican and Marshall 1997). Large lesions on the left commonly involve the left renal vein.

A careful history, physical examination, and chest X-ray or CT along with evaluation of the liver by the cross-sectional imaging modality used to evaluate the adrenal mass is often sufficient to evaluate a patient with adrenocortical carcinoma for metastatic disease. Further extent-of-disease work-up should be tailored to the signs and symptoms present. Complaints of bone pain from the patient should be carefully evaluated as bony metastases do occur (Table 53.3).

Treatment

Surgical treatment

The most effective treatment for adrenocortical carcinoma is complete resection. Surgery remains the only potentially curative treatment for this disease. For adrenocortical carcinomas less than 10 cm in size, a bilateral subcostal incision yields good exposure. This affords adequate access to the liver, omentum, peritoneum, and periaortic lymph nodes, which are common sites of involvement. Adrenocortical carcinomas commonly invade or are adherent to adjacent organs. *En bloc* excision of the kidney and regional lymph nodes may be required; however, routine removal of the adjacent kidney is not advocated. The right adrenal gland is exposed by mobilization of the hepatic flexure of the colon and performance of a Kocher maneuver. The inferior portion of the right triangular ligament is then incised and the liver mobilized cephalad to expose the right adrenal gland. The left adrenal gland may be approached via two techniques. It may be approached inferiorly through the lesser sac, where the inferior border of the body and tail of the pancreas is mobilized cephalad. This approach works quite nicely for smaller lesions. Alternatively, for larger lesions on the left side, the adrenal gland may be approached superiorly by mobilization of the splenic flexure of the colon and then the lateral attachments of the spleen. The spleen, stomach, pancreas, and left colon are then retracted medially *en bloc* to visualize the left adrenal gland.

For larger lesions (> 10 cm), a thoracoabdominal approach should be considered for better access. The patient is placed in a modified lateral decubitus position. The incision is then made starting in the midline from the umbilicus, curving through the costal margin, and on to the superior aspect of the ninth or tenth rib. The diaphragm is then incised, leaving a 1–2 cm cuff peripherally for reconstruction. This approach affords safer access for larger lesions and can afford simultaneous removal of ipsilateral lung metastases. It is important to recognize that the flank approach (or posterior approach), while technically feasible for smaller lesions, does not allow evaluation of all potential sites of metastases.

Some groups advocate the use of cardiac bypass techniques for lesions with intracaval extension, especially those that extend above the subhepatic vena cava into the right atrium (Hedican and Marshall 1997; Javadpour *et al.* 1978; Moul *et al.* 1991). Some alternatives to cardiac bypass include veno-veno bypass or simple suprahepatic venous control and intracaval extraction. Intracaval thrombus from adrenocortical carcinoma can be gelatinous and friable and attempts at extraction or clamping of the vena cava without knowledge of the superior extent of the lesion can result in massive tumor embolus. This can lead to hemodynamic instability via blockage of the pulmonary arteries as in classic pulmonary embolization or fragments can achieve independent vascularization and growth. On the left side, renal vein extension commonly stops as it passes over the aorta. It is possible to resect the left renal vein at the adrenal vein junction and keep the kidney allowing drainage via the left gonadal vein.

Patients with biochemically active tumors producing corticosteroids may have suppression of the contralateral gland. Careful attention must be given to corticosteroid coverage and replacement. These patients should receive 100 mg of hydrocortisone intravenously (IV) on call to the operating room and then every 8 hours thereafter. Depending on the degree of adrenal ablation and the recovery of the patient, the dose of hydrocortisone is tapered by 50–100 mg/day until a daily dose of 25–50 mg of hydrocortisone or its oral equivalent is reached. Patients who require long-term steroid maintenance will continue this daily dose. In patients with Cushing's syndrome, the contralateral adrenal gland may take up to 22 months to resume adequate steroid production (Bartagna and Orth 1981). Most patients, however, regain adequate adrenal function in a much shorter time.

Patients who undergo total adrenal ablation and require long-term steroid replacement should also be given mineralocorticoid replacement. Corticosteroids have some degree of mineralocorticoid action depending on the preparation; however, this may not be sufficient. The synthetic adrenocorticoid fludrocortisone acetate is given at an initial dose of 0.1 mg three times a week, and adjusted to serum electrolytes and patient weight up to a dose of 0.1 mg/day.

Medical treatment

The chemotherapeutic agent most used to treat adrenocortical carcinoma is mitotane. This agent was developed initially as an insecticide but was found to have activity in the adrenal cortex yielding necrosis. It is used in both primary and adjuvant therapy settings. Table 53.4 summarizes several studies that have evaluated the effectiveness of mitotane therapy on adrenocortical carcinoma. In general, a survival benefit with the use of mitotane is difficult to demonstrate in both primary and adjuvant settings.

Table 53.4 Response to mitotane therapy from reported series

Study	Institution/group	Number of patients	Response %	Response Type*
Venkatesh *et al.* 1989	M.D. Anderson	72	29	PR only
Luton *et al.* 1990	France	59	14	PR only
Pommier and Brennan 1991	Memorial Sloan–Kettering Cancer Center	29	24	PR only
Wooten and King 1993	English literature review	551	35	PR + CR
Haak *et al.* 1994	Holland	55	27	PR + CR

* CR, complete objective response; PR, partial response.

The report by Haak *et al.* (1994), however, did show a statistically significant increase in survival time in patients treated with very high doses of mitotane. This group of patients had disease that could not be completely resected and were treated with high doses of mitotane to keep their serum mitotane levels > 14 mg/l. Responses were found in 15/29 patients (55 per cent) in this subgroup with most of these only partial responses.

Significant toxicity is associated with mitotane therapy (Pommier and Brennan 1991). Almost all patients experience gastrointestinal symptoms consisting of nausea and anorexia. Neuromuscular toxicity, including lethargy, dizziness, somnolence, and depression, occurs in 40–60 per cent of patients undergoing mitotane therapy. Therapy often interferes with normal work or leisure activities. Adrenal insufficiency from the action of mitotane on normal adrenal tissue is almost universal and steroid replacement as outlined previously is routinely used.

Other chemotherapeutic agents have been evaluated against adrenocortical carcinoma but have been found to be even less efficacious (Norton 1997). Cisplatin, etoposide, and suramin show some activity in this disease and are sometimes used in unresectable patients who have failed mitotane therapy. These agents, however, are viewed as having low efficacy and high toxicity.

Several medications (in addition to mitotane) are useful in the treatment of symptoms caused by hormonal excess. Ketoconazole, aminoglutethimide, and metyrapone have been used to control the symptoms of glucocorticoid excess. These agents block various pathways in the synthesis of cortisol. Spironolactone, a competitive inhibitor for the aldosterone receptor, is used to control the symptoms of mineralocorticoid excess. It will usually correct hypokalemia but is infrequently adequate at controlling hypertension.

Radiation therapy

Radiotherapy is of very limited benefit in adrenocortical carcinoma. It does not prolong survival, but it does appear to provide significant palliation for pain from bone metastases (Norton 1997; Percapio and Knowlton 1976; Cohn *et al.* 1986).

Survival

The prognosis for patients with untreated adrenocortical carcinoma is very poor. In multiple large series, the overall 5-year survival in treated patients with adrenocortical carcinoma ranges from 16 to 37 per cent (Table 53.5). These series consist of patients who were treated with surgery and/or medical therapy, most often consisting of mitotane. In these series, if the patients underwent a complete resection of all evident tumor, the 5-year survival ranged from 38 to 62 per cent. If the patients were not completely resected, the 5-year survival ranged from 0 to 9 per cent. In the series of patients from Memorial Sloan–Kettering Cancer Center ($N = 113$), the 5-year survival of patients completely resected was 55 per cent and in patients incompletely resected it was 5 per cent (Fig. 53.4) It should be emphasized that 5-year survival is not equivalent to cure. Most patients surviving at 5 years are alive with disease, and 85 per cent of patients resected for cure will eventually develop recurrence or distant metastases (Pommier and Brennan 1991).

The studies reviewed in Table 53.5 have all identified early stage and curative resection as clinical factors of prognostic significance. Only one of the studies listed (Icard *et al.* 1992) found age

Table 53.5 Survival rates in patients with adrenocortical carcinoma from reported series

Study	Institution/group	Number of patients	5-year survival rate (%) Overall	5-year survival rate (%) Curative resection	5-year survival rate (%) Palliative resection
Soreide *et al.* 1992	Norway	99	16	62	0
Icard *et al.* 1992	France	156	34	42	0
Zografos *et al.* 1994	Roswell Park	53	19	38	0
Haak *et al.* 1994	Holland	96	27	49	9
Crucitti *et al.* 1996	Italy	129	35	48	7
Schulick and Brennan 1999	Memorial Sloan–Kettering Cancer Center	113	37	55	5

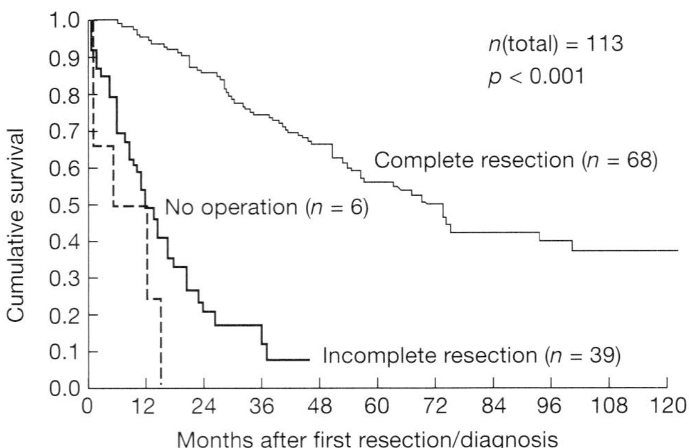

Fig. 53.4 Disease-specific survival of patients undergoing resection for adrenocortical carcinoma at Memorial Sloan–Kettering Cancer Center stratified by completeness of resection (Schulick and Brennan 1999).

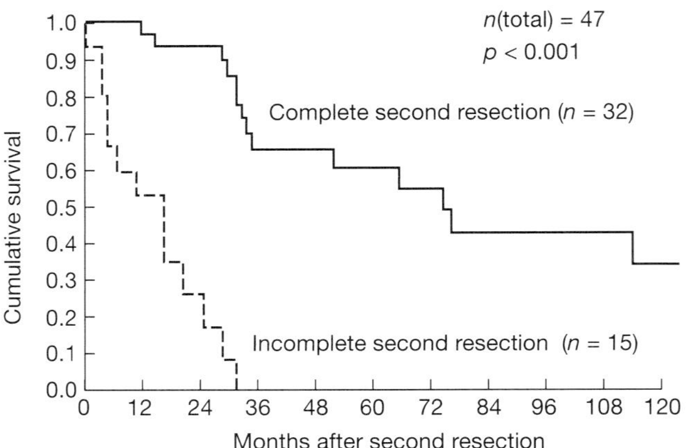

Fig. 53.5 Disease-specific survival of patients undergoing second resection for adrenocortical carcinoma at Memorial Sloan–Kettering Cancer Center stratified by completeness of second resection (Schulick and Brennan 1999).

or functional status of the lesion to be clinical factors of prognostic significance (younger patients and patients with androgen secretion had better survival).

In addition to identifying clinical factors, many studies have tried to identify pathologic factors of prognostic significance. A recent study at Memorial Sloan–Kettering Cancer Center reviewed 46 patients who had undergone curative resection (Harrison *et al.* 1999). Of 16 pathologic factors analyzed, tumor size, abnormal mitotic figures, and the presence of intratumoral hemorrhage were independent prognostic factors. Patients presenting with primary tumors measuring $\geq$ 12 cm had a worse outcome than those with smaller tumors (5-year survival, 23 versus 66 per cent). The presence of > 6 abnormal mitotic figures was a negative prognostic feature as compared to the presence of 0–6 abnormal mitotic figures per high-powered field (5-year survival, 13 versus 51 per cent). Hemorrhage into the tumor was also a negative prognostic factor as compared to patients without intratumoral hemorrhage (5-year survival, 22 versus 53 per cent). Patients with none of these risk factors had a 5-year survival of 83 per cent, whereas patients with all three risk factors had a 5-year survival of 0 per cent despite complete resection. Patients with one or two of the risk factors had intermediate 5-year survivals of 42 and 33 per cent, respectively.

Re-operative treatment

Recurrent and metastatic disease are extremely common even for patients who undergo complete resection. Resection of recurrent and metastatic disease when complete is associated with long-term survival and provides excellent palliation in patients with symptomatic steroid production. In a recent study from Memorial Sloan–Kettering Cancer Center (Schulick and Brennan 1999), 47 of 107 patients (primarily resected) underwent a second resection for locally recurrent or metastatic disease. As in primary resection, the main prognostic factor in patients undergoing a second operation was the ability to completely remove the lesion (Fig. 53.5). In this group of patients, some underwent a third, fourth, fifth, sixth, and even seventh resection for recurrent

disease. In total there were 83 repeat resections in this group of patients, 46 for metastatic disease, 30 for local recurrence, and 7 for both. Patients with distant metastases more often were able to undergo a complete resection of their recurrent disease. A majority of the repeat resections for distant metastases were for pulmonary lesions (55 per cent), liver lesions (28 per cent), or bone lesions (11 per cent). These 83 repeat resections were performed with a 30-day mortality of 3.6 per cent. It is clear that patients with locally recurrent or metastatic disease should undergo re-operation if they have potentially completely resectable disease and they are in otherwise good medical condition.

Follow-up

Recurrence and metastatic disease are common in adrenocortical carcinoma. Of patients undergoing complete resection, 85 per cent are expected to eventually develop local recurrence or metastatic disease (Pommier and Brennan 1991). Follow-up of these patients should be dependent on the ability to re-operate on recurrences found. As most surgeons would resect isolated local recurrence or resectable lung metastases in medically fit patients, an aggressive follow-up regimen incorporating chest X-ray and abdominal CT is recommended. Patients who are found to have elevated serum or urine markers prior to resection of the primary lesion should have these checked periodically. Follow-up should be continued indefinitely, as recurrences can occur very late.

References

Bartagna, C. and Orth, D.N. (1981). Clinical and laboratory findings and results of therapy in 58 patients with adrenocortical tumors admitted to a single medical center (1951–1978). *Am. J. Med.* **71**, 855–71.

Brennan, M.F. (1987). Adrenocortical carcinoma. *Cancer* **37**, 348–65.

Cohn, K., Gottesman, L., and Brennan, M.F. (1986). Adrenocortical carcinoma. *Surgery* **100**, 1170–7.

Crucitti, F., Bellantone, R., Ferrante, A., Boscherini, M., and Crucitti, P. The ACC Italian Registry Study Group (1996). The Italian registry for adrenal cortical carcinoma: analysis of a multiinstitutional series of 129 patients.

Surgery **119**, 161–70.

Egglin, T.K., Hahn, P.F., and Stark, D.D. (1988). MRI of the adrenal glands. *Sem. Roentgenol.* **23**, 280–7.

Haak, H.R., Hermans, J., van de Velde, C.J., Lentjes, E.G., Goslings, B.M., Fleuren, G.J., and Krans, H.M. (1994). Optimal treatment of adrenocortical carcinoma with mitotane: results in a consecutive series of 96 patients. *Br. J. Cancer* **69**, 947–51.

Hamwi, G.J., Serbin, R.A., and Kruger, F.A. (1957). Does adrenocortical hyperplasia result in adrenocortical carcinoma? *New Engl. J. Med.* **257**, 1153–7.

Harrison, L.E., Gaudin, P.B., and Brennan, M.F. (1999). Pathologic features of prognostic significance for adrenocortical carcinoma after curative resection. *Arch. Surg.* **134**, 181–5.

Hedican, S.P. and Marshall, F.F. (1997). Adrenocortical carcinoma with intracaval extension. *J. Urol.* **158**, 2056–61.

Henry, I., Grandjovans, S., Couillin, P., Barichard, F., Huerre-Jeanpierre, C., Glaser, T., Phillip, T., Lenoir, G., Chaussain, J.L., and Lunien, C. (1989). Tumor-specific loss of 11 15.5 alleles in del 11 p 13 Wilms tumor and in familial adrenocortical carcinoma. *Proc. Natl Acad. Sci., USA* **86**, 3247–51.

Icard, P., Chapuis, Y., Andreassian, B., Bernard, A., and Proye, C. (1992). Adrenocortical carcinoma in surgically treated patients: a retrospective study on 156 cases by the French Association of Endocrine Surgery. *Surgery* **112**, 972–80.

Javadpour, N., Woltering, E.A., and McIntosh, C.L. (1978). Thoraco abdominal-median sternotomy for resection of primary adrenal carcinoma extending into the inferior vena cava and hepatic vein. *Urology* **12**, 626–7.

Luton, J., Cerdas, S., Line, B., Thomas, G., Guilhaume, B., Betagna, X., Laudat, M., Louvel, A., Chapuis, Y., Blondeau, P., Bonnin, A., and Bricaire, H. (1990). Clinical features of adrenocortical carcinoma, prognostic factors, and the effect of mitotane therapy. *New Engl. J. Med.* **322**, 1195–201.

MacFarlane, D.A. (1958). Cancer of the adrenal cortex. The natural history, prognosis and treatment in a study of fifty-five cases. *Ann. R. Coll. Surg. Engl.* **23**, 155–86.

McNicol, A.M., Nolan, C.E., Struthers, A.J., Farauharson, M.A., Hermans, J., and Haak, H.R. (1997). Expression of p53 in adrenocortical tumours: clinicopathological correlations. *J. Pathol.* **181**, 146–52.

Moul, J.W., Hardy, M.R., and McLeod, D.G. (1991). Adrenal cortical carcinoma with vena cava tumor thrombus requiring cardiopulmonary bypass for resection. *Urology* **38**, 179–83.

National Cancer Institute (1975). Incidence data. In *Third national cancer survey*, pp. 75–787. National Cancer Institute, Bethesda, Maryland.

Norton, J.A. (1997). Adrenal tumors. In *Cancer: principles and practice of oncology*, 5th edn (ed. V.T. DeVita, S. Hellman, and S.A. Rosenberg), pp. 1659–77. Lippincott–Raven, Philadelphia.

Ohgaki, H., Kleihues, P., and Heitz, P.U. (1993). p53 mutations in sporadic adrenocortical tumors. *Int. J. Cancer* **54**, 408–10.

Peppercorn, P.D. and Reznek, R.H. (1997). State-of-the-art CT and MRI of the adrenal gland. *Eur. Radiol.* **7**, 822–36.

Percapio, B. and Knowlton, A.H. (1976). Radiation therapy of adrenal cortical carcinoma. *Acta Radiol. Ther. Phys. Biol.* **15**, 288–92.

Plager, J.E. (1984). Carcinoma of the adrenal cortex: clinical description, diagnosis, and treatment. *Int. Advan. Surg. Oncol.* **7**, 329–53.

Pommier, R.F. and Brennan, M.F. (1991). Management of adrenal neoplasms. *Curr. Prob. Surg.* **28**, 657–739.

Reincke, M. (1998). Mutations in adrenocortical tumors. *Horm. Metab. Res.* **30**, 447–55.

Ross, N.S. and Aron, D.C. (1990). Hormonal evaluation of the patient with an incidentally discovered adrenal mass. *New Engl. J. Med.* **323**, 1401–5.

Schulick, R.D. and Brennan, M.F. (1999). Long-term survival after complete resection and repeat resection in patients with adrenocortical carcinoma. *Ann. Surg. Oncol.* **6**, 719–26.

Soreide, J.A., Brabrand, K., and Thoresen, S.O. (1992). Adrenal cortical carcinoma in Norway, 1970–1984. *World J. Surg.* **16**, 663–8.

Tutuncu, N.B. and Gedik, O. (1999). Adrenal incidentaloma: report of 33 cases. *J. Surg. Oncol.* **70**, 247–50.

Venkatesh, S., Hickey, R.C., Sellin, R.V., Fernandez, J.F., and Samaan, N.A. (1989). Adrenal cortical carcinoma. *Cancer* **64**, 765–9.

Wooten, M.D. and King, D.K. (1993). Adrenal cortical carcinoma. *Cancer* **72**, 3145–55.

Yano, T., Linehan, M., Anglard, P., Lerman, M.I., Daniel, L.N., Stein, C.A., Robertson, C.N., LaRocca, R., and Zbar, B. (1989). Genetic changes in human adrenocortical carcinoma. *J. Natl Cancer Inst.* **81**, 518–23.

Zografos, G.C., Driscoll, D.L., Karakousis, C.P., and Huben, R.P. (1994). Adrenal adenocarcinoma: a review of 53 cases. *J. Surg. Oncol.* **55**, 160–4.

54. Pheochromocytoma

McClellan M. Walther, Graeme Eisenhofer, Karel Pacak, and W. Marston Linehan

Introduction

Pheochromocytomas are catecholamine-producing tumors known for their unpredictable and catastrophic course of malignant hypertension. The term pheochromocytoma was first coined by Pick in 1912 to describe an adrenal medullary tumor that developed a black-brown coloration after staining with dichromate-containing fixatives, so-called chromaffin cells. Pheochromocytomas can occur anywhere in the sympathetic nervous system—from the glomus jugulare at the base of the skull to the urinary bladder. The majority of pheochromocytomas, however, occur in the adrenal glands. Certain extra-adrenal pheochromocytomas, called paraganglia, are given unique names, such as glomus tumor derived from the glomus jugulare, chemodectoma from the carotid body, and organ of Zuckerkandl tumor named for that paraganglia. Familial forms of pheochromocytoma are thought to comprise about 10 per cent of cases.

Clinical signs and symptoms of pheochromocytoma arise from the excessive production of catecholamines by this tumor, with over half of patients developing marked hypertension. The prevalence of sustained essential hypertension has been estimated as 15 to 20 per cent of the adult population of Western countries (Manger and Gifford 1996; Epstein and Eckhoff 1967). Pheochromocytomas are thought to account for 0.05 to 0.3 per cent of these patients with sustained essential hypertension (Page 1976; Streeten *et al.* 1990). The diagnosis of pheochromocytoma in the general population is further compounded as about half of affected patients have only paroxysmal hypertension or are normotensive.

Pheochromocytomas are usually benign and curable if properly identified and removed, but can be fatal if undiagnosed or mistreated. Autopsy series, however, suggest that many pheochromocytomas are not suspected clinically and, in these patients, lead to a tragic outcome (Sutton *et al.* 1981).

Pathology

Pheochromocytoma cells appear similar to those of the normal adrenal medulla, but are more polyhedral in shape and often larger. Growth may occur in cords or alveolar patterns ('Zellballen') (Page *et al.* 1986). Adjacent nests of tumor cells are surrounded by richly vascular septa. Chromaffin cells can have marked pleomorphism or be small and regular. Cellular cytoplasm can vary from clear to granular, with eosinophilic or basophilic staining. Trabecular or diffuse patterns of growth may also occur, but maintain the rich vascular septa. Tumor necrosis, nuclear pleomorphism, increased mitotic atypia, or vascular invasion can also occur in benign tumors, making histologic determination of malignancy impossible (Page *et al.* 1986).

Malignant pheochromocytomas are defined clinically by the presence of metastases, which occur in 7–15 per cent of patients (Sutton *et al.* 1981; Remine *et al.* 1974; Melicow 1977; Ross and Griffith 1989; Ellison *et al.* 1988). Metastases should be identified as pheochromocytomas that occur at sites outside the location of normal sympathetic tissue where multifocal tumors could not arise. Clinical factors associated with malignant pheochromocytoma include preoperative elevations in plasma dihydroxyphenylalanine (dopa), 24-hour excretion of dopamine, extra-adrenal pheochromocytoma (28–65 per cent), tumor weight greater than 80 grams (more than about 5 cm diameter), increased MIB-1 labeling index, p53 mutations (40 per cent), and persistence of catecholamine elevations after surgery (John *et al.* 1999; Clarke *et al.* 1998; Yoshimoto *et al.* 1998; Proye *et al.* 1992; Nativ *et al.* 1992; Goldstein *et al.* 1986). Pheochromocytoma metastases usually present in the bone, lung, regional lymph nodes, liver, and brain (Remine *et al.* 1974; Proye *et al.* 1992; Schlumberger *et al.* 1992).

Clinical features

Women and men are similarly affected with pheochromocytoma. Sporadic pheochromocytomas most commonly present in the fourth through sixth decades of life (Sutton *et al.* 1981; Melicow 1977; Ross and Griffith 1989; Ellison *et al.* 1988; Modlin *et al.* 1979). Solitary adrenal pheochromocytomas occur in about 72–82 per cent of affected patients, bilateral adrenal pheochromocytoma in 3–11 per cent, and extra-adrenal tumors in 9–19 per cent (Sutton *et al.* 1981; Melicow 1977; Ross and Griffith 1989; Ellison *et al.* 1988; Modlin *et al.* 1979).

Patients may present with various signs or symptoms, but most present with hypertensive crisis, essential hypertension that responds poorly to conventional treatment, pallor, sweating, paroxysmal symptoms suggesting seizure disorder, or anxiety attacks (Ross and Griffith 1989; Modlin *et al.* 1979; Starkman *et al.* 1985).

Hypertension can be paroxysmal or sustained, with a similar occurrence of each, and is the primary finding, present in 61 to 100 per cent of patients with sporadic pheochromocytoma (Sutton *et al.* 1981; Remine *et al.* 1974; Ross and Griffith 1989; Ellison *et al.* 1988; Modlin *et al.* 1979). Marked blood pressure lability is characteristically observed, presenting as distinct crises in patients with sustained hypertension. These hypertensive crises can be severe and resistant to standard medications used in the setting of essential hypertension (Newell *et al.* 1988).

Hypertensive crises can occur as frequently as on a daily basis, or at intervals as long as weeks or months. Over time, the episodes usually tend to increase in frequency, duration, and severity. A typical crisis is sudden in onset, lasting from minutes to hours. Profuse sweating, palpitations, tachycardia, and headache are common (Table 54.1). Chest or abdominal pain, nausea and vomiting, or a feeling of apprehension or impending doom can also accompany these attacks (Ross and Griffith 1989). Episodes associated with marked vasoconstriction are associated with pallor or flushing. Cerebrovascular accident, myocardial infarction, congestive heart failure, cardiac arrhythmias, renal failure, hemorrhage into the tumor, or dissecting aortic aneurysms may result from a hypertensive crisis. Long-term exposure to pheochromocytoma has also been associated with catecholamine myocarditis, arteriosclerosis, and ischemic enterocolitis.

Catecholamine release from pheochromocytomas is not mediated by changes in neuronal activity, but thought to occur in association with tumor necrosis, changes in blood flow, or physical stimuli. An acute hypertensive crisis may be precipitated by surgery, physical activity, abdominal trauma, or, in patients with bladder pheochromocytoma, by voiding. Therefore, after removal of the tumor, a patient can develop hypotension, orthostatic hypotension, or shock during surgery. Elevated levels of plasma catecholamines result in vascular constriction with diminished plasma volume and elevations of hematocrit.

Lower elevations of catecholamines are present in patients with pheochromocytoma outside the times of crisis. These elevations can result in increased metabolic rate and weight loss. Elevated levels of catecholamines result in suppression of insulin production and increased hepatic glucose output, leading to hyperglycemia.

Table 54.1 Pheochromocytoma symptoms. Percentage of 324 sporadic pheochromocytoma patients affected with symptoms (from Walther *et al.* (1999c))

Symptom	Range (%)
Headache	43–80
Anxiety	15–72
Sweating	37–71
Palpitations	44–71
Abdominal pain	14–62
Chest pain	0–50
Pallor	42–44
Nausea	10–42
Dyspnea	15–39
Tremor	13–38
Weight loss	7–23
Flushing	4–19
Visual disturbance	11–22

Differential diagnosis

Patients with signs and symptoms related to pheochromocytoma can have a presentation similar to that of patients with essential or secondary hypertension, hypertension of pregnancy, renovascular hypertension, anxiety and panic attacks, hypertensive crises associated with withdrawal of some antihypertensive agents or drugs (cocaine), intracranial tumors, or after self-administration of sympathomimetic amines.

Patients with hypertension resistant to conventional therapy, newly diagnosed patients with hypertension, or patients with a familial syndrome associated with pheochromocytoma should be considered for evaluation for pheochromocytoma, with particular evaluation for the characteristic findings by history and physical examination. Patients with hereditary forms of pheochromocytoma should be evaluated before contemplating pregnancy as a high incidence of maternal or fetal death has been observed in undiagnosed patients with pheochromocytoma (Modlin *et al.* 1979; Page and Copeland 1968).

Special clinical situations

Epinephrine-producing tumors

Although adrenal medullary catecholamine production is 80–85 per cent epinephrine (adrenaline), norepinephrine (noradrenaline) is produced in excess in most pheochromocytomas (Page *et al.* 1986). Symptoms associated with epinephrine-producing tumors include headaches, panic attacks, leg and abdominal cramps, chest pain and palpitations, fever, and vomiting (Page and Copeland 1968). Sweating and impaired glucose tolerance are also seen in association with these tumors (Watson *et al.* 1990). The powerful beta-adrenergic effects of epinephrine can lead to hypotension and shock, especially after alpha-blockade (Page and Copeland 1968; Watson *et al.* 1990).

Malignant pheochromocytoma

Malignant pheochromocytomas are characterized by the development of tumors outside adrenal glands and the sympathetic nervous system. Many patients have slowly growing tumors, with a median survival greater than 10 years (Nativ *et al.* 1992). Elevations of catecholamine production are generally present (Proye *et al.* 1992; Schlumberger *et al.* 1992). Alpha- and beta-blockade with phenoxybenzamine are indicated to minimize symptoms and prevent catastrophic events. Metyrosine may be added if troublesome symptoms recur or persist.

No effective therapy currently exists for treatment of metastatic pheochromocytoma. Treatment of these often slowly growing tumors is usually reserved until symptoms are present. Therapeutic attempts using pheochromocytoma uptake of metaiodobenzylguanidine (MIBG) labeled with ^{131}I have had mixed results. Partial responses have been observed in up to a third of treated patients, with decreased hormonal secretion in more patients (Shapiro and Fig 1989; Loh *et al.* 1997). Reported median responses have been 19 months (Loh *et al.* 1997). Cyclophosphamide, vincristine, and dacarbazine chemotherapy has resulted in 57 per cent tumor response and 79 per cent biochemical response, although of limited duration (Averbuch *et al.* 1988). Radiation therapy has been useful in the palliation of bony metastases. Radiation therapy with therapeutic intent has been attempted using a range of doses. Higher doses have been associated with long-term responses in a small number of patients (Yu *et al.* 1996). Patients with isolated or slowly growing tumors treated with surgical resection have occasionally experienced long-term response (Schlumberger *et al.* 1992).

Associated diseases

Pheochromocytoma-associated paraneoplastic syndromes include hypercalcemia, erythrocytosis, and Cushing's syndrome (Modlin *et al.* 1979). Renal artery stenosis with elevated peripheral plasma renin values has also been occasionally observed (Hill *et al.* 1983). While removal of the pheochromocytoma is often curative, nephrectomy or renal artery reconstruction can be required. Cholelithiasis has been reported in 3–23 per cent of patients with pheochromocytoma (Remine *et al.* 1974; Ellison *et al.* 1988; Modlin *et al.* 1979).

Hereditary forms of pheochromocytoma

Patients with hereditary forms of pheochromocytoma have been described in association with von Hippel–Lindau disease (VHL), multiple endocrine neoplasia type 2 (MEN2), von Recklinghausen's neurofibromatosis, hereditary paraganglioma syndrome (PGL), and hereditary pheochromocytoma (Table 54.2) (Sutton *et al.* 1981; Modlin *et al.* 1979; Aguilo *et al.* 1991; Baysal *et al.* 1999).

Von Hippel–Lindau disease

VHL is an autosomal dominantly inherited disorder characterized clinically by the development of central nervous system hemangioblastoma, endolymphatic sac tumors, retinal angiomas, renal cysts and carcinomas, neuroendocrine tumors and cysts of the pancreas, epididymal cystadenomas, and/or pheochromocytoma (Linehan *et al.* 1995). The incidence of VHL disease has been estimated as 1 in 45 500 (Maddock *et al.* 1996).

The VHL gene is located on chromosome 3p25.5. Mean age at diagnosis was 29 years (range, 5–62 years) (Richard *et al.* 1994; Walther *et al.* 1999a). Twelve per cent of tumors were extra-adrenal and 1.6 per cent of patients developed metastases (Richard *et al.* 1994; Walther *et al.* 1999a). VHL patients with pheochromocytoma identified by screening family members infrequently (16 per cent) develop signs or symptoms of pheochromocytoma (Table 54.3) (Walther *et al.* 1999a). VHL pheochromocytomas are primarily norepinephrine-secreting (Eisenhofer *et al.* 1999).

Families with missense germline mutations in the VHL gene are at highest risk for the development of pheochromocytoma, extra-adrenal tumors, younger age at presentation, and metastatic disease (Walther *et al.* 1999a; Chen *et al.* 1996).

Multiple endocrine neoplasia type 2

MEN2A is clinically characterized by the presence of medullary thyroid cancer, parathyroid hyperplasia, and pheochromocytoma. Patients with MEN2B also develop mucosal ganglioneuromas, a

Table 54.2 Hereditary forms of pheochromocytoma (from Pacak *et al.* (2000))

Syndrome	Gene	Chromosome location
Multiple endocrine neoplasia type 2	RET oncogene	10q11
Von Hippel–Lindau disease	VHL tumor suppressor gene	3p25
Neurofibromatosis type 1	NF-1	17q11
Hereditary paraganglioma syndrome	PGL1	11q23

Table 54.3 Comparison of VHL and sporadic pheochromocytoma. Patients with hereditary forms of pheochromocytoma identified from screening affected families present at an earlier age, have less symptoms, function, and diagnostic tests, and have smaller tumors than patients with sporadic pheochromocytoma (from Pacak *et al.* (2000))

	VHL	Sporadic pheochromocytoma	*p*-value
Age (years)	29.9	39.7	0.0034
Symptoms	6/37	23/26	< 0.0001
Hypertension	3/37	24/26	< 0.0001
Diagnostic studies	23/27	26/26	0.00017
Volume (cm^3)	4.2	35.4	< 0.0001
Urine			
Epinephrine (g/24 hr)	6.5	14.1	0.0003
Metanephrine (mg/ 24 hr)	1.3	5.2	< 0.0001
VMA* (mg/24 hr)	7.6	19.3	< 0.0001

*VMA, vanillylmandelic acid.

less common phenotype. MEN2 results from the germline mutation of the RET protooncogene and is inherited in an autosomal dominant fashion. The incidence of MEN2 has been estimated as 1 in 30 000 (Stuhrmann and Arslan-Kirchner 1996).

As many as 85 per cent of MEN2A families have a mutation in codon 634, with a high association of pheochromocytoma (Raue 1998; Egawa *et al.* 1998; Eng *et al.* 1996). Mutations in codons 618 and 630, which are less clinically defined, may be less disposed to develop pheochromocytoma. Mean age at diagnosis has been 36.9 years (range, 18–73 years) (Howe *et al.* 1993; Walther *et al.* 1999*b*). As many as 52 per cent of affected patients were asymptomatic and 35 per cent hypertensive at initial diagnosis, although 91 per cent had demonstrable elevations of catecholamines (Pomares *et al.* 1998). Seventy per cent of affected patients have been reported to develop bilateral adrenal pheochromocytoma, and extra-adrenal tumors are rare (Howe *et al.* 1993; Pomares *et al.* 1998). In contrast to VHL-related pheochromocytoma, those in MEN2 display an adrenergic phenotype with production of both norepinephrine and epinephrine (Eisenhofer *et al.* 1999; Egawa *et al.* 1998).

Von Recklinghausen's neurofibromatosis

Von Recklinghausen's neurofibromatosis is inherited in an autosomal dominant fashion and is estimated to affect one in 3000 individuals (Walther *et al.* 1999*b*). Only patients with neurofibromatosis type 1, on chromosome 17q11.1, are thought to develop pheochromocytoma. From 0.1 to 5.7 per cent of affected patients develop clinical manifestations of pheochromocytoma. Mean patient age was 42 years (range, 1.5–74 years), 9.6 per cent had bilateral adrenal tumors, and 6.1 per cent extra-adrenal tumors (Walther *et al.* 1999*b*). Related symptoms or hypertension are reported in 61 per cent of patients. Pheochromocytoma secretion in these patients has been of both epinephrine and norepineprine. Malignant tumors have occurred in 11.5 per cent of patients. Of affected patients, 8.8 per cent also developed gastrointestinal carcinoid tumors.

Hereditary paraganglioma syndrome

PGL is characterized by paragangliomas of the head and neck region (glomus tumors or chemodectomas). The carotid body is most frequently affected and multiple tumors occur in about two-thirds of tumors (van Schothorst *et al.* 1998). PGL is subject to genomic imprinting, as children of affected men inherit the disorder in an autosomal dominant pattern, while children of affected women rarely develop the disease (Baysal *et al.* 1999). PGL has been estimated to have an incidence of 1 in 100 000 (van Schothorst *et al.* 1996) and has been linked to chromosome 11q23 (Baysal *et al.* 1999). PGL-related tumors are most frequently not functional (Bogdasarian and Lotz 1979; McCaffrey *et al.* 1994). Radiation has been associated with long-term cure in a number of patients (Skolyszewski *et al.* 1991).

Hereditary pheochromocytoma

Families with hereditary pheochromocytoma have been described who do not appear clinically to be associated with a previously described genetic disorder. Many of these families have missense mutations of the VHL gene and clinically manifest only subtle retinal angiomas or central nervous system hemangioblastomas associated with their pheochromocytoma (Richard *et al.* 1994; Tisherman *et al.* 1993; Ritter *et al.* 1996; Garcia *et al.* 1997). Pheochromocytoma-only phenotypes of MEN2 have not been described, as all families have had associated medullary thyroid cancer (Egawa *et al.* 1998; Lips *et al.* 1994). A small number of families with neither VHL nor RET mutations have been reported and are not well characterized genetically (Skoldberg *et al.* 1998).

Diagnostic evaluation

Functional studies

Norepinephrine is converted to epinephrine by the enzyme phenylethanolamine-N-methyl transferase (PNMT). Expression of PNMT is regulated by corticosteroid release in the adrenal cortex. Pheochromocytomas arising at these sites thus often secrete epinephrine in addition to norepinephrine. Tumors in other locations mainly secrete norepinephrine.

The diagnosis of pheochromocytoma has been classically made by the identification of elevated 24-hour urinary excretion of catecholamines and their metabolites. Proper preservation of collected urine is ensured by addition of acid to the container to be used and chilling until the evaluation is performed. Urine creatinine excretion determination can be performed to determine if an adequate collection was obtained.

Plasma catecholamine evaluation is more expensive and exhibits less sensitivity and specificity than urine studies, resulting in its infrequent use. Plasma free metanephrines determination is proving to be a more accurate test for pheochromocytoma (Eisenhofer *et al.* 1999; Lenders *et al.* 1995). Specificity of plasma catecholamine testing can be enhanced by suppressing sympathetic nervous activity with clonidine. Patients with essential hypertension and an active sympathetic nervous system will show suppression, whereas those with pheochromocytoma most often do not (Bravo 1991; Bravo *et al.* 1981). Provocative testing is used in patients with clinical suspicion of pheochromocytoma, but nondiagnostic catecholamine secretion. Glucagon stimulates release of catecholamines from pheochromocytoma and/or hypertension, but has no effect in patients with essential hypertension (Lawrence 1967; Siqueira-Filho *et al.* 1975). Plasma catecholamine determination, clonidine suppression, and glucagon stimulation are complementary and used as clinically indicated in patients where the diagnosis of pheochromocytoma is not clear (Bravo 1991; Grossman *et al.* 1991).

Localization studies

Computed tomography (CT) imaging is excellent in the identification of abdominal and thoracic pheochromocytomas (Ellison *et al.* 1988; Stewart *et al.* 1978). Magnetic resonance imaging (MRI) is a similarly sensitive test for pheochromocytoma (Maurea *et al.* 1993). T_2-weighted MRI yields a high-intensity signal from pheochromocytoma causing the tumor to appear very bright.

Arteriography has not been used in patients with pheochromocytoma because of the high incidence of hypertensive crisis (Christenson *et al.* 1976). Adrenal vein and random venous sampling for catecholamines or metanephrines may be informative if standard imaging is not informative (Chew *et al.* 1994; Newbould *et al.* 1991).

Metaiodobenzylguanidine (MIBG), an analog of norepinephrine, is taken up and stored in neural secretory granules. MIBG labeled with iodine-123 (^{123}I) allows better imaging of the adrenal medulla and pheochromocytoma than MIBG labeled with ^{131}I (Bomanji *et al.* 1987; Nakajo *et al.* 1983). MIBG-^{123}I scintigraphy is thus diagnostic for pheochromocytoma. Whole-body imaging with MIBG scintigraphy is useful for detecting extra-adrenal, metastatic, or recurrent pheochromocytoma (Maurea *et al.* 1993; Shapiro *et al.* 1985). Positron emission tomography (PET) imaging has shown promise as having better sensitivity in detecting pheochromocytoma than MIBG (Shulkin *et al.* 1999).

Current management

Preoperative blockade

Catecholamine release associated with anesthesia induction or tumor manipulation can lead to hypertensive crisis, arrhythmias, or stroke. Pheochromocytoma surgery without catecholamine blockade has historically been associated with a mortality ranging from 24 to 50 per cent (Levine and McDonald 1984; Pullerits *et al.* 1988). Recent adrenergic blockade of pheochromocytoma catecholamines has resulted in a significant decrease in mortality (Table 54.4). Phenoxybenzamine, 10 mg every 12 hours for 2 weeks prior to surgery, usually provides potent alpha-adrenergic blockade, contributing to vasodilatation and correction of constricted fluid volume. Blocked patients usually complain of a congested nose. A final preoperative loading dose is given at midnight the night before surgery. Patients are placed at bedrest with the side rails up because of associated orthostatic hypotension. Addition of a beta-blocker may be required to blunt the reflex tachycardia that can be associated with alpha-blockade.

An important contribution to the preoperative medical blockade of pheochromocytoma has been the addition of metyrosine, a tyrosine hydroxylase inhibitor (Perry *et al.* 1990; Atuk 1983). Metyrosine blocks the enzyme tyrosine hydroxylase that converts tyrosine to dopa, the rate-limiting step in the production of catecholamines (Pullerits *et al.* 1988). Metyrosine blockade can decrease tumor catecholamine content by 50–80 per cent. Metyrosine is started 2 weeks prior to surgery, 250 mg every 8 hours. After the first week, a single tablet may be added every 2 to 3 days as needed if additional blockade is needed. A 1 g dose is administered at midnight the night before surgery. Metyrosine use has resulted in less intraoperative medication needed to control blood pressure, lower intraoperative fluid requirements, and less blood loss (Perry *et al.* 1990). Metyrosine intolerance, manifested as excessive sedation, depression, hallucinations, extrapyramidal signs, sleep disturbances, or tremor, occurs in less than 10 per cent of patients. Doses greater than 4 g per day have been associated with urinary crystal formation. Alpha blockade and metyrosine inhibition of catecholamine formation, with a liberal salt diet, allow restoration of contracted plasma volume, making surgery safer.

Intraoperative management.

In addition to standard anesthetic monitoring, an arterial blood pressure monitoring line and two large-bore venous catheters are placed in the operating room. A Swan–Ganz catheter to monitor pulmonary capillary wedge pressure may be necessary in patients with cardiac disease. Special care is taken during intubation and manipulation of the tumors, as these maneuvers are particularly associated with the outpouring of catecholamines. Enflurane or isoflurane are commonly used as anesthetic agents, as they do not sensitize the heart to catecholamines.

After removal of the tumor and its associated catecholamines, hypotension can result if preoperative blockade was not adequate. Treatment of hypotension and re-expansion of plasma volume is performed using crystalloid replacement. Pharmacological efforts to support blood pressure are generally blunted by the preoperative blockade.

Surgery

Prior to the development of modern imaging techniques, full abdominal exploration and palpation were required to identify multifocal or extra-adrenal tumors (Orchard *et al.* 1993). CT and MRI have contributed to less intrusive open surgery, and made possible the use of laparoscopic surgery. After preoperative medical blockade, laparoscopic removal was the next major advance in the management of pheochromocytoma. Laparoscopic surgery has been reported to have lower narcotic requirements, shorter hospital stay, and more rapid return to normal activity, than open surgery (Vargas *et al.* 1997; Guazzoni *et al.* 1995; Walther 1997). The two surgical approaches have had no difference in hemodynamic changes or need for intraoperative antihypertensive

---

Table 54.4 Preoperative medical blockade of pheochromocytoma (from Walther *et al.* (1999c))

Two weeks before surgery

Oral phenoxybenzamine
- 10 mg two times daily
- Increase the dose 0.5 mg/kg/day in two divided doses to control blood pressure or symptoms

Beta-adrenergic blockers
- Administered to patients with tachycardia (pulse greater than 100) after adequate alpha blockade. Administration of propranolol before alpha blockade can worsen hypertension secondary to unopposed vasoconstriction

Metyrosine
- 250 mg every 6 hours
- Increase dosage by 250 to 500 mg per day to control blood pressure or symptoms (maximum dosage, 4 g/day)

Night before surgery
At 12 a.m. administer phenoxybenzamine, 1 mg/kg, and metyrosine, 1g. Patient put to bedrest with siderails up because of orthostatic hypotension

---

treatment (Vargas *et al.* 1997). Patients have similar operative time, blood loss, and transfusion rate by either approach (Vargas *et al.* 1997; Guazzoni *et al.* 1995; Reinig *et al.* 1986; Binkovitz *et al.* 1990). Laparoscopic removal of pheochromocytoma is safe and is replacing open surgery as the choice for management (Vargas *et al.* 1997; Guazzoni *et al.* 1995; Walther 1997; Gagner *et al.* 1997).

In contrast to sporadic pheochromocytoma, hereditary forms are frequently multifocal and recurrent. Partial adrenalectomy has been performed to preserve adrenal cortical function and maintain quality of life (Lee *et al.* 1996; Albanese and Wiener 1993; Telenius-Berg *et al.* 1989; de Graaf *et al.* 1999). Recently, laparoscopic partial adrenalectomy has been reported feasible (Janetschek *et al.* 1997; Walther *et al.* 2000).

Postoperative care

Removal of the pheochromocytoma can be associated with hypotension related to contracted plasma volume or orthostatic changes. Treatment requires fluid replacement to replenish intravascular volume and careful monitoring of blood pressure upon assuming upright position. Phenoxybenzamine has a half-life of 24 hours and metyrosine a half-life of 4 hours (Pullerits *et al.* 1988). Orthostasis and blunting of the effect of pressor drugs will occur until the preoperative blockade wears off, usually by 24 hours after surgery. Hypoglycemia related to increased insulin production from elevated levels of plasma catecholamines may also occur. Monitoring glucose levels and administration of 5 per cent intravenous dextrose will support the patient until normal physiologic responses return (Remine *et al.* 1974; Pullerits *et al.* 1988). After surgery patients may develop hypertension from overcorrection of fluid volume or pain.

Follow-up

Evaluation of patients after surgical removal of pheochromocytoma has demonstrated non-paroxysmal hypertension, attributed to essential hypertension, in 27–38 per cent (Remine *et al.* 1974; Ellison *et al.* 1988; Shapiro and Fig 1989; Pullerits *et al.* 1988). Reported 5-year survival after removal of benign pheochromocytoma is 84–96 per cent (Remine *et al.* 1974; Modlin *et al.* 1979; Levine and McDonald 1984; van Heerden *et al.* 1990). Long-term follow-up of patients with sporadic pheochromocytoma has shown a 4.5 per cent recurrence rate, usually associated with metastatic disease (van Heerden *et al.* 1990). Probability of recurrence in these patients has been estimated as 2 per cent at 10 years, 7 per cent at 15 years, and 9 per cent at greater than 20 years after surgery (van Heerden *et al.* 1990).

After removal of pheochromocytoma, patients are evaluated with plasma and urinary catecholamines and metanephrines about 6 weeks after surgery to confirm successful treatment. Patients with sporadic pheochromocytoma less than 5 cm in diameter are evaluated yearly for recurrence of symptoms or hypertension. Patients with larger sporadic tumors or bilateral adrenal tumors thought to be sporadic also have yearly catecholamine and free metanephrine determination based on elevated risk for metastases or recurrence.

Patients at risk for hereditary forms of pheochromocytoma are at high risk to develop multiple tumors over the course of their lives, and require closer follow-up. When no tumors are present, abdominal imaging with CT or MR and plasma and urinary catecholamine and free metanephrine determinations are performed yearly for 3 years. If findings compatible with pheochromocytoma are still not observed, patients are evaluated every 2 years.

Patients from families with hereditary forms of pheochromocytoma and a new or recurrent tumor suspicious for pheochromocytoma are evaluated every 6 months for related signs or symptoms, with appropriate imaging, and with plasma and urinary catecholamines and free metanephrines. MIBG may be performed as needed to characterize any tumor as pheochromocytoma, or before surgery. Provocative testing may be informative if other tests are not diagnostic. Surgery is recommended in patients with localized tumors, elevated catecholamine secretion, associated signs or symptoms, or when tumor size approached 4–5 cm in diameter. Patients with smaller tumors that appear destructive to the adrenal gland, who wish to undergo partial adrenalectomy, may require surgery when the tumor is smaller. Any affected patient from a hereditary pheochromocytoma family should be evaluated and treated before pregnancy or surgery is contemplated.

References

Aguilo, F., Tamayo, N., Vazquez-Quintana, E., *et al.* (1991). Pheochromocytoma: a twenty year experience at the University Hospital. *Puerto Rican Health Sci. J.* **10**, 135–42.

Albanese, C.T. and Wiener, E.S. (1993). Routine total bilateral adrenalectomy is not warranted in childhood familial pheochromocytoma. *J. Pediatr. Surg.* **28**, 1248–52.

Atuk, N.O. (1983). Pheochromocytoma: diagnosis, localization, and treatment. *Hosp. Pract.* **18**, 187–202.

Averbuch, S.D., Steakley, C.S., Young, R.C., *et al.* (1988). Malignant pheochromocytoma: effective treatment with a combination of cyclophosphamide, vincristine, and dacarbazine. *Ann. Intern. Med.* **109**, 267–73.

Baysal, B.E., van Schothorst, E.M., Farr, J.E., *et al.* (1999). Repositioning the hereditary paraganglioma critical region on chromosome band 11q23. *Hum. Genet.* **104**, 219–25.

Binkovitz, L.A., Johnson, C.D., and Stephens, D.H. (1990). Islet cell tumors in von Hippel–Lindau disease: increased prevalence and relationship to the multiple endocrine neoplasias. *Am. J. Roentgenol.* **155**, 501–5.

Bogdasarian, R.S. and Lotz, P.R. (1979). Multiple simultaneous paragangliomas of the head and neck in association with multiple retroperitoneal pheochromocytomas. *Otolaryngol. Head Neck Surg.* **87**, 648–52.

Bomanji, J., Levison, D.A., Flatman, W.D., *et al.* (1987). Uptake of iodine-123 MIBG by pheochromocytomas, paragangliomas, and neuroblastomas: a histopathological comparison. *J. Nucl. Med.* **28**, 973–8.

Bravo, E.L. (1991). Diagnosis of pheochromocytoma. Reflections on a controversy. *Hypertension* **17**, 742–4.

Bravo, E.L., Tarazi, R.C., Fouad, F.M., Vidt, D.G., and Gifford, R.W. Jr (1981). Clonidine-suppression test: a useful aid in the diagnosis of pheochromocytoma. *New Engl. J. Med.* **305**, 623–6.

Chen, F., Slife, L., Kishida, T., Mulvihill, J., Tisherman, S.E., and Zbar, B. (1996). Genotype–phenotype correlation in von Hippel–Lindau disease: identification of a mutation associated with VHL type 2A. *J. Med. Genet.* **33**, 716–17.

Chew, S.L., Dacie, J.E., Reznek, R.H., *et al.* (1994). Bilateral phaeochromocytomas in von Hippel–Lindau disease: diagnosis by adrenal vein sampling and catecholamine assay. *Quart. J. Med.* **87**, 49–54.

Christenson, R., Smith, C.W., and Burko, H. (1976). Arteriographic manifestations of pheochromocytoma. *Am. J. Roentgenol.* **126**, 567–75.

Clarke, M.R., Weyant, R.J., Watson, C.G., and Carty, S.E. (1998). Prognostic markers in pheochromocytoma. *Hum. Pathol.* **29**, 522–6.

de Graaf, J.S., Dullaart, R.P., and Zwierstra, R.P. (1999). Complications after bilateral adrenalectomy for phaeochromocytoma in multiple endocrine neoplasia type 2—a plea to conserve adrenal function. *Eur. J. Surg.* **165**, 843–6.

Egawa, S., Futami, H., Takasaki, K., *et al.* (1998). Genotype–phenotype correlation of patients with multiple endocrine neoplasia type 2 in Japan. *Jpn J. Clin. Oncol.* **28**, 590–6.

Eisenhofer, G., Lenders, J.W., Linehan, W.M., Walther, M.M., Goldstein, D.S., and Keiser, H.R. (1999). Plasma normetanephrine and metanephrine for detecting pheochromocytoma in von Hippel–Lindau disease and multiple endocrine neoplasia type 2. *New Engl. J. Med.* **340**, 1872–9.

Ellison, G.T., Mansberger, J.A., Wray, C.H., and Mansberger, A.R. (1988). Diagnosis and treatment of pheochromocytomas: Part I. Surgical rounds, pp. 39–54.

Eng, C., Clayton, D., Schuffenecker, I., *et al.* (1996). The relationship between specific RET proto-oncogene mutations and disease phenotype in multiple endocrine neoplasia type 2. International RET mutation consortium analysis. *J. Am. Med. Assoc.* **276**, 1575–9.

Epstein, F.H. and Eckhoff, R.D. (1967). The epidemiology of high blood pressure—geographic distributions and etiologic factors. In *The epidemiology of hypertension* (ed. J. Stamler, R. Stamler, and T.N. Pullman), pp. 155–66. Grune and Stratton, New York.

Gagner, M., Pomp, A., Heniford, B.T., Pharand, D., and Lacroix, A. (1997). Laparoscopic adrenalectomy. Lessons learned from 100 consecutive procedures. *Ann. Surg.* **226**, 238–47.

Garcia, A., Matias-Guiu, X., Cabezas, R., *et al.* (1997). Molecular diagnosis of von Hippel–Lindau disease in a kindred with a predominance of familial phaeochromocytoma. *Clin. Endocrinol.* (*Oxford*) **46**, 359–63.

Goldstein, D.S., Stull, R., Eisenhofer, G., *et al.* (1986). Plasma 3,4-dihydroxyphenylalanine (dopa) and catecholamines in neuroblastoma or pheochromocytoma. *Ann. Intern. Med.* **105**, 887–8.

Grossman, E., Goldstein, D.S., Hoffman, A., and Keiser, H.R. (1991). Glucagon and clonidine testing in the diagnosis of pheochromocytoma. *Hypertension* **17**, 733–41.

Guazzoni, G., Montorsi, F., Bocciardi, A., *et al.* (1995). Transperitoneal laparoscopic versus open adrenalectomy for benign hyperfunctioning adrenal tumors: a comparative study. *J. Urol.* **153**, 1597–600.

Hill, F.S., Jander, H.P., Murad, T., and Diethelm, A.G. (1983). The coexistence of renal artery stenosis and pheochromocytoma. *Ann. Surg.* **197**, 484–90.

Howe, J.R., Norton, J.A., and Wells, S.A. Jr (1993). Prevalence of pheochromocytoma and hyperparathyroidism in multiple endocrine neoplasia type 2A: results of long-term follow-up. *Surgery* **114**, 1070–7.

Janetschek, G., Lhotta, K., Gasser, R., Finkenstedt, G., Jaschke, W., and Bartsch, G. (1997). Adrenal-sparing laparoscopic surgery for aldosterone-producing adenoma. *J. Endourol.* **11**, 145–8.

John, H., Ziegler, W.H., Hauri, D., and Jaeger, P. (1999). Pheochromocytomas: can malignant potential be predicted? *Urology* **53**, 679–83.

Lawrence, A.M. (1967). Glucagon provocative test for pheochromocytoma. *Ann. Intern. Med.* **66**, 1091–6.

Lee, J.E., Curley, S.A., Gagel, R.F., Evans, D.B., and Hickey, R.C. (1996). Cortical-sparing adrenalectomy for patients with bilateral pheochromocytoma. *Surgery* **120**, 1064–70.

Lenders, J.W., Keiser, H.R., Goldstein, D.S., *et al.* (1995). Plasma metanephrines in the diagnosis of pheochromocytoma. *Ann. Intern. Med.* **123**, 101–9.

Levine, S.N. and McDonald, J.C. (1984). The evaluation and management of pheochromocytomas. *Advan. Surg.* **17**, 281–313.

Linehan, W.M., Lerman, M.I., and Zbar, B. (1995). Identification of the von Hippel–Lindau (VHL) gene. Its role in renal cancer. *J. Am. Med. Assoc.* **273**, 564–70.

Lips, C.J., Landsvater, R.M., Hoppener, J.W., *et al.* (1994). Clinical screening as compared with DNA analysis in families with multiple endocrine neoplasia type 2A. *New Engl. J. Med.* **331**, 828–35.

Loh, K.C., Fitzgerald, P.A., Matthay, K.K., Yeo, P.P., and Price, D.C. (1997). The treatment of malignant pheochromocytoma with iodine-131 metaiodobenzylguanidine (131I-MIBG): a comprehensive review of 116 reported patients. *J. Endocrinol. Invest.* **20**, 648–58.

Maddock, I.R., Moran, A., Maher, E.R., *et al.* (1996). A genetic register for von Hippel–Lindau disease. *J. Med. Genet.* **33**, 120–7.

Manger, W.M. and Gifford, R.W. (1996). *Clinical and experimental pheochromocytoma*. Blackwell Science, Cambridge, Massachusetts.

Maurea, S., Cuocolo, A., Reynolds, J.C., *et al.* (1993). Iodine-131-metaiodobenzylguanidine scintigraphy in preoperative and postoperative evaluation of paragangliomas: comparison with CT and MRI. *J. Nucl. Med.* **34**, 173–9.

McCaffrey, T.V., Meyer, F.B., Michels, V.V., Piepgras, D.G., and Marion, M.S. (1994). Familial paragangliomas of the head and neck. *Arch. Otolaryngol. Head Neck Surg.* **120**, 1211–16.

Melicow, M.M. (1977). One hundred cases of pheochromocytoma (107 tumors) at the Columbia-Presbyterian Medical Center, 1926–1976: a clinicopathological analysis. *Cancer* **40**, 1987–2004.

Modlin, I.M., Farndon, J.R., Shepherd, A., *et al.* (1979). Phaeochromocytomas in 72 patients: clinical and diagnostic features, treatment and long term results. *Br. J. Surg.* **66**, 456–65.

Nakajo, M., Shapiro, B., Copp, J., *et al.* (1983). The normal and abnormal distribution of the adrenomedullary imaging agent m-[I-131]iodobenzylguanidine (I-131 MIBG) in man: evaluation by scintigraphy. *J. Nucl. Med.* **24**, 672–82.

Nativ, O., Grant, C.S., Sheps, S.G., *et al.* (1992). Prognostic profile for patients with pheochromocytoma derived from clinical and pathological factors and DNA ploidy pattern. *J. Surg. Oncol.* **50**, 258–62.

Newbould, E.C., Ross, G.A., Dacie, J.E., Bouloux, P.M., Besser, G.M., and Grossman, A. (1991). The use of venous catheterization in the diagnosis and localization of bilateral phaeochromocytomas. *Clin. Endocrinol.* (*Oxford*) **35**, 55–9.

Newell, K.A., Prinz, R.A., Pickleman, J., *et al.* (1988). Pheochromocytoma multisystem crisis. A surgical emergency. *Arch. Surg.* **123**, 956–9.

Orchard, T., Grant, C.S., van Heerden, J.A., and Weaver, A. (1993). Pheochromocytoma—continuing evolution of surgical therapy. *Surgery* **114**, 1153–8.

Pacak, K., Linehan, W. M., Eisenhofer, G., Walther, M. M., and Goldstein, D. S. (2001). NIH Conference. Recent advances in genetics, diagnosis, localization, and treatment of pheochromocytoma. *Ann. Intern. Med.*, **134**, 315.

Page, D.L., DeLessis, R.A., and Hough, A.J. (1986). *Tumors of the adrenal. Pheochromocytoma*, Second Series, pp. 183–217. Armed Forces Institute of Pathology, Washington, DC.

Page, L.B. (1976). Epidemiologic evidence on the etiology of human hypertension and its possible prevention. *Am. Heart J.* **91**, 527–34.

Page, L.B. and Copeland, R.B. (1968). Pheochromocytoma. *Dis. Monthly* 1–40.

Perry, R.R., Keiser, H.R., Norton, J.A., *et al.* (1990). Surgical management of pheochromocytoma with the use of metyrosine. *Ann. Surg.* **212**, 621–8.

Pick, L. (1912). Das Ganglioma embryonale sympathicum (Sympathoma embryonale). *Berlin Klin. Wochenschr.* **49**, 16–22.

Pomares, F.J., Canas, R., Rodriguez, J.M., Hernandez, A.M., Parrilla, P., and Tebar, F.J. (1998). Differences between sporadic and multiple endocrine neoplasia type 2A phaeochromocytoma. *Clin. Endocrinol.* (*Oxford*) **48**, 195–200.

Proye, C., Vix, M., Goropoulos, A., Kerlo, P., and Lecomte-Houcke, M. (1992). High incidence of malignant pheochromocytoma in a surgical unit. 26 cases out of 100 patients operated from 1971 to 1991. *J. Endocrinol. Invest.* **15**, 651–63.

Pullerits, J., Ein, S., and Balfe, J.W. (1988). Anaesthesia for phaeochromocytoma. *Can. J. Anaesthesiol.* **35**, 526–34.

Raue, F. (1998). German medullary thyroid carcinoma/multiple endocrine neoplasia registry. German MTC/MEN Study Group. Medullary thyroid carcinoma/multiple endocrine neoplasia type 2. *Langenbecks Arch. Surg.* **383**, 334–6.

Reinig, J.W., Doppman, J.L., Dwyer, A.J., Johnson, A.R., and Knop, R.H. (1986). Adrenal masses differentiated by MR. *Radiology* **158**, 81–4.

Remine, W.H., Chong, G.C., van Heerden, J.A., Sheps, S.G., and Harrison, E.G. Jr (1974). Current management of pheochromocytoma. *Ann. Surg.* **179**, 740–8.

Richard, S., Beigelman, C., Duclos, J.M., *et al.* (1994). Pheochromocytoma as the first manifestation of von Hippel–Lindau disease. *Surgery* **116**, 1076–81.

Ritter, M.M., Frilling, A., and Crossey, P.A., *et al.* (1996). Isolated familial pheochromocytoma as a variant of von Hippel–Lindau disease. *J. Clin. Endocrinol. Metab.* **81**, 1035–7.

Ross, E.J. and Griffith, D.N. (1989). The clinical presentation of phaeochromocytoma. *Quart. J. Med.* **71**, 485–96.

Schlumberger, M., Gicquel, C., Lumbroso, J., *et al.* (1992). Malignant pheochromocytoma: clinical, biological, histologic and therapeutic data in a series of 20 patients with distant metastases. *J. Endocrinol. Invest.* **15**, 631–42.

Shapiro, B. and Fig, L.M. (1989). Management of pheochromocytoma. *Endocrinol. Metab. Clin. N. Am.* **18**, 443–81.

Shapiro, B., Copp, J.E., Sisson, J.C., Eyre, P.L., Wallis, J., and Beierwaltes, W.H. (1985). Iodine-131 metaiodobenzylguanidine for the locating of suspected pheochromocytoma: experience in 400 cases. *J. Nucl. Med.* **26**, 576–85.

Shulkin, B.L., Thompson, N.W., Shapiro, B., Francis, I.R., and Sisson, J.C. (1999). Pheochromocytomas: imaging with 2-[fluorine-18]fluoro-2-deoxy-D-glucose PET. *Radiology* **212**, 35–41.

Siqueira-Filho, A.G., Sheps, S.G., Maher, F.T., Jiang, N.S., and Elveback, L.R. (1975). Glucagon-blood catecholamine test: use in isolated and familial pheochromocytoma. *Arch. Intern. Med.* **135**, 1227–31.

Skoldberg, F., Grimelius, L., Woodward, E.R., *et al.* (1998). A family with hereditary extra-adrenal paragangliomas without evidence for mutations in the von Hippel–Lindau disease or ret genes. *Clin. Endocrinol.* (*Oxford*) **48**, 11–16.

Skolyszewski, J., Korzeniowski, S., and Pszon, J. (1991). Results of radiotherapy in chemodectoma of the temporal bone. *Acta Oncol.* **30**, 847–9.

Starkman, M.N., Zelnik, T.C., Nesse, R.M., and Cameron, O.G. (1985). Anxiety in patients with pheochromocytomas. *Arch. Intern. Med.* **145**, 248–52.

Stewart, B.H., Bravo, E.L., Haaga, J., Meaney, T.F., and Tarazi, R. (1978). Localization of pheochromocytoma by computed tomography. *New Engl. J. Med.* **299**, 460–1.

Streeten, D.H., Anderson, G.H. Jr, and Wagner, S. (1990). Effect of age on response of secondary hypertension to specific treatment. *Am. J. Hypertens.* **3**, 360–5.

Stuhrmann, M. and Arslan-Kirchner, M. (1996). Genetic changes associated with multiple endocrine neoplasia type 2A. In *Hereditary cancer*, 1st edn (ed. H.S.R.W.W. Muller), pp. 99–101. Karger, Basel.

Sutton, M.G., Sheps, S.G., and Lie, J.T. (1981). Prevalence of clinically unsuspected pheochromocytoma. Review of a 50-year autopsy series. *Mayo Clin. Proc.* **56**, 354–60.

Telenius-Berg, M., Ponder, M.A., Berg, B., Ponder, B.A.J., and Werner, S. (1989). Quality of life after bilateral adrenalectomy in MEN 2. *Henry Ford Hosp. Med. J.* **37**, 160–3.

Tisherman, S.E., Tisherman, B.G., Tisherman, S.A., Dunmire, S., Levey, G.S., and Mulvihill, J.J. (1993). Three-decade investigation of familial pheochromocytoma. An allele of von Hippel–Lindau disease? *Arch. Intern. Med.* **153**, 2550–6.

van Heerden, J.A., Roland, C.F., Carney, J.A., Sheps, S.G., and Grant, C.S. (1990). Long-term evaluation following resection of apparently benign pheochromocytoma(s)/paraganglioma(s). *World J. Surg.* **14**, 325–9.

van Schothorst, E.M., Jansen, J.C., Bardoel, A.F., *et al.* (1996). Confinement of PGL, an imprinted gene causing hereditary paragangliomas, to a 2-cM interval on 11q22-q23 and exclusion of DRD2 and NCAM as candidate genes. *Eur. J. Hum. Genet.* **4**, 267–73.

van Schothorst, E.M., Jansen, J.C., Grooters, E., *et al.* (1998). Founder effect at PGL1 in hereditary head and neck paraganglioma families from the Netherlands. *Am. J. Hum. Genet.* **63**, 468–73.

Vargas, H.I., Kavoussi, L.R., Bartlett, D.L., *et al.* (1997). Laparoscopic adrenalectomy: a new standard of care. *Urology* **49**, 673–8.

Walther, M.M. (1997). Laparoscopic surgery for adrenal disease. *Principles and Practice of Oncology Updates* **11**, 1–9.

Walther, M.M., Reiter, R., Keiser, H.R., *et al.* (1999*a*). Clinical and genetic characterization of pheochromocytoma in von Hippel–Lindau families. Comparison with sporadic pheochromocytoma gives insight into natural history of pheochromocytoma. *J. Urol.* **162**, 659–64.

Walther, M.M., Herring, J., Enquist, E., Keiser, H.R., and Linehan, W.M. (1999*b*). von Recklinghausen's disease and pheochromocytomas. *J. Urol.* **162**, 1582–6.

Walther, M.M., Keiser, H.R., and Linehan, W.M. (1999*c*). Pheochromocytoma: evaluation, diagnosis, and management. *World J. Urol.* **17**, 35–9.

Walther, M.M., Herring, J., Choyke, P.L., and Linehan, W.M. (2000). Laparoscopic partial adrenalectomy in patients with hereditary forms of pheochromocytoma. *J. Urol.*, **164**, 14.

Watson, J.P., Hughes, E.A., Bryan, R.L., Lawson, N., and Barnett, A.H. (1990). A predominantly adrenaline-secreting phaeochromocytoma. *Quart. J. Med.* **76**, 747–52.

Yoshimoto, T., Naruse, M., Zeng, Z., *et al.* (1998). The relatively high frequency of p53 gene mutations in multiple and malignant phaeochromocytomas. *J. Endocrinol.* **159**, 247–55.

Yu, L., Fleckman, A.M., Chadha, M., Sacks, E., Levetan, C., and Vikram, B. (1996). Radiation therapy of metastatic pheochromocytoma: case report and review of the literature. *Am. J. Clin. Oncol.* **19**, 389–93.

55. Congenital adrenal hyperplasia: 21-hydroxylase deficiency and 11β-hydroxylase deficiency

Maria I. New

Introduction

Congenital adrenal hyperplasia (CAH) is a family of autosomal recessive disorders involving impaired enzymatic function at any of the various steps in the synthesis of cortisol from cholesterol by the adrenal cortex. Blocks in cortisol synthesis impair the negative feedback control of adrenocorticotropin (ACTH) secretion, which leads to chronic stimulation of the adrenal cortex by ACTH. The enzyme deficiencies in CAH act as a dam behind which steroid precursors accumulate, which are then shunted through uninhibited pathways and result in excessive steroidogenesis. It is primarily the excess androgens and steroid precursors that determine the clinical presentation.

Over 90 per cent of CAH cases are caused by 21-hydroxylase deficiency. The second most common cause is 11β-hydroxylase deficiency, and less frequent causes are 3β-hydroxysteroid dehydrogenase deficiency, 17α-hydroxylase/17,20-lyase deficiency, and mutations in the gene for the steroidogenic acute regulatory (StAR) protein (causing congential lipoid adrenal hyperplasia) (New and White 1995; New *et al.* 1982; Lin *et al.* 1995).

21-Hydroxylase deficiency can occur in a classical (simple virilizing or salt-wasting) or a nonclassical form. In classical CAH due to 21-hydroxylase deficiency (21-OHD), prenatal exposure of female urogenital tissues to potent androgens such as testosterone and Δ⁴-androstenedione at a critical stage of differentiation results in ambiguous external genitalia in genetic females. Up to 75 per cent of these patients will be salt wasters as well, lacking adequate aldosterone production (New *et al.* 1995*a*). In the nonclassical form of adrenal hyperplasia, patients are born with normal genitalia and, with a moderate enzyme deficiency, they present with signs of hyperandrogenism in childhood or later.

11β-Hydroxylation is an enzymatic function necessary for the biosynthesis of cortisol by the zona fasciculata (ZF) of the adrenal cortex. Defects in this step lead to the abnormally increased production by the ZF of the steroid 11-deoxycorticosterone (DOC), a moderately potent mineralocorticoid, which causes sodium retention and volume expansion that result in hypertension. Further, the excess production of adrenal androgens leads to virilization, prenatally in the genetic female and postnatally in both sexes.

Steroidogenesis

Aldosterone, cortisol, and testosterone are derived from cholesterol and utilize many of the same enzymes for their synthesis in the adrenal cortex (Fig. 55.1). Therefore, defects in any of the enzymes that are common to the synthesis pathway of these hormones can result in the loss of a combination of some or all of their production, or unchecked negative feedback loops can lead to overproduction. In the case of 21-OHD and 11β-OHD, steroid precursors accumulate where the enzyme deficiency blocks their path, which then overflow into blocked biosynthetic pathways, resulting in the production of excess androgens.

The adrenal cortex produces cortisol and aldosterone by specific and largely separate regulatory systems. The cortex is divided into three distinct zones—the outer zona glomerulosa (ZG), the middle zona fasciculata (ZF), and the inner zona reticularis (ZR)—defined by their different cellular arrangements and distinct functionally. Mineralocorticoids are synthesized in the zona glomerulosa, glucocorticoids are produced by the zona fasciculata/reticularis, and androgenic steroids are synthesized in the zona reticularis.

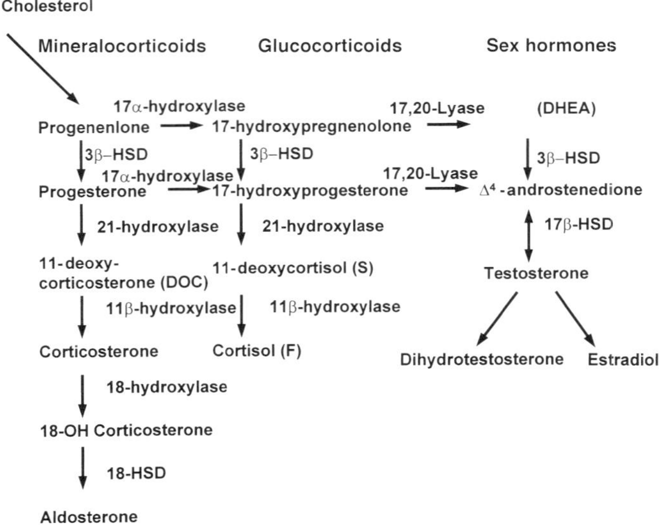

Fig. 55.1 Pathways of steroid biosynthesis. HSD, Hydroxysteroid dehydrogenase; DHEA, dehydroepiandrosterone.

The production of cortisol in the ZF occurs in five steps: cleavage of the cholesterol side chain by the cholesterol desmolase enzyme, cytochrome P450scc, to yield pregnenolone; conversion of pregnenolone by 3β-dehydrogenation (with accompanying $\Delta^{5,4}$-isomerization) to progesterone by the short-chain dehydrogenase family enzyme 3β-hydroxysteroid dehydrogenase (3β-HSD); and successive hydroxylations at the 17α, 21, and 11β positions, each mediated by a distinct cytochrome P450, resulting in cortisol (Fig. 55.1) (New and White 1995).

Cortisol synthesis is regulated by a negative feedback loop in which high serum levels of cortisol inhibit the release of ACTH from the pituitary, while low serum levels of cortisol stimulate the release of ACTH. This defines the hypothalamo–pituitary–adrenal axis. The central nervous system determines the hypothalamic set point for the plasma cortisol level, so that plasma cortisol levels lower than the hypothalamic–pituitary set point will increase the secretion (negative feedback regulation). The adrenal 21-OH or 11β-OH enzyme deficiencies, causing impaired synthesis and decreased secretion of cortisol, thus lead to chronic elevations of ACTH with overstimulation and consequent hyperplasia of the adrenal cortex.

Fetal development

Male genital differentiation in embryonic and fetal life is dependent upon two functions of the testes (Jost 1971): (1) the secretion from Leydig cells of sufficient quantities of testosterone to direct the formation of the internal male genital structures and external genitalia (after it has undergone peripheral conversion to dihydrotestosterone (DHT)); (2) the secretion from Sertoli cells of the nonsteroidal anti-Müllerian hormone (AMH) glycoprotein to suppress development of the Müllerian ducts, so that normal males are born without a uterus and fallopian tubes.

Since there is no anomalous production of AMH in the gonadally normal female with CAH, and the 21-OHD or 11β-OHD is only in the adrenal and not in the gonads, females presenting with even extreme virilization from DHT overexposure will have normal development of their internal reproductive structures. With proper treatment and reparative surgery of the external genitalia, child-bearing is possible.

21-Hydroxylase deficiency

Clinical manifestations

The 21-hydroxylase deficiency syndrome presents in three forms: classical simple virilizing; classical salt-wasting; and nonclassical.

Classical simple virilizing
Excess adrenal androgen production coincides with the time of sexual development of the fetus and will result in varying degrees of genital ambiguity in newborn genetic females with classical CAH. In extreme cases, the urethra opens at the tip of the phallus and cannot be distinguished from that of a normal male. In most cases, however, the excess androgens result in an enlarged clitoris with fusion of the labioscrotal folds, resulting in a urogenital sinus. For both extreme or milder cases, the female internal genitalia are normal with normal development of ovaries and Müllerian structures.

Males affected with 21-OHD are born with normal genitalia, although there may be excess pigmentation of the scrotal skin. After birth, both females and males develop signs of androgen excess such as precocious development of pubic and axillary hair, acne, phallic enlargement, rapid growth and musculoskeletal development, and advanced epiphyseal age. Though initial growth in the young child with CAH is rapid, potential height is reduced and short adult stature results due to premature epiphyseal fusion. Diagnosis is often delayed in males, as the genital ambiguity that leads to diagnosis at birth in females is absent in males. However, even if diagnosis is not delayed and adrenal androgen excess is controlled from birth, patients do not generally achieve their target height.

Classical salt-wasting
Depending on the severity of the loss of 21-hydroxylase function, adrenal aldosterone secretion may not be sufficient for sodium reabsorption by distal renal tubules. Patients with aldosterone deficiency suffer from salt-wasting 21-OHD. These patients are as virilized as those with simple virilizing 21-OHD and also have the potential of adrenal crisis (azotemia, vascular collapse, shock, and death) due to renal salt-wasting. Adrenal crisis can occur as early as 1–4 weeks of life. Affected males are at high risk of salt-wasting adrenal crisis since their normal genitalia do not flag their condition; they are sometimes discharged from the hospital at birth without diagnosis and suffer an adrenal crisis at home.

Nonclassical
Nonclassical 21-OHD (NC21-OHD) may present at any time postnatally—in infancy, childhood, adolescence, or adulthood. Symptoms of NC21-OHD are those of androgen excess, including acne, premature development of pubic hair, advanced bone age, accelerated linear growth velocity, and, as in classical 21-OHD, reduced adult stature due to premature epiphyseal fusion.

Females affected with NC21-OHD are born with normal genitalia, though postnatal symptoms may include hirsutism, temporal baldness, severe cystic acne, delayed menarche, menstrual irregularities, and infertility. A subset of female patients with NC21-OHD develop polycystic ovaries. Boys manifesting NC21-OHD may have early beard growth, acne, early growth spurt, premature pubic hair, an enlarged phallus, advanced bone age resulting in short adult stature, and reduced fertility. Proportionately small testes as compared to the phallus is a reliable indication of adrenal androgen excess as opposed to testicular androgen excess. Adrenal androgen excess in men is not easily detectable and may only be manifested by short stature or oligozoospermia and diminished fertility.

No clinical signs are present in a limited number of males and females who are affected with NC21-OHD, as discovered during family studies. However, biochemically they compare to affected patients.

Epidemiology

Analysis of CAH incidence data from almost 6.5 million newborns screened in the general population worldwide has demonstrated a consistent overall incidence of 1:15 000 live births for the severe classic form of CAH (Pang and Clark 1990, 1993; Pang *et al.* 1988). The incidence of CAH in either homogeneous or heterogeneous general populations has been as high as one in 7500 live births (Brazil).

The overall frequency of nonclassic 21-OHD is high. The study of Speiser *et al.* (1985), assessing the population genetics of the nonclassical disorder, found NC21-OHD to be the most common human autosomal recessive disease trait. The disease frequency in the general heterogeneous population of New York City was 1/100. The highest ethnic specific frequency was found among Ashkenazic Jews at 1/27. Other specific ethnic groups also exhibited high disease frequency: 1/40 Hispanics, 1/50 Slavs, and 1/300 Italians. These results have also been confirmed by other reports (Sherman *et al.* 1988; Zerah *et al.* 1990).

Molecular genetics

The gene for adrenal 21-hydroxylase, *CYP21*, is located about 30 kb from an inactive cognate gene, *CYP21P* (P for pseudogene), on chromosome 6p in the area of HLA genes. The high degree of sequence similarity (96–98 per cent) between *CYP21* and *CYP21P* apparently permits two types of recombination events: (1) unequal crossing-over during meiosis, which results in complementary deletions/duplications of *CYP21* and the possible transmission of a null allele; (2) nine non-correspondences between the pseudogene and the coding gene (Higashi *et al.* 1986; White *et al.* 1986) that, if transferred by 'gene conversion', result in deleterious mutations. Deletions generally account for 20–25 per cent of classic 21-OHD alleles, and small deletions and point mutations make up the rest.

Approximately 40 mutations in the *CYP21* gene causing 21-OHD have been identified thus far (Krawczak and Cooper 1997) and, of those, eight mutations (nine including deletions) account for 90–95 per cent of mutated alleles. Specific mutations may be correlated with a given degree of enzymatic compromise and the clinical form of 21-OHD (Werkmeister *et al.* 1986; Mornet *et al.* 1991; Higashi *et al.* 1991; Speiser *et al.* 1992*a*; Wedell *et al.* 1992; White *et al.* 1994*a*; New *et al.* 1996). The genotype for the classical form of CAH is predicted to be a severe mutation on both alleles at the 21-OH locus, with completely abolished enzymatic activity generally associated with salt-wasting. The point mutation A (or C) to G near the end of intron 2, which is the single most frequent mutation in classic 21-OHD, causes premature splicing of the intron and a shift in the translational reading frame (Higashi *et al.* 1991, 1988). Most patients who are homozygous for this mutation have the salt-wasting form of the disorder (Speiser *et al.* 1992*b*; Wilson *et al.* 1995*a*). One mutation in exon 4 (I172N), specifically associated with simple virilizing 21-OHD (Amor *et al.* 1988), has been shown in *in vitro* cell transfection assay to result in 1 per cent of normal enzyme activity (Tusie-Luna *et al.* 1990). Adrenal production of aldosterone is normally in the range of 1/100–1/1000 that of cortisol. The very low residual activity of the I172N mutation apparently is still able to allow aldosterone synthesis and thus prevent significant salt-wasting in most cases of the simple virilizing form of 21-hydroxylase deficiency.

Patients with NC21-OHD are predicted to have mild mutations on both alleles or one severe and one mild mutation of the 21-OH locus (compound heterozygote). Missense mutations in exon 1 (P30L) and exon 7 (V281L), which are predominantly associated with this form of the disease, reduce enzymatic activity in cultured cells to 20–50 per cent of normal (Tusie-Luna *et al.* 1990). These patients do not have salt-wasting.

In 1995 we published a study of genetic and clinical findings of over 200 patients with 21-OHD (Wilson *et al.*, 1995*a*). We carefully assessed phenotypic characteristics by: (1) genital status with respect to virilization in females; (2) ACTH stimulation tests to evaluate secretion of androgens and 17-hydroxyprogesterone; (3) salt deprivation studies (whenever safe) to precisely describe the phenotype with respect to aldosterone deficiency and salt-wasting. After dividing our patients into 26 mutation-identical groups, we found that, in 11 groups, the genotype did not always predict the phenotype. One example of this nonconformity is the following: the V281L/Del genotype group consisted of 13 patients; while they had identical mutations, 11 were nonclassical, one was a simple virilizer, and one was a salt-waster. Another example we found of nonconcordance of genotype to phenotype is illustrated in patients with exon1 (P30L)/intron2 (A or C to G) mutations, as some have the salt-wasting form, while the others have the nonclassical form. This unexplained phenotypic variability within each mutation group has important implications for prenatal diagnosis and treatment.

Hormonal diagnosis

For classical 21-hydroxylase deficiency, progesterone, 17-hydroxyprogesterone (17-OHP), androstenedione, and testosterone are secreted in excess. The urinary excretion of the metabolites of these steroids is also increased. Hormonal diagnosis of 21-OH deficiency of any degree is best achieved by an ACTH stimulation test, which involves taking a blood sample to measure the serum 17-OHP concentration before and 60 minutes after intravenous administration of 0.25 mg synthetic ACTH$_{1-24}$ (Cortrosyn). Testing should be done early in the morning since serum 17-OHP concentrations are elevated at this time (measuring morning salivary also correlates with serum concentration). Random basal serum concentrations may not differ from that of normal in nonclassical patients. As seen in Fig. 55.2, nomogram plots of baseline versus stimulated 17-OHP concentrations result in three distinguishable groups: classical, nonclassical, and an overlap of heterozygotes and genetically unaffected. It should be noted that serum 17-OHP may be elevated in premature infants and infants under stress, which can result in false-positives.

11β-Hydroxylase deficiency

Clinical features and pathophysiology

11β-Hydroxylase deficiency, like 21-OHD, occurs late in cortisol synthesis, causing a shunting of accumulating precursor steroids

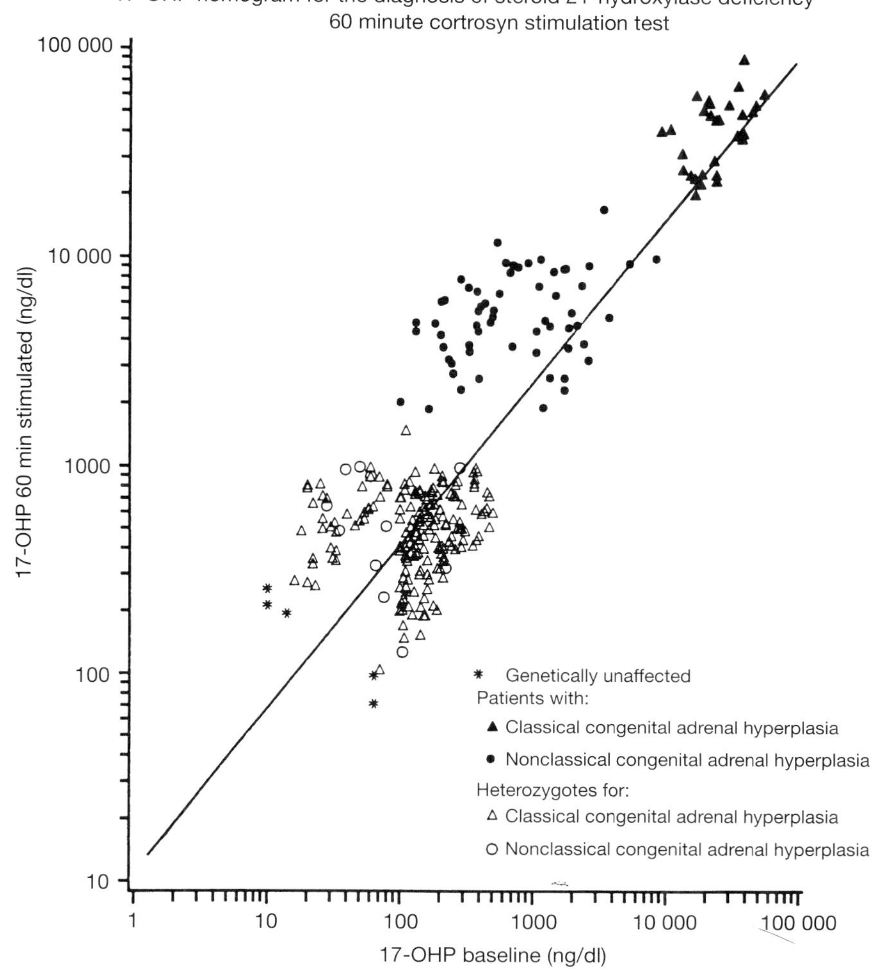

Fig. 55.2 Nomogram relating baseline to corticotropin-stimulated serum concentrations of 17-OHP. Scales are logarithmic. A regression line for all data points is shown.

into pathways of androgen biosynthesis, producing genital ambiguity in affected girls and postnatal hyperandrogenism in both sexes. Different types of imbalance in salt metabolism and fluid volume distinguish 21-OHD from 11β-OHD: in the former, deficient aldosterone synthesis causes salt-wasting and hypovolemia, whereas in the latter, an excess of mineralocorticoid causes expanded fluid volume and hypertension. As with 21-OHD, cases of mild, late-onset forms of 11β-OHD have also been reported.

Hypertension occurs in about 2/3 of untreated patients with 11β-OHD, appearing only infrequently in infancy and variably in later childhood (Mimouni *et al.* 1985). The deficiency of this enzyme results in an accumulation of precursors in the steroidogenic pathway, including deoxycorticosterone (DOC) and 11-deoxycortisol (Fig. 55.1). The abnormal adrenal steroid serum profile exerts a net mineralocorticoid effect, which alters renal function and causes sodium retention and volume expansion. Potassium depletion develops concomitantly with sodium retention; hypokalemia is variable. Plasma renin activity (PRA) production is suppressed secondary to mineralocorticoid-induced sodium retention and volume expansion, though hyporeninemia varies widely in degree, and in at least two cases has been absent (New *et al.* 1989). Aldosterone production is low secondary to low plasma renin. Accumulation of the late-pathway steroid intermediates increases their availability as substrates for the enzymes of androgen synthesis, causing excess adrenal androgen secretion.

It should be noted that it is not confirmed that DOC is the only factor in the development and maintenance of hypertension in 11β-OHD. In fact, blood pressure and DOC levels have not been well-correlated in some patients (Gandy *et al.* 1960; Green *et al.* 1960; Blunck 1969; Glenthoj *et al.* 1980), and administration of the steroid to both humans and animals has had only weak mineralocorticoid activity. Hence, it is possible that other metabolites of mineralocorticoid are responsible for the development of hypertension.

Epidemiology

The prevalence of 11β-hydroxylase deficiency is approximately 1 in 100 000 births in the general population (Zachmann *et al.* 1983). It accounts for 5–8 per cent of cases of congenital adrenal hyperplasia (CAH) (Rosler and Leiberman 1984; White *et al.* 1994*b*). The incidence is much higher in Israel (1 in 5000 to 7000 births) due to a clustering of cases traced to Jewish families of North African origin, particularly from Morocco and Tunisia (Rosler and Leiberman 1984; Rosler *et al.* 1992).

Molecular genetics

The *CYP11B1* gene, which encodes the 11β-hydroxylase enzyme, is comprised of 9 exons. Approximately 30 mutations in *CYP11B1* have been identified in cases of 11β-OH deficiency (Krawczak and Cooper 1997). It is located on chromosome 8q22, about 40 kb from the highly homologous gene *CYP11B2*, which encodes aldosterone synthase. Mutations in the *CYP11B1* gene have been identified throughout the coding region, but there is clustering around exons 2, 6, 7, and 8, suggestive of mutational hot spots (Merke *et al.* 1998). While gene conversions do occur between *CYP11B1* and *CYP11B2* (Merke *et al.* 1998; Mulatero *et al.* 1998), the majority of the mutations found in *CYP11B1* are random point mutations (White *et al.* 1991). These mutations have been identified from diverse ethnic backgrounds, with the highest incidence among a highly inbred group of Moroccan (Sephardic) Jews (Rosler and Leiberman 1984; Rosler *et al.* 1992).

Diagnosis

Oversecretion of the salt-retaining hormone DOC results in low-renin hypertension. The important diagnostic hormones are DOC, 11-deoxycortisol, and adrenal androgens, which are elevated. PRA is markedly suppressed (Rosler and Leiberman 1984).

Treatment

Treatment of CAH due to 21-hydroxylase deficiency has been ongoing since 1950. Glucocorticoid replacement therapy not only replaces the deficient hormone but also reduces the overstimulation of the adrenal cortex by reducing the release of ACTH, thereby suppressing the overproduction of adrenal androgens. Monitoring of 21-OHD should consist of measuring levels of 17-OHP and obtaining a simple adrenal profile (testosterone for females and prepubertal boys, and Δ^4-androstenedione for both males and females).

Hydrocortisone (cortisol) is the most often used compound for replacement therapy for 21-OH and 11β-OH deficiencies. Proper replacement therapy in 21-OH and 11β-OH deficiencies prevents further virilization, slowing accelerated growth and bone age advancement to a more normal rate, and allowing a normal onset of puberty. In 11β-OHD, glucocorticoid treatment suppresses the oversecretion of DOC and leads to the remission of hypertension. Excessive glucocorticoid administration can cause cushingoid facies, growth retardation, and inhibition of epiphyseal maturation. Some cases of long-standing hypertension in 11β-hydroxylase deficiency have responded to treatment (White *et al.* 1994*b*; New *et al.* 1995*b*), yet malignant hypertensive changes and considerable mortality are evident in some clinical surveys. Serum concentrations of DOC, PRA, and androgens are hormonal monitors of control, which should be combined with growth and skeletal age to obtain the best therapeutic outcome.

Hydrocortisone is a physiologic hormone and therefore minimizes complications. Oral administration is the usual mode of treatment, conventionally given daily in divided doses, as it is believed divided doses better suppress the production of adrenal androgens. Two equally divided doses of 10–20 mg/m^2 daily are adequate for the otherwise healthy child or, alternatively, a higher dosage can be given in the evening to suppress the morning ACTH surge (for example, 10 mg/m^2 in the morning and 15 mg/m^2 in the evening). The dosage may have to be increased for a few days to 2 to 3 times that of the normal daily dosage during times of non-life-threatening illness or stress. Families should be given injection kits of hydrocortisone (50 mg for young children; 100 mg for older patients) for times of emergency. Up to 5 to 10 times the daily dosage may be required during surgical procedures. Patients who show a poor response to the standard dosage of hydrocortisone may have their dosage increased to 20–30 mg/m^2 per day, or their regimen may have to be changed to a synthetic hormone analog such as prednisone or dexamethasone. The use of these analogs requires critical dosage adjustment since they are more potent and longer-acting. After puberty when final growth is achieved, treatment can be switched to dexamethasone, which is more convenient for the patient as it only needs to be taken once a day.

Patients with salt-wasting CAH may also require mineralocorticoid replacement. A cortisol analog, 21-acetyloxy-9α-fluorohydrocortisone (Florinef: 9α-FF), is used for its potent mineralocorticoid activity. A combination of hydrocortisone and Florinef has proven to be quite effective in treatment of patients with salt-wasting 21-OH deficiency. Florinef can be given to simple virilizers also as it reduces the amount of hydrocortisone necessary (and thus may reduce the side-effects of excess steroid use in children).

Patients with nonclassical 21-OHD and 11β-OHD are treated with glucocorticoids if they manifest symptoms of androgen excess. In cases of excess ovarian androgen production, women may have to be treated with progestational and estrogenic agents which act by suppression of the release of gonadotropin. Other anti-androgen agents that may help include spironolactone and cyproterone acetate, and the androgen receptor blocker, flutamide. The aim of treatment in these patients is to minimize symptoms without giving rise to glucocorticoid side-effects.

Prenatal diagnosis and treatment

Prenatal diagnosis of 21-OHD has been performed for several decades (Speiser *et al.* 1994). Diagnosis by 17-OHP levels and HLA serotyping were attempted but found to be diagnostically limited and inaccurate. The method generally used at the present time is direct DNA analysis of the 21-OH gene (*CYP21*) with molecular genetic techniques.

An algorithm has been developed for prenatal diagnosis and treatment (Fig. 55.3). Dexamethasone (20 μg/kg/day) is administered to the pregnant mother as early as 4 weeks gestation but not later than the ninth week, blind to the affected status of the fetus, to suppress excess adrenal androgen secretion and prevent virilization should the fetus be an affected female. Diagnosis by DNA analysis requires chorionic villus sampling in the eighth to tenth weeks gestation, or later, in the second trimester, by sampling of amniotic fluid cells obtained by amniocentesis (weeks 15–18). The fetal DNA is then used for specific amplification of the *CYP21*

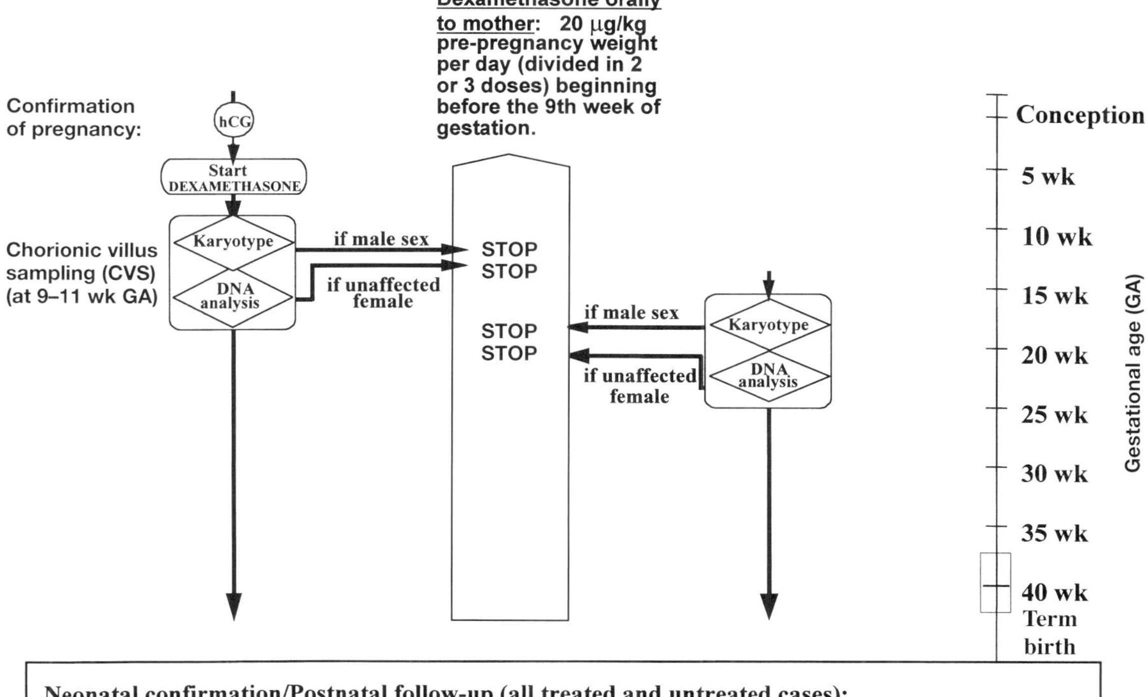

Neonatal confirmation/Postnatal follow-up (all treated and untreated cases):
   1. Clinical - Recording of birth weight, birth length, head circumference, developmental assessment, and other pertinent physical findings.
   2. Hormonal - Measurement of 17-hydroxyprogesterone levels (cord blood); post-72 hour blood sample, either dried blood spot on filter paper or whole blood (serum); electrolytes and plasma renin activity (PRA) for affected infants.
   3. Molecular - Blood sample (peripheral blood) for DNA analysis.

Fig. 55.3 Algorithm depicting prenatal management of pregnancy in families at risk for a fetus with 21-OHD. GA, Gestational age; HCG, human chorionic gonadotropin.

gene utilizing the polymerase chain reaction (PCR). The PCR products are dot blotted, followed by hybridization with radio-labeled allele-specific probes. We developed a method that only requires PCR with allele-specific primers, which reduces the time for prenatal diagnosis from about 2 weeks to only a few days, thus allowing unnecessary prenatal treatment to be terminated promptly (Wilson *et al.* 1995*b*).

If the fetus is determined to be a male upon karyotype or an unaffected female upon DNA analysis, treatment is discontinued. Otherwise, treatment is continued to term. When properly administered, dexamethasone is effective in preventing ambiguous genitalia in the affected female, and also is generally well-tolerated by both the mother and by the fetus (Mercado *et al.* 1995; Carlson *et al.* 1999). The largest human studies have shown no congenital abnormalities and that the birth weight, birth length, and head circumference were not different in offspring of dexamethasone-treated pregnancies and those not treated (Mercado *et al.* 1995; Carlson *et al.* 1999; Forest *et al.* 1989, 1993), provided patients and physicians adhered to the recommended therapeutic protocol.

In 11β-OHD CAH, the experience in prenatal treatment is limited compared to the experience with 21-OHD prenatal diagnosis and treatment. In 1989, Bouchard reported the first attempt at prenatal treatment with dexamethasone of an affected female with 11β-OHD, though it failed to prevent ambiguous genitalia in the newborn (Bouchard *et al.* 1989). Subsequently four additional families were reported to have undergone prenatal diagnosis for 11β-OHD. In three of the cases, the fetus was either a heterozygote or unaffected: Two families were reported by Curnow *et al.* (1993), one by Geley *et al.* (1996), and another by Cerame *et al.* (1999*a*). In 1999, Cerame *et al.* (1999*b*) reported the first prenatal diagnosis and treatment of an affected female with 11β-OHD CAH. The treatment was successful, as the newborn had normal female external genitalia.

Acknowledgement
I wish to express my appreciation to Laurie Vandermolen for her extensive editorial assistance.

References

Amor, M., Parker, K.L., Globerman, H., New, M.I., and White, P.C. (1988). Mutation in the CYP21B gene (Ile-172-Asn) causes steroid 21-hydroxylase deficiency. *Proc. Natl Acad. Sci., USA* **85**, 1600–7.

Blunck, W. (1969). Die beta-ketolischen Cortisol und Corticosteron-metaboliten sowie die 11-Oxy- und 11-Desoxy-17-ketosteroide im Urin von Kindern. *Acta Endocrinol.* **59** (suppl. 134), 9–112.

Bouchard, M., Forest, M.G., David, M., Dechaud, H., and Juif, J.G. (1989). [Familial congenital adrenal hyperplasia caused by 11 beta-hydroxylase. Failure of prevention of sexual ambiguity and prenatal diagnosis]. *Pediatrie* **44** (8), 637–40.

Carlson, A.D., Obeid, J.S., Kanellopoulou, N., Wilson, R.C., and New, M.I. (1999). Congenital adrenal hyperplasia: update on prenatal diagnosis and treatment. *J. Steroid Biochem. Mol. Biol.* **69**, 19–29.

Cerame, B.I., Newfield, R.S., Wilson, R.C., and New, M.I. (1999*a*). Prenatal diagnosis and treatment of 11beta-hydroxylase deficiency congenital adrenal hyperplasia. In *Diagnosis and treatment of the unborn child* (ed. M.I. New), pp. 175–8. Idelson–Gnocchi Ltd, Reddick, Florida.

Cerame, B.I., Newfield, R.S., Pascoe, L., Curnow, K.M., Nimkarn, S., Roe, T.F., New, M.I., and Wilson, R.C. (1999*b*). Prenatal diagnosis and treatment of 11beta-hydroxylase deficiency congenital adrenal hyperplasia resulting in normal female genitalia. *J. Clin. Endocrinol. Metab.* **84** (9), 3129–34.

Curnow, K.M., Slutsker, L., Vitek, J., Cole, T., Speiser, P.W., New, M.I., White, P.C., and Pascoe, L. (1993). Mutations in the CYP11B1 gene causing congenital adrenal hyperplasia and hypertension cluster in exons 6, 7, and 8. *Proc. Natl Acad. Sci., USA* **90** (10), 4552–6.

Forest, M.G., Betuel, H., and David, M. (1989). Prenatal treatment in congenital adrenal hyperplasia due to 21-hydroxylase deficiency: update 88 of the French multicentric study. *Endocr. Res.* **15**, 277–301.

Forest, M.G., David, M., and Morel, Y. (1993). Prenatal diagnosis and treatment of 21-hydroxylase deficiency [review]. *J. Steroid Biochem. Mol. Biol.* **45** (1–3), 75–82.

Gandy, H.M., Keutmann, E.H., and Izzo, A.J. (1960). Characterization of urinary steroids in adrenal hyperplasia: isolation of metabolites of cortisol, compound S, and deoxycorticosterone from a normotensive patient with adrenogenital syndrome. *J. Clin. Invest.* **39**, 364–77.

Geley, S., Kapelari, K., Johrer, K., Peter, M., Glatzl, J., Vierhapper, H., Schwarz, S., Helmberg, A., Sippell, W.G., White, P.C., *et al.* (1996). CYP11B1 mutations causing congenital adrenal hyperplasia due to 11 beta-hydroxylase deficiency. *J. Clin. Endocrinol. Metab.* **81** (8), 2896–901.

Glenthoj, A., Nielsen, M.D., and Starup, J. (1980). Congenital adrenal hyperplasia due to 11 beta-hydroxylase deficiency: final diagnosis in adult age in three patients. *Acta Endocrinol.* (*Copenhagen*) **93** (1), 94–9.

Green, O.C., Migeon, C.J., and Wilkins, L. (1960). Urinary steroids in the hypertensive form of congenital adrenal hyperplasia. *J. Clin. Endocrinol. Metab.* **20**, 929–46.

Higashi, Y., Yoshioka, H., Yamane, M., Gotoh, O., and Fujii-Kuriyama, Y. (1986). Complete nucleotide sequence of two steroid 21-hydroxylase genes tandemly arranged in human chromosome: a pseudogene and a genuine gene. *Proc. Natl Acad. Sci., USA* **83** (9), 2841–5.

Higashi, Y., Tanae, A., Inoue, H., Hiromasa, T., and Fujii-Kuriyama, Y. (1988). Aberrant splicing and missense mutations cause steroid 21-hydroxylase [P-450 (C21)] deficiency in humans: possible gene conversion products. *Proc. Natl Acad. Sci., USA* **85** (20), 7486–90.

Higashi, Y., Hiromasa, T., Tanae, A., Miki, T., Nakura, J., Kondo, T., Ohura, T., Ogawa, E., Nakayama, K., and Fujii, K.Y. (1991). Effects of individual mutations in the P-450 (C21) pseudogene on the P-450 (C21) activity and their distribution in the patient genomes of congenital steroid 21-hydroxylase deficiency. *J. Biochem.* **109** (4), 638–44.

Jost, A. (1971). Embryonic sexual differentiation. In *Hermaphroditism, genital anomalies and related endocrine disorders* (ed. H.W. Jones and W.W. Scott), p. 16. Wilkins and Wilkins, Baltimore.

Krawczak, M. and Cooper, D.N. (1997). The human gene mutation database. *Trends Genet.* **13**, 121–2.

Lin, D., Sugawara, T., Strauss, J.F.R., Clark, B.J., Stocco, D.M., Saenger, P., Rogol, A., and Miller, W.L. (1995). Role of steroidogenic acute regulatory protein in adrenal and gonadal steroidogenesis. *Science* **267**, 1821–31.

Mercado, A.B., Wilson, R.C., Cheng, K.C., Wei, J.Q., and New, M.I. (1995). Extensive personal experience: prenatal treatment and diagnosis of congenital adrenal hyperplasia owing to steroid 21-hydroxylase deficiency. *J. Clin. Endocrinol. Metab.* **80**, 2014–20.

Merke, D.P., Tajima, T., Chhabra, A., Barnes, K., Mancilla, E., Baron, J., and Cutler, G.B. Jr (1998). Novel CYP11B1 mutations in congenital adrenal hyperplasia due to steroid 11 beta-hydroxylase deficiency. *J. Clin. Endocrinol. Metab.* **83** (1), 270–3.

Mimouni, M., Kaufman, H., Roitman, A., Morag, C., and Sadan, N. (1985). Hypertension in a neonate with 11 beta-hydroxylase deficiency. *Eur. J. Pediatr.* **143** (3), 231–3.

Mornet, E., Crete, P., Kuttenn, F., Raux-Demay, M.C., Boue, J., White, P.C., and Boue, A. (1991). Distribution of deletions and seven point mutations on CYP21B genes in three clinical forms of steroid 21-hydroxylase deficiency. *Am. J. Hum. Genet.* **48** (1), 79–88.

Mulatero, P., Curnow, K.M., Aupetit-Faisant, B., Foekling, M., Gomez-Sanchez, C., Veglio, F., Jeunemaitre, X., Corvol, P., and Pascoe, L. (1998). Recombinant CYP11B genes encode enzymes that can catalyze conversion of 11-deoxycortisol to cortisol, 18-hydroxycortisol, and 18-oxocortisol. *J. Clin. Endocrinol. Metab.* **83** (11), 3996–4001.

New, M.I. and White, P.C. (1995). Genetic disorders of steroid metabolism. In *Genetic and molecular biological aspects of endocrine disease. Bailliere's clinical endocrinology and metabolism* (ed. R.V. Thakker), pp. 525–54. Bailliere Tindall, London.

New, M.I., Dupont, B., Grumbach, K., and Levine, L.S. (1982). Congenital adrenal hyperplasia and related conditions. In *The metabolic basis of inherited disease*, 5th edn (ed. J.B. Stanbury, J.B. Wyngaarden, D.S. Fredrickson, J.L. Goldstein, and M.D. Brown), pp. 973–1000. McGraw-Hill, New York.

New, M.I., Nemery, R.L., Chow, D.M., Kaufman, E.D., Stoner, E., Zerah, M., Crawford, C., and Speiser, P.W. (1989). Low-renin hypertension of childhood. In *The adrenal and hypertension: from cloning to clinic, Ares–Serona Symposium* (ed. E.G. Biglieri, C.R.W. Edwards, J.W. Funder, F. Mantero, T. Saruta, B.A. Scoggins, R. Takeda, and M.B. Vallotton), pp. 323–43. Raven Press, Tokyo.

New, M.I., Ghizzoni, L., and Speiser, P.W. (1995*a*). Update on congenital adrenal hyperplasia. In *Pediatric endocrinology*, 3rd edn (ed. F. Lifshitz), Chapter 16, pp. 305–20. Marcel Dekker, New York.

New, M.I., Crawford, C., and Virdis, R. (1995*b*). Low-renin hypertension in childhood. In *Pediatric endocrinology*, 3rd edn (ed. F. Lifshitz), pp. 775–89. Marcel Dekker, New York.

New, M.I., Crawford, C., and Wilson, R.C. (1996). Genetic disorders of the adrenal steroidogenic enzymes. In *Principles and practice of medical genetics*, 3rd edn (ed. A.E.H. Emery and D. Rimoin), pp. 1441–76. Churchill Livingstone, New York.

Pang, S. and Clark, A. (1990). Newborn screening, prenatal diagnosis, and prenatal treatment of congenital adrenal hyperplasia due to 21-hydroxylase deficiency. *Trends Endocrinol. Metab.* **1**, 300–7.

Pang, S. and Clark, A. (1993). Congenital adrenal hyperplasia due to 21-hydroxylase deficiency: newborn screening and its relationship to the diagnosis and treatment of the disorder. *Screening* **2**, 105–39.

Pang, S.Y., Wallace, M.A., Hofman, L., Thuline, H.C., Dorche, C., Lyon, I.C., Dobbins, R.H., Kling, S., Fujieda, K., and Suwa, S. (1988). Worldwide experience in newborn screening for classical congenital adrenal hyperplasia due to 21-hydroxylase deficiency. *Pediatrics* **81** (6), 866–74.

Rosler, A. and Leiberman, E. (1984). Enzymatic defects of steroidogenesis: 11beta-hydroxylase deficiency congenital adrenal hyperplasia. In *Adrenal diseases in childhood: pathophysiologic and clinical aspects* (ed. M.I. New and L.S. Levine), Vol. 13, pp. 47–71. S. Karger, Basel.

Rosler, A., Leiberman, E., and Cohen, T. (1992). High frequency of congenital adrenal hyperplasia (classic 11 beta-hydroxylase deficiency) among Jews from Morocco. *Am. J. Med. Genet.* **42** (6), 827–34.

Sherman, S.L., Aston, C.E., Morton, N.E., Speiser, P., and New, M.I. (1988). A segration and linkage study of classical and nonclassical 21-hydroxylase deficiency. *Am. J. Hum. Genet.* **42**, 830–8.

Speiser, P.W. and New, M.I. (1994). Prenatal diagnosis and treatment of congenital adrenal hyperplasia. *J. Pedatr. Endocrinol.* **7** (3), 183–91.

Speiser, P.W., Dupont, B., Rubinstein, P., Piazza, A., Kastelan, A., and New, I.M. (1985). High frequency of nonclassical steroid 21-hydroxylase deficiency. *Am. J. Hum. Genet.* **37**, 650–67.

Speiser, P.W., Dupont, J., Zhu, D., Serrat, J., Buegeleisen, M., Tusie, L.M., Lesser, M., New, M.I., and White, P.C. (1992*a*). Disease expression and molecular genotype in congenital adrenal hyperplasia due to 21-hydroxylase deficiency. *J. Clin. Invest.* **90** (2), 584–95.

Speiser, P.W., New, M.I., Tannin, G.M., Pickering, D., Yang, S.Y., and White, P.C. (1992*b*). Genotype of Yupik Eskimos with congenital adrenal hyperplasia due to 21-hydroxylase deficiency. *Hum. Genet.* **88** (6), 647–8.

Tusie-Luna, M., Traktman, P., and White, P.C. (1990). Determination of functional effects of mutations in the steroid 21-hydroxylase gene (CYP21) using recombinant vaccinia virus. *J. Biol. Chem.* **265** (34), 20916–22.

Wedell, A., Ritzen, E.M., Haglund, S.B., and Luthman, H. (1992). Steroid 21-hydroxylase deficiency: three additional mutated alleles and establishment of phenotype–genotype relationships of common mutations. *Proc. Natl Acad. Sci., USA* **89** (15), 7232–6.

Werkmeister, J.W., New, M.I., Dupont, B., and White, P.C. (1986). Frequent deletion and duplication of the steroid 21-hydroxylase genes. *Am. J. Hum. Genet.* **39** (4), 461–9.

White, P.C., New, M.I., and Dupont, B. (1986). Structure of the human steroid 21-hydroxylase genes. *Proc. Natl Acad. Sci., USA* **83**, 5111–15.

White, P.C., Dupont, J., New, M.I., Leiberman, E., Hochberg, Z., and Rosler, A. (1991). A mutation in CYP11B1 (Arg-448—-His) associated with steroid 11 beta-hydroxylase deficiency in Jews of Moroccan origin. *J. Clin. Invest.* **87** (5), 1664–7.

White, P.C., Tusie-Luna, M.T., New, M.I., and Speiser, P.W. (1994*a*). Mutations in steroid 21-hydroxylase (CYP21). *Hum. Mutat.* **3** (4), 373–8.

White, P.C., Curnow, K.M., and Pascoe, L. (1994*b*). Disorders of steroid 11beta-hydroxylase isozymes. *Endocr. Rev.* **15** (4), 421–38.

Wilson, R.C., Mercado, A.B., Cheng, K.C., and New, M.I. (1995*a*). Steroid 21-hydroxylase deficiency: genotype may not predict phenotype. *J. Clin. Endocrinol. Metab.* **80** (8), 2322–9.

Wilson, R.C., Wei, J.Q., Cheng, K.C., Mercado, A.B., and New, M.I. (1995*b*). Rapid DNA analysis by allele-specific PCR for detection of mutations in the steroid 21-hydroxylase gene. *J. Clin. Endocrinol. Metab.* **80** (5), 1635–40.

Zachmann, M., Tassinari, D., and Prader, A. (1983). Clinical and biochemical variability of congenital adrenal hyperplasia due to 11beta-hydroxylase deficiency. *J. Endocrinol. Metab.* **56**, 222–9.

Zerah, M., Ueshiba, H., Wood, E., Speiser, P.W., Crawford, C., McDonald, T., Pareira, J., Gruen, D., and New, M.I. (1990). Prevalence of nonclassical steroid 21-hydroxylase deficiency based on a morning salivary 17-hydroxyprogesterone screening test: a small sample study. *J. Clin. Endocrinol. Metab.* **70** (6), 1662–7.

56. The surgical management of congenital adrenal hyperplasia

G. Bino Rucker and Dix P. Poppas

Introduction

Congenital adrenal hyperplasia (CAH) is an enzymatic defect of steroid synthesis transmitted in an autosomal recessive pattern. CAH refers to a group of disorders that manifest with varying degrees of physical stigmata including virilization of female patients. The degree of stigmata differs according to the underlying enzyme deficit altering cortisol formation in the adrenal gland. The most commonly encountered defect is that of the 21-hydroxylase enzyme. Our attention will be focused on the surgical management of the virilized female with 21-hydroxylase deficiency since this is the most common type of CAH patient encountered (New and Newfield 1997).

Surgical treatment of infants born with ambiguous genitalia has evolved continuously since Hendren and Crawford (1969) described the management of adrenogenital syndrome. Several types of repair exist. The exact method of reconstruction depends on the anatomy of the patient. When a child is born with ambiguous genitalia, a multidisciplinary approach to diagnosis and management is essential because the clinical issues presented have much social and medical significance. Urologic and endocrine consultations should be obtained immediately. A thoughtful approach to the dilemma must be maintained in order to instil confidence in the parents and to avoid parental confusion. The actual gender assignment must be reserved until adequate biochemical and anatomical information is obtained (Lee and Donahoe 1997).

Intersex disorders can be classified into three major categories based on etiology. The first group is gonadal dysmorphogenesis. This group includes pure gonadal dysgenesis, mixed gonadal dysgenesis, and true hermaphroditism. The second group is undervirilized males also referred to as male pseudohermaphrodites. This category encompasses defects in testosterone synthesis, androgen resistance syndromes, and 5-alpha reductase deficits. The third group is our primary focus, virilized females. This group includes congenital adrenal hyperplasia, maternal virilization disorders, and iatrogenic etiologies such as *in utero* exposure to progestins and androgens (Lee and Donahoe 1997).

During evaluation of the child born with ambiguous genitalia, the first step is a thorough history including any prenatal maternal illnesses or possible exposure to androgens. A family history should be obtained directed toward relatives with genital anomalies, infant deaths, amenorrhea, or infertility. The physical examination is performed with special attention to evidence of dysmorphic features or any anomalies potentially related to an adrenogenital syndrome. The examiner should note the presence or absence of gonadal symmetry with respect to location and appearance. Also important are any evidence of labioscrotal fusion, the size of the phallus, presence of chordee, and the position of the urethra. Ultrasonography by an experienced sonographer is often employed to visualize the presence of Müllerian structures or abdominal gonads. A retrograde dye injection into the urogenital sinus is an accepted method of delineating the anatomy of the urethra and vagina. Such a study can also establish whether the vagina enters proximally or distally to the external urethral sphincter.

Essential laboratory studies that should be obtained are serum electrolytes, serum 17-hydroxyprogesterone levels, and a timed urine collection for pregnenetriol and 17-ketosteroids. Also essential is a complete karyotype of peripheral leukocytes. Further laboratory work can be tailored to the specific entity being considered.

Fifty per cent of intersex patients are identified as virilized females with CAH; three-quarters of these patients have a 21-hydroxylase deficiency. Fortunately, when medical and surgical evaluations are carried out properly, these children are afforded an excellent potential for normal female sexual and reproductive health (Lee and Donahoe 1997).

Pathophysiology

The most common enzymatic defect observed in CAH is that of the 21-hydroxylase enzyme. Also common are 11β-hydroxylase and 3β-hydroxysteroid dehydrogenase defects. In Fig. 56.1, the normal cortisol synthesis pathway is illustrated. When a defect occurs in this pathway, cortisol, the end product, is deficient. Adrenocorticotropin (ACTH) becomes elevated due to impairment of the negative feedback loop. A build-up of steroid synthesis intermediaries occurs along with excess products of alternate adrenal hormonal pathways. Subsequently, the adrenal achieves a state of hyperstimulation known as hyperplasia (Lee and Donahoe 1997). 21-hydroxylase and 11β-hydroxylase enzyme deficits both result in hyperstimulation of adrenal androgen pathways. Also important to realize is that severe forms of 21-hydroxylase deficiency result in a salt-wasting variant of CAH. The 21-hydroxylase deficit and its variants account for 75 per cent of all cases of CAH (Lee and Donahoe 1997).

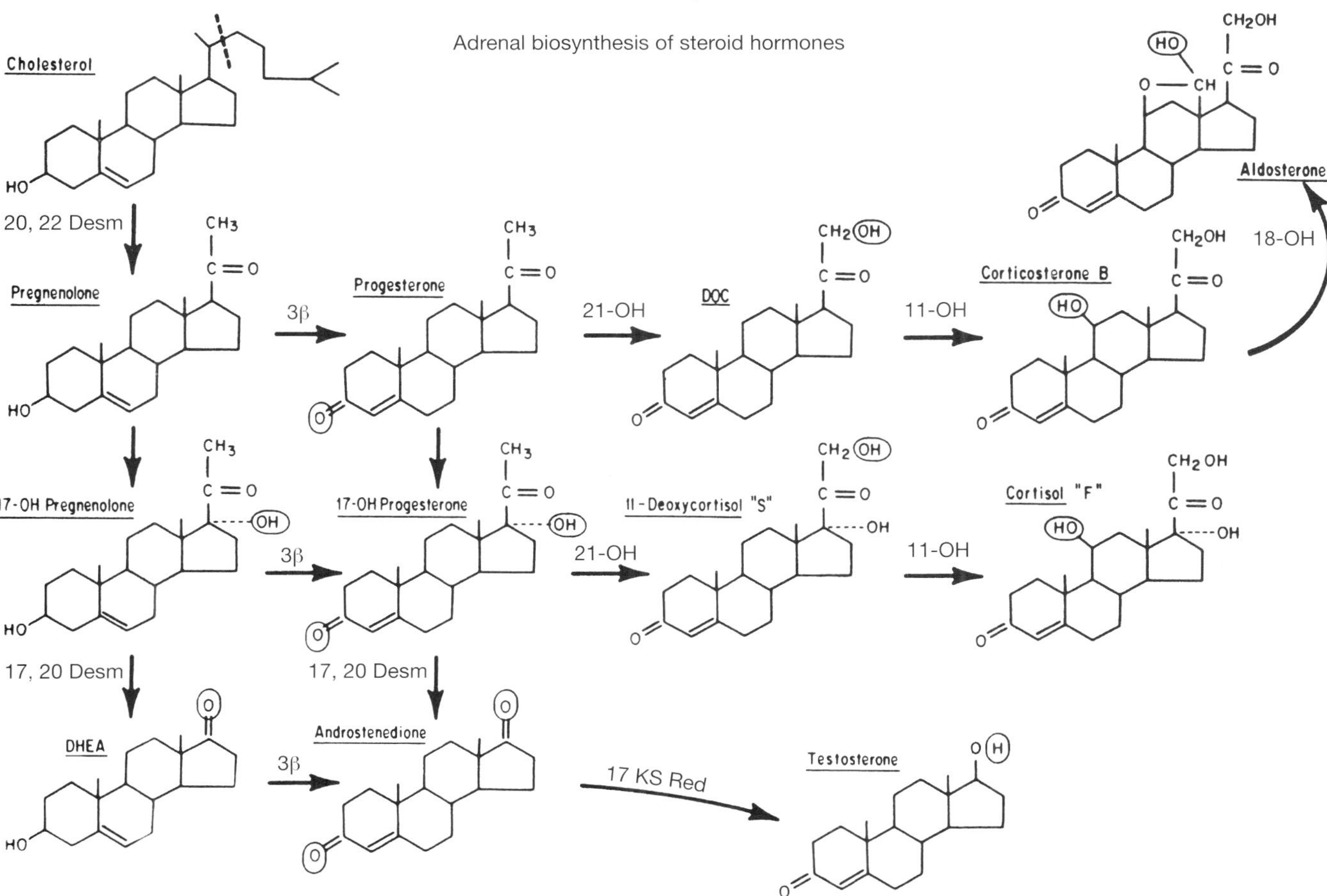

Fig. 56.1 Biosynthesis pathways of adrenal steroid hormones. (Desm = Desmolase, DHEA = Detosteroid Dihydroepiandrosterone)

Embryology

In CAH, adrenal androgen excess occurs *in utero* as early as the seventh to eighth week of gestation resulting in a virilized female. Normal female reproductive development is a product of the paired fusion of the Müllerian or paramesonephric ducts. The proximal unfused portions become the fallopian tubes, while the distal Müllerian ducts join to form the uterus and proximal vagina. A complex interaction between the Müllerian ducts, urogenital sinus, and cloaca allow the vagina to separate from the urethra distally. The Müllerian ducts are found lateral to the Wolffian ducts during the sixth week of gestation. The Müllerian ducts continue to grow inferiorly, until they juxtapose the caudal portion of the Wolffian ducts at which point they fuse. This fused terminal end of the Müllerian duct continues to grow until the posterior wall of the urogenital sinus is reached at which point the Müllerian tubercle is formed (Meyers 1997).

The primitive hindgut or cloaca is the precursor of the urogenital sinus and the dorsal hindgut. The dorsal hindgut evolves into the rectum and anus, while the urogenital sinus forms the bladder and urethra. Additionally, a pair of endodermal proliferations termed the sinovaginal bulbs grow to form the vaginal plate. As the solid vaginal plate grows toward the perineum, it pulls the urethra and vaginal introitus with it into their orthotopic location. When the urogenital sinus persists, the vagina and urethra are joined, the Müllerian tubercle does not form properly, and there is no formation of a vaginal plate. Thereby, the vagina does not descend and open into the perineum as is the case with adrenal hyperplasia (Meyers 1997).

Treatment

The major cause of morbidity and mortality in children with adrenal hyperplasia is the salt-wasting crisis. The enzyme defects most commonly associated with mortality are the salt-wasting 21-hydroxylase defect and the 3β-hydroxysteroid dehydrogenase deficiency (New and Newfield 1997). Fatalities were commonplace in the past because this syndrome went unrecognized. In Hendren and Crawford's landmark 1969 paper, all seven patients described were salt-wasting CAH females who were inappropriately assigned as males. The diagnosis was only established when each child underwent an adrenal crisis in the first month of life (Hendren and Crawford 1969).

Identification of a salt-wasting component is essential, and consultation with a pediatric endocrinologist is necessary to implement proper treatment. Glucocorticoids are given to replace the absent cortisol. Steroid replacement is also required to suppress ACTH so that additional excess androgen production is avoided. In females with CAH, glucocorticoid replacement is also necessary to prevent the stigmata of hyperandrogenism such as alopecia, acne, irregular menses, and infertility (Lee and Donahoe 1997).

Surgical treatment

Once a child with adrenal hyperplasia has undergone medical evaluation and begun necessary treatment, the reconstructive aspects of care can be addressed. In conjunction with surgery, the patient and their family should undergo counseling to help both the parents and child cope with physical and developmental anomalies caused by the syndrome (New and Newfield 1997).

The type of surgical repair performed must be tailored according to each individual patient's anatomy. The first important issue is the timing of the reconstruction. This remains a controversial area. The majority of surgical reconstructions are performed at an early age rather than delaying until adolescence. Reconstruction is generally initiated between the ages of 4 and 12 months (New and Newfield 1997; Mathews and Gearheart 1998; DeJong and Boemers 1995). An early one-stage repair has been recommended because of the belief that female patients are able to undergo a more natural psychological and sexual development when they have a normal appearing vagina (Hendren and Atala 1995). However, in our center, we will routinely perform the clitoral recession early and will only perform the vaginoplasty in the patient who has a low vaginal entrance. With few exceptions, those patients with high vaginal entrance do not undergo vaginal reconstruction until menarche.

The major features of reconstructive genitoplasty are clitoral recession, labioscrotal reduction, and vaginal exteriorization. Clitoral recession is also referred to as clitoroplasty (New and Newfield 1997).

Females who present with adrenal hyperplasia have a wide range of anatomic findings. The mildest variety of the syndrome is the presence of a low vagina (Hendren and Atala 1995). The severe end of the spectrum is the virilized child with a high vagina entering into a masculine appearing urethra at the area of a false verumontanum. Here the vagina enters proximally to the external urethral sphincter. The surgical approaches to the low and high vaginal entry are different and shall be described in detail (Hendren and Atala 1995).

Preoperative preparation

In preparation for surgery, a pelvic sinogram should be performed on patients. The most important information to be gained from this study is the anatomical relationship of the vagina to the urethra and external urethral sphincter. These data are crucial in determining the type of vaginal repair to be employed (Hendren and Atala 1995; Belman *et al.* 1992). Cystoscopy should be performed at the time of surgery. Though the sinogram provides important anatomical detail, the cystoscopy is required to confirm all findings. Cystoscopy also expedites catheterization of the vaginal introitus, which makes intraoperative identification of pertinent anatomy easier.

All children undergoing genitoplasty of any form should undergo preoperative antimicrobial prophylaxis. Additionally, some patients with 21-hydroxylase deficiency may need stress dose steroids preoperatively if the enzymatic defect blunts the physiologic adrenal response to surgical stress (New and Newfield 1997).

In the distant past clitorectomy was a recommended procedure, but this should never be considered today. It was initially advocated because those virilized females whose clitoris was left intact had erectile tissue that became painfully enlarged upon sexual arousal later in life (Mathews and Gearheart 1998). Instead, clitoral recession is performed with the following goals in mind. The erectile bodies are defunctionalized to prevent painful erections, the dorsal neurovascular bundles are preserved, and the clitoris is left intact. We rarely reduce the size of the clitoris (glans) during this reconstruction. In the past, wedge resections were often performed to reduce the size of the clitoris. We believe that patients with adequate steroid control will not have persistent enlargement of the clitoris and that surgical excision may remove or damage potentially sensitive tissue.

Surgical technique

For patients with low entering vaginas the most commonly used technique is initiated with an inverted U-shaped perineal incision (Fig. 56.2) (Mathews and Gearheart 1998). This incision is carried superiorly into the ventral aspect of the phallus while preserving the ventral mucosal groove. The phallus is degloved completely with preservation of the preputial skin. The dorsal aspect of the preputial skin is divided in the midline in order to create Byars' flaps that are used to form labia minora (Fig. 56.3) (Lee and Donahoe 1997). Next, the nerovascular bundles are isolated dorsolaterally over the corporal bodies. The corporal bodies are ligated at their bases and dissected from the clitoris and removed. The glans is reapproximated to the corporal stumps. The newly reduced clitoris is sutured to the skin of the mons pubis while the dorsal Byars' flaps are advanced posteriorly to construct labia minora (Lee and Donahoe 1997; Mathews and Gearheart 1998).At this point, if the glans is still too large, lateral wedge resections can be performed to effect further reduction (Passerini-Glazel 1989).

Our technique differs in several facets from those commonly described in the past. Once the phallic skin has been reduced, we make a ventral incision under each corporal body and elevate the neurovascular bundles widely to include all of the lateral tissue. We do not elevate or disturb the bundles dorsally and leave them intact over the tunica albugenia. Once the proximal corporal bodies are ligated the tunica albuginea and corporal tissue is excised laterally and ventrally leaving the dorsal tunica intact to support the bundles. The lateral edges of the tunica are approximated in the ventral midline.

Once the clitoral reduction is performed, attention is turned to the vaginoplasty. The type of vaginal repair used is strictly based on each individual's anatomy.

The mildest anomaly is that of the patient who presents with a vaginal introitus adjacent to the opening of the urogenital sinus (Mathews and Gearheart 1998; Belman *et al.* 1992). This anomaly can be idiopathic with no relation to any type of virilizing syndrome. As illustrated in Fig. 56.4, a midline incision is made in the perineum. The skin is closed in a transverse fashion. This type

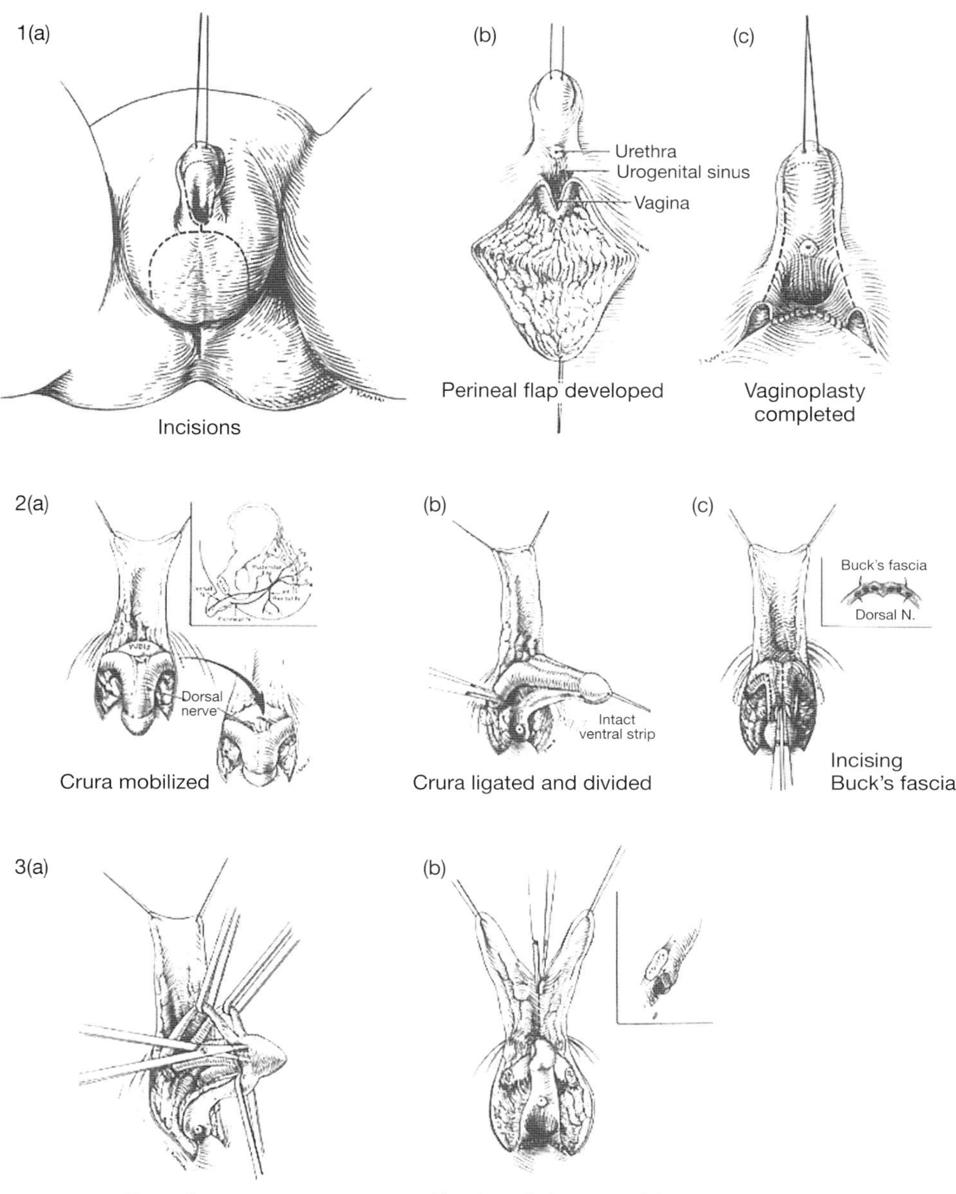

Fig. 56.2 Illustration of clitoral recession technique used in low vaginal repair. (Taken with permission from Mathews and Gearheart (1998).)

of plasty is called the Heineke–Mikulicz technique (Hendren and Donahoe 1983).

The next degree of virilization is that of the patient who presents with a vaginal opening distal to the urethral sphincter (low vagina). Here a flap vaginoplasty technique should be used (Hendren and Donahoe 1983). This is the most common technique utilized because the low vagina is the most common presentation of the adrenogenital syndrome. After cystoscopy has been performed to delineate anatomy, the opening of the urogenital sinus is incised in a posterior direction. Great care is taken to preserve the urethra and the integrity of the external urethral sphincter (Hendren and Donahoe 1983). Once the urethra has been properly identified, a Foley catheter is advanced into the bladder and the balloon of the catheter is inflated. Next, an inverted

U-shaped perineal flap is raised. The apex of the incision is joined to the posterior incision of the urogenital sinus. The skin outlined by this incision is raised as a flap. The skin flap is rounded at the apex in order to maximally preserve vascular supply (Mathews and Gearheart 1998). As the flap is raised, the subcutaneous fatty tissue should remain adherent in order for further vascular preservation to overlying skin. The posterior wall of the vagina can be visualized beneath this perineal flap. A finger can be placed into the rectum at this point to avoid entry into the rectum while dissecting the vagina. The posterior wall of the vagina is identified, and incised in a caudal direction. The length of the posterior incision in the vagina depends on the degree of vaginal shortening. Extremely short vaginas may require extension of the incision to the cervical os. Next the perineal skin flap is sutured to the pos-

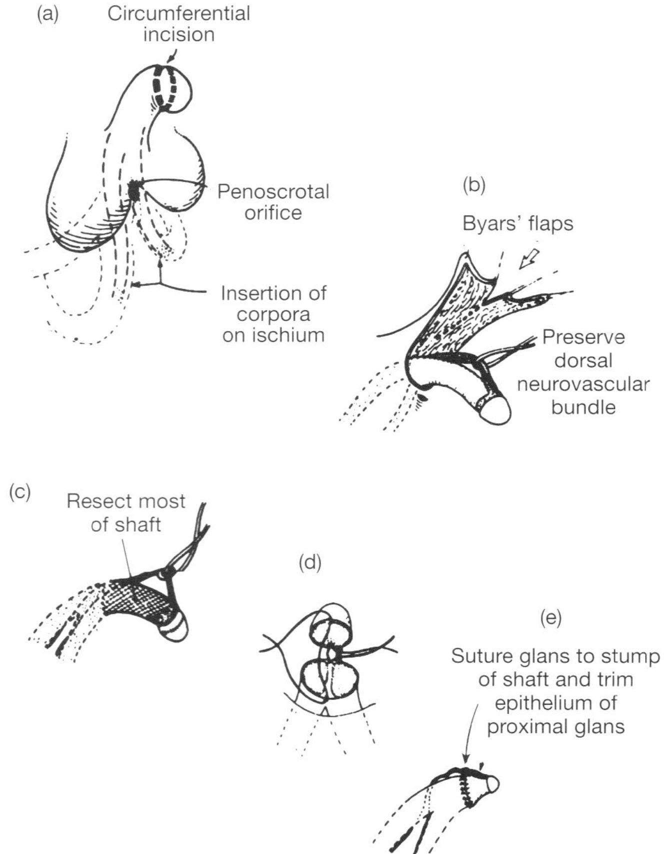

Fig. 56.3 Use of Byar's flaps to reconstruct female phallus. (Taken with permission from Lee and Donahoe (1997).)

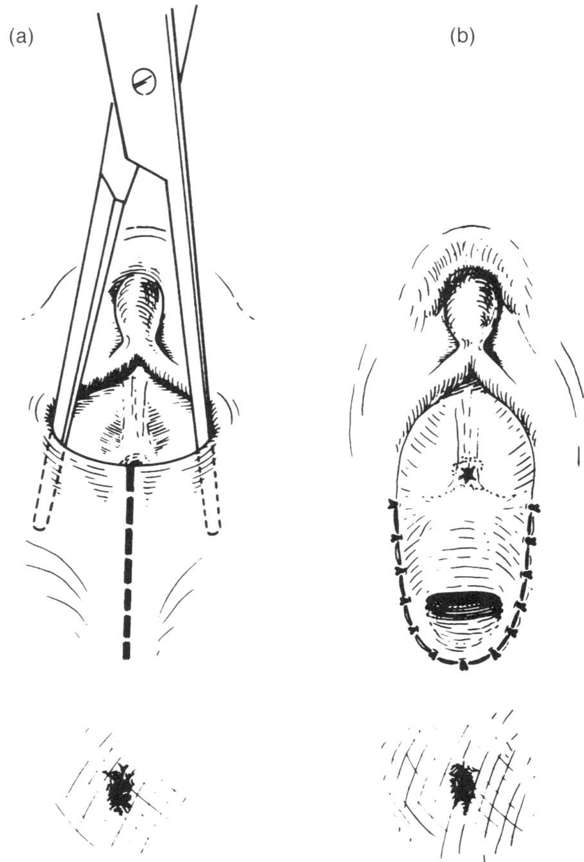

Fig. 56.4 Repair of mildest type of virilization anomaly. (Taken with permission from Hendren and Donahoe (1983).)

terior aspect of the vaginal incision using Y–V plasty (illustrated in Fig. 56.5) (Snyder *et al.* 1983). Vaginal dilatation may be required postoperatively to prevent stenosis (Hendren and Donahoe 1983).

A further degree of virilization is present in the patient with the high vagina. Here the vagina enters into the urethra proximal to the external urethral sphincter (Fig. 56.6) (Hendren and Atala 1995). Flap vaginoplasty is not feasible in this situation because of the risk of transection of the urethral sphincter (Hendren and Donahoe 1983). The patient is prepared for surgery by undergoing standard bowel prep with Golytely and oral antibiotics. Preoperative cystoscopy is performed and betadine-soaked packing is placed into the rectum. Next, a Fogarty catheter is inserted into the high vagina using cystoscopic guidance. An inverted U-shaped perineal incision is made anterior to the anus (Fig. 56.7). A finger is placed into the rectum and the vagina is dissected from the urethral sphincter and anterior wall of the rectum. At this point, the vagina is identified by palpating the Fogarty balloon in the vagina. Gentle intermittent traction upon the Fogarty catheter allows the surgeon to identify the precise location of the vaginal–urethral junction. The vaginal wall is now incised over the balloon catheter. The catheter is removed, and a metal sound is passed into the bladder. The urethro–vaginal junction is identified through the vaginal incision. The vagina is now

completely transected away from the urethra while a vaginal cuff of 1–2 mm is left behind on the urethra. This cuff is left behind so that the urethral lumen is not narrowed. After urethral closure, the sound is removed and a urethral catheter is passed into the bladder. The balloon of the catheter is inflated and will remain for 1 week. The vagina is mobilized from the urethra, bladder, and bladder neck. Even with an ideal dissection, the vagina is usually too short to reach the perineum at this point. Perineal skin flaps compensate the remainder of the distance to the perineum. The posterior U-shaped flap that was previously mobilized is sutured to the posterior wall of the vagina. Another U-shaped flap is created anteriorly and this is sutured to the anterior wall of the vagina. Now the longitudinal portions of each perineal incision are sewn together as illustrated in Fig. 56.7. The wound is drained with a small suction bulb, and a loose packing is left in the vagina. Just as described in low vaginal repairs, vaginal dilatations are to begin 2 weeks after the surgery. Monthly dilatation is recommended until the child matures and becomes sexually active.

For the most severely masculinized females, the Passerini-Glazel single-stage clitorovaginoplasty can be used (Passerini-Glazel 1989). Here the enlarged phallus is incised circumferentially below the glans and degloved. Once the phallus is degloved with the preputial skin remaining intact, the dorsal neurovascular bundle is dissected from the corporal body dorsally, and the urogenital

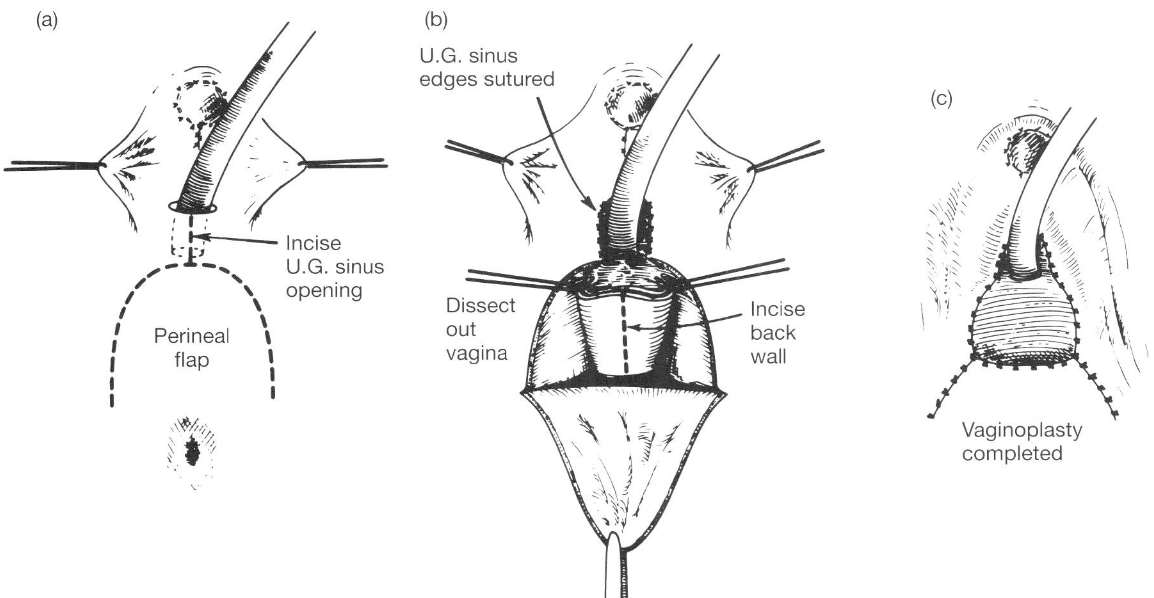

Fig. 56.5 Flap vaginoplasty technique used to repair low vagina. (Taken with permission from Snyder *et al.* (1983).)

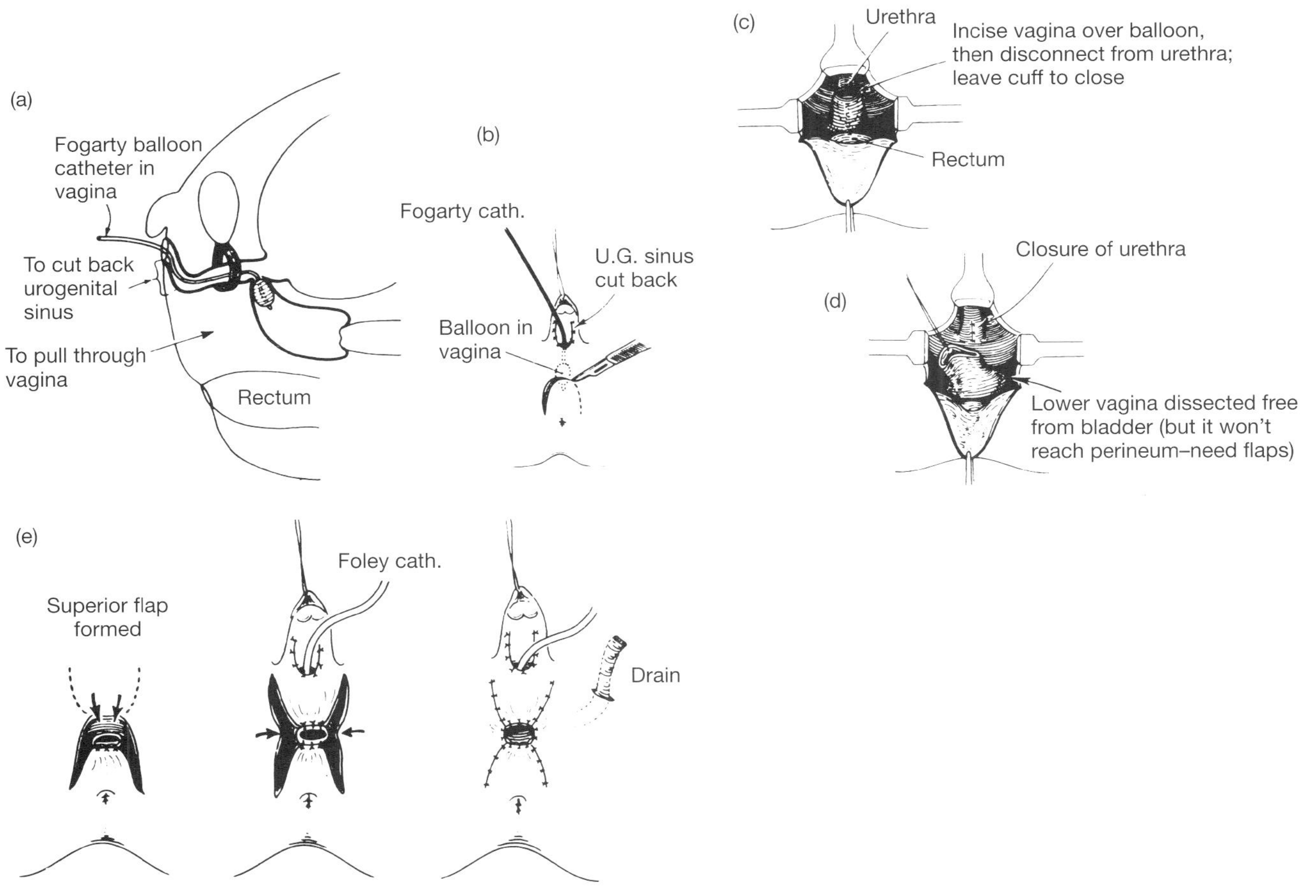

Fig. 56.6 Schematic illustration of high vaginal repair. (Taken with permission from Hendren and Atala (1995).)

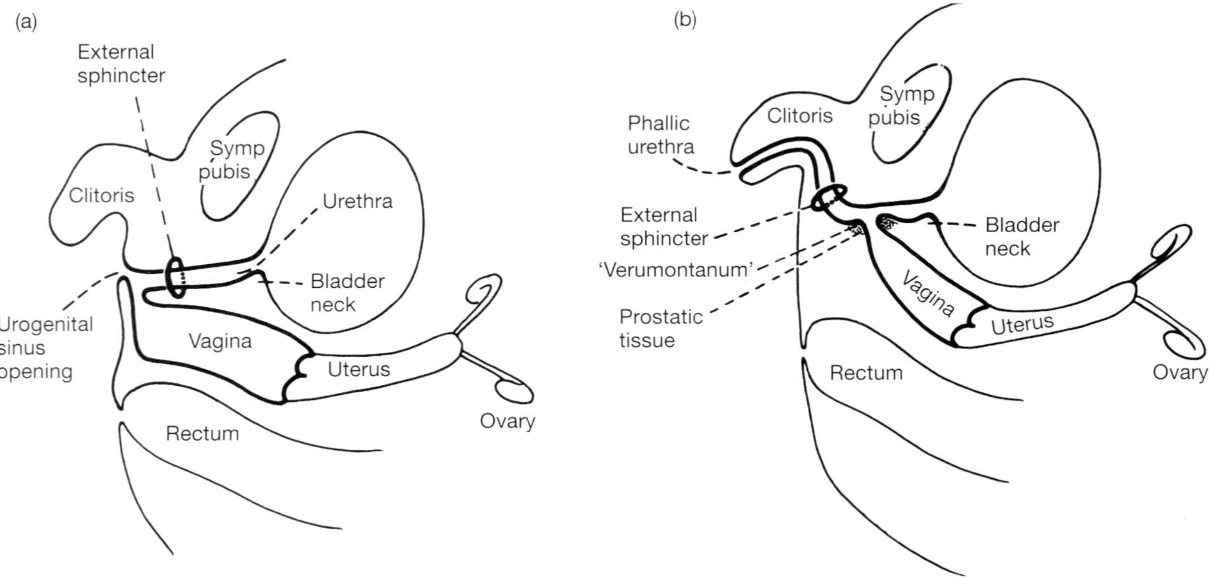

Fig. 56.7 Diagram illustrating anatomical differences between (a) low vagina and (b) high vagina. (Taken with permission from Hendren and Atala (1995).)

sinus is separated from the corpora ventrally. Now the corpora cavernosa are ligated proximally at the divergence of the corporal bodies, and divided $\frac{1}{2}$ cm above the ligation just below the glans. The neurovascular bundle is completely preserved throughout the procedure with great effort made to not place any traction upon the bundle. The remaining proximal corporal stumps are reanastomosed to the glans (Snyder *et al.* 1983). Next the corona of the glans is sutured posteriorly to the skin of the mons pubis. The preserved preputial skin is now divided in the midline ventrally and dorsally with the incision carried back to the labioscrotal folds. The urogenital sinus is now incised dorsally with the creation of a small dorsal flap at the proximal end of the incision.

Null allele subset of congenital adrenal hyperplasia

The majority of children with CAH will possess some ability to produce cortisol. In a small subset of patients, there is a total annihilation of the 21-hydroxylase enzyme. In this subset of patients, steroid replacement therapy has enjoyed only limited success because complete suppression of the pituitary-adrenal axis has proven difficult. The dose of glucocorticoid required to adequately suppress ACTH in these females is often supraphysiologic. The result is an iatrogenic hypercortisolism with its associated obesity and Cushingoid features. Furthermore, with complete 21-OH deficiency, adrenal suppression is often not complete despite the elevated doses of steroid. As a result, 21-hydroxylase deficient females must endure, to varying degrees, both the effects of the adrenal androgens and the side-effects of iatrogenic hypercortisolism.

Bilateral adrenalectomy has been proposed as a treatment for those females with CAH due to a complete absence of the 21-hydroxylase enzyme. This would eliminate androgen and 17-OHP overproduction and the need to suppress the pituitary– adrenal axis. Glucocorticoid dose would be reduced to the physiologic range, and the side-effects of iatrogenic hypercortisolism would be avoided. Androgen-induced virilization would be eliminated. Normal 17-OHP would allow for regular menses and fertility. Surgical adrenalectomy places females with a complete absence of 21-hydroxylase at no additional future risk because their adrenal glands do not produce cortisol or aldosterone and they are fully dependent on exogenous steroids from the time of birth. Genetic analysis can accurately identify this subgroup of females who would most benefit from surgical adrenalectomy.

We have performed transperitoneal laparoscopic bilateral adrenalectomy on two patients. There was a significant reduction in serum androgens and 17-OHP in both patients after adrenalectomy. Steroid requirements in both patients have been reduced to physiologic levels. Physical appearance is improved in both with a reduction in acne and hirsutism. Both patients report a weight loss between 10 and 6 kg. Spontaneous menses at regular intervals commenced at 5 and 2 months postoperatively.

Although dramatic improvements in our two patients were observed, the appropriate time to perform adrenalectomy remains controversial and must be further defined.

Conclusion

Treatment of children with congenital adrenal hyperplasia presents a complex clinical situation that requires a multidisciplinary approach. The surgical treatments described here are reliable approaches with few complications. However, before any treatment is undertaken, the surgeon must have an accurate picture of the patient's anatomy in order to tailor the proper repair.

Continued advances in prenatal care may one day obviate the need for reconstructive surgery. The administration of prenatal steroids to the mother is an accepted modality of treating CAH prenatally. Dexamethasone is given to the mother from the fifth week of pregnancy until delivery (David and Forest 1984; Pang 1997). When dexamethasone is begun early in the first trimester, effective prevention of virilization is accomplished 86 per cent of the time (Pang 1997). Still, 14 per cent of infants become virilized despite treatment and not all at-risk pregnancies can be identified prenatally. Better prenatal screening will be accomplished as more detailed molecular characterization of the underlying genetic defects is achieved. Also, because of continued biochemical advances, more efficient *in utero* treatment of infants with CAH will occur.

Since some infants fail prenatal treatment and others are born unwittingly, the surgical aspects of treatment are an important aspect of care for children with CAH. One-half of all intersex births are eventually diagnosed as virilized females with CAH; three-quarters of these patients have a 21-hydroxylase deficiency (New and Newfield 1997). We have described various approaches to genitoplasty depending upon the degree of virilization present.

When medical and surgical treatments are performed appropriately in this group of patients, a normal physiologic, emotional, and sexual development can be achieved.

References

Belman, A.B., Kelalis, P.P. and King, L.R. (ed.) (1992). *Clinical pediatric urology*, Vol. 1, p. 986. W.B. Saunders, Philadelphia.

David, M. and Forest, M.G. (1984). Prenatal treatment of congenital adrenal hyperplasia resulting from 21-hydroxylase deficiency. *J. Pediatr.* **105**, 799.

De Jong, T.P.V.M. and Boemers, T.M.L. (1995). Neonatal management of female intersex by clitorovaginoplasty. *J. Urol.* **154**, 830.

Hendren, W.H. and Atala, A. (1995). Repair of the high vagina in girls with severely masculinized anatomy from the adrenogenital syndrome. *J. Pediatr. Surg.* **30** (1), 91–4.

Hendren, W.H. and Crawford, J. (1969). Adrenogenital syndrome: the anatomy of the anomaly and its repair. Some new concepts. *J. Pediatr. Surg.* **4**, 49–58.

Hendren, W.H. and Donahoe, P. (1980). Correction of congenital abnormalities of the vagina and perineum. *J. Pediatr. Surg.* **15**, 751–63.

Lee, M. and Donahoe, P. (1997). The infant with ambiguous genitalia. In *Current endocrinology* (ed. Bardin), pp. 216–23.

Mathews, R. and Gearheart, J. (1998). Techniques of feminizing genitoplasty. In *American Urological Association update series* (ed. T.J. Ball), Vol. XVII, lesson 8. American Urological Association, Inc., Houston.

Meyers, R. (1997). Congenital anomalies of the vagina and their reconstruction. *Clin. Obstet. Gynecol.* **40** (1), 168–80.

New, M.N. and Newfield, R. (1997). Congenital adrenal hyperplasia. In *Current endocrinology* (ed. Bardin), pp. 179–86.

Pang, S. (1997). Congenital adrenal hyperplasia. *Endocrinol. Metab. Clin. N. Am.* **26** (4), .

Passerini-Glazel, G. (1989). A new 1-stage procedure for clitorovaginoplasty in severely masculinized female pseudohermaphrodites. *J. Urol.* **142**, 565–7.

Snyder, H. III, Retik, A.B., Bauer, S.B., and Colodny, A.H. (1983). Feminizing genitoplasty: a synthesis. *J. Urol.* **129**, 1024–5.

57. Open adrenalectomy: indications and surgical options

E. Darracott Vaughan Jr

Introduction

We are fortunate to be operating in an era where we have precise biochemical tests that, coupled with radiographic localization techniques, allow us to identify accurately patients who warrant adrenalectomy (Vaughan and Blumenfeld 1998).

Successful treatment of patients who require open adrenalectomy necessitates a clear understanding of adrenal physiology, anatomy, the metabolic consequences of the specific adrenal diseases, and potential perioperative complications. Moreover, the surgeon must master a variety of surgical techniques since the approach is often tailored either to the patients' underlying problems or to the patients' anatomy.

Currently, the vast majority of patients with surgical adrenal disorders undergo a laparoscopic adrenalectomy (Terachi *et al.* 2000). For those of us schooled in the nuances of adrenal surgery it has been with pleasure that we've seen the evolution of elegant laparoscopic techniques since the original cases reported by Gagner *et al.* (1992).

The complication rate of laparoscopic technique is low, 6 per cent in 370 cases, including complications that did not require surgical intervention. Conversion to open surgery only occurred in 3.5 per cent (Terachi *et al.* 2000).

Table 57.1 Possible errors in patient preparation for adrenal surgery

Primary aldosteronism
   Potassium repletion
   Blood pressure control
Cushing's syndrome
   Inhibition of glucocorticoid production using metapyrone when there are
     severe manifestations
   Control of diabetes
   Preoperative antibiotics
   Operative steroid administration
Incidentalomas
   Anesthetic preparation for pheochromocytoma—5% have negative
     diagnostic studies
Adenal carcinoma
   Consent for adjacent organ removal
   Failure to identify IVC involvement
Pheochromocytoma
   Preoperative catechole blockade
   Volume expansion
   Anesthesia consultation

However, remaining indications for open adrenalectomy include selected patients with adrenal carcinoma, patients with large pheochromocytoma where the blood pressure may be difficult to control, and patients requiring simultaneous abdominal procedures. Moreover, there are medical indications including bleeding disorders, morbid obesity, and patients who have had multiple previous abdominal procedures who require an open procedure.

In addition, if the surgeon understands specific complications that can occur with open adrenal surgery, the surgeon will be aware of their existence and will be prepared to react even if a patient is undergoing a laparoscopic adrenalectomy. For example, it has been demonstrated that there is significant catecholamine and cytokine response to laparoscopic adrenal surgery in patients with pheochromocytoma (Kanauchi *et al.* 2000).

This chapter will review the major aspects of adrenal surgery including preoperative preparation and intraoperative and postoperative problems that can occur.

Adrenal surgery

Adrenalectomy is the treatment of choice in most patients who have undergone appropriate metabolic evaluation and have been found to have a surgical lesion (Vaughan and Blumenfeld 1998). However, the surgeon must be aware that there are unique aspects to the care of these patients including specific preoperative management as outlined in Table 57.1. Accordingly, patients with hyperaldosteronism who are generally healthy require spironolactone 10–400 mg/day to restore their potassium supply. Patients with Cushing's syndrome have severe systemic effects from the hyperglucocorticoidism. They are often obese, have diabetic tendencies, are poor wound healers, easily sustain bony fractures, and are susceptible to infection. Thus, they are at a high risk for complications. In selected patients with markedly elevated cortisol levels the preoperative use of metabolic blockers such as metyrapone is required to reverse some of the clinical findings prior to adrenalectomy. Certainly glucocorticoid replacement is required throughout the surgical procedure and postoperatively until the function of the contralateral adrenal gland occurs. Finally, in patients with a pheochromocytoma, adrenergic blockade generally with dibenzyline is required and at times the blockade of catecholamine production with metyrosine is also useful as previously

Table 57.2 Surgical options*

Disease	Approach
Primary hyperaldosteronism	Posterior (left or right)
	Modified posterior (right)
	Eleventh rib (left > right)
	Posterior transthoracic
Cushing's adenoma	Eleventh rib (left or right)
	Thoracoabdominal (large)
	Posterior (small)
Cushing's disease	Bilateral posterior
Bilateral hyperplasia	Bilateral eleventh rib (alternating)
Adrenal carcinoma	Thoracoabdominal
	Eleventh rib
	Transabdominal
Bilateral renal ablation	Bilateral posterior
Pheochromocytoma	Transabdominal chevron
	Thoracoabdominal (large—usually right)
	Eleventh rib
Neuroblastoma	Transabdominal
	Eleventh rib

* From Vaughan (1996).

discussed as well as the use of other drugs (see Chapter 53). The additional preoperative evaluation that is mandatory in patients with pheochromocytoma is consultation with the anesthesiologist who should be familiar with the patient and can plan strategy for management (Malhotra 1995)

Thus the management of patients with an adrenal disorder is approached on a team basis involving experienced endocrinologists, radiologists, anesthesiologists, and urologists or general surgeons.

Numerous open approaches can be made to the adrenal gland (Table 57.2). The proper approach depends on the underlying cause of adrenal pathology, the size of the adrenal, the site of the lesion, the habitus of the patient, and the experience and preference of the surgeon. In addition to the surgical options, a laparoscopic approach can be utilized, particularly for smaller adrenal tumors. In most cases there are a number of different options available and a careful review of all the variables is required before a choice is made. Thus each case should be considered individually although some approaches are preferable for a given disease. For example, in patients with large adrenal tumors a thoracoabdominal approach is often utilized. In contrast, a posterior or modified posterior approach is preferred for small localized lesions. Finally a patient with multiple lesions, either extra-adrenal or bilateral, will be explored using a transabdominal chevron incision. Potential operative complications are shown in Table 57.3.

Before describing the specific techniques a number of unifying concepts warrant attention. First, adequate visualization is imperative; the adrenal glands lie high in the retroperitoneum and quite posterior. Therefore, the use of a headlight by both the surgeon and first assistant is critical and hemostasis should be maintained rigorously. The operator should bring the adrenal down by initially exposing the cranial attachments and dividing the right blood supply between either right-angled clips or utilizing a forceps cautery (Fig. 57.1. (a), (b)). If available, the harmonic scalpel (as used in laparoscopic surgery) is very useful for both

Table 57.3 Operative complications of adrenal surgery

Hemorrhage
  IVC
  Adrenal vein
  Lumbar vein
  Hepatic vein
Vascular
  Ligation of renal artery branch
  Ligation of mesenteric artery
  IVC involvement
Adjacent organ injury
  Pneumothorax
  Pancreas
  Liver
  Spleen
  Stomach
  Colon
  Kidney

dissection and coagulation. Thus, it is often simplest to begin the dissection laterally, identifying the vascular supply and working around the cranial edge of the gland. The posterior surface is generally devoid of vasculature and, after the gland is freed superiorly with gentle traction on the kidney, the gland can be brought inferiorly for control of the adrenal vein. The only tumor that would be handled in a different fashion would be a pheochromocytoma where the intent should be to obtain control of the adrenal vein early so as to stabilize the patient from a burst of catecholamine release during manipulation. The adrenal gland is extremely friable and fractures easily, which can cause troublesome bleeding. Therefore, tension or traction should be maintained on the

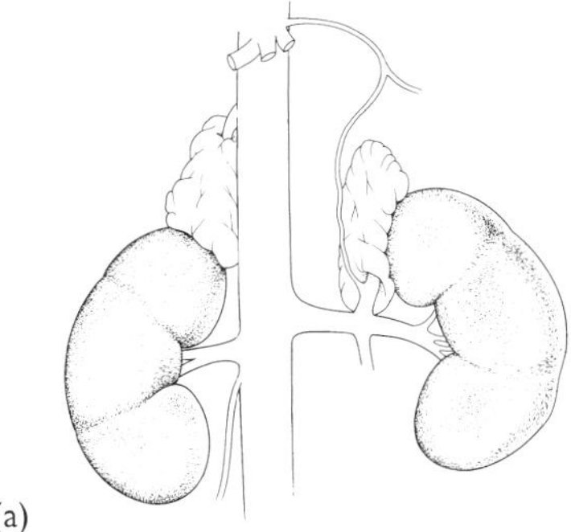

(a)

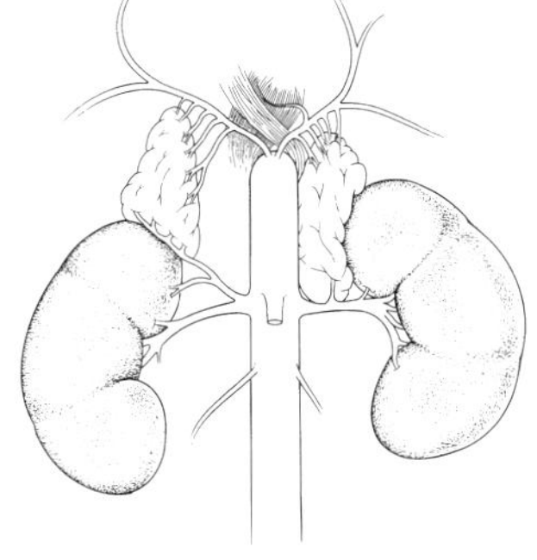

(b)

Fig. 57.1 (a) Venous drainage from both adrenals showing the presence of both the left adrenal vein and the phrenic branch and also showing the short, stubby posterior arising right adrenal vein. (b) Arterial supply to the adrenal.

kidney or surrounding structures and not on the adrenal itself. The concept has been expressed as 'the patient should be dissected from the tumor', a view that is particularly true in patients with pheochromocytomas where the gland should not be manipulated.

Posterior approach

The posterior approach can be used for either bilateral adrenal exploration or unilateral removal of small tumors. The bilateral approach is rarely utilized today because of our excellent localization techniques. It is now utilized primarily for ablative total adrenalectomy. The options for incisions are shown in Fig. 57.2; generally, rib resection is preferable in order to gain high exposure. After a standard subperiosteal rib resection, care should be taken with the diaphragmatic release; the pleura should be avoided and the diaphragm swept cranially.

The fibrofatty tissues with Gerota's fascia are swept away from the paraspinal musculature, exposing a subdiaphragmatic 'open space' that is at the posterior apex of the resection. The liver within the peritoneum is dissected off the anterior surface of the adrenal and the cranial blood supply is divided. Medially on the right, the inferior vena cava (IVC) is visualized. The short, high adrenal vein entering the cava in the dorsolateral position is identified and can be clipped or ligated. The adrenal can then be drawn caudally by traction on the kidney. The adrenal arteries will issue from under and from behind the IVC and these must be carefully clipped; otherwise, troublesome bleeding can occur.

Finally, the adrenal is removed from the superior aspect of the kidney and care must be taken to avoid apical branches of the renal artery. On the left, the approach is similar with division of the splenorenal ligament giving lateral exposure.

The posterior approach can be modified for a transthoracic adrenal exposure to the diaphragm (Novick *et al.* 1989); however, this more extensive approach is rarely necessary for small adrenal tumors.

Modified posterior approach

Although the posterior approach has the advantage of rapid adrenal exposure and low morbidity, there are definite disadvantages. This approach may impair respiration, the abdominal contents are compressed posteriorly, and the visual field is limited. In addition, if bleeding occurs it is difficult to extend the incision to gain a better exposure. Therefore, we have developed a modified posterior approach for right adrenalectomy utilizing the Gil-Vernet position (Gil-Vernet 1965).

The approach is based on the anatomical relationship with the right adrenal which lies deeply posterior and high in the retroperitoneum behind the liver (Fig. 57.3). In addition, the short, stubby right adrenal vein enters the IVC posteriorly at the apex of the adrenal. Hence, we utilize an approach that is posterior, but

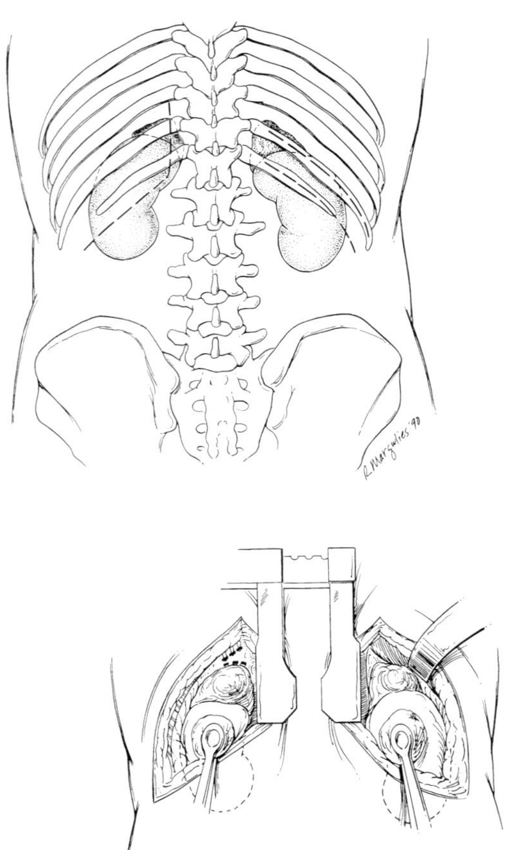

Fig. 57.2 Posterior approach to the adrenal; dotted lines show different incisions.

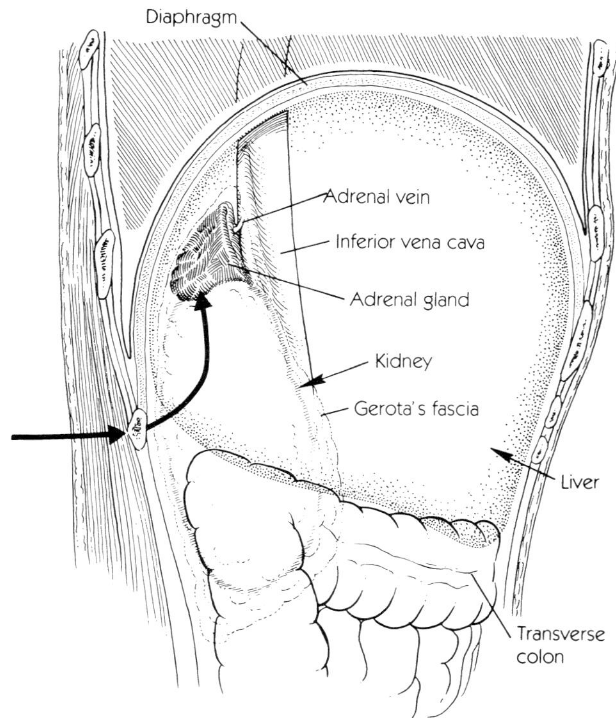

Fig. 57.3 Anatomical relationship of right adrenal and liver.

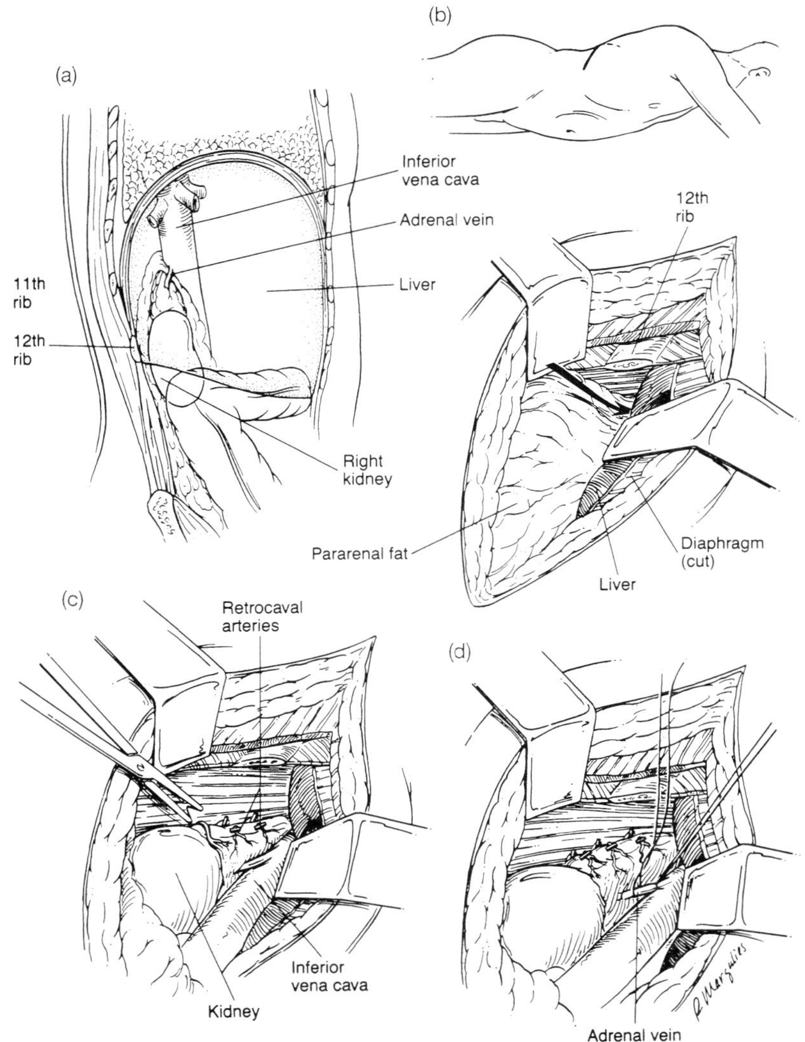

Fig. 57.4 Exposure of the right adrenal vein from the modified posterior approach. If the vein is injured, an Alis clamp can be placed at its origin and the cava oversewn.

the patient is in a modified position, similar to that used for a Gil-Vernet dorsal lumbotomy incision (Fig. 57.4) (Vaughan and Phillips 1987). The patient is first placed in a formal lateral flank position and then allowed to fall forward into the modified posterior position. Subsequently, the eleventh or twelfth rib is resected with care to avoid the pleura. The diaphragm then is dissected off the underlying peritoneum and liver in order to gain mobility. Similarly, the inferior surface of the peritoneum, loosely associated with the liver, is sharply dissected from Gerota's fascia, which is gently retracted inferiorly. It is of note that the adrenal gland is not identified during the early portion of the dissection and, because of the modified posterior approach, the surgeon can become disoriented if not thoroughly familiar with anatomical relationships.

The adrenal will become visible in the depth of the incision as the final hepatic attachments are divided. The lateral, empty space can be found exposing the posterior abdominal musculature and often the IVC. Multiple, small arteries course behind the IVC and emerge over the paraspinal muscles and these arteries are clipped and divided.

At this point the adrenal usually can be moved posteriorly against the paraspinal muscles exposing the anterior surface of the IVC below the adrenal gland.

The major advantage of this approach is that the adrenal vein is easily identified because it emerges from the exposed segment of the IVC and courses up to the adrenal, which now rises toward the surgeon. In other flank or anterior positions, the adrenal vein resides in its posterior relationship, requiring caval rotation and the chance of adrenal vein avulsion. After adrenal vein exposure, it is doubly tied and divided or clipped with right-angled clips and divided.

The remaining removal of the adrenal is as was previously described for the posterior approach.

On the left side we do not use this modified approach and use a standard flank approach with a fairly small incision.

We have used the modified posterior approach for all patients with right adrenal aldosterone-secreting tumors and for other patients with benign adenomas of less than 6 cm. We do not recommend the approach for patients with large lesions or malignant adrenal neoplasms. The approach has been used for patients with relatively small pheochromocytomas.

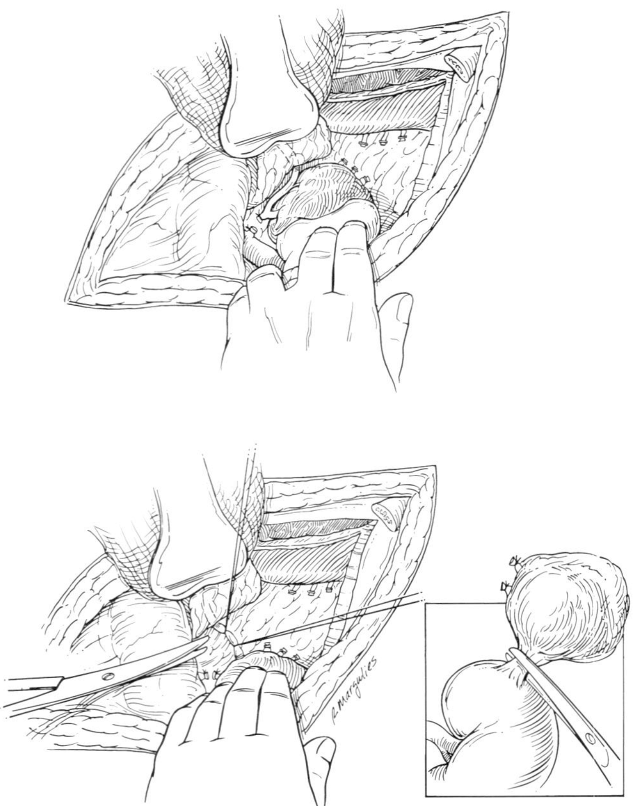

Fig. 57.5 Exposure of the left adrenal.

Flank approach

The standard extrapleural, extraperitoneal eleventh rib resection is excellent for either left or right adrenalectomy. After completion of the incision, the lumbocostal arch is utilized as a landmark showing the point of attachment of the posterior diaphragm to the posterior abdominal musculature. Gerota's fascia, containing the adrenal and kidney, can be swept medially and inferiorly, giving exposure to the splenorenal ligament on the left, which should be divided to avoid splenic injury (Fig. 57.5). Working anteriorly on the left, the spleen and pancreas within the peritoneum can be lifted cranially, exposing the anterior surface of the adrenal gland.

On the right side, a similar maneuver is used to lift the liver within the peritoneum off the anterior surface of the adrenal. Quite often, the adrenal gland cannot be identified precisely until these maneuvers are performed. One should not attempt to dissect into the body of the adrenal or to dissect the inferior surface of the adrenal off the kidney. The kidney is useful for retraction. The dissection should continue from lateral to medial along the posterior abdominal and diaphragmatic musculature, with precise ligation or clipping of the small but multiple adrenal arteries. While the operator clips these arteries with one hand, the opposite hand is employed to retract both adrenal and kidney inferiorly. With release of the superior vasculature, the adrenal is visualized. On the left medially, the phrenic branch of the venous

drainage must be carefully clipped or ligated (Fig. 57.1). This vessel is not noted in most atlases but can cause troublesome bleeding if divided. The medial dissection along the crus of the diaphragm and aorta will lead to the renal vein; finally, the adrenal vein is controlled, doubly tied, and divided. The adrenal is then removed from the kidney with care to avoid the apical branches of the renal artery.

On the right side, the dissection is similar. However, after release of the adrenal from the superior vasculature, it is helpful to expose the IVC and divide the medial arterial supply. This maneuver allows mobilization of the cava for better exposure of the high posterior adrenal vein, which is doubly tied or clipped and divided. Patients with large adrenal carcinomas may require *en bloc* resection of the adrenal and kidney following the principles of radical nephrectomy (Fig. 57.5).

A major deviation from this technique is used for the patient with pheochromocytoma, in whom the initial dissection should be aimed toward early control and division of the main adrenal vein on either side. Obviously, in this setting, the anesthesiologist should be notified when the adrenal vein is divided because a marked drop in blood pressure often occurs, even when the patient is adequately hydrated.

After removal of the adrenal, inspection should be made for any bleeding and for pleural tears of the diaphragm. The kidney should also be inspected. The incision is closed without drains with interrupted 0 polydioxanone sutures.

Thoracoabdominal approach

The thoracoabdominal ninth or tenth rib approach is utilized for large adenomas, for some large adrenal carcinomas, and for well-localized pheochromocytomas. The incision and exposure is standard, with a radial incision through the diaphragm and a generous intraperitoneal extension. The techniques described for adrenalectomy with the eleventh rib approach are used.

Transabdominal approach

The transabdominal approach is commonly selected for patients with pheochromocytomas, for children, and for some patients with adrenal carcinomas. The concept is to have the ability for complete abdominal exploration to identify either multiple pheochromocytomas or adrenal metastases.

I use the transverse or chevron incision, which I believe gives better exposure of both adrenal glands than a midline incision. The rectus muscles and lateral abdominal muscles are divided, exposing the peritoneum. Upon entering the peritoneal cavity, the surgeon should gently palpate the para-aortic areas and the adrenal areas. Close attention is given to blood pressure changes in an attempt to identify any unsuspected lesions if the patient has a pheochromocytoma. This maneuver is less important today because of the excellent localization techniques previously discussed. In fact, with precise preoperative localization of the offending tumor, the chevron incision does not need to be completely symmetrical and may be limited on the contralateral side.

If the patient has a lesion on the right adrenal, the hepatic flexure of the colon is reflected inferiorly. The incision is made

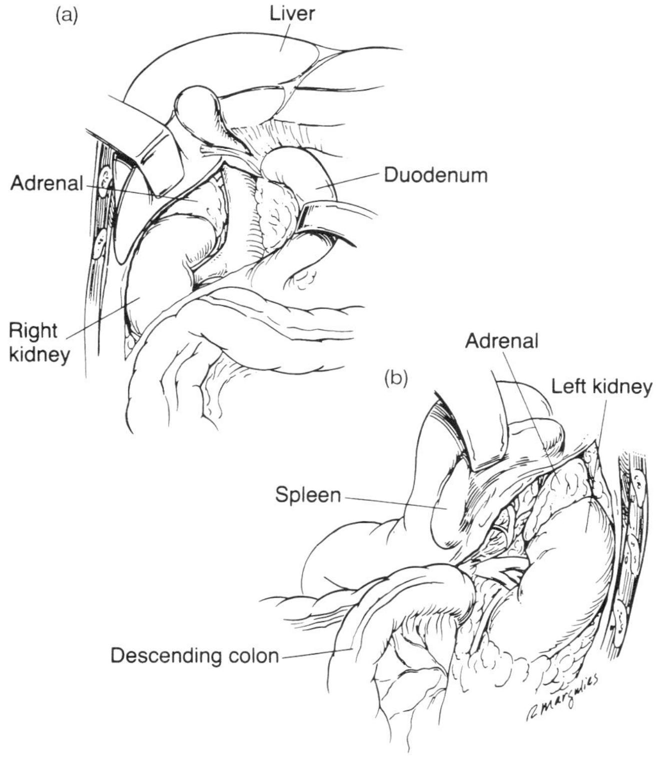

Fig. 57.6 Relationship of the adrenal to intraabdominal organs. Care should be taken to avoid injury to the spleen, splenic vein, and pancreas on the left and the liver and duodenum on the right.

in the posterior peritoneum lateral to the kidney and carried superiorly, allowing the liver to be reflected cranially (Fig. 57.6). Incision in the peritoneum is carried downward, exposing the anterior surface of theIVC to the entrance of the right renal vein. Once the cava is cleared, one or two accessory hepatic veins are often encountered, which should be secured. These veins are easily avulsed from the cava and may cause troublesome bleeding. Ligation of these veins gives 1 to 2 cm of additional caval exposure, which is often useful during the exposure of the short posterior right adrenal vein. Small accessory adrenal veins may also be encountered or the adrenal and a hepatic vein may enter the cava with a common trunk. The cava is then rolled medially, exposing the adrenal vein, which should be doubly tied or clipped and divided.

After control of the adrenal vein, it is simplest to proceed with the superior dissection, lifting the liver off the adrenal and securing the multiple small adrenal arteries arising from the inferior phrenic artery, which is rarely seen. The adrenal can be drawn inferiorly with retraction on the kidney, and the adrenal arteries transversing to the adrenal from under the cava can be secured with right-angled clips. The final step is removing the adrenal from the kidney.

The left adrenal vein is not as difficult to approach because it lies lower, partially anterior to the upper pole of the kidney, and the adrenal vein empties into the left renal vein. Accordingly, on

the left side, the colon is reflected medially, exposing the anterior surface of Gerota's capsule; the initial dissection should involve identification of the renal vein. In essence, the dissection is the same as for a radical nephrectomy for renal carcinoma. Once the renal vein is exposed, the adrenal vein is identified, doubly ligated, and divided. After this maneuver the pancreas and splenic vasculature are lifted off the anterior surface of the adrenal gland. Because of additional drainage from the adrenal into the phrenic system, I generally continue the medial dissection early to control the phrenic vein. I then work cephalad and lateral to release the splenorenal ligament and the superior attachments of the adrenal. The remainder of the dissection is carried out as previously described.

After removal of the tumor, regardless of size, careful inspection is made to ensure hemostasis and the absence of injury to adjacent organs. Careful abdominal exploration is carried out, after which the wound is closed with the suture material of choice. No drains are used.

Patients with multiple endocrine adenopathy or family histories of pheochromocytoma, as well as pediatric patients, should be considered at high risk for multiple lesions. Preoperative evaluation should identify these lesions but, regardless, a careful abdominal exploration should be carried out.

In patients with suspected malignant pheochromocytomas, *en bloc* dissections may be necessary to obtain adequate margins, a concept that also applies in patients with adrenal carcinomas. Evaluation with magnetic resonance imaging (MRI) to obtain transverse, coronal, and sagittal images is extremely useful to define clearly the adrenal relationships to the IVC and renal vessels as well as to localize the adrenal vein.

In patients with pheochromocytomas, postoperative management includes maintenance of arterial and venous lines in an intensive care setting until they are stable. Often, 24 to 48 hours is required for the full effect of phenoxybenzamine, the alpha-blocking agent commonly given, to wear off and for normal alpha-receptor activity to be restored (Table 57.4).

Table 57.4 Postoperative complications following adrenal surgery

Primary aldosteronism
Hypokalemia—secondary to continued potassium loss immediately postoperative
Hyperkalemia—secondary to failure of contralateral adrenal to secrete aldosterone
Cushing's syndrome
Inadequate steroid replacement leading to hypocorticoidism
Fracture secondary to osteoporosis
Poor wound healing
Increased risk of infection
Pheochromocytoma
Hypotension secondary to alpha-adrenergic blockade after tumor removal
Generic complications
Hemorrhage (IVC; adrenal arteries)
Pneumothorax
Pancreatitis
Pneumonia
Hiccoughs

Partial adrenalectomy

The standard treatment for patients with the adrenal lesions described has been total adrenalectomy. However, there is an excellent paper showing the utility of partial adrenalectomy in patients with primary hyperaldosteronism (Nakada *et al.* 1995). I have not used partial adrenalectomy in a patient with normal contralateral adrenal, but certainly have used the technique in patients with bilateral disease. Thus, in one patient with a pheochromocytoma on one side and a nonfunctioning adenoma on the other, the adenoma was simply enucleated from the adrenal. In a second patient with bilateral pheochromocytomas, the larger lesion was totally excised and partial adrenalectomy was utilized to remove the contralateral tumor. Care has to be taken to obtain thorough hemostasis when performing a partial adrenalectomy because of the vascular nature of the adrenal.

An additional appropriate use for partial adrenalectomy has been reported in patients known to have the potential for multiple adrenal lesions. The group at the US National Institute of Health reported 13 consecutive von Hippel–Lindau disease patients with pheochromocytoma who underwent 14 partial and 6 complete unilateral adrenalectomies (Walther *et al.* 1999). In addition, Mugiya *et al.* (1999) have utilized partial adrenalectomy in patients with multiple endocrine neoplasia type II A.

Summary

We are fortunate that our ability to diagnose the specific adrenal entities that mandate a surgical approach is extremely accurate. The combination of analytical methodology to measure the appropriate adrenocortical and medullary hormonal production and the radiologic techniques for localization is superb. The management of these adrenal disorders with precise surgical precision following localization is highly successful, resulting in a reversal of both metabolic abnormalities and the hypertension that often accompanies these diseases. Indeed, the evolution of these different techniques over the past 50 years is a true success story.

References

Gagner, M., Lacroix, A., and Bolte, E. (1992). Laparoscopic adrenalectomy in Cushing's syndrome and pheochromocytoma. *New Engl. J. Med.* **327**, 1033.

Gil-Vernet, J. (1965). New surgical concepts in removing renal calculi. *Urol. Int.* **20**, 255–62.

Kanauchi, H., Mimura, Y., Hiki, N., and Kaminishi, M. (2000). Catecholamine and cytokine response to laparoscopic adrenalectomy in patients with pheochromocytoma. *Biomed. Pharmacother.* **54**, 191s–202s.

Malhotra, V. (ed.) (1995). *Anesthesia for renal and genitourinary surgery*. McGraw Hill, New York.

Mugiya, S., Suzuki, K., Saisu, K., and Fujita, K. (1999). Unilateral laparoscopic adrenalectomy followed by contralateral retroperitoneoscopic partial adrenalectomy in a patient with multiple endocrine neoplasia type 2a syndrome. *J. Endourol.* **13**, 99–104.

Nakada, T., Kubota, Y., Sasagawa, I., *et al.* (1995). Therapeutic outcome of primary aldosteronism: adrenalectomy versus enucleation of aldosteron-production adenoma. *J. Urol.* **153**, 1775–80.

Novick, A.C., Strafon, R.A., and Kaylor, W. (1989). Posterior transthoracic approach for adrenal surgery. *J. Urol.* **141**, 254.

Terachi, T., Yoshida, O., Matsuda, T., *et. al.* (2000). Complications of laparoscopic and retroperitoneoscopic adrenalectomies in 370 cases in Japan: a multi-institutional study. *Biomed. Pharmacother.* **54**, 211s–212s.

Vaughan, E.D. Jr (1996). Adrenal surgery. In *Operative urology* (ed. F. Marshall). W.B. Saunders, Philadelphia. Chapter 24, 220–230.

Vaughan, E.D. Jr and Blumenfeld, J.D. (1998). The adrenals. In *Campbell's urology*, 7th edn (ed. P.C. Walsh, A.B. Retik, T.A. Stamey, and E.D. Vaughan Jr), Chapter 96. W.B. Saunders, Philadelphia.

Vaughan, E.D. Jr and Phillips, H. (1987). Modified posterior approach for right adrenalectomy. *Surg. Gynecol. Obstet.* **165**, 453–5.

Walther, M., Keiser, H., Choyke, P., *et al.* (1999). Management of hereditary pheochromocytoma in von Hippel–Lindau kindred with partial adrenalectomy. *J. Urol.* **161**, 395–8.

58. Partial adrenalectomy: indications and technique

Christian P. Pavlovich and McClellan M. Walther

Experience with organ-sparing techniques is growing as familial forms of adrenal tumors are increasingly recognized and the detrimental impact of bilateral adrenalectomy on quality of life is appreciated. Partial adrenalectomy has found specific applications in the setting of certain bilateral or hereditary adrenal tumors and in patients with tumors in a solitary adrenal gland. Partial adrenalectomy is feasible for adrenocortical or medullary lesions, and can be performed laparoscopically or in conventional open fashion. Several open approaches are used—posterior, flank, thoracoabdominal, or anterior—and laparoscopic access can be obtained via either transperitoneal or retroperitoneal routes. These approaches are described in detail elsewhere in this volume. We emphasize here the indications for and technical considerations relevant to partial adrenalectomy.

Indications

Partial adrenalectomy (PA) can be used to treat a variety of adrenal tumors. Since the 1980s, adrenal-sparing surgery has been reported for the treatment of pheochromocytomas, aldosteronomas, Cushing's adenomas, and carcinomas or solitary metastases. By the late 1990s, reports of laparoscopic PA appeared, starting with the enucleation of an aldosterone-producing adenoma by Janetschek *et al.* in 1997. Laparoscopic techniques have since been successfully applied to aldosteronomas, Cushing's adenomas, pheochromocytomas, and nonfunctioning tumors suspicious for malignancy. Pheochromocytomas do recur in a minority of patients with hereditary tumor syndromes, and are successfully managed with repeat surgery (van Heerden *et al.* 1984; Lee *et al.* 1996; Walther *et al.* 1999).

PA should be considered when the sparing of adrenal cortex would prevent lifelong steroid replacement, and when principles of cancer surgery are not compromised. Adrenal replacement therapy can have long-term complications related to fixed daily steroid overdosing (obesity, osteoporosis, and other manifestations of Cushing's syndrome) or to steroid underdosing in times of stress (Oelkers 1996; Zelissen *et al.* 1994). Of all patients undergoing bilateral adrenalectomy, acute adrenal insufficiency (which can rarely result in death) develops in 25–33 per cent, 30 per cent encounter significant fatigue, and 48 per cent consider themselves handicapped (Lairmore *et al.* 1993; Telenius-Berg *et al.* 1989). For patients with a solitary adrenal gland and for patients with bilateral tumors, PA is often preferable to total adrenalectomy. Whether the tumor(s) are manageable by partial resection and whether such an approach would be likely to result in complete resection with preservation of sufficient viable adrenal cortex must be determined. Patients with hereditary adrenal tumors may choose either to be cured by bilateral adrenalectomy and live with the associated morbidity, or to live with the risk of recurrence after partial adrenalectomy. Our bias has been to attempt PA in patients with hereditary pheochromocytoma to preserve adrenocortical tissue when the tumor can be completely excised. This bias is reinforced for patients at risk for recurrent tumors, such as those with multiple endocrine neoplasia type 2 (MEN2) or von Hippel–Lindau disease (VHL).

Aldosteronoma

Adrenalectomy has been the traditional treatment of choice for aldosterone-producing adenomas. While it is technically feasible to enucleate an isolated aldosteronoma, between 7 and 38 per cent of these tumors are associated with micro- or macronodular disease in neighboring areas of the gland (as reviewed by Ito *et al.* (1990)). As it is not currently possible to distinguish functioning from nonfunctioning nodules, adrenalectomy provides the best chance of cure when anything but a discrete, solitary tumor is present. PA has nevertheless been reported for discrete aldosteronomas (Nakada *et al.* 1995).

PA was first performed laparoscopically to treat Conn's syndrome in 1997, and several reports support its feasibility (Janetschek *et al.* 1997; Sasagawa *et al.* 1998; Suzuki *et al.* 1998; Walz *et al.* 1998; Imai *et al.* 1999). Imai *et al.* (1999) have pointed out that solitary aldosteronomas are the best suited tumor type for laparoscopic PA. These tumors are usually small and discrete, and are sometimes located in the extremity of the adrenal gland (Imai *et al.* 1999). The average tumor diameter was only 1.48 cm in a 35-patient aldosteronoma series (Weigel *et al.* 1994) An isolated report has shown a putative benefit of PA over unilateral adrenalectomy for aldosteronoma in terms of preserving patients' cortisol and aldosterone responses to provocative biochemical testing postoperatively (Nakada *et al.* 1995). The clinical relevance of this remains unclear, as patients with a solitary functional adrenal gland do no worse than patients with two (Vaughan and Blumenfeld 1998), and the number of patients actually cured of hypertension and hypokalemia by PA was not given.

Cushing's adenoma

Few resections of glucocorticoid-producing adrenal adenomas have been performed as PA. The adrenals become atrophic with an active Cushing's adenoma, and the adenoma is often several centimeters in size, making it a technical challenge to leave viable adrenal tissue in place. Walz *et al.* (1998) performed PA on four patients with 2–3 cm Cushing's adenomas, all of whom were cured but required steroid replacement at short published follow-up ($2\frac{1}{4}$ months). The remaining atrophic adrenal tissue usually requires more time to recover. The treatment of this form of Cushing's syndrome with PA might be considered in the hopes that, by preserving adrenal cortical parenchyma, the patient will have a greater chance of regaining enough functionality to allow a more rapid taper of steroid replacement. However, given that many of these lesions present when they are large and leave little viable adrenal around them, PA may continue to prove difficult and unrewarding.

Clinically, patients with Cushing's syndrome secondary to a small adrenal adenoma cannot be differentiated from those with a cortisol-producing adrenocortical cancer. The latter tumor, though rare, is best treated surgically with wide excision. A PA in the setting of an adrenocortical carcinoma stands to provide less satisfactory oncological results.

Pheochromocytoma

Pheochromocytoma is optimally managed with preoperative catecholamine blockade followed by surgical resection. This medical treatment has all but obviated the need for early control of the adrenal vein by open surgical approaches. Indeed, laparoscopic adrenalectomies, open PA, and laparoscopic PA for pheochromocytoma have been performed safely (van Heerden *et al.* 1985; Hamberger *et al.* 1987; Neumann *et al.* 1999; Vargas *et al.* 1997).

Partial adrenalectomies have been performed in patients with sporadic bilateral pheochromocytomas (Birnbaum *et al.* 1989), but are especially relevant to the treatment of pheochromocytomas in patients with hereditary tumor syndromes such as VHL or MEN2 (Lee *et al.* 1996; Neumann *et al.* 1999; Edstrom *et al.* 1999; Walther *et al.* in press). In these patients, the recurrence or metastatic spread of tumor is of particular concern (Carney *et al.* 1976), and the preservation of adrenal cortex is an important long-term issue. PA has been shown to preserve adrenocortical function in MEN2 patients with a 0–33 per cent risk of locally recurrent pheochromocytoma and 0 per cent metastasis over 54 to 88 months of follow-up (Lee *et al.* 1996; Lairmore *et al.* 1993; Albanese and Wiener 1993; Okamoto *et al.* 1996), which is similar to our experience with VHL patients (Walther *et al.* 1999). Fortunately, recurrent pheochromocytomas in VHL and MEN2 patients can be detected very early in their development with the advent of modern imaging (computerized tomography (CT), magnetic resonance imaging (MRI), and/or metaiodobenzylguanidine (MIBG) scanning) and highly sensitive biochemical testing (Stewart *et al.* 1978; Maurea *et al.* 1993; Shapiro *et al.* 1985; Eisenhofer *et al.* 1999). Thus, even subclinical pheochromocytomas of a few mm in diameter can be identified in remnant adrenals, and safely treated with repeat PA early in their development (Walther *et al.* 1999; Edstrom *et al.* 1999). While the average tumor diameter in a recent series was 2.3 cm, even tumors > 4 cm in diameter were successfully treated by PA (Walther *et al.* 1999). For patients with hereditary, localized pheochromocytomas, PA may be offered in an attempt to maintain quality of life at the cost of possible tumor recurrence.

Nonfunctioning tumor

The indications for PA in this subset of patients, which includes those with hormonally inactive or minimally active tumors, are variable. Sporadic nonfunctional lesions > 4–6 cm in diameter are at higher risk of malignancy and should be resected radically, usually by unilateral adrenalectomy with adequate margins. Smaller tumors can theoretically be excised by PA if viable cortex can be left *in situ*. Imai *et al.* (1999) reported on two cases of subclinical Cushing's syndrome caused by adrenal adenomas that were successfully treated with PA. Since the natural history of this syndrome is not well defined and its association with Cushing's syndrome is unclear, surgery may not be indicated for asymptomatic patients (Graham and McHenry 1998). Similarly, adrenal cysts and myelolipomas are benign lesions that need not be addressed unless size criteria or other suspicious findings on imaging studies suggest they should be resected. If the contralateral adrenal is normal and the patient has no evidence of a hereditary tumor syndrome, unilateral adrenalectomy is a time-tested approach for suspicious nonfunctioning tumors. As patients with one adrenal do not evidence difficulties with adrenal function (Vaughan and Blumenfeld 1998), the rationale for PA in solitary nonfunctioning tumors is in evolution at best. Nevertheless, PA has been performed in such cases, without reported recurrences or complications related to the adrenal-sparing procedure (Sasagawa *et al.* 1998; Walz *et al.* 1998).

Technical considerations

Laparoscopic and open approaches allow rapid access to the adrenal, more so on the right due to that gland's location just beneath the peritoneum adjacent to the vena cava. The incision is made (or the laparoscopic ports are placed) with the same considerations as for adrenalectomy, taking into account the preferences and experience of the operating surgeon as well as the location of the tumor. The procedure is performed in similar manner whether by laparoscopic or open means. Once the adrenal gland is exposed, lesions ≥ 1 cm should become readily apparent. For smaller lesions, or when there is a question of multiple lesions, intraoperative sonography is helpful.

Intraoperative ultrasound (IOUS) transducers of 7.5 MHz locate small adrenal tumors with relative ease if the area is irrigated to produce an appropriate transducing medium. For deeper lesions, the frequency can be decreased to 5 MHz. 10 mm laparoscopic IOUS probes are available at these frequencies and have been used to identify lesions in patients with a variety of adrenal pathologies (Imai *et al.* 1999; Heniford *et al.* 1997), including subcentimeter tumors in a VHL patient undergoing bilateral partial adrenalectomy (Fig. 58.1) (Walther *et al.* 2000).

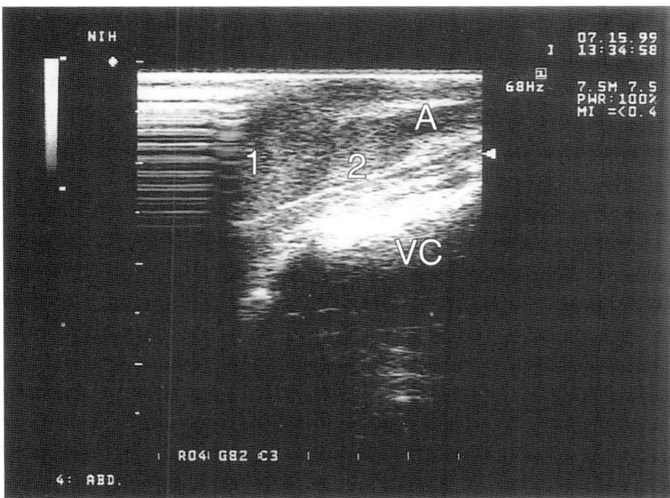

Fig. 58.1 This intraoperative sonogram demonstrates two adrenal nodules (1 and 2), as well as normal surrounding adrenal parenchyma (A) and vena cava (VC) in a von Hippel–Lindau disease patient. One of these lesions (2) was detected only by the sonogram. Both nodules were confirmed to be pheochromocytomas after partial adrenalectomy.

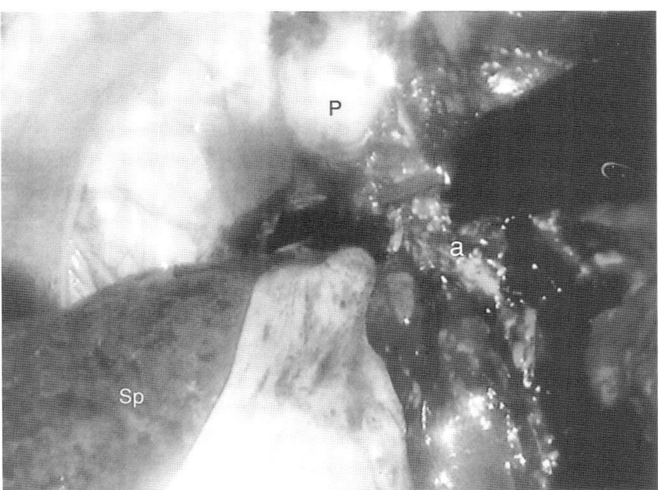

Fig. 58.2 A harmonic scalpel is being used to separate a pheochromocytoma (P) from adrenal parenchyma (a). The spleen (Sp) is seen at left.

Both open and laparoscopic PA require an understanding of the blood flow to and from the adrenal gland. The three-vessel blood supply to the adrenal glands (inferior phrenic, aorta, and renal artery) branches into smaller arteries that feed the adrenals circumferentially but generally leave the anterior and posterior surfaces avascular. Blood drains into a central vein, which enters the vena cava posteriorly on the right and the renal vein superiorly on the left. The tripartite arterial inflow to the adrenals is helpful in maintaining the viability of cortical tissue after PA.

As long as the rich periadrenal vascular supply is preserved, the main adrenal vein may be divided during PA. On the other hand, peripheral tumors may be excised with the vein left intact. Various authors advocate the latter, with the advantage that the remaining adrenal cortex stands to suffer less venous congestion if its outflow is not compromised (Sasagawa *et al.* 1998; Imai *et al.* 1999; Janetschek *et al.* 1998). Given the numerous smaller tributaries to and from the adrenal, it is doubtful that ligating the vein would cause complete venous disruption of remaining cortex, but many feel it is important to leave it intact. In a four-patient study of bilateral PA for pheochromocytomas in VHL patients, the adrenal vein was left intact in all cases with cure of pheochromocytoma as well as intact adrenal function at 2–24 months postoperatively (Neumann *et al.* 1999). A pragmatic approach that we favor is to attempt to preserve the vein, unless taking the vein would make the procedure substantially safer or allow a definite tumor margin (Walz *et al.* 1998; Walther *et al.* in press).

In order to bisect the adrenal at the point of choice, several techniques have been used with success. The clamp and suture method or vascular stapler effectively achieves hemostasis, while others advocate more gentle dissection with the harmonic scalpel or bipolar coagulation (Fig. 58.2) (Walz *et al.* 1998; Walther *et al.* 2000; Janetschek *et al.* 1998), with suture ligatures to complete the procedure. A suture ligature(s) (figure-of-eight or running) or a vascular stapler is appropriate for controlling bleeding from the subcapsular plexus, and surgical clips are also a helpful adjunct during PA (Sasagawa *et al.* 1998; Imai *et al.* 1999; Walther *et al.* in press). After laparoscopic resection, the tumor is placed in an endoscopic bag and removed through the largest port incision. Finally, insufflation pressure is decreased to 8 mm Hg for 5 minutes to check for bleeding prior to closure. Interestingly, Lee *et al.* (1996) were unable to correlate amount of adrenal left behind with subsequent endocrine functionality in their 30-year series of PA for hereditary pheochromocytoma. It has been suggested that at least 20 per cent of adrenal cortex be preserved in order to maintain endocrine functionality (Lee *et al.* 1996). Definitive studies are not available.

Summary

Partial adrenalectomy is a feasible parenchymal-sparing procedure that can be performed by a trained laparoscopist with relative ease. With preservation of enough viable adrenal cortex and (preferably) of the central adrenal vein, the endocrine function of the adrenal remnant can be maintained. The procedure is recommended for tumors that are relatively small and well-circumscribed, particularly for patients with a single adrenal gland or bilateral adrenal tumors. Most importantly, partial adrenalectomy is the procedure of choice for hereditary pheochromocytomas.

References

Albanese, C.T. and Wiener, E.S. (1993). Routine bilateral adrenalectomy is not warranted in childhood familial pheochromocytoma. *J. Pediatr. Surg.* **28**, 1248–52.

Birnbaum, J., Giuliano, A., and van Herle, A.J. (1989). Partial adrenalectomy for pheochromocytoma with maintenance of adrenocortical function. *J. Clin. Endocrinol. Metab.* **69** (5), 1078–81.

Carney, J.A., Sizemore, G.W., and Sheps, S.G. (1976). Adrenal medullary disease in multiple endocrine neoplasia, type 2: pheochromocytoma and its precursors. *Am. J. Clin. Pathol.* **66** (2), 279–90.

Edstrom, E., Grondal, S., Norstrom, F., Palmer, M., Svensson, K.-A., Widell, H., and Hamberger, B. (1999). Long term experience after subtotal adrenalectomy for multiple endocrine neoplasia type IIa. *Eur. J. Surg.* **165**, 431–5.

Eisenhofer, G., Lenders, J.W.M., Linehan, W.M., Walther, M.M., Goldstein, D.S., and Keiser, H.R. (1999). Plasma normetanephrine and metanephrine for detecting pheochromocytoma in von Hippel–Lindau disease and multiple endocrine neoplasia type 2. *New Engl. J. Med.* **340** (24), 1872–9.

Graham, D.J. and McHenry, C.R. (1998). The adrenal incidentaloma. *Surg. Oncol. Clin. N. Am.* **7** (4), 749–64.

Hamberger, B., Telenius-Berg, M., Cedermark, B., Grondal, S., Hansson, B.-G., and Werner, S. (1987). Subtotal adrenalectomy in multiple endocrine neoplasia type 2. *Henry Ford Hosp. Med. J.* **35**, 127–8.

Heniford, B.T., Iannitti, D.A., and Gagner, M. (1997). The role of intraoperative ultrasonography during laparoscopic adrenalectomy. *Surgery* **122** (6), 1068–74.

Imai, T., Tanaka, Y., Kikumori, T., Ohiwa, M., Matsuura, N., Mase, T., and Funahashi, H. (1999). Laparoscopic partial adrenalectomy. *Surg. Endosc.* **13**, 343–5.

Ito, Y., Fujimoto, Y., Obara, T., and Kodama, T. (1990). Clinical significance of associated nodular lesions of the adrenal in patients with aldosteronoma. *World J. Surg.* **14**, 330–4.

Janetschek, G., Lhotta, K., Gasser, R., Finkenstedt, G., Jaschke, W., and Bartsch, G. (1997). Adrenal-sparing laparoscopic surgery for aldosterone-producing adenoma. *J. Endourol.* **11** (2), 145–8.

Janetschek, G., Finkenstedt, G., Gasser, R., Waibel, U.G., Peschel, R., Bartsch, G., and Neumann, H.P.H. (1998). Laparoscopic surgery for pheochromocytoma: adrenalectomy, partial resection, excision of paraganglionomas. *J. Urol.* **160**, 330–4.

Lairmore, T.C., Ball, D.W., Baylin, S.B., and Wells, S.A. Jr (1993). Management of pheochromocytomas in patients with multiple endocrine neoplasia type 2 syndromes. *Ann. Surg.* **217** (6), 595–603.

Lee, J.E., Curley, S.A., Gagel, R.F., Evans, D.B., and Hickey, R.C. (1996). Cortical-sparing adrenalectomy for patients with bilateral pheochromocytoma. *Surgery* **120** (6), 1064–71.

Maurea, S., Cuocolo, A., Reynolds, J.C., Tumeh, S.S., Begley, M.G., Linehan, W.M., Norton, J.A., Walther, M.M., Keiser, H.R., and Neumann, R.D. (1993). Iodine-131-metaiodobenzylguanidine scintigraphy in preoperative and postoperative evaluation of paraganglionomas: comparison with CT and MRI. *J. Nucl. Med.* **34**, 173.

Nakada, T., Kubota, Y., Sasagawa, I., Yagisawa, T., Watanabe, M., and Ishigooka, M. (1995). Therapeutic outcome of primary aldosteronism: adrenalectomy versus enucleation of aldosterone-producing adenoma. *J. Urol.* **153**, 1775–80.

Neumann, H.P.H., Reincke, M., Bender, B.U., Elsner, R., and Janetschek, G. (1999). Preserved adrenocortical function after laparoscopic bilateral adrenal sparing surgery for hereditary pheochromocytoma. *J. Clin. Endocrinol. Metab.* **84** (8), 2608–10.

Oelkers, W. (1996). Adrenal insufficiency. *New Engl. J. Med.* **335**, 1206–12.

Okamoto, T., Obara, T., Ito, Y., Yamashita, T., Kanbe, M., Iihara, M., Hirose, K., and Yamazaki, K. (1996). Bilateral adrenalectomy with autotransplantation of adrenocortical tissue or unilateral adrenalectomy: treatment options for pheochromocytomas in multiple endocrine neoplasia type 2a. *Endocrinol. J.* **43**, 169–75.

Sasagawa, I., Suzuki, H., Tateno, T., Izumi, T., Shoji, N., and Nakada, T. (1998). Retroperitoneoscopic partial adrenalectomy using an endoscopic stapling device in patients with adrenal tumor. *Urol. Int.* **61**, 101–3.

Shapiro, B., Copp, J.E., Sisson, J.C., Eyre, P.L., Wallis, J., and Beierwaltes, W.H. (1985). Iodine-13 metaiodobenzylguanidine for the locating of suspected pheochromocytoma: experience in 400 cases. *J. Nucl. Med.* **26**, 576.

Stewart, B.H., Bravo, E.L., Haaga, J., Meaney, T.F., and Tarazi, R. (1978). Localization of pheochromocytoma by computed tomography. *New Engl. J. Med.* **299**, 460.

Suzuki, K., Sugiyama, T., Saisu, K., Ushiyama, T., and Fujita, K. (1998). Retroperitoneoscopic partial adrenalectomy for aldosterone-producing adenoma using an ultrasonically activated scalpel. *Br. J. Urol.* **82**, 138–9.

Telenius-Berg, M., Ponder, M.A., Berg, B., Ponder, B.A.J., and Werner, S. (1989). Quality of life after bilateral adrenalectomy in MEN-2. *Henry Ford Hosp. Med. J.* **37**, 160.

van Heerden, J.A., Sizemore, G.W., Carney, J.A., Grant, C.S., Remine, W.H., and Sheps, S.G. (1984). Surgical management of the adrenal glands in the multiple endocrine neoplasia type II syndrome. *World J. Surg.* **8**, 612–21.

van Heerden, J.A., Sizemore, G.W., Carney, J.A., Brennan, M.D., and Sheps, S.G. (1985). Bilateral subtotal adrenal resection for bilateral pheochromocytomas in multiple endocrine neoplasia, type IIa: a case report. *Surgery* **98** (2), 363–5.

Vargas, H.I., Kavoussi, L.R., Bartlett, D.L., Wagner, J.R., Venzon, D.J., Fraker, D.L., Alexander, H.R., Linehan, W.M., and Walther, M.M. (1997). Laparoscopic adrenalectomy: a new standard of care. *Urology* **49** (5), 673–8.

Vaughan, E.D. Jr and Blumenfeld, J.D. (1998). The adrenals In *Campbell's urology*, 7th edn (ed. P.C. Walsh, A.B. Retik, E.D. Vaughan Jr, and A.J.Wein), pp. 2915–72. W.B. Saunders, Philadelphia.

Walther, M.M., Keiser, H.R., Choyke, P.L., Rayford, W., Lyne, J.C., and Linehan, W.M. (1999). Management of hereditary pheochromocytoma in von Hippel–Lindau kindreds with partial adrenalectomy. *J. Urol.* **161**, 395–8.

Walther, M.M., Herring, J., Choyke, P.L., and Linehan, W.M. (2000). Laparoscopic partial adrenalectomy in patients with hereditary forms of pheochromocytoma. *J. Urol.* **164**, 14–17.

Walz, M.K., Peitgen, K., Saller, B., Giebler, R.M., Lederbogen, S., Nimtz, K., Mann, K., and Eigler, F.W. (1998). Subtotal adrenalectomy by the posterior retroperitoneoscopic approach. *World J. Surg.* **22**, 621–7.

Weigel, R.J., Wells, S.A., Gunnells, J.C., and Leight, G.S. (1994). Surgical treatment of primary hyperaldosteronism. *Ann. Surg.* **219** (4), 347–52.

Zelissen, P.M., Croughs, R.J.M., Van Rijk, P.P., *et al.* (1994). Effect of glucocorticoid replacement therapy on bone mineral density in patients with Addison's disease. *Ann. Intern. Med.* **120**, 207–10.

59. Lateral transperitoneal laparoscopic adrenalectomy

Steven Shichman, R. Ernest Sosa, and E. Darracott Vaughan, Jr

Introduction

Laparoscopic adrenalectomy has recently become the standard technique for the surgical removal of the adrenal gland. Gagner *et al.* (1992) first reported laparoscopic adrenalectomy. Since then, many reports have confirmed the advantages of laparoscopic adrenalectomy over open surgery: Laparoscopy offers a shorter length of stay (LOS) in hospital, a decrease in postoperative pain, a shorter time to return to preoperative activity level, and improved cosmesis, and reduces complications in the fragile Cushingoid patient (MacGillivary *et al.* 1996; Gagner 1996; Gagner *et al.* 1996, 1997).

Various laparoscopic approaches to the adrenal gland have been described. Amongst these are the lateral transabdominal, anterior transabdominal, and lateral retroperitoneal and posterior retroperitoneal approaches (Gagner *et al.* 1992; Brunt *et al.* 1996; Prinz 1996; Lee and Chung 1995; Gasman *et al.* 1998; Walz *et al.* 1996; Rutherford *et al.* 1995; Terachi *et al.* 1997). Each of these methods has specific advantages and disadvantages. Knowledge of the surgical anatomy and meticulous dissection techniques and hemostasis are paramount for successful laparoscopic adrenalectomy with minimal morbidity.

Lateral transperitoneal operative technique

All patients have a complete preoperative endocrine evaluation. Patients are placed on clear liquid diets and mechanical bowel preparation the day before surgery. General endotracheal anesthesia is used in all cases. A Foley catheter is employed to decompress the urinary bladder. Gastric decompression is achieved by an oral-gastric tube. Antiembolic stockings are used in all cases.

Standard laparoscopy equipment is used. In addition to electrocautery shears, we utilize a 5 or 10 mm harmonic scalpel and medium and large hemoclips. A fan or paddle retractor is used to retract the liver or spleen. A 30-degree laparoscope is used for all cases.

Patients are placed in the semilateral decubitus position with the side of the lesion elevated 45 degrees. The umbilical region is placed over the break in the table; the kidney rest is gently elevated and the table flexed. An axillary roll is used to protect the dependent brachial plexus. The upper arm is secured using a neuro arm support. Patients are secured to the table using 3-inch cloth tape across the shoulders and hips. In this position, rolling the table toward the side of the lesion achieves a near supine position for insertion of the umbilical Hasson trocar. Rolling the table in the opposite direction places the patient in the full flank position used for the majority of the dissection.

Patients are prepped and draped from their nipple line to the lower abdomen and well across the midline allowing for possible conversion to an open exposure. The Hasson trocar is inserted in the supraumbilical region. The peritoneal space is insufflated to 15 mm Hg using CO_2. The abdominal cavity is explored with a 30-degree laparoscope.

Right adrenalectomy

Three additional trocars are utilized for a right adrenalectomy. All ports should be 11 or 12 mm in size to allow insertion of the laparoscope, clip appliers, harmonic scalpel, and retractors. Two accessory ports are placed 2 cm below the costal margin at the midaxillary and anterior axillary lines. A third port is placed in the midclavicular line, halfway between the costal margin and umbilicus. Dissecting instruments are introduced via the two lateral trocars. The laparoscope and the retractor are inserted in the midclavicular and umbilical trocars, respectively.

The abdominal contents are initially explored to identify adhesions and other pathology. Adhesions, which will compromise exposure, are lysed. Most cases will not require mobilization of the hepatic flexure and ascending colon. The triangular ligaments of the liver are incised to facilitate gentle retraction of the liver medially. For this, a paddle retractor is inserted through the umbilical port once adequate room is established between the liver and the abdominal sidewall. The remainder of the triangular ligament and the anterior and posterior coronary ligaments are incised to release the right lobe of the liver from the diaphragm, exposing the bare area of the liver. The liver is mobilized until the vena cava is identified.

The posterior aspect of the right lobe of the liver may adhere to the anterior capsule of the adrenal gland and to the vena cava. In this situation, the anterior wall of the vena cava is identified close to the renal hilum and duodenum. Dissection along the anterior wall of the vena cava, in a cephalad direction, will release the right lobe of the liver. The accessory hepatic veins are identified and avoided. Meticulous dissection along the lateral vena cava will allow identification of the right adrenal vein. Once the vein is isolated, two or three hemoclips are applied on the caval side and one or two hemoclips on the adrenal side of the vein. Large hemoclips are frequently needed. The adrenal vein is sharply divided between the clips, releasing the medial aspect of the adrenal gland away from the vena cava.

The harmonic scalpel will facilitate the dissection and hemostatic division of numerous arterial branches coming off the aorta. These middle arterial vessels feeding the adrenal gland are usually small, but there can be a large vessel requiring hemoclips for control. As dissection continues cephalad, toward the diaphragm, the inferior phrenic vessels will be easily identified. These vessels can easily be controlled with hemoclips or with the harmonic scalpel. The natural tendency is to continue the dissection along the lateral aspect of the gland freeing it from the sidewall attachments. We do not recommend releasing the lateral attachments at this time. These attachments hold the gland lateral and cephalad, facilitating identification and control of the inferior vascular pedicle arising from the right renal hilum. Often, a large inferior adrenal artery originating from the right renal artery will be identified and require ligation with hemoclips. Care must be taken to avoid injury to the renal hilum. Once this inferior pedicle is released, the adrenal can easily be mobilized in a superior and lateral direction. The gland is retracted in an anterior and cephalad direction, away from the upper pole of the kidney, using a forceps to grasp Gerota's fascia overlying the adrenal gland. The harmonic scalpel or electrocautery shears is used to incise Gerota's fascia at the junction of the upper pole of the kidney and adrenal gland. Small adrenal vessels coming from the perinephric fat and renal capsule are controlled using the harmonic scalpel. The gland is completely mobilized except for the avascular lateral attachments, which are easily released. The paddle retractor is removed and a retrieval sack is inserted through the umbilical port. After the specimen is entrapped in the sack, it is placed on the kidney to allow inspection for hemostasis in the operative field. The paddle retractor is reinserted and the operative bed is irrigated and examined using low insufflation pressures to confirm adequate hemostasis. The specimen is then removed through the umbilical Hasson trocar site, which can be easily enlarged to accommodate large glands.

Left adrenalectomy

For removal of the left adrenal gland, the patient is placed in the right semilateral decubitus position. After insertion of the umbilical Hasson trocar, two accessory trocars are inserted approximately 2 cm below the costal margin in the midaxillary and anterior axillary. A third accessory trocar can be inserted in the midclavicular line, 3 to 4 cm cephalad to the umbilicus, to allow use of hemoclips, retractor or of a suction/irrigation device without removal of the operating instruments. If this third port is utilized, the laparoscope should be inserted through this site for optimal visualization of the operative field. All trocars should be at least 11mm in size to permit insertion of the various laparoscopic devices.

Diagnostic laparoscopy is performed to identify and incise adhesions that limit exposure to the left upper quadrant. The surgeon should identify the spleen, left lobe of the liver, splenic flexure, descending colon, and the underlying left kidney. The splenic flexure and spleen should be mobilized as a single unit off the kidney and abdominal sidewall. All splenic attachments to Gerota's fascia, the abdominal sidewall, and the diaphragm are released using the harmonic scalpel or electrocautery shears. Lateral splenic attachments are incised up to the level of the gastric fundus. If adequately mobilized, the spleen will fall medially out of harm's way without retraction. The plane between the tail of the pancreas and Gerota's fascia should be developed and the pancreas retracted with the spleen. If necessary, insertion of a paddle retractor will allow gentle medial retraction of the spleen and pancreas. The inferior phrenic vessels are identified, controlled using either clips or the harmonic scalpel, and transected. As on the right side, dissecting and releasing the avascular lateral attachments of the adrenal gland should be avoided at this time. These should be left intact, facilitating dissection along the medial aspect of the gland. Instead, working from the top of the adrenal, the dissection is carried along the medial aspect releasing small arterial branches coming from the aorta using either the harmonic scalpel or clips. After releasing all medial attachments, the adrenal vein can usually be identified, controlled with clips, and divided. Remaining lateral posterior and superior attachments are released using the harmonic scalpel. If the vein cannot be identified, the superior lateral attachments are released dissecting along the lateral aspect of the gland. Gerota's fascia is entered and the renal capsule is identified. Gerota's fascia overlying the adrenal is grasped and the gland is retracted away from the renal hilum. This maneuver will facilitate identification of the adrenal vein, for ligation and transection. The remaining posterior attachments are easily released and the gland is placed in a retrieval sac and placed on the kidney. The operative field is irrigated and examined under low insufflation pressures confirming adequate homeostasis. The gland is removed through the Hasson trocar site.

Patients are started on clear liquids immediately postoperation and their diet advanced as tolerated. Oral narcotics are started the evening of surgery and Foley catheters removed the evening of surgery or on postoperative day 1.

Lateral transperitoneal results

Between September 1993 and June 2000 we performed 84 lateral transperitoneal adrenalectomies. In 66 cases the adrenalectomy was unilateral and in 9 cases the adrenalectomy was bilateral. Indications for surgery included: Cushing's syndrome in 16, aldosteronoma in 13 patients; pheochromocytoma in 7 patients; non-functioning adenoma in 2 patients; Carney's syndrome in one patient; and a metastasectomy for colon cancer in one patient.

In the bilateral cases the mean age was 45 years. The mean height was 66 inches (range, 60–70 inches) and mean weight 177 pounds (range, 112–366 pounds). Average operating time was 486 minutes (range, 285–690 minutes) and mean blood loss was

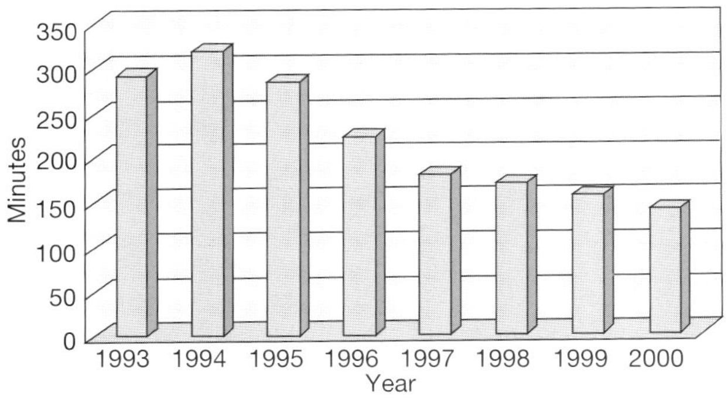

Fig. 59.1 Average operative times for unilateral transperitoneal adrenalectomies performed between 1993 and 2000.

Table 59.1 Indications (*Aldo* Aldosteronoma, *Pheo* Pheochromocytoma, *Cush* Cushing's, *Nonfunc* Nonfunctioning)

Transpeitoneal Ref	Aldo	Pheo	Cush Adenoma	Nonfunc Adenoma	Cush Syndrome	Other
Gagner	21	25	13	20	8	10
Terachi	41	8	0	22	21	8
Rutherford	48	3	1	7	0	1
Guazzoni	10	7	3	0	0	0
Brunt	6	11	1	0	2	4
Retroperitoneal						
Walz	5	7	7	4	3	1
Gasman	12	2	4	2	2	0

164 cubic centimeters. The average adrenal gland size was 7.5 cm (12 adrenals) and weighed 16.8 grams (range, 5–32 grams). There were no intraoperative complications. One patient required a two-unit blood transfusion postoperatively. All patients tolerated clear liquids the first postoperative day. The mean dose equivalent of narcotics was 2.8 parenterally and 2.6 orally (5 patients). The mean length of stay was 4 days.

For the unilateral cases, the mean age was 54 years. The average height was 66 inches (range, 60–73 inches) and mean weight was 178 pounds. The mean operative time for left cases was 221 minutes (range, 121–337 minutes) and for right cases 210 minutes (range, 135–355 minutes). A decrease in operative time was demonstrated on a yearly basis (Fig. 59.1). Intraoperative blood loss averaged 147 cubic centimeters and there were no intraoperative complications. The adrenal gland size averaged 6.8 cm (33 adrenals) and weighed 25.8 grams. (23 adrenals) A majority of patients began clear liquids on postoperative day one (29 on day one, 5 the day of surgery). An average of 5.2 doses of parenteral narcotic and 3.55 oral narcotic were administered postoperatively. The mean length of stay was 3 days.

Discussion

We consider laparoscopic adrenalectomy (LA) the procedure of choice for removal of the adrenal gland. Functional adrenal masses including aldosteronoma, glucocorticoid- and androgen/ estrogen-producing adenomas, and small- to moderate-sized solitary pheochromocytomas are all amenable to LA (see Table 59.1). In addition, selected cases of bilateral adrenal hyperplasia can be treated with bilateral laparoscopic adrenalectomy (if ectopic adrenocorticotropin (ACTH)-producing tumors cannot be located or pituitary tumor is unsuccessfully removed by transphenoidal hypophysectomy). Nonfunctional tumors larger than 3 cm demonstrating growth on serial imaging studies and tumors greater than 4–5 cm can be removed using LA. If the radiological characteristics of the tumor are strongly suggestive of malignancy, the experience and skill of the surgeon and specific anatomy of the tumor vasculature and surrounding viscera must be considered when deciding if the case can be approached laparoscopically. Recommendations regarding the maximum size of tumors that can be removed using a laparoscopic approach vary widely. As the size of the gland increases, the technical difficulties and operative risks increase. In addition, there is an increased risk of malignancy and the possibility of port site seeding as described with carcinoma of the gall bladder and colon. Gagner *et al.* (1996, 1997) have reported removal of a 14 cm adrenal mass. They use 15 cm as their size limit for laparoscopic approach. Brunt *et al.* (1996) advise caution when considering laparoscopic removal of adrenal masses greater than 6 cm in size. We do not have an absolute cut-off in size for adrenal masses we will approach laparoscopically. The largest mass we have removed was 8 cm in diameter and 14 cm long. Tumors greater than 6 cm in size should be considered on an individual basis, taking into account the increase in level of difficulty, the operating times, the limited exposure, aberrant retroperitoneal vasculature, and potential risk of local invasion.

Few absolute contraindications to LA exist. Invasive adrenal-cortical carcinomas requiring *en bloc* resection of the kidney and perinephric fat, spleen, tail of pancreas, diaphragm, and lymph nodes should be managed via an open approach.

Pheochromocytomas that demonstrate malignant behavior with multiple sites or metastatic nodes should not be removed laparoscopically. However, our recent success with hand-assisted laparoscopic extirpative surgery for adrenal, renal, and ureteral pathology has caused us to reconsider this absolute limitation. Prior to magnetic resonance imaging (MRI) and meta-iodobenzylguanidine (MIBG) nuclear scans, all pheochromocytomas were approached via a large anterior incision to provide adequate exposure for bilateral adrenal and peri-aortic exploration.

Relative contraindications include prior intraabdominal trauma or surgery, morbid obesity, uncorrectable coagulapathies, and large pheochromocytomas.

Prior trauma and/or surgery involving the spleen, liver, kidney, or tail of pancreas may preclude a safe laparoscopic procedure. Dense adhesions can limit the surgeon's ability to obtain adequate exposure, vascular control, and safe dissection and removal of the adrenal gland.

Morbid obesity can require high intraabdominal insufflation pressures to obtain an adequate pneumoperitoneum, which may impede venous return. Large amounts of retroperitoneal fat add to the difficulty of the dissection. Instruments may not be long enough to dissect under the diaphragm in patients with thick abdominal walls.

Coagulopathies need to be completely evaluated and corrected during the perioperative period. Re-anticoagulation of the patient in the early postoperative course can result in a retroperitoneal hematoma.

Pheochromocytomas are associated with a higher incidence of complications requiring conversion to an open technique. These tumors tend to be larger than most functional cortical adenomas. Removal of pheochromocytomas requires minimal manipulation, movement, and traction of the adrenal gland to prevent intravascular surges of catecholamines and the associated hypertensive crisis and arryhthmias. In Gagner *et al.*'s (1996) series of 97 LA, 60 per cent of the postoperative complications occurred in the removal of 25 pheochromocytomas. Intraoperative hypertension was documented in 56 per cent of these 25 cases. Prinz (1996) reported his only two conversions to an open approach with two large right adrenal pheochromocytomas.

A variety of laparoscopic approaches have been described. Included in this list are lateral transperitoneal, anterior transperitoneal, lateral retroperitoneal, and posterior retroperitoneal accesses. The most popular technique reported in the literature to date is the lateral transperitoneal approach. All techniques require a thorough understanding of the retroperitoneal anatomy and the ability to appreciate the anatomy on a two-dimensional video monitor via a 30-degree laparoscope.

The lateral transabdominal approach is used most commonly. This approach has distinct advantages. Most advanced laparoscopic surgeons have extensive experience identifying dissecting and mobilizing intraabdominal viscera. Numerous landmarks are easily identified. With the patient in the full lateral position, gravity helps retract the medially mobilized spleen or liver allowing for wide exposure of the adrenal gland. This generous exposure enables dissection of large tumors and is particularly helpful when removing pheochromocytomas, allowing the surgeon to perform minimal manipulation and retraction of the adrenal gland before ligation of the adrenal vein. This technique is easier to learn than the retroperitoneal techniques. Moreover, the transperitoneal approach also allows access to other organ systems. In one of our patients we performed a cholecystectomy in addition

to adrenalectomy using the lateral transperitoneal approach. Disadvantages of this approach include dissection difficulties in patients with intraabdominal adhesions. Bilateral transabdominal adrenalectomies require time-consuming repositioning, reprepping, and redraping of the patient. We performed all of our adrenalectomies, including all unilateral and bilateral cases in this series, using this approach.

The anterior transabdominal approach is the most infrequently described approach in the literature. Lee and Chung's (1995) preferred true anterior approach places the patient in the supine position with legs abducted and a sandbag under the lumbar spine. Exposure of the adrenal gland using the anterior approach is difficult and offers limited working space. In contrast to the lateral transperitoneal and retroperitoneal approaches, additional trocars are necessary for insertion of multiple retractors. The surgeon works against gravity, having to retract adjacent organs rather than releasing them from their attachments and letting them fall away as occurs with the lateral transperitoneal approach. Other problems with this approach include the fact that the adrenal bed is in the most dependent position with the patient supine. This position allows the collection of blood, lymphatic fluid, and irrigant, which can obscure the operative field and lengthen the operative time. Advantages of this approach include clear anatomic landmarks and the ability to perform bilateral adrenalectomies without repositioning the patient.

Retroperitoneoscopy is an alternate technique for removal of small benign adrenal lesions. This approach mimics the treatment of small adrenal lesions by open posterior approaches before the era of laparoscopy. Gasman *et. al.* (1998) reported their experience using the lateral retroperitoneal approach to perform 23 adrenalectomies. Reported operating times ranged from 45 to 160 minutes, with an average of 97 minutes. However, reported times include only the insufflation time. Our series and most reported series report the operating time from the first incision to the placement of the dressings. Mean diameter of the excised glands ranged from 26 mm to 4 cm. Contraindications to retroperitoneal laparoscopy included adrenal glands greater or equal to 5 cm in size or previous lumbar incisions. The authors state that this approach is less traumatic than a transperitoneal approach, though the morbidity rates were similar to the rates reported in the transperitoneal studies (see Table 59.2).

Utilizing the posterior retroperitoneal approach, the patient is placed on the operating table in the prone position and the table is flexed creating the semi-jackknife position. A balloon dissector is inserted 2 cm lateral and inferior to the tip of the twelfth rib. After the retroperitoneal space is dilated, two to three additional trocars are inserted. The kidney is identified and retracted in a caudal direction, enlarging the retroperitoneal space and facilitating identification and dissection of the adrenal gland. The superior aspect of the gland is released, ligating and dividing the inferior phrenic vessels. The remaining exposure and dissection of the gland as well as technique for controlling the adrenal vasculature is similar to that described for the lateral trans-

Table 59.2 Results published from series involving > 20 cases. (No. proc. Number of Procedures, Op operative, Insuff Insufflation)

Transperitoneal Ref	No. Pts.	No. Proc.	Complication Rate (%)	Open (%) Conversion	Hospital Stay (days)	Size (Cm) avg	Size (Cm) range	Op time Avg (min)	Op range
Gagner	85	97	12	3	3	4.5	0.7–14	123	80–360
Terachi	99	100	15	3	7.2	NR	10.0–70	240	110–480
Rutherford	60	60	3	NR	NR	NR	NR	128	59–315
Guazzoni	20	20	5	0	3.4	NR	1.5–6.0	170	100–375
Brunt	24	24	17	NR	3.2	2.7	1.0–5.5	183	120–265
Retroperitoneal									
Walz	27	30	8	17	NR		1.0–7.0	124	45–225
Gasman	22	23	9	0	3.3	2.6	1.0–4.0	Insuff Only 97	45–160

abdominal approach. Using this technique, retraction of the liver or spleen is not required. The posterior approach does not require repositioning of the patient who needs a bilateral adrenalectomy.

Retroperitoneal approaches avoid adhesions from prior abdominal surgery, potentially reducing operating times and complication rates by eliminating the need for adhesiolysis. Disadvantages of the retroperitoneal approach include a small working space limiting the size of the gland that can be safely removed. The small space also limits instrument placement, and crossing of instruments can easily occur. Balloon dilatation can inadvertently place direct pressure on the adrenal gland and, in the case of a pheochromocytoma, cause catastrophic release of catecholamines. Identification of landmarks is limited, and dissection in obese patients with large amounts of retroperitoneal fat can be quite difficult. Other concerns include the increased risk of hypercapnea secondary to subcutaneous emphysema.

The adrenal gland's unique location in the retroperitoneum makes it amenable to a variety of transperitoneal and retroperitoneal approaches. We believe that the lateral transperitoneal technique offers distinct advantages to the laparoscopist, including improved visibility of familiar anatomical landmarks, easy access to other organ systems, the use of gravity to work in the surgeon's favor to retract the spleen and liver, a wide exposure that allows removal of large adrenal lesions, and a position that allows the natural application of new innovations such as the hand-assisted technique.

Conclusion

The adrenal gland is ideal for laparoscopic removal and a variety of approaches have been described. LA has distinct advantages over the traditional open adrenalectomy in terms of decreasing length of stay in hospital, postoperative analgesic requirement, return to preoperative activity level, and improved cosmesis. We favor the lateral transperitoneal approach and believe that a majority of adrenal pathology can be safely removed in a timely manner with this technique. In addition, on the basis of our recent experience with the hand-assisted technique, we believe that the open adrenalectomy may one day become obsolete.

References

Brunt, L.M., Doherty, G.M., Norton, J.A., Soper, N.J., Quasebarth, M.A., and Moley, J.F. (1996). Laparoscopic adrenalectomy compared to open adrenalectomy for benign adrenal neoplasms. *J. Am. Coll. Surg.* **183**, 1–10.

Gagner, M. (1996). Laparoscopic adrenalectomy. *Surg. Clin. N. Am.* **76**, 523–37.

Gagner, M., Lacroix, A., and Bolte, E. (1992). Laparoscopic adrenalectomy in Cushing's syndrome and pheochromocytoma. *New Engl. J. Med.* **327**, 1003–6.

Gagner, M., Breton, G., Pharand, D., and Pomp, A. (1996). Is laparoscopic adrenalectomy indicated for pheochromocytomas? *Surgery* **120** (6), 1076–80.

Gagner, M., Pomp, A., Heniford, B.T., Pharand, D., and Lacroix, A. (1997). Laparoscopic adrenalectomy: lessons learned from 100 consecutive procedures. *Ann. Surg.* **226**, 238–47.

Gasman, D., Droupy, S., Koutani, A., Salomon, L., Antiphon, P., Chassagnon, J., Choin, D.K., and Abbou, C.C. (1998). Laparoscopic adrenalectomy: the retroperitoneal approach. *J. Urol.* **159**, 1816–20.

Guazzoni, G., Montorsi, F., Bocciardi, A., Da Pozzo, L., Rigatti, P., Lanzi, R., and Pontiroli, A. (1995). Transperitoneal laparoscopic versus open adrenalectomy for benign hyperfunctioning adrenal tumors: a comparative study. *J. Urol.* **153**, 1597–600.

Lee, D.W.H. and Chung, S.C.S. (1995). Laparoscopic adrenalectomy. *Int. Surg.* **80**, 311–14.

MacGillivray, D.C., Shichman, S.J., and Ferrer, F.A. (1996). A comparison of open vs. laparoscopic adrenalectomy. *Surg. Endosc.* **10**, 987–90.

Prinz, R.A. (1996). Laparoscopic adrenalectomy [editorial]. *J. Am. Coll. Surg.* **183**, 71–3.

Rutherford, J.C., Gordon, R.D., Stowasser, M., Tunny, T.J., and Klemm, S.A. (1995). Laparoscopic adrenalectomy for adrenal tumours causing hypertension and for 'incidentalomas' of the adrenal on computerized tomography scanning. *Clin. Exp. Pharmacol. Physiol.* **22**, 490–2.

Terachi, T., Matsuda, T., Terai, A., Ogawa, O. Kakehi, Y., Kawakita, M., Shichiri, Y., Mikami, O., Takeuchi, H., Okada, Y., and Yoshida, O. (1997). Transperitoneal laparoscopic adrenalectomy: experience in 100 patients. *J. Endourol.* **11**, 361–5.

Walz, M.K., Peitgen, K., Hoermann, R., Giebler, R.M., Mann, K., and Eigler, F.W. (1996). Posterior retroperitoneoscopy as a new minimally invasive approach for adrenalectomy: results of 30 adrenalectomies in 27 patients. *World J. Surg.* **20**, 769–74.

60. Laparoscopic versus open adrenalectomy

Anoop M. Meraney and Inderbir S. Gill

Introduction

Rapid advances in adrenal surgery have occurred during the last decade. Increased utilization of minimally invasive surgical techniques has led to several centers worldwide adopting laparoscopic adrenalectomy as the standard of care. Since its initial description by Gagner and colleagues (1992), laparoscopic adrenalectomy has evolved rapidly and can now be performed employing varied approaches, each with their own technical nuances.

In this chapter we present an up-to-date comparison of open versus laparoscopic approaches to adrenalectomy. The expanding indications for laparoscopic adrenalectomy in the rapidly progressing field of minimally invasive surgery are outlined. The suitability of laparoscopic adrenalectomy for pheochromocytoma, incidentaloma, adrenal metastasis, and primary adrenal cancer is discussed. Furthermore, a comparison of various laparoscopic techniques for the adrenal gland and their results is highlighted. A cost analysis between open and laparoscopic adrenalectomy is presented. Finally, emerging advances in laparoscopic adrenalectomy, needlescopic adrenalectomy, and outpatient adrenalectomy are presented.

A comparison of laparascopic and open adrenalectomy

Open adrenalectomy has been performed through transperitoneal or retroperitoneal approaches employing various incisions: chevron, semi-chevron, midline, thoracoabdominal, posterior transthoracic, lumbotomy, and extraperitoneal flank incisions. The choice of the incision depends on the size of the gland, unilateral versus bilateral procedures, the patient's body habitus, the underlying adrenal pathology, and the preference of the operating surgeon. When appropriately selected, these incisions provide precise and direct access to the adrenal gland. However, because of the location of the adrenal gland in the upper reaches of the retroperitoneum, and the abundance of its vascularity, large skin incisions, usually including rib-resection, are often required. Issues related to intercostal nerve compromise and wound healing contribute to the considerable postoperative morbidity associated with open adrenalectomy.

Reduced postoperative morbidity and superior cosmetic result are well-recognized features of laparoscopic adrenalectomy.

Recent reports suggest that, for comparable specimen weights, laparoscopic adrenalectomy can be performed in comparable operative times, with minimal associated blood loss, when compared to open surgery (Sung *et al.* 1999). Winfield and colleagues (1998) compared the laparoscopic ($n = 20$) and open ($n = 17$) techniques for adrenalectomy. Laparoscopic adrenalectomy was associated with less blood loss (183 versus 266 cm^3), decreased analgesic requirement (32.7 versus 74.3 mg morphine equivalent), shorter hospital stay (2.7 versus 6.2 days), and a shorter convalescence (22 versus 45 days). Minor complications occurred less frequently in the laparoscopic group (29 versus 53 per cent). However, operative times were longer for the laparoscopic procedure (3.7 versus 2.3 hours). Thompson and colleagues (1997) from the Mayo Clinic compared 50 patients undergoing open adrenalectomy with 50 patients undergoing laparoscopic adrenalectomy. Laparoscopic adrenalectomy was performed transperitoneally and open adrenalectomy was performed utilizing the posterior approach. Operative times were 2.8 hours in the laparoscopic group and 2.1 hours in the open group. The laparoscopic group was associated with a lesser analgesic requirement (28 versus 48 mg morphine equivalent), shorter hospital stay (3.1 versus 5.7 days), shorter convalescence (26 versus 42 days), and a lower minor complication rate (6 versus 18 per cent). A significant number of the patients in the open group (54 per cent) had late incisional neuromuscular sequelae secondary to the posterior surgical approach: laxity of the oblique muscles (30 per cent), significant chronic pain (14 per cent), and bothersome flank numbness (10 per cent). A study by Buell and colleagues (1997) revealed that more than 80 per cent of patients undergoing posterior adrenalectomy for Cushing's disease suffered from chronic back pain syndromes.

Our more recent retrospective analysis comparing 110 laparoscopic adrenalectomies with 100 open cases is illustrative of the changing trends in favor of minimally invasive surgery (Gill *et al.* 1999*a*). Patients from both the laparoscopic and open surgical groups had comparable demographics: age of patients, specimen weight (29 versus 28.6 g), American Association of Anesthesiology (ASA) scores (2.8 versus 2.7), and body mass index (BMI) (29.6 versus 29.4). Of the laparoscopic procedures, 85 were performed transperitoneally and 24 retroperitoneally. The open procedures were performed utilizing various approaches: chevron, flank, thoracoabdominal, subcostal, posterior lumbotomy, and midline transabdominal. Operative time for the laparoscopic procedure averaged 188.6 min as compared to 219.3 min for the open group ($p = 0.002$). Blood loss was significantly lower with laparoscopy than with open surgery (124.8 versus 563.4 cm^3; $p < 0.0001$). More patients following the laparoscopic procedure could be extubated in the operating room (102 versus 73 patients; $p < 0.001$). Patients from the laparoscopic group required less postoperative narcotic analgesia (38.2 versus 471.6 mg; $p < 0.0001$). Fewer laparoscopic cases required admission to the intensive care unit compared to open cases (2.6 versus 10 per cent; $p = 0.003$). Though the incidence of intraoperative complications was comparable (6 per cent in the laparoscopic group versus 5 per cent in the open group; $p = 0.81$), the incidence of postoperative complications was lower for the laparoscopic group (10 versus 27 per cent; i < 0.0001)). Three patients in the laparoscopic group were converted to open surgery. Postoperative fluid intake was resumed at an average of 1.04 days for patients undergoing laparoscopic adrenalectomy, compared to 3.2 days following open surgery. Patients were more quickly ambulatory following the laparoscopic procedure (1.0 versus 1.7 days). Finally, hospital stay was significantly shorter following laparoscopic adrenalectomy (1.9 versus 7.6 days; $p < 0.0001$).

The magnification provided by the operating laparoscope enables unmatched visualization of the operative field and facilitates meticulous dissection thereby minimizing blood loss. Laparoscopy is associated with a steep learning curve. However, with increased experience, laparoscopic surgeons are becoming more facile resulting in reduced operating times and low postoperative morbidity.

Adrenal metastasis/cancer

It is imperative to obtain wide surgical margins during excision of any malignant tumor. This basic principle of cancer surgery must also be strictly adhered to during laparoscopic radical adrenalectomy. Radical adrenalectomy is indicated for solitary adrenal metastasis or primary adrenal cancer. Since solitary adrenal metastasis from an unknown extra-adrenal primary is often, but not always, small in size and confined within the adrenal gland, the laparoscopic approach is particularly appealing and, in our experience, eminently feasible for this indication. Primary adrenal cancer, on the other hand, is often larger in size and not infrequently locally infiltrative beyond the adrenal capsule. Since the technical goal of achieving negative surgical margins may require wide excision, occasionally with local lymphadenectomy and/or resection of contiguous organ structures, laparoscopy may not be as well suited as open surgery to achieve these goals at this writing.

Laparoscopic radical adrenalectomy may be performed either by the transperitoneal (Winfield *et al.* 1998; Elashry *et al.* 1997; Gagner 1996; Gill *et al.* 1998*b*) or the retroperitoneal approach (Gill *et al.* 1998*b*). During the transperitoneal approach a laparoscopic steerable ultrasound probe may be utilized intraoperatively to assess for concomitant intraabdominal metastasis (Heniford *et al.* 1997). As mentioned, patients with large (> 8–10 cm), or locally advanced tumors (local infiltration, venous involvement) present a formidable technical challenge, and may be optimally treated with open surgery. Nevertheless, for most patients with surgical adrenal metastasis, laparoscopic adrenalectomy appears to be a viable surgical option.

The recent suggestions that laparoscopic surgery may result in decreased compromise of the immune system as compared to that of open surgery implies that host surveillance for cancer cells may be better preserved following laparoscopic surgery (Allendorf *et al.* 1996).

In patients with adrenal metastasis or cancer, we compared laparoscopic ($n = 12$) and open adrenalectomy ($n = 22$) (Hobart *et al.* 1999). Either the retroperitoneal ($n = 5$) or the transperitoneal ($n = 7$) laparoscopic techniques were employed. On comparing the laparoscopic and open groups, mean operating room time (205 versus 240 min; $p = 0.12$), and specimen weight (47 versus 99 g; $p = 0.21$) were comparable. However, the laparoscopic group was superior with regard to blood loss (150 versus 650 cm^3; $p = 0.0007$), narcotic requirements (15.4 versus 266 mg morphine sulfate; $p = 0.0002$), and hospital stay (1.5 versus 7 days; $p < 0.0001$). One patient in the laparoscopic group had positive surgical margins, while two were electively converted to open surgery for locally infiltrative cancer. Histopathology in the laparoscopic group included metastatic renal cell carcinoma (RCC) (5), lung cancer (3), colon cancer (2), adrenal carcinoma (1), and metastatic melanoma (1). Four patients have developed metastatic disease, with one patient death from brain metastases of the melanoma at 14 months. In selected patients with smaller radiologically confined adrenal metastasis or primary cancer, laparoscopy can provide the expected benefits of minimally invasive surgery, while achieving a radical resection with wide margins. However, for large tumors, or tumors with evidence of local infiltration or presence of thrombus in the adrenal vein or inferior vena cava, open surgery is clearly the preferred technique.

Suzuki and colleagues (1997) reported a case of local recurrence in the adrenal bed with peritoneal dissemination 19 months after adequate *en bloc* laparoscopic adrenalectomy that included excision of periadrenal fat. Despite combination chemotherapy, the patient died 3 years later. The authors wondered whether the intraoperative use of the ultrasonic surgical system (harmonic scalpel) might possibly have contributed to local recurrence. In another patient, severe adhesions between the kidney and the adrenal metastasis led to open conversion of the laparoscopic procedure. The patient died from metastatic lung cancer 8 months postoperatively. However, in both these instances, it was not clear whether the laparoscopic procedure *per se* contributed to tumor recurrence. As is well documented, local recurrences occur even after open surgical excision of adrenocortical carcinomas, with 5-year survival rates of 50 per cent or less (Bodie *et al.* 1989).

Pheochromocytoma

Laparoscopic adrenalectomy for pheochromocytoma must be approached cautiously by an experienced surgical and anesthetic team. As in open surgery, meticulous preoperative patient preparation, careful intraoperative hemodynamic monitoring, and delicate intraoperative manipulation of the adrenal gland are critical for excellent operative outcomes. Every attempt should be made to control the main adrenal vein prior to manipulating the tumor. Occasionally, hypertensive crises can be triggered by mere induction of pneumoperitoneum, as was noted in one of our patients (Sprung *et al.* 2000).

A retrospective comparison of the anesthetic aspects of laparoscopic ($n = 14$) and open ($n = 20$) adrenalectomy for pheochromocytoma was conducted at our institute. The operating room time for the laparoscopic procedure averaged 177 ± 59 min, and was 196 ± 69 min for the open group. Laparoscopic adrenalectomy resulted in less blood loss (100 versus 400 cm^3; $p = 0.0001$), earlier resumption of oral feeds (1 versus 3.5 days; $p = 0.0001$), and shorter hospital stay (3 versus 7.5 days; $p = 0.0001$). The highest intraoperative blood pressures were not significantly different for laparoscopic adrenalectomy for pheochromocytoma compared to those for open surgery (194/106 versus 191/98 mm Hg; $p = 0.5$). Similarly, the number of hypertensive episodes per patient in the laparoscopic group was not significantly different from that in the open group (1 versus 0.5; $p = 0.5$). However, patients undergoing laparoscopic surgery had fewer hypotensive episodes (0 versus 2; $p = 0.005$), which were less severe ($98 \pm 19/57 \pm 8$ versus $88 \pm 14/ 50 \pm 13$ mm Hg; $p = 0.05$), with fewer patients requiring treatment (1 versus 9; $p = 0.02$). In addition, no major differences were detected in the intraoperative extremes of high (101 ± 24 versus 104 ± 15 beats per minute; $p = 0.78$) and low (60 ± 9 versus 61 ± 11 beats per minute; $p = 0.81$) heart rates between the laparoscopic and open groups, respectively (Sprung *et al.* 2000).

Janetschek and colleagues (1998) described their experience with laparoscopic adrenalectomy for pheochromocytoma in 19 patients. Mean operative times (150 min) were the same for left ($n = 5$) and right ($n = 8$) adrenalectomy. Estimated blood loss was 114 cm^3 during left and 150 cm^3 during right adrenalectomy. The mean length of hospital stay was 4.9 days for these patients. Patients undergoing bilateral adrenalectomy had an average operative time of 516 minutes and blood loss of 248 cm^3. Intraoperatively, 5 patients had a blood pressure of > 200 mm Hg, and 3 patients had a blood pressure of < 80 mm Hg (Janetschek *et al.* 1998).

Laparoscopy does not appear to increase the surgical risk in the patient with pheochromocytoma. In fact, catecholamine release during laparoscopic adrenalectomy for pheochromocytoma may be lower than during open surgery (Fernandez-Cruz *et al.* 1996*a*).

Incidentalomas

Management decisions about an incidentally detected adrenal mass are based on its biochemical activity, size, imaging characteristics, and patient age and preference. Adrenalectomy is recommended for all hormonally active tumors, tumors 5 cm or larger in size, and tumors with suspicious characteristics on computerized tomography (CT) scanning. Younger patients (< 50 years old) with a 3–5 cm adrenal mass may be better served by a laparoscopic or needlescopic adrenalectomy as compared to watchful waiting. This is based on the observation that a majority of adrenal nodules increase with age, and the lifetime cancer risk of a 3 cm nodule would seem to be greater in a younger than in an older patient (Staren and Prinz 1995). Furthermore, watchful waiting in a 30–50 year old patient would mandate at least an annual radiologic and biochemical testing for a long period of time. Nevertheless, observation is recommended for (1) all hormonally inactive tumors less than 3 cm in size, and (2) hormonally inactive tumors 3–5 cm in size in a patient aged greater than 50 years.

Although laparoscopic adrenalectomy is a minimally morbid procedure, its mere availability should not alter the decision algorithm for management of an adrenal incidentaloma. Laparoscopic adrenalectomy by itself comprises a major surgical procedure under general anesthesia, with the ever-present possibility of conversion to an open procedure and related complications.

Laparoscopic adrenalectomy: transperitoneal versus retroperitoneal

Existing laparoscopic approaches to the adrenal gland include transperitoneal and retroperitoneal laparoscopy (Bonjer *et al.* 1997).

Transperitoneal laparoscopic adrenalectomy

The transperitoneal technique is performed with the patient in the 60° oblique flank position. Pneumoperitoneum is obtained by either the Veress needle or the open technique. Four ports (10/11 mm) are typically arranged along the ipsilateral costal margin to enable optimal visualization and dissection in the quadrant of interest (Winfield *et al.* 1997).

Right adrenalectomy
The liver is retracted anteriorly and a transverse incision is made in the posterior parietal peritoneum parallel to and 1–2 cm below the inferior edge of the liver. Extending from the line of Toldt laterally, up to the inferior vena cava medially, this incision allows access into the retroperitoneum directly on to the anterior surface of the adrenal gland. Virtually no mobilization of the hepatic flexure of the colon is required. Typically, dissection is initiated between the medial border of the adrenal gland and the right lateral edge of the inferior vena cava, where the main adrenal vein is identified, clipped, and divided. Superiorly, the gland is dissected free from the under-surface of the diaphragm, where inferior phrenic vessels are encountered. Inferiorly, adrenal vessels arising from the renal hilum are controlled and the gland is completely freed. The gland is entrapped within an impermeable sac and extracted intact.

Left adrenalectomy
In contrast to the right adrenal, formal mobilization of the spleen, splenic flexure, descending colon, and often the tail of pancreas is necessary in order to access the left adrenal gland. The left renal vein is traced medially to identify and control the main left adrenal vein at its origin. Multiple aortic, phrenic, and renal hilar branches supplying the adrenal gland are meticulously controlled, freeing the adrenal gland completely.

Basso and colleagues (1999) reported the utilization of the direct supragastric approach for transperitoneal laparoscopic left adrenalectomy. Initially, the gastrophrenic ligament is divided to mobilize the gastric fundus. Subsequently, the fundus is pulled down, allowing exposure of the left crus of the diaphragm, superior pancreatic edge, and perirenal fat with the adrenal gland. In contrast to the conventional laparoscopic technique mobilization of the left colon, spleen, and pancreas is avoided.

Retroperitoneoscopic laparascopic adrenalectomy

Retroperitoneal adrenalectomy may be performed utilizing either the lateral or posterior approaches. The lateral approach is employed more commonly. During the posterior approach, the patient is placed prone in a semi jack-knife position, and three ports are placed directly along the undersurface of the twelfth rib (Duh *et al.* 1996; Walz *et al.* 1996; Baba *et al.* 1997). During the lateral approach with the patient in the 90° full flank position, retroperitoneoscopic access is established by the balloon dilatation technique. A primary 10 mm blunt-tip port is placed off the tip of the twelfth rib. Two secondary ports are placed using laparoscopic guidance: a port at the anterior axillary line 3 cm cephalad to the iliac crest, and another port posterior to the posterior axillary line, at the lateral border of erector spinae muscle.

Left adrenalectomy

Dissection is initiated in the area between the aorta and the adrenal gland /upper renal pole in an attempt to identify and control adrenal branches arising from the aorta. Subsequently, the upper renal pole is completely mobilized within Gerota's fascia, and dropped posteriorly on the psoas muscle. Dissection proceeds towards the renal hilum, between the medial aspect of the upper renal pole and the adrenal gland. A combination of blunt and sharp dissection may identify the main adrenal vein at this juncture, which is clipped (5-mm clips) and transected. Subsequently the adrenal gland is circumferentially mobilized.

Right adrenalectomy

The procedure for a retroperitoneoscopic right adrenalectomy is similar except for securing the main adrenal vein. The right adrenal vein is often visualized earlier in the procedure because of its comparatively posterior location in the retroperitoneoscopic dissection between the inferior vena cava and the adrenal gland.

Comparison of the two approaches

Takeda and colleagues (1997) compared transperitoneal ($n = 27$) and retroperitoneal ($n = 11$) laparoscopic approaches for adrenalectomy. Both approaches were comparable in terms of mean operative time (248 versus 232 min), blood loss (151 versus 155 cm^3), oral intake (1.6 versus 1.4 days postoperatively), and ambulation (2 versus 1.8 days postoperatively). Transperitoneal needlescopic adrenalectomy ($n = 15$) and the retroperitoneoscopic technique ($n = 11$) were compared in a retrospective analysis at the Cleveland Clinic Foundation. Both techniques were comparable in terms of operative time (169 versus 173 min), blood loss (61 versus 104 cm^3), hospital stay (1.1 versus 1.3 days) and convalescence (2.1 versus 1.9 weeks) (Sung *et al.* 1998). Bonjer and colleagues (1997) compared the conventional transperitoneal ($n = 9$) and retroperitoneal ($n = 12$) laparoscopic adrenalectomy. They reported that the transperitoneal approach, which was performed using standard laparoscopic ports and instruments, was associated with longer operative times (150 versus 75 min; $p = 0.005$), greater blood loss (150 versus 20 cm^3; $p = 0.01$), longer hospital stay (6 versus 4 days; $p = 0.03$), and increased narcotic analgesic requirements (96 vs 20 mg; $p = 0.0003$). In order to

better assess the two approaches, a prospective randomized comparison between the transperitoneal and retroperitoneal laparoscopic approaches is currently underway at our institution. In an analysis of the initial 36 patients in this prospective comparison no significant differences were noted between the transperitoneal and retroperitoneal approaches as regards operating room time.

Data on 147 transperitoneal laparoscopic procedures that were performed at several centers revealed that the mean operating time was 3.4 hours, estimated blood loss was 191 cm^3, postoperative intake was resumed within 1.5 days, and mean hospital stay was 2.9 days (Winfield *et al.* 1998; Thompson *et al.* 1997; Guazzoni *et al.* 1995; Suzuki *et al.* 1993; Staren and Prinz 1996). Convalescence averaged 16 days. Minor and major complications occurred in 20 and 3 per cent of the patients, respectively. Yoshida and colleagues (1997) from Japan evaluated the complications occurring in 369 laparoscopic adrenalectomies in a multi-institutional study performed in nine centers from January 1992 through September 1996. They reported 32 intraoperative complications in 31 patients (9 per cent). Vascular injuries occurred in 20 patients (5 per cent) and included injury to the inferior vena cava (2), renal vein (2), central adrenal vein (4), and other adrenal vessels (12). Organ injuries occurred in 11 patients (3 per cent) and included injury to the liver (4), spleen (3), pancreas (2), gall bladder (1), and the ipsilateral adrenal gland (1). Postoperative complications were seen in 24 patients (6.5 per cent) and included hemorrhage (6), wound infection (4), atelectasis (3), ileus (2), chylocele (1), asthma (1), pulmonary effusion (1), angina (1), hyperventilation (1), delirium (1), compartment syndrome (1), urinary retention (1), and peritonitis (1). There was no mortality. The majority of these complications could be managed either conservatively or laparoscopically. However, open conversion was necessary in 14 patients (3.8 per cent).

More than 166 patients have undergone retroperitoneoscopic adrenalectomy since 1995. Indications for adrenalectomy included aldosteroma, Cushing's syndrome, pheochromocytoma, and non-functioning adenoma. The lateral retroperitoneoscopic approach was employed in 107 patients (Fernandez-Cruz *et al.* 1996*b*; Heintz *et al.* 1996; Chiu *et al.* 1997; Gasman *et al.* 1998; Takeda *et al.* 1997), and the posterior retroperitoneoscopic approach in 59 patients (Duh *et al.* 1996; Walz *et al.* 1996; Baba *et al.* 1997). The mean operative time and blood loss were 2.8 hours and 105 ml, respectively. Hospital stay averaged 4 days and convalescence was 15.8 days. Complications occurred in 15 per cent of patients, and 7 per cent were converted to open surgery.

Indications for retroperitoneal laparoscopic adrenalectomy are no different than those for transperitoneal laparoscopic adrenalectomy. However, we prefer the retroperitoneal approach to the transperitoneal approach in patients who are morbidly obese and have a prior history of extensive abdominal surgery.

Drawbacks for the retroperitoneal approach include a somewhat difficult anatomic orientation during one's initial experience, a smaller working space, closer proximity of the port sites, and, primarily, a steeper learning curve. However, it seems to have specific advantages. Since the peritoneal cavity is avoided completely, bowel manipulation and mobilization are avoided. The retroperitoneoscopic approach is superior in patients with intraperitoneal adhesions due to prior abdominal surgery. Similarly, in markedly or morbidly obese patients, the retroperitoneoscopic approach is preferred since it gives a shorter and more direct access to the adrenal gland despite the increased amount of retroperitoneal fat in this patient population (Heniford *et al.* 1997; Allendorf *et al.* 1996). Critical to success in this situation is appropriate retroperitoneal balloon dilatation outside of and posterior to Gerota's fascia and the adrenal gland, along the undersurface of the diaphragm. In our experience the retroperitoneoscopic approach to the left gland is rather straightforward, because the longer left adrenal vein is easier to identify. However, as noted by others, it is also our subjective impression that, for a right adrenalectomy, the transperitoneal laparoscopic approach may be technically somewhat simpler for two reasons: (1) the short main right adrenal vein, and (2) virtually no colonic mobilization is necessary during a transperitoneal laparoscopic approach to the right adrenal gland.

We feel that the laparoscopic surgeon should be adept at both the transperitoneal and retroperitoneal laparoscopic approaches in order to be able to select the optimal minimally invasive approach for the individual patient with surgical adrenal disease.

Needlescopic adrenalectomy

Salient features

Needlescopic instruments and optics have an external diameter of 2 mm, which is comparable to that of a 14-gauge angiocatheter. Various diagnostic and therapeutic urologic procedures may be performed utilizing 2 mm instruments (Soble and Gill 1998).

Needlescopic adrenalectomy is typically performed employing two 2 mm ports and one 5 mm port along the costal margin (Gill *et al.* 1998*b*). In addition, a 10/12 mm port is placed within the superior umbilical crease, which is the site of specimen extraction ultimately. The solitary 5 mm port allows the interchangeable use of various 5 mm instruments (clip-applier, hook cautery, scissors, suction-irrigator) by the surgeon's dominant hand. This is critical since, currently, 2 mm versions of these necessary instruments are either unavailable or technically inadequate. The only clearly visible large skin incision following a needlescopic adrenalectomy is the one created by the 5 mm subcostal port, since insertion of the 2 mm ports creates only a skin puncture, and the 1.5–2 cm skin incision for ultimate intact specimen extraction is cosmetically concealed within the umbilicus. This umbilical incision is used to intraoperative advantage by placing a 10 mm, 45° laparoscope at that site. Laparoscopic adrenalectomy is performed using techniques similar to those employed during transperitoneal laparoscopic adrenalectomy. Currently, needlescopic adrenalectomy only partially incorporates 2 mm technology, in that one larger (5 mm) port is still used in the subcostal location. Anticipated advances in 2 mm instrumentation may render the continued use of larger instruments unnecessary. Needlescopic adrenalectomy is currently our technique of choice in suitable patients who are candidates for a transperitoneal laparoscopic adrenalectomy.

Needlescopic versus conventional laparoscopic adrenalectomy

In an analysis at the Cleveland Clinic Foundation, needlescopic ($n = 15$) and conventional laparoscopic ($n = 21$) adrenalectomy techniques were compared retrospectively (Gill *et al.* 1998*b*). The needlescopic group was associated with shorter operative times (169 versus 220 min) and less blood loss (61 versus 183 cm^3). However, it is likely that these data were reflective of an improvement in the learning curve gained by prior experience with laparoscopic adrenalectomy, rather than an advantage of the needlescopic technique. Nevertheless, the needlescopic technique was associated with a shorter hospital stay (1.1 versus 2.7 days; $p < 0.001$), quicker convalescence (2.1 versus 3.1 weeks; $p < 0.001$), and a superior cosmetic result compared to conventional laparoscopic adrenalectomy.

Financial analysis: laparoscopic versus open adrenalectomy

Laparoscopic procedures are often associated with longer operative times, and therefore, greater intraoperative hospital charges. Several studies have demonstrated higher overall costs incurred during laparoscopic procedures compared to similar open surgical procedures. Hospital charges were US $1000 greater for laparoscopic adrenalectomy ($7000) as compared to open surgery ($6000; $p = 0.05$), in a study conducted at the Mayo Clinic.

At the Cleveland Clinic, financial data of 15 patients undergoing needlescopic adrenalectomy were compared to those of 15 contemporary patients undergoing open adrenalectomy between January 1995 and May 1997 (Hobart *et al.* 1998). Baseline data and patient demographics were similar between the two groups including patient age, adrenal tumor size, and pathology. Operative time was longer for the needlescopic procedure (163 versus 136 min). However, hospital stay was shorter in the needlescopic group (1 versus 7 days). Financial data were adjusted for inflation to 1998 data (4 per cent annual rate). Needlescopic adrenalectomy resulted in an 18.1 per cent increase in intraoperative costs, and a 63.4 per cent reduction in postoperative costs. Labor and supply costs, including disposables, were significantly higher in the needlescopic; group ($p = 0.0001$). Nevertheless, overall costs for needlescopic adrenalectomy were 18 per cent lower as compared to open adrenalectomy. Similarly, Korman and colleagues (1997) reported that laparoscopic adrenalectomy resulted in lower direct costs (US $3645 versus $5752) and lower total costs ($8188 versus $12 840) compared to the costs of open surgery.

Outpatient laparoscopic adrenalectomy

Salient features

Several laparoscopic procedures across various surgical disciplines are now performed on an outpatient basis. Laparoscopic general surgical procedures such as cholecystectomy, inguinal herniorrhaphy, incidental appendectomy, and fundoplication and laparoscopic gynecologic procedures such as lysis of pelvic adhesions have been performed in an ambulatory setting with good results. At the Cleveland Clinic, since September 1998, 14 selected patients have been entered into our outpatient laparoscopic adrenalectomy protocol (Gill *et al.* 1999*b*). For inclusion in the study, each patient expressed an understanding and willingness to undergo the proposed procedure in an outpatient setting, as well as its postoperative follow-up. To be included in the study selected patients were aged 70 years or younger. Additionally, patients with the diagnosis of a pheochromocytoma or an adrenal tumor > 5 cm in size were not considered to be suitable candidates. Patients were discharged on the day of surgery provided the procedure was technically uncomplicated, completed by noon, and the patient was hemodynamically stable both intra- and postoperatively.

In our initial nine patients, laparoscopic adrenalectomy was performed in a prospectively randomized manner by either the transperitoneal needlescopic ($n = 4$) or retroperitoneal ($n = 5$) technique. All nine patients (six males, three females) successfully completed the protocol. Diagnosis included aldosteroma (7), enlarging, nonfunctioning adenoma (1), and myelolipoma (1).

Mean surgical time was 2.3 hours, blood loss 53 ml, and postoperative hospital stay 416 min. Mean adrenal tumor size was 2 cm and specimen weight 22 g. The only complication was a postoperative abscess necessitating drainage 2 weeks following the ambulatory procedure. This was unrelated to the outpatient protocol. Patients, residing outside the Cleveland metropolitan area ($n = 4$), were discharged to a guesthouse adjacent to our hospital from which they went home the next morning. The other patients were discharged directly home after outpatient adrenalectomy.

Pheochromocytoma surgery may be associated with dramatic intra- and postoperative hemodynamic episodes. The routine need for invasive, hemodynamic monitoring precludes safe outpatient laparoscopic adrenalectomy in this setting and outpatient adrenalectomy should constitute a clear contraindication in these patients. Larger (> 5 cm) adrenal tumors often require considerable intraabdominal dissection, and we feel that outpatient laparoscopic adrenalectomy should probably not be offered in this setting. Selected patients with nonfunctioning adenomas and small, suspected adrenal metastasis might be excised laparoscopically in the outpatient setting. In addition, patients with a unilateral aldosteroma who have only mild, medically controlled hypertension are reasonable candidates for ambulatory adrenalectomy. A serum potassium level is obtained prior to discharge since reactive hyperkalemia may occur.

In conclusion, outpatient laparoscopic adrenalectomy is feasible and safe in the selected patients with excellent patient satisfaction. Considerable surgeon experience with laparoscopic adrenal surgery is essential before embarking upon ambulatory adrenalectomy. Judicious patient selection, careful and objective pre-discharge evaluation, and meticulous follow-up are essential to ensure excellent patient outcomes.

References

Allendorf, J.D.F., Bessler, M., Whelan, R.L., *et al.* (1996). Better preservation of immune function after laparoscopic-assisted versus open bowel resection in a murine model. *Dis. Colon Rectum* **39**, S67–S72.

Baba, S., Miyajima, A., Uchida, A., Asanuma, H., Miyakawa, A., and Murai, M. (1997). A posterior lumbar approach for retroperitoneoscopic adrenalectomy: assessment of surgical efficacy. *Urology* **50**, 19–24.

Basso, N., Leo, A.D., Fantini, A., Genco, A., Rosato, P., and Spaziani, E. (1999). Laparoscopic direct supragastric left adrenalectomy. *Am. J. Surg.* **178**, 308–10.

Bodie, B., Novick, A.C., Pontes, J.E., Straffon, R.A., Montie, J.E., Babiak, T., Sheeler, L., and Schumacher, P. (1989). The Cleveland Clinic experience with adrenal cortical carcinoma. *J. Urol.* **141**, 257.

Bonjer, H.J., Lange, J.F., Kazernier, G., de Herder, W.W., Steyerberg, E.W., and Bruining, H.A. (1997). Comparison of three techniques for adrenalectomy. *Br. J. Surg.* **84**, 679–82.

Brunt, L.M., Doherty, G.M., Norton, J.A., Soper, N.J., Quasebarth, M.A., and Moley, J.F. (1996). Laparoscopic adrenalectomy compared to open adrenalectomy for benign adrenal neoplasms. *J. Am. Coll. Surg.* **183**, 1–10.

Buell, J.F., Alexander, H.R., Norton, J.A., Yu, K.C., and Fraker, D.L. (1997). Bilateral adrenalectomy for Cushing's syndrome: anterior versus posterior surgical approach. *Ann. Surg.* **225**, 63–8.

Chiu, A.W., Hsu, Y., Chen, K., and Chang, L.S. (1997). Retroperitoneoscopic adrenalectomy—comparison study between the initial 20 and later 20 cases [abstract P6-28]. *J. Endourol.* **11**, S130.

Duh, Q.Y., Siperstein, A.E., Clark, O.H., Schecter, W.P., Horn, J.K., Harrison, M.R., Hunt, T.K., and Way, L.W. (1996). Laparoscopic adrenalectomy: comparison of the lateral and posterior approaches. *Arch. Surg.* **131**, 870–5.

Elashry, O.M., Clayman, R.V., Soble, J.J., and McDougall, E.M. (1997). Laparoscopic adrenalectomy for solitary metachronous contralateral adrenal metastasis from renal cell carcinoma. *J. Urol.* **157**, 1217–22.

Fernandez-Cruz, L., Taura, P., Saenz, A., Benarroch, G., and Sabater, L. (1996*a*). Laparoscopic approach to pheochromocytoma: hemodynamic changes and catecholamine secretion. *World J. Surg.* **20**, 762–8.

Fernandez-Cruz, L., Saenz, A., Benarroch, G., Astudillo, E., Taura, P., and Sabater, L. (1996*b*). Laparoscopic unilateral and bilateral adrenalectomy for Cushing's syndrome: transperitoneal and retroperitoneal approaches. *Ann. Surg.* **224**, 727–34.

Gagner, M. (1996). Laparoscopic adrenalectomy. *Surg. Clin. N. Am.* **76**, 523–37.

Gagner, M., Lacroix, A., and Bolte, E. (1992). Laparoscopic adrenalectomy in Cushing's syndrome and pheochromocytoma [letter]. *New Engl. J. Med.* **327**, 1033.

Gasman, D., Droupy, S., Koutani, A., Salomon, L., Antiphon, P., Chassagnon, J., Chopin, D.K., and Abbou, C.C. (1998). Laparoscopic adrenalectomy: the retroperitoneal approach. *J. Urol.* **159**, 1816–20.

Gill, I.S., Arca, M., Soble, J.J., Sung, G.T., and Heniford, B.T. (1998*a*). Laparoscopic adrenalectomy for cancer [abstract P18-9]. *J. Endourol.* **12**, S207.

Gill, I.S., Soble, J.J., Sung, G.T., Winfield, H.N., Bravo, E.L., and Novick, A.C. (1998*b*). Needlescopic adrenalectomy—the initial series: comparison with conventional adrenalectomy. *Urology* **52**, 180–6.

Gill, I.S., Sung, G.T., Schweizer, D., Nelson, D., Ochoa, R., Gagner, M., Winfield, H.N., Novick, A.C., and Bravo, E.L. (1999*a*). Laparoscopic versus open adrenalectomy: Cleveland Clinic experience with 210 cases. *J. Endourol.* **13**, PS 9-2.

Gill, I.S., Hobart, M.G., Schweizer, D., and Bravo, E.L. (1999*b*). Outpatient adrenalectomy. *J. Endourol.* **13**, PS 9-5.

Guazzoni, G., Montorsi, F., Bocciardi, A., Da Pozzo, L., Rigatti, P., Lanzi, F., and Pontiroli, A. (1995). Transperitoneal laparoscopic versus open adrenalectomy for benign hyperfunctioning adrenal tumors: a comparative study. *J. Urol.* **153**, 1597–600.

Heintz, A., Walgenbach, S., and Junginger, T. (1996). Results of endoscopic retroperitoneal adrenalectomy. *Surg. Endosc.* **10**, 633–5.

Heniford, B.T., Lannitti, D.A., Hale, J., and Gagner, M. (1997). The role of intraoperative ultrasonography during laparoscopic adrenalectomy. *Surgery* **122**, 1068–73.

Hobart, M., Schweizer, D., and Gill, I.S. (1998). Financial analysis of needlescopic versus open adrenalectomy [abstract P14-4]. *J. Endourol.* **12**, S184.

Hobart, M.G., Bravo, E.L., Schweizer, D., and Gill, I.S. (1999). Minimally invasive approach to the potentially malignant adrenal gland greater than 5 cm. *J. Endourol.* **13**, PS 9-6.

Janetschek, G., Finkenstedt, G., Gassser, R., Waibel, U.G., Peschel, R., Bartsch, G., and Neumann, H.P.H. (1998). Laparoscopic surgery for pheochromocytoma: adrenalectomy, partial resection , excision of paragangliomas. *J. Urol.* **160**, 330–4.

Korman, J.E., Ho, T., Hiatt, J.R., and Phillips, E.H. (1997). Comparison of laparoscopic and open adrenalectomy. *Am. Surg.* **63**, 908–12.

Soble, A. and Gill, I.S. (1998). Needlescopic urology: incorporating 2 mm instruments in laparoscopic surgery. *Urology* **52**, 187–94.

Sprung, J., O'Hara, J.F., Gill, I.S., Abdelmalak, B., Sarnaik, A., and Bravo, E.L. (2000). Anesthetic aspects of laparoscopic and open adrenalectomy for pheochromocytoma. *Urology* **55**, 339–43.

Staren, E.D. and Prinz, R.A. (1995). Selection of patients with adrenal incidentalomas for operation. *Surg. Clin. N. Am.* **75**, 499–510.

Staren, E.D. and Prinz, R.A. (1996). Adrenalectomy in the era of laparoscopy. *Surgery* **120**, 706–11.

Sung, G.T., Gill, I.S., Soble, J.J., and Bravo, E.L. (1998). Laparoscopic adrenalectomy: comparison of transperitoneal needlescopic versus retroperitoneoscopic approaches [abstract P18-3]. *J. Endourol.* **12**, S205.

Sung, G.T., Gill, I.S., Hobart, M., Soble, J., Schweizer, D., and Bravo, E.L. (1999). Laparoscopic adrenalectomy: prospective randomized comparison of transperitoneal versus retroperitoneal approaches. *J. Urol.* **161**, A69.

Suzuki, K., Kageyama, S., Ueda, D., Ushiyama, T., Kawabe, K., Tajima, A., and Aso, Y. (1993). Laparoscopic adrenalectomy: clinical experience with 12 cases. *J. Urol.* **150**, 1099.

Suzuki, K., Ushiyama, T., Mugiya, S., Kageyama, S., Saisu, K., and Fujita, K. (1997). Hazards of laparoscopic adrenalectomy in patients with adrenal malignancy. *J. Urol.* **158**, 2227.

Takeda, K., Go, K., Watanabe, R., Kurumada, S., Obara, K., Takahashi, E., Komeyama, T., Imai, T., and Takahashi, K. (1997). Retroperitoneal laparoscopic adrenalectomy for functioning adrenal tumors: comparison with conventional transperitoneal laparoscopic adrenalectomy. *J. Urol.* **157**, 19–23.

Thompson, G.B., Grant, C.S., van Heerden, J.A., Schlinkert, R.T., Young, W.F. Jr, Farley, D.R., and Ilstrup, D.M. (1997). Laparoscopic versus open posterior adrenalectomy: a case-control study of 100 patients. *Surgery* **122**, 1132–6.

Walz, M.K., Peitgen, K., Hoermann, R., Giebler, R.M., Mann, K., and Eigler, F.W. (1996). Posterior retroperitoneoscopy as a new minimally invasive approach for adrenalectomy: results of 30 adrenalectomies in 27 patients. *World J. Surg.* **20**, 769–74.

Winfield, H.N., Hamilton, B.D., and Bravo, E.L. (1997). Technique of laparoscopic adrenalectomy. *Urol. Clin.* **24**, 459.

Winfield, H.N., Hamilton, B.D., Bravo, E.L., and Novick, A.C. (1998). Laparoscopic adrenalectomy: the preferred choice? A comparison to open adrenalectomy. *J. Urol.* **160**, 325–9.

Yoshida, O., Terachi, T., Matsuda, T., *et al.* (1997). Complications in 369 laparoscopic adrenalectomies: a multi-institutional study in Japan [abstract 1098]. *J. Urol.* **157**, 282.

61. Laparoscopic adrenalectomy by the posterior lumbar approach

Shiro Baba and Masatsugu Iwamura

Introduction

Laparoscopy today is a procedure well past its learning curve and a standard part of the urologic armamentarium. Since laparoscopic adrenalectomy by transperitoneal anterior (Go 1993; Higashihara *et al.* 1993) and lateral approaches (Gagner *et al.* 1993) was reported in 1993, this procedure has gradually become the primary treatment option for benign adrenal diseases. Its success is due primarily to improvements in instrumentation and the rapid acquiring of laparoscopic anatomy by urologists. Operating in the retroperitoneum across the peritoneal cavity, however, necessitates considerable retraction of intraperitoneal organs. This implies the necessity for thorough bowel preparation and to make extra ports for retractors, which may increase perioperative morbidity and operative cost. Laparoscopic adrenalectomy, once confined to the transperitoneal approach, can now be performed by a completely extraperitoneal approach under a retroperitoneoscope that is introduced via the lateral flank or lumbodorsal area into a working space created in the posterior pararenal fossa. The lumbodorsal or posterior lumbar approach to the adrenal gland is probably the simplest method and takes the shortest way to the adrenal gland among the various laparoscopic or retroperitoneoscopic approaches. As in open surgery, the advantages of the lumbodorsal approach include the rapidity of the procedure, earlier access to and control of the adrenal vessels, and relative lack of morbidity. The procedure normally requires only one surgeon and one assistant, which can be further reduced to a single operator, if a voice-controlled robot arm is installed. Despite the technical simplicity, there are factors such as limited working space and paucity of clear anatomic landmarks that may defy the attempt to localize the adrenal gland. Other disadvantages include the required prone jack-knife position of the patient, relatively small skin area for trocar positioning, and risk of injury to the pleura or diaphragm by trocar insertion, resulting in tension pneumothorax. But these disadvantages seem to be outweighed by the advantages of this procedure, which leads to more cost-effective management by reducing operation time and manpower. The technical principles and pitfalls of this approach are described and our clinical results from retroperitoneoscopic adrenalectomy using the posterior lumbar approach with and without robot camera holder are discussed.

Materials and methods

From November 1992 to April 2000, 79 patients (42 females, 37 males) underwent laparoscopic or retroperitoneoscopic adrenalectomy. The procedure was performed by the transperitoneal anterior approach in 37 patients, by the transperitoneal lateral approach in 10 patients, by the extraperitoneal flank approach in 2 patients, and by the posterior lumabar approach in 30 patients. The clinical and pathologic diagnosis for the 30 patients (mean age $\pm$ SD, 45.4 $\pm$ 10.3 years; right adrenalectomy, 11 patients; left adrenalectomy, 19 patients) who underwent retroperitoneoscopic adrenalectomy by the posterior lumbar approach includes primary aldosteronism in 18, Cushing's syndrome in 8, virilizing adenoma in 1, pheochromocytoma in 1, endocrine-inactive adenoma in 1, and myelolipoma in 1. The body mass index (BMI; body weight/height^2) of these 30 patients ranged from 17.8 to 30.0 kg/m^2 (24.1 $\pm$ 3.4 kg/m^2, mean $\pm$ SD). In 21 patients, the procedure was performed with one operator and one assistant who manipulated the camera. The assistant (fourth-year resident) varied with every two cases. In 9 patients, the AESOP™ (Automated Endoscopic System for Optional Positioning) robotic arm(Computer Motion Inc., Goleta, CA, USA) for camera control was used to facilitate solo surgery by the same operator. The efficiency of this robot was compared with that of the most recent series of 10 cases in which a human assistant was used. The correlation between BMI and procedure time by the posterior lumbar approach was examined by Spearman rank correlation and simple regression analysis.

Surgical technique

The procedure was originally described by Baba *et al.* (1997). All patients underwent a mechanical bowel preparation 1 day prior to the surgery. Patients were typed and cross-matched for 2 units of blood. A nasogastric tube and urethral catheter were placed, with the patient under general intubated anesthesia. The patient was placed in the prone position with the kidney rest under the inferior margin of the anterior rib, and the table was flexed to a modified jack-knife position at about 30° (Fig. 61.1). The arms were kept extended, and cushions were placed under each shoulder to help appropriate excursion of the chest wall. The lower extremities were wrapped in a pair of garments that provides

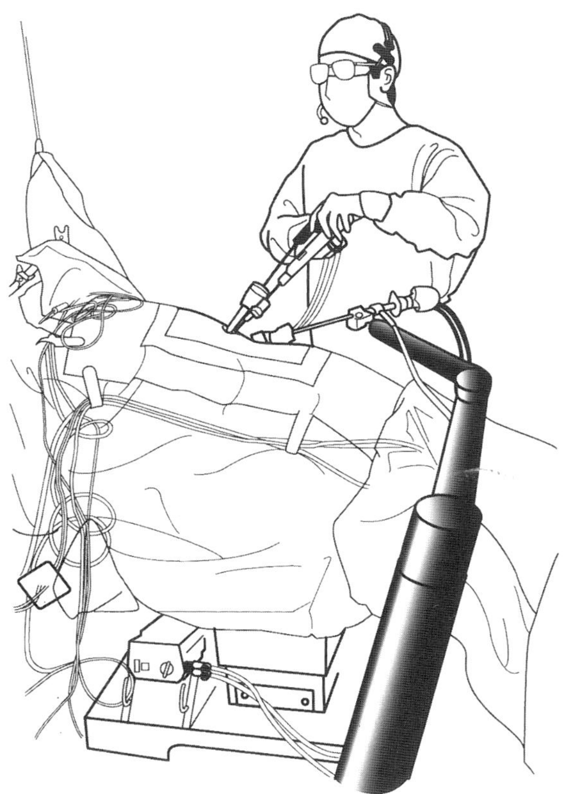

Fig. 61.1 The patient is placed in the prone position, and the relevant lumbar area is flexed on a kidney rest. The robotic arm is clamped on the side rail of the operating table opposite to the operator.

them with automatic sequenced pressure to facilitate active venous return during the operation. The table head was then elevated at 30°, and the tumor side was lowered at 15° to allow the kidney to slide away from the area of interest during dissection. A bean bag was used to hold the patient in this position. The operator stands on the same side of the diseased adrenal gland with an assistant. The procedure normally requires only three ports, including the camera port. To perform solo surgery, the human assistant is replaced with the AESOP™ robotic arm for camera control. In this case, the device was mounted on the railing of the operating table on the opposite side to the operator near the patient's knee joint (Fig. 61.1).

The skin incision for the first port was made 3 cm below the tip of the twelfth rib, and deepened to the transversalis fascia by bluntly dividing the abdominal muscle layers. The fascia was sharply incised under direct vision, and the posterior pararenal fossa was bluntly dissected with an index finger. A working space was then created with a dilatation balloon inflated up to 600 to 800 ml of air (Gaur 1992). A balloon-equipped 10 mm trocar was inserted in the first port, which was used as the camera port. The pneumoretroperitoneum was started under the maximum pressure of 10 mm Hg. The second port was made on the lateral margin of the sacrospinalis muscle and 2 to 3 cm below the twelfth rib (Fig. 61.2). A 12-mm trocar can be inserted either under retroperitoneoscopic guidance, or guided by the surgeon's

finger placed in the working space before starting pneumo-retroperitoneum (bimanual method). Another option is to use an optical surgical obturator (Optiview™, Ethicon USA; Visiport™, Autosuture USA) with a sheath that makes it possible to visually guide the tip of the trocar through the muscular layers and pararenal fat tissue (Connolly *et al.* 1995) on the way to the working space. The third trocar (5 mm) was inserted on the posterior axillary line in the eleventh intercostal space. Care must be taken to avoid the possible injury to the subcostal nerve, vessels, pleura, and the medial crus of the diaphragm. An additional 5-mm port can be made 3 cm below this port on the posterior axillary line, if retraction of the upper pole of the kidney becomes necessary as in some cases of adrenal tumor on the left side. The scope was usually inserted into the most caudal end of the working space, pointing to the dome of the diaphragm, which was not directly visible but completely covered with Gerota's fascia at this phase. The Gerota's fascia was subsequently opened and detached from the diaphragm by transversely dissecting its most cranial aspect along the rib, which helped to further enlarge the working space. Care was taken to avoid any injury to the peritoneum, which constitutes the lateral half of the floor of the working space. When sufficient working space was established, the Gerota's fascia was longitudinally incised along the psoas muscle and medial crus of the diaphragm, starting from the most medial side of the already opened Gerota's fascia down to the level of the renal pedicle. To expose the adrenal hilum and renal pedicle, the use of an ultrasonic aspirator (CUSA™: Valley-Lab, USA, or USU™: Olympus, Japan) made it possible to skeletonize these vessels within a significantly short period of time.

On the right side, the dissection of the adrenal gland itself was not started, until adrenal arteries and veins on the medial aspect of the gland were clipped and divided. The adrenal arteries were exposed just beneath the Gerota's fascia, while the adrenal veins were identified more ventral to this arterial layer. Adrenal arteries

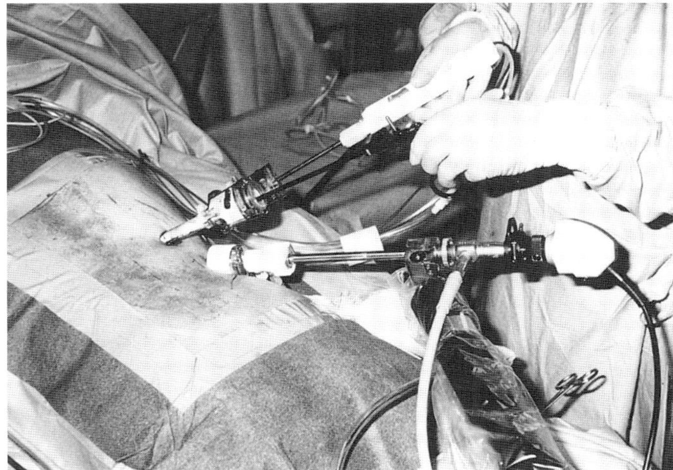

Fig. 61.2 The port sites for the right adrenalectomy. The camera port is made 3 cm below the tip of the twelfth rib. The second port is made 3 cm below the twelfth rib on the lateral margin of the sacrospinalis muscle. The third port is created in the eleventh intercostal space on the posterior axillary line.

penetrated the medial crura of the diaphragm that cover the abdominal aorta on both sides above the level of renal arteries, and were easily cauterized along the crura. On the right side, the posterior wall of the vena cava was directly identified beneath the arterial layer. Once the vena cava was identified, the posterior aspect was carefully dissected along its course starting from the diaphragm down to the level of the overlying renal artery. The right central adrenal vein draining into the vena cava postero-laterally was easily identified below the medial margin of the adrenal gland, and was secured with clips and transected. Care was taken to identify any short hepatic vein that occasionally drained into the vena cava in the vicinity of the right adrenal vein. Once the central vein was secured and transected, the lower aspect of the adrenal gland was dissected from the upper pole of the right kidney. The inferior and posterior adrenal vessels arising from the renal pedicle and capsule were secured and transected, and the lateral margin of the adrenal was then dissected upward to reach the superior adrenal artery and vein near the diaphragam. At this phase, the ventral aspect of the gland was dissected from the parietal peritoneum. The upper margin of the gland was finally clipped and divided from the peritoneum.

On the left side, the inferior phrenic vein was identified below the adrenal arterial layer. The upper pole of the left kidney was then dissected widely from the perirenal fatty tissue. Because the left kidney was more cranial than the right kidney and the left adrenal gland lay more ventral to the kidney than the right counterpart, the dissection of the left adrenal gland was started from its most lateral aspect toward the body of the gland along the upper pole of the kidney. To mobilize the adrenal gland from the kidney, the kidney was retracted toward the lateral side of the working space, while the tissue between the adrenal gland and the kidney was bluntly dissected toward the medial side, using an ultrasonic tissue aspirator placed along the margin of the renal capsule. The closer the second port was placed to the rib, the easier it was to undermine the lower margin of the left adrenal gland. The left renal artery and the inferior phrenic vein were the most important anatomic landmarks to start the dissection of the left middle adrenal artery and vein. The left middle adrenal vein was totally embedded deep within the adipose tissue of the triangular space that was surrounded by the inferior phrenic vein medially, the renal artery caudally, and the medial aspect of the left kidney laterally.

Once the adrenal gland was free, hemostasis was verified by irrigation and aspiration. If the adrenal tumor was larger than 3 cm in diameter, the camera port was changed to the most medially placed trocar, so that the gland entrapped in a self-expansible plastic pouch could be evacuated through the primary incisional wound that was relatively more spacious than the other punctured port sites.

Postoperative care

The nasogastric tube was removed on the day of surgery if the patient did not suffer from nausea. Chest and abdominal scout films are taken regularly after the operation to rule out any evidence of pneumothorax or free air caught in the peritoneal cavity, which may result from a peritoneum tear during the dissection. Oral intake is started in the morning of the first postoperative day. Most of the patients will tolerate the postoperative pain with a few doses of pentazocine injection.

Results

The BMI ranged from 17.9 to 29.6 kg/m^2, which indicates a wide variation of obesity among the patients. The placement of the trocars ,however, was without difficulty in all the patients and the retroperitoneoscopic observation within the posterior pararenal space was excellent even in obese patients. The procedure was successful in all except one case. This patient was converted to open surgery by a standard posterior approach with the rib resection, due to a sudden onset of tension pneumothorax caused by an inadvertent injury to the right medial crus of the diaphragm. The conversion rate by the posterior lumbar approach is, therefore, 3.3 per cent in the present series. With the exception of this patient, carbon dioxide absorption was not a problem, and hypercarbia was successfully avoided by close ventilatory management in all the other patients. The history of upper abdominal surgery in 3 patients or lower abdominal surgery in 8 patients caused no problem for the procedure. Other postoperative complications by this approach included fever($>$ 38°C) in 20.7 per cent (due to linear atelectasis in 10.3 per cent), retroperitoneal hematoma requiring blood transfusion in 3.4 per cent, and shoulder pain due to persistent pneumoperitoneum in 6.8 per cent.

The number of trocars required for this approach averaged only 3.1, which was significantly less than that required for the transperitoneal approach in our hands. In three patients with left-sided adrenal tumors (17.6 per cent of the left adrenalectomies), retraction of the left renal upper pole was performed by using a snake-tail retractor that was inserted via an additional 5-mm port made on the posterior axillary line and 3 cm apart from the third port. The blood loss was 44 $\pm$ 64 ml, and the procedure time averaged 144 $\pm$ 33 min (mean $\pm$ SD). Mean times to unassisted ambulation and return to normal diet were 1.24 $\pm$ 0.6 days and 1.2 $\pm$ 0.6 days, respectively. Mean postoperative hospital stay for primary aldosteronism averaged 4.7 $\pm$ 0.6 days (mean $\pm$ SD). The procedure time with and without AESOP™ did not differ significantly (Table 61.1). Because this device had voice-recognition capabilities, a transparent surgeon–robot interface was easily established within a short time, providing the surgeon with the required target magnification by moving the laparoscope into the working space by vocal orders (Partin *et al* 1995). This robot made it possible to maintain the surgical point of interest of the operator always in the center of the video frame, minimizing the chance of losing the target that was occasionally observed with a human assistant. The number of lens smearing decreased to one-fourth of that observed with a human assistant. (The laparoscope tended to be unintentionally approached toward the target tissue by a human assistant which accounted for the lens smearing.) All procedures were completed successfully without technical mishaps. In one patient, however, use of the robotic arm was terminated before completion of the surgery, which required frequent movement of the camera in order to control arterial bleeding.

Table 61.1 Efficiency of AESOP use (mean ± SD)

	Surgeon aided by		
	AESOP	**Human assistant**	**p-value**
Length of procedure (min)	132.8 ± 34	136.8 ± 15.5	0.45
Number of lens smearings	1.6 ± 0.6	5.8 ± 4.3	0.04
Number of scope removals	1.8 ± 0.5	6.6 ± 4.2	0.03
Number of inadvertent movements	1.0 ± 0.8	3.6 ± 1.9	0.02

No significant correlation was observed between BMI and procedure time in this series of 30 patients (Spearman rank correlation; $p = 0.079$, $r = 0.374$).

Discussion

The impact of open adrenalectomy by the dorsal approach on convalescence of the patient and the benchmark data for this open surgery have been reported (mean operative time, 200 min; blood loss, 237 ml; hospital stay, 4.4 days), by which the effectiveness of laparoscopic adrenalectomy may be judged (Nash *et al.* 1995). The procedure time for retroperitoneoscopic adrenalectomy in the present series averaged 144 min with a mean estimated blood loss of 44 ml. After the initial learning curve, the procedure time has been further shortened to 137 min with a human assistant and 133 min with the AESOP™ robotic assistant. The mean procedure time required for open adrenalectomy in our institute is 153 min with a mean blood loss of 195 ml. According to a questionnaire to our patients, the time required to gain full activity was 34 days after the open adrenalectomy, while it was only 7.6 days after the retroperitoneoscopic adrenalectomy. The shorter procedure time and lesser morbidity with much earlier recovery make the adrenalectomy by the posterior lumbar approach more appealing. The main advantage of the posterior lumbar approach is to gain direct access to the adrenal hilar vessels without the necessity of retracting any organs or manipulating the fragile adrenal gland. Once identified, these vessels can become the most reliable anatomic landmark to the adrenal gland. Furthermore, the history of intraperitoneal surgery is not a problem for retroperitoneoscopic adrenalectomy, and full bowel preparation is not required, resulting in shorter and less invasive preoperative management. By this direct approach to the adrenal hilum, most adrenal cortical tumors that are less than 5 cm in diameter can be safely removed. Pheochromocytomas on the right side are most suitable for this approach, because the vascular control can be done without mobilizing the tumor. On the left side, this approach should be limited to relatively smaller pheochromocytomas with a diameter less than 3 cm, because some adrenal veins including the left posterior adrenal vein cannot be secured without retracting the caudal aspect of the left adrenal tumor if the pheochromocytoma is large.

For laparoscopic or retroperitoneoscopic surgery, an experienced assistant is often required, even if most of the time it is only to manipulate the camera. This means that the operator's vision is effectively delegated to another individual. It is ideal to have an assistant who knows the *modus operandi* of the operator intimately. When camera holders get distracted, they tend to bump into the tissue, which smears the lens. Most surgeons can be more efficient, if they do not have to keep thinking about or asking the camera holder to correct the positioning of the scope. The robotic arm increased stability of the image, reduced inadvertent smearing of the lens, and provided the operator with absolute consistency of quality of assistance. It decreased the number of times the scope needed to be removed, and definitely reduced the number of human assistants.

Retroperitoneoscopic adrenalectomy by the lumbodorsal approach (Baba *et al.* 1999) could be safely performed by a single surgeon without assistant. Solo surgery can be defined as performance of the operative procedure without the help of assistant, a nurse, or another surgeon. The posterior lumbar approach makes it possible to perform the adrenalectomy using only three ports in 90 per cent of the patients (100 per cent on the right side), because the scope and instruments are directly approached to the adrenal gland, and there are few organs in the retroperitoneum that have to be retracted with the patient placed in the prone position.

Conclusion

The shorter operative time and lesser morbidity by the posterior lumbar approach indicate that the retroperitoneoscopic adrenalectomy is acceptable as a standard technique in most patients with benign adrenal disorders. Experience in laparoscopic adrenalectomy by transperitoneal approaches, however, should still be valued, as no single approach is satisfactory in all patients with different adrenal disorders. Proper patient selection and the optimal strategy of the approach are the essentials in safely performing laparoscopic or retroperitoneoscopic adrenalectomies.

References

Baba, S., Miyajima, A., Uchida, A., Asanuma, H., Miyakawa, A., and Murai, M. (1997). A posterior lumbar approach for retroperitoneoscopic adrenalectomy: assessment of surgical efficacy. *Urology* **50** (1), 19–24.

Baba, S., Ito, K., Yanaihara, H., Nagata, H., Murai, M., and Iwamura, M.(1999). Retroperitoneoscopic adrenalectomy by a lumbodorsal approach: clinical experience with solo surgery. *World J. Urol.* **17**, 54–8.

Connolly, P.J., Yuan, H.A., Kolata, R.J., and Clem, M.F. (1995). Endoscopic approach to the lumbar spine using the insufflation technique. In *Atlas of endoscopic spine surgery* (ed. M.D. Regan), pp. 345–9. Quality Medical Publishing,Inc,St. Louis.

Gagner, M., Lacroix, A., Prinz, R.A., Bolte, E., Albala, D., Potvin, C., Hamet, P., Kuchel, O., Querin, S., and Pomp, A.(1993). Early experience with laparoscopic approach for adrenalectomy. *Surgery* **114** (6), 1120–4.

Gaur, D.D. (1992). Laparoscopic operative retroperitoneoscopy; use of a new device. *J. Urol.* **148**, 1137–9.

Go, H. (1993). Laparoscopic adrenalectomy. *Jpn J. Urol.* **84**, 1675–80.

Higashihara, E., Tanaka, Y., Horie, S., Aruga, S., Nutahara, K., Minowada, S., and Aso, Y.(1993). Laparoscopic adrenalectomy: the initial 3 cases. *J. Urol.* **149** (5), 973–6.

Nash, P.A., Leibovitch, I., and Donohue, J.P. (1995). Adrenalectomy via the dorsal approach: a benchmark for laparoscopic adrenalectomy. *J. Urol.* **154**, 1652–4.

Partin, A.W., Adams, J.B., Moore, R.G., *et al.* (1995). Complete robot-assisted laparoscopic urologic surgery: a preliminary report. *J. Am. Coll. Surg.* **181** (6), 552–7.

62. Acute and chronic interstitial cryotherapy of the adrenal

David A. Schulsinger, R. Ernest Sosa, Aaron P. Perlmutter, and E. Darracott Vaughan, Jr

Introduction

Unilateral adrenalectomy is indicated for patients with large adrenal lesions or functional tumors. Various open surgical approaches have been utilized. Laparoscopic adrenalectomy has now become an important surgical technique for the management of adrenal lesions (Takeda *et al.* 1994), including patients with primary aldosteronism (Conn's syndrome) or Cushing's adenoma, Cushing's disease, pheochromocytoma, and nonfunctioning tumors greater than 6 cm in size. Laparoscopy can be performed by transabdominal or retroperitoneal access. The advantage of laparoscopic adrenalectomy is the reduced postoperative discomfort, morbidity, and shorter hospital stay.

Recently, adrenal-sparing surgery for adrenal tumors has been used as an alternative to unilateral adrenalectomy (Schomer and Mohler 1995; Heniford *et al.* 1997; Nakada *et al.* 1995; Janetschek *et al.* 1997; Suzuki *et al.* 1998; Sasagawa *et al.* 2000; Vaughan and Blumenfeld 1998). In these cases, open (Nakada *et al.* 1995) or laparoscopic adrenal-sparing surgery (Janetschek *et al.* 1997; Suzuki *et al.* 1998; Sasagawa *et al.* 2000) was used in the treatment of aldosterone-producing adenoma. Others have reported on open enucleation of a pheochromocytoma (Vaughan and Blumenfeld 1998). In these situations, adrenal-sparing surgery can be utilized when preservation of the remnant adrenal is necessary.

Liquid air, iced saline solutions, and carbonic snow have been used to destroy advanced malignancies for palliative purposes for over 150 years (Amott 1845). Advances in cryosurgery began with the development of an automated cryosurgical apparatus cooled by liquid nitrogen early in the 1960s and, more recently, by an argon gas delivery system (Schulsinger *et al.* 1998). Cryoablation is currently used as a surgical alternative for the treatment of prostate (Bonney *et al.* 1983), lung, breast (Rand *et al.* 1985), brain, pharynx (Gage 1969), and liver tumors (Shafir *et al.* 1996). More recently, cryosurgery has been used in the treatment of small renal tumors by open (Gill *et al.* 1998a; Rodriguez *et al.* 1998; Delworth *et al.* 1996), laparoscopic (Gill *et al.* 1998a; Rodriguez *et al.* 1998), or percutaneous access (Uchida *et al.* 1995). Renewed interest in cryoablative surgery is due largely to improved delivery systems and ultrasound-based monitoring systems.

The use of cryosurgery has not been previously described in the treatment of adrenal tissue ablation. The purpose of this study was to determine if this energy form could be delivered to small areas in the adrenal gland in an effective, controllable, and repro-ducible way. We examine our experience of open and laparoscopic adrenal cryosurgery in the canine model.

Materials and methods

Acute cryosurgery

Eight female mongrel dogs (20.5 ± 1.1 kg) were utilized for these experiments. An institutional review board for animal research approved the protocol. Pentobarbital (25–30 mg/kg, intravenous (IV)) anesthesia was given and an endotracheal tube placed and connected to a volume ventilator set for an FiO_2 of 100 per cent. The respiratory rate was fixed at 16 breaths/min and the tidal volume adjusted to produce a Pa CO_2 of 30 mm Hg. A 12-F Foley catheter was placed in the bladder. Using an open, transabdominal approach, the peritoneum was reflected off of the adrenal with standard surgical equipment. A 2 mm cryoprobe (ENDOcare, Irvine, CA) was placed interstitially (1 cm) into the upper pole of the adrenal, whereas 0.032 inch thermocouples were cannulated into the ipsilateral adrenal artery and vein. Adrenal parenchymal temperature changes were measured using 0.032 inch thermocouples placed in a template at 0.4 and 0.8 cm intervals from the cryoprobe. Freezing of the tissue was performed with argon gas via the CRYOcare Cryosurgical Unit (ENDOcare, Irvine, CA) for a single 15 min treatment period. A passive thaw was performed and the cryoprobe was removed when the temperature increased to 0°C.

At the conclusion of the acute cryosurgery, the dogs were euthanized with sodium pentobarbital (120 mg/kg). The adrenals were removed, weighed, and placed in 10 per cent formalin for histologic analysis.

Chronic cryosurgery

Eighteen female mongrel dogs (20.0 ± 0.9 kg) were randomly divided into three groups (4, 6, and 8 week groups; $n = 6$/group). Animals were anesthetized (ketamine, 11 mg/kg IV/valium, 0.5 mg/kg IV, 1:1 mixture to effect; isofluorane/O_2) and an endotracheal tube was placed and connected to a volume ventilator set for an FiO_2 of 100 per cent. The respiratory rate was fixed at 16 breaths/min and the tidal volume adjusted to produce a Pa CO_2 of 30-mm Hg. A 12-F Foley catheter was placed in the bladder. The animal was placed in the right lateral decubitus position. The animal was prepped and draped in the usual sterile fashion. A Hassan trocar was inserted into the peritoneum at the umbilicus for abdominal insufflation. A CO_2 gas pneumoperitoneum was developed to 15 mm Hg with a laparoscopic insufflator (Olympus, Lake Success, NY). Three additional 10-mm laparoscopic trocars (Autosuture Corp., Norwalk, CT) were placed subcostally in the left lower, middle, and upper quadrant along the midclavicular line. A 10 mm, 30° laparoscope (Olympus) and laparoscopy instruments were introduced through these ports. The intra-abdominal pressure was continuously monitored with an Olympus insufflator. The peritoneum was reflected off of the adrenal gland with standard laparoscopic equipment.

A 2 mm cryoprobe (ENDOcare, Irvine, CA) was placed interstitially (1 cm) into the upper pole of the adrenal. Freezing of the tissue was performed with argon gas via the CRYOcare Cryosurgical Unit (ENDOcare, Irvine, CA) for a single 15 min treatment period. A passive thaw was performed and the cryoprobe was removed when the temperature increased to 0°C.

At the conclusion of the cryosurgical procedure, the trocars were removed, the abdomen was desufflated and the entry sites sutured with 0-chromic sutures. Postoperatively, the animal's vitals were monitored biweekly. At the conclusion of the 4-, 6-, or 8-week study, the dogs were euthanized with sodium pentobarbital (120 mg/kg). Both adrenals were removed, weighed, and placed in 10 per cent formalin for histologic analysis.

Results

Acute cryosurgery

Interstitial cryoprobe temperatures decreased from 33.1 ± 1.9°C to −148 ± 1.2°C following 15 min of freezing. Cryoablation of adrenal tissue achieved temperatures of −41.8 ± 5.7°C and −21.8 ± 1.0°C at distances of 0.4 and 0.8 cm from the cryoprobe, respectively. Following 1 and 6 minutes of freezing, tissue was frozen to −20°C at a radius of 0.4 and 0.8 cm, respectively. There were no significant changes in venous or arterial adrenal temperatures during the entire cryosurgery period. These results are summarized in Fig. 62.1.

Histologically, there is a clear demarcation between viable and nonviable tissue (see Fig. 62.2(a)). The nonviable tissue includes areas of pyknosis, suggestive of cell death (see Fig. 62.2(b)). In addition, there are areas of diffuse hemorrhage.

Chronic cryosurgery

Adrenal tissue temperatures were reduced from a baseline of 33.3 ± 1.1°C to −157.7 ± 0.8°C following 15 min of freezing (see Fig. 62.3). There was no statistical difference in the weight of the adrenal gland undergoing cryoablation and that of the contralateral gland. Macroscopic examination of the adrenal demonstrated a firm lesion.

Gross evaluation of the adrenal gland demonstrated a central coagulated zone and a peripheral white zone. The coagulated zone had a volume of 0.15 ± 0.08 cm^3 and the whitish zone was 0.53 ± 0.17 cm^3. There was no evidence of gross hemorrhage

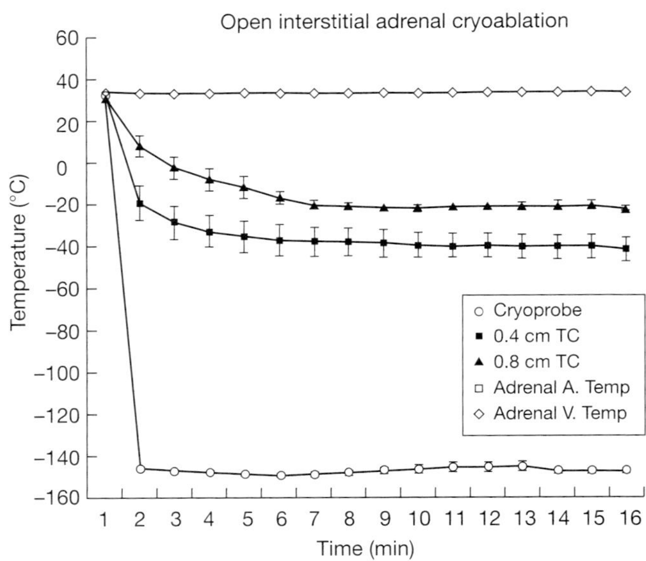

Fig. 62.1 Relationship between freezing time and adrenal parenchyma and adrenal vessel temperatures following acute cryoablation. TC, thermocouple; A, artery; V, vein; Temp, temperature.

after 4 weeks of cryoablation. The adrenal lesions measured 0.69 ± 0.14 cm^3, 0.59 ± 0.12 cm^3, and 0.52 ± 0.09 cm^3 at 4, 6, and 8 weeks, respectively (Fig. 62.3). These differences were not statistically significant.

Four-week group
Histologically, there was a well-defined area of total tissue necrosis (zone 1), inflammation (zone 2), fibrosis (zone 3), and viable/normal tissue (zone 4) (see Fig. 62.2(c), (d)). In zone 1, this area represents the epicenter of tissue destruction with no evidence of viable tissue (see Fig. 62.2(c)). In zone 2, this region contains areas of inflammation, scattered hemorrhage, and hemosiderin (see Fig. 62.2(c)). Zone 3 contains significant areas of fibrosis (see Fig. 62.2(c), (d)). Zone 4 contains normal adrenal tissue (see Fig. 62.2(d)). No histologic changes were observed in the untreated portion of the ipsilateral and contralateral adrenal gland.

Eight-week group
Histologically, the central area of necrosis (zone 1) had resolved and was replaced by fibrotic tissue. There was a larger zone of fibrosis, replacing the necrotic zone and zone 3. There was a minimal area of inflammation. In the fourth and final zone, there is normal adrenal tissue. No histologic changes were observed in the untreated portion of the ipsilateral and contralateral adrenal gland.

Discussion

Cryoablation of the adrenal can be delivered in a safe, effective, controllable, and reproducible manner. This controllable energy form may provide a new treatment modality for tissue destruc-

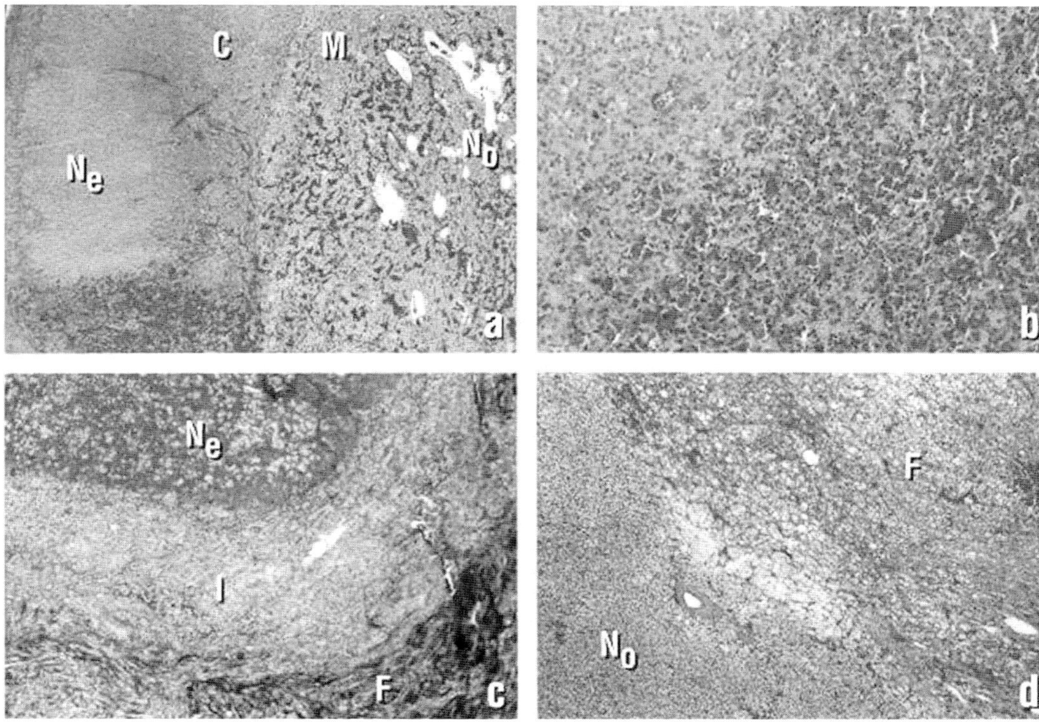

Fig. 62.2 Photomicrographs demonstrating histologic changes in the adrenal following (a, b) acute and (c, d) chronic cryoablation. (a) Line of demarcation between necrotic (N_e) and viable (N_o) tissue (hematoxylin and eosin (H & E), 20×). (b) Pyknosis and hemorrhage (H & E, 100×). (c) Trichrome stain demonstrating areas of necrosis (N_e), inflammation (I), fibrosis (F) (100×). (d) The two zones demonstrating defined areas of normal (N_o) tissue and fibrosis (F) (H & E, 40×).

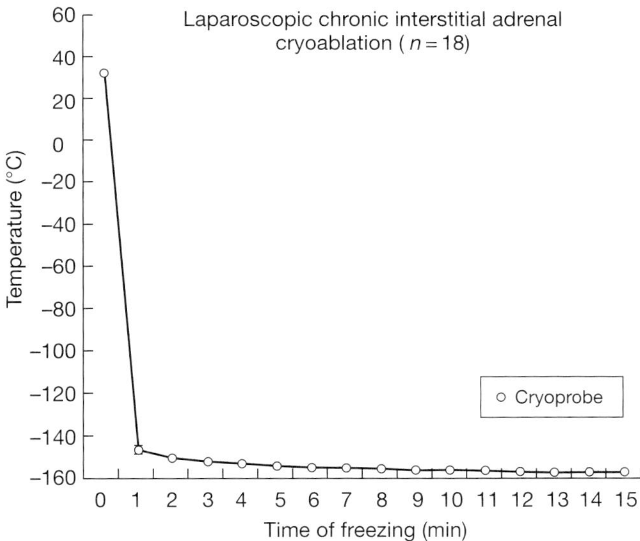

Fig. 62.3 Relationship of adrenal tissue temperature to time during the 15 min of cryosurgery.

tion where adrenal gland preservation is necessary and can be performed by the laparoscopic approach.

The enthusiasm over cryodestruction developed on the basis of the nontoxic nature of cold temperatures. Furthermore, this technique allows maximum sparing of uninvolved tissue, as only a small margin surrounding the cryoablated tissue is affected by the freezing temperature. Our study demonstrates that cryoablation is safe and effective and that destruction of adrenal tissue is reproducible. Although histologic evidence suggests a clear, well-defined region of total tissue necrosis, represented by zone 1 (Fig. 62.2(a), (b)), one can only speculate that the lesion size could be larger if: (1) larger cryoprobes were used; (2) multiple probes were placed to overlap frozen areas; (3) colder temperatures were achieved; (4) multiple freeze–thaw cycles were utilized; (5) longer freezing times were used. This study was limited by the use of a single, 2 mm probe. In the mongrel dog model, we are limited by the small size of the adrenal gland, precluding the use of multiple sticks.

This report represents the first published study utilizing argon gas as the cryogen for cryosurgery in the adrenal gland. Among the various cryogens, no other agent has the freezing capacity of liquid nitrogen (−196°C). Argon achieves relatively warmer freezing temperatures (−187.5°C) (Baust *et al.* 1997) than liquid nitrogen, but is more than sufficient in achieving cryodestruction in its effectiveness in ablating bulky tumor needs to be determined and requires further investigation.

In addition, the repetition of the freeze/thaw cycle allows cells to undergo the same deleterious effects, including a longer hypothermic period, which adds a greater degree of certainty to the destruction process. The present study, however, demonstrated that a single freeze–thaw cycle is effective at causing tissue necrosis. A single freeze–thaw cycle demonstrated tissue destruction without cellular regeneration by 8 weeks. Tissue destruction without cellular regeneration would be the goal of treatment, especially if tumor destruction were required. Future studies should address the histologic evidence of tissue destruction utilizing multiple freeze/thaw cycles.

The range of critical temperatures ensuring tissue destruction is wide. Experimental and clinical reports demonstrate that temperatures between −40°C and −50°C are necessary to be certain of cell death, which is of critical importance in the treatment of cancer (Baust *et al.* 1997). However, Nakada *et al.* (1997) have shown that cryotherapy is a means of soft-tissue destruction whereby cells are frozen below −20°C. In the present study, after 1 and 6 min of freezing, tissue was frozen to adequate levels at a radius of 0.4 and 0.8 cm, respectively, to achieve tissue ablation. Adrenal tissue temperatures were reduced to −40°C at a diameter of 0.8 cm by 10 min and were maintained at that temperature until the thaw process commenced at 15 min. In this study, care was taken to standardize the thermocouple placement since a 1 mm difference in placement produces a 15°C difference in tissue temperature measurement (Gage 1982). The critical temperature for tissue destruction was reached by 10 min; however, further investigations need to correlate the histologic findings with freezing temperatures.

Histologically, there are four distinct zones following adrenal cryoablation. Green (1977) and associates noted that cell membrane breakdown produced a 'ghostlike' appearance of prostatic tissue. This correlates to our findings of 'zone 1' or the region of total tissue necrosis (see Fig. 62.2(a)). There is a clear line of demarcation between this zone and zone 2, the region of inflammation. In this region, there is a large number of inflammatory cells, but with small areas of hemorrhage and hemosiderin (see Fig. 62.2(c)). Albin and Reddy (1977) also found that a necrotic zone is surrounded by an inflammatory zone consisting of lymphocytic aggregates, suggesting a cellular immune response (Bonney *et al.* 1983). One important question remains: how does adrenal cryoablation cause the gross and histopathologic changes? Some authors speculate that the intracellular ice formation disrupts intracellular organelle membranes resulting in a breakdown of intracellular machinery (Mazur 1977). Other authors suggest that osmotic fluctuations by freezing results in membrane malfunction and eventual destruction (Farrant *et al.* 1977). The exact mechanism of cellular destruction in the adrenal gland requires further investigation.

In the current study, there was a reduction (not statistically significant) in the adrenal lesion size between 4 and 8 weeks post-cryoablation (Fig. 62.4). The decrease in lesion size over time

following cryoablation is not unique to the adrenal, as this phenomenon has been seen in other organ systems. Similar findings of reduction in lesion size have been demonstrated following renal cryoablation in both human (Gill *et al.* 1998b) and animal (Schulsinger *et al.* 1999) studies. Gill *et al.* (1998b) showed that postoperative magnetic resonance imaging (MRI) evaluation of patients undergoing laparoscopic renal cryoablation demonstrated a decrease in the size of the cryoablated renal tumor of 21, 33, and 41 per cent at 1, 2, and 3 months, respectively. Schulsinger *et al.* (1999) showed that there was a 39 per cent decrease in renal lesion size between 4 and 8 weeks following laparoscopic renal cryoablation in the canine model. Similar findings of lesion size reduction were demonstrated in the prostate and liver lesions. In the present study, despite a smaller lesion size, there was an increase in the amount of fibrotic deposition. This increase in fibrosis and scar formation may explain the reduction in cryolesion size. The reduction in lesion size suggests that this may be the 'normal' physiological response following tissue injury. Thus, an *increase* in lesion size following cryoablation may suggest incomplete cryoablation or cryoresistant tissue of the tumor. Additional studies evaluating cryoablated tissue will need to address this issue.

The advantage of interstitial application of the cryoprobe is that it provides deeper freezing, but it has the disadvantage of producing a wound that bleeds, even substantially. In the present study, significant bleeding was not identified. The advantage of small interstitial probes is the reduced theoretical risk of bleeding. In addition, cracking of the iceball, as a cause of bleeding, was not observed in this study.

Infectious complications of cryosurgery are seldom reported. In one series of hepatic cryoablation, the procedure-related infection rate was 7.6 per cent (Riley *et al.* 1997). We have noted no morbidity related to cryoablation in any animal in our series. In the present study, there was no evidence of infection; however, we advocate the prophylactic use of antibiotics.

Unilateral adrenalectomy has been traditionally performed by open surgical technique. Recently, laparoscopic adrenalectomy by a transabdominal or retroperitoneal approach has been utilized for the treatment of aldosteronoma, adrenal hyperplasia (Cushing's disease), nonfunctioning (secretory) tumors, Cushing's adenoma, pheochromocytoma, and adrenal myelolipoma. This surgical modality is considered safe, with a reduced morbidity, convalescence time, and hospitalization. The use of transperitoneal laparoscopic access to the adrenal for cryosurgery provides a direct route for tissue ablation. Interstitial placement of the cryoprobe was easily assisted with standard laparoscopic equipment. Future studies via a retroperitoneoscopic or lumboscopic approach for direct cryoprobe access should be studied for comparison.

Despite the advantages of laparoscopy, the complication rate of 7.5 per cent and the conversion rate of 9 per cent (Chiu *et al.* 1997) continue to raise questions and concerns. The interstitial placement of cryoprobe via laparoscopic access should reduce the operating time and manipulation of the adrenal gland and may reduce the overall complication and conversion rates.

Adrenal-sparing surgery has been used in selected patients with adrenal tumors (Nakada *et al.* 1995; Janetschek *et al.* 1997; Suzuki

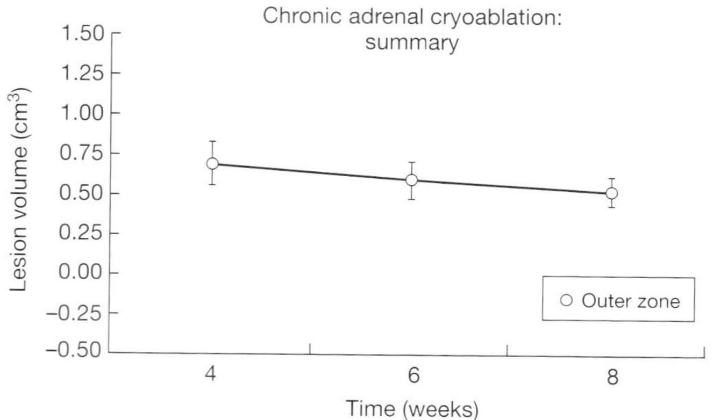

Fig. 62.4 Summary of change in lesion volume (cm³) over time (weeks) following adrenal cryoablation (mean ± SE).

et al. 1998; Sasagawa *et al.* 2000; Vaughan and Blumenfeld 1998). Partial adrenalectomy has been used successfully in the treatment of patients with primary hyperaldosteronism (Nakada *et al.* 1995; Janetschek *et al.* 1997; Suzuki *et al.* 1998) and pheochromocytoma (Vaughan and Blumenfeld 1998). The indication for adrenal-sparing surgery may be considered in patients with a solitary adrenal gland, bilateral adrenal tumors, adrenal tumor, and a contralateral nonfunctioning adenoma (Vaughan and Blumenfeld 1998). Adrenal-sparing surgery has been performed either by open enucleation (Schomer and Mohler 1995; Nakada *et al.* 1995; Vaughan and Blumenfeld 1998) or laparoscopic surgery (Heniford *et al.* 1997; Janetschek *et al.* 1997; Suzuki *et al.* 1998; Sasagawa *et al.* 2000). There were no recurrent adrenal lesions in a series of 26 patients undergoing open partial adrenalectomy for aldosterone-producing adenoma with a mean follow-up of 5 years (Nakada *et al.* 1995). Alternatively, this study has shown that cryosurgery can be delivered effectively by laparoscopic access. Cryosurgery may offer a surgical alternative to adrenal-sparing surgery in treating selected patients with an adrenal tumor by this minimally invasive approach.

Cryoablation is a safe, effective, controllable, and reproducible energy form for ablating localized adrenal tissue *in situ*. Tissue destruction is achieved and healed in a nonpathological way. Advanced unresectable adrenal tumors, bilateral adrenal tumors, or small, nonfunctioning lesions represent a challenge to the urologist and surgeon treating these patients. Understanding the effect of adrenal cryoablation may allow us to treat select patients with adrenal tumors where organ preservation is necessary.

Conclusion

This study was intended to demonstrate whether cryosurgery is an efficacious means of tissue destruction and nonpathological healing. Cryoablation of adrenal tissue achieves adequate freezing temperatures within a defined area necessary for tissue destruction. Cryosurgery of the adrenal can be delivered in an effective, controllable, and reproducible manner. Cryotherapy, coupled with the universal trend towards minimally invasive surgery, may provide a new treatment modality for tissue destruction where adrenal gland preservation is necessary.

References

Albin, R.J. and Reddy, K.P. (1977). Cryosurgery of the monkey (macaque) prostate. II. Apparent immunopathologic alterations following cryo-stimulation. *Cryobiology* **14**, 205–14.

Amott, J. (1845). *On the present state of therapeutic inquiry*. Churchill, London.

Baust, J., Gage, A.A., Ma, H., and Zhang, C.M. (1997). Minimally invasive cryosurgery. *Tech. Advan. Cryobiol.* **34**, 373–84.

Bonney, W.W., Fallon, B., Gerber, W.L., Hawtrey, C.E., *et al.* (1983). Cryosurgery in prostatic cancer: elimination of local lesion. *Urology* **22**, 8–15.

Chiu, A.W., Hsu, Y.S., Chen, K.K., and Chang, L.S. (1997). Retroperitoneoscopic adrenalectomy—results comparison study between the initial and later 20 cases. *J. Endourol.* **11**, S130.

Delworth, M.G., Pisters, L.L., Fornage, B.D., and von Eschenbach, A.C. (1996). Cryotherapy for renal cell carcinoma and angiomyolipoma. *J. Urol.* **155**, 252–5.

Farrant, J., Walter, C.A., Lee, H., and McGann, L.E. (1977). Use of two-step cooling procedures to examine factors influencing cell survival following freezing and thawing. *Cryobiology* **14**, 273–86.

Gage, A.A. (1969). Cryosurgery for oral and pharyngeal carcinoma. *Am. J. Surg.* **118**, 669–72.

Gage, A.A. (1982). Current issues in cryosurgery. *Cryobiology* **19**, 219–22.

Gill, I.S., Novick, A.C., Soble, J.J., Sung, G.T., O'Malley, C., and Hale, J. (1998*a*). Laparoscopic (retroperitoneal) renal cryoablation: initial clinical experience. *J. Urol.* **159**, 151A

Gill, I.S., Novick, A.C., Soble, J.J., Sung, G.T., Remer, E.M., Hale, J., and O'Malley, C.M. (1998*b*). Laparoscopic renal cryoablation: initial clinical series. *Urology* **52**, 543–51.

Green, N.A. (1977). Cryosurgery of the prostate gland. *Ann. R. Acad. Surg. Eng.* **59**, 288–97.

Heniford, B.T., Iannitti, D.A., Hale, J., and Gagner, M. (1997). The role of intra-operative ultrasonography during laparoscopic adrenalectomy. *Surgery* **122**, 1068–73.

Janetschek, G., Lhotta, K., Gasser, R., Finkenstedt, G., Jaschke, W., and Bartsch, G. (1997). Adrenal-sparing laparoscopic surgery for aldosterone-producing adenoma. *J. Endourol.* **11**, 145–9.

Mazur, P. (1977). The role of intracellular freezing in the death of cells cooled at supraoptimal rates. *Cryobiology* **14**, 251–72.

Nakada, S.Y., Chosy, S., Lee, F.T. Jr, and Warner, T.F. (1997). Thermosensor-monitored renal cryosurgery in swine: assessment of various predictors of tissue necrosis. *J. Endourol.* **11**, S55.

Nakada, T., Kubota, Y., Sasagawa, I., Yagisawa, T., Watanabe, M., and Ishigooka, M. (1995). Therapeutic outcome of primary aldosteronism: adrenalectomy versus enucleation of aldosterone-producing adenoma. *J. Urol.* **153**, 1775–80.

Rand, R.W., Rand, R.P., Eggerding, F.A., *et al.* (1985). Cryolumpectomy for breast cancer: an experimental study. *Cryobiology* **22**, 307–18.

Riley, D.K., Babinchak, T.J., Zemel, R., Weaver, M.L., and Rotheram, E.B. (1997). Infectious complications of hepatic cryosurgery. *Clin. Infect. Dis.* **24**, 1001–3.

Rodriguez, R., Bishoff, J.T., Chen, R.B., and Marshall, F.F. (1998). Renal ablative cryosurgery in select patients with peripheral renal masses. *J. Urol.* **159**, 151A.

Sasagawa, I., Suzuki, H., Iaumi, T., Suzuki, Y., Tateno, T., and Nakada, T. (2000). Posterior retroperitoneoscopic partial adrenalectomy using ultrasonic scalpel for aldosterone-producing adenoma. *J. Endourol.* **14**, 573–6.

Schomer, N.S. and Mohler, J.L. (1995). Partial adrenalectomy for renal cell carcinoma with bilateral adrenal metastates. *J. Urol.* **153**, 1196–8.

Schulsinger, D.A., Perlmutter, A.P., Sosa, R.E., Marion, D., and Vaughan, E.D. Jr (1998). Temperature monitoring and histologic evaluation following acute interstitial renal cryoablation in the canine model. *Surg. Forum* **49**, 680–1.

Schulsinger, D.A., Sosa, R.E., Perlmutter, A.P., Ravizzini, P.I., Guarnizo, E., Marion, D., Nguyen, H.P., and Vaughan, E.D. Jr (1999). Biochemical and histological evaluation of the kidney following chronic laparoscopic interstitial renal cryoablation in the canine model *J. Urol.* **161**, 2A.

Shafir, M., Shapiro, R., Sung, M., Warner, R., Sicular, A., and Klipfel, A. (1996). Cryoablation of unresectable malignant liver tumors. *Am. J. Surg.* **171**, 27–31.

Suzuki, K., Sugiyama, T., Saisu, K., Ushiyama, T., and Fujita, K. (1998). Retroperitoneoscopic partial adrenalectomy for aldosterone-producing adenoma using an ultrasonically activated scalpel. *Br. J. Urol.* **82**, 138–9.

Takeda, M., Go, H., Imai, T., and Komeyama, T. (1994). Experience with 17 cases of laparoscopic adrenalectomy: use of ultrasonic aspirator and argon beam coagulator. *J. Urol.* **152**, 902–5.

Uchida, M., Imaide, Y., Sugimoto, K., Uehara, H., and Watanabe, H. (1995). Percutaneous cryosurgery for renal tumors. *Br. J. Urol.* **75**, 132–7.

Vaughan, E.D. Jr and Blumenfeld, J.D. (1998). Adrenal glands. In *Campbell's urology*, 7th edn (ed. P.C. Walsh, A.B. Retik, T.A. Stamey, and E.D. Vaughan Jr), pp. 2915–72. W.B. Saunders, Philadelphia.

Index